Personalized and Precision
Integrative Cardiovascular Medicine

Wolters Kluwer

Philadelphia • Baltimore • New York • London
Buenos Aires • Hong Kong • Sydney • Tokyo

Personalized and Precision
Integrative Cardiovascular Medicine

EDITOR:

Mark C. Houston MD, MS, MSc, FACP, FAHA, FASH, FACN, FAARM, ABAARM, DABC

Director, Hypertension Institute and Vascular Biology
Medical Director of Division of Human Nutrition and Clinical Research
Saint Thomas Medical Group, Saint Thomas Hospital
Nashville, Tennessee

Clinical, Instructor in the Department of Physical Therapy and Health Care Sciences at George Washington
University (GWU) School of Medicine and Health Science
Associate Clinical Professor of Medicine,
Vanderbilt University Medical School (1990-2012)

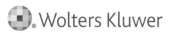 . Wolters Kluwer

Philadelphia • Baltimore • New York • London
Buenos Aires • Hong Kong • Sydney • Tokyo

Senior Acquisitions Editor: Sharon Zinner
Development Editor: Ashley Fischer
Editorial Coordinator: Dave Murphy
Production Project Manager: David Saltzberg
Design Coordinator: Terry Mallon
Manufacturing Coordinator: Beth Welsh
Prepress Vendor: TNQ Technologies

9 8 7 6 5 4 3 2 1

Printed in China

Library of Congress Cataloging-in-Publication Data

ISBN-13: 978-1-975115-28-9

Cataloging in Publication data available on request from publisher.

shop.lww.com

Preface

The New Cardiovascular Medicine

Despite aggressive guidelines and applications of advanced technology in cardiovascular (CV) medicine, the morbidity and mortality from coronary heart disease (CHD) is not declining worldwide. The traditional evaluation, prevention, and treatment strategies for the top five CHD risk factors still result in a CHD gap. This means that about 50% of patients still have CHD or a myocardial infarction despite "normal" levels of these CHD risk factors as presently defined in the medical literature. There are important details within each of these top five risk factors that are not being optimally addressed or applied clinically for the prevention and treatment of CHD. This suggests in all likelihood that we have reached a limit in our capacity to reduce CHD with our traditional approaches in cardiovascular medicine.

An evolved strategy is now required. It is time to redefine cardiovascular medicine and institute a "**new**" **cardiovascular medicine** paradigm. This "new" CV medicine can be interpreted or defined by a variety of terms such as "functional," "metabolic," "integrative," "personalized," "individualized," or "precision." Regardless of the language that we choose, the salient point is that we need to modernize our approach if we expect to have a positive impact on CV disease. Several key points need to be emphasized:

1. The traditional risk factor–induced development of CHD emphasizes only on the top five CHD risk factors of hypertension, dyslipidemia, diabetes mellitus, obesity, and smoking and their relationship to CV target organ damage. This strategy has severe limitation, specifically, the "cholesterol-centric" approach.
2. Recent results from clinical trials such as NAVIGATOR, ACCORD, and ROADMAP suggest that we have reached a limit in terms of reducing CV events by solely controlling these top five CHD risk factors.
3. New approaches, new testing, genetics, and other ancillary treatments will be necessary if we hope to reduce CHD in the future.
4. It is required that we understand, measure, prevent, and treat the downstream mediators of the CHD risk factors. The CHD risk factors lead to specific mediators of vascular disease that create a "snowball-like" effect that may be difficult to interrupt or reverse once initiated. Therefore, early evaluation of the risk factors and mediators coupled with aggressive prevention and treatment programs is mandatory.
5. The blood vessel has only three finite responses to an infinite number of insults. These responses are inflammation, oxidative stress, and immune vascular

dysfunction and imbalance. This model of cardiovascular medicine is shown in the figure below.

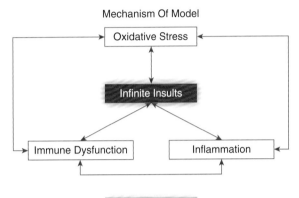

6. The blood vessel responds acutely to internal and external insults that are "correct and normal," but these chronic insults result in "a chronic exaggerated and dysregulated vascular dysfunction" with preclinical then clinical CVD due to maladaptation.
7. The subsequent environmental-gene expression patterns produce downstream mediators that damage the arteries.
8. Proper assessment, comprehension, and treatment of the top five and other numerous CHD risk factors and the downstream mediators is required.
9. The vascular system is the innocent bystander.
10. CVD needs to be approached within a systems biology analysis and with the knowledge of the various organ system interconnections.
11. Environmental-genetic interactions, CV genetics, nutragenomics, proteomics, and metabolomics provide important connections to advanced CV testing that will provide optimal individual responses.

Healthcare providers must provide quality, patient satisfaction, and value that is patient-centered and provides the best cardiovascular outcomes at the lowest cost. We must move away from a cardiovascular disease orientation to a process and prevention orientation. The education and training of physicians to provide unique cardiovascular centers of excellence is paramount in this endeavor. This transformation of cardiovascular medicine will require much time and effort, but it must be done.

This cardiovascular textbook was written to address all of these concepts in the **New Cardiovascular Medicine**. Leading experts in their respective fields have written the most comprehensive chapters on cardiovascular medicine that are available, which will appeal to internists, family physicians, osteopathic physicians, naturopathic physicians, cardiologists and cardiovascular specialists, and many others.

It has been my honor and privilege to serve as editor of this cardiovascular medicine textbook. I have learned much from my special colleagues. It is my hope that you will also learn and apply the information in this textbook and you will help to change the way that we practice cardiovascular medicine.

Mark Houston, MD, MS, MSc, FACP, FAHA, FASH,
FACN, FAARM, ABAARM, DABC
Editor

Contributors

George L. Bakris, MD

Professor of Medicine
Director
AHA Comprehensive Hypertension Center
The University of Chicago Medicine
Chicago, Illinois

Jeffrey S. Bland, PhD, FACN, FACB

President
Personalized Lifestyle Medicine Institute
Bainbridge Island, Washington

Nathan S. Bryan, PhD

Dept of Molecular and Human Genetics
Baylor College of Medicine
Houston, Texas

Alfred S. Callahan III, MD

Adjunct Associate Professor
Neurology
Meharry Medical College
Nashville, Tennessee

Jill C. Carnahan, MD, ABIHM, ABoIM, IFMCP

Flatiron Functional Medicine
Louisville, Colorado

Don Chomsky, MD

Cardiologist, Saint Thomas Medical Partners
Medical Director
Saint Thomas Mechanical Circulatory Support Program
Saint Thomas West Hospital
Nashville, Tennessee

Jay N. Cohn, MD

Professor of Medicine
University of Minnesota
Minneapolis, Minnesota

Jeanne Drisko, MD, CNS, FACN

Professor Emeritus
Department of Internal Medicine
University of Kansas Medical Center
Kansas City, Kansas

Daniel Duprez, MD, PhD

Donald and Patricia Garofalo Chair in Preventive
  Cardiology
Professor of Medicine/Cardiology
Cardiovascular Division/ Department of Medicine
University of Minnesota
Minneapolis, Minnesota

Jørn Dyerberg, MD, DMSc, DHC

Professor Emeritus
University of Copenhagen
Copenhagen, Denmark

Sergio Fazio, MD, PhD

The William and Sonja Connor Chair of Preventive
  Cardiology
Professor of Medicine and Physiology & Pharmacology
Director
Center for Preventive Cardiology
Knight Cardiovascular Institute
Oregon Health & Science University
Portland, Oregon

Dante J. Graves, MD, FACC

Director, Noninvasive Cardiology
Saint Thomas Heart West
Nashville, Tennessee

Mimi Guarneri, MD, FACC

President, Academy of Integrative Health and Medicine
Medical Director, Guarneri Integrative Health
Adjunct Faculty, University of California San Diego
San Diego, California

Thomas G. Guilliams, PhD

Adjunct Assistant Professor
University of Wisconsin School of Pharmacy -Madison,
  Wisconsin
Founder: The Point Institute. Stevens Point, Wisconsin
VP Science. Ortho Molecular Products- Stevens Point,
  Wisconsin

Andrew Heyman, MD, MHSA

Medical Director of Integrative Medicine
Department of Health Sciences
George Washington University
Director of Academic Affairs
Boca Raton, Florida
CEO, Metabolic Code
Mission Viejo, California

Mark C. Houston, MD, MS, MSc, FACP, FAHA, FASH, FACN, FAARM, ABAARM, DABC

Director, Hypertension Institute and Vascular Biology
Medical Director of Division of Human Nutrition and
    Clinical Research
Saint Thomas Medical Group, Saint Thomas Hospital
Nashville, Tennessee
Clinical, Instructor in the Department of Physical Therapy
    and Health Care Sciences at George Washington
    University (GWU) School of Medicine and Health Science
Associate Clinical Professor of Medicine, Vanderbilt
    University Medical School (1990-2012)

Gregori M. Kurtzman, DDS, MAGD, FPFA, FACD, FADI, DICOI, DADIA, DIDIA

General Practitioner
Silver Spring, Maryland

Joseph J. Lamb, MD

Physician/Owner
Personalized Lifestyle Medicine Center by Metagenics
Gig Harbor, Washington
Medical Director
The Hughes Center for Research and Innovation
Nature's Sunshine Products
Lehi, Utah

James B. LaValle, RPh, DHM, MS, CCN, ND (trad)

Founder
Progressive Medical of California
Chairman of the Board
Metabolic Intelligence

Tieraona Low Dog, MD

Director, Medicine Lodge Ranch
Chair: US Pharmacopeia Dietary Supplements Admissions
    Joint Standard Setting Sub-Committee
Pecos, New Mexico

Erik Lundquist, MD, ABFM, AboIM, IFMCP

Medical Director
Temecula Center for Integrative Medicine
Temecula, California

Deanna M. Minich, MS, PhD, FACN, CNS, IFMCP

Faculty, Human Nutrition and Functional Medicine
University of Western States
Portland, Oregon

Tom O'Bryan, DC, CCN, DACBN

Adjunct Faculty, The Institute for Functional Medicine,
Adjunct Faculty, The National University of Health
    Sciences,
Adjunct Faculty, Integrative and Functional Nutrition
    Academy
Chief Medical Officer, Sun Horse Energy
Clinical Consultant on Functional Medicine -NuMedica,
    Inc.
Clinical Consultant on Functional Medicine-Vibrant
    America
Editorial Review Board-Alternative Therapies in Health and
    Medicine
Medical Advisory Board, Functional Medicine Coaching
    Academy
Medical Advisory Board, Functional Medicine University
Medical Advisory Board, Cancer Schmancer
Medical Advisory Board, Institute for Functional Nutrition
Medical Advisory Board, Nutritional Therapy Association
Medical Advisory Board-National Association of
    Nutritional Professionals
Scientific Advisory Board-International and American
    Association of Clinical Nutritionists

Annalouise O'Connor, BS, PhD

Senior Manager, Research & Development
Metagenics
Gig Harbor, Washington

Bjarki J. Olafsson, MD, FACC

Cardiologist
Saint Thomas West
Nashville, Tennessee

Joseph Pizzorno, ND

Editor-in-Chief
Integrative Medicine, A Clinician's Journal
Bastyr University
Kenmore, Washington

Norbert W. Rainford, MD, FACC, FACP

Attending Cardiologist
Department of Medicine, Subsection Cardiology
Montefiore Nyack Hospital
Nyack, New York

James C. Roberts, MD, FACC, FAARFM
Comprehensive Heart Care
Toledo, Ohio

Joseph T. Shen, MD
Founder/Manager
Premier Heart, LLC
Port Washington, New York

Raffi B. Shen, BA
Director of Production and Quality Assurance
Premier Heart, LLC
Port Washington, New York

Stephen T. Sinatra, MD, FACC, FACN, CNS
Assistant Clinical Professor of Medicine
Department of Medicine
University of Connecticut School of Medicine
Farmington, Connecticut

Pamela W. Smith, MD, MPH, MS
Director
Center for Personalized Medicine
Founder
The Fellowship in Anti-Aging, Regenerative, and
    Functional Medicine
Grosse Pointe Farms, Michigan
Co-director
Master's Program in Metabolic and Nutritional Medicine
Morsani College of Medicine
University of South Florida
Tampa, Florida

Hillel Sternlicht, MD
AHA Comprehensive Hypertension Center
Department of Medicine
Section of Endocrinology, Diabetes, and Metabolism,
The University of Chicago Medicine
Chicago, Illinois

Shyamia Stone, ND, MPH
Naturopathic Doctor
Integrative Medicine
Guarneri Integrative Health
La Jolla, California

Ashley Swanson, MS
The Drs. Wolfson
Paradise Valley, Arizona

Douglas Thompson, DDS, FAAMM, ABAAHP
Faculty
The Kois Center
Seattle, Washington
Founder: The Wellness Dentistry Network

Filomena Trindade, MD, MPH, ABOIM, IFMCP, FAARM, ABFM
Metabolic Medical Institute
IFM
Private Practice
Capitola California

Ernst R. von Schwarz, MD, PhD, FESC, FACC, FSCAI
Clinical Professor of Medicine
David Geffen School of Medicine at UCLA
Cedars Sinai Medical Center
Los Angeles, California
University of California Riverside
Riverside, California
Medical Director
Southern California Hospital Heart Institute
Culver City, California

Jack M. Wolfson, DO, FACC
Wolfson Integrative Cardiology
Paradise Valley, Arizona

Andrew O. Zurick III, MD, FACC, FASE, FSCMR
Medical Director
Cardiovascular MRI & CT
Staff Cardiologist
St. Thomas West Hospital
Nashville, Tennessee

Contents

Section 7 **SPECIAL POPULATIONS AND CARDIOVASCULAR DISEASE 197**

Section 8   Additional Topics   442

Section 1

An Introduction to Functional, Metabolic and Integrative Cardiovascular Medicine

Chapter 1   **The Future of Functional Cardiovascular Medicine**
Jeffrey S. Bland, PhD, FACN, FACB

The Future of Functional Cardiovascular Medicine

Jeffrey S. Bland, PhD, FACN, FACB

Cardiovascular disease (CVD) still remains the leading cause of death in the United States with more than 610,000 people dying annually. Even with the advancements made in preventive cardiology over the past 30 years, there are more than 735,000 heart attacks annually. It is apparent that new approaches to the prevention and management of CVD that would reduce its burden would be an important step forward in decreasing both morbidity and preventable mortality. One approach that is gaining momentum that could accomplish this objective is seen through the prism of, and framed from, the advancements being made in systems biology and functional cardiology. The word "functional" when applied to cardiology a decade ago was mostly associated with psychosomatic and posttraumatic relationships to cardiovascular symptoms.[1] Charles Darwin during most of his adult life was chronically ill and had symptoms of cardiac disease that were attributed to him suffering from posttraumatic stress disorder.[2] He had experienced a painful, sudden death of his mother when he was 8 years old, seeing operations without anesthetics at a young age and witnessing the death of three of his children. His ill health was attributed at the time to an "irritable heart." The context of this connection of emotion to cardiovascular symptoms became classified as a member of the conditions termed "functional somatic syndromes" in 1999.[3,4] In the last 10 years, the use of the term "functional" in cardiovascular medicine, however, has changed considerably. It is recognized that the physiological function of the cardiovascular system can have influence on many other organs including the brain, liver, gastrointestinal, endocrine, and immune systems.[5] These new discoveries are redefining CVD that results from a complex set of physiological processes that modulate multiorgan systems which, in turn, influence the function of the vascular system.

We are witnessing the application of systems biology to cardiovascular medicine which focuses on the etiology of CVD resulting from the impact of altered physiological function among organ systems.[6] This systems medicine approach to both research and clinical development has provided the opportunity to better understand the etiology of complex cardiovascular-related disorders.[7] In this new systems biology application to CVD, the interaction of the functional status of the immune, endocrine, nervous, gastrointestinal microbiome, and hepatic detoxification systems is important in personalizing the treatment plan and making it more precise.[8] Functional status of the cardiovascular system is a result of the interaction of the organ systems that impact cardiovascular health and disease. The functional status of the cardiovascular system is determined by the unique interaction of the individual's genome with their lifestyle and environment throughout their lifetime. Functional cardiology then becomes the study of the dynamic factors that influence the plasticity and resilience of the cardiovascular system through the lens of systems biology.

The application of function of the cardiovascular system from this new perspective includes both assessment and intervention. Genomic evaluation coupled with lipid assessment, for example, provides a methodology for looking at CVD from a functional physiological perspective and can guide early intervention.[9] It is now recognized that several hundred different coronary heart disease (CHD) risk factors have been identified, and many new CHD-associated biomarkers and noninvasive cardiovascular (CV) tests are under evaluation for inclusion in routine practice The CV tests include high-sensitivity C-reactive protein (hsCRP), endothelial function and endothelial dysfunction (ED), arterial elasticity and compliance, pulse waveform analysis (PWA), pulse wave velocity (PWV), augmentation index (AI), central arterial blood pressure (CBP), 24-hour ambulatory blood pressure monitoring (ABPM), carotid artery duplex, micronutrient testing (MNT), cardiovascular toxicology, autonomic function testing (AFT) and heart rate variability, plethysmography, magnetocardiography, gene expression testing, ankle-brachial index, cardiopulmonary exercise testing (CPET), ECHO and exercise ECHO, computerized tomography angiography (CTA), cardiac magnetic resonance imaging/angiogram (MRI/MRA), positron emission tomography (PET) scans, nuclear medicine scans, and coronary artery calcium (CAC) score. These emergent biomarkers and noninvasive CV tests allow interrogation of the fundamental pathophysiological processes that have been identified to be involved in the understanding of the complex etiology of CVD. Many potential insults to the cardiovascular system have been identified, but only three finite physiological vascular responses to these insults result in disturbance of cardiovascular function that is associated with CVD. These three finite vascular responses are inflammation, oxidative stress, and vascular immune dysfunction.

Functional cardiology assessment has advanced because of multiple discoveries in radiology, bioinformatics, and physiology. Functional assessment using fractional flow reserve (FFR) and quantitative flow reserve has found application in coronary stenosis.[10] It has also been applied to evaluation of microvascular function related to CVD and patients with nonobstructive CHD.[11,12] New developments in the assessment of vascular function provide an accurate determination for the risk of atrial fibrillation and its prevention.[13] Functional cardiovascular assessment is now applied to evaluating outcomes in patients with transcatheter aortic valve replacement.[14] Evaluation of cardiovascular function has been used to determine the efficacy and safety of new cardiovascular medications as well as performing comparator studies on differing cardiovascular therapies.[15,16] As a consequence of progress made in functional MRI, better understanding of the unique cardiovascular pathology of the patient has been achieved allowing for greater therapeutic precision.[17-20]

In fetal and pediatric cardiology, functional MRI has resulted in noninvasive approaches to the understanding of cardiac pathology.[21-23]

These are examples of the advances made in the field of diagnostic functional cardiology. Similarly, progress has been made in interventional functional cardiology. Function can be segmented into four subcategories: structural, physiological, cognitive, and behavioral.

Structural functional features of the cardiovascular system are now being applied to the understanding of various CVDs.[24] Physical changes in cardiac function due to the deposition of amyloid plaque are being assessed using cardiac magnetic resonance and echocardiography.[25] Microcirculatory dysfunctions are now being assessed as contributors to CVD.[26]

Cardiovascular physiological function is being assessed as a result of the application of lipoprotein fractionation, particle number, particle size, low-density lipoprotein (LDL) modification and oxidation (oxLDL), and high-density lipoprotein (HDL) functionality.[27] Evaluation of the impact of the physiological influence of inflammation, oxidative stress, and vascular immune dysfunction on cardiovascular function and structure, in both the myocardium and the coronary arteries, is being explored.[28] The physiological functional impact of the diet and specific nutrients preoperatively and on recovery after cardiac surgery is now recognized as important.[29,30]

The relationship between cognitive function and CVD is now being examined looking at the influence of blood pressure, lipids, dysglycemia, obesity and homocysteine on vascular dementia, cerebral white matter disease (CWMD), microcerebral infarcts, memory, cognitive issues, and learning functions.[31] Lastly behavioral function as it relates to the risk to and recovery from CVD has become a major area of investigation.[32,33]

Conclusions

It has become apparent that the use of the term "functional cardiology" has changed over the past 20 years from that of a functional somatic connotation to that of a forward-looking indicator of systems biology understanding of cardiovascular dynamics. The future developments in functional cardiology will allow for both earlier assessment of risk to CVD and more precise personalized interventions that improve both clinical outcome and safety. The field of functional cardiology will be driven by advancements in data derived from real-time monitoring of cardiovascular function such as wearable devices, noninvasive radiological and noninvasive assessment technologies, advanced genomics/transcriptomics/metabolomics, gene expression testing, microbiome analysis and advanced CHD risk factor, mediators, and phenotypic biomarkers. The information provided by these sources of data will all be aggregated in a personal data cloud and then analyzed by new bioinformatics. Early and aggressive functional and structural diagnostic testing including endothelial function, arterial compliance, AFT, heart rate variability, AI, PWV, ECHO, carotid intimal medial thickness, and cardiac MRI/MRA are examples of new technologies that allow for a more meticulous and precise understanding of cardiovascular function. Aggressive focus on CVD prevention and treatment based upon this systems biology approach to functional cardiology will reduce both cardiovascular morbidity and increase preventable mortality.

References

1. Testa A, Giannuzzi R, Sollazzo F, et al. Psychiatric emergencies (part 1): psychiatric disorders causing organic symptoms. *Eur Rev Med Pharmacol Sci*. 2013;17(suppl 1):55-64.

2. Heyse-Moore L. Charles Darwin's (1809–1882) illness – the role of post-traumatic stress disorder. *J Med Biogr*. 2019;27(1):13-25.

3. Barsky AJ, Borus JF. Functional somatic syndromes. *Ann Intern Med*. 1999;130(11):910-921.

4. Henningsen P, Zipfel S, Herzog W. Management of functional somatic syndromes. *Lancet*. 2007;369(9565):946-955.

5. Chiavarino C, Bianchino C, Brach-Prever S, et al. Theory of mind deficit in adult patients with congenital heart disease. *J Health Psychol*. 2015;20(10):1253-1262.

6. Trachana K, Bargaje R, Glusman G, et al. Taking systems medicine to heart. *Circ Res*. 2018;122(9):1276-1289.

7. Lamb J, Bland J. The heart and medicine: exploring the interconnectedness of cardiometabolic-related concerns through a systems biology approach. *Glob Adv Health Med.* 2012;1(2):38-45.

8. Bland J. Defining function in the functional medicine model. *Integr Med (Encinitas).* 2017;16(1):22-25.

9. Rodriguez A, Pajukanta P. Genomics and systems biology approaches in the study of lipid disorders. *Rev Invest Clin.* 2018;70(5):217-223.

10. Cesaro A, Gragnano F, Di Girolamo D, et al. Functional assessment of coronary stenosis: an overview of available techniques. Is quantitative flow ratio a step to the future?. *Expert Rev Cardiovasc Ther.* 2018;16(12):951-962.

11. Lee JM, Doh JH, Nam CW, et al. Functional approach for coronary artery disease: filling the gap between evidence and practice. *Korean Circ J.* 2018;48(3):179-190.

12. Widmer RJ, Samuels B, Samady H, et al. The functional assessment of patients with non-obstructive coronary artery disease: expert review from an international microcirculation working group. *EuroIntervention.* 2019;14:1694-1702.

13. Przewlocka-Kosmala M, Jasic-Szpak E, Rojek A, et al. Association of central blood pressure with left atrial structural and functional abnormalities in hypertensive patients. Implications for atrial fibrillation prevention. *Eur J Prev Cardiol.* 2019;26(10):1018-1027. doi:10.1177/2047487319839162.

14. Fukui M, Gupta A, Abdelkarim I, et al. Association of structural and functional cardiac changes with transcatheter aortic valve replacement outcomes in patients with aortic stenosis. *JAMA Cardiol.* 2019. [Epub ahead of print].

15. Sabri MR, Shoja M, Shoja M, Hosseinzadeh M. The effect of tadalafil on functional capacity and echocardiographic parameters in patients with repaired Tetralogy of Fallot. *ARYA Atheroscler.* 2018;14(4):177-182.

16. Campbell BCV, Majoie CBLM, Albers GW, et al. Penumbral imaging and functional outcome in patients with anterior circulation ischaemic stroke treated with endovascular thrombectomy versus medical therapy: a meta-analysis of individual patient-level data. *Lancet Neurol.* 2019;18(1):46-55.

17. Katbeh A, Ondrus T, Barbato E, et al. Imaging of myocardial fibrosis and its functional correlates in aortic stenosis: a review and clinical potential. *Cardiology.* 2018;141(3):141-149.

18. Wang Y, Zhang Y, Xuan W, et al. Fully automatic segmentation of 4D MRI for cardiac functional measurements. *Med Phys.* 2019;46(1):180-189.

19. Miki T, Miyoshi T, Watanabe A, et al. Anomalous aortic origin of the right coronary artery with functional ischemia determined with fractional flow reserve derived from computed tomography. *Clin Case Rep.* 2018;6(7):1371-1372.

20. So A, Wisenberg G, Teefy P, et al. Functional CT assessment of extravascular contrast distribution volume and myocardial perfusion in acute myocardial infarction. *Int J Cardiol.* 2018;266:15-23.

21. Tsuritani M, Morita Y, Miyoshi T, et al. Fetal cardiac functional assessment by fetal heart magnetics resonance imaging. *J Comput Assist Tomogr.* 2019;43(1):104-108.

22. Zhou Z, Han F, Yoshida T, et al. Improved 4D cardiac functional assessment for pediatric patients using motion-weighted image reconstruction. *MAGMA.* 2018;31(6):747-756.

23. Barczuk-Falecka M, Malek LA, Krysztofiak H, et al. Cardiac magnetic resonance assessment of the structural and functional cardiac adaptations to soccer training in school-aged male children. *Pediatr Cardiol.* 2018;39(5):948-954.

24. Cui Y, Luo F, Li B, et al. Structural, functional and histological features of a novel ischemic heart failure model. *Front Biosci (Landmark Ed).* 2019;24:723-734.

25. Knight DS, Zumbo G, Barcella W, et al. Cardiac structural and functional consequences of amyloid deposition by cardiac magnetic resonance and echocardiography and their prognostic roles. *JACC Cardiovasc Imaging.* 2018;12(5):823-833. [Epub ahead of print].

26. Mejia-Renteria H, Lee JM, Lauri F, et al. Influence of microcirculatory dysfunction on angiography-based functional assessment of coronary stenoses. *JACC Cardiovasc Interv.* 2018;11(8):741-753.

27. Rowland CM, Shiffman D, Caulfield M, et al. Association of cardiovascular events and lipoprotein particle size: Development of a risk score based on functional data analysis. *PLoS One.* 2019;14(3):e0213172.

28. Gorbunova O, Panove T, Chernysheva E, Popov E. The level of protection from oxidative stress and three-year dynamics of structural and functional changes of the myocardium in chronic ischemic heart disease in men. *Georgian Med News.* 2018;(285):63-69.

29. Ogawa M, Izawa KP, Satomi-Kobayashi S, et al. Effects of postoperative dietary intake on functional recovery of patients undergoing cardiac surgery. *Nutr Metab Cardiovasc Dis.* 2019;29(1):90-96.

30. Katano S, Hashimoto A, Ohori K, et al. Nutritional status and energy intake as predictors of functional status after cardiac rehabilitation in elderly inpatient with heart failure – a retrospective cohort study. *Circ J.* 2018;82(6):1584-1591.

31. O'Caoimh R, Gao Y, Svendrovski A, et al. Effect of visit-to-visit blood pressure variability on cognitive and functional decline in mild to moderate alzheimer's disease. *J Alzheimers Dis.* 2019;68(4):1499-1510. [Epub ahead of print].

32. Beishon LC, Panerai RB, Robinson TG, et al. The assessment of cerebrovascular response to a language task from the Addenbrooke's cognitive examination in cognitive impairment: a feasibility functional transcranial Doppler ultrasonography study. *J Alzheimers Dis Rep.* 2018;2(1):153-164.

33. Rozanski A. Behavioral cardiology. *J Am Coll Cardiol.* 2014;64:100-110.

Section 2

Foundational Basics in Vascular Medicine

Vascular Biology and Vascular Aging for the Clinician

Nathan S. Bryan, PhD and Ernst R. von Schwarz, MD, PhD, FESC, FACC, FSCAI

Brief Introduction

Cardiovascular disease (CVD) remains the number one killer of men and women worldwide. In 2015, there were an estimated 422.7 million cases of CVD and nearly 18 million of these people died of CVDs, with 85% being due to myocardial infarction and stroke. This represented 31% of all global deaths.[1] This is up 30% since 1990 when there were 12.59 million deaths due to CVD. The people who survive or live with CVD cost the United States alone over $200 billion annually. This total includes the cost of health care services, medications, and lost productivity. CVD will cost the United States over $1 trillion in medical expenses (direct costs) and lost productivity (indirect costs) by 2035 (unpublished report from American Heart Association [AHA]). This is simply unacceptable given that the scientific community knows without a doubt what causes CVD, the loss of production of nitric oxide (NO). CVD is mainly caused by endothelial dysfunction,[2] and one of the main functions of the endothelium is to produce NO.[3] The functional loss of NO production by the vascular endothelium precedes the structural changes of arteriosclerosis and atherosclerosis by many years, sometimes decades.[4] Therefore, clinicians need to recognize and appreciate endothelial NO function in their patients and restore and maintain NO production. The onset and progression of CVD cannot and will not be managed, treated, or prevented without first correcting NO production.

Purpose of the Chapter

This chapter is designed and written to inform clinicians and health care providers on the mechanisms of vascular disease, risk factors and mechanisms of risks, effective methods of diagnosing endothelial dysfunction or NO deficiency, the earliest events in CVD, and evidence-based strategies for restoring vascular function to cure, treat, or prevent CVD.

It is abundantly clear that treatment of CVD over the past 50 years has been unsuccessful by focusing on treating disease states rather than on prevention. Therefore, a new paradigm is prudent. Focusing on restoration of NO in healthy patients without CVD, patients at risk for CVD, or even patients with apparent CVD should be the first-line consideration by clinicians. This chapter will provide the clinician with all the tools to diagnose and recognize NO insufficiency, early vascular dysfunction, as well as safe and effective treatments and preventative measures for CVD.

Pathophysiology of Cardiovascular Disease

The vascular endothelium is the organ system that maintains the integrity of the cardiovascular system. The endothelium is the single layer of cells lining various organs of the body, especially the blood vessels, heart, and lymphatic vessels. The endothelium is the largest endocrine organ and makes up over 14,000 square feet of surface area within the human body, enough cells to cover 6.5 tennis courts. The endothelium is responsible for a number of fundamental physiological functions. The endothelium serves a critical role as a barrier and primary sensor of physiological and chemical changes in the blood stream. Endothelial cells are highly specialized to detect diverse physical, chemical, and mechanical stimuli (blood pressure, pulsatile flow, shear stress). They are also involved in the regulation of blood flow through continuous modulation of vascular tone, primarily through the production of NO. When the endothelium is intact and functional, the cardiovascular system maintains its integrity and is protected from CVD. When the endothelium becomes dysfunctional, the cardiovascular system fails and CVD ensues. The manifestation of CVD, primarily atherosclerosis, is a reaction to injury and inflammation within the arterial wall only after the endothelium has lost its ability to maintain structure and function. The

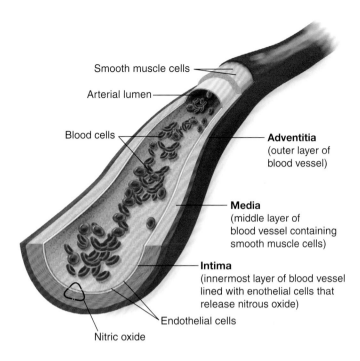

Smooth muscle cells

Arterial lumen

Blood cells

Adventitia
(outer layer of
blood vessel)

Media
(middle layer of
blood vessel containing
smooth muscle cells)

Intima
(innermost layer of blood vessel
lined with enothelial cells that
release nitrous oxide)

Endothelial cells

Nitric oxide

Figure 2.1 *The anatomy of a blood vessel. The endothelial cells produce NO that interacts with red blood cells in the lumen as well as the smooth muscle cells outside the intima. NO acts as an autocrine, paracrine, and endocrine mediator.*

integrity of the endothelium affects the structure and function of the other parts of the blood vessel including the intima and smooth muscle (see Figure 2.1). There are three finite responses by the vascular endothelium to the infinite number of insults it encounters all of which decrease NO production. These three finite responses are inflammation, oxidative stress, and immune dysfunction. One or all three of these are found and associated with all forms of CVD. However, they are more than associations and there is sufficient evidence that these are causal for CVD. Oxidative stress reduces vascular NO production.[5] Inflammation, specifically microvascular inflammation, is due to insufficient NO production and the consequential sequelae of leukocyte adhesion, emigration, and immune dysfunction.[6,7] The immune dysfunction that also occurs leads to a further dysregulation and production of NO. The inflammation that ensues also leads to further reduction in NO production creating a feed-forward mechanism exacerbating the vascular disease phenotype.[8] In most cases, loss of NO production occurs as a result of oxidative stress and oxidation of tetrahydrobiopterin (BH4), which causes the endothelial nitric oxide synthase (eNOS) enzyme uncoupling.[9]

Vascular Aging

Loss of functional endothelial NO production, termed endothelial dysfunction, precedes the structural changes in the vasculature by many years, sometimes decades, and correlates with cardiovascular risks.[2] Aging and hypertension are established and validated cardiovascular risk factors.[10,11] The functional and structural vascular changes that lead to the complication of CVD are similar in older healthy subjects and younger adults who have had hypertension most

of their life.[12] There are finite symptoms and conditions that result from vascular aging. These are shown in Table 2.1. The pathways of aging and vascular aging are identical, which allows the clinician to provide drugs, supplements, and lifestyle

Table 2.1

SYMPTOMS AND CONSEQUENCES OF VASCULAR AGING

1. Arterial stiffness with reduced elasticity and compliance with increased pulse wave velocity and augmentation index
2. Inflammation
3. Oxidative stress (NADPH oxidase, xanthine oxidase, uncoupled mitochondria)
4. Immune vascular dysfunction
5. Thrombosis
6. Growth and hypertrophy
7. Permeability (microalbuminuria)
8. Reduced angiogenesis
9. Impaired "circadian clock" genes
10. Increased sympathetic and decreased parasympathetic nervous system activity (SNS > PNS)
11. Vasoconstriction
12. Vascular calcification

changes and nutrition to improve or slow down the aging process. Furthermore, the vascular changes seen in essential hypertension appear to be an accelerated progressive form of vascular structure and function seen with normal aging.[13] Young healthy individuals have normal and sufficient endothelial production of NO through L-arginine. However, as we age, we lose our ability to synthesize NO from L-arginine; this is termed endothelial dysfunction. Most of the work on the production of NO in cells, tissues, and humans agree that the bioavailability or the generation of NOS-derived NO decreases with aging. Increased oxidative stress through production of superoxide can scavenge NO thereby reducing its effective concentrations and signaling actions in cells.[14] Aging also causes a decrease in the expression of the NOS enzyme.[15,16] Concomitantly, there is an upregulation of arginase (an enzyme that degrades the natural substrate for NOS, L-arginine) in the blood vessels with age that also causes a reduction in NO production[17] owing to a shuttling of L-arginine away from the NOS enzyme. Aging causes a gradual decline in NO production with a greater than 50% loss in endothelial function in some aged populations.[18] Some studies show a more than 75% loss of NO in the coronary circulation in patients in their 70s and 80s compared with young, healthy 20-year-old persons.[19] In fact, age may be the most significant predictor of endothelium-derived NO production[20] and loss of NO may be responsible for age-related disease, including CVD. These data clearly demonstrate that NO production from L-arginine declines as we get older. This is due to uncoupling of the NOS enzyme, which is then unable to convert L-arginine into NO. This process can be accelerated or decelerated depending on diet and lifestyle. The majority of studies reveal that loss of NO production was clearly evident by 40 years of age. However, the vasodilation to exogenous NO (endothelium-independent vasodilation) does not change over time with aging, illustrating that the body does not lose its ability to respond to NO, it only loses its ability to generate it with age. Vascular aging is characterized by progressive arterial stiffness, loss of arterial elasticity and arterial compliance, increase in pulse wave velocity and pulse pressure, and mechanosensitive gene expression from a myriad of structural and functional changes in the endothelium and vascular media and adventitia with altered gene expression. These include increased extracellular matrix, endothelial dysfunction loss of NO, increase cytokines and chemokines, altered vascular smooth muscle, altered adventitia, inflammation, loss of elasticity, and increased elastase and collagen along with calcium deposition.[21]

The control of blood pressure and the integrity of the cardiovascular system are critically dependent on NO, but there are also other vasoactive substances and mediators that affect the onset and progression of CVD. Another major player is angiotensin II. NO is a vasodilator, whereas angiotensin II is a vasoconstrictor. Angiotensin II is a hormone that binds to the angiotensin I receptor, which then mediates effects on the central nervous system to regulate renal sympathetic nerve activity, renal function, and, therefore, blood pressure. Angiotensin also stimulates the release of aldosterone from

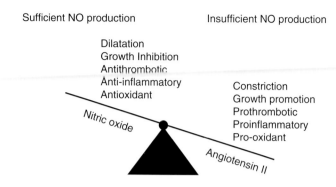

Figure 2.2 *Endothelial nitric oxide (NO) production maintains vascular health and integrity. Loss of NO causes all pathological conditions conducive to CVD.*

the adrenal cortex to promote sodium retention by the kidneys causing an increase in volume and subsequent increase in blood pressure. Maintaining the balance of NO with angiotensin II is vital to protecting the cardiovascular system. The loss of NO tips the balance of a healthy endothelium and cardiovascular system to one that becomes pro-oxidant, proinflammatory, proliferative, and constrictive, which becomes driven primarily by angiotensin II (**Figure 2.2**). These are hallmark conditions of CVD. These observations allow scientists and physicians to conclude that reduced production of NO occurs as we age and this creates the environment that is conducive to the onset and progression of CVD. The functional loss of NO leading to the structural changes in advanced vascular disease is illustrated in **Figure 2.3**.

Known Risk Factors for CVD and Mechanisms of Increased Risks

There are a number of known risk factors for CVD. Risk factors are conditions or habits that make a person more likely to develop CVD and/or increase the chances that the existing disease will get worse. Known and important risk factors for CVD are high blood pressure (hypertension), hyperlipidemia (increased levels of certain lipoproteins), diabetes and prediabetes, smoking, being overweight or obese, physical inactivity, family history of early heart disease, unhealthy diet, periodontal disease, and age (55 years or older for women). There are others, but these are the primary risk factors. All of these risk factors are modifiable with the exception of family history and age. However, mechanistically the risks of increased age can be mitigated by NO, so realistically, family history is truly the only nonmodifiable risk factor. All of the known risk factors have a common denominator that is responsible for increased risk of CVD. That commonality is loss of NO production. It is known that if you can eliminate these known risk factors, your chances of developing CVD are much less and in fact perhaps even eliminated. We will discuss the pathophysiology of each risk factor and how to restore to normal physiology.

Hypertension, the number one modifiable risk factor for the development of CVD is often times not sufficiently

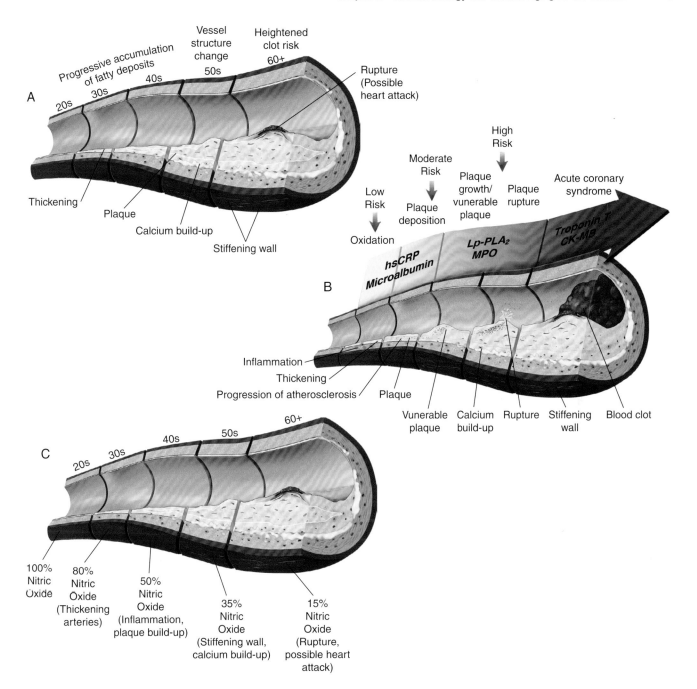

Figure 2.3 *(Left) Fat deposition and increased thickness of the media along with plaque formation occurs as we age. (Upper right) Specific blood biomarkers correlate with different stages of vascular disease and/or plaque vulnerability. (Lower right) Loss of endothelial NO production precedes presence of biomarker and structural changes that occur during progression of CVD. CK-MB, creatine kinase-MB; hsCRP, high-sensitivity C-reactive protein; Lp-PLA2, lipoprotein-associated phospholipase A2; MPO, myeloperoxidase.*

managed. In the United States, about 78 million (one of every three) people have high blood pressure or hypertension. Another one of three have prehypertension (CDC fact sheet). That puts over 150 million Americans at risk for heart disease. Despite major advances in understanding the pathophysiology of hypertension and availability of antihypertensive drugs, suboptimal blood pressure control is still the most important risk factor for cardiovascular mortality. According to the AHA 2015 Statistics Fact Sheet, of 75% of people who know they have hypertension and take medication for their

high blood pressure, only about half are adequately managed. Because blood pressure remains elevated in approximately half of all treated hypertensive patients,[22,23] new safe and cost-effective solutions are desperately needed. We now know from the Systolic Blood Pressure Intervention trial (SPRINT) that better management of blood pressure reduces all-cause mortality.[24] Additional drug therapy is not the solution. Loss of NO production and signaling is the cause of hypertension.[25,26] Because hypertension is primarily responsible for structural changes in the vasculature that increase the risk of myocardial infarction and stroke, a primary focus should be on normalizing blood pressure through the restoration of NO production.[27]

Hyperlipidemia or an elevation in specific lipids is a known risk factor for CVD. Lipids refer to a number of fat particles or proteins, including cholesterol, lipoproteins, and triglycerides. Although routine lipid screening plays an important role in cardiovascular risk assessment, it does not provide a complete picture of your health. In fact, nearly 50% of all myocardial infarctions and strokes occur in patients with "normal" cholesterol levels.[28-30] This suggests that many people at risk are presumed low risk because they have normal or controlled cholesterol levels. Therefore, routine cholesterol tests may fail to fully identify people at risk for myocardial infarction and stroke. However, oxidized low-density lipoprotein (LDL) (OxLDL) is a more sensitive biomarker than total LDL. OxLDL detects the amount of protein damage due to the oxidative modification of the ApoB subunit on LDL cholesterol. This is part of the three finite responses. The oxidation of LDL cholesterol (LDL-C) inhibits NO production and is one of the first steps in the development of atherosclerosis.[31] Briefly, LDL-C enters the artery wall where it becomes oxidized. OxLDL is then recognized by scavenger receptors on macrophages, which engulf OxLDL, resulting in foam cell formation, vascular inflammation, and the initiation of atherosclerosis. Providing an exogenous source of NO can reduce OxLDL, oxidative stress, and atherogenesis.[32,33] Therefore, loss of the protective NO leads to oxidative stress, increased OxLDL, and increased progression of atherosclerosis, and providing an exogenous source of NO appears to inhibit oxidative stress, reduce OxLDL, and inhibit the progression of CVD.

Diabetes has become a major epidemic around the globe. Clinical diabetes mellitus is a syndrome of disordered metabolism with inappropriate hyperglycemia due either to an absolute deficiency of insulin secretion or a reduction in the biologic effectiveness of insulin or both. The prevalence of diagnosed and undiagnosed diabetes in the United States is 25.8 million, or 8.3% of the population, according to the 2011 National Diabetes Fact Sheet. In 2005 to 2008, 67% of adults aged 20 years or older with self-reported diabetes had blood pressure greater than or equal to 140/90 mm Hg or used prescription medications for hypertension. Type 2 diabetes mellitus accounts for 80% to 90% of diabetes cases in the United States and is associated with an increased risk for a number of life-threatening complications. These include heart disease and stroke, high blood pressure, blindness, kidney disease, nervous system disease, amputation, and complications of pregnancy and surgery. Probably not coincidental, all of the above-mentioned complications are associated with insufficient NO production.[34] Endothelial dysfunction with reduced NO generation and bioavailability plays a key role in the pathogenesis of diabetic vascular disease and complications and likely serves as the key link between metabolic disorders and CVD.[35] A number of previous experimental studies have demonstrated impaired endothelial function in animal models of diabetes mellitus.[36-39] In addition, numerous clinical studies[40,41] have clearly documented severe endothelial dysfunction in people with diabetes mellitus. Polymorphisms in the eNOS gene have predictive value for the development of diabetic complications.[42] The dysfunctional NO pathway in people with diabetes is thought to be the cause of the increased incidence of cardiovascular complications.[43] The potential mechanisms that may account for attenuated eNOS function and a reduction in endothelial NO synthesis in diabetics are numerous. The increases in circulating glucose, insulin, and cytokines that occur in type 2 diabetes have all been independently shown to impair eNOS enzyme activity in experimental studies.[38,39] All of these conditions acting independently or in unison could render the eNOS enzyme dysfunctional (**Figure 2.4**). Mice without the genes that make NO become insulin resistant and diabetic.[44] This suggests that loss of NO may be causal for insulin-resistant diabetes. The physiological significance of impaired eNOS function and reductions in vascular NO bioavailability may serve to reduce blood flow to various organs in patients with diabetes mellitus as well as disrupt insulin-dependent glucose uptake. Restoring the functionality of NO-based signaling can improve glucose uptake and correct vascular dysfunction in diabetes.[45,46]

Smoking represents one of the most important preventable risk factors for the development of atherosclerosis. Vascular dysfunction induced by smoking is initiated by reduced NO production and/or bioavailability and further by the increased expression of adhesion molecules and subsequent endothelial dysfunction. For the past decades, it has been clear that smoking is an important (and modifiable) risk factor for CVDs; according to World Health Organization data, smoking is responsible for 10% of all CVD cases. Smoking reduces flow mediated dilatation (FMD) in systemic arteries in healthy young adults.[47] Several other experimental

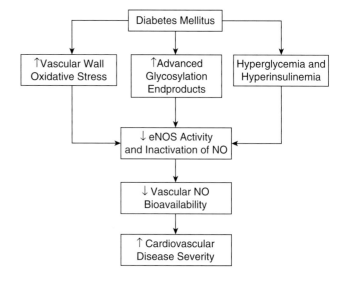

Endothelial Nitric Oxide Synthase (eNOS) and Diabetes

Figure 2.4 *Diabetes increases oxidative stress, inflammation, and immune dysfunction along with hyperglycemia and hyperlipidemia, all of which lead to decreased production of NO and increased risk for CVD.*

studies suggested a link between proatherogenic cellular and molecular effects of cigarette smoke and initiation of CVD.[48] Smoking-induced increased adherence of platelets and macrophages provokes the development of a procoagulant and inflammatory environment.[49] In addition to direct physical damage to endothelial cells, smoking induces tissue remodeling and prothrombotic processes together with activation of systemic inflammatory signals, all of which contribute to atherogenic vessel wall changes. Restoring the function of eNOS enzyme through treatment of chronic smokers with BH4 (cofactor of endothelial NO-synthase) and/or vitamin C improved smoking-impaired vasodilatation.[50,51] Smoking-induced impairment of FMD can be improved by simultaneous consumption of red wine, probably because of its antioxidant properties,[52] which will thereby improve NO production. Smoking cessation is the most effective measure for reversing damage that has already occurred and preventing fatal cardiovascular outcomes. At the very least, restoring NO production in smokers may mitigate many of the adverse effects of smoking.

Obesity (defined as a body mass index [BMI] of ≥30 kg/m²) is a risk factor for CVD. It is estimated that the relative risk of coronary heart disease in obesity is approximately 1.5 even after adjusting for all other traditional coronary heart disease risk factors that often comigrate with obesity (eg, hyperlipidemia, hypertension).[53] Increasing BMI actually predicts impaired endothelial NO function.[54] It is even more pronounced in patients with visceral obesity and insulin resistance.[55] The impact of and association between excess weight and endothelial dysfunction can present as early as childhood.[56] Obesity is thought to affect endothelial function predominately via comorbidities, such as insulin resistance and dyslipidemia. Obese individuals are resistant to the vasodilator actions of insulin.[57] Furthermore, hyperglycemia and hyperlipidemia, which are almost always present in obesity, are known to decrease NO-dependent vasodilation.[58,59] Adipose tissue itself plays an important role in the release of vasoactive substances.[60] Adiponectin accumulates in the vessel wall where it has anti-inflammatory effects and increases NO production.[61] Obesity is associated with relative adiponectin deficiency, which causes a loss of endogenous activator of NO production contributing to impaired endothelial function. Other cytokines such as interleukin 6 (IL-6) and fatty acids are thought to decrease NO production and so contribute to impaired endothelial function in obesity. Lastly, adipose-derived components of the renin-angiotensin system also contribute directly to fluid retention, vasoconstriction, and hypertension.[62] Given that excess body weight now affects more than 300 million persons worldwide, prevention and treatment of obesity should be considered one of the cornerstones for the prevention of CVD or at least the physiological consequences of obesity such as loss of NO production should be corrected.

Regular physical activity reduces the risk of dying prematurely from CVD. It also helps prevent or delay the development of diabetes, helps maintain weight loss, and reduces hypertension, all previously mentioned risk factors for CVD.

Higher levels of physical fitness appear to delay all-cause mortality primarily owing to lowered rates of CVD and cancer.[63] Physical inactivity is a significant risk factor for CVD itself. It ranks similarly to cigarette smoking, high blood pressure, and elevated cholesterol. It is estimated that twice as many adults in the United States are physically inactive than the number of people who smoke cigarettes. The benefits of exercise are indisputable. Long-term physical exercise improves endothelium-dependent vasorelaxation through an increase in the production of NO in both normotensive and hypertensive subjects.[64] The ability to generate NO during exercise predicts your exercise capacity and endurance.[65] To the contrary, patients with endothelial dysfunction or with known CVD risk factors fail to produce NO during exercise.[66,67] Exercise is medicine because it increases NO production. Therefore, lack of exercise causes loss of NO production and increased risk of CVD.

Diet or food patterns have been shown to be associated with a substantial proportion of deaths from heart disease, stroke, and type 2 diabetes.[68] Recent prospective epidemiologic studies show that green leafy vegetables are among the most protective foods against coronary heart disease and ischemic stroke risk.[69,70] Probably not coincidental, these foods contain relatively high amounts of nitrate and nitrite, which when consumed and metabolized generate NO.[27,71] The Dietary Approaches to Stop Hypertension (DASH) studies found that diets rich in vegetables (ie, 8-10 servings) and low-fat dairy products could lower blood pressure to an extent similar to single hypotensive medications.[72,73] The blood pressure lowering effect of this diet was hypothesized to be attributable to the high calcium, potassium, polyphenols, and fiber content and low sodium and animal protein content[74]; however, we now understand that the food choices of the DASH diet contain sufficient inorganic nitrate that may be responsible for the blood pressure lowering effects.[75] The typical Japanese diet, known for its protection against cancer and CVD, is enriched in nitrate sufficient to lower blood pressure.[76] What is clear is that diets or foods that contain sufficient nitrate and/or nitrite are protective from CVD and those that do not offer no protection. To the contrary, high-salt diets increase blood pressure and increase the risk of CVD and high–glycemic index diets cause oxidative stress and inflammation and reduce NO thereby increasing the risk of CVD.

Periodontal disease and poor oral health are known to increase the risk of all-cause mortality, including CVD.[77,78] Salivary uptake and concentration of inorganic nitrate from consumption of green leafy vegetables and subsequent bacterial reduction to nitrite and NO provides a viable and effective pathway for maintaining NO homeostasis and thus preventing cardiovascular risk.[79] This pathway in humans appears to serve as an alternative pathway that can provide an endothelium-independent source of bioactive NO compensating for insufficient host NO production. This pathway is dependent on commensal oral bacteria of the tongue to perform the first step (two-electron reduction) because mammals lack a functional nitrate reductase. There is significant evidence in the literature that these bacterial communities provide the host a source of NO that may be able to overcome insufficient NO production from the endothelium.[80] The bacteria associated with periodontal diseases are predominantly gram-negative anaerobic bacteria. Toxins produced by the bacteria in plaque irritate the gums. The toxins stimulate a chronic inflammatory response, in which the body in essence turns on itself and the tissues and bone that support the teeth are broken down and destroyed, also causing systemic inflammation. The presence of these pathogenic bacteria outcompetes the good nitrate-reducing bacteria that are responsible for producing the cardioprotective NO.[81] An effective strategy to therapeutically promote NO production and overcome conditions of NO insufficiency may be to focus on understanding specific oral bacterial communities and the optimal conditions for efficient oral nitrate reduction and addressing the underlying periodontal disease causing the oral dysbiosis.

The risk factors for the development of CVD all are known to disrupt NO production. Loss of NO is the first event in the onset and progression of CVD. Risk factors are difficult to manage in patients because it requires compliance and often a change in lifestyle and habits. As you increase the number of risk factors, this leads to a stepwise reduction in NO production.[82] The best management strategy for your patients, especially if you cannot convince them to change their diet, stop smoking, start exercising, go see a good dentist, or lose weight, is to start them on a regimen that will restore their NO production pathways. There are now safe and effective, evidenced-based methods for restoring NO in patients. It is imperative for all patients to have NO support.

Clinical Presentation

Patients suffering from insufficient NO production will have diverse clinical presentations. One of the early signs and symptoms of NO deficiency can present as erectile dysfunction (ED) in men[83] because NO is required for engorgement of blood into the penis for optimal erections.[84] Loss of NO in women will also present as female sexual arousal disorder because NO is also required for dilation of blood vessels of the clitoris to increase blood flow and increase pressure required for orgasm. It is important for clinicians to recognize this symptom as NO deficiency. ED in men is associated with endothelial dysfunction, atherosclerosis, peripheral artery disease, heart failure, hypertension, and coronary artery disease.[85] Therefore, ED should be considered the "canary in the coalmine" and an early sign of NO deficiency that must be corrected, or patients will progress to CVD, myocardial infarction, and stroke at a much faster pace than those without ED. Most patients who are deficient in NO will be hypertensive because NO is the primary vasodilator that maintains normal blood pressure. Because NO is protective from atherosclerosis, patients without adequate NO will have advance atherosclerotic disease. Platelets have their own NOS enzyme,[86] and loss of functional production of NO will cause platelets to become hyperactive leading to coagulopathies. NO controls and regulates mitochondrial biogenesis

Table 2.2

CLINICAL CONSEQUENCES OF INSUFFICIENT NO PRODUCTION

Hypertension	Atherosclerosis
Alzheimer disease (vascular dementia)	Thrombosis
Metabolic syndrome	Diabetes
Peripheral artery disease	Erectile dysfunction
Immune dysfunction—recurrent infections	Chronic fatigue
Uncontrolled cell proliferation—cancer	Chronic inflammation
Inability to adapt to altitude (hypoxia)	Exercise intolerance
Inability to heal (nonhealing ulcers)	Poor circulation

and mitochondrial ATP production.[87,88] Therefore, loss of NO will cause a disruption in cellular energy production and will manifest as chronic fatigue syndrome in many patients. Because NO is a ubiquitous signaling molecule involved in the regulation of many essential cellular functions, loss of NO production will affect a host of organ systems, resulting clinical symptoms. Table 2.2 highlights some of the most common clinical presentations that are directly due to insufficient NO production. The objective is to educate physicians so that NO can be a serious consideration in the diagnosis and treatment of these disorders that are commonly seen in clinical practice. Recommending or prescribing methods that are known to restore and produce NO will remedy many if not all of the above-mentioned symptoms. What might seem like completely unrelated symptoms with multiple etiologies may simply be a lack of NO.

Early Diagnosis of Vascular Dysfunction Is Key to Prevention and Effective Treatment

Early detection of endothelial dysfunction and recognition of the loss of NO before the onset of progression of symptoms and disease is essential and necessary for the prevention of CVD. Prevention is much more cost-effective than treatment. A fundamental question in primary care is how to detect NO insufficiency in patients. The major pathway for NO metabolism is the stepwise oxidation to nitrite and nitrate. For years, both nitrite (NO_2^-) and nitrate (NO_3^-) (collectively, NOx) have been used as surrogate markers of NO production in biological tissues, but there have not been any new developments in the use of NO biomarkers in the clinical setting for diagnostic or prognostic utility. A report by Kleinbongard et al.[82] demonstrated that plasma nitrite levels in humans progressively decrease with increasing cardiovascular risk load.

Risk factors considered included age, hypertension, smoking, and hypercholesterolemia, conditions all known to reduce the bioavailability of NO. However, NO status is still not part of the standard blood chemistry routinely used for diagnostic purposes. There are now salivary test strips on the market (N-O Indicator strips, HumanN, Inc., Austin, TX) that detect salivary nitrite as a proxy for total body NO bioavailability.[89] This is a nice tool to have in your tool box as a point-of-care indication of NO status. Additional diagnostic laboratories should include panels of inflammation that include high-sensitivity C-reactive protein, myeloperoxidase, lipoprotein associated phospholipase A2, oxidized LDL, asymmetric dimethyl L-arginine, and symmetric dimethyl L-arginine. F2-isoprostanes (F2-IsoPs) are prostaglandin-like compounds formed from the free radical–mediated oxidation of arachidonic acid[90] and are the "gold standard" for measuring oxidative stress in the body. F2-IsoPs also have potent biological effects associated with inflammation and therefore may mediate chronic disease initiation and progression. Additionally, F2-IsoPs may also act as potent vasoconstrictors[91] via thromboxane formation in the endothelium, which can promote platelet activation resulting in thrombus formation.[92] Lower F2-IsoPs are associated with a lower risk of CVD. These and all laboratories should be supported with additional functional measurements of NO. The only true measure of endothelial NO production (endothelial function) is through FMD. FMD is a noninvasive ultrasound-based method in which arterial diameter is measured in response to an increase in shear stress, which causes release of NO from the endothelium and consequent endothelium-dependent dilatation. FMD has been shown to correlate with invasive measures of endothelial function, as well as with the presence and severity of the major traditional vascular risk factors.[93] Endothelial dysfunction is an accurate predictor of future cardiovascular events (CVD) and target organ damage, such as coronary heart disease, myocardial infarction, stroke, and congestive heart failure. For each 1% improvement in endothelial function by FMD there is an 8% decrease in CVD risk. This is particularly true in low-risk hypertensive patients and less so in the late stages of CVD.[94] There is also nonischemic plethysmography used for structural measurements in blood vessels to detect arterial stiffness. The Max Pulse test is noninvasive and uses a photoelectric clip on the fingertip. By measuring the blood at the fingertip, the Max Pulse can graph the heart beat as it moves through systolic and diastolic pressure waves. If a patient's arterials are flexible, the pressure at the fingertip has lots of small deviations as the arteries flex. If the patient's arteries are stiff, the graph becomes tight and regular. The result is an assessment of arterial hardening that is accurate. In addition to providing an accurate assessment of arterial hardening, the final report also shows an index for circulation, indicating if circulation is compromised owing to insufficient NO production. There is a separate result for large arteries, small arteries, and capillaries. This information is also valuable to a practitioner for assessing risks in patients. The device also performs an accurate heart rate variability test and prints an autonomic nervous system analysis, showing if the person is overstressed and the sympathetic nervous system is dominant, or in some cases showing that the person is inhibited or suppressed and the parasympathetic system is dominant. These types of Food and Drug Administration (FDA)-cleared medical devices that are also reimbursed by most insurance companies provide a valuable noninvasive measurement of vascular function. These must be used to accurately assess vascular NO function in individual patients. These devices can also determine optimal therapy for personalized medicine and track progress on patient compliance and therapeutic success.

Prevention and Treatment Strategies Using Nutrition, Nutritional Supplements, Lifestyle, and Drugs

There is not a single action more important than employing safe and effective methods to restore and maintain NO production in any patient. As described earlier, all known risk factors are risk factors because they all lead to dysregulation or disruption in NO production. The earliest event in the onset and progression of CVD, the number one killer of men and women worldwide, is the loss of NO production. Therefore, it is not only logical but scientifically validated to focus on NO as the first-line therapy for any and all patients. Patients cannot and will not get better until NO-based signaling is restored. The only FDA-approved drug therapy that has NO as a mechanism of action are organic nitrates such as nitroglycerin or isosorbide. These drugs are effective for short-term use for angina pectoris but are not safe to be used long term because of tachyphylaxis[95] and worsening of endothelial function.[96,97] Therefore, they have very limited utility for long-term management of patients. It is always best to use diet and lifestyle as the first-line therapy for patients at risk for CVD, but many times, drug therapy may be necessary. First-line drug therapy considerations for cardiovascular symptoms include angiotensin converting enzyme inhibitors and angiotensin I receptor type I blockers. These drugs will mitigate the negative effects of the renin angiotensin system but will not be most effective unless the NO production pathways are corrected. Another drug consideration may be diuretics (potassium-sparing diuretics are preferred) to remove excess fluid and volume due to disruption of RAS and overproduction of aldosterone. Calcium channel blockers can be used sparingly as the second- or third-line consideration, and only if necessary beta-blockers can be considered. Nebivolol is preferred because it has known effects on NO signaling.[98] It is important for the clinician to recognize that drug therapy typically does not correct the underlying pathology that leads to CVD but rather temporarily addresses important symptoms. Focus must be emphasized on restoring NO production pathways, which will then correct many of the cardiovascular symptoms and underlying pathology.

There are now a number of nutritional and dietary supplements that can be used to restore NO-based signaling. Inorganic nitrate such as found in beetroot can be used, and there are a number of published studies showing safety and efficacy of inorganic nitrate. This is a different molecule with a mechanism of action different from that of organic nitrates.[99] There are a number of products on the market that contain nitrate that are marketed as NO dietary supplements or nutritional products. At the doses found in food and tested in randomized controlled clinical trials in humans, there appears to be very little if any toxicity. In fact, there are several clinical trials showing remarkable efficacy of inorganic nitrate in the treatment of hypertension,[100,101] peripheral artery disease,[102] heart failure with reduced ejection fraction,[103] heart failure with preserved ejection fraction,[104] nonischemic dilated cardiomyopathy,[105] vascular function in hyperlipidemia,[106] and even a rare form of muscular dystrophy[107] with little or no unwanted side effects. Interestingly there are a number of human clinical studies showing no response or improvement using inorganic nitrate.[108-113] This should be expected given the requirements for metabolic nitrate activation to nitrite and NO. Inorganic nitrate is inert in humans because humans lack a functional nitrate reduction gene.[114] Nitrate is taken up in the proximal intestine, and approximately 25% is transported and concentrated in the salivary glands.[115] Up to 20% of the salivary nitrate is reduced to nitrite by oral nitrate-reducing bacteria.[81,116,117] This metabolism and reduction of nitrate can lead to salivary nitrite levels that reach millimolar concentrations.[118] Use of antiseptic mouthwash and antibiotics inhibit the blood pressure lowering effects of nitrate and the increase in salivary and plasma levels of nitrite.[79,119] Once nitrite-enriched saliva is swallowed and reaches the acid environment of the stomach, nitrite becomes protonated and becomes NO oxide in the lumen of the stomach.[120,121] The blood pressure lowering effects of oral nitrite are abolished by use of proton pump inhibitors (PPIs).[122] Therefore, there are a number of requirements necessary for inorganic nitrate to have a therapeutic and physiological effect in humans. All three of the following steps are necessary and sufficient for use of nitrate as a therapeutic agent. If one or more steps are missing, inorganic nitrate, either from diet or supplements, will be of no therapeutic value.

1. Must have sufficient nitrate ingestion (roughly 300-400 mg as a bolus)
2. Must have the correct nitrate reducing bacteria in the oral cavity
3. Must have sufficient stomach acid production

These requirements create a problem with the use of nitrate as a therapeutic agent. Over 180 million Americans use mouthwash on a daily basis, and in 2015 alone, approximately 269 million antibiotics were prescribed from physicians in the United States, enough for five of every six people to receive one antibiotic prescription each year. At least 30% of these antibiotic prescriptions were unnecessary.[123] Use of both antiseptic mouthwash and antibiotics disrupts the oral microbiome and leads to a complete lack of nitrate reduction or at least a decreased efficiency of nitrate reduction. Also given the diversity and variability of the oral microbiome between certain individuals and cultures, it is uncertain how many people have the correct nitrate reducing bacteria.[81] With prevalence of antibiotic and antiseptic mouthwash use in the United States along with periodontal disease and poor oral hygiene, it would

not be surprising if over half of the population is unable to reduce dietary nitrate. The other problem is the use of PPIs. Studies consistently find that PPIs are overprescribed globally in both primary and secondary care. In 2016, over 115 million prescriptions were written for PPIs. This is not counting the number of people taking an over-the-counter PPI. Combing the number of people taking antiseptic mouthwash or antibiotics with those taking PPIs, one can easily imagine conditions in which inorganic nitrate would have no effect in the majority of the population. So, although there is growing evidence on the benefits of inorganic nitrate in a number of human diseases and conditions, it is highly unlikely that it will have a consistent effect across different populations owing to these metabolic requirements and social norms.

A more practical approach to overcome patient variability is a product designed to overcome any limitations in NO production. The design of the commercial product (Neo40, HumanN) is in the form of an orally disintegrating tablet. By design, it has a specific and slow dissolution rate when placed in the oral cavity. This allows for dissipation of the lozenge so that the natural product components containing inorganic nitrite along with an active nitrite reductase can come together and generate NO gas. The lozenge generates 20 to 30 ppm NO gas as it dissolves in the oral cavity. This technology is protected by over a dozen issued US and international patents. To demonstrate the safety and efficacy of this approach a number of randomized controlled clinical trials have been conducted. This technology is designed to do two things: (1) If the patient is unable to produce NO because of the underlying pathology, then the lozenge generates NO itself providing an exogenous source of bioactive NO. (2) Recouple the NOS enzyme so that endogenous production of NO is restored. To date, the clinical data suggest that the lozenge does in fact accomplish those two objectives. In subjects over the age of 40 years with two or more cardiovascular risk factors, taking the NO lozenge twice daily for 30 days leads to a significant reduction in triglycerides, reduction in inflammation, and lowering of blood pressure.[124] In another double-blinded, randomized, placebo-controlled study of subjects with prehypertension (BP 120-139 mm Hg systolic and 80-89 mm Hg diastolic), taking the lozenge twice daily for 30 days reduced systolic blood pressure by 12 mm Hg and reduced diastolic blood pressure by 6 mm Hg. Subjects on the lozenge were able to walk significantly further on a 6-minute walk test after 30 days, demonstrating an improvement in functional capacity. These subjects also reported an improved quality of life in both a physical and mental composition score (SF-36).[125] To demonstrate the bioactivity of the acute effects of the NO release in the oral cavity, a double-blind, placebo-controlled crossover study was conducted in unmedicated subjects with hypertension (BP > 140/90 mm Hg). Administration of a single lozenge lead to a statistically significant reduction in both systolic and diastolic blood pressures after 20 minutes and further significant reduction in both systolic and diastolic pressures after 60 minutes. After 10 minutes there was a significant increase in dilation of the carotid artery as measured by ultrasound. On average carotid artery dilation increased by 13%. A 13% increase in blood vessel diameter translates into a 35% increase in blood flow through the carotids. Furthermore, after 30 minutes there was a significant improvement in arterial compliance and improvement in arterial stiffness. After 4 hours from administration of the lozenge, there was a significant 15% improvement in endothelial function[126], demonstrating an improvement in eNOS-derived NO from the lozenge. In a study of a rare genetic inborn error in metabolism, argininosuccinic aciduria (ASA), the NO lozenge was able to normalize blood pressure, kidney function, and cognitive function and reverse heart disease in a single 15-year-old patient,[127] when all other medications had failed. This is based on the now known clear mechanism of the disruption of NO production in patients with ASA.[128] The NO lozenge has also been shown to reduce the burden of carotid plaque in a pilot study of 10 patients with stable plaque. Using the lozenge twice daily for 6 months leads to a 11% regression of plaque in the carotid artery as determined by ultrasound.[129] Using the same lozenge with 70 mg of added caffeine in a double-blinded placebo-controlled study has been shown to improve cycling time-trial performance by 2.1% in 15 moderately trained athletes.[130] Collectively this demonstrates that providing a source of NO and restoring the function of endogenous NO production can restore NO-based signaling, modify risk factors, and perhaps prevent, treat, or cure CVD. Obviously, more studies are needed, but the future looks bright.

Summary

CVD cannot and will not be adequately managed, treated, or cured without correcting NO production or NO-based signaling. This single disruption of NO production and NO-based signaling is responsible for the onset and progression of CVD.

Employing methods to diagnose NO insufficiency in patients early in the disease process is key to proper management of patients to prevent myocardial infarctions and strokes. The science is clear, mechanisms are known, and proven strategies are available to restore NO production in patients. The burden of CVD will only be improved by proper strategies to restore NO production in patients. We can and we must do better.

Future Challenges

Despite the over 160,000 published studies on NO, a Nobel Prize for its discovery in 1998, and its clearly defined role as the root cause of CVD, many if not most physicians, clinicians, and health care practitioners are uninformed on how to diagnose or correct conditions of NO deficiency. We do not need more research. The science is clear. The major challenge in the fight against CVD is education and the employment of the science and knowledge around NO to patient care. Education about NO in medical school and allied health schools is a must. Clinicians must become more comfortable utilizing new tools for diagnosing endothelial dysfunction and recommending dietary supplements or nutritionals before prescribing drug therapy. Our challenge is education, perhaps not just educating clinicians but educating the public, the patients. As William Mayo has said "The aim of medicine is to prevent disease and prolong life; the ideal of medicine is to eliminate the need of a physician." The word "doctor" is derived from the Latin, docco, which means "teach." If we accomplish our job as teachers and educate the masses on the importance of NO in health and medicine, then perhaps we can accomplish what Sir William Osler described as "One of the first duties of the physician is to educate the masses not to take medicine." The practice of medicine must change from a reactive approach to a proactive approach. Applied physiology is always superior to applied pharmacology.

References

1. Roth GA, Johnson C, Abajobir A, et al. Global, regional, and national burden of cardiovascular diseases for 10 causes, 1990 to 2015. *J Am Coll Cardiol.* 2017;70(1):1-25.
2. Vita JA, Treasure CB, Nabel EG, et al. Coronary vasomotor response to acetylcholine relates to risk factors for coronary artery disease. *Circulation.* 1990;81(2):491-497.
3. Furchgott RF, Zawadzki JV. The obligatory role of endothelial cells in the relaxation of arterial smooth muscle by acetylcholine. *Nature.* 1980;288(5789):373-376.
4. Keaney JF Jr, Vita JA. Atherosclerosis, oxidative stress, and antioxidant protection in endothelium-derived relaxing factor action. *Prog Cardiovasc Dis.* 1995;38(2):129-154.
5. Harrison DG. Endothelial function and oxidant stress. *Clin Cardiol.* 1997;20(11 suppl 2):II-11-7.
6. Granger DN, Kubes P. The microcirculation and inflammation: modulation of leukocyte-endothelial cell adhesion. *J Leukoc Biol.* 1994;55(5):662-675.
7. Pauletto P, Rattazzi M. Inflammation and hypertension: the search for a link. *Nephrol Dial Transpl.* 2006;21(4):850-853.
8. Suematsu M, Suzuki H, Delano FA, et al. The inflammatory aspect of the microcirculation in hypertension: oxidative stress, leukocytes/endothelial interaction, apoptosis. *Microcirculation.* 2002;9(4):259-276.
9. Landmesser U, Dikalov S, Price SR, et al. Oxidation of tetrahydrobiopterin leads to uncoupling of endothelial cell nitric oxide synthase in hypertension. *J Clin Invest.* 2003;111(8):1201-1209.
10. Lakatta EG, Yin FC. Myocardial aging: functional alterations and related cellular mechanisms. *Am J Physiol.* 1982;242(6):H927-H941.
11. Kannel WB, Gordon T, Schwartz MJ. Systolic versus diastolic blood pressure and risk of coronary heart disease. The Framingham study. *Am J Cardiol.* 1971;27(4):335-346.
12. Ross R. Atherosclerosis–an inflammatory disease. *N Engl J Med.* 1999;340(2):115-126.
13. Soltis EE. Effect of age on blood pressure and membrane-dependent vascular responses in the rat. *Circ Res.* 1987;61(6):889-897.
14. van der Loo B, Labugger R, Skepper JN, et al. Enhanced peroxynitrite formation is associated with vascular aging. *J Exp Med.* 2000;192(12):1731-1744.
15. Pie JE, Baek SY, Kim HP, et al. Age-related decline of inducible nitric oxide synthase gene expression in primary cultured rat hepatocytes. *Mol Cells.* 2002;13(3):399-406.
16. Zhou XJ, Vaziri ND, Zhang J, Wang HW, Wang XQ. Association of renal injury with nitric oxide deficiency in aged SHR: prevention by hypertension control with AT1 blockade. *Kidney Int.* 2002;62(3):914-921.

17. Berkowitz DE, White R, Li D, et al. Arginase reciprocally regulates nitric oxide synthase activity and contributes to endothelial dysfunction in aging blood vessels. *Circulation.* 2003;108(16):2000-2006.

18. Taddei S, Virdis A, Ghiadoni L, et al. Age-related reduction of NO availability and oxidative stress in humans. *Hypertension.* 2001;38(2):274-279.

19. Egashira K, Inou T, Hirooka Y, et al. Effects of age on endothelium-dependent vasodilation of resistance coronary artery by acetylcholine in humans. *Circulation.* 1993;88(1):77-81.

20. Gerhard M, Roddy M-A, Creager SJ, Creager MA. Aging progressively impairs endothelium-dependent vasodilation in forearm resistance vessels of humans. *Hypertension.* 1996;27(4):849-853.

21. Ungvari Z, Kaley G, de Cabo R, Sonntag WE, Csiszar A. Mechanisms of vascular aging: new perspectives. *J Gerontol A Biol Sci Med Sci.* 2010;65(10):1028-1041.

22. Wang YR, Alexander GC, Stafford RS. Outpatient hypertension treatment, treatment intensification, and control in Western Europe and the United States. *Arch Intern Med.* 2007;167(2):141-147.

23. Cutler JA, Sorlie PD, Wolz M, Thom T, Fields LE, Roccella EJ. Trends in hypertension prevalence, awareness, treatment, and control rates in United States adults between 1988-1994 and 1999-2004. *Hypertension.* 2008;52(5):818-827.

24. Wright JT Jr, Wright JT, Williamson JD, et al. A randomized trial of intensive versus standard blood-pressure control. *N Engl J Med.* 2015;373(22):2103-2116.

25. Arnold WP, Mittal CK, Katsuki S, Murad F. Nitric oxide activates guanylate cyclase and increases guanosine 3':5'-cyclic monophosphate levels in various tissue preparations. *Proc Natl Acad Sci USA.* 1977;74(8):3203-3207.

26. Bryan NS, Bian K, Murad F. Discovery of the nitric oxide signaling pathway and targets for drug development. *Front Biosci.* 2009;14:1-18.

27. Bryan NS. Functional nitric oxide nutrition to combat cardiovascular disease. *Curr Atheroscler Rep.* 2018;20(5):21.

28. Fernandez-Friera L, Fuster V, López-Melgar B, et al. Normal LDL-cholesterol levels are associated with subclinical atherosclerosis in the absence of risk factors. *J Am Coll Cardiol.* 2017;70(24):2979-2991.

29. Ravnskov U, de Lorgeril M, Diamond DM, et al. LDL-C does not cause cardiovascular disease: a comprehensive review of the current literature. *Expert Rev Clin Pharmacol.* 2018;11(10):959-970.

30. Sachdeva A, Cannon CP, Deedwania PC, et al., Lipid levels in patients hospitalized with coronary artery disease: an analysis of 136,905 hospitalizations in get with the guidelines. *Am Heart J.* 2009;157(1):111-117 e2.

31. Tanner FC, Noll G, Boulanger CM, et al. Oxidized low density lipoproteins inhibit relaxations of porcine coronary arteries. Role of scavenger receptor and endothelium-derived nitric oxide. *Circulation.* 1991;83(6):2012-2020.

32. Napoli C, Ackah E, de Nigris F, et al. Chronic treatment with nitric oxide-releasing aspirin reduces plasma low-density lipoprotein oxidation and oxidative stress, arterial oxidation-specific epitopes, and atherogenesis in hypercholesterolemic mice. *Proc Natl Acad Sci USA.* 2002;99(19):12467-12470.

33. Hacker A, Müller S, Meyer W, Kojda G. The nitric oxide donor pentaerythritol tetranitrate can preserve endothelial function in established atherosclerosis. *Br J Pharmacol.* 2001;132(8):1707-1714.

34. Potenza MA, Gagliardi S, Nacci C, Carratu M, Montagnani M. Endothelial dysfunction in diabetes: from mechanisms to therapeutic targets. *Curr Med Chem.* 2009;16(1):94-112.

35. Huang PL. eNOS, metabolic syndrome and cardiovascular disease. *Trends Endocrinol Metab.* 2009;20(6):295-302.

36. Pieper GM, Langenstroer P, Siebeneich W. Diabetic-induced endothelial dysfunction in rat aorta: role of hydroxyl radicals. *Cardiovasc Res.* 1997;34(1):145-156.

37. Pieper GM, Gross GJ. Oxygen free radicals abolish endothelium-dependent relaxation in diabetic rat aorta. *Am J Physiol.* 1988;255(4 pt 2):H825-H833.

38. Pieper GM, Meier DA, Hager SR. Endothelial dysfunction in a model of hyperglycemia and hyperinsulinemia. *Am J Physiol.* 1995;269(3 pt 2):H845-H850.

39. Tesfamariam B, Cohen RA. Free radicals mediate endothelial cell dysfunction caused by elevated glucose. *Am J Physiol.* 1992;263(2 pt 2):H321-H326.

40. Williams SB, Cusco JA, Roddy M-A, Johnstone MT, Creager MA. Impaired nitric oxide-mediated vasodilation in patients with non-insulin dependent diabetes mellitus. *J Am Coll Cardiol.* 1996;27(3):567-574.

41. de Tejada IS, Goldstein I, Azadzoi K, Krane RJ, Cohen RA. Impaired neurogenic and endothelium-mediated relaxation of penile smooth muscle from diabetic men with impotence. *N Engl J Med.* 1989;320(16):1025-1030.

42. Cilensek I, Mankoč S, Globočnik Petrovič M, et al. The 4a/4a genotype of the VNTR polymorphism for endothelial nitric oxide synthase (eNOS) gene predicts risk for proliferative diabetic retinopathy in Slovenian patients (Caucasians) with type 2 diabetes mellitus. *Mol Biol Rep.* 2012;39(6):7061-7067.

43. Loscalzo J, Welch G. Nitric oxide and its role in the cardiovascular system. *Prog Cardiovasc Dis.* 1995;38(2):87-104.

44. Shankar RR, Wu Y, Shen HQ, Zhu JS, Baron AD. Mice with gene disruption of both endothelial and neuronal nitric oxide synthase exhibit insulin resistance. *Diabetes.* 2000;49(5):684-687.

45. Jiang H, Torregrossa AC, Potts A, et al. Dietary nitrite improves insulin signaling through GLUT4 translocation. *Free Radic Biol Med.* 2014;67:51-57.

46. Carlstrom M, Larsen FJ, Nyström T, et al. Dietary inorganic nitrate reverses features of metabolic syndrome in endothelial nitric oxide synthase-deficient mice. *Proc Natl Acad Sci USA.* 2010;107(41):17716-17720.

47. Celermajer DS, Sorensen KE, Georgakopoulos D, et al. Cigarette smoking is associated with dose-related and potentially reversible impairment of endothelium-dependent dilation in healthy young adults. *Circulation.* 1993;88(5 pt 1):2149-2155.

48. Messner B, Bernhard D. Smoking and cardiovascular disease: mechanisms of endothelial dysfunction and early atherogenesis. *Arterioscler Thromb Vasc Biol.* 2014;34(3):509-515.

49. Ichiki K, Ikeda H, Haramaki N, Ueno T, Imaizumi T. Long-term smoking impairs platelet-derived nitric oxide release. *Circulation.* 1996;94(12):3109-3114.

50. Heitzer T, Just H, Munzel T. Antioxidant vitamin C improves endothelial dysfunction in chronic smokers. *Circulation.* 1996;94(1):6-9.

51. Heitzer T, Brockhoff C, Mayer B, et al. Tetrahydrobiopterin improves endothelium-dependent vasodilation in chronic smokers: evidence for a dysfunctional nitric oxide synthase. *Circ Res.* 2000;86(2):E36-E41.

52. Karatzi K, Papamichael C, Karatzis E, et al. Acute smoking induces endothelial dysfunction in healthy smokers. Is this reversible by red wine's antioxidant constituents? *J Am Coll Nutr.* 2007;26(1):10-15.

53. Bogers RP, Bemelmans WJ, Hoogenveen RT, et al. Association of overweight with increased risk of coronary heart disease partly independent of blood pressure and cholesterol levels: a meta-analysis of 21 cohort studies including more than 300 000 persons. *Arch Intern Med.* 2007;167(16):1720-1728.

54. Olson TP, Schmitz KH, Leon AS, Dengel DR. Vascular structure and function in women: relationship with body mass index. *Am J Prev Med.* 2006;30(6):487-492.

55. Darvall KA, Sam RC, Silverman SH, Bradbury AW, Adam DJ. Obesity and thrombosis. *Eur J Vasc Endovasc Surg.* 2007;33(2):223-233.

56. Pena AS, Wiltshire E, MacKenzie K, et al. Vascular endothelial and smooth muscle function relates to body mass index and glucose in obese and nonobese children. *J Clin Endocrinol Metab.* 2006;91(11):4467-4471.

57. Eringa EC, Stehouwer CDA, Roos MH, Westerhof N, Sipkema P. Selective resistance to vasoactive effects of insulin in muscle resistance arteries of obese Zucker (fa/fa) rats. *Am J Physiol Endocrinol Metab.* 2007;293(5):E1134-E1139.

58. Makimattila S, Virkamäki A, Groop PH, et al. Chronic hyperglycemia impairs endothelial function and insulin sensitivity via different mechanisms in insulin-dependent diabetes mellitus. *Circulation.* 1996;94(6):1276-1282.

59. Vogel RA, Corretti MC, Plotnick GD. Effect of a single high-fat meal on endothelial function in healthy subjects. *Am J Cardiol.* 1997;79(3):350-354.

60. Guzik TJ, Mangalat D, Korbut R. Adipocytokines – novel link between inflammation and vascular function? *J Physiol Pharmacol.* 2006;57(4):505-528.

61. Brook RD. Obesity, weight loss, and vascular function. *Endocrine.* 2006;29(1):21-25.

62. Rocchini AP, Key J, Bondie D, et al. The effect of weight loss on the sensitivity of blood pressure to sodium in obese adolescents. *N Engl J Med.* 1989;321(9):580-585.

63. Blair SN, Kohl HW III, Paffenbarger RS Jr, et al. Physical fitness and all-cause mortality. A prospective study of healthy men and women. *JAMA.* 1989;262(17):2395-2401.

64. Higashi Y, Sasaki S, Kurisu S, et al. Regular aerobic exercise augments endothelium-dependent vascular relaxation in normotensive as well as hypertensive subjects: role of endothelium-derived nitric oxide. *Circulation.* 1999;100(11):1194-1202.

65. Rassaf T, Lauer T, Heiss C, et al. Nitric oxide synthase-derived plasma nitrite predicts exercise capacity. *Br J Sports Med.* 2007;41(10):669-673; discussion 673.

66. Lauer T, Heiss C, Balzer J, et al. Age-dependent endothelial dysfunction is associated with failure to increase plasma nitrite in response to exercise. *Basic Res Cardiol.* 2008;103(3):291-297.

67. Rassaf T, Heiss C, Mangold S, et al. Vascular formation of nitrite after exercise is abolished in patients with cardiovascular risk factors and coronary artery disease. *J Am Coll Cardiol.* 2010;55(14):1502-1503.

68. Micha R, Peñalvo JL, Cudhea F, Imamura F, Rehm CD, Mozaffarian D. Association between dietary factors and mortality from heart disease, stroke, and type 2 diabetes in the United States. *JAMA.* 2017;317(9):912-924.

69. Joshipura KJ, et al. Fruit and vegetable intake in relation to risk of ischemic stroke. *JAMA.* 1999;282(13):1233-1239.

70. Joshipura KJ, Hu FB, Manson JE, et al. The effect of fruit and vegetable intake on risk for coronary heart disease. *Ann Intern Med.* 2001;134(12):1106-1114.

71. Bryan NS, Ivy JL. Inorganic nitrite and nitrate: evidence to support consideration as dietary nutrients. *Nutr Res.* 2015;35(8):643-654.

72. Appel LJ, Moore TJ, Obarzanek E, et al. A clinical trial of the effects of dietary patterns on blood pressure. DASH Collaborative Research Group. *N Engl J Med.* 1997;336(16):1117-1124.

73. Sacks FM, Svetkey LP, Vollmer WM, et al. Effects on blood pressure of reduced dietary sodium and the Dietary Approaches to Stop Hypertension (DASH) diet. DASH-Sodium Collaborative Research Group. *N Engl J Med.* 2001;344(1):3-10.

74. Most MM. Estimated phytochemical content of the dietary approaches to stop hypertension (DASH) diet is higher than in the control study diet. *J Am Diet Assoc.* 2004;104(11):1725-1727.

75. Hord NG, Tang Y, Bryan NS. Food sources of nitrates and nitrites: the physiologic context for potential health benefits. *Am J Clin Nutr.* 2009;90(1):1-10.

76. Sobko T, Marcus C, Govoni M, Kamiya S. Dietary nitrate in Japanese traditional foods lowers diastolic blood pressure in healthy volunteers. *Nitric Oxide.* 2010;22(2):136-140.

77. Joshy G, Arora M, Korda RJ, Chalmers J, Banks E. Is poor oral health a risk marker for incident cardiovascular disease hospitalisation and all-cause mortality? Findings from 172 630 participants from the prospective 45 and up study. *BMJ Open.* 2016;6(8):e012386.

78. Duncan C, Li H, Dykhuizen R, et al. Protection against oral and gastrointestinal diseases: importance of dietary nitrate intake, oral nitrate reduction and enterosalivary nitrate circulation. *Comp Biochem Physiol A Physiol.* 1997;118(4):939-948.

79. Petersson J, Carlström M, Schreiber O, et al. Gastroprotective and blood pressure lowering effects of dietary nitrate are abolished by an antiseptic mouthwash. *Free Radic Biol Med.* 2009;46(8):1068-1075.

80. Bryan NS, Tribble G, Angelov N. Oral microbiome and nitric oxide: the missing link in the management of blood pressure. *Curr Hypertens Rep.* 2017;19(4):33.

81. Hyde ER, Andrade F, Vaksman Z, et al. Metagenomic analysis of nitrate-reducing bacteria in the oral cavity: implications for nitric oxide homeostasis. *PLoS One.* 2014;9(3):e88645.

82. Kleinbongard P, Dejam A, Lauer T, et al. Plasma nitrite concentrations reflect the degree of endothelial dysfunction in humans. *Free Radic Biol Med.* 2006;40(2):295-302.

83. Archer SL, Gragasin FS, Webster L, Bochinski D, Michelakis ED. Aetiology and management of male erectile dysfunction and female sexual dysfunction in patients with cardiovascular disease. *Drugs Aging.* 2005;22(10):823-844.

84. Rajfer J, Aronson WJ, Bush PA, Dorey FJ, Ignarro LJ. Nitric oxide as a mediator of relaxation of the corpus cavernosum in response to nonadrenergic, noncholinergic neurotransmission. *N Engl J Med.* 1992;326(2):90-94.

85. Rodriguez JJ, Al Dashti R, Schwarz ER. Linking erectile dysfunction and coronary artery disease. *Int J Impot Res.* 2005;17(suppl 1):S12-S18.

86. Radomski MW, Palmer RM, Moncada S. An L-arginine/nitric oxide pathway present in human platelets regulates aggregation. *Proc Natl Acad Sci USA.* 1990;87(13):5193-5197.

87. Cleeter MW, Cooper JM, Darley-Usmar VM, Moncada S, Schapira AHV. Reversible inhibition of cytochrome c oxidase, the terminal enzyme of the mitochondrial respiratory chain, by nitric oxide. Implications for neurodegenerative diseases. *FEBS Lett.* 1994;345:50-54.

88. Nisoli E, Clementi E, Paolucci C, et al. Mitochondrial biogenesis in mammals: the role of endogenous nitric oxide. *Science.* 2003;299(5608):896-899.

89. Bryan NS. The potential use of salivary nitrite as a marker of NO status in humans. *Nitric Oxide.* 2015;45:4-6.

90. Morrow JD, Hill KE, Burk RF, Nammour TM, Badr KF, Roberts LJ. A series of prostaglandin F2-like compounds are produced in vivo in humans by a non-cyclooxygenase, free radical-catalyzed mechanism. *Proc Natl Acad Sci USA.* 1990;87(23):9383-9387.

91. Morrow JD, Minton TA, Roberts LJ III. The F2-isoprostane, 8-epi-prostaglandin F2 alpha, a potent agonist of the vascular thromboxane/endoperoxide receptor, is a platelet thromboxane/endoperoxide receptor antagonist. *Prostaglandins.* 1992;44(2):155-163.

92. Minuz P, Andrioli G, Degan M, et al. The F2-isoprostane 8-epiprostaglandin F2alpha increases platelet adhesion and reduces the antiadhesive and antiaggregatory effects of NO. *Arterioscler Thromb Vasc Biol.* 1998;18(8):1248-1256.

93. Patel S, Celermajer DS. Assessment of vascular disease using arterial flow mediated dilatation. *Pharmacol Rep.* 2006;58 suppl:3-7.

94. Yang Y, Xu J-Z, Wang Y, Tang X-F, Gao P-J. Brachial flow-mediated dilation predicts subclinical target organ damage progression in essential hypertensive patients: a 3-year follow-up study. *J Hypertens.* 2014;32(12):2393-2400; discussion 2400.

95. Elkayam U, Kulick D, McIntosh N, Roth A, Hsueh W, Rahimtoola SH. Incidence of early tolerance to hemodynamic effects of continuous infusion of nitroglycerin in patients with coronary artery disease and heart failure. *Circulation.* 1987;76(3):577-584.

96. Caramori PR, Adelman AG, Azevedo ER, Newton GE, Parker AB, Parker JD. Therapy with nitroglycerin increases coronary vasoconstriction in response to acetylcholine. *J Am Coll Cardiol.* 1998;32(7):1969-1974.

97. Gori T, Mak SS, Kelly S, Parker JD. Evidence supporting abnormalities in nitric oxide synthase function induced by nitroglycerin in humans. *J Am Coll Cardiol.* 2001;38(4):1096-1101.

98. Jiang H, Polhemus DJ, Islam KN, et al. Nebivolol acts as a S-nitrosoglutathione reductase inhibitor: a new mechanism of action. *J Cardiovasc Pharmacol Ther.* 2016;21(5):478-485.

99. Omar SA, Artime E, Webb AJ. A comparison of organic and inorganic nitrates/nitrites. *Nitric Oxide.* 2012;26(4):229-240.

100. Kapil V, Khambata RS, Robertson A, Caulfield MJ, Ahluwalia A. Dietary nitrate provides sustained blood pressure lowering in hypertensive patients: a randomized, phase 2, double-blind, placebo-controlled study. *Hypertension.* 2015;65(2):320-327.

101. Webb AJ, Patel N, Loukogeorgakis S, et al. Acute blood pressure lowering, vasoprotective, and antiplatelet properties of dietary nitrate via bioconversion to nitrite. *Hypertension.* 2008;51(3):784-790.

102. Bock JM, Treichler DP, Norton SL, Ueda K, Hughes WE, Casey DP. Inorganic nitrate supplementation enhances functional capacity and lower-limb microvascular reactivity in patients with peripheral artery disease. *Nitric Oxide.* 2018;80:45-51.

103. Coggan AR, Leibowitz JL, Spearie CA, et al. Acute dietary nitrate intake improves muscle contractile function in patients with heart failure: a double-blind, placebo-controlled, randomized trial. *Circ Heart Fail.* 2015;8(5):914-920.

104. Zamani P, Rawat D, Shiva-Kumar P, et al. Effect of inorganic nitrate on exercise capacity in heart failure with preserved ejection fraction. *Circulation*. 2015;131(4):371-380; discussion 380.

105. Kerley CP, O''Neill JO, Reddy Bijjam V, Blaine C, James PE, Cormican L. Dietary nitrate increases exercise tolerance in patients with non-ischemic, dilated cardiomyopathy-a double-blind, randomized, placebo-controlled, crossover trial. *J Heart Lung Transpl* 2016;35(7):922-926.

106. Velmurugan S, Gan JM, Rathod KS, et al. Dietary nitrate improves vascular function in patients with hypercholesterolemia: a randomized, double-blind, placebo-controlled study. *Am J Clin Nutr*. 2016;103(1):25-38.

107. Nelson MD, Rosenberry R, Barresi R, et al. Sodium nitrate alleviates functional muscle ischaemia in patients with Becker muscular dystrophy. *J Physiol*. 2015;593(23):5183-5200.

108. Gilchrist M, Winyard PG, Aizawa K, Anning C, Shore A, Benjamin N. Effect of dietary nitrate on blood pressure, endothelial function, and insulin sensitivity in type 2 diabetes. *Free Radic Biol Med*. 2013;60:89-97.

109. Bescos R, Ferrer-roca V, Galilea PA, et al. Sodium nitrate supplementation does not enhance performance of endurance athletes. *Med Sci Sports Exerc*. 2012;44(12):2400-2409.

110. Nabben M, Schmitz JPJ, Ciapaite J, et al. Dietary nitrate does not reduce oxygen cost of exercise or improve muscle mitochondrial function in patients with mitochondrial myopathy. *Am J Physiol Regul Integr Comp Physiol*. 2017;312(5):R689-R701.

111. Siervo M, Oggioni C, Jakovljevic DG, et al. Dietary nitrate does not affect physical activity or outcomes in healthy older adults in a randomized, cross-over trial. *Nutr Res*. 2016;36(12):1361-1369.

112. Hirai DM, Zelt JT, Jones JH, et al. Dietary nitrate supplementation and exercise tolerance in patients with heart failure with reduced ejection fraction. *Am J Physiol Regul Integr Comp Physiol*. 2017;312(1):R13-R22.

113. Schiffer TA, Larsen FJ, Lundberg JO, Weitzberg E, Lindholm P. Effects of dietary inorganic nitrate on static and dynamic breath-holding in humans. *Respir Physiol Neurobiol*. 2013;185(2):339-348.

114. Lundberg JO, Weitzberg E, Cole JA, Benjamin N. Nitrate, bacteria and human health. *Nat Rev Microbiol*. 2004;2(7):593-602.

115. Eisenbrand G, Spiegelhalder B, Preussmann R. Nitrate and nitrite in saliva. *Oncology*. 1980;37(4):227-231.

116. Duncan C, Dougall H, Johnston P, et al. Chemical generation of nitric oxide in the mouth from the enterosalivary circulation of dietary nitrate. *Nat Med*. 1995;1(6):546-551.

117. Li H, Duncan C, Townend J, et al. Nitrate-reducing bacteria on rat tongues. *Appl Environ Microbiol*. 1997;63(3):924-930.

118. Govoni M, Jansson EÅ, Weitzberg E, Lundberg JO. The increase in plasma nitrite after a dietary nitrate load is markedly attenuated by an antibacterial mouthwash. *Nitric Oxide*. 2008;19(4):333-337.

119. Kapil V, Haydar SMA, Pearl V, Lundberg JO, Weitzberg E, Ahluwalia A. Physiological role for nitrate reducing oral bacteria in blood pressure control. *Free Radic Biol Med*. 2013;55:93-100.

120. McKnight GM, Smith LM, Drummond RS, Duncan CW, Golden M, Benjamin N. Chemical synthesis of nitric oxide in the stomach from dietary nitrate in humans. *Gut*. 1997;40(2):211-214.

121. Benjamin N, O'Driscoll F, Dougall H, et al. Stomach NO synthesis. *Nature*. 1994;368(6471):502.

122. Montenegro MF, Sundqvist ML, Larsen FJ, et al. Blood pressure-lowering effect of orally ingested nitrite is abolished by a proton pump inhibitor. *Hypertension*. 2017;69(1):23-31.

123. Fleming-Dutra KE, Hersh AL, Shapiro DJ, et al. Prevalence of inappropriate antibiotic prescriptions among us ambulatory care visits, 2010–2011. *JAMA*. 2016;315(17):1864-1873.

124. Zand J, Lanza F, Garg HK, Bryan NS. All-natural nitrite and nitrate containing dietary supplement promotes nitric oxide production and reduces triglycerides in humans. *Nutr Res*. 2011;31(4):262-269.

125. Biswas OS, Gonzalez VR, Schwarz ER. Effects of an oral nitric oxide supplement on functional capacity and blood pressure in adults with prehypertension. *J Cardiovasc Pharmacol Ther*. 2015;20(1):52-58.

126. Houston M, Hays L. Acute effects of an oral nitric oxide supplement on blood pressure, endothelial function, and vascular compliance in hypertensive patients. *J Clin Hypertens (Greenwich)*. 2014;16(7):524-529.

127. Nagamani SC, Campeau PM, Shchelochkov OA, et al. Nitric-oxide supplementation for treatment of long-term complications in argininosuccinic aciduria. *Am J Hum Genet*. 2012;90(5):836-846.

128. Erez A, Nagamani SCS, Shchelochkov OA, et al. Requirement of argininosuccinate lyase for systemic nitric oxide production. *Nat Med*. 2011;17(12):1619-1626.

129. Lee E. Effects of nitric oxide on carotid intima media thickness: a pilot study. *Altern Therapies Health Med*. 2016;22(S2):32-34.

130. Lee J, Kim HT, Solares GJ, Kim K, Ding Z, Ivy JL. Caffeinated nitric oxide-releasing lozenge improves cycling time trial performance. *Int J Sports Med*. 2015;36(2):107-112.

3

Atherosclerotic Oxidative Stress: A Maladaptive Immune System Response to Perceived Intimal Infection

James C. Roberts, MD, FACC, FAARFM

Oxidative stress occurs when superoxide generation exceeds the ability of our innate enzymatic and diet-derived antioxidant defenses to neutralize this reactive oxygen species (ROS) and its physiologic second messenger H_2O_2, allowing the generation of longer-lived and vasculopathic ROS and RNS (reactive nitrogen species). Oxidative stress is the driving force of atherosclerosis, a pathophysiology that we can understand and contain.

This chapter covers the causes and consequences of intimal oxidative stress, as well as strategies to prevent and counter its adverse effects (particularly the Th1/Th17-led acquired immune system attack against oxidized LDL and other altered intimal proteins). Let us start with a step-by-step review of atherosclerosis, with particular focus on steps mediated by oxidative and (secondary) inflammatory stress and immune dysregulation.

Focal Endothelial Activation and Lipid Infiltration

Atherosclerosis begins when apo-B 100–containing lipoproteins (LDL, Lp(a), and remnants) infiltrate the artery wall at sites of endothelial activation. This focal perturbation in endothelial barrier function occurs beyond branch points, where low laminar flow combined with high oscillatory shear leads to reduced eNOS (generates nitric oxide) and Nrf-2 (antioxidant enzyme transcription) expression, combined with upregulated NADPH oxidase, xanthine oxidase, and Ang II activity. An intimal local environment is thus created where reactive oxygen and nitrogen derived species (ROS and RNS) are not counterbalanced by nitric oxide and intrinsic enzymatic antioxidant defenses. As flotsam and jetsam accumulate beyond a bend in the river, so will atherosclerosis initiate beyond arterial branch points.

Lipid particles traverse the endothelial cell monolayer via diffusion. The greater the number of lipid particles, and the smaller their particle size, the greater will be the level of passive lipid translocation. Systemic hypertension favors this process, as will other factors, including toxins, that promote systemic endothelial activation (adaptive in our response to true infection but when maladaptively present in atherosclerosis we term this phenomenon endothelial dysfunction).

This initial lipid intimal translocation is not by itself immunopathologic, as apo-B 100 is composed of amino acid sequences to which the innate and acquired immune system is not intolerant. LDL itself is food. It is a transport vehicle for the biosynthetic raw material cholesterol. Every cell of the intima expresses the molecular LDL receptor, at a level commensurate with its perceived need for free cholesterol. If the cell perceives a need for free cholesterol, the receptor will be expressed. If not, the LDL receptor is not expressed. LDL will not be taken up (your stomach is full so you put down your knife and fork).

Once oxidized, LDL cannot be taken up via the molecular LDL receptor; it is no longer biochemically useful. Thus, LDL carries with it antioxidant protection (lipid-soluble antioxidants such as tocopherol, beta-carotene, and coenzyme Q_{10}, which can be "recharged" by water-soluble vitamin C). This defense is typically sufficient to protect LDL within the relatively reductive plasma environment. The extracellular intimal compartment, however, is more pro-oxidative (a thousand times more so than plasma). Standard LDL antioxidant defense levels may not provide sufficient protection. This should not be an issue, as "unneeded" LDL particles, those not ligated by an open LDL receptor, will freely diffuse back into the circulation, and find an open LDL receptor elsewhere. In the absence of infection/inflammation, LDL will be internalized by cells only when and if it is needed for biosynthetic activity (steroid hormones, bile salts, vitamin D synthesis, etc.).

Physiologic intimal LDL give and take, a demand and supply phenomenon, has worked well for Man over our 4-million-year history. Mother Nature promotes hyperlipidemia and focal infiltration of lipids beyond homeostatic synthetic need only when these processes are needed to defend against Man's natural predator, which is infectious. Primitive Man experienced oxidative and inflammatory stress only in relation to infection. Modern Man experiences a pseudoinfectious pathophysiology in a progressive, age-related fashion, in relation to our ROS-generating diet, lifestyle, expanding waist line, and cumulative toxin burden—thus lipid metabolism is deranged!

To fight infection, we need more cholesterol (leukocyte cell membrane synthesis), we need ROS and RNS "bullets" (fired by WBCs to kill the invaders), and we need an activated endothelium (expressing adhesion molecules and elaborating chemotactic signals to pull immune cells into the breach). HMG Co-A reductase, the rate-limiting enzyme in cholesterol biosynthesis, thus upregulates, generating copious quantities of needed cholesterol, along with isoprenoid signaling molecules, which upregulate NADPH Oxidase, our most powerful superoxide generator, and downregulate eNOS, activating the endothelium. Oxidative stress means that "we are at war"!

Oxidative and inflammatory byproducts of Western living, false flags for chronic infection, thus lead to an age-related increase in circulating cholesterol, a progressively activated and thus leaky endothelium, and a biochemical milieu characterized by oxidative stress and dysregulated (Th1/Th17 rich and Treg poor) immune activation.

Thus, we have hyperlipidemia and endothelial activation, particularly beyond branch points. Lipids will infiltrate the endothelium at these stress points, but again, if they are not needed, if there are no open LDL receptors, then they will diffuse out. With respect to pathological atherosclerosis, the first thing to "really go wrong" is lipid retention within the subendothelial space. Retained lipid particles cannot diffuse out and are thus subject to pre-atherosclerotic oxidative modification.

LDL Modification, Trapping, and Oxidation

LDL cholesterol is composed of cholesterol and cholesterol ester (food), containing a small number of single-use nonenzymatic antioxidants (protectors), surrounded by the apo-B 100 protein, which is studded with phosphatidylcholine molecules. The rheological characteristics of a given LDL particle relate to the status of its surface phospholipids (the initial composition of which, in turn, relates to relative dietary intake of saturated vs. unsaturated fatty acids).

Phospholipase enzymes, the expression of which is upregulated in relation to systemic and focal inflammation (which itself relates to systemic and focal oxidative stress; as we will discuss), can alter LDL surface phospholipids, causing them to clump together, and bind irreversibly to intimal

proteoglycan (rich in chondroitin sulfate) matrix material. Sphingomyelinase (S-Smase), degrades LDL surface phospholipids, and this alteration leads to LDL particle adhesion and clumping. Lipoprotein lipase (LPL), present on the luminal endothelial surface, breaks large lipid particles down into smaller versions, favoring their diffusion across the endothelium (working in our favor within the liver, helping to clear circulating lipid particles, but working against us at vulnerable arterial branch points). All cells of the intima (endothelial cells, vascular smooth muscle cells, and especially activated mononuclear cells) can synthesize LPL. The role of this subendothelial LPL is to bind LDL to proteoglycan. Bound LDL cannot diffuse back out into the circulation. By generating LPL, intimal cells can "keep their food close at hand." Phospholipase A2 (PLA2) splits a fatty acid (typically arachidonic acid in Industrialized Man) from the second carbon position of LDL surface phosphatidylcholine, to generate lysophosphatidylcholine (LysoPc) and one arachidonic acid molecules. The latter is subject to enzymatic (cyclooxygenase) and nonenzymatic (oxidative) conversion into downstream pro-inflammatory mediators (such as thromboxane A2). Lysophosphatidylcholine itself leads to endothelial activation. Its presence within the subendothelial space means that "something is wrong." LysoPc (and other downstream products of phospholipid degradation such as diacylglycerol and platelet-activating factor) stimulates endothelial cells to express adhesion molecules (VCAM and ICAM), such that circulating monocytes can be drawn in to investigate this initial perturbation of intimal homeostasis (from Mother Nature's perspective, likely another infectious breach). As with the case of S-Smase alteration, LDL particles containing PLA2-modified membrane phospholipids will adhere and clump together on proteoglycan (Figure 3.1). Clumped LDL particles will no longer "fit" into an open LDL receptor. They may appear as "debris" and thus are subject to ligation

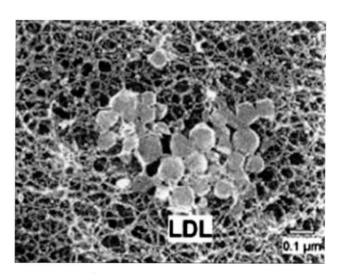

Figure 3.1 *Modified LDL particles trapping to intimal proteoglycan. (From Tabas I, Williams KJ, Borén J. Subendothelial lipoprotein retention as the initiating process in atherosclerosis. Update and therapeutic implications.* Circulation. *2007;116:1832-1844.)*

by the scavenger receptor of resident tissue macrophages (roving monocytes that have wandered into the subintimal space looking for microbes or cellular debris), with subsequent endocytosis, followed by macrophage activation.

Altered (termed minimally oxidized, or MM-LDL) and now immobilized LDL particles will be subject to further oxidative alteration by free radical species generated within the subintimal space (initially with superoxide generated during normal oxidative metabolism and later with superoxide and secondary ROS/RNS species generated by pathologically upregulated NADPH oxidase [NOX], xanthine oxidase [XO], angiotensin II—angiotensin receptor type 1 (AT1R) trafficking, and HMG Co-A reductase expression).

Carbon to carbon double bonds on LDL particle surface area are polyunsaturated fatty acids (PUFAs), susceptible to oxidative alteration, convert into reactive aldehydes, which form adducts with exposed lysine and arginine of the apolipoprotein B100, altering LDL particle configuration and charge. The now heightened negative charge of the oxidized LDL particle (oxLDL) allows tighter binding to the positive charge of proteoglycan sulfate and carboxyl groups as well as to the scavenger receptor of tissue mononuclear cells, favoring its immobilization and uptake, respectively. Of greater consequence, this "acquired mutation" of apo-B 100 creates a protein sequence, or more precisely a protein shape, to which developing T lymphocytes were not exposed to during their maturation within the thymus. Oxidized apo-B 100 thus appears as a foreign molecule, an invader, a microbial "look alike" that must be killed or neutralized by the full force of Mother Nature's anti-infectious defense mechanisms.

Oxidized LDL Phagocytosis and Innate Immune System Activation

At this point we have trapped LDL molecules that are being oxidized, and an activated, nitric acid–poor, endothelial surface that is nonspecifically pulling in monocytes (termed macrophages upon entrance into the intima). Macrophages, as do all cells of the intima, bear LDL receptors. Oxidized LDL is not ligated by the native LDL receptor; it no longer fits. Rather the scavenger receptor expressed by mononuclear cells recognizes oxidized LDL as a microbe or cellular debris. Oxidized LDL is thus taken in. Having captured this nonnative and thus threatening particle, the macrophage activates. We kill microbes with superoxide and downstream ROS and RNS, and thus their production within the macrophage is increased. More scavenger receptors are elaborated. The activated macrophage will also express nonphagocytic threat receptors (such as TLR4, the Toll-like receptor, and cytokine receptors), such that it can better sense its local environment and carry out its search and destroy mission. ROS that cross into the local environment serve to hasten oxidation of adjacent immobilized but not-yet-oxidized LDL particles. The activated macrophage releases chemotactic molecules (such as MCP-1, monocyte chemotactic protein), creating a chemoattractant trail to lead mononuclear cells

that ligated endothelial adhesion molecules to actively translocate to the point of perceived infection, and activation signals, such as MCSF (monocyte colony stimulating factor), stimulating the translocating mononuclear cells to "lock and load," upregulating ROS/RNS generation and scavenger and threat receptor expression.

Intimal infection has been diagnosed. The endothelium further activates. Monocytes, along with second wave monocular defenders (dendritic cells and T memory cells), swarm in, more cholesterol is oxidized, and more oxidized cholesterol is phagocytosed (Figure 3.2). At this point, the activated macrophages contain more cholesterol than it needs for biosynthetic purposes, and thus its native LDL receptor should be withdrawn. That is not the case. As will be discussed in more detail later, inflammatory cytokines, the products of nuclear factor kappa beta (NF-κB) translocation, stimulate the conversion of free cholesterol into cholesterol ester (storing fuel for the infectious winter to come). As expression of the native LDL receptor relates to the level of free, not esterified cholesterol within the cell, the LDL receptor remains expressed even though the activated macrophage is chock full of phagocytosed oxidized LDL. The activated macrophage, eager to nonspecifically rid the local environment of all potential threats, not just the threat it perceives from oxidized LDL, begins to pinocytose adjacent molecules, including nonoxidized LDL particles.

We now have an activated macrophage, loaded to the gills with oxidized cholesterol, sending out distress signals to attract and activate fellow first-line defenders. Although later arriving, innate immune defenders can leave this inflamed intimal environment to warn the adaptive immune system as to the specific nature of the oxLDL threat, the early arriving and now cholesterol choked macrophage inactivates, transforming into a lipid-laden foam cell. Apoptosis and coalescences of foam cells create the fatty streak, the initial histologic manifestation of atherosclerosis.

This process, of course, is reversible. When a microbial threat has been neutralized, a wave of nonactivated macrophages (M2 macrophages) will infiltrate the previously inflamed region and phagocytose the dead first-line defenders, allowing function and histology to return to normal (termed catabasis). This process is programmed to occur. When Mother Nature initiates an inflammatory response, the biological clock begins to tick, and a few days later the immune response shifts from search and destroy to inflammation resolution, as the cytokine milieu shifts from Th1/Th17 (IL-1β, TNFα, IL-6, IL-17, IL-23) to Treg (IL-10 and TGF-β). This programmed shift from infiltration to catabasis will occur, of course, only if the infectious threat is indeed neutralized. If microbes continue to breach the endothelial barrier, the inflammatory response is not called off, and inflammation resolution will not occur. In the setting of human atherosclerosis, if the level of lipid particles diffusing into vulnerable endothelial sites decreases, then the foam cells will be resorbed. In contrast, if cholesterol infiltration continues (the situation in Industrialized Man), then catabasis will not occur, more foam cells will be created, apoptosis

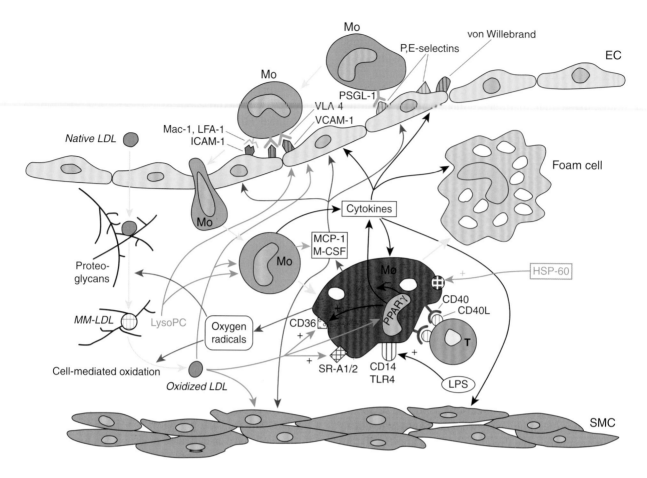

Figure 3.2 *Phagocytosis of intimal oxidized LDL activates mononuclear cells into infection battle mode. (From Osterud B, Bjorklid E. Role of monocytes in atherogenesis.* Physiol Rev. *2003;83(4):1069-1112.)*

will give way to tissue necrosis, and we now have a mass of coalesced lipid droplets and crystals within the vascular wall, the lipid core of the developing plaque.

Even before we get to this point, of atheroma development, and well afterward, we do have a means of removing cholesterol, and reversing LDL oxidation, within the intimal environment. Mother Nature (evolution or the creator, depending on your perspective) knew that our corrective response to endothelial microbial breach in the setting of infection-induced hyperlipidemia could lead to macrophage lipid engorgement and subsequent apoptosis. Thus she (or he, again depending on your perspective) created the HDL system. The HDL-associated enzyme lecithin cholesterol acyltransferase (LCAT) esterifies free or deesterified cholesterol from mononuclear and intimal cells with linoleic acid, and then loads up the newly formed cholesterol-linoleate into the HDL particle, for transport back to the liver. Paraoxonase, another HDL-associated enzyme, removes lipid peroxides from mononuclear cells, intimal cells, and lipoproteins, essentially reversing LDL oxidation (and why stimulating HDL reverse cholesterol transport and antioxidant function protects against disease progression and adverse events).

Anatomic atherosclerosis begins with the fatty streak. If cholesterol levels fall, then catabasis and reverse cholesterol transport can occur, and the fatty streak will resorb. If cholesterol continues to breach the endothelium, then more mononuclear cells will be brought in, and the fatty streak gives way to the slowly growing atheroma. The focal absence of endothelial-derived nitric oxide allows vascular smooth muscle cells to proliferate and migrate into the endothelial zone, adding bulk to the atheroma. At some point the lesion will become visible on angiography.

So far, we have confined ourselves to the innate immune response, how pattern receptors on mononuclear cells react to perceived environmental threat. But atherosclerosis is a maladaptive response of the acquired immune system to perceived infection of the arterial wall with oxidized LDL and other perceived nonnative entities. How do we go from LDL oxidation to the Th1/Th17-rich, Treg-poor intimal environment where interferon-gamma stimulates macrophages to release matrix metalloproteinases to degrade the fibrous cap and precipitate an acute coronary event? A review of immune system dynamics is thus warranted.

Immune System Basics

Immune system effector cells, both innate and adaptive, originate within the bone marrow from a common hematopoietic progenitor stem cell line. Innate immune cells sense threat in a nonspecific fashion; they respond to abnormal shapes.

They sound an alarm and stimulate an adaptive or acquired immune response against a specific invader (in true infection, a snippet of bacterial protein; in atherosclerosis, initially an 8- to 20-amino-acid-long snippet of oxidized apo-B 100).

Innate immune cells sample the environment. A large surface area facilitates this function, and thus they send out cytoplasmic pseudopods (hence the generic term dendritic cells), coated with receptors that recognize nonnative shapes. PAMPs (pathogen-activated molecular receptors) recognize lipopolysaccharide of gram-negative microbes and like molecules expressed by gram-positive bacteria. DAMPs (damage-activated molecular receptors) recognize debris of apoptotic cells or particulate matter and oxLDL. In fact, oxLDL is the most common DAMP. Monocytes serve as circulating dendritic cells. Upon entry into the intima or other tissue compartments they transform into macrophages. Kupffer cells (liver), microglia (brain), Langerhans cells (skin) are all dendritic cells that have specialized to sense threats found within these specific tissue environments.

So, a microbe breaches our skin, or an oxidized LDL protein forms within the intima. PAMPs on the first in dendritic cell ligate the nonnative shape in question. The structure is then phagocytosed into a lysosome, where it is degraded into its component parts, including snippets of its protein structure. Having captured an invader, the roving dendritic cell now migrates to the nearest lymph node or lymph organ (liver or spleen), to inform the adaptive immune system as to the specific threat faced, aiming to initiate a rapidly amplifying immune response (antibodies and cytokine elaborating T helper cells) directed against the specific invader. In this process the dendritic cell, functionally an antigen capture cell, converts itself into an antigen-presenting cell (APC), prepared to present what it caught on a MHC II molecule, to display co-stimulatory molecules, and to secrete co-stimulatory cytokines, all in an effort to awaken a naïve T helper cell, to serve its one and only function, to activate, proliferate, and then direct an overwhelming immune response to a specific threat.

The lymphocyte population of the acquired immune response consists of B cells and T cells. B cells generate antibodies, only in response to T cell instruction, aiming to immobilize or damage invaders that are not destroyed via the mechanism of macrophage phagocytosis. B cells play little role in atherosclerosis and will not be discussed further. Nascent T cells leave the bone marrow, and migrate to the thymus, where they are "educated." Within the thymus, T cells will be exposed to antigenic determinants (8- to 20-amino-acid-long snippets of native protein) that they will see within their lives within the specific human. T cells that react with normal proteins will be culled via apoptosis. The trillion different T cells that survive thymic maturation can "read" antigenic determinants presented on MHC molecules. No surviving T cells should react to a self-molecule (clinical auto-immunity occurs only when a self-molecule has been altered, such as in myocardial infarction, or when chronic, unrelenting oxidative and inflammatory stress overstimulates the immune system, such that it begins to indiscriminately

misrecognize self as foreign). Following thymic maturation, naïve, nonactivated T cells migrate from the thymus to peripheral lymph organs, where they do nothing until they are awakened from biochemical slumber by an activated innate immune cell that bears an antigenic determinant, on an MHC II molecule, that is a specific match for the T cell receptor of the resting T cell.

Innate immune cells thus awaken dormant T helper cells by presenting antigenic determinants on an MHC II molecule. What are MHC molecules? What are T cell receptors? How does the acquired immune system activate to legitimate infection, or pathologically to oxidized LDL or troponin?

MHC (major histocompatibility) molecules are flag poles that can fly different flags. Cell membrane–bound MHC molecules "present" 12- to 20-amino-acid-long protein snippets, designed to inform adjacent or roving T cells as to the proteins contained within them.

Nonimmune, somatic cells bear MHC I molecules. Their job is to inform and activate natural killer T cells and CD8 self-surveillance T cells if their cell has undergone malignant transformation or viral invasion. Our cells generate specific proteins, in relation to which genes are being transcribed within the nucleus, when specific mRNA molecules are translated into specific amino acid sequences at the level of the ribosome. Transcribed proteins contribute to cell structure and function. After a period of time each cell protein will be degraded, thus allowing for an adaptive turn over in cellular protein, in relation to which genes are being translated, related to differing intracellular conditions, related to differing signals the cell is receiving from its outside local and systemic environment. Intracellular proteins are degraded within proteosomes, which will cut the protein into 12- to 20-amino-acid-long antigenic determinants, which are then attached to MHC I molecules to be expressed on the cell membrane. CD8 and T killer cells are monitoring this situation. If all intracellular proteins are native, then the antigenic determinants presented on MHC I molecules are something that they have seen before, something to which they are tolerant, and no action is taken.

However, if the cell has been hijacked, say by a virus, and is now cranking out nonnative, viral proteins, or if the cell has undergone malignant conversion and is generating inappropriate proteins, then nonnative antigenic determinants will be expressed on the MHC I molecules. Roving natural killer and CD8 T cells will recognize this anomaly, bind to the now rogue cell within an immune synapse, and then destroy it (clinical cancer occurs only when this monitoring process breaks down).

Antigen Capture and Presentation

Cells of the innate immune, first-line defenders, also bear MHC II molecules, designed to "show off" the microbes that they have captured. Say you are a Kupffer cell in the liver or a macrophage or dendritic cell that has just phagocytosed an oxidized LDL molecule. Pattern receptor ligation with these entities tells you that something is wrong, that some form of invasion has occurred, so you gobble up the target entity, begin to degrade it within your phagolysosomes, and then leave the site of antigenic capture and make your way to the nearest lymph organ, to "sound the alarm." As your travel you transform yourself from an antigen capture cell into an APC. You mount antigenic determinants derived from the bacteria or oxLDL protein that you took in on to an MHC II molecule, and "show it off" to resting T cells within the lymph organ. If your antigenic determinant is an exact match to the configuration of the T cell receptor on one of the trillion T helper cells previously released by the thymus, then an acquired immune synapse will occur.

The initial immune synapse, at least 100 "lock in key" MHC II–antigenic determinant–T cell receptor molecular couplings between the APC and naïve T cell, is necessary to initiate an acquired immune response directed against the specific antigenic determinant (and the microbe from which it was derived), but by itself is not sufficient. The APC must elaborate co-stimulator molecules and co-stimulatory cytokines to "fully wake up" the resting naïve T cell. Stated otherwise, the APC must be "alarmed and angry" if it to fully "lock and load" the resting T cell (in this fashion, we will not mount an acquired immune response to a normal protein that was accidentally internalized by a first-line defender). Interleukins released by the APC awakens the slumbering naïve T cell. As it is activating, the previously naïve T cell will likewise release cytokines to further activate the APC to stimulate its own clonal proliferation. The greater the level of mutual co-stimulation, the greater will be the level of T cell activation and clonal proliferation.

CD80 and CD86 (often referred to as B7) on the APC will interact with CD28 on the resting T cell. The now activating T cell will express CD40L, which will interact with CD40 on the APC. CD4 on the T cell (T helper cells are all CD4 while T cells that eliminate rogue native cells are termed CD8) coordinates the interaction between an antigenic determinant bearing MHC II molecule on the APC and the TCR (T cell receptor) on the resting T cell.

Mother Nature thus created a number of checks and balances (which we can understand and therapeutically manipulate) with respect to whether or not the immune system will activate against a specific antigenic determinant, as well as to the direction and magnitude of any specific immune response to follow.

Naïve T cells activate into one of four lineages. If an antigen capture cell is bearing news of a large invader, such as a parasite, that cannot be phagocytosed by immune cells, then it will elaborate cytokine IL-4, which directs the activating T cell to differentiate within the Th2 lineage. Th2 cells instruct specific clones of B cells to generate antibodies to neutralize and kill the critter. If the first-line defender instead has captured a bacterium which can be phagocytosed by mononuclear cells, then it will activate within the Th1 or Th17 framework. These T helper cells secrete stimulatory cytokines and bear membrane signaling molecules designed to activate mononuclear cells to phagocytose and kill bacterial invaders. Not all antigens captured by innate immune cells

are an appropriate target of an immune response. Antigens derived from inhaled or ingested molecules ideally should not lead to an immune response; in this situation we would become immunologically reactive to molecules that we breathe in or take in within our diet. Thus, the biochemical milieu within immune organs in the upper respiratory and GI tract promotes activation of T cells into the Treg lineage. Treg cell membrane–expressed CTLA-4 binds tightly to co-stimulatory molecules expressed by the APC, turning down the APC's activation state. Soluble Treg-generated cytokines such as IL-10 and TGF-β turn down APC and T helper cell activity (stable plaques contain Treg cells; this inhibition is lost in unstable lesions).

Above and beyond the characteristic of the protein snippet presented to the resting, inactive T cell, and the location at which the immune synapse is occurring, the internal biochemical milieu of the lymph organ plays a role in determining the route into which the T cell will develop. Vitamin D, for example, alters the characteristics of the APC, such that the co-stimulating molecules that it elaborates will encourage the newly stimulated T helper cell to take an immune downregulating Treg course (consider the link between vitamin D sufficiency/insufficiency and the incidence of multiple sclerosis, which involves autoimmune attack against self-protein).

The cytokine and redox status of the lymph organ will greatly influence the lineage of a newly activated T cell (**Figure 3.3**). One's immune history, in a sense, determines one's immune future. If you are a chronic allergy sufferer, you bear Th2 cells that secrete IL-4 and stimulate B cells to make antibodies (unfortunately for you) to the pollen that you just inhaled (not enough Treg cells and too many Th2 cells and thus allergy occurs). Allergy begets more allergy, as the more IL-4 within the lymph organs, the more likely will you mount an undesirable Th2 response to newly presented protein snippets. Conversely, lots of IL-12 within the lymph organ skews new immune responses to newly presented antigenic determinants down the Th1 pathway. If you suffer from recurrent bacterial invasion, as did primitive man, then

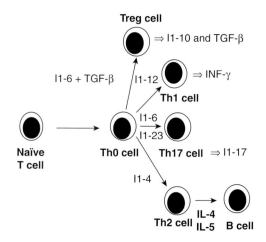

Figure 3.3 *Cytokine milieu influences direction of naïve T cell differentiation.*

the lymph node is rich in IL-12, and you tend toward a Th1 response. Recurrent infection adds IL-17 to the mix, stimulating T cells to mature within the Th17 lineage (essentially a more powerful version of the TH1 cell).

Oxidative stress trumps all other T lineage determinants and promotes maturation down the Th1 and Th17 pathways. The immune response to oxidized LDL, and other abnormal intimal proteins, as well as to troponin and other myocardial molecules to which a deleterious T cell response occurs in heart failure, is Th1 and Th17 driven. CV disease is characterized by skewing of the immune response, toward Th1/Th17 and away from Th2/Treg. Oxidative stress initially skews the immune response, these T cells release inflammatory mediators that lead to more oxidative stress, and the viscous, self-stimulating cycle of oxidative stress and immune dysregulation that drives CV disease follows.

Once activated by an upregulated innate immune cell that bears an antigenic determinant that matches its T cell receptor, the T cell assumes its role as a T effector cell. The cell line proliferates (generating IL-2 and a high affinity IL-2 receptor, leading to oligoclonal proliferation of this specific T helper cell line) and the daughter cells migrate to the periphery, aiming to kill their target (microbe in infection and oxidized LDL in atherosclerosis) at the site of initial stimulation of the innate immune system and at all other points in the body.

The previously naïve T cell bearing a T cell receptor specific for a protein snippet of a microbe (in this example bacteria or a snippet of oxLDL) has activated and proliferated. Millions if not billions of these activated T helper cells are soon swarming the circulation, seeking to help macrophages and other innate defenders phagocytose and kill the invaders (before they can kill us).

T Helper Cell Homing and Reactivation

How do the T cells know where to go? Although the initially activated (within the lymph organ closest to the site of initial infection) Th1 helper cell can access any site within the vasculature, it makes more sense if they can be drawn into the region where the innate immune system initially identified the focal breach. This will be an area where activated immune cells (macrophages and dendritic cells) have generated ROS/RNS and inflammatory cytokines, such that the local endothelium has activated, generating chemokines (MCP-1) to pull circulating mononuclear cells toward the site of infection as well as adhesion molecules (ICAM and VCAM) to tether the mononuclear cells to the site of endothelial activation, making it easier for the cells to enter the subintimal space (where their target, invading bacteria or oxLDL snippets, reside). The first T helper cell bearing a T cell receptor specific to a protein snippet derived from the invader (microbe or oxLDL) has now been drawn into the area of infection.

Along with the newly activated T helper cell line, our circulation also contains T memory cells, allowing the acquired immune system to rapidly respond to recurrent infection.

After a microbe has been eradicated (a joint effort between the innate and acquired immune systems), local ROS/RNS generation tails off, T cells specific to the target cease to proliferate, and most then die of senescence. A few persist, as T memory cells. They "remember" the threat, continue to bear TCRs specific to the threat (the specific antigenic determinant), and exist in a dormant state. However, upon reinfection, reexposure to "their" remembered antigenic determinant, they can fire up rapidly, undergo oligoclonal proliferation, and "return to the breach." With your initial exposure to a specific microbe you may be sick for a week, the time needed to mount an effective acquired immune response to the specific organism. Upon reexposure, you may be sick for 1 to 2 days or not at all, as you now possess an at least partial "immunity" to the invader.

Vaccination creates T memory cells to specific potential invaders. Antigenic determinants derived from microbes or inactivated microbes are administered along with adjuvants (pro-inflammatory substances such a thimerosal) that stimulate innate immune cells to activate, internalize the exogenous protein, and then transform into an APC and initiate an acquired immune response to the potential invader. If the CDC accurately predicts which flu strains will dominate in a given year, then they will create a flu vaccine that generates T memory cells that will recognize and eradicate the incoming viruses. If they predict incorrectly, the flu vaccine will not protect you, as the flu virus is constantly mutating, trying to outwit mankind's defenses (our T memory cell repertoire).

The circulation contains T memory cells, related to prior invasion, and newly activated T helper cells specific for the new infection (or pseudoinfection with oxLDL in atherosclerosis or altered myocardial molecules in heart failure). All of these T cells, along with circulating dendritic cells, will be attracted to and pulled into a region of endothelial activation, where infection resides, or (pathologically) at coronary branch points where ROS/RNS generation has activated the endothelium, allowing entry of LDL molecules that subsequently became trapped, oxidized, and internalized by mononuclear cells. All of these infiltrating T cells will sample the local intimal environment. If there are no activated intimal cells (macrophages or dendritic cells initially but within the oxidative milieu of an activated plaque smooth muscle and endothelial cells can transform into APCs) expressing "their" specific antigenic determinant, then they will return to the circulation, to see if they can be useful elsewhere.

If instead they undergo a second, lock in key interaction, with an intimal dendritic cell expressing "their" specific antigenic determinant, then a secondary, immune reactivation will occur. The job of the locally reactivated T helper cell is to help other cells in its vicinity to destroy the invader. Cell to cell contact (CD40L-CD40 or membrane bound TNF-TNF receptor) or secretory (interferon-gamma, IL-1β, and TNF) stimulate the APC into a phagocytic frenzy, generating more MHC II molecules and more lethal ROS/RNS. Although the interaction between the T helper cell and the APC is specific to a specific antigenic determinant, the cytokines released as a result of this antigenic determinant–specific interaction will affect the general inflammatory status of all cells in the vicinity. The greater the number of individual skirmishes (T helper cells activating macrophages to kill a specific target), the greater will be the potential to damage, and potentially scar, the tissue battlefield.

Thus, the number and type of immunoreactive antigenic determinants within a local intimal environment (and the corresponding number and type of ligating T cells) will determine its overall activation state. If the molecules within the intima are normal, self in nature, then its T cell repertoire will consist of Treg cells, which release IL-10 and TGF-β, which downregulate, or temper the level of immune activation. An activated plaque contains few Treg cells, and 20 to 40 clones of T helper cells that have undergone local oligomeric proliferation in response to reactivation against 20 to 40 specific antigenic determinants. The local milieu will be inflammatory (Th1 and Th17 cytokines) and oxidative (these cytokines stimulate endothelial, smooth muscle cells, and infiltrating mononuclear cells to generate ROS/RNS).

The Links Between Infection and Atherosclerosis

20 to 40 clones of T helper cells reacting to 20 to 40 specific antigenic determinants! What are the determinants, from what proteins were they derived, and how did they get into the intima? We can qualitatively identify the T cell repertoire in plasma, within a plaque, within any region of the body. The T cells are harvested, and in vitro reacted with antigenic determinants derived from specific microbes or specific proteins. If T cells proliferation occurs (you measure radiolabeled thymidine incorporation), you can infer that T cells bearing TCRs specific for that microbe/protein snippet were present in the tissue sampled (and if you are dealing with an atherosclerotic plaque, that the same microbe/protein snippet was present within the plaque, at some time point). In the absence of infection, plasma will contain small numbers of T memory cells specific to any infection that you have experienced, a bell-shaped curve or polyclonal distribution of lymphocytes. If you contract an infection, say pneumonia, you will see skewing of the T cell repertoire, with oligoclonal proliferation of T memory cells specific to the invader or previously naïve, newly activated T helper cells reacting to a newly identified microbial antigenic determinant. As the infection clears, T cells specific to the microbe will die of senescence, and the polyclonal distribution will return. The T cell repertoire within a plaque relates to the age of the lesion, infectious activity elsewhere in the body, and local and systemic levels of ROS/RNS and cytokine milieu. 10% of the T cells within any plaque will react to oxLDL. A similar number will react to intimal structural proteins such as beta-2 glycoprotein and heat shock protein (HSP). Stressed cells, human and microbial, translocate mitochondrial HSPs to the cell membrane, aiming to stabilize their cytoskeleton (you are under attack, so circle your wagons). Intimal HSP expression is negligible within the healthy intima, low level

within an early lesion, and extensive within a complicated lesion. But these are self-proteins. Why should they be subject to an acquired immune response? These proteins can be oxidized, rendered immunogenic, just as in the case of oxidized LDL. Also, in the presence of overwhelming ROS/RNS/cytokine stimulation, the frenzied acquired immune system can "break tolerance," misrecognizing self-proteins (that are at the wrong place at the wrong time) as nonself (consider the link between intestinal hyperpermeability and autoimmune disease; with chronic cytokine stimulation the immune system starts making mistakes).

If you carry out incidental atherectomy of a noninflamed, nonculprit, 60% RCA narrowing in your patient who presents with chest pain and ST segment depression on the basis of an inflamed 95% LAD lesion, you will find that the T cell repertoire and immune histology of these two lesions are quite different. To paraphrase Tip O'Neil, atherosclerotic immune activation is local. The smooth nonculprit narrowing will contain macrophages, dendritic cells, and T helper cells, certainly some specific for oxLDL protein and other altered intimal proteins. Within a stable plaque, there will also be Treg cells, elaborating IL-10 and TGBF, aiming to neutralize the interferon-gamma and other Th1 cytokines being released from plaque Th1 helper cells, keeping plaque inflammation in check. Nitric oxide inhibits vascular smooth muscle cell (VSMC) growth and proliferation. Nitric oxide was lost long age, and proliferated VSMCs, along with fibroblasts, have generated a stabilizing fibrous cap, sequestering lesional atheromatous gruel and inflammatory activity from the vessel lumen. Such lesions, if they obstruct the lumen sufficiently, may produce effort-induced ischemia. If adjacent vessels are not severely diseased, and if local nitric oxide is available, then the pressure differential between the patent and diseased vessel will lead to the elaboration of a protective collateral network. Stable plaques, characterized by a low ROS/RNS/inflammatory cytokine burden, will not rupture/erode to precipitate ischemic injury (as a therapeutic corollary, if we can convert an inflamed plaque into a stable plaque, ischemic event risk will attenuate).

The culprit plaque demonstrates a quite different immune histology. Along with T helper cells specific for oxLDL and other altered intimal proteins, you will find 20 to 40 clones of T cells specific to a wide variety of microbes. You are aware of the link between infectious history and atherosclerosis. The greater the number of microbes to which you display immune experience (reactive T cells or IgG antibody levels), the greater is your atherosclerotic risk (and risk of disease recurrence following revascularization).

How does this link work? Are the microbes invading the intima, or is the link indirect? Recall that an active plaque is constantly elaborating chemotactic signals and adhesion molecules, aiming to pull in mononuclear help (Mother Nature is fighting what she perceives as infection, initially with oxLDL). Let us say you bear a chronic bacterial infection (gum disease being the most common). Mononuclear cells infiltrate the gum tissue, gobble up the corresponding microbes, and digest them within phagolysosomes. Some hightail it to the nearest lymph node, generating a proliferation of Th1/Th17 cells specific to the invader, while some return to the circulation. If that mononuclear cell happens to traverse a coronary vessel containing an active plaque, it may be nonspecifically pulled into the lesion. There it may display gum microbe antigenic determinants to gum microbe sensitized T cells (T memory cells) that have also been nonspecifically pulled into the lesion, reactivating them to battle mode. As long as gum disease is present and the plaque remains active, more and more gum bacterial antigenic material will enter the plaque, and thus the immune system will be mounting an inflammatory response against gum disease within the active plaque. Nearly all plaques contain T cells sensitized to gingival invaders such as *Porphyromonas gingivalis*. Common pulmonary pathogens such as *Chlamydia pneumoniae* and *Mycoplasma pneumoniae*, frequently encountered viruses such as EBV and CMV, and GI and GU microbes will also be represented. In fact, virtually any infection can do this, such as bacterial, viral, fungal, TB, parasite, and other infections. As long as the plaque is active, focal infection elsewhere will contribute to plaque immune dysregulation. Keep this principle in mind the next time you attend a meeting in Las Vegas, where you might be tempted to interact with the wrong sort of people without proper protection. Do you want those sorts of microbial proteins within your coronary intima? The link between infection and atherosclerosis led to antibiotic intervention trials, which for the most part were unsuccessful. This is because the bacteria within the intima are long dead. Within the coronary vasculature T cells are reactivating to their antigenic determinants, not to the microbes themselves. Preventing chronic infection (and thus chronic immune stimulation) by killing the microbes where they reside, however, will be helpful (thus resolution of gum disease reduces your coronary risk). Also, recurrent bacterial infection will lead to skewing of the immune response toward Th1/Th17 and away from Th2/Treg, creating a cytokine milieu that drives atherosclerosis and heart failure. Heat shock protein (HSP) molecular mimicry is another link between extravascular infection and atherosclerosis. The HSP concept has worked well in evolution, for man and microbes. The HSP amino acid sequence of man and his common pathogens are little different. In response to infection, let us say with *C. pneumonia*, we will mount an immune response against antigenic determinants derived for this organism. The invaders feel the heat, and thus elaborate HSPs on their outer surface. We then respond by generating an immune response against *C. pneumonia* HSP, hastening clearance of the invader. Healthy endothelial cells do not express HSP; unhealthy cells (smokers, diabetics, individuals bearing a toxin burden) do, as do atherosclerotic cells, at a level commensurate with the degree of local immune dysregulation. Smokers experience more MIs in the winter than in the summer, in part related to immune cross-reactivity between endothelial and microbial HSPs.

Plaque Activation

The atheromatous core of a stable plaque is contained by a fibrous cap. In response to dietary/lifestyle change and/or appropriate pharmaceutical/nutraceutical intervention, ROS/RNS generation will have curtailed, Treg cells will be neutralizing Th1/Th17 activity, and endothelial nitric oxide production may return. This plaque will not progress and it will not activate.

The active or vulnerable plaque demonstrates quite dissimilar cytology and histology. The plaque will be infiltrated, particularly at its shoulder region, with activated mononuclear cells, all elaborating pro-inflammatory cytokines, ROS, and RNS. Plaque-derived chemokines are pulling in mononuclear cells bearing antigenic determinants from distant sites; foreign wars are now being conducted locally, and we see oligoclonal proliferation of 20 to 40 clones or Th1/Th17 cell lines within the plaque. Ongoing, intense inflammation leads to Treg cell regression (we do not want Treg cells turning down our Th1/Th17 defenses when we are fighting chronic infection). The character of the T cell response also changes. Recall that initial cell activation and T memory cell reactivation requires "lock in key" co-stimulatory as well specific antigenic determinant–T cell receptor interaction. In response to chronic re-activation to its specific antigenic determinant, T helper cells mutate such that their co-stimulatory receptor, CD 28, drops off. These cells (CD4+CD28^{null}) spontaneously express IL-12 receptors and may activate in response to their antigenic determinate, or simply to IL-12. Thus, immune activation elsewhere, which might lead to IL-12 generation, can activate these cells within the unstable plaque (another link between winter infection and MI). CD4+CD28^{null} cells are long-lived, spontaneously generate interferon-gamma, and are cytotoxic to endothelial cells. These cells may egress the activated plaque, may infiltrate distant intimal sites, and "splash" the vasculature with interferon-gamma. If you bear a 50% carotid plaque, it is far more likely to itself activate over the 2 years following an ACS (acute coronary event) than over a corresponding time period pre-ACS (you can think of this as metastatic plaque activation). The greater the percentage of plaque and circulating T cells that are CD4+CD28^{null} in character, the greater is the likelihood of subsequent ACS (and conversely, the greater will be your gain with anti-atherosclerotic therapy).

Large plaques may neovascularize. Hemorrhage within the plaque releases free iron, which catalyzes the Fenton reaction (discussed in more detail later), converting relatively benign H_2O_2 into 1000-fold more damaging hydroxyl anion. ROS-stimulated NLRP3 pathway activation (discussed in the Colchicine and NLRP3 section) also plays a role in plaque activation. "Frustrated phagocytosis" of crystalline cholesterol leads to a polymorphonuclear cell–led inflammatory response that activates NF-κB–generated pro-cytokines, precipitating plaque activation.

Atherosclerosis begins at points of intimal oxidative stress. Oxidative stress drives plaque progression and activation. Our goal, therapeutically, is not just to lower cholesterol (which rises with age in relation to oxidative status), but to lower oxidative stress, and with it inflammation and the dysregulated, Th1/Th17-skewed immune response that drives vascular disease. A discussion of oxidative stress, how it relates to atherosclerotic risk factors, and how to attenuate it is thus in order.

The Oxidative Cascade

Generation of superoxide (SO) and its second messenger hydrogen peroxide (H_2O_2) is constitutive and necessary for normal cellular function. Their synthesis can be physiologically upregulated to deal with infection and trauma.

Oxidative stress (OS) occurs when the production of these reactive oxygen species (ROS) is chronically and inappropriately increased, overwhelming our innate enzyme-based and dietary small molecule antioxidant defenses, allowing their conversion into more long-lived and damaging ROS and reactive nitrogen species (RNS) such as peroxynitrite (ONOO), hydroxyl (OH), and hypochlorous acid (HOCL) (**Figure 3.4**). When underdefended intimal ROS/RNS generation leads to endothelial activation, lipid trapping, and oxidation, and secondary Th1/Th17 skewed immune dysregulation, we experience intimal oxidative distress, followed by atherosclerosis and its sequelae.

Free radical species, ROS and RNS, are reactive electrophiles; they are electronically imbalanced. ROS such as SO contain an unpaired electron within their outer orbital shell. Absent a neutralizing electron donor (an antioxidant), a ROS will snatch an electron from an adjacent structure, quenching its electron thirst, but creating a new radical species. A biochemical chain reaction occurs, with resultant damage to cellular lipids, proteins, and nucleic acids.

Antioxidant enzymes (mineral dependent) convert a ROS to a less toxic metabolite. "Spent" antioxidant enzymes must then be recharged by a secondary antioxidant enzyme, or be resynthesized. Diet-derived antioxidant molecules "donate" an electron to the ROS, quenching its electron thirst, rendering it nonreactive. "Spent" antioxidants can be recharged by other antioxidants. Mother Nature designed us to maintain a dynamic and adaptive balance between ROS generation and antioxidant neutralization.

Primitive Man did not experience inappropriate or chronic oxidative stress. When faced with infection, microbicidal ROS/RNS generation was transiently increased, allowing for threat eradication. Modern Man is experiencing chronic oxidative stress, rarely because of chronic infection, but endemically because of errors of modern living, such as diabesity, intestinal hyperpermeability, chronic emotional stress, and age-related accumulation of radical-producing metal and organic pollutant toxins, phenomena not anticipated by evolution. Risk factors for atherosclerosis are either a cause or a consequence of inappropriate ROS/RNS generation.

The primary source of constitutive SO production is the mitochondria, where 1% to 2% of inhaled oxygen is incompletely reduced to SO, designated as a free radical as SO contains an unpaired electron in it outer orbital shell (molecular oxygen contains two, and is chemically far less reactive). Housekeeping enzyme systems (protein generation, digestion, and nutrient assimilation) generate lesser quantities of SO. SO is short-lived, but if not converted into H_2O_2 by superoxide dismutase (SOD) it can react with nitric oxide (NO) to generate peroxynitrite (ONOO).

Intimal ONOO generation, outside of our response to infection, is 100% maladaptive, as are the other "atherosclerotic bastard" descendants of SO and H_2O_2 (OH, HOCL, and lipid radicals). They fill no homeostatic need, they are not neutralized by endogenous antioxidant enzymes, they oxidize indiscriminately, and in this manner they initiate and drive atherosclerosis, malignancy, and neurodegenerative disease states.

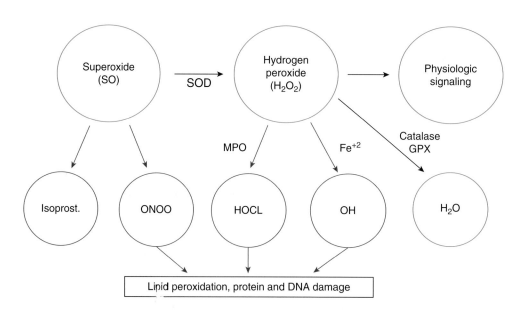

Figure 3.4 *Uncontrolled oxidative cascade leading to peroxidation of lipids, proteins, and DNA.*

As stated above, ROS generation is constitutive, a necessary byproduct of oxidative metabolism. Low-level H_2O_2 trafficking is also necessary for multiple cellular housekeeping functions, including protein folding, and appropriate cell growth and differentiation. Mother Nature generates and needs ROS, at a low level tonically, and at a high level transiently, when dealing with infection. Keeping SO and H_2O_2 under control, and preventing their conversion into ONOO, OH, and HOCL, is the responsibility of our mineral-based antioxidant defense enzymes, backed up, as needed, by diet-derived small molecule antioxidants.

Superoxide dismutase (SOD), present as three-cell compartment-specific isomers, rapidly converts SO into H_2O_2. If SO generation is not pathologically (or appropriately in infection) upregulated, SOD will convert SO into H_2O_2, and ONOO will not be generated. Copper and zinc-dependent SOD1 neutralizes SO within the cytoplasm. Manganese-dependent SOD2 degrades SO that is generated within the mitochondria. SOD3 (often referred to as extracellular SOD) is present on the endothelial surface or released into the intimal space; SOD3 protects these compartments against NO to ONOO conversion. Adequate mineral nutriture (not the rule in Western Man) is obviously important here. Some, but not all, diet-derived antioxidants, if at the right place at the right time, may assist in SO neutralization (vitamin C, coenzyme Q_{10}, and melatonin but not vitamin E).

Conversion of SO into H_2O_2 is thus a good thing, protecting against ONOO formation, and we do need low-concentration H_2O_2 for homeostatic signaling. Excessive SO to H_2O_2 trafficking must also be dealt with, and here Mother Nature has provided a redundant defense.

Single-purpose and single-use catalase (CAT) rapidly neutralizes H_2O_2 into H_2O. New CAT enzymes then must be transcribed via the Nrf-2 pathway. Dual-purpose glutathione peroxidase (GPX) transfers an electron from reduced glutathione (GSH) to H_2O_2, also generating H_2O (GPX can also neutralize lipid radicals). Now "spent" or oxidized glutathione (GSSG) is "recharged" into GSH by glutathione reductase (GSR), with an electron derived from NADPH, itself generated within the pentose phosphate biochemical pathway. A similar enzyme system, peroxiredoxin (PRX), also neutralizes H_2O and is "recharged" with an electron transferred from NADPH by the thioredoxin (TRX) system.

If our enzymatic and small molecule antioxidant defense systems cannot contain SO and H_2O_2, then bad things happen. Arachidonic acid (split off from LDL phosphatidylcholine by PLA_2) can be nonenzymatically converted into pro-inflammatory isoprostane molecules. The Fenton reaction, catalyzed by reduced iron (Fe^{2+}) or copper (Cu^{2+}), converts SO and H_2O_2 into hydroxyl anion (OH), a ROS with 1000-fold more destructive power (why we wish to avoid iron overload, why premenopausal status confers protection against atherosclerosis, and why low-dose vitamin C, which reduces Fe^{3+} to Fe^{2+}, might work against us in the situation of iron overload). OH readily abstracts an electron from the double bond of cell membrane or organelle membrane polyunsaturated fatty acids, to create a lipid peroxide radical, which reacts with an adjacent double bond, setting up a membrane damaging chain reaction (generating oxLDL, malondialdehyde, hydroxyenol, and other lab markers, and mediators, of oxidative distress).

Lipophilic vitamin E (tocopherols and tocotrienols), found within the cell or organelle membrane, will react with lipid peroxides, fortunately 1000-fold faster than the lipid radical can react with an adjacent double bond, breaking the chain reaction. Spent vitamin E will then be recharged by hydrophilic vitamin C within the circulation or cytoplasm, and spent vitamin C can be recharged by diet-derived bioflavonoids.

Myeloperoxidase (MPO) converts H_2O_2 into microbicidal hypochlorous acid (HOCL). HOCL, essentially bleach, is great to have around during infection, but in the setting of inappropriate oxidative stress, is particularly damaging. MPO expression is upregulated, in turn, by upregulated H_2O_2 expression, because, as you appreciate, Mother Nature regards high-level H_2O_2 expression as a sign of infection. If MPO remains chronically elevated because of chronic infections, it will cause HDL to become dysfunctional, increase CHD plaque rupture, open calcium channels in the arteries, and increase blood pressure.

Paraoxonase (generated in the liver and associated with HDL within the circulation) excises oxidized regions within cell membranes, and within LDL and HDL particles. Paraoxonase thus mediates the antioxidant, or oxLDL neutralizing effect, of HDL. MPO is a physiologic antagonist of PON, degrading PON and oxidizing HDL, whereas PON degrades MPO and reverses lipoprotein oxidation. PON activity is uniquely upregulated by pomegranate juice, in part mediating the vasoprotective properties of this diet-derived polyphenol antioxidant.

The cartoons below describe the appropriate systemic response to infection, and how oxidative and inflammatory cues, artifacts of Western living, have hijacked these systems to generate what we refer to as risk factors for atherosclerosis (**Figure 3.5**). Let us explore these links, starting with endothelial dysfunction.

Oxidative Endothelial Dysfunction

Endothelial dysfunction is a key determinant of outcome in all stages of atherosclerosis and in heart failure (**Figure 3.6**). This is because endothelial dysfunction is both a sign and a mediator of intimal and myocardial oxidative stress, the key driving force in CV disease. Before we discuss endothelial activation, an adaptive response to infection, let us discuss how endothelial chemistry works in a physiologic, reductive environment (stated otherwise, when Mother Nature does not perceive infection). Endothelial nitric oxide synthase (eNOS, or NOS3) converts arginine into nitric oxide (NO), which then diffuses within the cell and across the endothelial cell membrane, to activate soluble guanylate cyclase (sGC) in adjacent platelets and vascular smooth muscle cells. sGC in turn activates cAMP-dependent processes, which lead to

Adaptive Response to Infection

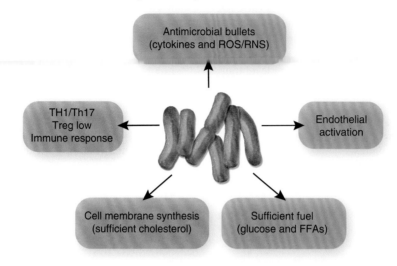

Oxidative Stress = Infection

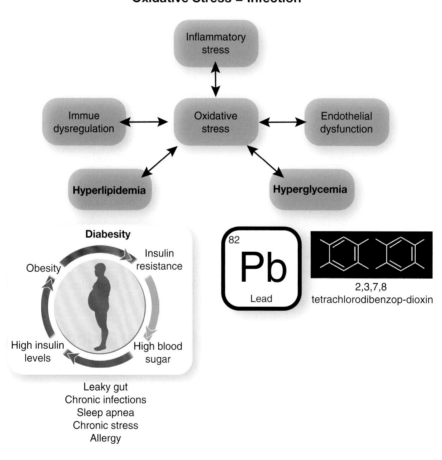

Figure 3.5 *Adaptive and microbiocidal in infection, inappropriate oxidative stress mediates endothelial dysfunction, inflammation, and immune dysregulation.*

vascular smooth muscle relaxation, with subsequent vasodilatation, and reduced platelet adherence and activation. NO inhibits vascular smooth muscle cell proliferation and hypertrophy (preventing hypertension and muscle cell encroachment within the intima). NO restrains the endothelial cell

from elaborating adhesion molecules and chemoattractant signals that would pull leukocytes into the intima. NO also inhibits nuclear translocation of NF-kB, our primary inflammation amplification pathway, and generator of nascent IL-1β and IL-18, and activation of the NLRP3 inflammasome,

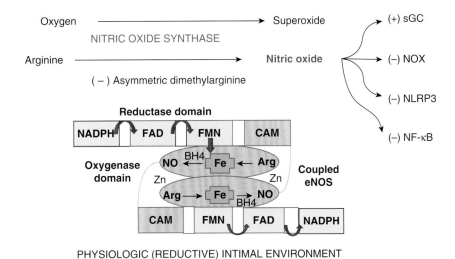

Figure 3.6 *Nitric oxide formation via eNOS and the needed cofactors for production of NO.*

which activates the nascent cytokines and generates an inhibitor of endothelial tone. NADPH oxidase (NOX), the key pathologic source of intimal superoxide (SO), is directly inhibited by NO. When eNOS is functioning properly, we maintain appropriate vasodilation, platelets are not sticky, and we inhibit enzyme systems that would, if unrestrained, lead to intimal oxidative stress, inflammation, atherosclerosis, and plaque destabilization.

Within an oxidative intimal environment, not only are these vascular protections lost, but eNOS itself becomes an SO generator (**Figure 3.7**). Adaptively, in infection, and maladaptively, in the setting of chronic, acquired oxidative stress, SO generation is upregulated, outpacing the rate at which it can be converted to H_2O_2 by SOD. SO reacts with NO three times more rapidly than it does with SOD, creating the long-lived pro-oxidant peroxynitrite (ONOO). ONOO

is not constitutively generated; it has no physiologic role other than to kill microbes. Thus, ONOO is not subject to degradation by our endogenous antioxidant enzymes systems. ONOO is not neutralized by vit E, but it can be neutralized by taurine, N-acetylcysteine, methyl-folate, and pharmaceutically, by hydralazine. ONOO, a reactive nitrogen species (RNS), will activate (via tyrosine nitration) pro-inflammatory enzyme systems. With respect to endothelial function, ONOO degrades BH4, the key co-factor of NOS. NOS then splits into its monomeric form, stops generating NO, and instead starts converting oxygen into SO. Restraint on NOX is lost, leading to more SO, which along with the SO generated by now uncoupled eNOS combines with what little NO we have left to form more ONOO. Restraint of NF-κB (and a related inflammation amplification pathway, activator protein-1) is lost; thus, pro-inflammatory cytokines and

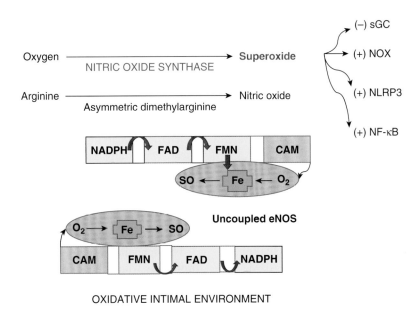

Figure 3.7 *Uncoupled or dysfunctional eNOS becomes a superoxide generator.*

endothelial adhesion molecules and chemokines will be elaborated. Restraint on the NLRP3 inflammasome is lost. This enzyme complex (discussed in the Colchicine and NLRP3 section) promotes maturation of nascent NF-κB–generated IL-1β and IL-8, unleashing their inflammatory potential, and directly compromises endothelial tone. This intimal metabolic shift works in our favor when we are dealing with infection (the leading cause of death in Primitive Man), particularly if trauma is involved (saber tooth tiger bite). Here you want vasoconstriction, platelet activation, endothelial activation within the infected region, and bullets (cytokines, SO, ONOO, HOCL, and OH). iNOS, or inducible NOS, is present in phagocytic cells and upregulates its response to infection, here generating NO to combine with SO to form ONOO, to help kill the invaders. Our clinical problem, in the treatment of CV disease, is that Mother Nature interprets oxidative stress as a sign of infection, and thus chronic, inappropriate oxidative stress converts eNOS into a mediator of inflammatory atherosclerosis.

eNOS activity is modulated by two other redox sensitive phenomena: differential shear stress and the ADMA to arginine ratio. Physiologic laminar shear stress (5-20 dynes/cm^2) upregulates transcription of eNOS and Nrf-2 (which controls transcription of our innate antioxidant enzymes). Low laminar flow, just beyond branch points and on bends, creates focal points of reduced NO and antioxidant intimal protection. Oscillatory shear, present beyond branch points, upregulates expression of intimal SO-generating enzymes systems (NADPH oxidase and xanthine oxidase). Focal insufficiency of NO in the presence of excessive SO thus explains the focal initiation of atherosclerosis just beyond branch points, and secondarily along curves. Saphenous vein grafts last, on average, 7 years, whereas 90% of left internal mammary (LIMA) grafts remain patent at 10 years, also in relation to differential intimal redox status. The LIMA is a long straightaway, and thus nonhypertensive flow creates a reductive, atherosclerosis-resistive LIMA intimal environment. The thin wall of the saphenous vein is designed for nonpulsatile venous flow; SO is not generated here and little NO is needed. Placing the SV within the high-pressure arterial circuit leads to upregulated SO generation, and thus rapidly developing SV graft atherosclerosis. Physiologic laminar flow promotes a reductive intimal environment, whereas excessive laminar shear (>20 dynes/cm^2), on the basis of hypertension, turns up NADPH oxidase, creating an oxidative intimal environment, essentially the link between hypertension and atherosclerosis.

eNOS enzymatic activity is also governed by the ratio between its raw material, the amino acid arginine, and its physiologic, competitive inhibitor, asymmetric dimethylarginine (ADMA). ADMA is generated at a constant, constitutive rate, in relation to protein degradation. ADMA is metabolized by dimethylarginine dimethylaminohydrolase (DDAH). When DDAH is functioning normally, ADMA is broken down rapidly, the ADMA to arginine ratio is low, and if eNOS has not been oxidatively inhibited, arginine will be converted into NO. DDAH is inhibited by essentially all atherosclerotic risk factors, via the common mechanism of (you guessed it) oxidative stress. The more risk factors you bear, the more compromised will be DDAH function, the greater will be your ADMA to arginine ratio, the less NO you will generate. It is not the absolute level of ADMA that governs eNOS activity, but rather the ratio of ADMA to arginine; an imbalance here can be rectified with arginine supplementation.

Cumbersome methodologies have been utilized to measure endothelial function (intracoronary acetyl choline, forearm plethysmography, brachial artery flow–mediated vasodilation). Peripheral artery tonometry (EndoPAT) provides a low-cost (typically insurance-covered) office assessment of endothelial tone. Endothelial dysfunction is covered in greater detail elsewhere, but from the redox perspective we can address endothelial dysfunction with targeted antioxidant support (taurine and methyl-folate to neutralize ONOO and vit C and N-acetylcysteine to neutralize SO), neutralization of intimal SO generators (ARBs, HMG Co-A reductase inhibitors, berberine, or hydralazine to downregulate NADPH oxidase, and allopurinol to inhibit xanthine oxidase), and arginine (2-4 g tid). As we normalize endothelial function, we will also be turning down NF-κB, AP-1, NLRP3, and NADPH oxidase activity.

Oxidative Stress Promotes NF-κB Translocation

Microbes divide rapidly, and thus we need to keep up, with the rapid generation of microbicidal, pro-inflammatory cytokines and endothelial adhesion molecules. Our primary pathway of inflammation amplification is the nuclear factor kappa beta (NF-κB) transcription pathway. Under resting, reductive conditions, NF-κB is sequestered within the cytoplasm, complexed with IKBα (inhibitor of kappa beta). Ligation of threat receptors on immune response cells activates a chain reaction of serine kinases (ERK $1/2$, p38MAPK, c-Jun N-terminal kinase), which converge to activate inhibitor of kappa beta kinase (IKK), which degrades IKBα, allowing NF-κB to translocate to the nucleus and transcribe the appropriate defense molecules. LPS (bacterial cell wall lipopolysaccharide) appropriately activates this pathway, as will molecules found in the presence of legitimate infection (IL-1β, Ang II, CD40L).

These "threat molecules" (and other NF-κB agonists such as free fatty acids) upregulate pathologically, in relation to the pro-oxidant and pro-inflammatory cues present in Western Man (leaky gut, visceral adiposity, toxins, etc.) such that NF-κB is constantly on the move (NF-κB upregulates 10-fold within unstable plaques), cranking out pro-atherogenic molecules.

NO upregulates IKBα expression, and thus blunts NF-κB trafficking within the intima. This restraint is lost in the presence of endothelial dysfunction (**Figure 3.8**). H_2O_2, in excess, will activate IKK to degrade IKBα, shunting NF-κB to the nucleus. Stated otherwise, you do not need real infection, or

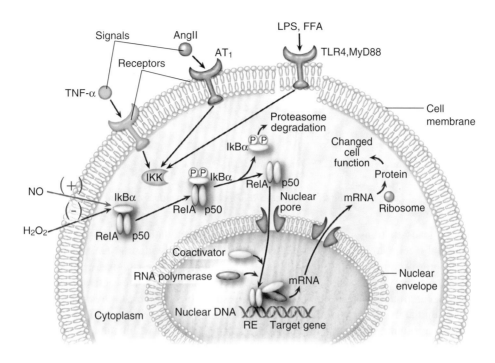

Figure 3.8 *Nitric oxide deficiency and hydrogen peroxide excess both promote NF-κB activation.*

the presence of infection signaling molecules, to activate the pro-inflammatory genes under NF-κB control; all you need is oxidative stress. Why? Primitive Man experienced oxidative stress only in relation to infection. Thus, our physiology interprets oxidative stress as "another infection" and translocates NF-κB, leading to the generation of hundreds of pro-inflammatory mediators.

Although episodic oxidative stress typically triggers a balancing, rebound generation of antioxidant molecules (via Nrf-2, to be discussed later), a downstream action of NF-κB is to inhibit Nrf-2 translocation (in legitimate infection we do not want antioxidant molecules; we want ROS/RNS bullets).

When circulating markers of inflammation, such as CRP or fibrinogen, are elevated, we often intervene with anti-inflammatory therapies, such as fish oil or turmeric. While these agents are helpful, a more expedient and complete approach would be to neutralize oxidative stress, as oxidative stress precedes and drives inflammatory stress.

The Hyperlipidemia of Pseudoinfection

In response to legitimate infection, HMG-Co-A reductase (the rate-limiting step in cholesterol generation) upregulates. This makes sense, as you need cholesterol to manufacture cell membranes for the rapidly proliferating leukocytic defenders. It also helps if you can activate the endothelium, making it easier for the defenders to access infected tissues, and to generate ROS/RNS bullets to kill the microbes.

HMG Co-A reductase generates cholesterol through a system of intermediate molecules, including the isoprenoids farnesyl and geranylgeranyl pyrophosphate. They activate

(via prenylation) the signaling molecules Rac, Rho, and Ras, which in turn upregulate SO production, activate the endothelium, and upregulate Ang II receptor expression. These actions generate more ROS, which in turn promotes NF-κB translocation, to generate more pro-inflammatory cytokines (a virtuous cycle to deal with infection).

This system worked great for Primitive Man. Genomic hyperlipidemia thus arose as a defense against perinatal sepsis, the leading cause of death in the history of mankind. A minority of us carry these traits, accounting for the infrequently encountered situation of familial hyperlipidemia (good for your ancestors but bad for you). As a corollary, if your bear sickle cell genes, you will not die of malaria (Mother Nature never does anything without a good reason).

In the rest of us HMG Co-A reductase is not genomically upregulated, and when we are young our cholesterol levels are low. However, in Western Man, cholesterol values start to rise in our 20s, and continue to rise with aging. Why is this occurring? What factors determine the level of expression of HMG Co-A reductase?

HMG-Co-A reductase transcription is governed by the cell's perceived need for free cholesterol. When intracellular free cholesterol is adequate, the free cholesterol sensor Insig sequesters SREBP (sterol regulatory element binding protein) within the endoplasmic reticulum (**Figure 3.9**). When free cholesterol is low, Insig releases SCAP (Sterol Regulating Element Binding Protein Cleavage Activating Protein) to transport SREBP to the Golgi apparatus, where it is enzymatically modified, promoting its translocation into the nucleus, where it binds the sterol regulatory element (SRE), the promoter site for the three key genomic sequences involved in cholesterol homeostasis.

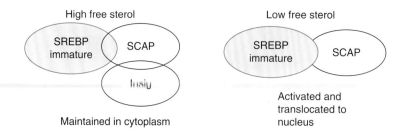

Figure 3.9 *Low cellular free sterol triggers SREBP activation to induce cholesterol synthesis.*

Activation of the SRE leads to transcription of HMG Co-A reductase, such that the cell can generate more cholesterol, and of LDL receptor protein, enabling the cell to pull more cholesterol out of the circulation. Cholesterol biosynthesis and uptake occurs mainly in the liver, and as Mother Nature does not want the liver to hog all the cholesterol, SRE activation also leads to the generation of PCSK9 (Proprotein Convertase Subtilisin/Kexin type 9), a counterbalancing protein that degrades the hepatic LDL receptor, maintaining serum cholesterol to meet the needs of other cells.

In the presence of legitimate infection (lipopolysaccharide) or inflammation, acetyl Co-A acyl transferase (ACAT) expression upregulates, promoting cholesterol esterification (to store cholesterol raw material for the upcoming infectious winter). As Insig senses only free cholesterol, HMG Co-A reductase and PCSK9 transcription increase, even though total intracellular cholesterol is rising. Intracellular and circulating cholesterol thus rise with age. This does not relate directly to dietary cholesterol (in our 20s we consumed pizza and beer and our cholesterol values were low) but rather to the progressive accumulation of pro-oxidant and pro-inflammatory phenomena (visceral fat, leaky gut, metals, organic pollutants, etc.) that lead to maladaptive HMG Co-A reductase and PCSK9 transcription.

HMG Co-A reductase does not generate cholesterol; it generates mevalonate, which converts to cholesterol, through the intermediate isoprenoid molecules farnesyl and geranylgeranyl pyrophosphate (**Figure 3.10**). These molecules activate (via prenylation) a series of GTPase signaling molecules that activate pathways critical to the response to infection, but which in our patients add to their oxidative/inflammatory burden.

Rac prenylation activates rho kinase, which translocates the NADPH oxidase (NOX) regulatory element Rac to the cell membrane, enabling assembly and activation of NOX. Infection appropriate activation of phagocytic NOX is responsible for the SO "respiratory burst," whereas within the intima NOX generated SO is likely to react with NO to form ONOO, or within the diabese liver to downstream ROS/RNS that promote NF-κB translocation and heightened insulin insensitivity.

Rho prenylation downregulates eNOS activity, compromising NO generation, whereas Ras activation increases angiotensin receptor type I expression (ATR1), through which Ang II leads to NF-κB translocation and further NOX activation.

Avoiding or resolving the age- and diet-related oxidative/inflammatory cues that increase HMG Co-A reductase transcription is the best approach here. But if the patient is unable or unwilling to take these steps, or if we do not have the luxury of time, then interventions to inhibit HMG Co-A reductase activity will lower cholesterol and reduce trafficking through the NOX, ATR1, and NF-κB pathways. This can be achieved with statin drugs; nutraceutical "green statins" such as red yeast rice extract, bergamot, and amla; tocotrienols which hasten degradation of the enzyme; and AMP-sensitive protein kinase (AMPK) agonists such as berberine, which physiologically (via phosphorylation) downregulate the enzyme. It really does not matter how you inhibit flow through HMG Co-A reductase, but if you do so cholesterol generation will fall, and oxidative stress and inflammation will attenuate.

The indication for intervention is not a specific cholesterol level, but rather the presence of inflammation and oxidative stress in the presence of atherosclerosis,

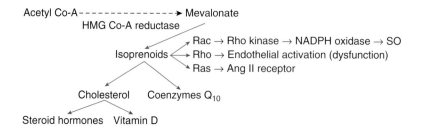

Figure 3.10 *The cholesterol pathway with downstream production of steroid hormones, vitamin D, and Co-Q$_{10}$.*

endothelial dysfunction, or other factors, suggesting that HMG Co-A reductase is inappropriately upregulated. There will be little gain in a 30-year-old woman with an LDL of 130 and an otherwise pristine risk profile, but tremendous gain in her diabese grandfather who sustained his second MI because graft failure, whose LDL is at a similar level. On the negative side, coenzyme Q, steroid hormone, vit D, and vit K generation will also be compromised. Thus, if we intervene against HMG Co-A reductase, we must also be ready to measure and replace these physiologic substances. We also need to remember that Mother Nature created countless other oxidative stress and inflammation upregulation pathways, so if we rely on statin therapy alone, we will not be covering all the necessary bases of atherosclerosis protection. As a consequence of HMG Co-A reductase inhibition, PCSK transcription will inevitably increase (why you have to keep increasing the statin dose). Berberine blunts this process, and will thus synergize nicely with any HMG Co-A reductase inhibition strategy (stated otherwise you can get the job done with a lower statin drug dose).

Oxidative Stress Promotes Insulin Insensitivity and Hyperglycemia

Insulin mediates and governs cellular glucose homeostasis. Insulin ligation of the insulin receptor leads to tyrosine phosphorylation of the insulin receptor substrate (IRS) and downstream signaling molecules (PI3-K/Akt), leading to appropriate glucose uptake and utilization. Serine kinases (such as IKK, the same molecule that shoots Nf-κB to the nucleus), upregulated in relation to oxidative and inflammatory stress, mediate antagonistic serine phosphorylation of IRS molecules, leading to insulin insensitivity, impaired glucose utilization, and hyperglycemia. This is helpful when fighting infection (leukocytes need glucose), but chronic disruption of insulin signaling leads to the progressive hyperglycemia, diabesity, and hyperlipidemia that characterizes Western Man. The inability to take up and utilize glucose leads to increased use of fatty acids in mitochondrial energy generation, which in turn leads to increased mitochondrial superoxide and hydrogen peroxide generation, which leads to more NF-κB translocation (and you know what follows), more inflammation.

Oxidative stress is damaging to mitochondrial DNA, leading to mitochondrial apoptosis and loss of energy generation (limited exercise capacity, difficulty in weight control). Insulin upregulates eNOS activity; this tonic upregulation in endothelial tone is lost in the setting of insulin insensitivity. Exogenous insulin and insulin sensitizing agents inhibit NOX, upregulate IKBA, and blunt NF-κB translocation, with a secondary reduction in endothelial adhesion molecules, MCP-1, and PAI-1. Conversely, glycated molecules (AGEs, advanced glycation end products) will ligate RAGE (receptor for AGEs) on the mononuclear cell membrane, stimulating NF-κB translocation.

Impaired glucose utilization leads to inappropriate triglyceride synthesis, and this leads to fatty liver. Here, chronic inflammation leads to cholesterol esterification, a fall in free cholesterol, such that SREBP is shunted to the nucleus, to generate more HMG Co-A reductase and PCSK9. Impaired skeletal muscle glucose uptake and impaired mitochondrial function leads to fatigue. Fatigued people do not exercise. They eat more, sit around, and put on visceral fat. Visceral fat is hypoperfused and distressed; the sick adipocytes release chemokines that lead to mononuclear infiltration, the generation of inflammatory cytokines, leading to increased lipid synthesis, and more fatty liver and insulin insensitivity. An imbalance between NO and SO within the myocardium compromises calcium flux across the sarcolemma, compromising energy generation, leading to the diastolic and later systolic dysfunction of diabetic cardiomyopathy.

Diabesity, uncommon two generations ago, is rapidly becoming the norm, and is Western Man's most important cause of avoidable oxidative stress. Conversely, diabetics have the most to gain with antioxidant strategies.

Hypertension is the consequence of long-standing intimal oxidative stress. Insufficient NO generation leads to hypertrophy and proliferation of vascular smooth muscle cells, and "hardening of the arteries." The resultant non-physiologic elevation in shear stress upregulates intimal NOX and XO, leading to more endothelial dysfunction and more oxidative stress.

Oxidative stress shunts the immune response to Th1/Th17 and away from Th2/Treg, not what we want in our patients with atherosclerosis or heart failure.

Oxidative and inflammatory stress, a 4-million-year-old response to life (and species) threatening infection, is being chronically and inappropriately activated by the diet, toxic milieu, and lifestyle of modern man, creating the viscous cycle that drive atherosclerosis and age-related disease in general. Our job as individuals is to avoid these unnatural oxidative burdens. Our job as clinicians is to counsel our patients as to how to do that, and to intervene, at a level appropriate to the patient's age and disease burden, with pharmaceutical and nutraceutical antioxidant interventions.

Risk factors are a cause and consequence of oxidative stress (**Figure 3.11**). If we lower oxidative stress, atherosclerotic risk factors will improve. If we attenuate one risk

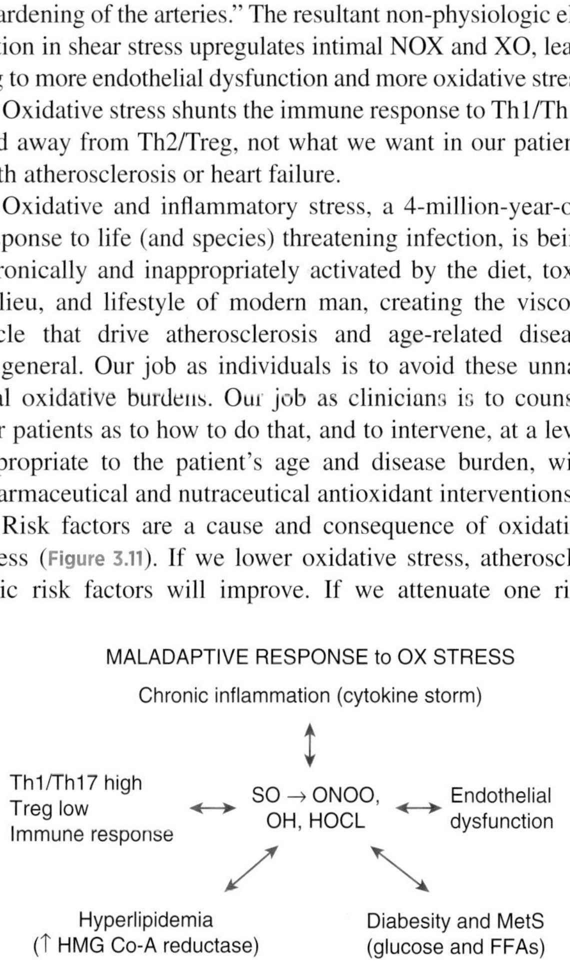

MALADAPTIVE RESPONSE to OX STRESS

Chronic inflammation (cytokine storm)

Th1/Th17 high
Treg low
Immune response

SO → ONOO,
OH, HOCL

Endothelial
dysfunction

Hyperlipidemia
(↑ HMG Co-A reductase)

Diabesity and MetS
(glucose and FFAs)

Figure 3.11 *Maladaptive oxidative stress induces the risk factors for atherosclerosis.*

factor, oxidative stress and the other risk factors will likewise improve. Our goal as clinicians, stated otherwise, is to replace vicious with virtuous metabolic cycles. For strategies, see section on the Free Radical Cascade.

The Free Radical Cascade

All ROS and RNS descend from superoxide (SO), the sole free radical species that we de novo generate. **Figure 3.12** depicts the pathways of superoxide generation. Constitutive processes, depicted in blue, generate the SO we need to provide the low level H_2O_2 requisite for cellular signaling. With adequate mineral nutriture, our antioxidant enzymes can detoxify any H_2O_2 in excess to H_2O. In red are the metabolic sins of Modern Man, the key causes of age-related acquired oxidative stress. Without supra-normal small molecule antioxidant support, SO and H_2O_2 overload will occur. ONOO, OH, HOCL, and lipid peroxides will be generated and oxidative distress will follow. As Mother Nature recognizes oxidative stress as evidence of (another) infection, additional superoxide generating systems (NOX, XO, MPO, NLRP3), depicted in black, will be activated, furthering self-inflicted intimal injury. Chronic infection and Th1/Th17 immune response skewing are also causes and consequences of oxidative stress. Vicious cycles are initiated, we get sick, and eventually we die, well before we should.

We do not want unnecessary sickness, and we certainly do not want to die before our time. Thus, we need to block these cascades. We cannot let H_2O_2 "get out of the barn." The common sense approach here is to avoid and/or resolve the three key metabolic sins:

1. **Maintain an ideal body weight and take in a clean diet.**
2. **Organic pollutants generate ROS as our body tries (often without success) to excrete them.** Nonbiotransformable pollutants (PCB, dioxins, and TCDD, the toxin in Agent Orange) travel within the LDL particle and ligate the aryl hydrocarbon receptor (the expression of which upregulates in atherosclerosis) within monocytes. Strategies exist to measure and resolve an organic pollutant burden (detox supplements, far infrared sauna, and ionic footbath therapy).
3. **Toxic metals catalyze free radical chemistry, displace nutritional minerals, and inhibit our antioxidant enzymes systems.** Metal detox is thus of value in the attenuation of oxidative stress and should have salutary effects in disease states driven by ROS/RNS overload. The benefit of EDTA-based lead detoxification in chronic kidney disease has been demonstrated in three separate studies. The Trial to Assess Chelation Therapy (TACT) demonstrated that EDTA-based metal detoxification improved outcome in infarct survivors already on standard medical therapy (which, as we will discuss, blocks SO generating systems), with particular benefit in diabetics (greater baseline ROS burden).

Patients typically present with active atherosclerosis, the result of decades of ROS-generating diabesity, poor diet, and toxin accumulation. Resolving these factors is important, and

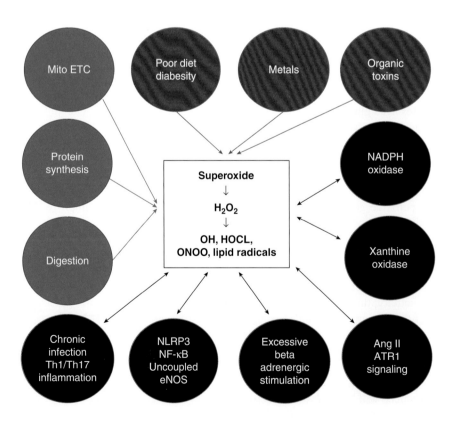

Figure 3.12 *This shows all of the causes of oxidative stress and the bidirectional processes.*

in theory could arrest the atherosclerotic process. However, most patients are unable or unwilling to address these issues, and in unstable or symptomatic patients we do not enjoy the luxury of time. Thus, we need to intervene with measures to block ROS-generating enzyme systems, while concomitantly upregulating antioxidant defense capacity.

Before taking aim at oxidative stress, we need to assess its severity. Thus, our first step will be a metabolic survey. Lab analysis will tell us where oxidative damage is occurring and will quantitate its severity:

Lipid oxidation markers include oxidized LDL, lipid peroxides, malondialdehyde (MDA), 4-hydroxynonenol (4-HNE), and isoprostanes.

- Protein oxidation markers include 3-nitrotyrosine and protein carbonyls.
- DNA oxidation results in the formation of 8-hydroxyguanosine (8-OHdG).
- Depleted glutathione, coenzyme Q_{10}, vitamin C, and vitamin E levels provide us with a mirror image as to the degree of oxidative stress the patients is currently experiencing.
- Endothelial function assessment will give us an intimal redox assessment.

We do not need to measure all of the above markers, but some form of baseline assessment is appropriate (obtain the studies that your preferred lab reports and become comfortable with their analysis). The studies can be repeated periodically to guide our therapeutic efforts.

Antioxidant supplementation has an important role to play and will be discussed. However, antioxidant supplementation does not address the causes of oxidative stress, and the supplemented molecules may not reach all sites of concern (circulating LDL oxidation is blunted by vit E, but plaque LDL is unaffected). The allopathic approach to atherosclerosis prevention and treatment is to utilize pharmaceutical agents (and in some cases we can use nutraceuticals) to blunt SO generating systems that are inappropriately upregulated.

NADPH oxidase (NOX) is Mother Nature's most powerful superoxide (SO) generator (see **Figure 3.13**). In infection, phagocytic NOX upregulates appropriately to generate the SO "respiratory burst" needed to kill microbes. Genomic NOX downregulation leads to chronic granulomatous disease,

with impaired clearing of microbes, whereas genomic upregulation of NOX is associated with an increased risk of atherosclerosis (from our perspective, NADPH oxidase is an obNOXious enzyme). Intimal cells, as well as infiltrating leukocytes, all transcribe NOX. NOX is composed of six subunits. Cytochrome b, a complex of gp91^{phox} and p22^{phox}, is permanently embedded within the cell or organelle membrane. Chemical warfare agents kill via overwhelming oxidative injury. These agents are inherently unstable. Thus, their components are generated at different sites, and brought together only immediately prior to their deployment (an action that our spy satellites can detect). Likewise, Mother Nature does not want the full oxidizing fury of NOX to be released outside of the intended response to infection. Thus, NOX components p47^{phox}, p40^{phox}, and p67^{phox} are sequestered within the cytosol. Stimuli that activate NOX phosphorylate Rac, which then translocates the cytoplasmic components to membrane-embedded cytochrome b. Activated NOX transfers electrons from cytoplasmic NADPH to generate SO from O_2.

NOX's job is to protect us from microbial death. As atherosclerosis is a maladaptive response of the innate and acquired immune systems to perceived infection with oxLDL, it is not surprising that risk factors and mediators of atherosclerosis lead to upregulated intimal NOX expression.

Direct and Indirect NOX Activators:
- HMG Co-A reductase flux
- Ang II–ATR1 Ligation
- Intima shear > 20 or < 5 dynes/cm^2
- Th1 cytokines, OxLDL, FFAs, AGEs, endothelin
- Aldosterone, growth factors, and chemokines

Not all NOX activation is pathologic. Low-level NOX SO generation likely plays a role in the physiologic (<100 nM) generation of H_2O_2 needed for cell signaling, growth, and development. Thus, growth factors and insulin play a role in NOX homeostasis. Mediators of pathologic NOX upregulation, leading to SO generation with subsequent high level (>250 nM) H_2O_2 conversion, may activate Rac directly or indirectly via the mechanism of upregulated ATR1 expression.

Rac prenylation, downstream from HMG Co-A reductase, activates rho kinase, which phosphorylates Rac to activate NOX (thus HMG Co-A reductase inhibition lowers SO

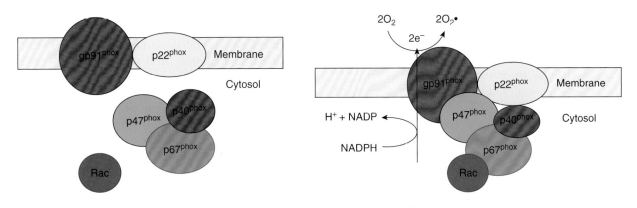

Figure 3.13 *NADPH oxidase assembly leads to superoxide generation.*

generation). ATR1 ligation by Ang II increases NOX transcription (ATR1 transcription is upregulated by prenylation of Rho, also downstream from HMG Co-A reductase). NOX activation on the basis of oscillatory shear explains the focal initiation of atherosclerosis and likely plays a role in lesion progression (the tighter the narrowing, the greater the oscillatory stress, so more focal SO and less NO). Aldosterone activates NOX in a manner distinct from ATR1 ligation. Other mediators of oxidative and inflammatory stress, as listed above, may directly or indirectly activate NOX.

NOX-generated oxidative stress will activate xanthine oxidase, a key ROS generator in diabesity, atherosclerosis, and heart failure, and NLRP3, which mediates plaque activation in relation to "frustrated phagocytosis" of intimal crystalline cholesterol. NOX-generated SO will combine with NO to form ONOO, to convert eNOS itself into an SO generator, and will convert to H_2O_2 at a level sufficient to translocate NF-κB to the nucleus, generating inflammatory mediators and inhibiting rebound activation of Nrf-2.

NOX activation recapitulates our response to infection. This is war! Mother Nature has had 4 million years to get this right. When Western Man lives incorrectly, we generate an oxidative chemical warfare attack against ourselves.

The best approach to NOX is the best approach to HMG Co-A reductase and to the other pathways of intimal distress—eat and live the way Mother Nature intended. In our patients, we do not have this luxury of time, and thus pharmaceutical and nutraceutical NOX blockade is appropriate. HMG Co-A reductase inhibition, ARB, lipophilic ACEI, aldosterone blockade, hydralazine, nebivolol, and colchicine all blunt intimal NOX assembly or activity. Berberine and polyphenols have activity against NOX. Standard antioxidants do not, but assist by scarfing up the ROS/RNS generated by upregulated NOX.

Xanthine Oxidase Inhibition With Allopurinol

$$\text{Adenosine} + \text{Oxygen (2)} \xrightarrow{\text{Xanthine Oxidase}} \text{Uric acid} + \text{Superoxide}$$

Allopurinol inhibits xanthine oxidase (XO), NADPH oxidase's partner in intimal oxidative crime. Xanthine oxidoreductase (XDH) degrades end products of purine metabolism. In a reductive environment, XDH functions as a reductase, utilizing NAD+ as a co-factor, generating uric acid and NADH. In an oxidative environment, sulfhydryl groups on XDH are oxidatively modified, converting XDH into XO. XO utilizes two molecules of oxygen to generate uric acid and superoxide.

In the setting of energy failure (ischemia, heart failure, diabesity, fatty liver) AMP cannot be recycled to ADP and ATP, and degrades to adenosine. Adenosine converts to xanthine and hypoxanthine, the direct substrates of XO. Conditions associated with adenosine excess stimulate transcription of XDH, and conditions associated with oxidative stress convert XDH to XO (recall that XO upregulation in

relation to oscillatory shear plays a role in the focal initiation of atherosclerosis). Mother Nature interprets these stimuli as evidence of microbial invasion, and thus XO's contribution to the ROS/RNS pool is greatly appreciated.

Clinical gout involves a (NLRP3-mediated) innate immune system inflammatory response to the presence of crystalline uric acid within joints. Allopurinol blocks uric acid generation and thus can be used in the prevention of gout. We can use allopurinol to block oxidative stress anywhere in the body, as at these sites XO will be pathologically upregulated.

In stable angina, allopurinol decreases angina frequency and increases treadmill time and time to ST depression. Allopurinol has no effect on HR and BP; rather this agent works by preventing the heart from wasting precious oxygen to generate SO. Thus, allopurinol attenuates symptoms while also favorably effecting the disease process. XO upregulates 10-fold (just like ACE) in acute coronary syndromes (ACS). Irrespective of how ACS is treated, allopurinol begun in the emergency room improves short- and long-term outcome (why not—the driving force here is too much SO). Allopurinol pretreatment reduces arrhythmia and pump dysfunction following on-pump bypass surgery (as will antioxidants, statins, ARBs, and beta-blockers) by blunting the ischemia-reperfusion pathophysiology inherent in this procedure. Diabesity and metabolic syndrome are associated with oxidative stress. ROS/RNS overload are causes and consequences of diabesity and metabolic syndrome. Allopurinol lowers oxidative markers in these settings, and provides a modest glucose lowering effect (remember, H_2O_2 activates IKK which serine phosphorylates IRS molecules, leading to insulin insensitivity). Endothelial function and carotid intima-media thickness are favorably affected by allopurinol therapy. While uric acid serves an antioxidant function within the circulation, cellular uptake of uric acid leads to mitochondrial oxidative stress. The kidneys retain filtered uric acid, and thus it is not surprising that low-dose allopurinol therapy delays disease progression in patients with renal insufficiency with a concomitant reduction in CV event rate.

Allopurinol thus seems to be of universal value in the treatment and prevention of CV and renal disease. The standard dose of allopurinol is 300 mg/d, but in the literature doses up to 900 mg/d have been utilized. There is a dose-related, nonallergic toxicity to allopurinol, characterized by pruritis, rash, malaise, and fever, which will attenuate with a dose reduction. As allopurinol is cleared via the kidneys, preexistent renal insufficiency, along with small stature and female gender, is associated with an increased sensitivity to this agent.

The indication for allopurinol is to lower oxidative stress, not to lower uric acid. As a general rule, the greater the baseline uric acid level, the greater will be the benefit of allopurinol therapy, but elevated uric acid was not a selection requirement in most of the clinical trials demonstrating benefit. For example, if you are experiencing angina on the basis of 95% circumflex narrowing, there is not much arterial surface area on which XO will generate uric acid and SO. Systemic uric acid will not be elevated, but if we blunt

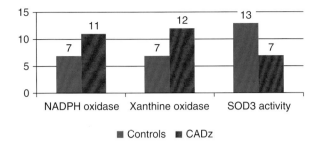

Figure 3.14 *Intimal redox status.*

inappropriate conversion of oxygen to uric acid and SO at that site, then angina will attenuate.

Allopurinol can be initiated at 100 mg/d, and advanced in 100 mg/d monthly increments, with a reassessment of oxidative stress markers and serum uric acid at the 3 months point. Increasing allopurinol from 300 to 600 mg/d provides a greater incremental improvement in endothelial function than going from nil to 300 mg/d. Thus, if markers of oxidative stress or endothelial tone have not normalized, the dose can be cautiously, and incrementally increased. Patients with preexistent renal disease have much to gain from allopurinol, but in this population a little allopurinol will go a long way and thus the starting dose will be 50 mg qod, with slow dose advancement. With any hint of toxicity, the dose can be incrementally decreased to a previously well tolerated level.

Patients with CADz and CHF demonstrate upregulated NOX and XO activity. ROS created by NOX converts XDH to XO, generating more SO, leading to SOD3 depletion (**Figure 3.14**).

Intimal Angiotensin II–ATR1 Interaction

Activation of the RAAS (renin, angiotensin, and aldosterone system) is a primary defense against tissue hypoperfusion. Salt and/or water deficiency were common problems for Primitive Man (**Figure 3.15**). Pathologic vasodilation on the basis of infection threatened to shut down his organ systems. As pathologic upregulation of the RAAS plays a role in hypertension and heart failure, ACEI, ARB, and aldosterone blockade are recognized as mainstay treatments in these disorders.

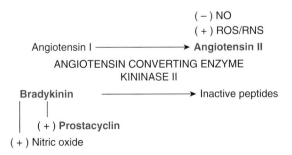

Figure 3.15 *ACE degrades bradykinin and generates Ang II leading to endothelial oxidative stress.*

From the perspective of atherosclerosis, we need to appreciate that 90% of ACE is intracellular. ACEI expression is inducible, and rises 10-fold in unstable plaques, generating Ang II, which upregulates NOX. While low-level ROS generation mediates physiologic growth and differentiation, upregulated NOX and Ang II–ATR1 trafficking leads to vascular smooth muscle proliferation with endothelial intrusion, medial hypertrophy, and left ventricular hypertrophy; stated otherwise, "hardening of the arteries." ANG II–ATR1 signaling translocates NF-κB, which generates IL-6, which stimulates the liver to make more angiotensinogen, creating a pathologic feed forward loop. NF-κB–generated COX and PGE2 activation leads to matrix metalloproteinase formation, predisposing to fibrous cap rupture. We need to address this. What processes lead to excess intimal Ang II–mediated oxidative stress?

ACE converts Ang I, an inactive precursor, into Ang II, which leads to vasoconstriction, aldosterone generation, and sodium retention. ACE has another role (for which it has another name, kininase II). ACE as kininase II degrades bradykinin into inactive peptides. From the atherosclerosis perspective, bradykinin works in our favor, stimulating eNOS and prostacyclin (to generate NO and vasodilating prostaglandins, respectively).

Standard hydrophilic ACE inhibitors (lisinopril, enalapril, and captopril) work well in hypertension and CHF management. As these agents do not penetrate the intima, they will have no beneficial effect in atherosclerosis (other than lowering excessive intimal shearing stress that would otherwise upregulate NOX and XO). Lipophilic ACEIs (quinapril and ramipril) will work in hypertension and CHF. They will also blunt Ang II generation within the intima, and from the atherosclerosis perspective are clearly preferred.

There is also an intimal RAS, whereby chymase and tryptase convert Ang I into Ang II, an action that is not blocked by lipophilic ACEI. This led to the development of selective angiotensin type I receptor (ATR1) blockade. When Mother Nature opens up a pro-inflammatory, pro-oxidative pathway, she also opens up the door for a counterbalancing mechanism. While ligation of ATR1 with Ang II is pro-atherosclerotic, ligation of ATR2 leads to an equal and opposite, endothelial restorative effect. Thus, if we block ATR2 with an ARB (angiotensin receptor blocker, all of which are lipophilic), then Ang II becomes our vasodilating friend (and why combined ACEI and ARB therapy is counterproductive).

Whether lipophilic ACEI or ARB therapy is preferable is a matter of debate. Increased generation of bradykinin leads to the nuisance ACEI cough, and shifts the scale toward ARB therapy. ACEI and ARB therapy may lead to hyperkalemia, and with excessive dosing hypotension and/or renal hypoperfusion. Either agent may produce the uncommon side effect of angioedema, with swelling of the lips and oral mucosa.

As lipophilic ACEI/ARB therapy lowers ROS/RNS generation, you would expect this approach to be effective in the primary and secondary prevention of atherosclerosis. The HOPE study demonstrated a benefit of ramipril in the primary prevention of atherosclerotic events (22% event reduction at 2 years), not on the basis of BP control (DBP fell only 2 mm Hg). And at the time puzzling co-benefit was an attenuation in new onset diabetes and in diabetic consequences. This makes sense to us now, as oxidative stress is both a cause and consequence of DM2. Lipophilic ACEI improves outcome following MI and CABG. Adding lipophilic ACEI or an ARB to a preexistent statin/aspirin regimen in nonhypertensive, stable atherosclerotic patients did not cause symptomatic hypotension, but did lower circulating levels of ROS, IL-6, TNF-alpha, and endothelial adhesion molecules. We care about inflammation in the circulation, but we care more about what is going on within active plaques. Lipophilic ACEI/ARB therapy added to the preoperative regimen of individuals scheduled for elective carotid endarterectomy led to a beneficial effect on plaque biochemistry and histology. Plaque lipid content was decreased, with a concomitant increase in smooth muscle and collagen. There were fewer monocytes and T helper cells, less oxLDL and CRP, and lower expression COX, PGE2, and MMP. Bypass surgery leads to profound oxidative stress. We can blunt this with antioxidant therapies such as vitamin C and coenzymes Q_{10}, but these agents are off limits in the hospital setting. Here we can blunt post-bypass ROS/RNS/inflammation with statins, ARB/ACEI, and allopurinol, in synergistic fashion.

If risk factors for atherosclerosis are present, then Ang II–ATR1 trafficking is likely upregulated. Ras prenylation downstream from HMG CoA reductase upregulates AT1R expression. ATR1 stimulation upregulates Rac expression, favoring NOX activation. Sympathetic stimulation leads to renin release, whereas ATR1 ligation facilitates norepinephrine release from sympathetic nerve endings. As is the case with NF-κB, NO inhibits ATR1 signaling; thus, with endothelial dysfunction ATR1 expression increases. No wonder that Ang II expression is 10-fold upregulated within unstable plaques.

Lipophilic ACEI/ARB intervention makes biologic sense as a first-line treatment of hypertension. In patients with known atherosclerosis, unless hypotension is present, blockade of intimal Ang II–ATR1 trafficking assists in the return of the intima to an anti-atherosclerotic reductive environment.

Third Generation β Blockade

Catecholamines, norepinephrine and epinephrine, effect change in CV physiology via ligation of adrenergic receptors (**Figure 3.16**). Norepinephrine preferentially ligates α_1 and β_1, whereas epinephrine at physiologic levels interacts only with β receptors.

With respect to oxidative stress and endothelial tone, nonspecific β blockade (propranolol or nadolol), via control of hypertension (which increases NOX expression) and inhibition of renin release (which leads to Ang II which increases NOX), will lower intimal oxidative stress. As Th1 lymphocytes bear β receptors, β blockade leads to a desirable shift in immune bias away from Th1 and toward Treg. However, as β_2 ligation mediates smooth muscle relaxation, an undesirable increase in peripheral resistance will occur. β_2- and β_3-mediated eNOS stimulation will be lost, also working against us.

The second-generation β_1 specific agents (metoprolol or atenolol) will lower HR, contractility, and renin release, but are less likely to increase afterload, compromise endothelial tone, and precipitate bronchospasm, and were thus a step forward. Third-generation agents (carvedilol and nebivolol) provide the standard benefits of β blockade, while adding direct antioxidant protection.

Carvedilol is a nonselective adrenergic blocker (**Figure 3.17**). Undesirable inhibition of β_2-mediated vasodilation is neutralized by blockade of norepinephrine-mediated α_1 vasoconstriction. While loss of β_3-related eNOS upregulation is undesirable, the carbazole side chain of carvedilol provides a counterbalancing antioxidant effect, 10-fold greater than vitamin E. By squelching ROS, NO loss to ONOO is prevented, and endothelial tone improves.

Oxidative stress is a cause and consequence of heart failure. CHF driving forces (RAAS, catecholamines, inflammatory cytokines, pressure overload) all increase myocardial ROS/RNS generation. Conversely, interventions in our CHF arsenal that improve outcome work, at least in part, by attenuating myocardial oxidative stress. The failing heart is also an overworked heart. The greater the workload, the greater the electron leak from the stressed electron transport chain, the greater the SO generation, the less NADPH available to recharge our backup enzyme-based antioxidant enzymes (GSR, PRX, TRX). Endothelial dysfunction, a sign of intimal oxidative stress, portends a poor outcome in heart failure because SO > NO in the arteries is also SO > NO in the myocardium.

Myocardial ATPase enzymes pump ions across membranes, to coordinate and fuel myocyte contraction and

	α1	β_1	β_2	β_3
HR and contractility		↑		↓
Vasoconstriction	↑		↓	↓
Renin release		↑	↑	
eNOS activity			↑	↑

Figure 3.16 *Vascular effects mediated by adrenergic receptors.*

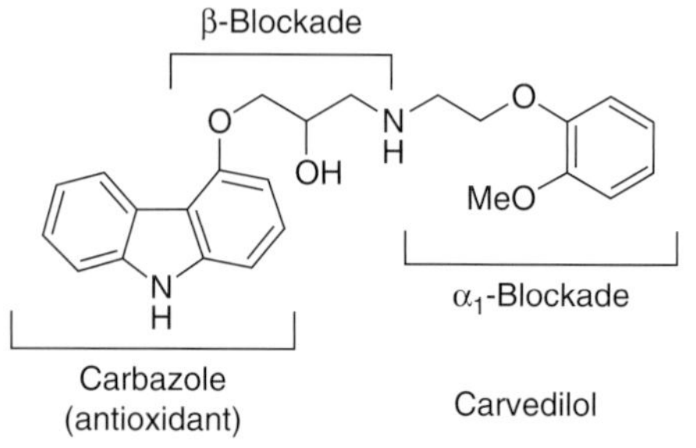

Figure 3.17 *Carvedilol contains an antioxidant moiety.*

relaxation; all are subject to oxidative inhibition and damage. Sarcolemmal Ca^{2+}-ATPase (SERCA) pumps calcium ions in and out of the sarcoplasmic reticulum. SERCA is inhibited by oxidative stress, as is its transcription. In vitro H$_2$O$_2$-mediated downregulation in SERCA mRNA and protein expression is abrogated by clinically relevant concentrations of carvedilol and N-acetylcysteine (both of which "mop up" ROS), but not by metoprolol or propranolol. Furthermore, in the absence of oxidative stress, carvedilol increases SERCA transcription fivefold (carvedilol interacts with the SERCA gene promoter, unrelated to its beta-blocker or antioxidant activity).

For these reasons (ROS-scavenging, blockade of α-vasoconstriction, SERCA agonism) carvedilol is preferred in the treatment of heart failure. Circulating oxidative and inflammatory stress markers (oxLDL, MDA, inflammatory cytokines) fall, in concert with improving functional status and ejection fraction. In patients with dilated cardiomyopathy, the addition of carvedilol (mean dose 22 mg/d) to prior therapy with ACEI/ARB, digitalis, and diuretics leads to a 40% reduction in myocardial 4-HNF (a tissue lipid oxidation marker). These myocardial benefits are dose-related. Thus, we start carvedilol at 3.1 mg twice a day, and slowly work up to 25 mg twice a day.

With respect to creating a reductive intimal environment, nebivolol takes us a step further. Nebivolol (5-40 mg/d) is by far the most β$_1$ specific agent. Thus, loss of β$_2$ vasodilation and eNOS upregulation is not an issue. Furthermore, nebivolol is a β$_3$ agonist, stimulating eNOS activity. Nebivolol also directly inhibits NOX, blunting de novo SO formation.

As you would expect, in trials comparing carvedilol and nebivolol to bioequivalent doses (same effect on HR and BP) of metoprolol or atenolol, the third-generation agents provide unique benefits. Lab markers of oxidative stress, such as oxLDL, malondialdehyde, and 8-isoprostanes, fall, and endothelial function is more likely to improve. Animal models demonstrate improved intimal and myocardial histology, with attenuated muscle cell hypertrophy, proliferation, and fibrosis. Nuisance side effects such as fatigue and weight gain are also less likely to occur.

If β blockade is clinically indicated (angina, hypertension, arrhythmia), the third-generation agents will get the job done, with concomitant neutralization of the oxidative distress and impaired endothelial tone that underlie CV disease states.

Colchicine and NLRP3

NLRP3, the pathomechanism of acute gout, plays a key role in plaque destabilization. In a sense, you can think of ACS as "gouty arteritis". In gout, uric acid crystals slowly and silently build up within joint tissue. Gouty attacks typically follow an inflammatory incident, such as infection, fever, or a night on the town.

The NLRP3 inflammasome (**Figure 3.18**) acts as an intracytoplasmic mediator of sterile inflammation. Mononuclear

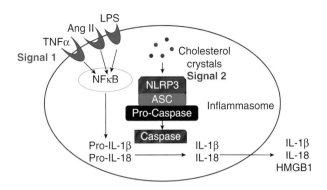

Figure 3.18 *Inflammasome activation generates inflammatory cytokines, compromises endothelial function, and precipitates plaque activation.*

cells can phagocytose and degrade microbes, but they cannot dissolve rocks. To clear particulate matter (asbestos, silica, and crystalline uric acid and cholesterol) a "flushing" sterile inflammatory response is needed.

Recall that NF-κB transcribes over 100 pro-inflammatory mediators. Interleukin 1β (IL-1β) and IL-18 are actually transcribed in nascent form. To exert their inflammatory potential, they must first be activated by caspase, which is generated within the activated NLRP3 inflammasome. Activated IL-1β and IL-18 lead to further NF-κB activation (another feed forward loop). NLRP3 also generates a specific mediator of endothelial activation (HMG box protein). Polymorphonuclear leukocyte will be pulled in, NOX will activate, and a "respiratory burst" of SO will follow.

With gout, crystals of uric acid have built up. NLRP3 is activated, but in the absence of NF-κB translocation, there is no nascent IL-1β or IL-8 to activate. Then the fever, or other cause of NF-κB activation, and all of a sudden you have a hot red toe.

The same phenomenon is occurring in the coronaries. The majority of lesional cholesterol is cholesterol ester, but a portion exists in crystalline form. NLRP3 activates, silently at first, but then you experience fever, infection, or smoke one too many cigarettes. NF-κB activates, caspase unleashes the inflammatory power of IL-1β and IL-8, HMG box protein creates endothelial dysfunction, PMNs are pulled in, and plaque activation occurs.

This process can be attenuated with colchicine. Colchicine blocks tubulin formation, which is needed to assemble both NLRP3 and NOX. As colchicine concentrate 50-fold in leukocytes, doses nontoxic to other organ systems can prevent or ameliorate gout, vascular inflammation, and plaque activation.

Coronary sinus (reflecting coronary artery specific production) IL-1β, IL-8, and IL-6 (the latter reflecting secondary activation of NF-κB) are increased in ACS patients. 1.5 mg of colchicine given 1 day precatheterization reduces coronary sinus IL-1β, IL-8, and IL-6 to levels found in patients with stable angina. Adding colchicine to standard therapy in stable patients will lower CRP. In a study of 500 Australians with known coronary disease, the addition of colchicine 0.6 mg/d to standard therapy (statin, ACEI/ARB, beta-blocker, and an antiplatelet agent) lowered 3-year event rate (ACS, CVA, cardiac arrest) by 66% (75% in those who remained on colchicine over the entire study period). In heart failure, colchicine lowers inflammatory markers but does not improve outcome. Colchicine does not prevent restenosis post PTCA, but it does attenuate neointimal proliferation is diabetics s/p bare-metal stent placement. Colchicine decreases atrial fib recurrence early post–fib ablation and is of excepted value in dealing with pericarditis and postcardiotomy inflammation. The standard dose of colchicine is 0.6 mg/d, but in some studies a dose of 1.2 mg/d was used. The key side effect of colchicine is dose-related diarrhea, which typically resolves with a reduction to every other day or every third day dosing. As colchicine concentrate in leukocytes and has a 2 day half-life, intermittent dosing will still provide persistent protection. One can make a case for colchicine add-on therapy for all patients with significant atherosclerosis, especially when inflammatory mediators, such as CRP, are elevated.

Hydralazine and Nitrate Tolerance

Three decades ago, the direct vasodilator hydralazine was in common use, in BP control and to provide "afterload reduction" in heart failure, typically paired with a "preload reducing" long-acting nitrate. This concept made hemodynamic sense but did not work well in practice. Hydralazine vasodilation led to reflex sympathetic activation, increasing HR, and the potential for coronary ischemia. Hydralazine also stimulates renin release, with consequent activation of the RAAS. Long-acting nitrates provide an endogenous NO boost, certainly of short-term benefit, but curiously we had to keep increasing the dose to obtain the desired effect, a phenomenon termed "nitrate tolerance." Later it was learned that long-acting nitrate therapy was associated with an increased ischemic event rate, termed "nitrate toxicity." Stated otherwise, long-acting nitrates reduced symptoms but accelerated the disease. We now understand the problem. As mitochondrial aldehyde dehydrogenase converts a long-acting nitrate to NO, NOX is activated, generating SO, which combines with NO to form ONOO, converting eNOS into an SO factory. The 1986 V-Heft study showed no reduction in mortality with hydralazine/nitrate therapy in CHF, and its use was phased out. African American V-Heft subjects, however, did benefit (African Americans experience less RAAS activation vs. Caucasians). This observation led to A-Heft, which randomized African American CHR patients on standard therapy to hydralazine 75 mg tid and isosorbide dinitrate 40 mg tid versus double placebo. BP fell only 2 to 3 mm Hg, but quality-of-life scores improved and event rate fell by 33%.

Why is hydralazine working better now? Well, most A-Heft subjects were receiving a beta-blocker, to blunt reflex SNS activation, an anti-RAAS agent, and diuretics were on board to blunt vasodilatory induced fluid retention. The key redox benefit is that hydralazine directly scavenges ROS, particularly ONOO, and it inhibits assembly of NOX. Stated otherwise, like nebivolol, hydralazine blunts NOX

SO generation and sops up ROS/RNS created by other maladaptively activated enzyme systems. Provided we cover for reflex SNS/RAAS stimulation, we can make good use of hydralazine as an afterload reducing, radical squelching, NOX inhibitor. Hydralazine is initiated at 10 mg qid, and can be increased to 50 mg qid. Drug-induced lupus is an uncommon side effect and will not show itself for 6 months (and resolves with drug discontinuation). Reversible hydralazine-induced hepatotoxicity has also been described.

Other direct or indirect NOX inhibitors will ameliorate nitrate tolerance/toxicity, as will small molecule antioxidant supplements. Some, such as N-acetylcysteine, which supports both glutathione and hydrogen sulfide expression, will synergize with nitrates to attenuate symptoms while also improving outcome.

Taurine, N-Acetylcysteine, and Hydrogen Sulfide (the New NO)?

Like NO, hydrogen sulfide (H_2S) is enzymatically generated and serves as a short-lived physiologic governor (**Figure 3.19**). NO nitrosylates, while H_2S sulfhydrates, cysteine moieties on enzymes and signaling molecules (which might otherwise be oxidized by ROS/RNS). NO and H_2S work together to oppose oxidative stress, and thus protect against CV and other ROS/RNS-driven disease states. H_2S upregulates eNOS, and NO protects H_2S from degradation.

Along the gradient from healthy controls to individuals with risk factors, to those with stable versus unstable angina, we see a progressive decrease in H_2S. As H_2S appears to be NO's partner in CV protection, efforts to increase H_2S expression are warranted. As outlined above, H_2S is derived from homocysteine, within a serine and P-5-P–dependent pathway that also produces GSH. Co-synthesized cysteine and taurine also increase production of H_2S, helping to explain their across-the-board benefit in CV disease states.

N-acetylcysteine (NAC) supplementation upregulates GSH expression, and in doses of 500 to 2000 mg/d has been shown to be of value in hepatic, renal, and pulmonary disease states. NAC ameliorates nitrate toxicity, improves endothelial function, synergizes with ACEI in BP control, and assists

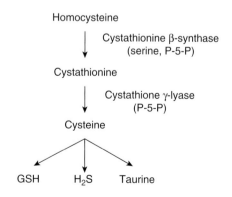

Figure 3.19 *Hydrogen sulfide and taurine biosynthetic pathway.*

in homocysteine clearance (splitting free homocysteine from its sequestering protein).

Taurine is the most abundantly conserved sulfur-containing amino acid in the heart. Taurine buffers ions, and thus protects the heart from Ca^{2+} deficiency or excess, conserves Mg^{2+}, and protects against digitalis toxicity. Taurine scavenges free radicals, and (unlike vit E) protects against HOCL-induced lipid oxidation. Taurine improves endothelial function in smokers and diabetics, attenuates angina (uncontrolled study), and with or without Co-Q supplementation relieves symptoms and improves outcome in CHF and in the post-MI setting. Taurine is helpful in BP control and in some individuals will assist in lipid control.

NAC and taurine are inexpensive and nontoxic. In the setting of endothelial dysfunction, known CV disease, or oxidative stress, taurine at 1000 mg bid and NAC at 500 mg bid can do no wrong and a lot of good.

Pentoxifylline to Shift Th1 to Treg

Pentoxifylline (PTX) is not a direct antioxidant. Rather, PTX shifts immune bias away from Th1 and toward Treg, with a resultant reduction in inflammatory cytokine and ROS/RNS generation. PTX has been shown to be of value in Th1-driven states, ranging from psoriasis to renal disease to fatty liver.

Heart failure, irrespective of the cause, is associated with cytokine and/or T cell–mediated immune attack against the myocardium. PTX has been shown to attenuate symptoms and/or improve pump function in ischemic, hypertensive, postpartum, and idiopathic cardiomyopathic states. In hypertensive type 2 diabetics, PTX lowers markers of inflammation and increases GSH. PTX improves treadmill time in stable angina, improves outcome in patients undergoing stent placement for ACS, and protects against vein graft failure. PTX is inexpensive and nontoxic. The most common side effect is dose-related nausea or malaise that typically attenuates over time. A case can be made to utilize PTX, starting at 400 mg daily, and titrating up to 400 mg tid, in patients with CV disease states, particularly if inflammatory markers are elevated.

Berberine

Like pentoxifylline, berberine is not a direct antioxidant. Berberine interacts with complex 1 of the electron transport chain, creating a biochemical illusion of energy deficiency on the basis of caloric deprivation. Because caloric restriction lowers ROS/RNS generation and promotes life extension, the metabolic health benefits of berberine are not surprising.

Berberine activates AMP-sensitive protein kinase (AMPK), which mediates "burn and do not build" signaling. AMPK physiologically downregulates HMG Co-A reductase, along with the enzymes involved in triglyceride and glycogen synthesis. Berberine protects LDL receptor mRNA from degradation; thus more LDL receptor protein makes it to the hepatocyte membrane. Berberine enters the nucleus and blunts transcription of PCSK9. Thus berberine synergizes with all other means of cholesterol generation inhibition. Berberine increases insulin receptor expression and blunts IKK-mediated serine phosphorylation (and thus downregulation) of IRS proteins, protecting against inflammation-aggravated hyperglycemia. IKK is the same enzyme that shunts NF-κB to the nucleus, and thus we are not surprised that berberine blunts generation of inflammatory cytokines. Berberine promotes translocation of Nrf-2 (which codes for our antioxidant and detox enzymes), blunts activation of NOX, improves endothelial tone, and has a favorable effect on the GI microbiome (the first recorded use of berberine was in the treatment of bacterial dysentery).

Berberine is thus of value in the prevention of atherosclerosis, and via its ability to attenuate ROS/RNS/cytokine generation, berberine also helps us deal with its consequences. As in the case of PTX, adding berberine to standard therapy lowers inflammation and improves short-term outcome in ACS patients undergoing PCI. A Chinese study (berberine is a standard therapy in the Orient) demonstrated attenuation of arrhythmia, improved pump function, and reduced mortality when berberine was added to standard anti-CHF therapy.

Berberine is inexpensive and nontoxic. Nuisance GI side effects, primarily constipation or diarrhea, occur in 5% to 10% of us, and typically resolve with a 50% dose reduction. Berberine itself will not cause hypoglycemia, but if added to insulin or sulfonylurea therapy a reduction in drug dose may be required. The literature includes one case report of berberine-induced bradycardia. The greater the dose or lipid-lowering effect of statin therapy, the greater will be the rise in PCSK9, and thus the greater will be the benefit, and dose-requirement, of add-on berberine therapy. The standard dose of berberine is 500 mg bid; the dose can be advanced to 1000 mg bid, GI tolerance permitting.

Iron Status and Fenton Chemistry

Iron is constitutive in multiple enzymatic steps and is needed for heme synthesis. Iron deficiency is not uncommon and is looked for in routine lab screening. Iron assists in the battle against infection, catalyzing the conversion of H_2O_2 into microbicidal OH. Primitive man was constantly dealing with infection and red meat was not always available.

H_2O_2 not neutralized to H_2O will be converted, in the presence of ferrous (Fe^{2+}) iron, into OH. OH serves no homeostatic function (other than to kill microbes) and indiscriminately attacks lipids, protein, and DNA. Iron excess will thus lead to intimal oxidative distress, in relation to baseline SO and H_2O_2 generation, enzymatic antioxidant defense status, and haptoglobin genotype.

Our physiology stores iron as ferritin. Iron excess (ferritin >200 ng/mL) is a risk factor for atherosclerosis, synergizing statistically with a rising LDL. Menstrual cycling limits the potential for iron overload, explaining in part the protective nature of premenopausal status (also, estradiol upregulates NO and H_2S expression). Iron status relates to dietary iron intake interacting with iron absorptive ability and haptoglobin genotype. Iron deficiency was likely an issue for primitive man, as many of us bear genomic variants coding for heightened iron absorption. Homozygous status for these variants leads to hemochromatosis, with secondary liver, myocardial, and endocrine (oxidative) failure. Heterozygous status or possession of less powerful iron absorption traits leads to the not uncommon finding (12% of us) of iron excess.

In nonanemic individuals with iron excess, periodic blood donation, aiming for a ferritin in the 100s, makes sense. Deferoxamine chelates iron and can be used when phlebotomy is not possible. The greater the baseline level of oxidative stress, the greater should be the benefit of iron removal. Of interest to our discussion, irrespective of baseline iron status, IV deferoxamine will acutely improve endothelial function in smokers and diabetics.

With respect to atherosclerosis and endothelial tone, iron itself is not the problem, but rather the availability of redox active iron within the intima and in proximity to circulation lipoproteins, which in turn relates to haptoglobin genomic and hemoglobin glycosylation status.

Hemoglobin Glycosylation and Haptoglobin Genotype

Why Vitamins Do Not (Always) Work

Direct small molecule antioxidant supplementation is an intuitive approach to oxidative stress. If LDL oxidation is the problem, and vit E (rechargeable with vit C) serves as a key defense against LDL particle oxidation (Co-Q_{10} and other lipophilic antioxidants are also involved), then why not supplement?

Vitamin E inhibits LDL oxidation in vitro and in vivo and is protective in animal models (all wild type for haptoglobin and typically normoglycemic). In Industrialized (and now progressively hyperglycemic) Man, primary and secondary intervention with vit E has been shown to be protective in some, but not in all trials. In some studies harm with vit C is suggested.

These discrepant and counterintuitive findings can be explained, at least in part, in relation to hemoglobin glycosylation and haptoglobin genomic status.

Total body iron is not the culprit. Rather it is redox active (reduced or ferrous) Fe^{2+} iron, in proximity to lipid particles or within the intima, that catalyzes pro-atherosclerotic H_2O_2 to OH conversion. Degenerating RBCs release hemoglobin, exposing the circulation to redox active iron. Haptoglobin, generated by the liver, ligates free hemoglobin and facilitates its clearance (90% hepatic and 10% via mononuclear uptake). Extravascular hemoglobin or heme iron will be cleared by tissue macrophages (which within an active plaque are redox active, churning out their own SO and H_2O_2).

Haptoglobin exists in two genomic forms, wild type (Hp1) and a variant (Hp2) form, with impaired Hb binding. 16% of us are Hp1/1, 36% Hp1/2, and 48% of us are blessed (from the perspective of iron-deficient primitive man battling infection) or cursed (from the perspective of atherosclerotic man) with Hp2/2 status.

Hp2/2 status compromises Hb clearance and iron shielding, as does hemoglobin glycosylation. Diabetics also generate excessive SO and H_2O_2, and if downregulated for Hp function, then more redox active iron is available to convert these ROS into OH. The poorly cleared Hp2/2-glcoHb complex ligates and oxidizes HDL. HDL thus becomes dysfunctional, with reduced antioxidant and reverse cholesterol transport function.

Given that Hp2/2 status compromises iron clearance, it is not surprising that in men (but not women) iron and ferritin status relate to Hp genomic status (Table 3.1).

Iron, Hp genomic status, and hyperglycemia all interact. Vitamin E will influence the oxidation status of circulating LDL, but does not affect (at least at 6 weeks) advanced plaque (atherectomy specimen analysis) vit E or lipid oxidation status. With this understanding of redox biology and vit E kinetics let us revisit the vit E intervention trials.

CHAOS randomized 2002 subjects with newly identified CADz (abnormal angiograms; most with angina or positive stress ECG studies) to placebo versus vit E (natural source alpha-tocopherol) 400 IU or 800 IU per day. 8% were diabetic, and in this 1996 study pharmaceutical interventions designed to blunt ROS generation were not extensively employed (36% on atenolol and ACEI/statin use was not recorded). 510-day MI risk fell by 77% with vit E (4.2% vs. 1.4%). The majority of CV deaths occurred early in the study, and here vit E had no effect.

SPACE randomized 196 hemodialysis patients with preexistent CV disease (note that dialysis itself generates copious ROS) to vit E 800 IU (natural source alpha-tocopherol) or placebo. Diabetes prevalence was 43%, and in this 2000 study ACEI therapy was employed in 17%, β blockade in 20%, and 14% were receiving (type not specified) lipid-lowering therapy. At 519 days, an adverse CV event occurred in 33% of placebo subjects versus 16% in the vit E group, a 53% risk reduction.

In contrast, vit E 400 IU per day did not improve outcome in the 2000 HOPE study. 9541 subjects with stable atherosclerosis (80% coronary, 43% peripheral, and 11% cerebral) or diabetes with one other risk factor (36% of participants) received either placebo or vit E 400 IU. 39% were on a

Table 3.1

HP2 GENOMIC STATUS MEDIATES MONOCYTE IRON RETENTION

	Hp1/1	Hp1/2	Hp2/2
Serum iron (µmol/L)	18.6	19.2	22.6
Serum ferritin (µg/L)	66	77	128
Monocyte ferritin (µg/g)	326	366	687

Increased iron with increased CHD. All of these labs and genomics should be measured.

beta-blocker and 29% lipid-lowering therapy (none were on ACEI as another arm of HOPE looked at the effect of ramipril, a lipophilic ACEI). 510-day event rate was 16% with vit E and 15.5% with placebo.

Likewise, the 1999 GISSI study showed no benefit at 3.5 years of vit E 400 IU per day in 11,324 recent infarct survivors (46% on ACEI, 4% β blockade, and 29% lipid-lowering therapy).

In trying to reconcile these studies, we can make two observations:

1. **The greater the level of baseline oxidative stress (not measured but presumable greater in the CHAOS and SPACE vs. the stable HOPE subjects), the greater the benefit of vit E antioxidant intervention.**
2. **The greater the use of drugs that block ROS generation (statins, ACEI/ARB, and beta-blockers), the lower the relative benefit of vit E.**

Our analysis becomes more complex, and more informative, if we also consider Hb glycosylation and Hp genomic status. HDL obtained from Hp2/2 diabetics is highly susceptible to in vitro oxidation, a process that is ameliorated by vit E. Hp1/1 status is protective, especially in diabetics. Hp1/1 status is associated with relative protection against diabetic nephropathy, better outcome post-PCI or post-MI, and better collateral flow. The Strong Heart case-control epidemiology study demonstrated 5-fold and 2.3-fold increased risk for prevalent CV disease among diabetics with 2/2 and 1/2 versus 1/1 Hp status. Among nondiabetics, relative risk was less, with 2.3- and 1.4-fold increased risk.

HOPE study data retrospective analysis revealed a greater event rate in placebo-treated diabetic Hp2/2 versus diabetic Hp1/1 subjects, whereas vit E intervention in the diabetic Hp2/2 subjects led to 43% and 55% reductions in MI and CV death. ICARE randomized Hp2/2 diabetic subjects to vit E 400 IU per day versus placebo. Hp1/1 and Hp1/2 diabetic subjects were not treated but were monitored for adverse events. ICARE was halted at 18 months, because of the findings of a 2.2% event rate with vit E versus 4.7% with placebo. Event rate in diabetic Hp2/2 subjects treated with vit E was similar to that of diabetic Hp1/1 and Hp1/2 subjects followed within the ICARE registry. Stated otherwise, vit E neutralized the pro-oxidant risk associated with Hp2/2 genotype. Looking at the DM/Hp2/vit E interaction from another angle, post-ICARE subjects coming off vit E were 4.5 times more likely to experience an adverse during the 18 months postintervention versus subjects discontinuing placebo.

Extrapolating these findings to the real world of patient care, it is estimated that administering vit E to the 42% of diabetics who are homozygous for Hp2 will extend their life 3 years. Treating 1000 diabetic Hp2/2 diabetics with vit E over 50 years should prevent 75 MI admits, 31 CABG, and 19 PCI procedures, a risk reduction similar to that of smoking cessation (and superior to that of lifetime statin therapy in high-risk patients and of BP and glucose control in DM2).

How does Hp genotype interact with vitamin C? The 2004 WAVE study randomized postmenopausal women with abnormal angiograms to bid vit E 400 IU and vit C 500 mg versus bid double placebo. Angiography was repeated at a mean interval of 18 months and change in minimal lumen diameter recorded. Antioxidant supplementation was protective against disease progression in Hp1/1 subjects, particularly in Hp1/1 diabetic subjects. Conversely, there was a trend toward increased disease progression in Hp2/2 subjects, also more pronounced in Hp2/2 diabetics.

Wait a minute? We just said that Hp2/2 diabetics benefit greatly from vit E. Now WAVE is telling us that vit E + vit C intervention may accelerate atherosclerosis in the Hp2/2 population.

In vitro HDL oxidation in Hp2/2 diabetics is inhibited by vit E, whereas it is accelerated by vit C. Vit C reduces iron to its redox active, ferrous status, accelerating conversion of H_2O_2 to OH. Thus the pro-oxidative effect of vit C overwhelms the ROS-neutralizing benefit of vit E (in these in vitro studies, high concentration vit C was less pro-oxidative, presumably via the mechanism of SO neutralization, such that less H_2O_2 was available for conversion into OH).

A lot of numbers and a lot of biochemistry. How can we use this understanding of redox biochemistry to reduce risk in our patients? Keeping in mind that other factors will affect decision making, consider the following guidelines:

- **Measure ferritin in all patients.** If persistently elevated (ferritin may rise transiently as an acute phase reactant), take measures to reduce iron burden (blood donation or iron chelation). This is particularly important in diabetics and in others with intrinsically increased ROS generation.
- **Genotype for Hp.** Vit E supplementation (400 IU per day) makes sense in Hp2/2 individuals, particularly in the setting of DM2. Low-dose vit C monotherapy may cause harm in individuals with intrinsically increased ROS generation, elevated iron stores, or DM2-Hp2/2 status, and is best avoided (at least until these pro oxidant phenomena have been addressed).

Optimizing Our Innate Enzymatic Antioxidant Defense

Nrf-2 Translocation, Minerals, GliSODin, and Pomegranate

Watching the Green Bay Packers defeat the Detroit Lions, my Father told me "remember son, a strong defense wins championships." Father Nature might say "remember Doctor, an optimally expressed mineral-based antioxidant enzyme system is a strong defense against ONOO and OH formation." How can we achieve this strong defense?

Antioxidant enzyme expression, at any given time point, relates to demand and resupply. SOD and catalase are single-use enzymes. SOD levels are low in CHF and CADz because SO generation is persistently high. GPX and PRX can be recharged by GSR and TRX, but these systems also require periodic resynthesis.

Resupply relates to the extent of Nrf-2 (nuclear factor-2 erythroid factor-2) nuclear translocation and ARE (antioxidant receptor element) promoter ligation (Figure 3.20). Nrf-2 codes for all antioxidant enzymes, as well as 250 other proteins involved in cell defense and life protection (phase II detox, cell repair, cell cycle arrest, apoptosis, and more Nrf-2). Nrf-2 is constitutively transcribed. Cytoplasmic Nrf-2 is sequestered by Keap1, which promotes its ubiquitination and degradation. The half-life of Nrf-2 is short (in a physiologic, reductive environment, ≈ 30 minutes). Keap1 contains cysteine residues with exposed sulfhydryl (SH) groups. SH oxidation by H_2O_2 leads to Keap1-Nrf-2 dissociation, allowing Nrf-2 to translocate to the nucleus and ligate ARE promoters. As long as oxidative stress persists, Nrf-2 will generate antioxidant defense molecules and more Nrf-2. As oxidative stress resolves (from Mother Nature's perspective after infection has cleared) Keap1 SH group oxidation ceases, transcribed Nrf-2 is again sequestered, and antioxidant enzyme synthesis downregulates.

Primitive Man experienced only intermittent oxidative stress, and here the Nrf-2 system allowed for redox homeostasis. Atherosclerotic Modern Man experiences constant oxidative bombardment (Detroit Lions scenario), and thus stands to benefit from Nrf-2 translocation support.

Exercise improves endothelial function. Recall that pulsatile, laminar flow (exercise or EECP) stimulates eNOS and Nrf-2 transcription. Strenuous exercise also leads to load-dependent ROS generation (muscle soreness correlates with ROS-induced muscle damage). Daily runs from Marathon to Sparta could oxidatively shorten your life, but episodic exercise, with longer periods of Nrf-2 rebound (vigorous workouts 2-4 days per week), leads to increased antioxidant/ARE gene expression and health enhancement.

Plants do not wish to be eaten; thus they generate bitter in taste, insecticidal compounds. Man can derive nourishment from bitter plants as these plant "toxins" precipitate Nrf-2 translocation, and thus the enzymes needed to neutralize them. Sulforaphane (found in cruciferous vegetables), curcumin, rosemary, thyme, and other plant compounds translocate Nrf-2. Some appear to cause a brief, oxidative stress, altering SH groups on Keap1, whereas others (berberine and melatonin) somehow directly enhance Nrf-2 nuclear transport. Nutraceutical firms provide plant compound blends designed to optimize Nrf-2 trafficking (several can provide documentation of efficacy).

To prevent oxidative distress, atherosclerosis, and malignancy, a program of regular exercise and dietary plant intake makes sense. In patients with established disease or manifest oxidative stress, Nrf-2 pro-translocation supplementation should lessen SO/H_2O_2 to ONOO/OH conversion.

Antioxidant (and essentially all other) enzyme systems require mineral co-factors (Mn, Zn, Se, I, Zn, and Cu). It is intuitive that mineral deficiency will compromise antioxidant enzyme status and conversely that repletion will be ameliorative, a position that is supported by epidemiology and the (albeit limited) clinical trial data available.

Pharmaceuticals often deplete minerals, toxic metals antagonize their effects (cadmium displaces zinc and lead and mercury knock out selenium), and the processed Western diet is mineral deficient. Thus mineral repletion makes clinical sense, but which minerals and at what doses? A best answer to this question would require periodic biopsy of our organs with mineral dose titration to optimize enzyme activity in relation to ROS generation. We cannot do this, but as we understand the science we can make sound recommendations.

Acknowledging that excessive dosing of a single mineral can have undesirable consequences (eg, high-dose iodine can adversely affect thyroid function and high-dose zinc can deplete copper and vice versa), multimineral supplementation is nontoxic and inexpensive and certainly has a role in the prevention and resolution of oxidative stress. Dosing can relate to laboratory assessment of nutrient and ROS status, whereas a simple approach in the patient with atherosclerosis would be to approximate the mineral content of the TACT-1 (Trial to Assess Chelation Therapy-1) supplement (discussed below).

GliSODin consists of melon-derived SOD, bound to a molecule of gliadin, rendering it absorbable. GliSODin attenuates oxidative stress in vitro and in animal models. In humans, GliSODin (the standard dose is 250 mg bid) protects against HBO-induced oxidative DNA damage and increases SOD expression while reducing CRP in competitive athletes (rowers). In middle-aged French men and women with risk factors for atherosclerosis, GliSODin supplementation over 3 years lowered MDA, increased SOD and GPX expression, and regressed IMT (thus providing a demonstrable anti-atherosclerotic effect). GliSODin is nontoxic (the gliadin moiety appears to be inactive, but tolerance in celiac disease has not been specifically studied) and serves as another member of our SO defense squad.

Dietary intake of plant polyphenolic flavonoids, (colorless) anthoxanthins and (pigmented) anthocyanins (red wine, green and black tea, and in general a plant-based diet), relates inversely to atherosclerosis prevalence. The pomegranate tree is said to have flourished in the Garden of Eden (where Adam and Eve did well without statins),

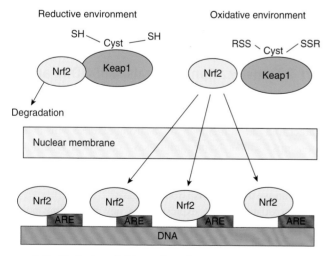

⇒ Antioxidant, phase II detox, cell repair, etc.

Figure 3.20 *NRF2 plays a major role in detoxification and antioxidant effects.*

and its products have been used in the folk medicine of diverse cultures. Pomegranate (POM) polyphenols neutralize ROS and (demonstrated in vitro) inhibit NOX and Nf-κB expression. Relating to this discussion, POM increases transcription and expression of the paraoxonase (PON) antioxidant enzymes. Intracellular PON2 interacts with Co-Q$_{10}$ to contain mitochondrial SO. PON1, synthesized in the liver, associates with HDL within the circulation, using this platform to excise oxidized lipids within lipoproteins. Stated otherwise, PON1 prevents and reverses LDL oxidation. Different forms and doses of POM have been utilized in the (relatively small) intervention trials to date, but these studies have shown that pomegranate:

- Increases PON1 expression, lowering (in vivo and in vitro) lipid oxidation in the circulation.
- Enters established plaque, thereby lowering lipid oxidation and preserving GSH.
- Favorably affects IMT progression (the greater the baseline disease burden, the more powerful the effect), while decreasing carotid flow velocities (suggesting macroscopic disease regression).
- Attenuates stress-induced ischemia (as assessed by stress perfusion imaging). PON has as second (also POM-enhanced) function, promoting the clearance of lipophilic organic pollutants and homocysteine thiolactone (homocysteine is another cause and consequence of oxidative stress).

The best approach to POM supplementation is not certain, but four ounces a day of pomegranate juice is certainly a tasty way to enhance PON expression.

Antioxidant Supplementation

Antioxidant supplementation has become an area of controversy in terms of the studies selected and socialized to the community of practitioners of Integrative Medicine regarding "vitamins don't work."

We understand that vitamins do not (always) work, when used in noncomprehensive fashion, as a drug-like mono-therapy versus the complicated ROS/RNS oxidative cascade, and we understand that in certain conditions (iron overloaded or Hp2/2 diabetics), vit C monotherapy could work against us. However, as practitioners of Integrative Medicine (we can use drugs,

nutritionals, interventions, and anything else that might help and will not hurt), with an awareness of human physiology, we can make good use of antioxidants, because we understand that:

- Antioxidants do not decrease SO generation; they serve only to mitigate the downstream toxic effects of SO excess.
- No single vitamin can neutralize all ROS/RNS (vit E neutralizes lipid radicals but has no activity against SO or HOCL).
- No single vitamin is active within all cellular compartments (lipophilic molecules are inactive in the cytoplasm while vit C alone cannot protect lipid membranes).
- Vitamins may not enter all sites of concern (vit E will blunt LDL oxidation in the circulation but not within an advanced plaque).
- Antioxidants work within our physiology as a team (C recharges E and lipoic acid and bioflavonoids recharge C). Intervening with a single antioxidant is biologically unreasonable.

Thus, if our patients are to benefit from antioxidant supplementation, it must be comprehensive (mimicking Mother Nature's designs), and it should supplement (not replace) SO generation and ONOO/OH conversion inhibition strategies. The literature supports this comprehensive approach.

The Antioxidant Supplementation Atherosclerosis Prevention Study (ASAP) looked at IMT progression (**Figure 3.21**) in relation to antioxidant supplementation in 510 asymptomatic Finns with cholesterol > 193 mg/dL. Subjects received daily vitamin E 272 IU, sustained release vitamin C 500 mg, both, or placebo. In healthy Americans, CCA mean-IMT progresses at 0.01 mm/y, whereas in the Finnish ASAP population, IMT progression on placebo was 0.02 mm/y. With vitamin E or vitamin C monotherapy, IMT progression was attenuated by 5%/y, whereas combination therapy blunted progression by 35%/y. Combination therapy provided greater benefit in smokers versus nonsmokers (64% vs. 34% reduction). You understand why—the greater the baseline level of oxidative stress (DM, CHF, MI, or smoking as in ASAP), the greater the relative antioxidant need and thus the greater the upside potential of antioxidant support.

The Indian Experiment of Infarct Survival randomized 125 acute MI patients (all receiving standard therapy) to a 28-day program (IV days 1-3 and then PO) of vitamins C, E, A and beta

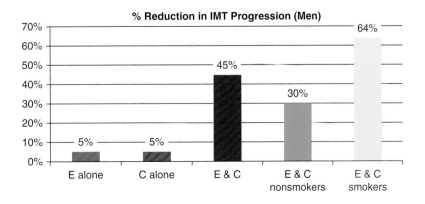

Figure 3.21 *Relative protection against IMT progression in relation to antioxidant supplementation.*

Table 3.2

TACT MULTI—SIX PILLS PROVIDES

Vit A	25,000 IU	Vit B_6	50 mg	Magnesium	500 mg	Potassium	99 mg
Vit C	12,000 mg	Folate	800 µg	Zinc	20 mg	Inositol	50 mg
Vit D_3	100 IU	Vit B_{12}	100 µg	Selenium	200 µg	PABA	50 mg
Vit E	400 IU	Biotin	300 µg	Copper	2 mg	Boron	2 mg
Vit K_1	60 µg	Vit B_5	400 mg	Manganese	20 mg	Vanadium	39 µg
Thiamine	100 mg	Calcium	500 mg	Chromium	200 µg	Citrus bioflavonoids	100 mg
Niacin	200 mg	Iodine	150 µg	Molybdenum	150 µg		

carotene versus placebo. Infarct size (judged by CK release and QRS score) was reduced and 28-day adverse event rate fell from 31% to 21%. Similar results were obtained in a Polish acute MI trial involving a 28-day program of vit C 2000 mg and vit E 600 mg, and in post-MI trials involving Co-Q_{10} with/without other antioxidants.

These studies were carried out one to two decades ago, before the widespread adoption of pharmaceutical ROS inhibition. Will combination antioxidant therapy be of value when added to standard (SO generation suppression) therapy (how we are going to use it)? The best guidance comes from TACT-1 (Trial to Assess Chelation Therapy-1) (see Table 3.2).

TACT-1 randomized 1708 infarct survivors on standard therapy (73% statin, 72% beta-blocker, 63% ACEI/ARB, and 84% ASA) to 40 weekly sessions of IV Mg-EDTA (to remove pro-oxidant metals) and/or a three-pill bid broad-spectrum antioxidant vitamin and mineral supplement (to attenuate residual oxidative stress). Metal detoxification led to an 18% reduction in 5-year event rate (38%-33%). Greater protection was afforded to subjects s/p anterior as opposed to inferior MI (greater injury and presumably greater subsequent oxidative stress), with a 37% risk reduction, and in diabetics, in whom event rate fell by 39%. Antioxidant monotherapy reduced 5-year event rate a nonsignificant 11% (37%-34%). Metal detox and antioxidant support demonstrated event reducing synergy that was not statistically significant, but the best and worst outcomes were recorded in the double-active and double-placebo groups, respectively. Synergy was more pronounced in the diabetics; here double-active therapy reduced 5-year death rate by 50%. Among subjects not receiving a statin, antioxidant support decreased event risk by 38% (36%-23%).

Special Teams—Mixed Tocopherols and Tocotrienols

In CHAOS (Table 3.3) vit E (400 or 800 IU/d) decreased 510-day nonfatal MI risk by 77% (4.2% placebo vs. 1.4% vit E). Vit E works, at least in part, by blunting oxidation of circulating LDL. CHAOS utilized two vit E dosing levels. Thinking about vit E the way we think about drugs, more should be better. CHAOS reminds us that nutrients are not drugs; specifically that more α-tocopherol is not better (MI rate 2% with E 800 vs. 0.61% with E 400). How can we explain this?

Tocopherol exists as four homologues (α, β, γ, and δ), differing only in orientation and extent of methyl binding at C5 and C7 of its chromanol nucleus. In man, the majority of tocopherol exists as the α-homologue, and thus a decision was made to use pure α-tocopherol in clinical cardiovascular research. The other three homologues exist in nature and seem to play specific roles within our physiology, roles that cannot be filled by α-tocopherol at any dose. Specifically, γ-tocopherol, but not its α-homologue, can neutralize ONOO, and thus is a good thing to have around.

Tocopherols and tocotrienols share a common, and saturable, GI tract absorption pathway. High-dose α-tocopherol will blunt absorption of dietary (and supplemental) β, γ, and δ-tocopherol and tocotrienols, robbing us of their unique benefits. To get around this problem, mixed tocopherol supplements have been designed, and while not yet subject to clinical trial assessment, when vit E support is indicated their use makes sense, with or without separate α-tocopherol (Figure 3.22).

Now the plot speeds up (at least within lipid membranes). In contrast to tocopherols, tocotrienols contain three double bonds within their lipophilic side chain. As is the case with saturated versus unsaturated fatty acids, the double bonds increase mobility within lipid membranes. Thus tocotrienols provide 40-fold greater lipid radical quenching versus their less mobile tocopherol cousins.

Tocopherols blunt lipid LDL oxidation. Tocotrienols blunt LDL oxidation and they blunt LDL generation, via two pathways not related to their antioxidant activity (Figure 3.23).

Table 3.3

CHAOS TRIAL—NONFATAL MI RATE

Placebo	Vit E	Vit E 800	Vit E 800
4.2%	1.35%	2%	0.61%

HO—R'

CH₃ CH₃ CH₃

Tocopherols

α: R' = CH₃, R" = CH₃

β: R' = CH₃, R" = H

γ: R' = H, R" = CH₃

δ: R' = H, R" = H

HO—R'

Tocotrienols

Figure 3.22 *Comparative structures of tocopherols and tocotrienols.*

HMG Co-A reductase (HMG) transcription is under Insig/SCAP free cholesterol sensing control. Posttranslational enzyme activity is governed at two additional levels. Berberine and other AMPK agonists promote HMG phosphorylation, which decreases enzyme activity. HMG ubiquitination and proteosomal catabolism increases in relation to rising free cholesterol and/or free sterol levels within the cytoplasm. Tocotrienols (but not tocopherols) shunt isoprenoid molecules (which increase NOX and ATR1 and decrease eNOS expression) to their free sterol homologues, thereby accelerating HMG degradation.

Statin drugs and like-acting nutraceuticals are competitive inhibitors of HMG (they look like acetyl-Co-A and gum up enzyme activity). They reduce cytoplasmic free cholesterol and shoot SREBP into the nucleus. LDL receptor mRNA is transcribed and translated into membrane LDL receptors, and LDL is cleared from the circulation. The problem here is that SREBP also codes for PCSK9, which degrades the LDL receptor, and for HMG itself. Thus statins set up their own failure (so we keep increasing the dose). We mitigate the PCSK problem with berberine, which blunts PCSK9 transcription. Tocotrienols (but not tocopherols) destabilize HMG mRNA, so less "rebound" HMG is translated.

Clinical trials demonstrate LDL reduction with tocotrienol supplementation, and (as you would expect) synergy with statin agents. Tocotrienols combine LDL reduction with a powerful lipid radical neutralizing effect. Tocotrienols available in supplement form are derived from rice bran, the annatto plant, and palm oil. A 1997 Malaysian study randomized 50 subjects with symptomatic carotid disease to palm oil tocotrienol (240 mg α and γ) or placebo. Plaque burden was stratified as 0% to 15%, 16% to 49%, 50% to 79%, and 80% to 99%. Over 2 years, 6/25 placebo subjects progressed one level and 4 by two. Conversely, in the tocotrienol group, only 2 of 25 experienced one level progression; 6 regressed by one level, and 1 subject by two.

This is a small study, but if our goal is to lower LDL and quench lipid peroxides, then tocotrienol supplementation makes sense, particularly in patients who require HMG inhibition/berberine therapy.

Summary and Plan of Action

Atherosclerosis is a maladaptive response of the immune system to what it perceives as infection of the artery wall with oxidized lipids. To prevent/attenuate this process we work to achieve physiologic lipid levels and optimal endothelial tone, with concomitant blunting of intimal lipid trapping, lipid oxidation, and secondary immune dysregulation. ROS/RNS overload drives each of these steps. Heart failure, irrespective of etiology, also involves Th1/Th17-led immune attack against the myocardium and a ROS/RNS-driven impairment in contractility. Stated otherwise:

SO > NO + hyperlipidemia = CV disease

For a plan to prevent/resolve oxidative stress, please see Table 3.4.

For a list of abbreviations used throughout this chapter, please see Table 3.5.

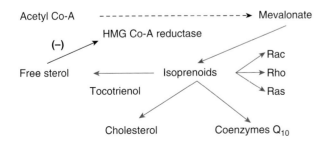

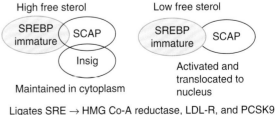

Figure 3.23 *HMG Co-A reductase (HMG) transcription is under Insig/SCAP free cholesterol sensing control.*

Table 3.4

PREVENT/RESOLVE OXIDATIVE STRESS

A. **Baseline measures of oxidative stress and its pathologic expression**
   1. Lab markers such as oxLDL, MDA, 8-OHdG, GSH, and Co-Q$_{10}$
   2. Physiologic markers such as endothelial function and carotid IMT
B. **Identify and resolve nonphysiologic causes (and consequences) of oxidative distress**
   1. Visceral fat, smoking, poor diet, lack of exercise, sleep apnea, chronic infection, etc.
   2. Insulin insensitivity/DM2
   3. Hypertension
   4. Iron excess (particularly with Hp2/2 genotype)
   5. Toxic metals and organic pollutants
   6. Mineral depletion consequent to drug therapy
C. **Pharmaceutical/nutraceutical measures to blunt upregulated ROS generating systems**
   1. HMG Co-A reductase (drug and nondrug statins + berberine + tocotrienols)
   2. NADPH oxidase (HMG inhibition, ACEI/ARB, spironolactone, nebivolol, hydralazine, berberine, colchicine, and polyphenols)
   3. Xanthine oxidase (allopurinol)
   4. NLRP3 (colchicine)
   5. β-Adrenergic blockade (carvedilol and nebivolol provide additional antioxidant support)
   6. Pentoxifylline to shunt the immune response away from Th1 and toward Treg
D. **Remeasure markers of oxidative stress**
   1. If endothelial dysfunction persists, intervene with arginine, taurine, and NAC
   2. If oxidative stress persists:
      a. Strengthen enzymatic antioxidant defenses with mineral, Nrf-2, GliSODin™, and pomegranate supplementation
      b. Antioxidant supplementation, beginning with a TACT-like multiaugmented with special team players (taurine to neutralize HOCL and generate HS, NAC to neutralize ONOO and generate HS, γ-tocopherol to neutralize ONOO, tocotrienols for lipid peroxide neutralization, and Co-Q$_{10}$ for mitochondrial support)
E. **Repeat baseline measures and apply the above principles until redox status has normalized**
F. **Always keep in mind that SO > NO + hyperlipidemia = CV disease**

Table 3.5

ABBREVIATIONS

4-HNE	4-Hydroxynonenol	CD4	T helper cells
8-OHdG	8-Hydroxyguanosine	CD40L	CD40-CD40L APC-T cell co-stimulatory pair
ADMA	Asymmetric dimethylarginine	CD8	T surveillance cells
AGE	Advanced glycation end product	CD80/86	APC co-stimulatory molecules
AMPK	AMP sensitive protein kinase	COX	Cyclooxygenase
Ang II	Angiotensin II	CTLA-4	Turns down APC activity
AP-1	Activator protein-1	DAMP	Damage activated molecular receptor
APC	Antigen presenting cell	DDAH	Dimethylaminohydrolase
ARE	Antioxidant receptor element	eNOS	Endothelial nitric oxide synthase
ATR1	Ang II receptor type 1	GPX	Glutathione peroxidase
CAT	Catalase	GSR	Glutathione reductase
CD28	T cell CD80/86 receptor	H_2O_2	Hydrogen peroxide
CD28^{null}	CD4+28^{null} T helper cells are autonomous and do not require co-stimulation to activate	HMG	HMG Co-A reductase

(Continued)

Table 3.5

ABBREVIATIONS—CONT'D

HOCL	Hypochlorous acid	OH	Hydroxyl
Hp	Haptoglobin	ONOO	Hydroxynitrite
HS	Hydrogen sulfide	OS	Oxidative stress
Ifn	Interferon gamma	oxLDL	Oxidized LDL
IKBα	Inhibitor of kappa beta	PAMP	Pathogen activated molecular receptor
IKK	Inhibitor of kappa beta kinase	PCSK9	Proprotein convertase subtilisin/kexin type 9
IL-1β	Interleukin-1 beta	PGE2	Prostaglandin E2
IL-6	Interkleukin-6	PLA2	Phospholipase A2
IRS	Insulin receptor substrate	POM	Pomegranate
Keap1	Kelch-like ECH-associated protein	PON	Paraoxonase
LCAT	Lecithin chol acyl transferase	PRX	Peroxiredoxin
LDL-R	LDL receptor	PTX	Pentoxifylline
LIMA	Left internal mammary artery	Rac	Activates NADPH
LPL	Lipoprotein lipase	RAGE	Receptor for AGEs
LPS	Lipopolysaccharide	Ras	Increases ATR1 expression
LysoPC	Lysophosphatidylcholine	Rho	Activated endothelium
MCP-1	Monocyte chemotactic protein	RNS	Reactive nitrogen species
MCSF	Mono colony stimulating factor	SCAP	SREBP cleavage activating protein
MDA	Malondialdehyde	SERCA	Sarcolemmal Ca^{2+}-ATPase
MHC	Major histocompatibility molecule	SO	Superoxide
MMP	Matrix metalloproteinase	SRE	Sterol regulating element
MPO	Myeloperoxidase	SREBP	Sterol regulating element binding protein
NAC	N-acetylcysteine	S-Smase	Sphingomyelinase
NF-κB	Nuclear factor kappa beta	SV	Saphenous vein
NLRP3	Nucleotide-binding oligomerization domain-like receptor, pyrin domain-3 inflammasome	TGF-β	Transforming Growth Factor beta
NO	Nitric oxide	TLR	Toll-like receptor
NOX	NADPH oxidase	TNF	Tumor necrosis factor alpha
Nrf-2	Nuclear factor-2 erythroid factor-2	TRX	Thioredoxin

Bibliography

Atherogenesis

1. Hansson G, Robertson AK, Söderberg-Nauclér C. Inflammation and atherossclerosis. *Annu Rev Pathol Mech Dis*. 2006;1:297-329.
2. Robertson A, Hansson G. T cells in atherogenesis. For better or for worse? *ATVB*. 2006;26:2421-2432.
3. Periera I, Borba E. The role of inflammation, humoral and cell mediated autoimmunity in the pathogenesis of atherosclerosis. *Swiss Med Wkly*. 2008;138(37-38):534-539.
4. Osterud B, BJorklid E. Role of monocytes in atherogenesis. *Physiol Rev*. 2003;83:1069-1112.
5. Ross R. Atherosclerosis – an inflamatory disease. *NEJM*. 1999;340(2):115-126.
6. Tabas I, Williams KJ, Borén J. Subendothelial lipoprotein retention as the initiating process in atherosclerosis. Update and therapeutic implications. *Circulation*. 2007;116:1832-1844.
7. Aviram M. Macrophage foam cell formation during early atherogenesis is determined by the balance between pro-oxidants and anti-oxidants in arterial cells and blood lipoproteins. *Antioxid Redox Signaling*. 1999;1(4):585-594.
8. Aukrust P, Otterdal K, Yndestad A, et al. The complex role of T-cell-based immunity in atherosclerosis. *Curr Atheroscler Rep* 2008, 10:236-243.
9. Tabas I, Lichtman A. Monocyte-macrophages and T Cells in atherosclerosis. *Immunity*. 2017;47(4):621-634.

10. De Palma R, Del Galdo F, Abbate G, et al. Patients with acute coronary syndrome show oligoclonal T-cell recruitment with unstable plaque evidence for a local, intracoronary immunologic mechanism. *Circulation.* 2006;113:640-646.

11. Van der Meer JJ, van der Wal AC, Teeling P, Idu MM, van der Ende A, de Boer OJ. Multiple bacteria contribute to intraplaque T-cell activation in atherosclerosis. *Eur J Clin Invest.* 2008;38(11):857-862.

Oxidative Stress

12. Poljsak B. Strategies for reducing or preventing the generation of oxidative stress. *Oxidative Med Cell Longevity.* 2011;2011:194586.

13. Martin-Ventura J, Rodrigues-Diez R, Martinez-Lopez D, Salaices M, Blanco-Colio LM, Briones AM. Oxidative stress in human atherothrombosis: sources, markers, and therapeutic targets. *Int J Mol Sci.* 2017;18:2315.

14. Yang X, Li Y, Li Y, et al. Oxidative stress-mediated atherosclerosis: mechansims and therapies. *Front Physiol.* 2017;8:600.

15. Sena C, Leandro A, Azul L, Seiça R, Perry G. Vascular oxidative stress: impact and therapeutic approaches. *Front Physiol.* 2018;9:1668.

16. Kattoor A, Pothineni NVK, Palagiri D, Mehta JL. Oxidative stress in atherosclerosis. *Curr Atheroscler Rep.* 2017;19:42.

17. Schieber M, Chanel N. ROS function in redox signaling and oxidative stress. *Curr Biol.* 2014;24(10):R453-R462.

18. Ottaviano F, Handy DE, Loscalzo J. Redox regulation in the extracellular environment. *Circ J.* 2008;72:1-16.

19. Bubici C, Papa S, Dean K, Franzoso G. Mutual cross-talk between reactive oxygen species and nuclear factor-kappa B: molecular basis and biological significance. *Oncogene.* 2006;25:6731-6748.

20. Sack MN, Fyhrquist FY, Saijonmaa OJ, Fuster V, Kovacic JC. Basic biology of oxidative stress and the cardiovascular system. Part 1 of a 3-part series. *JACC.* 2017;70:196-211.

21. Camici GG, Maack C, Bonetti NR, Fuster V, Kovacic JC. Impact of oxidative stress on the heart and vasculature. Part 2 of a 3-part series. *JACC* 2017;70:212-229.

22. Rohrbach S, Miller MR, Newby DE, Fuster V, Kovacic JC. Oxidative stress and cardiovascular risk: obesity, diabetes, smoking, and pollution. Part 3 of a 3-part series. *JACC.* 2017;70:230-251.

Endothelial Function and Oxidative Stress

23. Beckman J, Koppenol W. Nitric oxide, superoxide, and peroxynitrite: the good, the bad, and the ugly. *Am J Physiol.* 1996;271(5 pt 1):C1424-C1437.

24. McNally J, Davis ME, Giddens DP, et al. Role of xanthine oxidoreductase and NAD(P)H oxidase in endothelial superoxide production in response to oscillatory shear stress. *Am J Physiol Heart Circ Physiol.* 2003;285(6):H22907.

25. Antoniades C. 5-methyltetrahydrofolate rapidly improves endothelial function and decreases superoxide production in human vessels: effects on vascular tetrahydrobiopterin availability and endothelial nitric oxide synthase coupling. *Circulation.* 2006;114(11):1193-1201.

26. Cooke J, Dzau V. Nitric oxide synthase: role in the genesis of vascular disease. *Annu Rev Med.* 1997;48:489-509.

27. Arrignoni F, Ahmetaj B, Leiper J. The biology and therapeutic potential of the DDAH/ADMA pathway. *Curr Pharm Designs.* 2010;16:4089-4102.

28. Davignon J, Ganz P. Role of endothelial dysfunction in atherosclerosis. *Circulation.* 2004;109(suppl III):III-27-III-32.

29. Rubbo H, Trostchansky A, Botti H, Batthyány C. Interactions of nitric oxide and peroxynitrite with low-density lipoprotein. *Biol Chem.* 2002;383(3):547-552.

30. Topper J, Cai J, Falb D, Gimbrone MA Jr. Identification of vascular endothelial genes differentially responsive to fluid mechanical stimuli: cyclooxygenase-2, manganese superoxide dismutase, and endothelial cell nitric oxide synthase are selectively up-regulated by steady laminar shear stress. *Proc Natl Acad Sci.* 1996;93:10417-10422.

31. Takabe W, Warabi E, Noguchi N. Anti-atherogenic effect of laminar shear stress via Nrf2 activation. *Antioxid Redox Signal.* 2011;15(5):1415-1426.

32. Cooke J. Does ADMA cause endothelial dysfunction? *Artioscler Thromb Vasc Biol.* 2000;20:2032-22037.

33. Landmesser U, Hornig B, Drexler H. Endothelial function a critical determinant in atherosclerosis? *Circulation.* 2004;109(suppl II):II-27-II-33.

HMG Co-A Reductase

34. Shishebor M, Brennan ML, Aviles RJ, et al. Statins promote potent systemic antioxidant effects through specific inflammatory pathways. *Circulation.* 2003;108:426-431.

35. Scheonbeck U, Libby P. Inflammation, immunity, and HMG-CoA reductase inhibitor. Statins as antiinflammatory agents? *Circulation.* 2004;109(suppl II):II-18-II-26.

36. Mason R, Walter MF, Jacob RF. Effects of HMG-CoA reductase inhibitors on endothelial function. Role of microdomains and oxidative stress. *Circulation.* 2004;109(suppl II):II-34-II-41.

37. Yoshida M. Potential role of statins in inflammation and atherosclerosis. *J Atheroscler Thromb.* 2003;10:140-144.

38. Wassmann S, Laufs U, Müller K, et al. Cellular antioxidant effects of atorvastatin in vitro and in vivo. *Arterioscler Thromb Vasc Biol.* 2002;22:300-305.

39. Okuyama H, Langsjoen PH, Hamazaki T, et al. Statins stimulate atherosclerosis and heart failure: pharmacological mechanism. *Expert Rev Clin Pharmacol.* 2015;8(2):189-199.

Diabesity

40. Dandona P, Aljada A, Mohanty P, et al. Insulin inhibits intranuclear nuclear factor κB and stimulates IκB in mononuclear cells in obese subjects: evidence for an anti-inflammatory effect? *J Clin Endocrinol Metab.* 2001;86:3257-3265.

41. Tan B, Norhaizan ME, Liew WP. Nutrients and oxidative stress: friend or foe. *Oxidative Med Cell Longevity Vol.* 2018;2018:971958.

42. Ilkun O, Boudina S. Cardiac dysfunction and oxidative stress in the metabolic syndrome: an update on antioxidant therapies. *Curr Pharm.Des.* 2013;19(27):4806-4817.

43. Pitocco D, Zaccardi F, Di Stasio E, et al. Oxidative stress, nitric oxide, and diabetes. *Rev Diabetic Stud.* 2010;7:15-25.

NADPH Oxidase

44. Singel K, Segal B. NOX2-dependent regulation of inflammation. *Clin Sci (Lond).* 2016;130(7):479-490.

45. Guzik T, West NE, Black E, et al. Vascular superoxide production by NAD(P)H oxidase. *Circ Res.* 2000;86(9):E85-E90.

46. Schramm A, Matusik P, Osmenda G, Guzik TJ. Targeting NADPH oxidases in vascular pharmacology. *Vasc Pharmacol.* 2012;56:216-231.

47. McNally J, Davis ME, Giddens DP, et al. Role of xanthine oxidoreductase and NAD(P)H oxidase in endothelial superoxide production in response to oscillatory shear stress. *Am J Physiol Heat Circ Physiol.* 2003;285:H2290-H2297.

48. De Keulenaer G, Chappell DC, Ishizaka N, Nerem RM, Alexander RW, Griendling KK. Oscillatory and steady laminar shear stress differentially affect human endothelial redox state: role of a superoxide-producing NADH oxidase. *Circ Res.* 1998;82(10):1094-1101.

49. Hwang J, Saha A, Boo YC, et al. Oscillatory shear stress stimulates endothelial production of O From p47[phox]-dependent NAD(P)H oxidases, leading to monocyte adhesion. *J Biol Chem.* 2003;278(47):47291-47298.

50. Selemidis S, Dusting GJ, Peshavariya H, Kemp-Harper BK, Drummond GR. Nitric oxide suppresses NADPH oxidase-dependent superoxide production by S-nitrosylation in human endothelial cells. *Cardiovasc Res.* 2007;75:349-358.

Xanthine Reductase and Allopurinol

51. Saavedra W, Paolocci N, St John ME. Imbalance between xanthine oxidase and nitric oxide synthase signaling pathway underlies mechanoenergetic uncoupling in the failing heart. *Circ Res.* 2002;90:297-304.

52. Doehner W, Tarpey MM, Pavitt DV, et al. Elevated plasma xanthine oxidase activity in chronic heart failure: sources of increased oxygen radical load and effect of allopurinol in a placebo controlled, double blinded treatment study. *JACC.* 2003;41(6):1184-1281.

53. Cappola T, Kass DA, Nelson GS, et al. Allopurinol improves myocardial efficiency in patients with idiopathic dilated cardiomyopathy. *Circulation.* 2001;104:2407-2411.

54. George J, Carr E, Davies J, Belch JJ, Struthers A. High-dose allopurinol improves endothelial function by profoundly reducing vascular oxidative stress and not by lowering uric acid. *Circulation.* 2006;114:2508-2516.

55. Yiginer O, Ozcelik F, Inanc T, et al. Allopurinol improves endothelial function and reduces oxidant-inflammatory enzyme of myeloperoxidase in metabolic syndrome. *Clin Res Cardiol.* 2008;97:334-340.

56. Takir M, Kostek O, Ozkok A, et al. Lowering uric acid with allopurinal improves insulin resistance and systemic inflammation in asymptomatic hyperuricemia. *J Investig Med.* 2015;63:924-929.

57. Norman A, Ang DS, Ogston S, Lang CC, Struthers AD. Effect of high-dose allopurinol on exercise in patients with chronic stable angina: a randomised, placebo controlled crossover trial. *Lancet.* 2010;375(9732):2161-2167.

58. Liu P, Wang H, Zhang F, Chen Y, Wang D, Wang Y. The effects of allopurinol on the carotid intima-media thickness in patients with type 2 diabetes and asymptomatic hyperuricemia: a three-year randomized parallel-controlled study. *Intern Med.* 2015;54:2129-2137.

59. Higgins P, Walters MR, Murray HM, et al. Allopurinol reduces brachial and central blood pressure, and carotid intima-media thickness progression after ischaemic stroke and transient ischaemic attack: a randomised controlled trial. *Heart.* 2014;100:1085-1092.

60. Goicoechea M, de Vinuesa SG, Verdalles U, et al. Effects of allopurinol in chronic kidney disease (CKD) progression and cardiovascular risk. *Clin J Am Soc Nephrol.* 2010;5:1388-1393.

61. Goicoechea M, Garcia de Vinuesa S, Verdalles U, et al. Allopurinol and progression of CKD and cardiovascular events: long-term follow-up of a randomized clinical trial. *Am J Kidney Dis.* 2015;65(4):543-549.

62. De Abajo F, Gil MJ, Rodríguez A, et al. Allopurinol use and risk of non-fatal acute myocardial infarction. *Heart.* 2015;101:679-685.

63. Huang Y, Zhang C, Xu Z, et al. Clinical study on efficacy of allopurinol in patients with acute coronary syndrome and its functional mechanism. *Hellenic J Cardiol.* 2017;58:1-6.

64. Separham A, Ghaffari S, Najafi H, Ghaffari R, Ziaee M, Babaei H. The impact of allopurinol on patients with acute ST elevation myocardial infarction undergoing thrombolytic therapy. *J Cardiovasc Pharmacol.* 2016;68:265-268.

65. Sisto T, Paajanen H, Metsä-Ketelä T, Harmoinen A, Nordback I, Tarkka M. Pretreatment with antioxidants and allopurinol diminishes cardiac onset events in coronary artery bypass grafting. *Ann Thorac Surg.* 1995;59:1519-1523.

Renin-Angiotensin-Aldosterone System

66. Braiser A, Recinos A III, Eledrisi MS. Vascular inflammation and the renin-angiotensin system. *Arterioscler Thromb Vasc Biol.* 2002;22:1257-1266.

67. Mehta PK, Griendling KK. Angiotensin II cell signaling: physiological and pathological effects in the cardiovascular system. *Am J Physiol Cell Physiol.* 2007;292:C82-C97.

68. Chang Y, Wei W. Angiotensin II in inflammation, immunity, and rheumatoid arthritis. *Clin Exp Immunol.* 2014;179:137-145.

69. Cipollone R, Fazia M, Iezzi A, et al. Blockade of the angiotensin II type 1 receptor stabilizes atherosclerotic plaques in humans by inhibiting prostaglandin E2-dependent matrix metalloproteinase activity. *Circulation.* 2004;109:1482-1488.

70. Gage J, Fonarow G, Hamilton M, et al. Beta blocker and angiotensin-converting enzyme inhibitor therapy is associated with decreased Th1/Th2 cytokine ratios and inflammatory cytokine production in patients with chronic heart failure. *NeuroImmuneModulation.* 2004;11:173-180.

71. Sattler K, Woodrum JE, Galili O, et al. Concurrent treatment with renin-angiotensin system blockers and acetylsalicylic acid reduces nuclear factor κB activation and C-reactive protein expression in human carotid artery plaques. *Stroke.* 2005;36:14-20.

72. Khan B, Navalkar S, Khan QA, Rahman ST, Parthasarathy S. Irbesartan, an angiotensin type 1 receptor inhibitor, regulates the vascualar oxidative state in patients with coronary artery disease. *JACC.* 2001;38:1662-1667.

73. Heart Outcomes Prevention Evaluation Study Investigators, Yusuf S, Sleight P, Pogue J, Bosch J, Davies R, Dagenais G. Effects of an angiotensin-converting-enzyme inhibitor, ramipril, on cardiovascular events in high-risk patients. *NEJM.* 2000;342:145-153.

β-Adrenergic Blockade

74. Conti V, Russomanno G, Corbi G, Izzo V, Vecchione C, Filippelli A. Adrenoreceptors and nitric oxide in the cardiovascular system. *Front Physiol.* 2013;4:311.

75. Yasunari K, Maeda K, Nakamura M, Watanabe T, Yoshikawa J, Asada A. Effects of carvedilol on oxidative stress in polymorphonuclear and mononuclear cells in patients with essential hypertension. *Am J Med.* 2004;116(7):460-465.

76. Maggi E. Protective effects of carvedilol, a vasodilating beta-adrenergic blocker, against in vivo low density lipoprotein oxidation in essential hypertension. *J Cardiovasc Pharmacol.* 1996;(4):52208.

77. Koitabashi N, Arai M, Tomaru K, et al. Carvedilol effectively blocks oxidative stress-mediated downregulation of sarcoplasmic reticulum Ca^{+2}-ATPase 2 gene transcription through modification of Sp1 bindings. *Biochem Biophysical Res Commun.* 2005;328:116-124.

78. Feuerstein G, Yue T-L, Ma X, Ruffolo RR. Novel mechanisms in the treatment of heart failure: inhibition of oxygen radicals and apoptosis by carvedilol. *Prog Cardiovasc Dis.* 1998;41(1 suppl 1):17-24.

79. Nakamura K, Kusano K, Nakamura Y, et al. Carvedilol decreases elevated oxidative stress in human failing myocardium. *Circulation.* 2002;105:2867-2871.

80. Dandora P, Ghanim H, Brooks DP. Antioxidant activity of carvedilol in cardiovascular disease. *J Hypertens.* 2007;25:731-741.

81. Kurum T, Tatli E, Yuksel M. Effects of carvedilol on plasma levels of pro-inflammatory cytokines. *Tex Heart Inst J.* 2007;34:52-59.

82. Coats A, Jin S. Protective effects of nebivolol from oxidative stress to prevent hypertension-related target organ damage. *J Hum Hypertens.* 2017;31:376-381.

83. Pasini A, Garbin U, Nava MC, et al. Nebivolol decreases oxidative stress in essential hypertensive patients and increases nitric oxide reducing its oxidative inactivation. *J Hypertens.* 2005;23:589-596.

Colchinine and NLRP3

84. Nidorf S, Verma S. Is there a role for colchicine in acute coronary syndromes? *J Am Heart Assoc.* 2015;4:e00237.

85. Martínez GJ, Robertson S, Barraclough J, et al. Colchicine acutely suppresses local cardiac production of inflammatory cytokines in patients with an acute coronary syndrome. *J Am Heart Assoc.* 2015;4:e002128.

86. Nidorf N, Thompson P. Effect of colchicine (0.5 mg twice daily) on high-sensitivity C-reactive protein independent of aspirin and atorvastatin in patients with stable coronary artery disease. *Am J Cardiol.* 2007;99(6):805-807.

87. Nidorf S, Eikelboom JW, Budgeon CA, Thompson PL. Low-dose colchicine for secondary prevention of cardiovascular disease. *JACC.* 2013;61:404-410.

88. Deftereos S, Giannopoulos G, Raisakis K, et al. Colchicine treatment for the prevention of bare-metal stent restenosis in diabetic patients. *JACC.* 2013;61:1679-1685.

89. Deftereos S, Giannopoulos G, Kossyvakis C, et al. Colchicine for prevention of early atrial fibrillation recurrence after pulmonary vein isolation. *JACC.* 2012;60:1790-1796.

90. Chappey ON, Niel E, Wautier J-L, et al. Colchicine disposition in human leukocytes after single and multiple oral administration. *Clin Pharmacol Ther*. 1993;54:360-367.

91. Varghese G, Folkersen L, Strawbridge RJ, et al. NLRP3 inflammasome expression and activation in human atherosclerosis. *J Am Heart Assoc*. 2016;5:e003031, doi:10.1161/JAHA.115.003031.

92. Zhang Y, Li X, Pitzer AL, Chen Y, Wang L, Li PL. Coronary endothelial dysfunction induced by nucleotide oligomerization domain-like receptor protein with pyrin domain containing 3 inflammasome activation during hypercholesterolemia: beyond inflammation. *Antioxid Redox Signal*. 2015;22:1084-1096.

93. Galea J, Armstrong J, Gadsdon P, Holden H, Francis SE, Holt CM. Interleukin-1β in coronary arteries of patients with ischemic heart disease. *Arteriosclerosis, Thromb Vascular Biol*. 1996;16:1000-1006.

94. Jo E-K, Kim JK, Shin D-M, Sasakawa C. Molecular mechanism regulating NLRP3 inflammasome activation. *Cell Mol Immunol*. 2016;13:148-159.

Hydralazine

95. Daiber A. Hydralazine is a powerful inhibitor of peroxynitrite formation as a possible explanation for its beneficial effects on prognosis in patients with congestive he art failure. *Biochem Biophys Res Commun*. 2005;338(4):1865-1874.

96. Hare J. Nitroso-redox balance in the cardiovascular system. *NEJM*. 2004;351:2112-2114.

97. Münzel T, Kurz S, Rajagopalan S, et al. Hydralazine prevents nitroglycerin tolerance by inhibiting activation of a membrane-bound NADH oxidase. A new action for an old drug. *J Clin Invest*. 1996;98(6):1465-1470.

98. Tayor A, Ziesche S, Yancy C, et al. Combination of isosorbide dinitrate and hydralazine in blacks with heart failure. *NEJM*. 2004;351:2049-2057.

99. Munzel T, Camici GG, Maack C, et al. Impact of oxidative stress on the heart and vasculature. *JACC*. 2017;70(2):212-229.

Taurine and N-Acetylcysteine

100. DiNicolantonio J, OKeefe JH, McCarty MF. Supplemental N-acetylcysteine and other measures that boost intracellular glutathione can downregulate interleukin-1β signaling: a potential strategy for preventing cardiovascular events. *Open Heart*. 2017;4 e000599.

101. Tan B, Jiang D-J, Huang H, et al. Taurine protects against low-density lipoprotein-induced endothelial dysfunction by the DDAH/ADMA pathway. *Vascul Pharmacol*. 2007;46(5):338-345.

102. Abee W, Mozaffari M. Role of taurine in the vasculature: and overview of experimental and human studies. *Am J Cardiovasc Dis*. 2011;1(3):293-311.

103. DiNicolantonio J, O'Keefe JH, McCarty MF. Boosting endogenous production of vasoprotective hydrogen sulfide via supplementation with taurine and N-acetylcysteine: a novel way to promote cardiovascular health. *Open Heart*. 2017;4:e000600.

104. Xu Y, Arneja AS, Tappia PS, Dhalla NS. The potential health benefits of taurine in cardiovascular disease. *Exp Clin Cardiol*. 2008;13(2):57-65.

105. Khaledifar A, Mobasheri M, Kheiri S, Zamani Z. Comparison of N-acetylcysteine and angiotensin converting enzyme inhibitors in blood pressure regulation in hypertensive patients. *ARYA Atheroscler*. 2015;11(1):5-13.

Pentoxifylline

106. Fernandes J, de Oliveira RTD, Mamoni RL, et al. Pentoxifylline reduces pro-inflammatory and increases anti-inflammatory activity in patients with coronary artery disease-A randomized placebo-controlled study. *Atherosclerosis*. 2008;196:434-442.

107. Insel J, Halle AA, Mirvis DM. Efficacy of pentoxifylline in patients with stable angina pectoris. *Angiology*. 1988;39(6):514-519.

108. Angelides N, Minas C. Can aortocoronary and peripheral venous bypass graft patency be improved by the administration of Pentoxifylline on a long-term basis? *Cardiologia*. 1999;44(12):1059-1064.

109. Maiti R, Agrawal NK, Dash D, Pandey BL. Effect of pentoxifylline on inflammatory burden, oxidative stress, and platelet aggregability in hypertensive type 2 diabetes mellitus patients. *Vasc Pharmacol* 2007;47:118-124.

Vitamin E and Haptoglobin Genotype

110. Blum S, Vardi M, Brown JB, et al. Vitamin E reduces cardiovascular disease in individuals with diabetes mellitus and the haptoglobin 2-2 genotype. *Pharmacogenomics*. May 2010;11(5):678-684.

111. Blum S, Vardi M, Levy NS, Miller-Lotan R, Levy AP. The effect of vitamin E supplementation on cardiovascular risk in diabetic individuals with different haptoglobin phenotypes. *Atherosclerosis*. 2010;211(1):25-27.

112. Levy A, Hochberg I, Jablonski K, et al. Haptoglobin phenotype is an independent risk factor for cardiovascular disease in individuals with diabetes: the Strong Heart Study. *J Am Coll Cardiol*. 2002;40:1984-1990.

113. Boaz M, Smetana S, Weinstein T, et al. Secondary prevention with antioxidants of cardiovascular disease in endstage renal disease (SPACE): randomised placebo-controlled trial. *Lancet*. 2000;356:1213-1218.

114. Stephens N, Parsons A, Brown MJ, et al. Randomized controlled trial of vitamin E in patients with coronary disease: cambridge Heart Antioxidant Study (CHAOS). *Lancet*. 1996;347:781-786.

115. Yusuf S, Dagenais G, Pogue J, Bosch J, Sleight P. Vitamin E supplementation and cardiovascular events in high-risk patients (HOPE). *N Eng J Med*. 2000;342(3):156-160.

116. Levy A, Friedenberg P, Lotan R, et al. The effect of vitamin therapy on the progression of coronary artery atherosclerosis varies by haptoglobin type in postmenopausal women. *Diabetes Care*. 2004;27:925-930.

117. Langlois MR, Martin ME, Boelaert JR, et al. The haptoglobin 2-2 phenotype affects serum markers of iron status in healthy males. *Clin Chem*. 2000;46(10):1619-1625.

118. Hochberg I, Roguin A, Nikolsky E, Chanderashekhar PV, Cohen S, Levy AP. Haptoglobin phenotype and coronary artery collateral in diabetic patients. *Atherosclerosis*. 2002;161(2):441-446.

119. Milman U, Blum S, Shapira C, et al. Vitamin E supplementation reduces cardiovascular events in a subgroup of middle-aged individuals with both type 2 diabetes mellitus and the haptoglobin 2-2 genotype: a prospective double-blinded clinical trial. *Arterioscler Thromb Vasc Biol*. 2008;28:341-347.

120. Dietary supplementation with n-3 polyunsaturated fatty acids and vitamin E after myocardial infarction: results of the GISSI-Prevenzione trial. *Lancet*. 1999;354:447-455.

121. Micheletta F, Natoli S, Misuraca M, Sbarigia E, Diczfalusy U, Iuliano L. Vitamin E supplementation in patients with carotid atherosclerosis. *Artioscler Thromb Vasc Biol*. 2004;24:136-140.

122. Bernard D, Christophe A, Delanghe J, Langlois M, De Buyzere M, Comhaire F. The effect of supplementation with an antioxidant preparation on LDL-oxidation is determined by haptoglobin polymorphism. *Redox Rep*. 2003;8(1):41-46.

123. Levy AP, Levy JE, Kalet-Litman S, et al. Haptoglobin genotype is a determinant of iron, lipid peroxidation, and macrophage accumulaiiotn in the atherosclerotic plaque. *Arterioscler Thromb Vasc Biol*. 2007;27:134-140.

124. Asleh R, Levy A. Divergent effects of alpha-tocopherol and vitamin C on the generation of dysfunctional HDL associated with diabetes and the Hp 2-2 genotype. *Antioxid Redox Signal*. 2010;12:209-218.

125. Levy A, Moreno P. Intraplaque hemorrhage. *Curr Mol Med*. 2006;6:6479-6488.

126. Fukami K, Yamagishi S, Iida S, Matsuoka H, Okuda S. Involvement of iron-evoked oxidative stress in smoking related endothelail dysfucntion in healthy young men. *PLoS One*. 2014;9(2):1-16.

127. Upston J, Terentis AC, Morris K, Keaney JF, Stocker R. Oxidized lipid accumulates in the presence of α-tocopherol in atherosclerosis. *Biochem J*. 2002;363:753-760.

Glisodin

128. Cloarec M, Caillard P, Provost JC, Dever JM, Elbeze Y, Zamaria N. GliSODin®, a vegetal SOD with gliadin, as preventative agent vs. atherosclerosis as confirmed with carotid ultrasound-B imaging. *Eur Ann Allergy Clinical Immunol.* 2007;39(2):45-50.
129. Skarpanska A, Pilaczynska-Szczesniak L, Basta P, Deskur-Smielecka E, Woitas-Slubowska D, Adach Z. Effects of oral supplementation with plant superoxide dismutase extract on selected redox parameters and an inflammatory marker in a 2,000-m rowing-ergometer test. *Int J Sport Nutr Exerc Metab.* 2011;21:124-134.
130. Vouldoukis I, Conti M, Krauss P, et al. Supplementation with gliadin-combined plant superoide dismutase extract promotes antioxidant defense and protects against oxidative stress. *Phytother Res.* 2004;18:957-962.
131. Romao S. Therapeutic value of oral supplementation with melon superoxide dismutase and wheat gliadin combination. *Nutrition.* 2015;31:430-436.

Pomegranate and Paraoxonase

132. Aviram M, Rosenblat M. Pomegranate protection against cardiovascular diseases. *Evid Based Complement Altern Med.* 2012;2012:382763.
133. Fuhrman B, Volkova N, Aviram M. Pomegranate juice polyphenols increase recombinant paraoxonase-1 binding to high-density lipoprotein: studies in vitro and in diabetic patients. *Nutrition.* 2010;26:359-366.
134. Rock W, Rosenblat M, Miller-Lotan R, Levy AP, Elias M, Aviram M. Consumption of wonderful variety pomegranate jucie amd extract by diabetic patients increases paraoxonase 1 association with high-density lipoprotein and stimulates its catalytic activities. *J Agric Food Chem.* 2008;56:8704-8713.
135. Rosenblat M, Hayek T, Aviram M. Anti-oxidative effects of pomegranate juice (PJ) consumption by diabetic patients on serum and on macrophages. *Athrsoclerosis.* 2009;187:363-371.
136. Litvinov D, Mahini H, Garelnabi M. Antioxidant and anti-inflammatory role of paraoxonase 1: implication in arteriosclerosis diseases. *N Am J Med Sci.* 2012;4(11):523-532.
137. Huang Y, Wu Z, Riwanto M, et al. Myeloperoxidase, paraoxonase-1, and HDL form a functional ternary complex. *J Clin Invest.* 2013;123(9):3815-3828.

Antioxidant Support

138. Salonnen R, Nyyssönen K, Kaikkonen J, et al. Six-year effect of combined vitamin C and E supplementation on atherosclerotic progression: the antioxidant supplementation in atherosclerosis prevention (ASAP) study. *Circualtion.* 2003;107(7):947-953.
139. Issa O, Roberts R, Mark DB, Effect of high-dose oral multivitamins and minerals in participants not treated with statins in the randomized Trial to Assess Chelation Therapy (TACT). *Am Heart J.* 2018;195:70-77.
140. Farbstein D, Kozak-Blickstein A, Levy AP. Antioxidant vitamins and their use in preventing cardiovascular disease. *Molecules.* 2010;15:8098-8110.
141. Hodis H, Mack WJ, LaBree L, et al. Serial coronary angiographic evidence that antioxidant vitamin intake reduces progression of coronary artery atherosclerosis. *JAMA.* 1995;273(23):1849-1854.
142. Lamas G, Boineau R, Goertz C, et al. EDTA chelation therapy alone and in combination with oral high-dose multivitamns and minerals for coronary disease: the factorial group results of the trial to assess chelation therapy. *Am Heart J.* 2014;168(1):37-44.
143. Lamas G, Boineau R, Goertz C. Oral high-dose multivimans and minerals after myocardial infarction. *Ann Intern Med.* 2013;159:797-804.
144. Tan BBL. Norhaizan ME, Liew WP. Nutrients and oxidative stress: friend or foe? *Oxid Med Cell Longev.* 2018;2018:9719584.
145. Moser M, Chun O. Vitamin C and heart health: a review based on findings from epidemiologic studies. *Int J Mol Sci.* 2016;17:1328.

Tocotrienols

146. Meganathan P, Fu J-Y. Biological properties of tocotrienols: evidence in human studies. *Int J Mol Sci.* 2016;17:1682.
147. Ramanathan N, Tan E, Loh LJ, Soh BS, Yap WN. Tocotrienol is a cardioprotective agent against ageing-associated cardiovascular disease and its associated morbidities. *Nutr Metab (Lond).* 2018;15:6.
148. Quereshi A, Sami SA, Salser WA, Khan FA. Synergistic effect of tocotrienol-rich faction (TRF(25)) of rice bran and lovastatin on lipid parameters in hypercholesterolemic humans. *J Nutr Biochem.* 2001;(6):318-329.
149. Tomeo A. Antioxidant effects of tocotrienols in patients with hyperlipidemia and carotid stenosis. *Lipids.* 1995;30(12):1179-1183.
150. Kooyenga D, Geller M, Watkins TR, Gapor A, Diakoumakis E, Bierenbaum ML. Palm oil antioxidant effects in patients with hyperlipidemia and carotid stenosis-2 year experience. *Asia Pac J Nutr.* 1997;6(1):7205.

Melatonin

151. Reiter R. Mitochondria: central organelles for melatonin's antioxidant and anti-aging actions. *Molecules* 2018;23:509.
152. Korkmaz A, Reiter RJ, Topal T, Manchester LC, Oter S, Tan DX. Melatonin: an established antioxidant worthy of use in clinical trials. *Mol Med.* 2009;15(1-2):43-50.

Metals and Oxidative Stress

153. Patra R, Rautray AK, Swarup D. Oxidative stress in lead and cadmium toxicity and its amelioration. *Vet Med Int.* 2011;2011:457327.
154. Ni Z, Hou S, Barton CH, Vaziri ND. Lead exposure raises superoxide and hydrogen peroxide in human endothelial and vascular smooth muscle cells. *Kidney Int.* 2004;66:2329-2336.

Section 3

Nutrition and Cardiovascular Disease

4

The Role of Food Patterns, Nutrition, and (Phyto)Nutrients in Cardiovascular Disease: The Clinical Trials, Their Implications, and Clinical Application for the Prevention and Treatment of Cardiovascular Disease, Coronary Heart Disease, Stroke, Hypertension, Dyslipidemia, and Diabetes Mellitus

Deanna M. Minich, MS, PhD, FACN, CNS, IFMCP

Introduction

Currently, there is a global health crisis and accompanying financial burden related to lifestyle-induced chronic disease, which largely encompasses cardiovascular disease (CVD) and type 2 diabetes. Fortunately, the cause of these related conditions is also part of the solution. Regardless of population stratifications like gender or ethnicity, it is generally accepted that about 80% of CVD can be prevented with a combination of nutrition and lifestyle therapies.[1] Owing to their shared etiologies, cardiovascular and diabetic conditions are often approached with similar nutritional interventions.[2] Epidemiological studies have consistently shown that there is an association between whole food-based, plant-rich dietary patterns, such as the Mediterranean diet, and lowered risk of cardiometabolic concerns, including total mortality, CVD mortality,[3] hemoglobin A1C,[4] inflammatory markers,[4] endothelial function,[4] systolic blood pressure, and arterial stiffness.[5]

Purpose

In this chapter, a concise overview of the recent science on dietary patterns, specific classifications of components such as macronutrients and micronutrients, and select whole foods will be discussed as they relate to cardiovascular and metabolic conditions. In addition to the detailed summary the reader will be provided, it is imperative to acknowledge the application of these findings within a personalized therapeutic plan that considers genotype, phenotype, toxin exposure and overall toxin load, age, gender, ancestry, environment, and pregnancy.[6] These will not be extensively addressed within this short chapter. It is becoming increasingly recognized and appreciated that an individual's responses to foods must be evaluated within the context of one's entire exposome,[7] suggesting that the way a meal is received physiologically is not independent but dependent on several variables, including, but not limited to, socioeconomic status.

There is heightened clinical focus on the translation of nutrigenomics to dietary recommendations. As part of developing a therapeutic plan for the patient, the clinician needs to consider gene polymorphisms, such as those involved with one-carbon metabolism (often referred to as methylation), familial hypercholesterolemia, salt sensitivity, hypertension (angiotensinogen, ß2-adrenergic receptor, and kallikrein),[6,8] and Apolipoprotein E (APOE). These will not be discussed in this chapter, but it is worthwhile to mention these as features to incorporate in designing a therapeutic plan that is truly individualized.

Further to nutrition, lifestyle behaviors such as sleep, relationships, stress level, and physical activity can all alter how one responds to nutrients. Nine modifiable risk factors (both food and lifestyle) were reported in the INTERHEART study[9] to account for over 90% of the risk of an initial acute myocardial infarction, which suggests that the clinician would serve the patient best by developing a comprehensive food and lifestyle plan consistent with the 21st century concepts of personalized medicine. This chapter will be specific to providing an overview of the recent science on whole foods, whole food patterns, and food constituents as they relate to CVD and metabolic dysfunction.

Dietary Patterns: Looking at the Whole of Food

Even though specific food components such as meat, dairy, and vegetables have long been the cornerstone of nutrition science recommendations for cardiometabolic disorders, the trend for research has been to examine the entire food pattern one eats.[10,11] After all, people do not specifically eat certain types of fats or carbohydrates but a matrix of foods that may combine in synergistic or antagonistic ways.[12] Further to this point, it is clinically practical as well as relevant to discuss foods rather than specific nutrients with patients.[13]

There are a host of established and emerging dietary patterns for cardiometabolic dysfunction that have been researched and/or reviewed for their efficacy. Perhaps the two classic food patterns, at least for CVD risk reduction, have been the Mediterranean diet and the Dietary Approaches to Stop Hypertension (DASH) diet. There have also been hybridized dietary patterns discussed that incorporate cultural context and tradition such as the "MediterrAsian" diet[14] and, most recently, the "MedÉire" diet.[15]

Aside from the trending dietary patterns and their evolving nomenclature, it is essential to investigate the nutritional framework of what makes these and other diets helpful in the prevention and treatment of cardiovascular and diabetic conditions. This framework can be viewed in two ways: one as what is important to include in the diet and the other as what needs to be excluded. For the former, "prudent," healthy dietary patterns have been generally described as primarily plant-based foods such as fruits, herbs, legumes, nuts, olive oil, seeds, spices, vegetables, and whole grains. On the contrary, foods that seem to warrant caution include high amounts of red and processed meats, solid fats, and foods with little to no nutrient reserves, such the category of processed carbohydrates, which includes refined sugars, sugar-sweetened beverages, desserts, and refined (ready-to-eat) cereals.[16]

Relevant to the discussion in this chapter, healthful dietary patterns may help favorably modulate the profile of cardiometabolic parameters such as body weight, fat mass, body mass index (BMI), waist circumference, systolic and diastolic blood pressure, plasma insulin and glucose, homocysteine, cholesterol (total, high-density lipoprotein [HDL], and low-density lipoprotein [LDL]), and inflammatory markers such as high-sensitivity C-reactive protein (hsCRP),[17-20] together with lowering the risk of morbidity and mortality from CVD and the incidence of myocardial infarction (MI),[21] stroke,[22] atherosclerosis,[23] and diabetes.[24]

A Cultural Eating Pattern: The Mediterranean Diet

A recent literature search on the "Mediterranean diet" at the time of writing this chapter reveals over 4000 published articles in PubMed.[25] This diet has been purported to have benefit for several chronic lifestyle-induced conditions, including CVD, metabolic syndrome and type 2 diabetes, cancer, liver disease, depression, and anxiety.[3] Based on the quantity of articles published, the Mediterranean diet could be considered the most "well-studied" diet, even though its scientific recognition roughly began only 2 decades ago when it was observed that people living on the Greek island of Crete had reduced risk of CVD.[26] In addition to being one of the most researched dietary patterns, it is shared by multiple countries in the Mediterranean basin within the context of varying populations of people living within different degrees of industrialization of food production. As a result of the intercountry differences, it has become necessary to more specifically define the contents of this dietary pattern for research purposes.

Although it varies to some degree, the broad definition of the traditional Mediterranean diet has been deemed to have these characteristics[27]:

- Plant-based (cereals, fruits, vegetables, legumes, spices, tree nuts, seeds, and olives)
- Olive oil as the main dietary fat
- High to moderate intakes of fish and seafood
- Moderate consumption of eggs, poultry, and dairy products (cheese and yogurt)
- Low consumption of red meat
- Moderate intake of alcohol (primarily red wine during meals)

For maintaining consistency and for research study purposes, a quantitative and qualitative research tool has been developed to assess a percentage compliance to the Mediterranean diet.[28] Such a questionnaire may be valuable for patients who are following this way of eating so that the clinician can better assess their adherence to the dietary program. Several studies[29] indicate that various levels of adherence (from first quartile to fourth) are associated with differing health benefits (eg, reduced risk for metabolic syndrome) with the highest compliance being associated with greatest benefit.[30] Factors that may determine compliance include the following: dietitian involvement, education, goal setting, mindfulness, recipe books and other materials such as meal plans, consistent contact with staff, clinic visits, and recipes.[3]

Numerous studies tout the efficacy of the Mediterranean diet for cardiovascular and metabolic benefit, specifically being protective against ischemic stroke, MI, and vascular death.[31] A 10% lower incidence of nonfatal and fatal CVD was documented for each two-unit increment in the Mediterranean diet score in a meta-analysis and review of prospective cohort studies.[32] With greater adherence to this dietary pattern, there was a 56% lower incidence of fatal CVD in a Dutch cohort compared with the group who had lower adherence over an almost 12-year period.[33]

Furthermore, the Mediterranean diet has been shown to be superior in its ability to produce clinically relevant shifts in body weight, BMI, blood pressure, fasting glucose, total cholesterol, and hsCRP compared with the long-standing, widely recognized and advocated low-fat diet.[34] The well-known PREDIMED trial indicated that a Mediterranean diet in conjunction with nuts or olive oil led to a 30% reduction in major cardiovascular events compared with a low-fat diet.[35]

An overall summary of the cardiovascular and metabolic benefits of the Mediterranean diet include the following as based on the review article by Houston et al.[1]:

- Lowers blood pressure
- Improves serum lipids: lowers total cholesterol, LDL, triglycerides; increases HDL; lowers oxidized low-density lipoprotein (oxLDL) and Lp(a) lipoprotein. Shifts LDL size and decreases LDL-P to a less atherogenic profile
- Improves type 2 diabetes and dysglycemia
- Improves oxidative defense and reduces oxidative stress: F-2 isoprostanes and 8-Oxo-2'-deoxyguanosine
- Reduces inflammation: lowers hsCRP, interleukin 6 (IL-6), soluble vascular cell adhesion molecule, and soluble cell adhesion molecule
- Reduces thrombosis and factor VII after meals
- Decreases brain natriuretic peptide
- Increases nitrates/nitrites
- Improves membrane fluidity
- Reduces MI, coronary heart disease (CHD), and cerebrovascular accident (CVA)
- Reduces homocysteine

The Dietary Approaches to Stop Hypertension Dietary Pattern

The DASH diet was unlike the Mediterranean diet in that it had no cultural underpinning, but it was unique for its time because it emphasized a pattern of eating instead of simply avoiding certain foods, which was the nutritional trend at that time.[36] The DASH diet was conceived in the 1990s to create an evidence-based dietary prescription to reduce the incidence of hypertension.[37]

The DASH diet is similar to the Mediterranean diet. It touts high intake of fruits, vegetables, whole grains, low-fat dairy foods, legumes, and nuts; moderate intake of poultry and fish; and low intake of sodium, sweetened beverages, and red and processed meat.[38] In general, it was designed to reduce cholesterol, saturated fat, trans fat, salt, and added sugars, and, at the same time, increase minerals such as potassium, magnesium, and calcium, along with protein and fiber.[39] There were two versions of the DASH diet: DASH 1 had a sodium content of about 3100 mg per day,[40] whereas DASH 2 had about half as much sodium at 1500 mg daily.[41] As one might anticipate, the second version was more effective in reducing blood pressure.[41]

Although the DASH diet was designed for hypertension specifically, its implementation has led to significant improvements in cardiovascular risk factors, such as vascular and autonomic function (pulse wave velocity, baroreflex sensitivity), reduced left ventricular mass, and a lowering of total cholesterol and LDL-cholesterol.[42] A meta-analysis[43] of 12 prospective cohort studies (n = 548,632) with 5.7 to 24 years of follow-up found that greater adherence to the DASH diet was related to a reduced risk of stroke (relative risk, 0.88), with a greater benefit in Asian compared with Western populations. For each four points in the DASH diet score, there was a 4% risk reduction in total stroke events. Additionally, a meta-analysis of prospective studies found that the DASH diet, along with the Mediterranean diet and Alternative Healthy Eating Index, reduced the risk of type 2 diabetes.[44]

In contrast, the DASH diet has led to no effect on triglycerides and a reduction in HDL-cholesterol.[42] Additional effects include reductions in homocysteine, C-reactive protein (CRP), and IL-6[45,46] and an even better blood pressure lowering response in those who are carriers of the *A* allele of the β2-adrenergic receptor.[8,47]

Proposed mechanisms for reduction in cardiovascular risk include[1]:

1. Increased nitric oxide and plasma nitrate
2. Natriuresis
3. Decreased oxidative stress and increased oxidative defense
4. Reduced urinary F2-isoprostanes
5. Improved endothelial function
6. Decreased pulse wave velocity and augmentation index
7. Reduced arterial stiffness

Vegetarian/Vegan Dietary Patterns

The sum of current evidence would suggest that vegetarian diets are beneficial for cardiometabolic health. Plant-based diets have been touted for both the prevention and treatment of heart failure, cerebrovascular disease, and CHD.[48] For decades, Dean Ornish has studied their efficacy, together with lifestyle strategies, for the reversal of CHD.[49,50] Vegetarian dietary patterns can reduce the risk of metabolic syndrome, type 2 diabetes, and CHD (by 40%),[48] in addition to being able to lower blood pressure, blood lipids, and reduce platelet aggregation over nonvegetarian diets. In a prospective investigation[51] of 131,342 participants from both the Nurses' Health Study and Health Professionals Follow-up Study, it was found that high plant protein intake was negatively associated with all-cause and cardiovascular mortality (hazard ratio [HR], 0.90 per 3% energy increment; 95% confidence interval [CI], 0.86-0.95; *P* for trend < .001, and HR, 0.88 per 3% energy increment; 95% CI, 0.80-0.97; *P* for trend = .007, respectively), whereas animal protein intake was positively correlated with cardiovascular mortality. Substituting plant protein for animal protein (processed or unprocessed red meat, and eggs) led to lower mortality.

Depending on the type of vegetarian diet, there may be certain nutrients that require additional supplementation[52] such as vitamins B12 and D, omega-3 fatty acids, the minerals iron and zinc, L-carnitine, and possibly some high-quality amino acids, especially sulfur-containing amino acids, and protein.

Gluten-Free Diets

Avoiding gluten-containing foods, including select whole grains and even processed foods and beverages, has been on the rise for a variety of reasons. Traditionally, it is held that following a gluten-free diet is a necessity for individuals with celiac disease, an autoimmune condition that leads to gastrointestinal and systemic dysfunction in response to the intake of the gluten protein commonly found in wheat, barley, and rye. However, there is awareness of the potential health effects of dietary gluten in nonceliac populations. Laboratory testing is available to detect nonceliac gluten sensitivity (NCGS), which is associated with the dysfunctional effects on gastrointestinal tight junctions through the protein zonulin.[53]

With respect to cardiometabolic health, there is some emerging research in the literature. In a review of published studies on celiac disease and cardiovascular conditions,[54] the authors noted that there were studies on the relationship between celiac disease and cardiomyopathy (33 studies), thrombosis (27 studies), cardiovascular risk (17 studies), atherosclerosis (13 studies), stroke (12 studies), arterial function (11 studies), and ischemic heart disease (11 studies). They concluded that there can be cardiovascular issues in those with celiac disease, particularly if they are untreated.

Some concern has been raised about the quality of a gluten-free diet and whether it may result in decreased intake of vitamins and minerals and increased exposure to environmental toxins such as arsenic (which is high in rice, an alternate grain in the gluten-free diet).[55] In a systematic review[55] of the literature of the gluten-free diet and cardiometabolic parameters (blood pressure, glycemia, BMI, waist circumference, and serum lipids), it was noted that most studies were done in those with celiac disease and there were consistent increases in total cholesterol, HDL, fasting blood glucose, and BMI.

Moreover, one study[56] in 185 patients with celiac disease found an increased risk of developing both metabolic syndrome (3.24% before gluten-free diet and 14.59% after

the gluten-free diet) and hepatic steatosis after following a gluten-free diet (1.7% at the time of diagnosis and 11.1% after the gluten-free diet). The authors report that several criteria of metabolic syndrome were increased after the gluten-free diet compared with baseline at celiac disease diagnosis, including elevated waist circumference and BMI >25, hypertension, hyperglycemia, hypercholesterolemia, and lowered HDL-cholesterol.

However, more studies are required to look more specifically at NCGS and the exact dietary composition, as there can be a wide spectrum of unhealthy and healthy gluten-free diets.[57]

Calorie and Food Restriction Patterns

Presently, the timing of eating and the amount of food eaten, along with patterns of caloric cycling, have been gaining traction in the cardiovascular and diabetic arenas. Indeed, there are a plethora of animal studies to suggest that fasting to the point of maintaining normal body weight in the absence of malnutrition may be highly beneficial for extending lifespan and enhancing cardiovascular and metabolic health[58,59] by reducing oxidative stress, inflammation, and atherosclerosis.[60] Although limited, some clinical studies suggest that these benefits may translate to humans as well.[61] In general, preliminary and observational clinical studies indicate that several cardiovascular and diabetic risk factors may improve with some degree of caloric restriction, from body composition to inflammation, blood pressure, and insulin sensitivity.[62]

Similar effects, such as weight loss and reductions in cardiometabolic parameters such as CRP, cholesterol fractions, triglycerides, and blood pressure,[63-65] are being reported with alternate-day (fasting 1 day and eating ad libitum the next) or intermittent fasting (typically described as a 12- to 16-hour nightly fast), which has become popular within certain nutrition-focused groups.

Whether it is caloric restriction, food restriction, or some pattern of food withdrawal and fasting, it is best to advise patients to plan for engaging in such a protocol to the extent that when they are eating, they are eating nutrient-dense foods such as fruits, vegetables, nuts, seeds, and other high-quality protein- and fat-containing foods so as to ensure they are not becoming nutritionally depleted, hungry, or not feeling satiated, all of which can affect compliance to the regimen.[66]

Cooked Food Patterns: Avoiding Advanced Glycation End Products

Eating cooked food has advantages of improving digestibility and, at the same time, the downside of creating glycosylated protein compounds known as advanced glycation end products (AGEs). This acronym provides an effective way for patients to remember the effect of these deleterious compounds that cause premature aging,[67] like what is seen in cardiometabolic conditions, especially type 2 diabetes.[68]

AGEs are formed endogenously, such as the case with hemoglobin A1C (a glycosylated protein), or taken in exogenously through the diet, primarily though cooked foods as heat facilitates this inflammatory complex of carbohydrate and protein (known as the Maillard reaction). Often, patients will be able to recognize the presence of AGEs in food as it can appear as the "browning" of food through broiling, frying, grilling, roasting, and searing.[69] A list of AGE content in a wide array of foods can be found in the practical guide by Uribarri et al.[69] It is of note that animal-based foods high in fat and protein (eg, bacon, fried chicken) tend to be high in AGE content, whereas vegetables, fruits, whole grains, and even milk (with some cheeses as exceptions) contain relatively less AGEs, even with heat methods applied. Although cooking is one of the primary drivers of AGE formation, some foods are naturally high in AGEs and should be reduced in the diet. High-fat and aged cheeses are among the highest in AGE levels, so choosing a lower-fat cheese or one that has not been cured as long would be preferred.[69]

Eating less AGEs in the diet directly translates to lower circulating AGE levels in serum, along with lower inflammatory cytokines.[70] A single meal consisting of a chicken breast, potatoes, carrots, tomatoes, and vegetable oil caused significant postprandial endothelial function and oxidative stress in type 2 diabetic patients when the meal underwent frying or broiling rather than when it was steamed or boiled.[71] In a crossover design with healthy subjects fed for 1 month a meal containing either high AGEs formed by cooking with high temperatures or low AGEs through mild steaming, it was reported that the high-AGE meals caused lower insulin sensitivity, omega-3 fatty acids, and vitamins C and E and increased cholesterol and triglycerides.[72] In contrast, diabetic patients following a low-AGE diet had lower inflammation and oxidative stress compared with those eating a standard diet.[73]

Clinically, in some cases, it may be easier to effect change in a patient's eating by first starting with altering cooking methods rather than asking them to shift the foods in their dietary pattern. From a therapeutic perspective, there is great benefit in doing so, and it can be easily done. One way to reduce AGEs in foods is by foregoing the high-heat methods of cooking such as frying and grilling and substituting with slow, moist, lower-heat methods including boiling, poaching, steaming, and stewing.[74] Or, if cooking with heat, preferentially use water to steam, and as a second tier to use an oil with a higher smoke point such as olive oil or avocado oil. Oil use over butter led to 50% to 75% less AGE formation.[69] The second way is to reduce or avoid foods high in AGEs, such as full-fat cheeses, whole milk, meats, and highly processed foods (eg, crackers, French fries, potato chips).

An Alkaline Dietary Pattern

A cornerstone concept recognized in naturopathic medicine and discussion on Paleolithic dietary principles is that of an alkaline versus an acidic diet.[75] More specifically, diet-induced "low-grade" metabolic acidosis translates to the imbalance between foods in the diet due to their differing electrolyte content. Potassium alkali salts found primarily in vegetables and fruits would be desirable and essentially reduce the dietary net acid load, whereas eating foods that are low in essential minerals and rich in either amino "acids" and/or fatty "acids" such as animal products would lead to increased acid (low alkaline) load.[76,77] The general basis for this concept in nutritional medicine seems to have come, in part, from exploration into the Paleolithic diet by Loren Cordain[78] and others,[76] as it would have featured high-fiber, wild-cultivated, highly alkalizing plant foods and less of the more "acidic" foods that came into being with the agricultural revolution such as cereal grains, dairy products, and meats.

Although it may be difficult to discern if the therapeutic benefit of eating more "alkaline" is simply because of eating more fruits and vegetables, a large, prospective, population study with 22,034 men and women aged 39 to 78 years did find that urinary pH shifted to more alkaline with a diet higher in fruits and vegetables.[79] With respect to cardiovascular markers, Murkami et al.[80] demonstrated that higher dietary acid load was associated with CVD risk factors such as blood pressure, total and LDL-cholesterol, and body composition metrics, including BMI and waist circumference. Furthermore, lowering risk of hypertension has been noted in some studies utilizing dietary acid load, although results are not consistent.[81,82] There is also an indication that diet-induced acidosis may perturb insulin sensitivity and, ultimately, CVD risk.[83]

Quite simply, although the science for such positioning is not as compelling, the outcome or therapeutic approach is in line with what has been discussed previously. It entails an approach that is like that of both the Mediterranean and DASH diets, both of which are high in plant-based, "alkalizing" foods and lower in animal-based, "acidifying" foods.

Macronutrients

As each section for the individual macronutrients (carbohydrate, fats and oils, protein) is discussed, please note that it is often difficult to isolate and attribute a result to a particular macronutrient because of the complex variety of compounds that foods contain.[84] As is well recognized, food components may interact in unacknowledged ways or means that cannot be accounted for; therefore, please keep this point in mind as each category is detailed as they each relate to the trending studies on cardiometabolic parameters. Furthermore, unlike it is portrayed in nutrition media at large, there does not seem to be a single culprit or offender in the development of chronic disease. Much depends on the larger context of food, including quantity, quality, and variety.

Dietary Carbohydrates

Because of its implication in blood glucose balance, dietary carbohydrate is often seen as a significant macronutrient for type 2 diabetes, whereas dietary fat is typically associated with

CVD. However, dietary carbohydrate quality and quantity are essential for both type 2 diabetes and CVD. In some nutrition-oriented protocols, there is discussion that a patient should have no carbohydrate whatsoever. Yet, there are many forms of carbohydrate that need to be acknowledged and assessed as there is sufficient evidence that whole-food sources of plant-based carbohydrates, including fruits, legumes, vegetables, and whole grains, may not only be suitable for those with type 2 diabetes and/or CVD but also actually be therapeutic and serve as part of a treatment protocol. Hence, there is no need to vilify the entire class of carbohydrates when instructing a patient.

The role of carbohydrate quantity has been evaluated in several studies, one of which was a meta-analysis by Hu et al.[85] who surveyed the impact of either a low-carbohydrate or low-fat diet on cardiometabolic parameters in 2788 participants from 23 trials. Low-carbohydrate diets were better at lowering total cholesterol, LDL-cholesterol, and triglycerides, and, at the same time, improving HDL-cholesterol, compared with the low-fat diets. These findings are not always consistent, however, as Nordmann et al.[86] did a meta-analysis with five trials consisting of 447 overweight individuals and found that the low-fat diet led to better reductions in total cholesterol and LDL-cholesterol (but not triglycerides or HDL-cholesterol). Another meta-analysis published by Santos et al.[87] found similar mixed results with the low-carbohydrate diet lowering systolic and diastolic blood pressure, plasma triglycerides, and raising HDL-cholesterol, but there was no significant change in the primary CVD marker of LDL-cholesterol. In a review by Jung and Choi,[88] high-carbohydrate diets were found to be comparable with low-carbohydrate diets on metabolic parameters in patients with type 2 diabetes. Indeed, as explained previously, the discrepancies within these studies may be due to the quality of carbohydrate that was consumed, the glycemic index, glycemic load, and even the phytochemicals the food contains.

GLYCEMIC INDEX AND GLYCEMIC LOAD

One of the most popularized concepts within carbohydrates is that of the glycemic index. Glycemic index (GI) refers to the ability of a standardized amount of carbohydrate to alter blood glucose levels, whereas glycemic load (GL) takes the GI into account with the total amount of food consumed. Foods that are high in GI/GL are thought to lead to greater glucose levels in the blood and, consequently, a greater need for insulin, which is undesirable over decades of chronic consumption. A review of 73 scientific articles published between 2006 and 2018 on glycemic index, glycemic load, diabetes, CVD, body weight, satiety, and obesity resulted in the finding that there is an equivocal relationship between GI/GL and disease outcome.[89] Although this is an important concept to consider, it may be that there are several variables that can determine an individual's glycemic response at each feeding.[90] GI/GL may not be as predetermined as originally thought, based on newer research involving the microbiome.

Although there may be other factors to consider, there are, however, studies that would suggest increased risk of CVD with higher GI/GL. One of the more significant and recent studies was a meta-analysis by Ma et al.,[91] in which 14 studies with a total of 229,213 participants were analyzed. They reported that women were more at risk than men. Similar to what was identified by Ma et al.,[91] Dong et al.[92] assessed eight prospective studies with the sum of 220,050 subjects and found not only that dietary GI and GL were responsible for an increased risk for CHD but that women had a greater risk of 69%.

Although there could be several mechanisms as to why GI and GL could potentially be associated with cardiometabolic indications, one of the proposed routes is through inflammation. A low-GI diet has been shown to favorably reduce CRP.[93,94] The FUNGENUT study reported that two types of carbohydrate-containing meals both equal in caloric load had varying effects in individuals with metabolic syndrome. The rye pasta (low GI) group had lesser upregulation of genes related to inflammation, stress, and immunity after 12 weeks compared with the group eating the high-GI oat-wheat-potato meal.[95] This breakthrough study indicates the impact of glycemic index and specific carbohydrate types on gene expression within 12 weeks of consumption.

FIBER

Fiber is one of the constituents of carbohydrate-containing foods that can help in reducing the release of dietary glucose into the systemic circulation, thereby beneficially altering the GI of a food or meal. It may explain, to some extent, why high-carbohydrate diets may be beneficial in some studies investigating cardiometabolic health as discussed earlier. High-fiber foods tend to be plant based and include fruits, legumes, vegetables, and whole grains, all of which, as discussed, have favorable effects on cardiometabolic health, such as reducing body weight, blood lipids, blood glucose, blood pressure, and inflammatory cytokines.[96-98]

There have been studies that have attempted to distinguish the effects of different fiber types on cardiometabolic risk. In general, there is a preponderance of studies that suggest that there is an inverse association between dietary fiber intake and CVD risk, especially for cereal fiber, which outperforms fruit or vegetable fiber.[96] Soluble fiber, from sources such as fruits, vegetables, whole grains, guar gum, konjac, pectin, and psyllium, most likely owing to its adsorbent characteristics, is therapeutic for cardiometabolic outcomes, such as lowering systolic and diastolic blood pressure.[99] Yet, there are some indications that high-fiber foods may be beneficial not just for their fiber content but also for some of the other constituents, such as the phytochemicals, caffeic acid, p-coumaric acid and ferulic acid, and secoisolariciresinol diglucoside.[100-102]

Recommendations for fiber intake are 14 g per 1000 kcal consumed as per the Dietary Guidelines for Americans 2015-2020, equating to roughly 28 and 35 g for women and men, respectively.[103]

SWEETENERS

There is consistent alignment among the breadth of nutrition research findings that daily high intake of added sugars, such as sucrose, fructose, high-fructose corn syrup, and the overwhelming intake of high-calorie, nonnutritious sugar-sweetened beverages are detrimental to cardiometabolic health.[104] Added sugar intake displaces nutrient-dense foods and increases the risk chronic diseases such as diabetes and CVD through multiple mechanisms, including metabolic dysfunction, obesity, immune dysregulation, dyslipidemia, inflammation, and oxidative stress.[105,106] As a result, opinion-leading organizations[6] such as the American Heart Association have suggested reductions in added sugar intake.[107]

Dietary fructose is controversial. When it is included in fruit sources, it does not seem to have the same consequences as when it is part of high-fructose corn syrup (HFCS), most likely because of the beneficial additional components in fruit and the absence of healthy compounds in processed foods containing HFCS.[108] The amount ingested may also need to be considered, as there appears to be a threshold at which fructose (according to the meta-analysis by Livesey and Taylor,[109] ≤90 g daily for acceptable levels of hemoglobin A1C; <50 g daily for fasting triglycerides; ≤100 g daily for body weight) may lose its effectiveness and, instead, be implicated in metabolic derangement.[109,110] Mechanistically, excessive dietary fructose can be concerning for cardiometabolic risk because of its ability to increase triglycerides and uric acid.[105] This is a case where investigating a patient's single nucleotide polymorphisms to determine their propensity to metabolize fructose might be warranted (eg, as in cases of hereditary fructose intolerance).[111]

When it comes to HFCS, sugar-sweetened beverages (SSBs) are thought to be implicated in metabolic health. Indeed, there are studies that indicate a relationship between SSBs and hypertension.[112-114] Participants in the Framingham Heart Study cohort[114] who drank one or more SSBs daily had a higher incidence of hypertension, hypertriglyceridemia, and low HDL-cholesterol. Specific patient populations might be more at risk as high intakes of sugars (fructose, glucose, sucrose) are associated with more pronounced effects in men than in women, those who eat a low-fiber diet, and those who are sedentary, are overweight, or already have metabolic syndrome.[115-118]

Regarding artificial or nonnutritive sweeteners, there are limited data to suggest that they may cause metabolic dysfunction, possibly through nutrient signaling[119] and/or via changes they may create in the gastrointestinal tract, particularly through the gut microbiome.[120] Overall, it would seem prudent to avoid artificial sweeteners entirely because of their negative effects on the microbiome, decreased satiety signals, alterations in glucose homeostasis, and overall increase in calorie intake and weight gain.[121]

Dietary Fats and Oils

Among the three classes of macronutrients, dietary fats and oils have been most scrutinized for their implication in CVD risk and, to some degree, cardiometabolic dysfunction. The same principle mentioned in the section on carbohydrates would apply here: that the universal guideline of quality and quantity needs to be considered. As Harvard epidemiologist Walter Willett[122] suggested, the amount of total fat in the diet is likely not as important as the diet itself. Along similar lines, there is complexity within the different fatty acids, including a variety of carbon chain lengths, single or double bonds, and configuration (cis- and trans-).

For the most part, dietary fat provides a substantial source of energy (9 kcal/g), and fatty acids comprise the bilayer membrane of the cell, which implies that they can be responsible for the activity of receptor sites and cell signaling cascades that could ultimately lead to inflammation, insulin resistance, and stress response intracellularly.[123]

POLYUNSATURATED FATS: THE ESSENTIAL OMEGA-3 AND OMEGA-6 FATTY ACIDS

Polyunsaturated fatty acids (PUFAs) have two or more carbon-carbon double bonds and are often found in liquid fats and oils. Overall, diets containing PUFAs translate to CVD risk reduction[124]: a 5% increase in caloric energy has resulted in a 10% CVD risk reduction.[125] Substituting saturated fat with PUFAs has been shown to lead to favorable effects compared with monounsaturated fats and carbohydrate.[122] Specifically, when replacing dietary saturated fat with PUFAs, compensatory decreases in total, LDL-, and HDL-cholesterol have been documented.[126,127]

Within this category of PUFAs, there are two main fatty acid families to consider as it relates to inflammatory-induced chronic diseases such as diabetes and CVD: omega-6 and omega-3 fatty acids. Omega-6 fats tend to be found in nuts, seeds, whole grains, and vegetable oils, whereas fish, seafood, nuts, seeds, and leafy vegetables are good sources of omega-3 fatty acids.

Essential fatty acids are specific fatty acids that are not made endogenously and, therefore, must be taken in the diet for system-wide regulation of cell membrane fluidity, cell receptors, and processes such as inflammation via prostaglandin synthesis. An imbalance in the ratio of the essential omega-6 to the omega-3 fatty acids is one of the underlying mechanisms associated with dysregulation of inflammation, the foundation of both CVD and diabetes.[128] A patient's essential fatty acid status can readily be determined from a simple dried blood spot test or from a blood sample. Established percentages are defined for each fatty acid measured, often 64 total; however, only a select few of them are in the essential fatty acid category. Research by William Harris[129] has demonstrated that levels of omega-3 fatty acids (specifically the sum of eicosapentaenoic acid [EPA] and docosahexaenoic acid [DHA]) at 8% of the total amount are consistent with lower rates of CVD. Levels below 4% are associated with increased CVD.

Larsson et al.[130] studied 34,670 Swedish women over a mean of 10.4 years in a prospective study and reported an inverse relationship between dietary omega-3 PUFA intake and risk of stroke. Furthermore, a more recent and larger analysis[131] of omega-3 intake (18 randomized controlled trials [RCTs] with a cumulative 93,000 subjects in addition to 16 prospective cohort studies comprising 732,000 participants) from foods or supplements revealed a nonstatistically significant 6% reduction in CHD risk with EPA and DHA. However, subgroup analyses of high-risk populations such as in those with elevated triglycerides and LDL-cholesterol had a statistically significant CHD risk reduction (14%-16%).

The cumulative benefits of omega-3 fatty acids for cardiovascular health include a number of effects[1]: a decrease in MI and coronary heart disease with concomitant use of statins, reduction in stent restenosis, post-MI mortality, coronary artery bypass graft, plaque formation, coronary artery calcification, atherosclerosis, and improve blood lipids, glucose, blood pressure, and insulin resistance.

Although the ratio of omega-6 to omega-3 fatty acids and, arguably, the omega-3 index, may be important for CVD risk reduction, it is difficult to translate these concepts into clinical application unless specific amounts of fatty acids are known for each food consumed (and in some cases, omega-3 supplements are used for this reason). Therefore, it is more plausible to focus on whole foods that are beneficial for the features of cardiometabolic health. At the time of writing, the American Heart Association recommends to consumers via its website to eat fish (particularly fatty fish) at least two times (two servings, each at 3.5 ounces as a cooked portion) per week.[132] Other recommendations have been made, including those from Lavie et al.,[133] in which EPA and DHA are suggested to be at least 800 to 1000 mg/d for those with known heart conditions. Although it is difficult to know the exact amount required for each individual, it would seem that assessing blood levels of the distinct fatty acids and altering the diet accordingly would be the first step, possibly followed by supplementation.

If a dietary supplement is to be used, the author prefers a balanced formulation of alpha linolenic acid (ALA), EPA, DHA, gamma linolenic acid (GLA), together with fat-soluble antioxidants such as tocopherols to prevent lipid peroxidation.[134] The matter of dietary supplementation remains an area of much debate owing to conflicting results for either the primary[133] or secondary prevention of CVD.[135] Mixed results could be due to several potential variables including the dose, quality of the supplement, quality of the diet, and even one's SNPs.

MONOUNSATURATED FATS

Monounsaturated fatty acid (MUFA)-rich diets, particularly those that tend to include olive oil, have been touted as being cardioprotective in that they reduce LDL-cholesterol without the downside of lowering HDL-cholesterol.[136] Substituting dietary MUFA for saturated fat has been shown to have favorable effects on reducing CHD risk and improving the blood lipid and lipoprotein profile, although not to the same degree as PUFAs.[137] For example, in the Nurses' Health Study (n = 84,628 women) and the Health Professionals Follow-up Study (n = 42,908 men), which involved decades of follow-up,

replacing saturated fat with MUFA was associated with a 15% lower risk of CHD, yet there was a 25% lower risk with PUFA substitution.

A meta-analysis by Jakobsen et al.[138] indicated somewhat unprecedented results a positive correlation between MUFA-rich diets and risk of coronary events (but not with risk of coronary deaths). Because these diets included all sources of MUFA and not just from olive oil, the quality of foods providing the MUFA would need to be further evaluated for greater understanding of the conflicting results. Along similar lines, Baum et al.[139] reported some questionable effects of MUFAs, specifically possible greater enrichment of LDL particles with cholesteryl oleate, an indicator of atherogenicity.[140-142]

Indeed, olive oil is heralded as the healthy source of MUFAs, along with avocadoes. Different types of olive oil have been extensively studied and collectively found to have desirable properties for cardiometabolic health as it is anti-inflammatory, antioxidant, and antithrombotic, particularly those varieties that are high in the phenol content (eg, hydroxytyrosol).[143,144] In fact, the phenol content may account for more of olive oil's therapeutic effect than most realize, as high-phenol olive oil was shown to impact more genes related to inflammatory pathways than the low-phenol variety.[145]

SATURATED FATS

Dietary saturated fats have long been associated with increased incidence of CVD owing to the early published research of Ancel Keys.[146] His research led to public health recommendations to reduce saturated fat and cholesterol intake because of its ability to increase LDL-cholesterol. Since that time, there have been other findings that have come to light, namely, that saturated fat also increases HDL-cholesterol. Thereby, the ratio of LDL-cholesterol to HDL-cholesterol, or even total cholesterol to HDL-cholesterol, both of which are regarded as significant CVD risk markers, would not seem to be impacted.[147]

Moreover, published studies in the past decades have revealed contradictory and inconclusive results,[148] and as a result, there has been confusion in the communication of the health effects of saturated fat to the public. Unfortunately, the broader context of examining the source, carbon length, replacement nutrient, genotype, and even microbiome composition has been largely overlooked within this consumer messaging.

Importantly, much of the effect will depend on what the saturated fat is being replaced with in the diet, or the source of the fat. For example, a higher intake of saturated fat from dairy was associated with a lower CVD risk, but a higher risk was found with intake from meat.[149] In fact, substituting just 2% of the calories from saturated fat derived from meat with saturated fat from dairy resulted in a 25% reduced CVD risk. Fermented dairy foods such as yogurt and cheese have pronounced anti-inflammatory effects that may result in subsequent CVD risk reduction.[150] This difference may be due to the probiotic content. It may also be from the different types of fatty acids contained in the foods. For example, odd-chain saturated fatty acids (SFAs) like 15:0 and 17:0, which are typically found in dairy-based foods, seem to be inversely associated with cardiometabolic risk.[151]

Similar to the complexity of PUFAs and MUFAs, fatty acids have varying effects on lipids, inflammation, thrombosis, and oxidative stress. For example, the long-chain, stearic acid (18:0), has a neutral effect, whereas the medium-chain, lauric acid (12:0), has a significant impact on increasing LDL- and HDL-cholesterol.[152] Furthermore, stearic acid (18:0) can be desaturated to MUFA (18:1n-9) through enzymatic activity by stearoyl-CoA Δ-9-desaturase, which can vary based on genotype.[153,154] Therefore, it is difficult to correlate dietary SFA intake with serum lipid incorporation and, ultimately, unreliable to assess whether dietary SFA intake is the underlying issue or if it is the high SFA content in serum cholesterol esters and erythrocytes.[155]

Additionally, the endogenous saturated fat content can be miscalculated owing to the conversion of carbohydrates to synthesis of palmitic acid (16:0). With less dietary carbohydrate, internally sourced saturated fat can be utilized for energy harvesting.[1] One of the disadvantages of long-chain SFA, however, is that they can enhance the gastrointestinal production of gram-negative bacteria and subsequent production of lipopolysaccharide, an endotoxin that can lead to a cascade of systemic inflammation-immune dysfunction.[156] Clinical dietary interventions to offset the effects of metabolic endotoxemia have been investigated.[157]

Overall, the essential takeaways regarding dietary saturated fat are the following, as modified from Houston et al.[1]:

1. It is best to replace dietary SFA with PUFA, MUFA, omega-6 FA, whole grains, and plant proteins to decrease CHD risk, but replacement with refined carbohydrate increases risk.
2. Note the source of the SFA, as not all sources are equal in their ability to increase CHD risk. Specifically, meat and animal-derived fat impart the greatest risk, yet the aspects of quality (eg, grass fed versus grain fed) have not been thoroughly evaluated.
3. The chain length of the saturated fatty acid is relevant. Available data would suggest that long-chain fatty acids (especially palmitic acid, or 16:0) are most likely associated with CHD risk. Medium-chain saturated fats may be associated with increased risk, whereas short-chain fatty acids, particularly owing to their different absorption route (portal vein versus lymphatic) do not seem to be problematic, although more studies are required for confirmation.
4. In addition to the chain length, the number of carbons, whether odd or even, may be relevant, with odd-number SFA seeming to have less risk than even-numbered SFA.

Coconut Oil

Owing to the increased popularity of coconut-derived products such as coconut oil (along with cocoa butter, coconut milk, and even coconut sugar) in some nutritional arenas, it is worthwhile to evaluate its effects on cardiometabolic health. Virgin coconut oil has a similar fatty acid profile to the copra coconut oil, but it contains slightly more nutrients such as vitamin E and even polyphenols.[158] From a fatty acid perspective, coconut oil is almost entirely SFA (92%), with a predominant concentration of lauric acid (12:0) and myristic acid (14:0). In general, medium-chain SFAs are more rapidly absorbed and oxidized than long-chain SFAs, and while they increase LDL-cholesterol, they also increase HDL-cholesterol to a greater extent.[159] A meta-analysis[160] with 8 clinical trials and 13 observational studies concluded that coconut oil raised total cholesterol and LDL-cholesterol more than PUFA-rich plant oils but to a lesser extent than butter. Cultural dietary patterns that include coconut flesh or coconut water do not appear to result in unfavorable cardiovascular outcomes; however, there are many other variables to consider. Unfortunately, at this time, there is a lack of sufficient data to be able to recommend coconut oil for cardiometabolic conditions.[158]

TRANS FATS

There are two types of trans fats (TFAs): those found naturally in meat and milk products derived from ruminants[161] and those produced through a human-made mechanized process involving hydrogenation or even via the refining of vegetable oils (often referred to as "industrially processed").[162,163] The latter have received much attention for the multitude of detrimental effects on cardiovascular and metabolic health combined, including increasing LDL-cholesterol, the risk of thrombogenesis, inflammation, triglycerides, and Lp(a) lipoprotein, while at the same time decreasing HDL-cholesterol.[164-169]

The clinical translation of these mechanisms is quite pronounced: one meta-analysis by Mozaffarian et al.[170] found that just a 2% increase in energy intake from TFAs was associated with a 23% increase in CHD. These results have led to changes in ingredient labeling in the food manufacturing industry, accompanied by increased consumer awareness of the issue. Studies on the consumption of naturally occurring TFAs are less conclusive. A clinician can measure circulating TFAs in the blood through an extensive fatty acid panel. It can be one way to assess whether the patient is compliant with a low processed-food diet.

Dietary Protein

Compared with dietary carbohydrate or fat, dietary protein often garners much less negative or conflicting attention in the cardiometabolic arena, except when there is discussion about the origin of dietary protein, whether from animal or vegetable sources, or to what extent it may replace other macronutrients. From a cardiometabolic perspective, proteins serve a host of functions as amino acids are integral to the structure of cell membranes that hold receptors to signal cellular action and, ultimately, DNA. Perhaps the most recognized role of protein within this field is through discussion on the precursor peptides that convert into angiotensin-converting enzyme (ACE) inhibitory compounds.

Although the quality of protein remains one of the largest questions, it also continues to be the least well studied. For example, how does what an animal eats impact the tissues and subsequent metabolism by humans? Does it matter if eggs are from free-range chickens or if red meat comes from cows that were grass or grain fed? What about the accumulation of biotoxins in the adipose tissue of animals because of the environmental exposure? How does the inefficient digestion of protein often seen with aging (referred to as hypochlorhydria or achlorhydria) relate to CVD or metabolic risk factors? Those pivotal questions lack strong data and may even be responsible for the conflicting results in the literature. Thus, with this disclaimer in mind, the best in scientific studies at the time of writing will be presented.

PROTEIN SOURCE: ANIMAL VERSUS VEGETABLE

It is difficult to discern in population-based studies whether plant-food consumption is associated with healthier lifestyles overall. There are several studies for various aspects of cardiometabolic health that would denote a slight favoring of plant-based protein over animal protein. One of the earlier and larger studies was on the Nurses' Health Study cohort, from which numerous publications were derived. Hu et al.[171] indicated a positive association between animal food intake (red meat, high-fat dairy products) and the risk of CHD compared with fish, low-fat dairy, and poultry, which all showed a lower risk in over 80,000 women followed over 14 years. Halton et al.[172] went further with this cohort to show that substituting protein (and fat) for dietary carbohydrate was favorable for reducing CHD risk. When lean beef was compared with poultry or fish consumption, a meta-analysis by Maki et al.[173] found no significant differences in total, LDL-, or HDL-cholesterol. As Cordain et al.[174] reported, field studies of hunter-gatherer tribes subsisting primarily (65%) on animal food did not display atherogenic symptomatology, most likely because of their active lifestyle.

When it comes to blood pressure, some observational studies would seem to conclude that there is a general trend toward improvement with plant protein[175-180]; however, there are also studies that would suggest no particular preference between the protein sources.[181,182] Rather than the source of protein, it might be more important to note whether the protein is replacing dietary carbohydrate.[182] Thus, ensuring that the patient is reducing GI/GL and including phytochemical-rich fiber with dietary protein might be an overall effective strategy.

A Note About TMAO

Trimethylamine N-oxide (TMAO) is an organic compound manufactured endogenously from the metabolism of animal-based products that contain choline (eg, red meat, fish, poultry, eggs) by the gut microbiota[183] and subsequent oxidation by hepatic enzymes. TMAO levels increase in blood after ingesting TMAO-rich foods. There is much recent interest in exploring TMAO as a link between gastrointestinal health and cardiometabolic indications.[184]

Wang et al.[185] showed that metabolism of phosphatidylcholine predicted CVD risk.[186] A systematic review and meta-analysis of prospective studies (n = 19,256) indicated that those with elevated concentrations of TMAO precursors (L-carnitine, choline, or betaine) were associated with a 1.3 to 1.4 times higher risk for major adverse CVD events and death compared with those who had low concentrations of these compounds.[183] It remains to be explored how TMAO levels can be modulated through the gut through nutrients, antibiotics, probiotics, prebiotic fibers, and even fecal transplantation.

SOY PROTEIN

One of the main plant-based dietary protein sources is soy. This is an area of great controversy in a variety of dietary discussions. When it comes to cardiometabolic health, there are studies[187] indicating that soy protein intake at 15 to 30 g daily produced favorable impacts in serum lipids (LDL- and HDL-cholesterol, triglycerides) compared with the group not consuming soy. Soy protein was shown to be superior to milk protein for reducing LDL-cholesterol and increasing HDL-cholesterol.[188]

Despite the seeming preponderance of data supporting soy, there has been substantial debate on whether the health claim on soy protein and heart health should be reconsidered owing to some diverse interpretations of the long-standing data, including potential variability in the population subgroups such as women who may or may not be menopausal.[189-191] It might be that the variability in soy products, combined with various genotypes or even hormonal status, could be responsible, at least in part, for the discrepancies, although that idea remains to be explored scientifically.

WHEY PROTEIN

Whey protein has notoriously been recognized for its blood pressure–lowering effects because it contains peptides for ACE inhibition. Long-term intake of several grams of whey protein (upwards of 20 g daily) has been shown to have therapeutic effects in lowering blood pressure[192-196] and may even have other cardiometabolic benefits such as reducing triglycerides, cholesterol, and inflammatory markers.[193,197] The type of whey protein used may play a role in efficacy, with hydrolyzed protein into the ACE-inhibitor peptides being most active.[192-194,198,199] Other preparations have been noted to cause a higher insulin response relative to other proteins.[200,201]

FISH

A preponderance of data supports fish intake for cardiovascular benefit.[202] One to two servings weekly translate into a 36% reduced risk of coronary death and a 17% reduction in total mortality.[170] The concern with fish consumption is the concurrent consumption of methylmercury,[170] which may attenuate the anti-inflammatory effects of the omega-3 fatty acids in the fish through effects such as increasing heart rate,[203] blood pressure,[204,205] and risk for MI.[206] There may be benefits to fish that surpass its omega-3 fatty acid content such as the presence of ACE-inhibitory peptides in bonito,[207] tuna,[208] and sardines.[209] Additionally, it is worthwhile to consider confounding variables related to those who eat fish, such as engaging in other positive health behaviors[210] like physical activity and eating a healthier diet, as well as even genetic factors relating to metabolism and clearance of methylmercury.[211-213] Despite all the factors to consider with fish, it has been suggested that the benefits outweigh the risks.[170]

EGGS

The subject of eggs has been a long-time issue of debate in nutrition, especially as it relates to cardiovascular health and, more recently, type 2 diabetes. The negative reputation around eggs most likely began decades ago when the American Heart Association recommended that dietary cholesterol consumption should be no more than 300 mg/d and that no more than three egg yolks should be consumed per week.[214] Since that time, there has been a gradual evolution of removing cholesterol-based guidelines, owing to subsequent studies showing a weak correlation between dietary cholesterol/egg consumption and CVD risk.[215]

An egg is a nutrient-dense food containing a complete complex of protein, fats, and micronutrients, all of which may be influenced by the constitution and environment of the hen. Generally, a medium-sized egg (50 g) contains 78 kcal, 6.3 g protein, 0.6 g carbohydrate, 5.3 g fat, of which 1.6 g is saturated, with 186 mg cholesterol.[215] A systematic review[216] investigating the relationship between egg intake and the risk for CVD in diabetics utilized six randomized, controlled clinical trials and found that egg consumption did not impact major CVD risk factors. More specifically, 6 to 12 eggs weekly had no effect on total cholesterol, LDL-cholesterol, triglycerides, fasting glucose, insulin, or CRP compared with control groups that had no eggs or less than two eggs weekly. HDL-cholesterol increases were seen in four of the six studies.

Moreover, in a small study with 37 men and women with metabolic syndrome, consuming three whole eggs daily on a carbohydrate-restricted diet compared with an egg substitute resulted in favorable changes in lipids and, in the egg group only, a reduction in the inflammatory marker, plasma tumor necrosis factor-α.[217] In a prospective study[218] of a large cohort of Swedish men (n = 39,610) followed for more than a decade for incident type 2 diabetes, there was no association with egg consumption; however, in an accompanying meta-analysis with 12 studies, it was only the United States–based studies that had a positive association between frequent egg consumption and higher risk of type 2 diabetes. These results may suggest there could be a general dietary pattern to consider when evaluating eggs. There may be an interaction between meat and eggs. A longitudinal study[219] with 55,851 participants of the Adventist Health Study 2 who were followed for 5.3 years showed that all stratifications of meat intake significantly increased the risk of type 2 diabetes compared

with no meat intake. Furthermore, egg intake on its own, as compared with no egg intake, was not associated with type 2 diabetes risk, but within the categories of egg intake, there was a rise in risk as meat intake increased. The converse was not true except for non-meat eaters consuming ≥5 eggs/wk.

In summary, egg intake needs to be personalized to the individual and within the context of a healthy diet, most likely lower in meat.

Foods

In this section, a variety of different foods for cardiometabolic health will be discussed.

Plant Foods

As mentioned previously, plant foods such as fruits, vegetables, whole grains, herbs, spices, nuts, and seeds have well-documented benefits for chronic diseases involving the cardiovascular and metabolic systems. A large component of healthful dietary patterns such as the Mediterranean diet, DASH diet, and vegetarian diets is the inclusion of these therapeutic plant-derived foods, which provide a plethora of important nutrients such as fiber, vitamins, minerals, and thousands of phytochemicals that act on cellular pathways of inflammation, oxidative stress, and insulin signaling.[220,221] They also act to displace less-desirable, highly processed foods. Increased intake of fruits and vegetables is associated with reduced coronary heart disease by 4% to 7% for each additional portion daily, as documented in a meta-analysis of 91,379 men and 129,701 women, respectively.[222] There are also benefits to higher intake in reducing risk of stroke[223] and improving endothelial function in hypertensive subjects.[224]

LEGUMES

Legumes include alfalfa, clover, soybeans, peanuts, pinto, kidney, lima beans, garbanzo beans, black beans, and peas such as split green peas or lentils, to name a few. This category of food is an integral part of the Mediterranean diet, with an average per capita consumption between 8 and 23 g daily.[225] In general, studies overall suggest cardiovascular-protective effects, although the range of benefits may be different depending on the legume. Each legume varies in its carbohydrate (eg, oligosaccharides), fiber, protein, and phytochemical content (eg, phytoestrogens, saponins, phenolic compounds).[225]

Owing to their composition of quality protein and low-glycemic, complex carbohydrates, they are often touted as a food for cardiometabolic health. More data suggest that this recommendation is justified. A prospective assessment of 3349 participants from the PREDIMED study followed for 4.3 years showed that those in the highest quartile of total legume and lentil intake had a lower risk of diabetes compared with the lowest quartile of intake (HR, 0.65; 95% CI, 0.43, 0.96; P-trend = 0.04; and HR, 0.67; 95% CI, 0.46-0.98;

P-trend = 0.05, respectively).[226] A borderline association was observed for chickpeas. The researchers suggested that substituting half a serving daily of legumes for bread, rice, baked potato, or eggs within the context of a Mediterranean diet could lead to a lower risk of diabetes.

WHOLE GRAINS

Like legumes, whole grains provide a substantial amount of nutrients such as insoluble and soluble fiber, vitamins and minerals, and select phytonutrients like ferulic acid that may help with oxidative stress, inflammation, hyperlipidemia, blood pressure, vascular function, and glycemic response.[187] Those consuming three to five servings of whole grains daily were shown to have an ~20% lower risk of CVD compared with those who rarely or never ate whole grains.[227] Adding whole grains to a hypocaloric diet resulted in a significant reduction in CRP and abdominal body fat in obese adults with metabolic syndrome compared with those who ate refined grains.[228] A systematic review and dose-response meta-analysis with 1,041,692 participants reported that, for each 28 g per day intake of whole grain, there was a 9% and 14% lower risk for total and CVD mortality, respectively.[229]

NUTS

Nuts are phytonutrient-rich foods that contribute protein, fiber, vitamins, minerals, tocopherols, and phytosterols. Clinical trials have shown that there are significant cardiovascular[230] and possibly metabolic[231] benefits to the inclusion of nuts in the diet with their abilities to reduce oxidative stress and inflammation and enhance vascular reactivity.[232] A meta-analysis of prospective studies[231] showed a 19% reduction of cardiovascular mortality, 20% to 34% reduction in CHD incidence, and 10% to 11% decrease in stroke. No association was found for risk of type 2 diabetes; however, a decrease of 0.08 to 0.15 mmol/L was noted in three meta-analyses of intervention studies. One concern, particularly for diabetic patients, is whether regular nut consumption increases body weight owing to the high fat content; however, some would argue that this is not a relevant issue.[231,233] Salas-Salvadó et al.[234] found that a Mediterranean diet supplemented with 30 g of nuts daily actually led to a decrease in the incidence of metabolic syndrome, mostly because of reduced visceral adiposity.

HERBS AND SPICES

One of the overlooked staples of the Mediterranean diet is that of the use of herbs and spices, which reduces the need for salt and oil, and at the same time, imparts medicinal benefit.[235] Some of the common herbs and spices belonging to this diet include anise, basil, bay, cardamom, cinnamon, chervil, chilis, chives, cloves, cumin, coriander, dill, fennel, fenugreek, garlic, marjoram, mint, nutmeg, oregano, peppers, rosemary, saffron, sage, tarragon and thyme,[236] and many others. Tsui et al.[236] provide a detailed review of the anti-inflammatory mechanisms by which herbs and spices may act as antiatherogenic agents as shown in vitro and in vivo.

COCOA

Cocoa in the form of a powder and incorporated into dark chocolate may have benefits for cardiovascular health, namely, improvements in flow-mediated dilatation and insulin resistance.[237] Combined data from seven population studies with a cumulative total of 114,009 participants indicated that a higher intake of chocolate was correlated with reducing heart disease, diabetes, and stroke incidence.[238] A systematic review and meta-analysis of RCTs that consisted of 1131 participants found that cocoa flavanol intake ranging from 166 to 2110 mg/d over 2 to 52 weeks significantly improved insulin sensitivity and select lipids and inflammatory markers (triglycerides, HDL-cholesterol, fasting insulin, HOMA, C-reactive protein, and vascular cell adhesion molecule 1).[239]

COFFEE AND TEA

Drinking both black and green teas has been associated with reducing risk of coronary heart disease and stroke by 10% to 20%.[240] Depending on genetics and whether one carries the slow allele of the cytochrome P-450 1A2 gene, caffeine may be beneficial or detrimental for one's cardiometabolic health and could explain why there are mixed results in a variety of studies.[241,242] Those who rapidly metabolize caffeine (estimated to be at 40%-45% of the population)[1,242,243] may even benefit from caffeinated beverages through blood pressure reduction and reduced risk of MI.[241] On the other hand, those who slowly metabolize caffeine could have higher blood pressure from consuming caffeinated coffee, along with other potential symptoms such as aortic stiffness, catecholamines, vascular inflammation, and tachycardia, to name a few.[242-246]

ALCOHOL

There are mixed opinions on the inclusion of alcohol into a cardiometabolic-protective dietary pattern, likely because of the context in which it is used. Of course, it is a well-known feature of the Mediterranean diet, especially deep red wines rich in polyphenols. Overall, there is a cumulative U-shaped relationship between alcohol intake and CHD with the base of the U correlated with the lowest risk of CHD.[247,248] A drink is typically defined as 14 g of ethanol or 0.6 fluid ounces of pure alcohol, equating to 1.5 ounces of hard liquor, a 5-ounce glass of table wine, and a 12-ounce beer. Light to moderate drinking, defined as one drink and two drinks per day for women and men, respectively, is associated with less CHD morbidity and mortality, type 2 diabetes, heart failure, and stroke, most likely due to the ability of alcohol to improve insulin resistance, raise HDL-cholesterol, and quell inflammation and clotting.[1]

A meta-analysis of six cohorts (n = 35,132) with intake analysis over a decade suggests that compared with consistently moderate drinkers (males: 1-168 g ethanol/wk; females: 1-112 g ethanol/wk), inconsistently moderate drinkers had a greater risk of incident CHD.[249] Another meta-analysis[250] examined the effect of alcohol on blood pressure reduction using 36 trials with 2865 participants. The researchers identified that people who drank two or fewer drinks daily did not experience a reduction in blood pressure with a reduction in alcohol, whereas those who drank more than two drinks per day had blood pressure–lowering benefit. The reduction was strongest for those drinking six or more drinks daily when they reduced their intake by 50%.

Phytonutrients

With the primary focus of nutrition research dedicated to macronutrients and micronutrients, the role of more than 25,000 noncaloric phytochemically derived bioactives[251] remains poorly understood with relationship to CVD and metabolic conditions. It has been suggested that they may be mechanistically important because of their anti-inflammatory and antioxidant effects.[252] Classes of phytochemicals include phenolics (eg, phenolic acids, flavonoids, lignans, coumarins, and stilbenes), alkaloids (eg, caffeine, theobromine), N-containing compounds (nitrates), organosulfur compounds (eg, indoles, isothiocyanates), phytosterols (eg, sitosterol, campesterol, stigmasterol, and respective stanols), and carotenoids (ie, several hundred varieties, including beta-carotene, lutein, lycopene, and astaxanthin).[253]

Carotenoids

Carotenoids comprise a family of compounds that impart colorful pigmentation to plants and to animals that eat these plants (eg, shrimp, salmon, krill, egg yolks). Although there are several hundreds of carotenoids, there are only a select few that have been well researched, including alpha-carotene, beta-carotene, lutein, lycopene, astaxanthin, and zeaxanthin. Some of them, like beta-carotene, can convert to vitamin A, yet they are pleiotropic in function. Their mechanisms of interest relating to cardiometabolic health would seem to primarily be their antioxidant and anti-inflammatory potential. Serum hsCRP concentrations were negatively associated with a prudent fruit and vegetable dietary pattern and carotenoid scores.[254] Furthermore, there is an inverse relationship between dietary carotenoids and intima-media thickness of common carotid artery wall.[255]

Using the National Health and Nutrition Examination Survey (NHANES) 2003-2006 dietary data (about 3000 men and women combined), Wang et al.[256] indicated an inverse relationship between LDL-cholesterol and dietary beta-carotene and lutein + zeaxanthin, and with total homocysteine for dietary beta-carotene, lycopene, and total carotenoids. HDL-cholesterol and dietary lutein + zeaxanthin were positively associated. In each case, these effects were mediated by serum carotenoid concentrations.

Of all the carotenoids, perhaps the most well featured for cardiovascular health is that of lycopene. Lycopene is the red pigment found in tomatoes, watermelon, guava, papaya, and pink grapefruit. There are studies[257-259] that would suggest tomatoes and tomato-based products (particularly cooked tomato products such as tomato paste and tomato sauce) may be beneficial for reducing inflammation and cardiovascular and cardiometabolic risk (eg, decreasing lipids, blood pressure, and endothelial dysfunction), likely because of the lycopene content.

Flavonoids

Flavonoids are ubiquitously found in plant foods, especially teas, apples, onions, cocoa, wine, citrus fruits, legumes, and whole grains.[260] Some flavonoids exert their cardioprotective activity through antioxidant function and by reducing platelet aggregation.[261] In a prospective cohort (n = 38,180 men and 60,289 women) followed for 7 years, total dietary flavonoid intake was associated with a lower risk of fatal CVD, particularly for five subclasses: anthocyanidins, flavan-3-ols, flavones, flavonols, and proanthocyanidins. The authors suggested that even relatively small amounts of flavonoid-containing foods may be all that is required for beneficial effect.[262] Finally, mounting evidence suggests that dietary naringenin, a flavonoid found in citrus fruits (eg, bergamot), may help to reduce CVD risk.[263-267]

Clinical Application

There is strong evidence to support using dietary intervention for the prevention and treatment of CVD (and aspects such as dyslipidemia, hypertension) and metabolic dysfunction (oxidative stress, body composition). In general, the goal would be to have overarching guidelines that model the Mediterranean diet with copious amounts of whole, unprocessed, plant foods as a foundation, together with quality fats and oils, including extra-virgin olive oil, and complete proteins such as nuts, seeds, cold-water, low-methylmercury fish, poultry, and lean meats. Foods to exclude or minimize include refined, high-GI carbohydrates and sugars, artificial sweeteners, sugar-sweetened beverages, and industrially produced trans fats. Eggs and (fermented) dairy foods are not associated with poor cardiometabolic outcomes. Insufficient data exist for making any recommendations on coconut oil, gluten-free diets, or soy. Personalization of the diet to the individual is essential for best and consistent outcomes. Identifying genetic polymorphisms will help to assess whether caffeine and/or alcohol may be contraindicated for certain populations.

Summary

- Nutrition and lifestyle are essential first-line therapies for the prevention and treatment of lifestyle-induced chronic diseases such as CVD and type 2 diabetes (Table 4.1).
- A whole-foods, plant-based diet with adequate protein and sufficient levels and ratios of dietary fats is best for most individuals, although there needs to be tailoring to one's genotype, symptoms, functional status, food preferences, environment, and even socioeconomic status.
- Plant-based foods rich in phytonutrients help to reduce the net dietary acid load with increased level of potassium relative to sodium.
- Whole grain intake seems to be compelling for reducing risk of chronic disease. Gluten-free diets may be helpful for some individuals, particularly those with celiac disease; however, a nutrient-dense selection of foods rather than simply replacing carbohydrates with gluten-free counterparts should be considered.

Table 4.1

NUTRITION RECOMMENDATIONS FOR CARDIOMETABOLIC HEALTH

Nutrient/Nutrition	General Recommendations
Preferred dietary patterns	Mediterranean diet, DASH diet, plant-based diet
Cooking method	Slow, low, moist methods; steaming or raw
Carbohydrates	Low glycemic index and glycemic load; high in fiber (14 g per 1000 kcal), little to no added sweeteners, refrain from artificial sweetener use
Fats	Aim for less animal-based fats; avoid all industrially produced trans fats; balanced omega-3 and omega-6 fats from plant-based foods (1:4 ratio); use fatty acid laboratory testing to assess levels and whether dietary supplementation is warranted
Protein	Aim for more plant than animal protein
Animal meat	Avoid processed red meat; aim for leaner cuts; eat together with plant foods whenever possible to reduce potential inflammatory effects
Dairy	Low-fat dairy and fermented dairy products (eg, yogurt, cheeses, kefir) are acceptable, 1-2 servings daily
Eggs	Choose eggs from free-range or pasture-raised chickens; 6-12 weekly
Fish	One to two times weekly of fatty fish with higher omega-3 fatty acid content (eg, wild salmon, herring, sardines, oysters); avoid shark, swordfish, king mackerel, tilefish, albacore tuna owing to high mercury content)
Fruits and vegetables	At a minimum of 5 servings daily; include plant foods from the entire color spectrum for the diversity of phytonutrients
Legumes	One serving daily, ensure variety
Extra-virgin olive oil (EVOO)	10-30 mL (about 2-6 tablespoons) of unrefined, unfiltered EVOO daily
Coconut oil	No recommendation owing to lack of evidence
Nuts	1 ounce (28 g) five times weekly as mixed nuts without additional oil and salt
Whole grains	Up to three servings daily; gluten-free whole grains for those with celiac disease or NCGS
Tea	Up to three cups daily
Alcohol	Evaluate based on regularity of use and context for drinking; 1-2 drinks/d for women, 2-4 drinks/d for men

NCGS, nonceliac gluten sensitivity.

- Animal protein and fat should not be the predominant feature of one's dietary pattern. If animal products are eaten, reduce toxin load by choosing organic, grass-fed varieties when available.
- Eggs and dairy products are not associated with increased risk of either CVD or type 2 diabetes; however, it is important to look at the context of the entire diet.
- Owing to the lack of evidence at this time, coconut oil is not recommended.
- Caffeine and alcohol intake need to be evaluated for the individual based on genetics, liver function tests, and detoxification enzyme status, as well as their lifestyle behaviors around use.

References

1. Houston M, Minich D, Sinatra ST, Kahn JK, Guarneri M. Recent science and clinical application of nutrition to coronary heart disease. *J Am Coll Nutr*. 2018;37(3):169-187. doi:10.1080/07315724.2017.1381053. [Epub 2018 January 9].
2. Badawi A, Klip A, Haddad P, et al. Type 2 diabetes mellitus and inflammation: prospects for biomarkers of risk and nutritional intervention. *Diabetes Metab Syndr Obes Targets Ther*. 2010;3:173-186.
3. Murphy KJ, Parletta N. Implementing a mediterranean-style diet outside the mediterranean region. *Curr Atheroscler Rep*. 2018;20(6):28. doi:10.1007/s11883-018-0732-z.
4. Esposito K, Maiorino MI, Bellastella G, Panagiotakos DB, Giugliano D. Mediterranean diet for type 2 diabetes: cardiometabolic benefits. *Endocrine*. 2017;56(1):27-32. doi:10.1007/s12020-016-1018-2. [Epub 2016 July 9].

5. Jennings A, Berendsen AM, de Groot LCPGM, et al. Mediterranean-style diet improves systolic blood pressure and arterial stiffness in older adults. *Hypertension.* 2019;73(3):578-586. doi:10.1161/HYPERTENSIONAHA.118.12259. [Epub ahead of print].

6. Minich DM, Bland JS. Personalized lifestyle medicine: relevance for nutrition and lifestyle recommendations. *Scientific World J.* 2013;2013:129841. doi:10.1155/2013/129841. Print 2013.

7. Prescott SL, Logan AC. Each meal matters in the exposome: biological and community considerations in fast-food-socioeconomic associations. *Econ Hum Biol.* 2017;27(pt B):328-335. doi:10.1016/j.ehb.2017.09.004. [Epub 2017 September 27].

8. Svetkey LP, Harris EL, Martin E, et al. Modulation of the BP response to diet by genes in the renin-angiotensin system and the adrenergic nervous system. *Am J Hypertens.* 2011;24(2):209-217. doi:10.1038/ajh.2010.223. [Epub 2010 November 18].

9. Yusuf S, Hawken S, Ounpuu S, et al; INTERHEART Study Investigators. Effect of potentially modifiable risk factors associated with myocardial infarction in 52 countries (the INTERHEART study): case-control study. *Lancet.* 2004;364(9438):937-952.

10. Jacobs DR, Tapsell LC. Food synergy: the key to a healthy diet. *Proc Nutr Soc.* 2013:1-7. [Epub ahead of print].

11. Bhupathiraju SN, Tucker KL. Coronary heart disease prevention: nutrients, foods, and dietary patterns. *Clin Chim Acta.* 2011;412(17-18):1493-1514. doi:10.1016/j.cca.2011.04.038. [Epub 2011 May 7].

12. Jacobs DR Jr, Steffen LM. Nutrients, foods, and dietary patterns as exposures in research: a framework for food synergy. *Am J Clin Nutr.* 2003;78(3 suppl):508S-513S. doi:10.1093/ajcn/78.3.508S. Review.

13. Mozaffarian D, Ludwig DS. Dietary guidelines in the 21st century–a time for food. *JAMA.* 2010;304(6):681-682. doi:10.1001/jama.2010.1116.

14. Pallauf K, Giller K, Huebbe P, Rimbach G. Nutrition and healthy ageing: calorie restriction or polyphenol-rich "MediterrAsian" diet? *Oxid Med Cell Longev.* 2013;2013:707421. doi:10.1155/2013/707421.

15. Tierney AC, Zabetakis I. Changing the Irish dietary guidelines to incorporate the principles of the Mediterranean diet: proposing the MedÉire diet. *Public Health Nutr.* 2018:1-7. doi:10.1017/S136898001800246X. [Epub ahead of print].

16. Wirfält E, Drake I, Wallström P. What do review papers conclude about food and dietary patterns? *Food Nutr Res.* 2013;57. doi:10.3402/fnr.v57i0.20523. [Epub 2013 March 4].

17. Olinto MT, Gigante DP, Horta B, Silveira V, Oliveira I, Willett W. Major dietary patterns and cardiovascular risk factors among young Brazilian adults. *Eur J Nutr.* 2012;51(3):281-291. doi:10.1007/s00394-011-0213-4. [Epub 2011 June 17].

18. Sadakane A, Tsutsumi A, Gotoh T, et al. Dietary patterns and levels of blood pressure and serum lipids in a Japanese population. *J Epidemiol.* 2008;18(2):58-67.

19. Paradis AM, Godin G, Pérusse L, Vohl MC. Associations between dietary patterns and obesity phenotypes. *Int J Obes (Lond).* 2009;33(12):1419-1426. doi:10.1038/ijo.2009.179.

20. Fung TT, Willett WC, Stampfer MJ, Manson JE, Hu FB. Dietary patterns and the risk of coronary heart disease in women. *Arch Intern Med.* 2001;161(15):1857-1862.

21. Lockheart MS, Steffen LM, Rebnord HM, et al. Dietary patterns, food groups and myocardial infarction: a case-control study. *Br J Nutr.* 2007;98(2):380-387. [Epub 2007 March 29].

22. Sherzai A, Heim LT, Boothby C, Sherzai AD. Stroke, food groups, and dietary patterns: a systematic review. *Nutr Rev.* 2012;70(8):423-435. doi:10.1111/j.1753-4887.2012.00490.x.

23. Millen BE, Quatromoni PA, Nam BH, O'Horo CE, Polak JF, D'Agostino RB. Dietary patterns and the odds of carotid atherosclerosis in women: the Framingham Nutrition Studies. *Prev Med.* 2002;35(6):540-547.

24. Khazrai YM, Defeudis G, Pozzilli P. Effect of diet on type 2 diabetes mellitus: a review. *Diabetes Metab Res Rev.* 2014;30 (suppl 1):24-33. doi:10.1002/dmrr.2515.

25. https://www.ncbi.nlm.nih.gov/pubmed/?term=%22mediterranean+diet%22. Accessed January 23, 2019.

26. Simopoulos AP. The Mediterranean diets: what is so special about the diet of Greece? The scientific evidence. *J Nutr.* 2001;131(11 suppl):3065S-3073S. doi:10.1093/jn/131.11.3065S.

27. Bach-Faig A, Berry EM, Lairon D, et al. Mediterranean diet pyramid today. Science and cultural updates. *Public Health Nutr.* 2011;14(12A):2274-2284. doi:10.1017/S1368980011002515. Review.

28. Gnagnarella P, Dragà D, Misotti AM, et al. Validation of a short questionnaire to record adherence to the Mediterranean diet: an Italian experience. *Nutr Metab Cardiovasc Dis.* 2018;28(11):1140-1147. doi:10.1016/j.numecd.2018.06.006. [Epub 2018 June 18].

29. Becerra-Tomás N, Blanco Mejía S, Viguiliouk E, et al. Mediterranean diet, cardiovascular disease and mortality in diabetes: a systematic review and meta-analysis of prospective cohort studies and randomized clinical trials. *Crit Rev Food Sci Nutr.* 2019:1-21. doi:10.1080/10408398.2019.1565281. [Epub ahead of print].

30. Godos J, Zappalà G, Bernardini S, Giambini I, Bes-Rastrollo M, Martinez-Gonzalez M. Adherence to the Mediterranean diet is inversely associated with metabolic syndrome occurrence: a meta-analysis of observational studies. *Int J Food Sci Nutr.* 2017;68(2):138-148. doi:10.1080/09637486.2016.1221900. [Epub 2016 August 25].

31. Gardener H, Wright CB, Gu Y, et al. Mediterranean-style diet and risk of ischemic stroke, myocardial infarction, and vascular death: the Northern Manhattan Study. *Am J Clin Nutr.* 2011;94(6):1458-1464. doi:10.3945/ajcn.111.012799. [Epub 2011 November 9].

32. Sofi F, Abbate R, Gensini GF, Casini A. Accruing evidence on benefits of adherence to the Mediterranean diet on health: an updated systematic review and meta-analysis. *Am J Clin Nutr.* 2010;92(5):1189-1196. doi:10.3945/ajcn.2010.29673. [Epub 2010 September 1]. Review.

33. Hoevenaar-Blom MP1, Nooyens AC, Kromhout D, et al. Mediterranean style diet and 12-year incidence of cardiovascular diseases: the EPIC-NL cohort study. *PLoS One.* 2012;7(9):e45458. doi:10.1371/journal.pone.0045458. [Epub 2012 September 28].

34. Nordmann AJ, Suter-Zimmermann K, Bucher HC, et al. Meta-analysis comparing Mediterranean to low-fat diets for modification of cardiovascular risk factors. *Am J Med.* 2011;124(9):841-851.e2. doi:10.1016/j.amjmed.2011.04.024.

35. Estruch R, Ros E, Salas-Salvadó J, et al. Primary prevention of cardiovascular disease with a Mediterranean diet. *N Engl J Med.* 2013;368(14):1279-1290. doi:10.1056/NEJMoa1200303. [Epub 2013 February 25]. Erratum in: *N Engl J Med.* 2014;370(9):886. Retraction in: *N Engl J Med.* 2018;378(25):2441-2442. Corrected and republished in: *N Engl J Med.* 2018;378(25):e34.

36. Sacks FM, Obarzanek E, Windhauser MM, et al. Rationale and design of the Dietary Approaches to Stop Hypertension trial (DASH). A multicenter controlled-feeding study of dietary patterns to lower blood pressure. *Ann Epidemiol.* 1995;5(2):108-118.

37. Champagne CM. Dietary interventions on blood pressure: the Dietary Approaches to Stop Hypertension (DASH) trials. *Nutr Rev.* 2006;64(2 pt 2):S53-S56. Review.

38. United States Department of Health and Human Services, National Institutes of Health, National Heart Lung, and Blood Institute. Your Guide Lowering Your Blood Press With DASH. Available at http://www.nhlbi.nih.gov/health/public/heart/hbp/dash. Accessed June 22, 2018.

39. National Heart, Lung, and Blood Institute (NHLBI). *Your Guide to Lowering Your Blood Pressure With DASH.* Washington DC: U.S. Dept. of Health and Human Services, National Institutes of Health, National Heart, Lung, and Blood Institute; 2006.

40. Appel LJ, Moore TJ, Obarzanek E, et al. A clinical trial of the effects of dietary patterns on blood pressure. DASH Collaborative Research Group. *N Engl J Med.* 1997;336(16):1117-1124.

41. Sacks FM, Svetkey LP, Vollmer WM, et al. Effects on blood pressure of reduced dietary sodium and the Dietary Approaches to Stop Hypertension (DASH) diet. DASH-Sodium Collaborative Research Group. *N Engl J Med.* 2001;344(1):3-10.

42. Blumenthal JA, Babyak MA, Hinderliter A, et al. Effects of the DASH diet alone and in combination with exercise and weight loss on blood pressure and cardiovascular biomarkers in men and women with high blood pressure: the ENCORE study. *Arch Intern Med.* 2010;170(2):126-135. doi:10.1001/archinternmed.2009.470.

43. Feng Q, Fan S, Wu Y, et al. Adherence to the dietary approaches to stop hypertension diet and risk of stroke: a meta-analysis of prospective studies. *Medicine (Baltimore)*. 2018;97(38):e12450.

44. Jannasch F, Kröger J, Schulze MB. Dietary patterns and type 2 diabetes: a systematic literature review and meta analysis of prospective studies. *J Nutr*. 2017;147(6).1174-1182. doi:10.3945/jn.116.242552. [Epub 2017 April 19].

45. Appel LJ, Miller ER III, Jee SH, et al. Effect of dietary patterns on serum homocysteine: results of a randomized, controlled feeding study. *Circulation*. 2000;102(8):852-857.

46. Fung TT, Chiuve SE, McCullough ML, Rexrode KM, Logroscino G, Hu FB. Adherence to a DASH-style diet and risk of coronary heart disease and stroke in women. *Arch Intern Med*. 2008;168(7):713-720. doi:10.1001/archinte.168.7.713. Erratum in: *Arch Intern Med*. 2008;168(12):1276.

47. Sun B, Williams JS, Svetkey LP, Kolatkar NS, Conlin PR. Beta2-adrenergic receptor genotype affects the renin-angiotensin-aldosterone system response to the Dietary Approaches to Stop Hypertension (DASH) dietary pattern. *Am J Clin Nutr*. 2010;92(2):444-449. doi:10.3945/ajcn.2009.28924. [Epub 2010 June 2].

48. Kahleova H, Levin S, Barnard ND. Vegetarian dietary patterns and cardiovascular disease. *Prog Cardiovasc Dis*. 2018;61(1):54-61. doi:10.1016/j.pcad.2018.05.002. [Epub 2018 May 22].

49. Ornish D, Brown SE, Scherwitz LW, et al. Can lifestyle changes reverse coronary heart disease? The Lifestyle Heart Trial. *Lancet*. 1990;336(8708):129-133.

50. Ornish D, Scherwitz LW, Billings JH, et al. Intensive lifestyle changes for reversal of coronary heart disease. *JAMA*. 1998;280(23):2001-2007.

51. Song M, Fung TT, Hu FB, et al. Association of animal and plant protein intake with all-cause and cause-specific mortality. *JAMA Intern Med*. 2016;176(10):1453-1463.

52. Ingenbleek Y, McCully KS Vegetarianism produces subclinical malnutrition, hyperhomocysteinemia and atherogenesis. *Nutrition*. 2012;28(2):148-153.

53. Sturgeon C, Fasano A. Zonulin, a regulator of epithelial and endothelial barrier functions, and its involvement in chronic inflammatory diseases. *Tissue Barriers*. 2016;4(4):e1251384.

54. Ciaccio EJ, Lewis SK, Biviano AB, Iyer V, Garan H, Green PH. Cardiovascular involvement in celiac disease. *World J Cardiol*. 2017;9(8):652-666. doi:10.4330/wjc.v9.i8.652.

55. Potter MDE, Brienesse SC, Walker MM, Boyle A, Talley NJ. Effect of the gluten-free diet on cardiovascular risk factors in patients with coeliac disease: a systematic review. *J Gastroenterol Hepatol*. 2018;33(4):781-791. doi:10.1111/jgh.14039. [Epub 2018 February 14].

56. Ciccone A, Gabrieli D, Cardinale R, et al. Metabolic alterations in celiac disease occurring after following a gluten-free diet. *Digestion*. 2018:1-7. doi:10.1159/000495749. [Epub ahead of print].

57. Melini V, Melini F. Gluten-free diet: gaps and needs for a healthier diet. *Nutrients*. 2019;11(1). pii:E170. doi:10.3390/nu11010170.

58. Fontana L. The scientific basis of caloric restriction leading to longer life. *Curr Opin Gastroenterol*. 2009;25(2):144-150. doi:10.1097/MOG.0b013e32831ef1ba. Review.

59. Omodei D, Fontana L. Calorie restriction and prevention of age-associated chronic disease. *FEBS Lett*. 2011;585(11):1537-1542. doi:10.1016/j.febslet.2011.03.015. [Epub 2011 March 12]. Review.

60. Weiss EP, Fontana L. Caloric restriction: powerful protection for the aging heart and vasculature. *Am J Physiol Heart Circ Physiol*. 2011;301(4):H1205-H1219. doi:10.1152/ajpheart.00685.2011. [Epub 2011 August 12].

61. Brown JE, Mosely M, Aldred S. Intermittent fasting: a dietary intervention for prevention of diabetes and cardiovascular disease?. *Br J Diabetes Vasc*. 2013;13(2):68-72.

62. Holloszy JO, Fontana L. Caloric restriction in humans. *Exp Gerontol*. 2007;42(8):709-712. [Epub 2007 March 31]. Review.

63. Varady KA, Hellerstein MK. Alternate-day fasting and chronic disease prevention: a review of human and animal trials. *Am J Clin Nutr*. 2007;86(1):7-13. Review.

64. Varady KA, Hudak CS, Hellerstein MK. Modified alternate-day fasting and cardioprotection: relation to adipose tissue dynamics and dietary fat intake. *Metabolism*. 2009;58(6),803-811. doi:10.1016/j.metabol.2009.01.018.

65. Varady KA, Bhutani S, Klempel MC, et al. Alternate day fasting for weight loss in normal weight and overweight subjects: a randomized controlled trial. *Nutr J*. 2013;12(1):146. doi:10.1186/1475-2891-12-146.

66. Rickman AD, Williamson DA, Martin CK, et al. The CALERIE Study: design and methods of an innovative 25% caloric restriction intervention. *Contemp Clin Trials*. 2011;32(6):874-881. doi:10.1016/j.cct.2011.07.002. [Epub 2011 July 8]. Review.

67. Del Turco S, Basta G. An update on advanced glycation end products and atherosclerosis. *Biofactors*. 2012;38(4):266-274. doi:10.1002/biof. 1018. [Epub ahead of print].

68. Stern DM, Yan SD, Yan SF, Schmidt AM. Receptor for advanced glycation end products (RAGE) and the complications of diabetes. *Ageing Res Rev*. 2002;1(1):1-15.

69. Uribarri J, Woodruff S, Goodman S, et al. Advanced glycation end products in foods and a practical guide to their reduction in the diet. *J Am Diet Assoc*. 2010;110(6):911-916.e12. doi:10.1016/j.jada.2010.03.018.

70. Lin RY, Choudhury RP, Cai W, et al. Dietary glycotoxins promote diabetic atherosclerosis in apolipoprotein E-deficient mice. *Atherosclerosis*. 2003;168(2):213-220.

71. Negrean M, Stirban A, Stratmann B, et al. Effects of low- and high-advanced glycation end product meals on macro- and microvascular endothelial function and oxidative stress in patients with type 2 diabetes mellitus. *Am J Clin Nutr*. 2007;85(5):1236-1243. Erratum in: *Am J Clin Nutr*. 2007;86(4):1256.

72. Birlouez-Aragon I, Saavedra G, Tessier FJ, et al. A diet based on high-heat-treated foods promotes risk factors for diabetes mellitus and cardiovascular diseases. *Am J Clin Nutr*. 2010;91(5): 1220-1226. doi:10.3945/ajcn.2009.28737. [Epub 2010 March 24].

73. Luévano-Contreras C, Garay-Sevilla ME, Wrobel K, Malacara JM, Wrobel K. Dietary advanced glycation end products restriction diminishes inflammation markers and oxidative stress in patients with type 2 diabetes mellitus. *J Clin Biochem Nutr*. 2013;52(1):22-26. doi:10.3164/jcbn.12-40. [Epub 2012 December 6].

74. Goldberg T, Cai W, Peppa M, et al. Advanced glycoxidation end products in commonly consumed foods. *J Am Diet Assoc*. 2004;104(8):1287-1291.

75. Schwalfenberg GK. The alkaline diet: is there evidence that an alkaline pH diet benefits health?. *J Environ Public Health*. 2011;2012:727630.

76. Frassetto L, Morris RC Jr, Sellmeyer DE, Todd K, Sebastian A. Diet, evolution and aging–the pathophysiologic effects of the post-agricultural inversion of the potassium-to-sodium and base-to-chloride ratios in the human diet. *Eur J Nutr*. 2001;40(5):200-213. Review.

77. Remer T, Manz F. Don't forget the acid base status when studying metabolic and clinical effects of dietary potassium depletion. *J Clin Endocrinol Metab*. 2001;86(12):5996-5997.

78. Eaton SB, Konner MJ, Cordain L. Diet-dependent acid load, Paleolithic [corrected] nutrition, and evolutionary health promotion. *Am J Clin Nutr*. 2010;91(2):295-297. doi:10.3945/ajcn.2009.29058. [Epub 2009 December 30].

79. Welch AA, Mulligan A, Bingham SA, Khaw KT. Urine pH is an indicator of dietary acid-base load, fruit and vegetables and meat intakes: results from the European Prospective Investigation into Cancer and Nutrition (EPIC)-Norfolk population study. *Br J Nutr*. 2008;99(6):1335-1343. [Epub 2007 November 28].

80. Murakami K, Sasaki S, Takahashi Y, Uenishi K; Japan Dietetic Students' Study for Nutrition and Biomarkers Group. Association between dietary acid-base load and cardiometabolic risk factors in young Japanese women. *Br J Nutr*. 2008;100(3):642-651. doi:10.1017/S0007114508901288. [Epub 2008 February 18].

81. Zhang L, Curhan GC, Forman JP. Diet-dependent net acid load and risk of incident hypertension in United States women. *Hypertension*. 2009;54(4):751-755.

82. Engberink MF, Bakker SJ, Brink EJ, et al. Dietary acid load and risk of hypertension: the Rotterdam Study. *Am J Clin Nutr.* 2012;95(6):1438-1444. doi:10.3945/ajcn.111.022343. [Epub 2012 May 2].

83. Souto G, Donapetry C, Calviño J, Adeva MM. Metabolic acidosis-induced insulin resistance and cardiovascular risk. *Metab Syndr Relat Disord.* 2011;9(4):247-253. doi:10.1089/met.2010.0108. [Epub 2011 February 25]. Review.

84. Jacobs DR, Tapsell LC. Food synergy: the key to a healthy diet. *Proc Nutr Soc.* 2013;72(2):200-206. doi:10.1017/S0029665112003011. [Epub 2013 January 14].

85. Hu T1, Mills KT, Yao L, et al. Effects of low-carbohydrate diets versus low-fat diets on metabolic risk factors: a meta-analysis of randomized controlled clinical trials. *Am J Epidemiol.* 2012;176(suppl 7):S44-S54. doi:10.1093/aje/kws264.

86. Nordmann AJ, Nordmann A, Briel M, et al. Effects of low-carbohydrate vs low-fat diets on weight loss and cardiovascular risk factors: a meta-analysis of randomized controlled trials. *Arch Intern Med.* 2006;166(3):285-293.

87. Santos FL, Esteves SS, da Costa Pereira A, Yancy WS Jr, Nunes JP. Systematic review and meta-analysis of clinical trials of the effects of low carbohydrate diets on cardiovascular risk factors. *Obes Rev.* 2012;13(11):1048-1066. doi:10.1111/j.1467-789X.2012.01021.x. [Epub 2012 August 21].

88. Jung CH, Choi KM. Impact of high-carbohydrate diet on metabolic parameters in patients with type 2 diabetes. *Nutrients.* 2017;9(4). pii: E322. doi:10.3390/nu9040322.

89. Vega-López S, Venn BJ, Slavin JL. Relevance of the glycemic index and glycemic load for body weight, diabetes, and cardiovascular disease. *Nutrients.* 2018;10(10). pii: E1361. doi:10.3390/nu10101361.

90. Zeevi D, Korem T, Zmora N, et al. Personalized nutrition by prediction of glycemic responses. *Cell.* 2015;163(5):1079-1094. doi:10.1016/j.cell.2015.11.001.

91. Ma XY, Liu JP, Song ZY. Glycemic load, glycemic index and risk of cardiovascular diseases: meta-analyses of prospective studies. *Atherosclerosis.* 2012;223(2):491-496. doi:10.1016/j.atherosclerosis.2012.05.028. [Epub 2012 June 6].

92. Dong JY, Zhang YH, Wang P, Qin LQ. Meta-analysis of dietary glycemic load and glycemic index in relation to risk of coronary heart disease. *Am J Cardiol.* 2012;109(11):1608-1613. doi:10.1016/j.amjcard.2012.01.385. [Epub 2012 March 20].

93. Neuhouser ML, Schwarz Y, Wang C, et al. A low-glycemic load diet reduces serum C-reactive protein and modestly increases adiponectin in overweight and obese adults. *J Nutr.* 2012;142(2):369-374. doi:10.3945/jn.111.149807. [Epub 2011 December 21].

94. Kelly KR, Haus JM, Solomon TP, et al. A low-glycemic index diet and exercise intervention reduces TNF(alpha) in isolated mononuclear cells of older, obese adults. *J Nutr.* 2011;141(6):1089-1094. doi:10.3945/jn.111.139964. [Epub 2011 April 27].

95. Kallio P, Kolehmainen M, Laaksonen DE, et al. Dietary carbohydrate modification induces alterations in gene expression in abdominal subcutaneous adipose tissue in persons with the metabolic syndrome: the FUNGENUT Study. *Am J Clin Nutr.* 2007;85(5):1417-1427.

96. Satija A, Hu FB. Cardiovascular benefits of dietary fiber. *Curr Atheroscler Rep.* 2012;14(6):505-514. doi:10.1007/s11883-012-0275-7.

97. Chuang SC, Vermeulen R, Sharabiani MT, et al. The intake of grain fibers modulates cytokine levels in blood. *Biomarkers.* 2011;16(6):504-510. doi:10.3109/1354750X.2011.599042. [Epub 2011 August 3].

98. Johansson-Persson A, Ulmius M, Cloetens L, Karhu T, Herzig KH, Onning G. A high intake of dietary fiber influences C-reactive protein and fibrinogen, but not glucose and lipid metabolism, in mildly hypercholesterolemic subjects. *Eur J Nutr.* 2013. [Epub ahead of print].

99. Khan K, Jovanovski E, Ho HVT, et al. The effect of viscous soluble fiber on blood pressure: a systematic review and meta-analysis of randomized controlled trials. *Nutr Metab Cardiovasc Dis.* 2018;28(1):3-13. doi:10.1016/j.numecd.2017.09.007. [Epub 2017 October 7].

100. Wang H, Wang J, Qiu C, et al. Comparison of phytochemical profiles and health benefits in fiber and oil flaxseeds (Linum usitatissimum L.). *Food Chem.* 2017;214:227-233. doi:10.1016/j.foodchem.2016.07.075. [Epub 2016 July 11].

101. Zhu Y, Sang S. Phytochemicals in whole grain wheat and their health-promoting effects. *Mol Nutr Food Res.* 2017;61(7). doi:10.1002/mnfr.201600852. [Epub 2017 March 17].

102. Okarter N, Liu RH. Health benefits of whole grain phytochemicals. *Crit Rev Food Sci Nutr.* 2010;50(3):193-208. doi:10.1080/10408390802248734.

103. Chapter 7 Carbohydrates. Dietary Guidelines for Americans 2005. https://health.gov/dietaryguidelines/dga2005/document/html/chapter7.htm. Accessed January 27, 2019.

104. Khan TA, Sievenpiper JL. Controversies about sugars: results from systematic reviews and meta-analyses on obesity, cardiometabolic disease and diabetes. *Eur J Nutr.* 2016;55(suppl 2):25-43.

105. Bray GA. Energy and fructose from beverages sweetened with sugar or high-fructose corn syrup pose a health risk for some people. *Adv Nutr.* 2013;4(2):220-225. doi:10.3945/an.112.002816.

106. Mucci L, Santilli F, Cuccurullo C, Davì G. Cardiovascular risk and dietary sugar intake: is the link so sweet? *Intern Emerg Med.* 2012;7(4):313-322. doi:10.1007/s11739-011-0606-7. [Epub 2011 May 5].

107. Johnson RK, Appel LJ, Brands M, et al; American Heart Association Nutrition Committee of the Council on Nutrition, Physical Activity, and Metabolism and the Council on Epidemiology and Prevention. Dietary sugars intake and cardiovascular health: a scientific statement from the American Heart Association. *Circulation.* 2009;120(11):1011-1020. doi:10.1161/CIRCULATIONAHA.109.192627. [Epub 2009 August 24].

108. Sharma SP, Chung HJ, Kim HJ, Hong ST. Paradoxical effects of fruit on obesity. *Nutrients.* 2016;8(10):633. Published 2016 October 14. doi:10.3390/nu8100633.

109. Livesey G, Taylor R. Fructose consumption and consequences for glycation, plasma triacylglycerol, and body weight: meta-analyses and meta-regression models of intervention studies. *Am J Clin Nutr.* 2008;88(5):1419-1437.

110. Sievenpiper JL, Chiavaroli L, de Souza RJ, et al. 'Catalytic' doses of fructose may benefit glycaemic control without harming cardiometabolic risk factors: a small meta-analysis of randomised controlled feeding trials. *Br J Nutr.* 2012;108(3):418-423. doi:10.1017/S000711451200013X. [Epub 2012 February 21].

111. Debray FG, Damjanovic K, Rosset R, et al. Are heterozygous carriers for hereditary fructose intolerance predisposed to metabolic disturbances when exposed to fructose? *Am J Clin Nutr.* 2018;108(2):292-299. doi:10.1093/ajcn/nqy092.

112. Nguyen S, Choi HK, Lustig RH, Hsu CY. Sugar-sweetened beverages, serum uric acid, and blood pressure in adolescents. *J Pediatr.* 2009;154:807-813.

113. Bremer AA, Auinger P, Byrd RS. Relationship between insulin resistance-associated metabolic parameters and anthropometric measurements with sugar-sweetened beverage intake and physical activity levels in US adolescents: findings from the 1999–2004 National Health and Nutrition Examination Survey. *Arch Pediatr Adolesc Med.* 2009;163:328-335.

114. Dhingra R, Sullivan L, Jacques PF, et al. Soft drink consumption and risk of developing cardiometabolic risk factors and the metabolic syndrome in middle-aged adults in the community. *Circulation.* 2007;116(5):480-488.

115. Lê KA, Tappy L. Metabolic effects of fructose. *Curr Opin Clin Nutr Metab Care.* 2006;9(4):469-475. Review.

116. Stanhope KL, Schwarz JM, Keim NL, et al. Consuming fructose-sweetened, not glucose-sweetened, beverages increases visceral adiposity and lipids and decreases insulin sensitivity in overweight/obese humans. *J Clin Invest.* 2009;119:1322-1334.

117. Fried SK, Rao SP. Sugars, hypertriglyceridemia, and cardiovascular disease. *Am J Clin Nutr.* 2003;78(4):873S-880S. Review.

118. Bantle JP, Raatz SK, Thomas W, Georgopoulos A. Effects of dietary fructose of plasma lipids in healthy subjects. *Am J Clin Nutr.* 2000;72:1128-1134.

119. Swithers SE. Not so sweet revenge: unanticipated consequences of high-intensity sweeteners. *Behav Anal.* 2015;38(1):1-17. doi:10.1007/s40614-015-0028-3. eCollection 2015 May.

120. Rodriguez-Palacios A, Harding A, Menghini P, et al. The artificial sweetener splenda promotes gut proteobacteria, dysbiosis, and myeloperoxidase reactivity in Crohn's disease-like ileitis. *Inflamm Bowel Dis*. 2018;24(5):1005-1020. doi:10.1093/ibd/izy060.

121. Pearlman M, Obert J, Casey L. The association between artificial sweeteners and obesity *Curr Gastroenterol Rep*. 2017;19(12):64. doi:10.1007/s11894-017-0602-9.

122. Willett WC. Dietary fats and coronary heart disease. *J Intern Med*. 2012;272(1):13-24. doi:10.1111/j.1365-2796.2012.02553.x.

123. Howitz KT, Sinclair DA. Xenohormesis: sensing the chemical cues of other species. *Cell*. 2008;133(3):387-391. doi:10.1016/j.cell.2008.04.019.

124. Anton SD, Heekin K, Simkins C, Acosta A. Differential effects of adulterated versus unadulterated forms of linoleic acid on cardiovascular health. *J Integr Med*. 2013;11(1):2-10. doi:10.3736/jintegrmed2013002.

125. Mozaffarian D, Micha R, Wallace S. Effects on coronary heart disease of increasing polyunsaturated fat in place of saturated fat: a systematic review and meta-analysis of randomized controlled trials. *PLoS Med*. 2010;7(3):e1000252.

126. Mensink RP, Katan MB. Effect of dietary fatty acids on serum lipids and lipoproteins. A meta-analysis of 27 trials. *Arterioscler Thromb*. 1992;12(8):911-919.

127. Siri-Tarino PW, Sun Q, Hu FB, Krauss RM. Meta-analysis of prospective cohort studies evaluating the association of saturated fat with cardiovascular disease. *Am J Clin Nutr*. 2010;91(3):535-546. doi:10.3945/ajcn.2009.27725. [Epub 2010 January 13].

128. Simopoulos AP. Omega-3 fatty acids in health and disease and in growth and development. *Am J Clin Nutr*. 1991;54(3):438-463. Review.

129. Harris WS. Omega-3 fatty acids and cardiovascular disease: a case for omega-3 index as a new risk factor. *Pharmacol Res*. 2007;55(3):217-223.

130. Larsson SC, Virtamo J, Wolk A. Dietary fats and dietary cholesterol and risk of stroke in women. *Atherosclerosis*. 2012;221(1):282-286. doi:10.1016/j.atherosclerosis.2011.12.043. [Epub 2012 January 8].

131. Alexander DD, Miller PE, Van Elswyk ME, Kuratko CN, Bylsma LC. A meta-analysis of randomized controlled trials and prospective cohort studies of eicosapentaenoic and docosahexaenoic long-chain omega-3 fatty acids and coronary heart disease risk. *Mayo Clin Proc*. 2017;92(1):15-29.

132. American Heart Associate. Fish and Omega-3 Fatty Acids. https://www.heart.org/en/healthy-living/healthy-eating/eat-smart/fats/fish-and-omega-3-fatty-acids?uid=1879. Accessed January 27, 2019.

133. Lavie CJ, Milani RV, Mehra MR, Ventura HO. Omega-3 polyunsaturated fatty acids and cardiovascular diseases. *J Am Coll Cardiol*. 2009;54(7):585-594. doi:10.1016/j.jacc.2009.02.084.

134. Houston M. The role of nutrition and nutraceutical supplements in the treatment of hypertension. *World J Cardiol*. 2014;6(2):38-66.

135. Kwak SM, Myung SK, Lee YJ, Seo HG; Korean Meta-analysis Study Group. Efficacy of omega-3 fatty acid supplements (eicosapentaenoic acid and docosahexaenoic acid) in the secondary prevention of cardiovascular disease: a meta-analysis of randomized, double-blind, placebo-controlled trials. *Arch Intern Med*. 2012;172(9):686-694. doi:10.1001/archinternmed.2012.262.

136. Mattson FH, Grundy SM. Comparison of effects of dietary saturated, monounsaturated, and polyunsaturated fatty acids on plasma lipids and lipoproteins in man. *J Lipid Res*. 1985;26(2):194-202.

137. Zock PL, Blom WA, Nettleton JA, Hornstra G. Progressing insights into the role of dietary fats in the prevention of cardiovascular disease. *Curr Cardiol Rep*. 2016;18(11):111.

138. Jakobsen MU, O'Reilly EJ, Heitmann BL, et al. Major types of dietary fat and risk of coronary heart disease: a pooled analysis of 11 cohort studies. *Am J Clin Nutr*. 2009;89(5):1425-1432.

139. Baum SJ, Kris-Etherton PM, Willett WC, et al. Fatty acids in cardiovascular health and disease: a comprehensive update. *J Clin Lipidol*. 2012;6(3):216-234. doi:10.1016/j.jacl.2012.04.077. [Epub 2012 April 13].

140. Rudel LL, Parks KS, Sawyer JK. Compared with dietary monounsaturated and saturated fat, polyunsaturated fat protects African green monkeys from coronary artery atherosclerosis. *Arterioscler Thromb Vasc Biol*. 1995;15:2101-2110.

141. Ma J, Folsom AR, Lewis L, Eckfeldt JH. Relation of plasma phospholipid and cholesterol ester fatty acid composition to carotid artery intima-media thickness: the Atherosclerosis Risk in Communities (ARIC) Study. *Am J Clin Nutr*. 1997;65(2):551-559.

142. Degirolamo C, Shelness GS, Rudel LL. Review LDL cholesteryl oleate as a predictor for atherosclerosis: evidence from human and animal studies on dietary fat. *J Lipid Res*. 2009;50 suppl:S434-S439.

143. Loued S, Berrougui H, Componova P, Ikhlef S, Helal O, Khalil A. Extra-virgin olive oil consumption reduces the age-related decrease in HDL and paraoxonase 1 anti-inflammatory activities. *Br J Nutr*. 2013:1-13. [Epub ahead of print].

144. Martín-Peláez S, Covas MI, Fitó M, Kušar A, Pravst I. Health effects of olive oil polyphenols: recent advances and possibilities for the use of health claims. *Mol Nutr Food Res*. 2013. doi:10.1002/mnfr.201200421. [Epub ahead of print].

145. Camargo A, Ruano J, Fernandez JM, et al. Gene expression changes in mononuclear cells in patients with metabolic syndrome after acute intake of phenol-rich virgin olive oil. *BMC Genomics*. 2010;11:253. doi:10.1186/1471-2164-11-253.

146. Keys A, Anderson JT, Grande F. Serum cholesterol response to changes in the diet: IV. Particular saturated fatty acids in the diet. *Metabolism*. 1965;14(7):776-787.

147. Siri-Tarino PW, Sun Q, Hu FB, Krauss RM. Saturated fatty acids and risk of coronary heart disease: modulation by replacement nutrients. *Curr Atheroscler Rep*. 2010;12(6):384-390. doi:10.1007/s11883-010-0131-6.

148. Hoenselaar R. Saturated fat and cardiovascular disease: the discrepancy between the scientific literature and dietary advice. *Nutrition*. 2012;28(2):118-123. doi:10.1016/j.nut.2011.08.017.

149. de Oliveira Otto MC, Mozaffarian D, Kromhout D, et al. Dietary intake of saturated fat by food source and incident cardiovascular disease: the Multi-Ethnic Study of Atherosclerosis. *Am J Clin Nutr*. 2012;96(2):397-404.

150. Tapsell LC. Fermented dairy food and CVD risk. *Br J Nutr*. 2015;113(suppl 2):S131-S135. doi:10.1017/S0007114514002359.

151. Yu E, Hu FB. Dairy products, dairy fatty acids, and the prevention of cardiometabolic disease: a review of recent evidence. *Curr Atheroscler Rep*. 2018;20(5):24. doi:10.1007/s11883-018-0724-z.

152. Mensink RP, Zock PL, Kester AD, Katan MB. Effects of dietary fatty acids and carbohydrates on the ratio of serum total to HDL cholesterol and on serum lipids and apolipoproteins: a meta-analysis of 60 controlled trials. *Am J Clin Nutr*. 2003;77(5):1146-1155.

153. DiNicolantonio JJ, Lucan SC, O'Keefe JH. The evidence for saturated fat and for sugar related to coronary heart disease. *Prog Cardiovasc Dis*. 2016;58(5):464-472.

154. Vessby B, Gustafsson IB, Tengblad S, Berglund L. Indices of fatty acid desaturase activity in healthy human subjects: effects of different types of dietary fat. *Br J Nutr*. 2013;110(5):871-879. doi:10.1017/S0007114512005934. [Epub 2013 February 18].

155. Ruiz-Núñez B, Kuipers RS, Luxwolda MF, et al. Saturated fatty acid (SFA) status and SFA intake exhibit different relations with serum total cholesterol and lipoprotein cholesterol: a mechanistic explanation centered around lifestyle-induced low-grade inflammation. *J Nutr Biochem*. 2014;25(3):304-312.

156. Netto Candido TL, Bressan J, Alfenas RCG. Dysbiosis and metabolic endotoxemia induced by high-fat diet. *Nutr Hosp*. 2018;35(6):1432-1440. doi:10.20960/nh.1792.

157. Brown BI. Nutritional management of metabolic endotoxemia: a clinical review. *Altern Ther Health Med*. 2017;23(4):42-54.

158. Wallace TC. Health effects of coconut oil-a narrative review of current evidence. *J Am Coll Nutr*. 2018:1-11. doi:10.1080/07315724.2018.1497562. [Epub ahead of print].

159. DeLany JP, Windhauser MM, Champagne CM, Bray GA. Differential oxidation of individual dietary fatty acids in humans. *Am J Clin Nutr*. 2000;72(4):905-911.

160. Eyres L, Eyres MF, Chisholm A, Brown RC. Coconut oil consumption and cardiovascular risk factors in humans. *Nutr Rev*. 2016;74(4):267-280. doi:10.1093/nutrit/nuw002. [Epub 2016 March 5].

161. Bauman DE, Mather IH, Wall RJ, Lock AL. Major advances associated with the biosynthesis of milk. *J Dairy Sci*. 2006;89(4):1235-1243.

162. Ledoux M, Juanéda P, Sébédio JL. Trans fatty acids: definition and occurrence in foods. *Eur J Lipid Sci Technol.* 2007;109(9):891-900.

163. Tasan M, Demirci M. Trans FA in sunflower oil at different steps of refining. *J Am Oil Chem Soc.* 2003;80(8):825-828.

164. Lopez-Garcia E, Schulze MB, Meigs JB, et al. Consumption of trans fatty acids is related to plasma biomarkers of inflammation and endothelial dysfunction. *J Nutr.* 2005;135(3):562-566.

165. van de Vijver LP, Kardinaal AF, Couet C, et al. Association between trans fatty acid intake and cardiovascular risk factors in Europe: the TRANSFAIR study. *Eur J Clin Nutr.* 2000;54(2):126-135.

166. Sun Q, Ma J, Campos H, et al. A prospective study of trans fatty acids in erythrocytes and risk of coronary heart disease. *Circulation.* 2007;115(14):1858-1865.

167. Estadella D, da Penha Oller do Nascimento CM, Oyama LM, Ribeiro EB, Dâmaso AR, de Piano A. Lipotoxicity: effects of dietary saturated and trans fatty acids. *Mediators Inflamm.* 2013;2013:137579. doi:10.1155/2013/137579. [Epub 2013 January 31].

168. Wymann MP, Schneiter R. Lipid signalling in disease. *Nat Rev Mol Cell Biol.* 2008;9(2):162-176. doi:10.1038/nrm2335.

169. do Nascimento CMO, Ribeiro EB, Oyama LM. Metabolism and secretory function of white adipose tissue: effect of dietary fat. *Anais da Academia Brasileira de Ciencias.* 2009l;81(3):453-466.

170. Mozaffarian D, Rimm EB. Fish intake, contaminants, and human health: evaluating the risks and the benefits. *JAMA.* 2006;296(15):1885-1899.

171. Hu FB, Stampfer MJ, Manson JE, et al. Dietary protein and risk of ischemic heart disease in women. *Am J Clin Nutr.* 1999;70(2):221-227.

172. Halton TL, Willett WC, Liu S, et al. Low-carbohydrate-diet score and the risk of coronary heart disease in women. *N Engl J Med.* 2006;355(19):1991-2002.

173. Maki KC, Van Elswyk ME, Alexander DD, Rains TM, Sohn EL, McNeill S. A meta-analysis of randomized controlled trials that compare the lipid effects of beef versus poultry and/or fish consumption. *J Clin Lipidol.* 2012;6(4):352-361. doi:10.1016/j.jacl.2012.01.001. [Epub 2012 January 21].

174. Cordain L, Eaton SB, Miller JB, Mann N, Hill K. The paradoxical nature of hunter-gatherer diets: meat-based, yet non-atherogenic. *Eur J Clin Nutr.* 2002;56(suppl 1):S42-S52.

175. Stamler J, Liu K, Ruth KJ, Pryer J, Greenland P. Eight-year blood pressure change in middle-aged men: relationship to multiple nutrients. *Hypertension.* 2002;39(5):1000-1006.

176. Alonso A, Beunza JJ, Bes-Rastrollo M, Pajares RM, Martínez-González MA. Vegetable protein and fiber from cereal are inversely associated with the risk of hypertension in a Spanish cohort. *Arch Med Res.* 2006;37(6):778-786.

177. Elliott P, Stamler J, Dyer AR, et al. Association between protein intake and blood pressure: the INTERMAP Study. *Arch Intern Med.* 2006;166(1):79-87.

178. Wang YF, Yancy WS Jr, Yu D, Champagne C, Appel LJ, Lin PH. The relationship between dietary protein intake and blood pressure: results from the PREMIER study. *J Hum Hypertens.* 2008;22(11):745-754.

179. Umesawa M, Sato S, Imano H, et al. Relations between protein intake and blood pressure in Japanese men and women: the Circulatory Risk in Communities Study (CIRCS). *Am J Clin Nutr.* 2009;90(2):377-384.

180. Altorf-van der Kuil W, Engberink MF, van Rooij FJ, et al. Dietary protein and risk of hypertension in a Dutch older population: the Rotterdam study. *J Hypertens.* 2010;28(12):2394-2400.

181. Rebholz CM, Friedman EE, Powers LJ, Arroyave WD, He J, Kelly TN. Dietary protein intake and blood pressure: a meta-analysis of randomized controlled trials. *Am J Epidemiol.* 2012;176(suppl 7):S27-S43. doi:10.1093/aje/kws245.

182. He J, Wofford MR, Reynolds K, et al. Effect of dietary protein supplementation on blood pressure: a randomized, controlled trial. *Circulation.* 2011;124(5):589-595. doi:10.1161/CIRCULATIONAHA.110.009159. [Epub 2011 July 18].

183. Heianza Y, Ma W, Manson JE, Rexrode KM, Qi L. Gut microbiota metabolites and risk of major adverse cardiovascular disease events and death: a systematic review and meta-analysis of prospective studies. *J Am Heart Assoc.* 2017;6(7):e004947. Published 2017 June 29. doi:10.1161/JAHA.116.004947.

184. Leustean AM, Ciocoiu M, Sava A, et al. Implications of the intestinal microbiota in diagnosing the progression of diabetes and the presence of cardiovascular complications. *J Diabetes Res.* 2018;2018:5205126. Published 2018 November 12. doi:10.1155/2018/5205126.

185. Wang Z, Klipfell E, Bennett BJ, et al. Gut flora metabolism of phosphatidylcholine promotes cardiovascular disease. *Nature.* 2011;472:57-63.

186. Erickson ML, Malin SK, Wang Z, Brown JM, Hazen SL, Kirwan JP. Effects of Lifestyle intervention on plasma trimethylamine N-oxide in obese adults. *Nutrients.* 2019;11:179.

187. Anderson JW, Bush HM. Soy protein effects on serum lipoproteins: a quality assessment and meta-analysis of randomized, controlled studies. *J Am Coll Nutr.* 2011;30(2):79-91.

188. Wofford MR, Rebholz CM, Reynolds K, et al. Effect of soy and milk protein supplementation on serum lipid levels: a randomized controlled trial. *Eur J Clin Nutr.* 2012;66(4):419-425. doi:10.1038/ejcn.2011.168. [Epub 2011 September 28].

189. Campbell SC, Khalil DA, Payton ME, Arjmandi BH. One-year soy protein supplementation does not improve lipid profile in postmenopausal women. *Menopause.* 2010;17(3):587-593. doi:10.1097/gme.0b013e3181cb85d3.

190. Roughead ZK, Hunt JR, Johnson LK, Badger TM, Lykken GI. Controlled substitution of soy protein for meat protein: effects on calcium retention, bone, and cardiovascular health indices in postmenopausal women. *J Clin Endocrinol Metab.* 2005;90(1):181-189. [Epub 2004 October 13].

191. Hodis HN, Mack WJ, Kono N, et al. Isoflavone soy protein supplementation and atherosclerosis progression in healthy postmenopausal women: a randomized controlled trial. *Stroke.* 2011;42(11):3168-3175. doi:10.1161/STROKEAHA.111.620831. [Epub 2011 September 8].

192. FitzGerald RJ, Murray BA, Walsh DJ. Hypotensive peptides from milk proteins. *J Nutr.* 2004;134(4):980S-988S.

193. Pins JJ, Keenan JM. Effects of whey peptides on cardiovascular disease risk factors. *J Clin Hypertens.* 2006;8(11):775-782.

194. Aihara K, Kajimoto O, Takahashi R, Nakamura Y. Effect of powdered fermented milk with Lactobacillus helveticus on subjects with high-normal blood pressure or mild hypertension. *J Am Coll Nutr.* 2005;24(4):257-265.

195. Sousa GT, Lira FS, Rosa JC, et al. Dietary whey protein lessens several risk factors for metabolic diseases: a review. *Lipids Health Dis.* 2012;11:67. doi:10.1186/1476-511X-11-67.

196. Pal S, Ellis V. Acute effects of whey protein isolate on blood pressure, vascular function and inflammatory markers in overweight postmenopausal women. *Br J Nutr.* 2011;105(10):1512-1519. doi:10.1017/S0007114510005313. [Epub 2011 January 28].

197. de Aguilar-Nascimento JE, Prado Silveira BR, Dock-Nascimento DB. Early enteral nutrition with whey protein or casein in elderly patients with acute ischemic stroke: a double-blind randomized trial. *Nutrition.* 2011;27(4):440-444.

198. Tavares T, Contreras Mdel M, Amorim M, Pintado M, Recio I, Malcata FX. Novel whey-derived peptides with inhibitory effect against angiotensin-converting enzyme: in vitro effect and stability to gastrointestinal enzymes. *Peptides.* 2011;32(5):1013-1019. doi:10.1016/j.peptides.2011.02.005. [Epub 2011 February 16].

199. Pins J, Keenan J. The antihypertensive effects of a hydrolyzed whey protein supplement. *Cardiovasc Drugs Ther.* 2002;16(suppl):68.

200. Mortensen LS, Holmer-Jensen J, Hartvigsen ML, et al. Effects of different fractions of whey protein on postprandial lipid and hormone responses in type 2 diabetes. *Eur J Clin Nutr.* 2012;66(7):799-805. doi:10.1038/ejcn.2012.48. [Epub 2012 May 16].

201. Esteves de Oliveira FC, Pinheiro Volp AC, Alfenas RC. Impact of different protein sources in the glycemic and insulinemic responses. *Nutr Hosp.* 2011;26(4):669-676. doi:10.1590/S0212-16112011000400002.

202. Park K, Mozaffarian D. Omega-3 fatty acids, mercury, and selenium in fish and the risk of cardiovascular diseases. *Curr Atheroscler Rep.* 2010;12(6):414-422. doi:10.1007/s11883-010-0138-z.

203. Valera B, Dewailly E, Poirier P. Association between methylmercury and cardiovascular risk factors in a native population of Quebec (Canada): a retrospective evaluation. *Environ Res.* 2013;120:102-108. doi:10.1016/j.envres.2012.08.002. [Epub 2012 September 5].

204. Valera B, Dewailly E, Poirier P. Environmental mercury exposure and blood pressure among Nunavik Inuit adults. *Hypertension.* 2009;54(5):981-986. doi:10.1161/HYPERTENSIONAHA.109.135046. [Epub 2009 October 5].

205. Choi AL, Weihe P, Budtz-Jørgensen E, et al. Methylmercury exposure and adverse cardiovascular effects in Faroese whaling men. *Environ Health Perspect.* 2009;117(3):367-372. doi:10.1289/ehp.11608. [Epub 2008 October 16].

206. Roman HA, Walsh TL, Coull BA, et al. Evaluation of the cardiovascular effects of methylmercury exposures: current evidence supports development of a dose-response function for regulatory benefits analysis. *Environ Health Perspect.* 2011;119(5):607-614. doi:10.1289/ehp.1003012. [Epub 2011 January 10].

207. Curtis JM, Dennis D, Waddell DS, MacGillivray T, Ewart HS. Determination of angiotensin-converting enzyme inhibitory peptide Leu-Lys-Pro-Asn-Met (LKPNM) in bonito muscle hydrolysates by LC-MS/MS. *J Agric Food Chem.* 2002;50(14):3919-3925.

208. Qian ZJ, Je JY, Kim SK. Antihypertensive effect of angiotensin i converting enzyme-inhibitory peptide from hydrolysates of Bigeye tuna dark muscle, Thunnus obesus. *J Agric Food Chem.* 2007;55(21):8398-8403. [Epub 2007 September 26].

209. Otani L, Ninomiya T, Murakami M, Osajima K, Kato H, Murakami T. Sardine peptide with angiotensin I-converting enzyme inhibitory activity improves glucose tolerance in stroke-prone spontaneously hypertensive rats. *Biosci Biotechnol Biochem.* 2009;73(10):2203-2209. [Epub 2009 October 7].

210. Wennberg M, Tornevi A, Johansson I, Hörnell A, Norberg M, Bergdahl IA. Diet and lifestyle factors associated with fish consumption in men and women: a study of whether gender differences can result in gender-specific confounding. *Nutr J.* 2012;11:101. doi:10.1186/1475-2891-11-101.

211. Sofi F, Fatini C, Sticchi E, et al. Fish intake and LPA 93C>T polymorphism: gene-environment interaction in modulating lipoprotein a concentrations. *Atherosclerosis.* 2007;195(2):e147-e154. [Epub 2007 July 2].

212. Wang Y, Goodrich JM, Gillespie B, Werner R, Basu N, Franzblau A. An investigation of modifying effects of metallothionein single-nucleotide polymorphisms on the association between mercury exposure and biomarker levels. *Environ Health Perspect.* 2012;120(4):530-534. doi:10.1289/ehp.1104079. [Epub 2012 January 9].

213. Schläwicke Engström K, Strömberg U, Lundh T, et al. Genetic variation in glutathione-related genes and body burden of methylmercury. *Environ Health Perspect.* 2008;116(6):734-739. doi:10.1289/ehp.10804.

214. American Heart Association. *The National Diet-Heart Study.* American Heart Association; 1968.

215. Kuang H, Yang F, Zhang Y, Wang T, Chen G. The impact of egg nutrient composition and its consumption on cholesterol homeostasis. *Cholesterol.* 2018;2018:6303810. Published 2018 August 23. doi:10.1155/2018/6303810.

216. Richard C, Cristall L, Fleming E, et al. Impact of egg consumption on cardiovascular risk factors in individuals with type 2 diabetes and at risk for developing diabetes: a systematic review of randomized nutritional intervention studies. *Can J Diabetes.* 2017;41(4):453-463. doi:10.1016/j.jcjd.2016.12.002. [Epub 2017 March 27].

217. Blesso CN, Andersen CJ, Barona J, Volk B, Volek JS, Fernandez ML. Effects of carbohydrate restriction and dietary cholesterol provided by eggs on clinical risk factors in metabolic syndrome. *J Clin Lipidol.* 2013;7(5):463-471.

218. Wallin A, Forouhi NG, Wolk A, Larsson SC. Egg consumption and risk of type 2 diabetes: a prospective study and dose-response meta-analysis. *Diabetologia.* 2016;59(6):1204-1213.

219. Sabaté J, Burkholder-Cooley NM, Segovia-Siapco G, et al. Unscrambling the relations of egg and meat consumption with type 2 diabetes risk. *Am J Clin Nutr.* 2018;108(5):1121-1128.

220. Holt EM, Steffen LM, Moran A, et al. Fruit and vegetable consumption and its relation to markers of inflammation and oxidative stress in adolescents. *J Am Diet Assoc.* 2009;109(3):414-421. doi:10.1016/j.jada.2008.11.036.

221. Flock MR, Kris-Etherton PM. Dietary guidelines for Americans 2010: implications for cardiovascular disease. *Curr Atheroscler Rep.* 2011;13(6):499-507. doi:10.1007/s11883-011-0205-0.

222. Dauchet L, Amouyel P, Hercberg S, Dallongeville J. Fruit and vegetable consumption and risk of coronary heart disease: a meta-analysis of cohort studies. *J Nutr.* 2006;136(10):2588-2593.

223. Dauchet L, Amouyel P, Dallongeville J. Fruit and vegetable consumption and risk of stroke: a meta-analysis of cohort studies. *Neurology.* 2005;65(8):1193-1197.

224. McCall DO, McGartland CP, McKinley MC, et al. Dietary intake of fruits and vegetables improves microvascular function in hypertensive subjects in a dose-dependent manner. *Circulation.* 2009;119(16):2153-2160. doi:10.1161/CIRCULATIONAHA.108.831297. [Epub 2009 April 13].

225. Bouchenak M, Lamri-Senhadji M. Nutritional quality of legumes, and their role in cardiometabolic risk prevention: a review. *J Med Food.* 2013;16(3):185-198. doi:10.1089/jmf.2011.0238. [Epub 2013 February 11].

226. Becerra-Tomás N, Díaz-López A, Rosique-Esteban N, et al. Legume consumption is inversely associated with type 2 diabetes incidence in adults: A prospective assessment from the PREDIMED study. *Clin Nutr.* 2018;37(3):906-913. doi:10.1016/j.clnu.2017.03.015. [Epub 2017 March 24].

227. Ye EQ, Chacko SA, Chou EL, Kugizaki M, Liu S. Greater whole-grain intake is associated with lower risk of type 2 diabetes, cardiovascular disease, and weight gain. *J Nutr.* 2012;142(7):1304-1313. doi:10.3945/jn.111.155325. [Epub 2012 May 30].

228. Katcher HI, Legro RS, Kunselman AR, et al. The effects of a whole grain-enriched hypocaloric diet on cardiovascular disease risk factors in men and women with metabolic syndrome. *Am J Clin Nutr.* 2008;87(1):79-90.

229. Zhang B, Zhao Q, Guo W, Bao W, Wang X. Association of whole grain intake with all-cause, cardiovascular, and cancer mortality: a systematic review and dose-response meta-analysis from prospective cohort studies. *Eur J Clin Nutr.* 2018;72(1):57-65. doi:10.1038/ejcn.2017.149. [Epub 2017 November 1].

230. Sabaté J, Ang Y. Nuts and health outcomes: new epidemiologic evidence. *Am J Clin Nutr.* 2009;89(5):1643S–1648S. doi:10.3945/ajcn.2009.26736Q. [Epub 2009 March 25]. Review.

231. Kim Y, Keogh J, Clifton PM. Nuts and cardio-metabolic disease: a review of meta-analyses. *Nutrients.* 2018;10(12):1935. Published 2018 December 6. doi:10.3390/nu10121935.

232. Kris-Etherton PM, Hu FB, Ros E, Sabaté J. The role of tree nuts and peanuts in the prevention of coronary heart disease: multiple potential mechanisms. *J Nutr.* 2008;138(9):1746S-1751S. Review.

233. Mattes RD. The energetics of nut consumption. *Asia Pac J Clin Nutr.* 2008;17(suppl 1):337-339. Review.

234. Salas-Salvadó J, Fernández-Ballart J, Ros E, et al. Effect of a Mediterranean diet supplemented with nuts on metabolic syndrome status: one-year results of the PREDIMED randomized trial. *Arch Intern Med.* 2008;168(22):2449-2458. doi:10.1001/archinte.168.22.2449.

235. Shen J, Wilmot KA, Ghasemzadeh N, et al. Mediterranean dietary patterns and cardiovascular health. *Annu Rev Nutr.* 2015;35:425-449. doi:10.1146/annurev-nutr-011215-025104..

236. Tsui PF, Lin CS, Ho LJ, Lai JH. Spices and atherosclerosis. *Nutrients.* 2018;10(11):1724. Published 2018 November 10. doi:10.3390/nu10111724.

237. Hooper L, Summerbell CD, Thompson R, et al. Reduced or modified dietary fat for preventing cardiovascular disease. *Cochrane Database Syst Rev.* 2012;5:CD002137. doi:10.1002/14651858.CD002137.pub3.

238. Buitrago-Lopez A, Sanderson J, Johnson L, et al. Chocolate consumption and cardiometabolic disorders: systematic review and meta-analysis. *BMJ.* 2011;343:d4488. doi:10.1136/bmj.d4488.

239. Lin X, Zhang I, Li A, et al. Cocoa flavanol intake and biomarkers for cardiometabolic health: a systematic review and meta-analysis of randomized controlled trials. *J Nutr.* 2016;146(11):2325-2333.

240. Bøhn SK, Ward NC, Hodgson JM, Croft KD. Effects of tea and coffee on cardiovascular disease risk. *Food Funct.* 2012;3(6):575-591. doi:10.1039/c2fo10288a.

241. Cornelis MC, El-Sohemy A, Kabagambe EK, et al. Coffee, CYP1A2 genotype, and risk of myocardial infarction. *JAMA.* 2006;295(10):1135-1141.

242. Palatini P, Ceolotto G, Ragazzo F, et al. CYP1A2 genotype modifies the association between coffee intake and the risk of hypertension. *J Hypertens*. 2009;27(8):1594-1601.

243. Cornelis MC, El-Sohemy A. Coffee, caffeine, and coronary heart disease. *Curr Opin Lipidol*. 2007;18(1):13-19.

244. Hu G Jou ilahti P Nissinen A, Bidel S, Antikainen R, Tuomilehto J. Coffee consumption and the incidence of antihypertensive drug treatment in Finnish men and women. *Am J Clin Nutr*. 2007;86(2):457-464.

245. Vlachopoulos CV, Vyssoulis GG, Alexopoulos NA, et al. Effect of chronic coffee consumption on aortic stiffness and wave reflections in hypertensive patients. *Eur J Clin Nutr*. 2007;61(6):796-802.

246. Mesas AE, Leon-Muñoz LM, Rodriguez-Artalejo F, Lopez-Garcia E. The effect of coffee on blood pressure and cardiovascular disease in hypertensive individuals: a systematic review and meta-analysis. *Am J Clin Nutr*. 2011;94(4):1113-1126.

247. Di Castelnuevo A, Costanzo S, Bagnardi V, et al. Alcohol dosing and total mortality in men and women: an updated meta-analysis of 34 prospective studies. *Arch Intern Med*. 2006;166(22):2437-2445.

248. Ronksley PE, Brien SE, Turner BJ, et al. Association of alcohol consumption with selected cardiovascular disease outcomes: a systematic review and meta-analysis. *BMJ*. 2011;342:d67.

249. O'Neill D, Britton A, Hannah MK, et al. Association of longitudinal alcohol consumption trajectories with coronary heart disease: a meta-analysis of six cohort studies using individual participant data. *BMC Med*. 2018;16(1):124. Published 2018 August 22. doi:10.1186/s12916-018-1123-6.

250. Roerecke M, Kaczorowski J, Tobe SW, Gmel G, Hasan OSM, Rehm J. The effect of a reduction in alcohol consumption on blood pressure: a systematic review and meta-analysis. *Lancet Public Health*. 2017;2(2):e108-e120.

251. Carlsen MH, Halvorsen BL, Holte K, et al. The total antioxidant content of more than 3100 foods, beverages, spices, herbs and supplements used worldwide. *Nutr J*. 2010;9:3. doi:10.1186/1475-2891-9-3.

252. Riccioni G, Speranza L, Pesce M, Cusenza S, D'Orazio N, Glade MJ. Novel phytonutrient contributors to antioxidant protection against cardiovascular disease. *Nutrition*. 2012;28(6):605-610. doi:10.1016/j.nut.2011.11.028. [Epub 2012 April 4].

253. Liu RH. Health-promoting components of fruits and vegetables in the diet. *Adv Nutr*. 2013;4:384S-392S. doi:10.3945/an.112.003517.

254. Wood AD, Strachan AA, Thies F, et al. Patterns of dietary intake and serum carotenoid and tocopherol status are associated with biomarkers of chronic low-grade systemic inflammation and cardiovascular risk. *Br J Nutr*. 2014;112(8):1341-1352. doi:10.1017/S0007114514001962.

255. Giordano P, Scicchitano P, Locorotondo M, et al. Carotenoids and cardiovascular risk. *Curr Pharm Des*. 2012;18(34):5577-5589.

256. Wang Y, Chung SJ, McCullough ML, et al. Dietary carotenoids are associated with cardiovascular disease risk biomarkers mediated by serum carotenoid concentrations. *J Nutr*. 2014;144(7):1067-1074. doi:10.3945/jn.113.184317. [Epub 2014 April 17].

257. Mozos I, Stoian D, Caraba A, Malainer C, Horbańczuk JO, Atanasov AG. Lycopene and vascular health. *Front Pharmacol*. 2018;9:521. Published 2018 May 23. doi:10.3389/fphar.2018.00521.

258. Rao AV. Lycopene, tomatoes, and the prevention of coronary heart disease. *Exp Biol Med (Maywood)*. 2002;227(10):908-913.

259. Cheng HM, Koutsidis G, Lodge JK, Ashor A, Siervo M, Lara J. Tomato and lycopene supplementation and cardiovascular risk factors: a systematic review and meta-analysis. *Atherosclerosis*. 2017;257:100-108. doi:10.1016/j.atherosclerosis.2017.01.009. [Epub 2017 January 13].

260. Chun OK, Chung SJ, Song WO. Estimated dietary flavonoid intake and major food sources of U.S. adults. *J Nutr*. 2007;137(5):1244-1252.

261. Faggio C, Sureda A, Morabito S, et al. Flavonoids and platelet aggregation: a brief review. *Eur J Pharmacol*. 2017;807:91-101. doi:10.1016/j.ejphar.2017.04.009. [Epub 2017 April 13].

262. McCullough ML, Peterson JJ, Patel R, Jacques PF, Shah R, Dwyer JT. Flavonoid intake and cardiovascular disease mortality in a prospective cohort of US adults. *Am J Clin Nutr*. 2012;95(2):454-464.

263. Yamada T, Hayasaka S, Shibata Y, et al. Frequency of citrus fruit intake is associated with the incidence of cardiovascular disease: The Jichi Medical School cohort study. *J Epidemiol*. 2011;21:169-175.

264. Knekt P, Kumpulainen J, Jarvinen R, et al. Flavonoid intake and risk of chronic diseases. *Am J Clin Nutr*. 2002;76:560-568.

265. Cassidy A, Rimm EB, O'Reilly EJ, et al. Dietary flavonoids and risk of stroke in women. *Stroke*. 2012;43:946-951.

266. Onakpoya I, O'Sullivan J, Heneghan C, Thompson M. The effect of grapefruits (Citrus paradisi) on body weight and cardiovascular risk factors: a systematic review and meta-analysis of randomized clinical trials. *Crit Rev Food Sci Nutr*. 2017;57:602-612.

267. Salehi B, Fokou PVT, Sharifi-Rad M, et al. The therapeutic potential of naringenin: a review of clinical trials. *Pharmaceuticals (Basel)*. 2019;12(1). pii: E11. doi:10.3390/ph12010011.

5

The Paleo Diet and Coronary Heart Disease

Jack M. Wolfson, DO, FACC and Ashley Swanson, MS

"Whatever is Contrary to Nature Cannot Be Fact."

Animals in the wild eat foods that are native to them. Lions, tigers, giraffes, baboons, and all animals, evolved over millions of years on a steady diet that is best summarized as *hunter-gatherer*. All animals are hunter-gatherers. All animals eat plant material. All animals eat other animals, seafood, and/or insects.

Nature needs no instruction and needs no input from the U.S. Department of Agriculture (USDA). Why should humans be any different? Why must we deliberate over what the best nutrition is for a man or woman? Baby humans enjoy the best health when they consume human milk. This is just common sense. The Paleo diet makes common sense. All societies in the history of the world ate meat, seafood, insects, or a combination thereof.

What Is the Paleo Diet?

In general terms, the Paleo diet refers to foods available to our ancient ancestors. Our ancestors were all hunter-gatherers. They would hunt animals, seafood, and insects. They would gather vegetables, fruit, tubers, nuts, seeds, and eggs. Foods not on our ancestral diet include cereal grains, such as wheat, oats, soy, corn, and other grasses, dairy, and sugar (aside from raw honey).

The word Paleo comes from the Greek word *palaios*, meaning "ancient." Paleolithic refers to a period of time before recorded history starting around 3 million years ago with the earliest use of stone tools and ending around 12,000 years ago with the advent of farming.

The word Paleo in reference to a diet has been used interchangeably with Caveman, Hunter-Gatherer, Primal, and Ancestral. Most would say that a Paleo diet falls more toward the "low-carb" side with higher consumption of fats and proteins. All would agree that Paleo foods are not processed and exist in their natural form.

There are modern societies of Paleo eaters, but their numbers are small. Explorers from Cook to Magellan documented the food selection of prehistoric man. Weston A. Price, a dentist from the early part of the 20th century, traveled around the world by boat with his wife. He documented the ill effects on human health for those who suffered from poor dentition, development disorders, and childhood disease.

Clearly, different populations around the world consume different Paleo foods. What Paleo food is available to islanders in the South Pacific is clearly different from that available to an Eskimo in Canada or an African Hadza tribesman.

Two modern TV shows seem to epitomize what life was like in the Paleolithic time period: *Survivor* and *Naked and Afraid*. In each program, human contestants are living off the land as hunter-gatherers. They are in a perpetual quest for shelter and food. But the food they are searching for is not plant material. There is plenty of greenery around them. They are searching for animal and seafood. Finding such is always a cause for celebration.

The 1950s and a New Diet Paradigm

Medical doctors, researchers, and epidemiologists realized that there was a dramatic rise in chronic diseases in the United States and in developed countries around the world. Morbidity and mortality from infectious diseases were dramatically reduced with the improvement in sanitation, access to clean water, and plentiful availability of food. People were now living longer in an industrialized society, but easy access to food would prove to be a double-edged sword.

Caloric intake was much higher in the 1900s than ever before. White flour, white sugar, and white rice provided a massive spike in caloric intake, with little nutritional value. Obesity was rampant and myocardial infarction, stroke, and cancer rates were exploding. There were many key people in what can only be described as a low fat, high carbohydrate revolution. But there was no bigger persona than Dr Ancel Keys.

Ancel Keys was apparently a brilliant man with a wide scope of interests and scientific degrees. He researched the effects of starvation on prisoners of war and eventually on "conscientious deserters" from war. He developed the food protocols for military personnel known as the K-ration. Eventually his research would lead him to believe cholesterol and saturated fat were the villains in the story of human health. Ultimately, Keys would publish his Diet-Lipid Heart Disease Hypothesis and lead a massive study known as the Seven Countries Study.[1] In short, foods rich in cholesterol and fats were condemned. Keys himself was a huge promoter of the Mediterranean diet and described his personal diet in a 1961 *Time* magazine article as "fish, chicken, calves' liver, Canadian bacon, Italian food, Chinese food, supplemented by fresh fruits, vegetables and casseroles."[2]

Keys and others in the low saturated fat camp would heavily influence US dietary guidelines in the 1970s that would culminate in the USDA Food Pyramid and other documents promoting the limitation of animal fats in favor of high-carbohydrate choices. Critics of the Seven Countries Study would point to the fact that Keys selected only seven countries to fit with his hypothesis. He excluded countries such as France, known to consume high amounts of saturated fats but with low cardiac morbidity and mortality, the so-called French Paradox. There is no paradox. Fat is not the problem.

Low Carb Fights Back

Not all doctors and nutrition authorities agreed with Ancel Keys. In fact, many outright disagreed. One of the most vocal critics of Keys dietary observation was Dr John Yudkin. He published a book in 1958 called *This Slimming Business* that blamed the current rise of cardiovascular disease on sugar. A movie based on his work was released in 1972, *Pure, White, and Deadly*. Yudkin had a different take from Keys on the increased incidence of cardiovascular disease and other chronic health conditions. He found that the increase in sugar consumption correlated with the alarming increase of myocardial infarctions in many countries during the first half of the 20th century. In a paper published in 1957,[3] Yudkin analyzed diets and coronary mortality in different countries for the year 1952 and also analyzed trends in diet, and trends in coronary mortality, in the United Kingdom between 1928 and 1954. His conclusion produced no evidence for the view that total fat, or animal fat, or hydrogenated fat was the direct cause of coronary thrombosis. Yudkin thought it was all from sugar.

There were many other contemporaries critical of the work of Ancel Keys, including Dr George Mann, Thomas Cleave, George Campbell, and Edward Ahrens, Jr. Then, in the 1970s, a radical dietary recommendation was espoused by Dr Robert Atkins, MD. In 1972, Atkins' book titled *Dr Atkins' Diet Revolution* was published. In his book, Atkins pushed for a low-carbohydrate, high-fat diet. His theories led to a generation of physicians, PhD's, and nutritionists promoting a high-fat, low-carbohydrate dietary plan. Ironically, Atkins died in 2003 from an intracranial bleed he suffered after a slip and fall on a patch of ice.

Paleo Reemerges As a Modern Dietary Recommendation

Dr Walter L. Voegtlin argues on the side of high fat, low carbohydrate in his book *The Stone Age Diet*, published in 1975.[4] Voegtlin was a gastroenterologist and asserted that humans are mostly carnivorous animals. The Stone Age diet was that of a carnivore—chiefly fats and protein, with only small amounts of carbohydrates. He notes that, like the carnivorous dog, man has canine teeth, ridged molars, and incisors in both jaws. His jaw is designed for crushing and tearing as it moves in vertical motions. His stomach holds two quarts, empties in three hours, rests between meals, lacks bacteria and protozoa, secretes large quantities of hydrochloric acid, and does not digest cellulose. His digestive tract is short relative to body length, his cecum is nonfunctional, and his appendix vestigial. His rectum is small, contains putrefactive bacterial flora, and does not contribute to the digestive process. The volume of feces is small; digestive efficiency borders on 100%. The gallbladder is an organ with one purpose: the digestion of fat. The above-mentioned fact is obviously in contrast to a cow, sheep, or any other ruminant animal.

S. Boyd Eaton, MD wrote an article in the *New England Journal of Medicine* in 1985 espousing the health benefits of Paleo nutrition.[5] Eaton graduated at the top of his class from Harvard Medical School and would practice radiology for 41 years. His book *Paleolithic Prescription* was released in 1988. The year 1999 saw the release of *Neander-thin* by Ray Audette, and then in 2001, Loren Cordain, a professor at Colorado State University, published his book titled *The Paleo Diet: Lose Weight and Get Healthy by Eating the Food You Were Designed to Eat.* With this publication, millions of people became Paleo acolytes. Paleo was recognized as our ancestral and evolutionary diet complete with macro- and micronutrients to optimize health and longevity.

Cordain and Eaton coauthored a paper published in the *American Journal of Clinical Nutrition* in 2000. They studied 229 different hunter-gatherer groups and found that, on average, two-thirds of net energy consumption was from animal foods, the other third coming from plants.[6] Many sources including Eaton and Weston A. Price document extraordinary health in these hunter-gatherer populations.

Paleo Proof

In the following sections, I will make the case that Paleo nutrition, the diet humans have consumed for millions of years, is the best food plan for optimal cardiovascular health and longevity. Finding evidence for what appears to be common sense is not easy.

Let us face it, there are not many people eating the way Voegtlin recommends.

At this point, I would like to discuss the difficulty with nutritional scientific study. Reviewing the literature as it pertains to Paleo nutrition reveals the paucity of quality data in randomized trials. The following represents the issues that continue to cause such debate among professionals and public alike in the dietary arena.

1. Randomized trials to assess long-term results are fraught with difficulty. It is difficult for a study group to stay on a recommended diet and even more difficult for researchers to account for study adherence.

2. Epidemiological and observational studies have substantial flaws, including the difficulty in accounting for possible confounding factors. For example, a group identified as eating less red meat may also smoke less, exercise more, and experience less stress. All of these are other factors known to be linked to cardiovascular risk.

3. Food surveys are imprecise. This method of research includes dietary recall to generate data points and is notoriously fraught with error.

4. Conflicts of interest are rampant in research. Suffice to say that just about every researcher has conflicts, including how studies are funded or personal bias.

5. Animal data do not necessarily apply to humans. For example, many cardiovascular studies are done on the rodent model. Rodents may be easy to study, but the applicability of the results to human is imprecise. Rodents in the wild eat a diet high in plant matter; therefore, feeding studies high in animal fat, animal protein, and cholesterol may not have much value.

6. All foods cannot be considered equal. Evidence shows that the nutritional makeup of pasture-raised animals differ from that of grain-fed, confined animals. Omega-3 ratios, fat, and other nutrient content differ.[7] Organic produce is different from pesticide and genetically modified plant materials. Wild seafood is nutritionally different from farm-raised fish.[175]

7. What exactly are Paleo foods, and in what percentages are fat, protein, and carbohydrates represented. What is the appropriate ratio of animal to plant-based foods?

With the aforementioned difficulties in mind, I will try to limit my review on Paleo nutrition to randomized trials and meta-analysis of such trials whenever possible, thus limiting observational studies. I will also try to limit my review to studies on humans, as animal research is not easily applicable to our purpose. For example, thousands of studies have used a rodent model for dietary assessment, yet rats and many other rodents do not have a gallbladder, an important organ for fat digestion.

Optimal Dietary Approach

Ultimately, each person is an individual. Although I believe that one's nutritional intake should mimic the ancestral region from which they came, this can be fine-tuned based on laboratory testing. When following any dietary pattern, testing is warranted for cardiovascular risk, including quantitative serum lipoprotein assessment; markers of inflammation and oxidative stress; blood sugar, insulin, and glycohemoglobin; 25-hydroxy vitamin D; homocysteine; and omega-3 indices. In addition, noninvasive measurements such a salivary nitric oxide, carotid intima-media thickness (CIMT), echo-cardiography, and heart rate variability and other parameters

will help us perfect the nutritional plan. Finally, continued research into areas of fasting and seasonal eating patterns will guide future health practitioners in the dietary optimization of their patients.

In the following review on Paleo and cardiovascular health, I will try to focus on data including Paleo versus other diets, low-carbohydrate versus low-fat, saturated fat intake, animal meat consumption, and seafood consumption as they relate to cardiovascular outcomes and risk factors.

Why Is Paleo the Best Diet for Cardiovascular Health?

The authors of a novel literature review entitled *Biological and Clinical Potential of Paleolithic Diet*, that spanned 17 years and encompassed 200 scientific journals concluded that the Paleolithic diet is the best diet for preventing Western diseases. This review highlighted the need to look to "evolutionary biology" and "evolutionary medicine" for preventing chronic diseases. Furthermore, the authors concluded that the diets of our ancestors would have been much higher in nutritional value and aided in the prevention of diseases such as atherosclerosis, stroke, heart disease, and insulin resistance. The authors of this article contend that Paleolithic nutrition promotes health, whereas, conversely, they argue that the components of the Standard American Diet (dairy, cereals, refined carbohydrates, and salt) cause disease.[8]

The author Geoffrey Rose indirectly and eloquently highlighted the importance of studying prehistoric populations for insight into health and disease. His article, entitled *Sick Individuals and Sick Populations*, called for a shift in how we view the etiology of disease. Rather than look at an individual's risk for disease, he contends it is more helpful to look at why certain populations remain healthy, whereas others get sick. As an example, he quotes, "We might achieve a complete understanding of why individuals vary, and yet quite miss the most important public health question, namely, 'Why is hypertension absent in the Kenyans and common in London?'. The answer to that question has to do with the determinants of the population mean; for what distinguishes the two groups has nothing to do with the characteristics of individuals, it is rather a shift of the whole distribution —a mass influence acting on the population as a whole. To find the determinants of prevalence and incidence rates, we need to study characteristics of populations, not characteristics of individuals." This population prevention strategy is more effective in mitigating chronic disease as it works to alter exposures to be more favorable in the whole population. This allows for more sustainable lifestyle and behavior changes on a large scale in society that need to take place to eradicate our modern diseases. It also allows us to be guided by evolutionary biology.[9]

Paleo and Mortality

The ultimate arbiter of any health outcome must be mortality. Unfortunately, there are no randomized trials dedicated to mortality on Paleo nutrition versus other diets. The closest trial we have is the 2017 REGARDS (Reasons for

Geographic and Racial Differences in Stroke) study assessing the diets of 21,423 participants. They looked at outcomes of quintiles based on adherence to a Paleo diet. The authors found a 23% lower risk of death in the group most adherent to Paleo nutrition principles versus the quintile with the lowest compliance, although other confounding factors were present. A 28% reduction in cancer deaths and a 22% reduction in cardiovascular death was noted in the high- versus low-adherence group.[10]

An excellent trial assessing mortality in reference to the type of fat intake was the Minnesota Coronary Experiment. In 2016, the long-term outcomes of people randomized to diets of either high saturated fat or high polyunsaturated fat from corn oil was released. This study was based on data acquired in the late 1960s and included human participants who were institutionalized. Adherence to study protocol was meticulous in this highly controlled population. What the authors found was quite the contradiction to common modern dietary recommendations. Although the polyunsaturated group had dramatically lower total cholesterol, mortality INCREASED (emphasis mine) as serum cholesterol was reduced. There was a 22% higher risk of death for each 30 mg/dL reduction in serum cholesterol.[11] The authors of the Minnesota Coronary Experiment study also added a meta-analysis of five other randomized trials and concluded a higher risk of death in groups randomized to polyunsaturated fat versus saturated fat. A large meta-analysis of observational studies assessing over 300,000 people confirmed that consumption of saturated fat does not lead to excess mortality, myocardial infarction, or stroke risk, as reported in the British Medical Journal.[12] Substituting saturated fat for polyunsaturated fat does not reduce mortality from cardiovascular disease according to data from the Sydney Diet Heart Study and additional meta-analysis.[13]

Meat/Seafood/Eggs and Mortality

A 2014 meta-analysis of meat consumption found that unprocessed red meat did not lead to excess mortality, although processed meat did. Again, this analysis was based on data from observational trials.[14] A 2010 meta-analysis including over 1,000,000 persons found no link to unprocessed red meat and cardiovascular mortality.[15] Processed meats likely increase risk because of several factors including preservatives, cooking methods, meat quality, and lifestyle behaviors of those who consume these foods.

Fish eaters enjoy a 12% lower risk of death compared with non-fish eaters in a meta-analysis of over 650,000 people.[16] Another recent meta-analysis of over 400,000 people found a 9% lower risk of death in men who consumed the most fish, 8% in women.[17] Of note, women who ate the most fish enjoyed 38% lower risk of mortality from Alzheimer disease. A study often used by those promoting a vegan nutrition plan is the data from the Seventh Day Adventists. Yet the group of Seventh Day Adventists with the lowest mortality were those in the pescatarian group. Fish-eaters enjoyed a 19% mortality reduction compared with the group described as nonvegetarian. Other variables were noted between groups, including differences in exercise, tobacco use, and alcohol

consumption.[18] Marital status and ethnicity may also play a role in results.

The food that seems to conjure the most critique among the diet gurus is the egg. The egg graced the cover of *Time* magazine in 1984 as the anticholesterol poster food. A 2017 study on over 40,000 people found that those who consumed the most eggs had a 12% reduction in overall mortality.[19] A recent article reviewing the massive amount of literature on eggs ended with the authors concluding, "The evidence suggests that a diet including more eggs than is recommended (at least in some countries) may be used safely as part of a healthy diet in both the general population and for those at high risk of cardiovascular disease, those with established coronary heart disease, and those with type 2 diabetes mellitus."[20]

Other Paleo Foods and Mortality

Coconut and coconut oil are often ridiculed and regarded as unhealthy by nutrition authorities including the American Heart Association.[21] Despite the health and wellness of island populations consuming coconut, there is a paucity of research regarding mortality. A recent review of palm oil consumption, an oil with a similar nutritional profile to coconut oil, found no increased risk of mortality in palm oil users.[22]

Nuts and seeds would fall into the category of paleolithic foods, although our ancestors would struggle to crack nuts from shells. Store-bought walnuts shelled into a bag is a lot easier to eat than cracking one by one. Seeds, dried out of a pumpkin or sunflower, were likely an easier proposition. People who consume the largest amount of nuts and seeds enjoy a much lower risk of dying. In one study, nut eaters of over three servings per week led to a 29% lower mortality than those who did not eat nuts/seeds.[23] Another study from 2016 displayed similar findings including lower total mortality and cardiovascular mortality in the group consuming the most servings of nuts per week.[24]

Paleo Lifestyle and Mortality

Paleo nutrition is the subject of this chapter as it pertains to cardiovascular risk and overall mortality, but nutrition is obviously only one part of overall lifestyle considerations. Other factors may be just as important as the food we eat including sleep, sun exposure, tobacco use, and physical activity.

The origins of diseases of affluence, as opposed to diseases of infection, have long been speculated. In 2008, a professor known as Johan Mackenbach published a short article in the *Journal of Epidemiology and Community Health*. He claimed that the pathogenesis of chronic disease in humans arises from two factors: (1) effects to the internal system of humans arising from interactions within the external environment and (2) effects to the internal system of humans arising from a failing of internal physiological mechanisms. This important contention highlights the fact that every single cell in our bodies is affected by the effects of both our internal and external environments. External environment can be diet, toxins, exposure to the sun, and even physical activity. It is what our bodies are exposed to on a daily basis.[25]

Another study further corroborates this contention, stating that disease is the direct result of both the health inside the body and the "healthy" or "unhealthy" exposures outside the body.[26]

This idea warrants questioning of how our environments have changed throughout evolution. Both the diet and lifestyle of our discordant Westernized society today is much different from that of hunter-gatherer societies of long ago. As a result, there are now "diseases of civilization," such as cardiovascular disease, that are the direct result of changes to the environment we live in. Thus, when looking for diet and lifestyle causes of cardiovascular disease, it is beneficial to examine the effects of the divergence from a traditional hunter-gatherer society to one rooted in agrarian ways.[27]

The modern world is burdened with increased antinutrients, toxins, pharmaceuticals, physical inactivity, and heightened levels of stress. These factors all take their toll on health over time. To prevent and reverse disease, one must alter these other lifestyle factors *along with diet* to achieve better health outcomes and reverse chronic disease rates.

Energy expenditure through physical activity was an important part of survival for the ancestral hunter-gatherers of long ago. Activities included foraging and hunting for food and water, creating shelter, interacting with others, and protecting themselves from predators. This highly active lifestyle is much different from the modern sedentary lifestyle we see in society today. In fact, the authors of one study make the case that the shift from the traditional "hunter-gatherer" lifestyle to one in which people are "sedentary, overfed and always indoors" is associated with the rise of disease, obesity, depression, and weakness experienced today. The primal link between energy intake and energy expenditure has been abolished owing to the modern world, and as a result the health of society has been drastically impacted.[28]

A "real world" field setting study analyzed activity patterns similar to those found during the Paleolithic period. Four healthy men were recruited to undertake a 12-day Alaskan backcountry hunting immersion. The results showed negative energy balance, along with reductions in body fat, total fat mass, visceral fat volume, and intrahepatic lipids. There was also a pattern of reduced low-density lipoprotein (LDL) cholesterol. Interestingly, lean tissue mass was preserved. This emulation of the hunter-gatherer lifestyle showed increased rates of total energy expenditure, improved lipid profiles, and beneficial metabolic effects.[29]

The Iowa Women's Health Study looked at nutrition AND other lifestyle factors as to their evolutionary concordance. They recruited and followed a population-based cohort of 41,837 postmenopausal women in Iowa from 1986 to 2012 to identify if diet, body fat distribution, and other risk factors increased the incidence of cancer and all-cause mortality. The findings of this research endeavor revealed that there was a significant inverse association between individuals following an "evolutionary-concordant" diet and lifestyle pattern and all-cause mortality.[30] The key here was the LIFESTYLE. What can be described as a Paleo diet versus Mediterranean did not matter. What mattered was the lifestyle.

Weston A. Price was a dentist who traveled the world studying groups of people who followed an ancestral nutrition and lifestyle pattern. He found health and wellness without the chronic disease states found in the developed world. For example, traditional hunter-gatherer-type diets like those of the aboriginal Arctic Eskimos were historically low in carbohydrate and high in protein. The traditional diet consisted of wild land and sea animals and fish and was found to be a complete source of essential nutrients despite limited selection. An article written in 1977 in the *American Anthropologist* concluded that the "modern" Eskimo, who has been exposed to dietary acculturation and has veered away from traditional diet and lifestyle, is known to experience the same chronic diseases that affect the US population, including obesity, cardiovascular disease, hypertension, and tooth decay.[31] Furthermore, a study published in the *American Journal of Clinical Nutrition* concluded that, "it is likely that no hunter-gatherer society, regardless of the proportion of macronutrients consumed, suffered from diseases of civilization." These diseases of civilization include obesity, cardiovascular disease, and type 2 diabetes (T2D), to name a few.[32]

A unique historical perspective review concluded that, although life expectancy has increased, there are still low levels of "healthy life expectancy," defined as less suffering from chronic disease before death. A review compared diet and lifestyle behaviors of primitive populations of the past with that of the modernized societies of today. The finding is that modern diets are drastically different from those of the past with less variability, a declining nutritional value, and an increased intake of calories, all of which impact total mortality and chronic disease risk. Furthermore, the review artfully concluded that the true difference in health outcomes is a result of differences in food intake. Hunter-gatherer populations focused on "eating to live," whereas Westernized societies of today have shifted to a focus of "living to eat" and this is where health problems have arisen.[33]

Paleo and Lipids

Foods common on the Paleolithic diet are considered by many to negatively impact the lipid profile. Meat, eggs, coconut, and other sources of saturated fat and/or dietary cholesterol have been vilified by many health authorities and promoted as foods to avoid. The reality is that these foods are beneficial for cardiovascular protection.

Much of the attack on red meat consumption centers on its association with abnormal cholesterol levels. But publicity and perception around this link may not be the reality. A recent meta-analysis of 24 randomized trials concluded that total red meat intake of ≥0.5 servings/d does not negatively influence cardiovascular disease risk factors, compared with those who consume red meat <0.5 servings/d. There were no significant differences in total cholesterol, LDL, high-density lipoprotein (HDL), or triglycerides.[34]

A 2004 trial comparing very low-carb to low-fat in human participants concluded, "The short-term hypoenergetic low-fat diet was more effective at lowering serum LDL-C, but the very low-carbohydrate diet was more effective at improving characteristics of the metabolic syndrome as shown by a decrease in fasting serum TAG, the TAG/HDL-C ratio, postprandial lipemia, serum glucose, an increase in LDL particle size, and also greater weight loss ($P < .05$)."[35]

In a 2-year Dietary Intervention Randomized Controlled Trial - Carotid (DIRECT-Carotid) study, participants were randomly assigned to a low-carbohydrate, low-fat, or Mediterranean treatment group. Authors looked at the effect of diet on serum lipoproteins. The Apo B to Apo A ratio may be the best conventional lipid marker used to assess cardiovascular risk.[36] The results showed a significant reduction in the ratio of apolipoprotein B(100) to apolipoprotein A1 in the low-carbohydrate group compared with the low-fat group. Over time, the low-carbohydrate group experienced the greatest significant increase of Apo A1 compared with the low-fat group. Furthermore, levels of Apo B100 were significantly increased in the low-fat group.[37]

Seafood has been recognized for millennia for its sustenance value. A review from the College of William and Mary in 1944 found that seafood, particularly shellfish, are a complete food. Seafood contains fat, protein, and limited carbohydrates including a full complement of minerals (best source of iodine) and vitamins, including A, B, D, E, and K. Only shellfish have appreciable levels of vitamin C.[38] A 2018 trial found that fatty fish consumption increases HDL particle number and size, both recognized as cardioprotective changes.[39] This is confirmed in multiple studies.[40]

Coconut and coconut oil have been vilified for years because of their high content of saturated fat. Despite this fact, islands in the South Pacific have very high consumption of coconut and enjoy excellent health.[41] A recent prospective randomized analysis compared coconut oil with butter and olive oil. Study participants were asked to consume 50 g of their assigned fat. Coconut oil was found to be neutral on LDL, increase HDL, and improve the total cholesterol (TC)/HDL ratio.[42] Another 2017 randomized trial among young men in Thailand found coconut oil at 30 mL/d had a nonsignificant effect on TC and LDL but led to a 5.72 mg/dL increase in HDL concentration.[43] Finally, a 2017 study on postmenopausal women found that coconut oil raised TC, LDL, and HDL, thus preserving the TC/HDL ratio. The study authors conclude coconut oil to be safe but also recommended that future studies use advanced lipoprotein analysis including particle numbers.[44]

Recent evidence has shown that saturated fat is cardioprotective and can change LDL particles from a small, dense size to large size.[45] Saturated fat can modify the particle size to a benign type that can actually reduce cardiovascular risk. A low-carbohydrate diet can promote positive changes on particle size, whereas the opposite is true for a low-fat diet.[46] A study of genetically predisposed children found that a high-carbohydrate, low-fat diet can induce a particle size change in LDL from large to small and dense.[47] In a study of men with a majority of large LDL particles, a low-fat diet had adverse effects. The low-fat diet shifted LDL particle size to small, reduced HDL concentrations, and increased triglyceride levels.[48]

Thirty-two participants were randomized to a Paleo diet versus the Dutch diet for 2 weeks. The Dutch diet has a similar macronutrient breakdown to the Mediterranean diet. In this short period of time, the Paleo group saw a significant reduction in total cholesterol and triglycerides and an increase in HDL versus the reference Dutch diet.[49]

Paleo bested the Diabetes diet in individuals with T2D. The study concluded that being on a Paleo diet short-term is beneficial for lipid profiles compared with an American Diabetes Association (ADA)-recommended diet (one rich in grains, added salt, and low-fat dairy).[50] A Paleo diet resulted in significant reductions of cardiovascular risk factors, including decreased triglycerides and increased HDL, as compared with a Diabetes diet.[51]

Paleo and Blood Pressure

A novel postulation published in 2018 in *Medical Hypotheses* stated that the hypertension of modern American society is the result of a diet that is low in potassium, depleted of antihypertensive phytochemicals, and high in sodium. The authors contend that the effects of this type of diet results in essential hypertension caused by oxidative stress and restricted nitric oxide bioavailability. They reveal that the current intake of potassium-to-sodium (in molar ratio) of Americans is less than or equal to 1. Conversely, our Paleolithic ancestors consumed molar ratios of potassium-to-sodium at levels of 5 to 10 or greater. Indeed, this highlights a dire need for increased potassium in the diet.[53] It is widely known that patients with a low dietary intake of potassium have an increased risk for hypertension and cardiovascular-related issues. Furthermore, the less-than-ideal ratios of potassium to sodium experienced in the Standard American diet (including a deficiency of potassium and surplus of sodium) contributes to intracellular acidity, a known risk factor for vascular endothelial dysfunction.[53]

Most health authorities agree that sodium consumption is causative of hypertension. The highest risk of hypertension is in those who consume high sodium, especially in relation to potassium intake. A study was done on chimpanzees and found that the addition of salt to the monkey diet led to progressive high blood pressure.[54]

In humans, a Paleo diet was compared with a Diabetic diet in those with T2D. The Paleo group enjoyed a significant blood pressure drop in this short-term trial. The Diabetes group did not.[51] Observational data on over 3000 people in Korea found that a low consumption of eggs and meat was linked to a higher risk of hypertension. Salted seafood consumption was also a risk factor for hypertension in this study.[55] Fish consumption is linked to lower blood pressure in several studies.[56] High cellular levels of omega-3 docosahexaenoic acid (DHA) demonstrated a 36% lower risk of hypertension.[57]

Impaired endothelial function is a risk factor for hypertension. A low-carbohydrate diet has been shown to improve carotid endothelial function. In the DIRECT-Carotid study, participants were randomly assigned to low-carbohydrate, low-fat, or Mediterranean diet treatment group and analyzed for changes to carotid artery thickness and carotid vessel volume. The results showed a regression of carotid vessel volume and a decrease in carotid artery thickness in all three treatment groups at 2 years.[37]

A recent 2019 randomized trial looked at subjects receiving varying levels of glycemic load and glycemic index foods on arterial stiffness. A diet with low-carbohydrate and low glycemic index was found to support healthy vascular tone.[58]

A study analyzed the effects of a very-low-carbohydrate diet on risk factors of cardiovascular disease including endothelial function. The study found that markers of endothelial function, including E- and P- selectin, ICAM1, plasminogen-activator inhibitor 1, and tissue-type plasminogen activator were significantly improved by a carbohydrate-restriction diet.[59]

Paleo and Blood Sugar/Metabolic Syndrome

Elevated blood sugar, diabetes, and the metabolic syndrome are all considered risk factors for cardiovascular disease. It would behoove us to find the best diet for glycemic control. The Standard American Diet tends to be rich in highly processed, empty calorie foods and as a result depleted of many essential nutrients required for health. It is often linked with the pathogenesis of postprandial dysmetabolism, including hypertriglyceridemia, elevated glucose, and elevated insulin. Postprandial dysmetabolism is associated with oxidative stress, inflammation, and subsequent atherogenic changes. Authors of a 2008 JACC study concluded that an anti-inflammatory and minimally processed diet along with a healthy lifestyle can play a role in the prevention of postprandial dysmetabolism.[60]

A 2018 randomized trial found that those participants placed on a high-fat diet versus high-carbohydrate enjoyed lower blood sugar during the fasted and postprandial state.[61] The Paleo diet exhibits fewer calories and lower glycemic index spikes and is more satiating, and as a result it causes greater decreases in weight and waist circumference and is favorable for reversing metabolic disease.[62]

Further studies corroborate beneficial effects on cardiovascular risk factors in T2D. Two groups were randomized to either a Paleolithic diet or the standard ADA diet. HbA1c and other parameters of the metabolic syndrome were markedly improved on Paleo versus ADA.[51]

Paleo was compared with Mediterranean in patients with coronary artery disease (CAD). Twenty-nine patients with CAD plus either glucose intolerance or T2D were randomized to receive (1) a Paleolithic diet (n = 14), based on lean meat, fish, fruits, vegetables, root vegetables, eggs and nuts; or (2) a Consensus (Mediterranean-like) diet (n = 15), based on whole grains, low-fat dairy products, vegetables, fruits, fish, oils, and margarines. Primary outcome variables were changes in weight, waist circumference, and plasma glucose AUC (area under curve) and plasma insulin AUC in OGTTs. The results were clearly in favor of Paleo. Over 12 weeks, there was a 26% decrease in AUC glucose in the Paleolithic group and a 7% decrease in the Consensus group. Weight circumference reduction was 2× greater in the Paleo group.[176]

A review study compared 28 reports of data on the diets, lifestyles, and metabolic effects of traditional hunter-gatherer

Australian Aborigines versus Westernized Aborigines. The results were striking. When Aboriginals lost their traditional hunter-gatherer lifestyle, they developed an increased rate of abdominal adiposity, obesity, impaired glucose tolerance, hyperinsulinemia, non-insulin-dependent diabetes, and hypertriglyceridemia, all of which are early and established risk factors for cardiovascular disease. Before Australia became colonized, Aborigines lived as traditional hunter-gatherers. The review concluded that there is no evidence that these traditional hunter-gatherer Aboriginals experienced any of the chronic diseases, or diseases of civilization, we see in the Western society today.[63] It has been shown that when Westernized Aborigines reverted to a traditional hunter-gatherer lifestyle for a short term (2 week) or long term (3 month) period, there are significant reductions of circulating insulin and triglyceride levels.[64,65]

In one study, agricultural versus hunter-gatherer societies were compared. Fifty-nine healthy Shuar Amerindian women living in five isolated communities in the Ecuadorian Amazonian rainforest were included in the study. Women who were from regions that were more dependent on agriculture had stark metabolic differences compared with traditional hunter-gatherer populations. These discrepancies show an increased risk of metabolic syndrome due to agricultural living as a result of increased fat mass, higher leptin, increased plasma insulin, and increased plasma triglycerides.[66]

Another study of Paleo versus Mediterranean found that Paleo was more satiating and led to lower calorie intake. Leptin, a hormone released from adipose tissue was lower in the Paleo group.[67] Leptin is implicated in the control of food intake via appetite suppression and may also stimulate oxidative stress, inflammation, thrombosis, arterial stiffness, angiogenesis, and atherogenesis.[68]

In a metabolically controlled study of obese patients with T2D, 14 participants were assigned to a Paleo diet and 10 were assigned to a conventional diet based on recommendations made by the ADA. The results revealed that those on a Paleo diet had greater improvements to glucose control and lipid profiles. Another astounding finding was that participants with the most insulin resistance had a significant increase of insulin sensitivity on the Paleo diet. Conversely, insulin-resistant participants on the conventional ADA diet did not experience significant improvements in insulin sensitivity.[50]

In a review of randomized control trials conducted thus far, the study found that the Paleo diet resulted in better improvements for the five components of metabolic syndrome (waist circumference, triglycerides, HDL, blood pressure, and fasting blood sugar) than the four control diets, which were all similar diets based on national nutritional guidelines.[69]

It has been concluded that the Western diet consisting of grains, sugar, and dairy promotes insulin resistance and disease pathogenesis through its pleiotropic effects on insulin/IGF-1 signaling (IIS). Up-regulation of IIS is associated with hyperglycemia, hyperinsulinemia, oxidative stress, and B-cell dysfunction, all of which lay the framework for T2D and cardiovascular disease. Although access to these hyperglycemic and insulinotropic foods became available roughly

10,000 years ago, it is proposed that our human genomes have not yet adapted to this type of diet and its increased activation of ISS. Dietary behaviors (elimination of sugar, grains, and dairy) such as those found on the Paleo diet can lower ISS and are speculated to reduce disease pathology as a result.[70]

T2D is associated with an increased risk for neurodegenerative disease including a decline in cognition. A clinical trial published in 2017 randomized T2D patients taking metformin to a Paleolithic diet with and without high-intensity exercise for 12 weeks. The study found that both interventions resulted in significant weight loss, improved insulin sensitivity, decreased HbA1C, reduced triglycerides, and increased oxygen uptake. Additionally, with both intervention groups there was increased BDNF, increased functional brain responses, and increased gray matter volume in the right hippocampus, all of which are neuroprotective and can stimulate synaptic plasticity.[71]

A clinical trial had 32 individuals with T2D follow the Paleo diet ad libitum for 12 weeks. They were then randomized to standard care exercise or supervised exercise training. Both groups had significant weight loss and reductions in fat mass. Additionally, the Paleo diet treatment resulted in significant decreases in liver fat and intramyocellular lipid content.[72] Fifty-eight overweight women were assigned to a Paleo or control diet for 24 months. Results showed that the Paleo diet surpassed the control diet with improved insulin sensitivity.[52]

Paleo Diet and Weight Management

Obesity is a significant risk factor for cardiovascular disease and overall mortality. In the general population, obesity increases overall mortality by 250% compared with an ideal body weight.[73] Research has shown that for traditional hunter-gatherer and subsistence farmer populations engaged in increased amounts of physical activity and with limited exposure to highly processed, high-calorie foods, there is little to no evidence of obesity or metabolic disorders.[74] The Physicians Health Study found that men had a 42% lower risk of cardiovascular events and women a 35% lower risk in the group with normal waist to hip ratio compared with the highest category.[75]

With the above-mentioned data on obesity risks, we should assume that most diets leading to a reduction in weight are likely beneficial. The results of a 3-week Paleo diet intervention in 14 healthy patients in Stockholm, Sweden, resulted in an average weight loss of 2.3 kg along with reduced body mass index (BMI), decreased waist circumference, and favorable effects on cardiovascular risk.[76] The journal *Nature* reported a study on 70 obese, postmenopausal women randomized to a Paleo diet versus a Nordic diet. Both groups lost weight, but Paleo excelled at the 6-month mark with lower weight and reduced waist circumference compared with Nordic Nutrition Recommendations diet.[77]

Leptin is a hormone produced by adipose tissue and is involved in fat storage regulation and appetite regulation. The more fat your cells carry, the more leptin will be produced. Obese individuals have higher levels of leptin. Leptin resistance, seen in overweight and obese individuals, is now thought to be a major biological contributor to obesity. Inflammation, increased serum fatty acids, and elevated levels of leptin contribute to leptin resistance. An article published in the *Journal of American College of Cardiology* revealed that increased circulating levels of leptin are an independent risk factor for cardiovascular disease. Additionally, the study further explains that leptin can potentially physically interact with the inflammatory molecule C-reactive protein (CRP), stimulating increased leptin resistance.[78]

There is research to show that following a Paleo diet significantly lowers fasting plasma leptin levels and helps to lower leptin resistance as a result. One mechanism could be due to the diet's ability to regulate inflammation.[79] A clinical trial showed that the Paleo diet was effective in lowering leptin over a 3-month period in participants with T2D.[79]

Caloric deficit is proven to lead to weight loss, but the difficulty is long-term adherence to a calorie-restricted diet. One mechanism of success in people on a higher-fat diet is likely due to increased satiety compared with a high-carbohydrate, low-fat diet.[80] Finally, according to Professor Loren Cordain, protein has a significantly greater thermic effect on food than either fat or carbohydrates, further contributing to energy balance.[81]

The Mediterranean diet is another low-carbohydrate nutritional model that has a similar emphasis on fish and seafood, leafy greens, nuts and legumes, and healthy fats. A 2019 study published data showing that the Mediterranean diet restores liver health and significantly improves body composition in patients with nonalcoholic fatty liver disease (NAFLD). Twenty patients with NAFLD and an average BMI of 30.9 were put on a Mediterranean diet treatment for 16 weeks. Mean body weight, mean waist circumference, and serum transaminase levels were all significantly decreased post intervention, alluding to the potential link between an anti-inflammatory diet and improved body composition and liver function.[82] Comparative studies show that Paleo trumps Mediterranean.

Additionally, weight loss on Paleo is likely to contribute to a reduction of sleep apnea, a metabolic condition independently associated with increased cardiovascular risk.[83]

Paleo and Inflammation

Inflammation is the response of the innate branch of the immune system triggered by noxious stimuli, microbial pathogens, and injury. An acute inflammatory response in the face of infection or injury is a beneficial adaptation. Chronic inflammation is detrimental and a sign that the body is "on fire." Markers of inflammation are linked with most disease states including cardiovascular disease, cancer, and brain disorders. Pharmaceuticals can lower inflammation, but at what cost? For example, prednisone lowers inflammation but led to a 200% increased risk of myocardial infarction in the first 30 days of use.[84] Let us say that the answer is to remove causative inflammatory factors. Diet is an easy place to start.

The REGARDS study of 2000 participants randomized to either a Paleo or Mediterranean diet found significant decreases in inflammation for each group. Mean high-sensitivity CRP (hs-CRP) level was reduced by 31% in those people who adhered to Paleo dietary recommendations the most. Both groups also reduced their oxidative stress levels as measured by an 11% reduction in F_2-isoprostane. Altering inflammation and oxidative balance levels reduces cardiovascular disease (CVD) risk.[85]

A review of in vitro and in vivo studies concluded that a withdrawal of cereal grains from the diet, based on Paleo diet principles, resulted in beneficial effects on health. Cereal grains contain "antinutrients," which the authors point out are compounds such as gluten and lectin. Antinutrients can cause disease by causing a proinflammatory immune response, increasing intestinal permeability and stimulating immune activation.[86]

A pilot study analyzing the effects of a Modified Paleo Diet Intervention (MPDI) on 17 patients with relapsing-remitting multiple sclerosis found improvements to health outcomes. The MDPI group was advised to eat nine cups of vegetables and some fruits and meat protein including organ meat and maintain complete abstinence from products containing gluten, dairy, potatoes, and legumes (beans, lentils, peanuts, soy, etc.). Patients on the MPDI experienced reductions in hs-CRP levels, 25%. Additionally, the MPDI resulted in a decrease of perceived fatigue in patients along with increased mental and physical functioning, all of which could be a result of lower levels of inflammation. Serum vitamin K levels increased significantly with the Paleo diet, which owing to vitamin K's unique effects, could result in lower oxidative stress, reduced inflammation, and decreased cell damage, the authors speculated.[87]

In a study performed on pigs, the group given Paleo foods had an 82% lower CRP than those given cereal-based swine feed. Diastolic blood pressure was 13% lower on Paleo versus a cereal diet.[88]

Studies have shown that the nutrients found on the Paleo diet (such as antioxidants like alpha lipoic acid and polyphenols) can inhibit the key inflammatory NF-KB pathway and decrease inflammation as a result.[89] A study found that a Paleo diet compared with the Western diet has higher intakes of protein and anti-inflammatory long-chain polyunsaturated fatty acids and lower intakes of inflammatory linoleic acid.[90]

Dietary factors associated with increased inflammation include a higher omega-6 to omega-3 fatty acid ratio[91] and a high intake of simple sugars.[92] A Paleo diet, which lowers sugar intake and balances omega fatty acid ratios, helps to improve dietary factors associated with lower inflammation and reduce disease pathology. Conversely, the Westernized diet has been associated with an increased risk for chronic inflammatory diseases such as obesity, diabetes, and inflammatory bowel disease due to an increased intake of dairy, processed meat, refined grains, sugar, and alcohol and a decreased intake of vegetables and fruits.[93]

Omega-3 fatty acids, an essential component of the Paleo diet, have been found to significantly reduce soluble intercellular adhesion molecule type, an inflammatory vascular biomarker and risk factor for cardiovascular diseases.

T2D and cardiovascular disease are linked, and inflammation is thought to play a role in both etiologies. A randomized study assigned patients with T2D to either a low-fat diet or a low-carbohydrate diet treatment group. At 6 months, the low-carbohydrate diet group experienced significant reductions of clinical inflammatory biomarkers along with improvements to glycemic control. Conversely, the low-fat diet group had an increase in markers of inflammation, including CRP, tumor necrosis factor, and interleukin 6.[94]

High white blood cell counts are indicative of systemic inflammation, stress, and disease. White blood cells are a biomarker used to detect inflammation. Results of a randomized, controlled, single-blinded 2-week pilot study with the Paleo diet resulted in lowered white blood cell counts, which is protective against CVD.[49]

Psoriasis is an inflammatory, immune condition. There is evidence to suggest a link between psoriasis and cardiovascular disease along with other disorders. A survey had 1206 patients with psoriasis report their dietary behaviors and motivation for diet change. About 86% of patients reported a need for dietary change to control their psoriasis with the most beneficial effects to skin seen after elimination of gluten, sugar, alcohol, and nightshades. The Paleo diet, Pagano diet, and vegan diet were the top three diets used by patients to manage psoriasis. The Paleo diet restores microbiota health, regulates inflammation, and can help to heal the intestinal lining.[95] All of these are risk factors for cardiovascular events.

Paleo and Congestive Heart Failure

Heart failure (HF) is a common and growing public health problem worldwide. At present, approximately 26 million people are living with HF in the world. In the United States, there were 5.8 million patients with HF in 2012, and this is expected to increase to 8.5 million by 2030.[96] Even with the best pharmacological and nonpharmacological therapies, the treatment of HF remains a challenge, and areas of improvement are available.

Part of the medical dietary dogma is the low-sodium prescription. Certainly, this is true for cardiovascular patients with hypertension and congestive heart failure. The recommendations of the American College of Cardiology are to follow a low-sodium diet for general cardiac health. Sodium limits for patients with moderate to severe congestive heart failure is stated to be less than 1500 mg. Whether this is beneficial is subject to debate, as seen in an article from 2015.[97]

No matter where you sit on the sodium spectrum of recommendations, Paleo nutrition would be considered on the lower side, certainly as compared with modern consumption. However, we should note that the salt trade has been prolific for thousands of years. Paleo people would have found salt by the sea and used it regularly. Paleo does include seafood and sea vegetables that are higher in sodium than other ancestral foods. Sardines and anchovies are also regularly added to a Paleo diet plan and contain significant sodium when packaged in a can or glass container. Nonetheless, Paleo sodium consumption was one-fifth that of our modern average consumption, as documented by Boyd Eaton in the 1980s. Given the standard diet full of processed foods loaded with sodium, this discrepancy is not a surprise.

There are no randomized trials of high-fat versus low-fat with patients with heart failure on mortality. There are no data specifically on Paleo nutrition in the prevention or treatment of heart failure. A 2017 study of 88 patients with heart failure randomized to low-carbohydrate versus a standard diet found that the low-carb group enjoyed better oxygen saturation, as the standard diet group worsened.[98] Rodent data are strongly in favor of high-fat versus low-fat in the prevention and treatment of heart failure. Multiple studies show that rats with HF enjoy longer survival, improved contractile function, and regression of left ventricular hypertrophy when fed a high-fat (60%) diet.[99]

Fish is a food that should be plentiful on a Paleo plate and appears to be beneficial in the prevention and treatment of HF. In 2005, Mozaffarian and colleagues reported a significant benefit to those who consumed fish regularly versus rarely. A total of 4738 adults free of HF were assessed by a food questionnaire. After a 12-year follow-up, fish consumption of 3 to 4 times/wk led to a 31% reduction in HF, compared with intake less than once a month.[100] Many studies have found that fish eaters enjoy lower levels of inflammation and oxidative stress, two findings common in the patient with HF.

Abundant data exist on the benefits of fish oil consumption and HF. Fish oil supplementation is easy and cheap for a randomized trial. The GISSI investigators randomized patients with heart failure to fish oil versus control. The fish oil group had lower mortality and a lower rate of hospital admissions for HF.[101] Fish oil supplementation improved left ventricular ejection fraction and endothelial function and lowered inflammation in patients with HF versus placebo.[102] Fish oil supplementation has been shown to limit the progression of cardiac fibrosis in rodent and cellular models.[103] Fish oil improves mitochondrial function, an achievement that can only be a positive finding for a patient with HF.[104] A 2017 meta-analysis including nine studies found that fish oil improved BNP and LVEF and decreased norepinephrine levels compared with placebo.[96] In summary, any diet plan that excludes seafood consumption is wrong (aside from those with seafood allergy).

Consumption of unprocessed red meat was not found to be a risk factor for HF in a study of over 2000 Swedish women. Processed meat intake was a risk factor.[105] The same outcome was found in a study of over 30,000 men.[106] Personally, I think the quality of processed meat matters. We have to assume that processed meat from pasture-raised animals, using natural preservatives such as sea salt and celery powder, is different from meat from grain-fed cattle and artificial preservatives such as butylated hydroxytoluene, citric acid, corn syrup, sodium nitrite, sodium ascorbate, and sodium benzoate.

Paleo and Atrial Fibrillation

Atrial fibrillation (AF) is a common finding among the elderly in Western societies. Its prevalence increases over age and mounts to 10% to 20% after the age of 80 years.

Its impact on an emotional, mental, and physical level is immense. Fortunately for the people studied in rural Africa, they do not share the same AF burden as Western societies. An epidemiological study on the incidence of atrial fibrillation was conducted in a traditional African population in the rural and impoverished Upper East Region of Ghana. Electrocardiograms were performed on 921 subjects aged 50 years and older. Of 921 participants, only 3 individuals (0.3%) had atrial fibrillation.[107] Likewise, in a rural Tanzanian population of individuals aged 70 years and older, the prevalence of atrial fibrillation was found to be 0.7%. Only 15 of 2232 individuals had AF.[108] The low prevalence of AF in these rural populations can be attributed to a decreased prevalence of established AF risk factors such as obesity, inflammation, insulin resistance, and clearly a lower exposure of environmental pollutants and unhealthy lifestyle behaviors.

Saturated fat consumption does not appear to be a risk factor for AF. In a 2017 paper, substitution of dietary saturated fat in favor of polyunsaturated fatty acids led to an 8% higher risk of atrial fibrillation. This finding was confirmed only in men.[109] Giving women their due respect, a 2015 paper found that women in the highest category of saturated fat intake enjoyed a 15% lower risk of paroxysmal atrial fibrillation.[109]

Omega-3 fatty acids from seafood have long been postulated to have antiarrhythmic properties. Among 3326 US men and women aged ≥65 years and free of AF at baseline, plasma phospholipid levels of eicosapentaenoic acid (EPA), docosapentaenoic acid (DPA), and DHA were measured. Incident AF (789 cases) was prospectively identified from hospital discharge records and study visit electrocardiograms. The relative risk in the top versus the lowest quartile of total n-3 PUFA (EPA + DPA + DHA) levels was 0.71 and of DHA levels, 0.77.[110] Not all data have shown that fish eaters enjoy a lower risk of AF. A 2017 meta-analysis of seven studies found fish consumption not protective for atrial fibrillation.[111] A 2014 study found that fish consumption and atrial fibrillation had a U-shaped curve, with the middle tertile of fish eaters at the lowest risk of AF.[112]

Nut consumption has many proven benefits, one of which is an 18% lower risk of atrial fibrillation in those who ate more than three servings of nuts per week.[113] Egg intake and atrial fibrillation has not been studied as a primary intake, but the Physicians Health Study data did not show statistical differences of AF in those who at two eggs per day versus less than one egg per week.[114]

Paleo and Cerebrovascular Accident

Not many things are more devastating than suffering a stroke. After the fear of cancer, brain disorders are second on the scare scale. There is great news for fish eaters.

In a *JAMA* article from 2001, women in the Nurses' Health Study enjoyed a 52% lower risk of stroke when they ate fish five or more times per week compared with women who rarely ate fish; two to four times per week consumers had a 27% lower stroke risk. These data were adjusted for other confounding factors.[115] Another study found that fish consumption lowers stroke risk from 12% to 19% depending on the type of fish.[116] The Japanese Atherosclerosis Society pushes seafood intake in their dietary guidelines to reduce cardiovascular disease risk.[117]

An analysis study followed 41,020 men aged 29 to 69 years old from Spain for a mean of 13.8 years. After multiple adjustments, unprocessed red meat, processed meat, and total red meat consumption were not correlated with incidence of total stroke or ischemic stroke in either men or women. The hazard ratios for unprocessed red meat and processed meat and risk of total stroke comparing the highest with the lowest quintiles were, respectively, 0.81 and 0.92 in men and 1.21 and 0.81 in women.

A meta-analysis from 2017 in the *Journal of the American Heart Association* found red meat consumption, processed and unprocessed, was linked to higher stroke risk, whereas white meat consumption led to a 13% lower stroke risk.[118]

Dietary cholesterol in multiple studies and a recent meta-analysis of seven trials with over 260,000 participants found no link between dietary cholesterol and stroke risk.[119]

A 2016 meta-analysis included 15 studies and over 476,569 individuals, and 11,074 strokes were included. A higher SFA intake was associated with a reduced overall stroke risk (relative risk [RR] = 0.89 [95% confidence interval (CI), 0.82-0.96]) and fatal stroke risk (RR = 0.75 [95% CI 0.59-0.94]).[120] A Japanese study published in the *American Journal of Clinical Nutrition* on 58,453 men and women found that the group in the highest quintile of saturated fat intake enjoyed a 42% lower ischemic stroke risk compared with the lowest intake of sat fat.[121]

Low-carbohydrate and low-calorie diets have been found to be neuroprotective. On prolonged ischemia, numerous metabolic pathways become activated. Although there are not currently any studies conducted on the Paleo diet and neuroprotection, research has shown that similar low-carbohydrate diets like the ketogenic diet confer protection to neurons.[122]

The Paleo diet provides the nutrients the brain needs. A recent clinical trial by Dr Terry Wahls has shown that the Paleolithic diet along with exercise and electrical stimulation as part of a 12-month multimodal intervention in patients with multiple sclerosis resulted in significant improvements. Patients on this intervention showed improved cognition, increased executive function, and decreased anxiety. Based on statistical analyses, improvements to cognition were more closely linked to the Paleo diet than to the other two interventions, highlighting the potential for this diet to be neuroprotective.[123]

In islands in the south Pacific, a subsistence lifestyle, uninfluenced by Western dietary habits, is still maintained. Tubers, fruit, fish, and coconut are dietary staples. With over 2000 people, there were 125 people between 60 and 96 years old. The frequencies of spontaneous sudden death, exertion-related chest pain, hemiparesis, aphasia, and sudden imbalance were assessed by semistructured interviews. No cases corresponding to stroke, sudden death, or angina pectoris were described by the interviewed subjects. Electrocardiograms were obtained. Stroke and ischemic heart disease appear to be absent in this population.[124]

Paleo and Overall CVD Risk

A unique, metabolically controlled study analyzed the effects of a Paleo diet on nonobese, sedentary healthy participants. They ensured no weight loss by measuring weight each day. The results showed that a Paleo diet reduced blood pressure, decreased total cholesterol and LDL cholesterol, decreased triglycerides, improved arterial distensibility (arterial elasticity), and improved insulin sensitivity and glucose tolerance independent of weight loss in healthy sedentary individuals. All cardiovascular risk factors improved upon a Paleo diet treatment.[125]

There is evidence that a Paleo diet aids in chronic disease prevention by reducing key risk factors of these diseases. A review of preliminary intervention studies elucidated the beneficial impacts of the Paleo diet on cardiovascular risk factors such as weight, waist circumference, CRP, blood pressure, lipid profiles, hbA1C, insulin sensitivity, and glucose tolerance.[126]

Research published in 2019 in the *Journal of the American Heart Association* assigned 22 overweight and obese patients with T2D to a Paleo diet with either standard care exercise recommendations or supervised exercise training for 3 hours per week. The Paleo diet with supervised exercise training had significant reductions in myocardial triglycerides, increased stroke volume, and improved left ventricle remodeling.[127]

A recent report published in 2018 in the *Journal of Clinical Lipidology* concluded that replacing saturated fats with carbohydrates (like previous antisaturated fat recommendations) does not lower the incidence of cardiovascular events.[128]

Recently, a trial of low-carbohydrate diets and coronary artery calcification (CAC), as assessed by computed tomography scans, was published. The authors report that following an animal-based low-carbohydrate diet was not linked to CAC prevalence, incidence, and progression.[129]

The novel Lugawala study, published in 1996, analyzed two Bantu village populations and their diets in rural Tanzania. A total of 618 people lived near a lake and consumed freshwater fish, whereas 645 people lived on a hill and were vegetarians. The two groups had similar genetics and lifestyles, yet their diet varied. The study found that the fish-consuming population had a decreased CVD risk owing to increased omega-3 fatty acids, lower blood pressure, lower cholesterol, reduced Lp(a), lower triglycerides, and lower leptin levels.[130]

A novel article published in the journal *Obesity Reviews* in 2018 highlighted the importance of evaluating data from hunter-gatherer and subsistence farmer populations to reveal evolutionary insights for understanding and treating the chronic diseases we see in industrialized society today. These populations had a diet free from processed, high-calorie foods along with increased levels of physical activity that seemed to correspond to low rates of obesity and chronic disease. Specifically, the authors note the exceptional level of cardiovascular health these groups experienced. In this review of prior research conducted and the authors' own unpublished data from their study of the Hadza, they make the case for why the hunter-gatherer populations should be models for attenuating disease. Their measurements of the Hadza revealed that there was a low prevalence of obesity. They also found the average BMI for both female and male Hadza to be around 20 to 22. Additionally, fasting blood glucose levels in the population were not above 85 mg/dL. As a result, there was little to no hypertension reported in the Hadza population and heart disease was undetectable.[74]

The !Kung are one of the last groups of people on earth to live as the ancient humans did 10,000 years ago. As a group of isolated hunter-gathers, the !Kung have been found to have no evidence of obesity, hypertension, or coronary artery disease. Surprisingly, on analysis, there was no classification of hypertension even in the aging cohort. For example, the average blood pressure for the 70- to 83-year-old age group was 120/67 compared with the control group of 70- to 83-year-olds in London with an average blood pressure of 168/90. The authors speculate that the rare and complete absence of hypertension in the society is because of low salt intake, low adiposity, and lack of mental stress. On further observation and electrocardiogram testing, they found no clinical evidence of coronary heart disease in any of the individuals. Interestingly, this group is known for smoking tobacco regularly. Additionally, serum cholesterol and triglyceride levels were found to be low, which is attributed to diet. The !Kung consume nuts rich in polyunsaturated fats along with wild game, which contain polyunsaturated fat and mild amounts of saturated fat. The low triglyceride levels are also likely due to the low-carbohydrate diet and reduced adiposity. They had adequate levels of iron, B12, and folate. The authors found no qualitative nutritional deficiencies in this population.[131,132]

Evidence reveals that hunter-gatherer societies derived the majority of their energy (roughly 65% of their calories) from animal-based foods. This information is based on the study of over 200 groups on indigenous peoples. Chronic disease is not present in these groups of Paleo people.[133]

Studies have pointed to the antiatherosclerotic properties of long-chain, polyunsaturated fatty acids.[134] Wild game was the main source of protein for hunter-gatherer populations. In his research, S. Boyd Eaton noted the compositional differences between wild game of the Paleo era and the domesticated animals of today. On review, he noted that today's domesticated livestock contain significantly more total fat and over five times less polyunsaturated fat per gram than wild game. Additionally, domesticated animals contain imperceptible amounts of omega-3 fatty acids, whereas the fat of wild game has been found to contain up to 4% of essential omega-3 fatty acids. Boyd concluded that, along with their nutrient profiles, wild, free-ranging animals also contain less calories and more protein per unit of weight further contributing to their health benefits.[5]

An imbalanced ratio of omega-6 to omega-3 fatty acids is correlated with cardiovascular events. Epidemiological studies have shown that our ancestors consumed a ratio of omega-6 to omega-3 of around one. Conversely, it has been found that Americans on a Standard American Diet consume an omega-6 to omega-3 ratio of about 15:1 to 16.7:1.[135] The disproportionate essential fatty acid ratio found with Western diets is highly proinflammatory and significantly associated with an increased risk for chronic diseases such as CVD.[136]

Paleo and Homocysteine

High levels of the amino acid homocysteine are linked to early development of cardiovascular disease. Vitamins B6, B12, and folate are key nutrients for lowering levels of homocysteine, and diminished intake is associated with elevated plasma homocysteine levels. A study of hunter-gatherer bushmen who consumed a diet rich in game meat and natural vegetation like the Stone-Age diet found that this population had adequate folate levels, normal to elevated B12 levels, and elevated B12-binding proteins. Furthermore, the authors concluded that B12 and folate deficiencies we see today would not have existed during the Stone Age. Rather, these essential micronutrient deficiencies are the result of a predominantly cereal-based diet.[137]

A study published in 2006 found that plasma homocysteine levels remain unchanged when participants were placed on an ad-libitum low-carbohydrate diet. This was despite increases in protein overall and the amino acid methionine, a precursor to homocysteine.[138] B6, B12, and folate levels were higher than baseline, 12 weeks after the start of low carbohydrate. Of note, calorie consumption was cut by 30% spontaneously, participants lost weight, improved lipids, and Lp(a) dropped by 11%.

Interestingly, omnivore populations have 30% lower homocysteine compared with vegans and almost triple the B12 levels. Folate levels are not statistically different between groups.[139]

Paleo and the Gut/Heart Connection

Over the last decade, we have witnessed an explosion of scientific literature about the gut-heart connection. Hundreds of articles document how gut bacteria influence cardiovascular health, including hypertension, lipids, and heart failure. In addition to awareness about gut bacteria, known as the microbiome, the awareness of intestinal permeability is pervasive in the medical community. Often referred to as Leaky Gut, intestinal hyperpermeability is linked to cardiovascular risk. I have often referred to this as the *Leaky Gut, Leaky Heart* connection.

Novel markers of intestinal permeability include zonulin, zonulin antibodies, antibodies to actin, and antibodies to lipopolysaccharide (LPS). Zonulin is a protein mainly found in the gastrointestinal lining that is responsible for tight junction permeability in the small intestine. Elevations of zonulin are linked to cardiovascular risk. A 2016 study found that plasma zonulin levels of patients with CAD were almost double that of age-matched controls.[140] Another study analyzed zonulin in centenarians versus people with acute myocardial infarction and their age-matched controls. Levels of zonulin were 4.0, 7.6, and 5.2 pg/mL respectively.[141] Another novel marker of intestinal hyperpermeability is the antiactin antibody. Actin is a major component of the sarcomere subunit of muscle tissue. Back in 2003, a study showed that antiactin antibodies were related to CIMT.[142] The data on serum endotoxemia as measured by LPS are extensive. LPS is found on the outside of the cell wall in gram-negative bacteria. Intestinal hyperpermeability is not the only source of LPS endotoxemia. The oral cavity is ripe with opportunity for bacterial translocation into the bloodstream,[143] and oral bacteria are found in samples of coronary artery plaque.[144]

It is now widely accepted that one of the mechanisms for how the Paleo diet benefits health is through its advantageous effects on gut health via elimination of wheat and other sources of grains. Gluten is a small protein found in grains such as wheat, barley, and rye. Gluten consumption is the cause of clinical manifestations of celiac disease, a condition linked to increased cardiovascular risk. Scientific evidence has shown that the consumption of wheat along with other gluten-containing cereal grains has detrimental impacts on intestinal permeability and is associated with chronic inflammation and autoimmune pathologies.[86]

The medical community appears to be missing gluten as a risk factor for CAD in millions of people with nonceliac gluten sensitivity.[145]

A novel article published by Canadian researcher Ian Spreadbury suggests that obesity and other Western diseases arise from dietary inflammation as a result of inflammatory microbes. He claims the health of your gut and your body all comes down to the density of the carbohydrates you are eating. The Western diet rich in flour, sugar, and processed foods contains acellular carbohydrates, which have a high carbohydrate density and are so processed that they do not contain any intact living cells. Carbohydrate density is the percent of food mass that is carbohydrate minus the fiber. In nature, it is not normal for the foods we eat to have a high carbohydrate density. The theory is that our gut never evolved to process these highly dense carbohydrate; therefore, microbial dysbiosis and production of LPS results. The article discusses ancestral diets, free from these highly processed carbohydrates, as the best tool to reverse and prevent disease. In fact, in his review of research, he concluded that this is why the Paleo diet (removal of grains and processed foods) has the most beneficial metabolic effects and often the most significant reductions in weight. Tubers, fruits, and plants (carbohydrate sources on Paleo diet) are cellular foods that are less dense and have the bulk of their weight from water. These living cell foods contain their carbohydrates in an inner storage unit that is not accessed until digestive processes act on it. Changing the diet to one that contains cellular carbohydrates helps to reduce inflammation of the gut, decrease leptin resistance, and improve metabolic markers.[146]

Dietary factors that promote intestinal permeability and the resultant inflammatory reactions are associated with the onset of metabolic diseases such as cardiovascular disease and T2D.[147] A randomized trial studied 18 people on the Paleo diet versus 14 people on the Dutch diet. One of the outcome measures was intestinal permeability (IP) based on the lactulose:mannitol urinary ratio. The Paleo group saw an improvement in IP, whereas the Dutch group actually had worse numbers at 2-week follow-up.[49]

The Paleo diet is rich in key preventative nutrients such as omega-3 fats, and it also eliminates harmful foodstuffs including refined sugar and processed additives that can wreak havoc on gut lining integrity. For example, a novel study showed that the consumption of 30% fructose solution for 8 weeks in a mouse model resulted in a loss of key tight junction proteins (occludin and zonula occludens) and an increase in bacterial endotoxin in the portal vein.[148] Food additives are also known to be causative of intestinal hyperpermeability and autoimmune disease.[149]

The most important factor for prevention of gut hyperpermeability appears to be the gut microbiome. The Hadza are one of the last remaining hunter-gatherer populations in Africa. This group of hunter-gatherers has been found to have a high level of bacterial diversity, a marker of health.[150] Higher microbial diversity has also been found in hunter-gatherer populations such as the Bantu compared with Westernized, industrialized societies.[151] Conversely, there has been a continual reduction in the microbial diversity of Western populations. It is now established that microbial diversity is disappearing in humans in Westernized countries. There is a dire need to preserve our ancestral microbiome. Urbanization and the shift to the Westernized diet have vastly altered the microbial ecology of humans, and it could have significant biomedical effects.[152] Comparisons of the fecal microbiota of children from Europe with those from rural Africa revealed higher levels of microbial diversity in the African children. The authors speculate that the reduction in microbial diversity is due to an increased amount of sugar and calorically dense foods found on a Western diet.[153]

One review reveals the main question raised by ancestral microbiome studies: *"is the westernized world losing crucial components of the gut microbiome irreversibly?"* The article points out that, although diet changes can help to restore microbial health, there are established dietary changes in industrialized society along with xenobiotics that could have lasting and potentially irreversible effects including a significant loss of microbial diversity.[152]

A novel experiment conducted in 2015 swapped the diets of urbanized African Americans with rural South Americans for 2 weeks. The diet changes revealed corresponding alterations in microbiome and mucosal biomarkers of colon cancer risk. These Westernized food changes in rural South Americans were associated with significant mucosal inflammation and cell proliferation, both of which are carcinogenic risk factors. Mucosal inflammation leads to gut barrier dysfunction and immune activation.[154]

An article published in 2018 reported that increased microbial diversity in women has been correlated with lower arterial stiffness.[177]

New research demonstrates that probiotic and prebiotic supplementation are beneficial in healing the leaky gut.[155] Omega-3 fish oil supplementation appears to protect the intestinal lining from increased permeability.[156]

Trimethylamine-N-oxide, or TMAO, is a gut microbial metabolite. TMAO is linked to an increased risk of coronary artery disease and can accelerate atherosclerosis. Increased

TMAO levels have been associated with an increased risk for all-cause mortality.[178] Specific types of high-TMAO-producing bacterial strains have been found to advance atherosclerosis in mice.[179] In a recent small study, women were randomized to either a Paleo diet or the Australian Guide to Healthy Eating (AGHE) diet for 4 weeks. Resistant starch (RS), which the Paleo diet is low in, is thought to reduce TMAO concentrations. Animal meat, which is found in increased amounts on the Paleo diet, is thought to raise TMAO. The results showed that despite a low level of RS and a high intake of animal protein on the Paleo diet, there was no significant difference in TMAO concentrations between the two diets.[180]

The way to control TMAO is to heal the gut microbiota. Studies have shown that RS diets do not actually improve TMAO levels.[181] Studies show that positively altering the gut microbiota could play a role in lowering TMAO concentrations and have cardioprotective effects. The gut microbiome, influenced by the diet, can play a significant role in cardiovascular disease pathogenesis. The composition of gut flora is determined by diet. A Paleo diet, which is rich in fiber and polyphenols, may be protective. Conversely, a Western diet is low in fiber and high in sugar and saturated fat and could play a role in increasing microbiota dysregulation, which is linked with TMAO production.[182] It is speculated that modulating TMAO levels can be achieved through positively altering intestinal bacteria.[183] Diet and supplementation are two good options for improving bacterial dysbiosis. For example, production of TMAO can be altered by probiotic supplementation.[184] Therefore, recommendations to alter diet and administer probiotic supplementation could aid in the prevention and treatment of atherosclerotic heart disease.[185]

Another mechanism for controlling TMAO activity is through flavin monooxygenase (FMO) regulation. The essential omega-3 fatty acid DHA has been found to increase metabolism of TMAO concentrations through FMO upregulation.[186]

Paleo and Dental Health

There is an established link between periodontal disease, atherosclerosis, and cardiovascular disease.[157] An analysis of the oral, gut and atherosclerotic plaques of 15 patients revealed that the pattern of bacterial phylotypes found in the mouth and gut of patients significantly correlated to those found in the arterial plaques of the same patients. These results elucidate the connection between oral, gut, and cardiovascular health.[157] Bacteria in both the oral cavity and the gut have been linked to atherogenic development.[157]

A study of the oral microbiomes of hunter-gatherers in the Philippines revealed greater oral microbial diversity including an excess of species often thought to be associated with oral disease. This species excess is likely a result of their diet. Yet, this hunter-gatherer population had better oral health and fewer dental caries compared with other traditional farming populations.[158]

The constituents of a Paleo-like diet such as low carbohydrates, increased omega-3 fatty acids, increased fiber, increased antioxidants, and increased vitamin C and vitamin D have been found to be preventative of gingival and periodontal inflammation because of the abilities of these nutrients to reduce inflammatory markers.

A study of the dental health of the Guaraní Indians of the State of Rio de Janeiro found that nearly 60% of the population experienced no periodontal disease. The Guarani Indians are the largest nomadic indigenous tribe in Brazil. Currently, their diet remains a mix of cultured and industrialized foods.[187]

Paleo Versus Keto

Over the last few years, a ketogenic diet has become popular as a way to optimize health. A keto diet is very high in fat, moderate in protein, and very low in carbohydrate. Keto allows for many dairy foods, while drastically limiting carbohydrates like fruit and potatoes, two items on our Paleolithic menu.

Ketosis is a natural state for the body when it is almost completely fueled by fat. This is normal during fasting, or when a person is on a very-low-carbohydrate diet. This is often called the Keto diet. Our Paleo ancestors would have spent significant time fasting, as finding food in prehistoric times may not have been that easy. The Keto diet looks for adherents to spend most of the time in ketosis.

The "keto" in the word ketosis comes from "ketones," the name of small fuel molecules in the body. This is an alternative fuel, produced from fat we eat and used when blood sugar (glucose) is in short supply. These ketones are produced when you eat very few carbs (the main source of blood sugar) and only moderate amounts of protein (excess protein is converted to blood sugar). Under these circumstances, fat is converted in the liver to ketones that then enter the bloodstream. Ketones are used as fuel by cells in the body, just like glucose. They can even be used by the brain.

Given that ketones easily cross the blood-brain barrier and are used for energy by the brain, many patients have experienced success for conditions such as epilepsy, cognitive disorders, and movement disorders like Parkinson disease. Most research on ketogenic diets have been in populations with these conditions and in other cohorts with advanced disease. The data on "Keto for Cardiac" is a limited but burgeoning area of research. No direct comparison has been done on Paleo versus Keto.

Keto Proof

Cholesterol

In 2006, a study was reported on 66 obese participants put on a carbohydrate restriction to under 20 g/d. The group had dramatic improvements in total cholesterol, LDL-C, and raised HDL-C.[159] One of the likely reasons is that ketosis leads to very low insulin. It is insulin that is strongly linked to LDL production,[160] and as insulin levels go up, so does cardiovascular risk.[161] A 2016 *British Journal of Nutrition* meta-analysis of studies looking at low carb versus low fat found that lipid parameters on low carbohydrate bested low fat.[162]

Inflammation

A 2008 study reported in the journal *Lipids* found that reduction in markers of inflammation were greater in the group assigned to a very-low-carbohydrate diet versus a low-fat diet.[163] A review on the anti-inflammatory effects of a ketogenic diet can be found in a 2018 article published in the journal *Antioxidants*.[164]

Blood Pressure

Very-low-carb dieting bested low fat for diastolic blood pressure reduction in a 2013 publication.[165] Very-low-carb nutrition led to an average drop in systolic pressure of 10 mm Hg in a 3-month period in a 2016 publication.[166]

Weight loss

A study randomized 58 obese people to two groups: one to a ketogenic diet and the other to a hypocaloric diet. After 6 months, weight loss occurred in both groups, but it was greater in the ketogenic diet group.[167] Other trials on low-carbohydrate dieting found similar results regarding weight loss.[168]

Blood Sugar

A 2014 study over a 24-week period divided 93 participants into a low-carbohydrate (under 50 g/d) and an energy-matched high-carbohydrate diet. Both groups adhered to their diets well. Both groups lost equal amounts of weight. Low carb had a significantly greater improvement in HbA1C by 27%.[169] Low-carbohydrate dieting led 14 obese subjects to lower blood glucose and improve insulin sensitivity in a 2013 study.[170]

Intermittent Fasting

One could imagine that food was not always plentiful in Paleolithic times. Obviously, there was not a grocery store on every corner with imported fruit and veggies from all over the world and a larger frozen food section. Major religions all discuss the virtues of fasting for health and wellness, in addition to any spiritual benefits. There are many different types of fasts, and their descriptions, benefits, and risks are beyond the scope of this chapter. However, I would like to highlight fasting as a Paleolithic behavior that has

evidence-based benefits. Surely, more data will come in the near future.

The oldest article in Pubmed.gov is from 1946. The authors studied rodents and found that intermittent fasting led to increased longevity.[171]

A review by Tinsley in 2015 found that intermittent fasting was linked to weight reduction, decreased fat mass, lower total cholesterol, and lower triglycerides.[172]

Cherif and colleagues found that intermittent fasting, along with burst aerobic activity, increased HDL-C.[173]

A 2019 study of a Muslim group who practiced intermittent fasting in observance of Ramadan found lower inflammation, weight loss, and improved lipid profiles at the end of the 30-day period.[174]

Conclusion

At this point of the chapter, my hope is that the reader is convinced that following the nutritional plan of our ancestors makes common sense and I have provided evidence to support Mother Nature. But the obvious next question is, how can one eat this ancestral diet in the 21st century? Sadly, following a Paleo diet in concordance with how our ancestors lived is close to impossible. Modern humans do not have easy access to wild game, wild seafood, and plant-based foods that grew purely from nature on a planet free from environmental contaminants. So now what?

We do the best we can in a modern society. The more you follow the Paleo food plan, the better and longer you will live.

In summary, the diet recommended by this author consists of:

1. Vegetables
2. Wild seafood
3. Pastured animal meat including organ cuts
4. Pastured eggs
5. Nuts and seeds
6. Avocado, coconut, and olives
7. Seasonal fruit
8. Potatoes
9. Herbs and spices
10. Occasional raw dairy

All organic, non-GMO, and pesticide-free. Occasional raw dairy from pastured animals.

Go Paleo! Everything else is just a fad.

References

1. https://www.sevencountriesstudy.com/.
2. Medicine: The Fat of the Land. *Time.* 1961;77(3):48. 8p.
3. Yudkin J. Diet and coronary thrombosis. Hypothesis and fact. *Lancet.* 1957;273:155-162.
4. Voegtlin WL. *The Stone Age Diet.* New York: Vantage Press; 1975.
5. Eaton SB, Konner M. Paleolithic nutrition. A consideration of its nature and current implications. *N Engl J Med.* 1985;312(5): 283-289.

6. Loren C, Miller JB, Eaton SB, Mann N, Holt SHA, Speth JD. Plant-animal subsistence ratios and macronutrient energy estimations in worldwide hunter-gatherer diets. *Am J Clin Nutr.* 2000;71(3):682-692. doi:10.1093/ajcn/71.3.682.
7. Cordain L, Watkins BA, Florant GL, Kelher M, Rogers L, Li Y. Fatty acid analysis of wild ruminant tissues: evolutionary implications for reducing diet-related chronic disease. *Eur J Of Clin Nutr.* 2002;56:181.

8. Lindeberg S, Cordain L, Boyd Eaton S. Biological and clinical potential of a palaeolithic diet. *J Nutr Environ Med*. 2003;13(3):149-160. doi:10.1080/13590840310001619397.

9. Rose G. Sick individuals and sick populations. *Int J Epidemiol*. 2001;30(3):427-432. doi:10.1093/ije/30.3.427.

10. Whalen KA, Judd S, McCullough ML, Flanders WD, Hartman TJ, Bostick RM. Paleolithic and mediterranean diet pattern scores are inversely associated with all-cause and cause-specific mortality in adults. *J Nutr*. 2017;147(4):612-620. doi:10.3945/jn.116.241919.

11. Ramsden CE, Zamora D, Majchrzak-Hong S, et al. Re-evaluation of the traditional diet-heart hypothesis: analysis of recovered data from Minnesota Coronary Experiment (1968-73). *BMJ*. 2016;353:i1246. Published 2016 April 12. doi:10.1136/bmj.i1246.

12. de Souza RJ, Mente A, Maroleanu A, et al. Intake of saturated and trans unsaturated fatty acids and risk of all cause mortality, cardiovascular disease, and type 2 diabetes: systematic review and meta-analysis of observational studies. *BMJ*. 2015;351:h3978. doi:10.1136/bmj.h3978.

13. Fairfield K. Review: replacing dietary saturated fatty acids with n-6 polyunsaturated fatty acids does not reduce mortality. *Ann Intern Med*. 2013;158:JC6. doi:10.7326/0003-4819-158-10-201305210-02006.

14. Larsson SC, Orsini N. Red meat and processed meat consumption and all-cause mortality: a meta-analysis. *Am J Epidemiol*. 2014;179(3):282-289. doi:10.1093/aje/kwt261. Epub 2013 October 22.

15. Micha R, Wallace SK, Mozaffarian D. Red and processed meat consumption and risk of incident coronary heart disease, stroke, and diabetes mellitus: a systematic review and meta-analysis. *Circulation*. 2010;121(21):2271-2283. doi:10.1161/CIRCULATIONAHA.109.924977. Epub 2010 May 17.

16. Zhao LG, Sun JW, Yang Y, Ma X, Wang YY, Xiang YB. Fish consumption and all-cause mortality: a meta-analysis of cohort studies. *Eur J Clin Nutr*. 2016;70(2):155-161. doi:10.1038/ejcn.2015.72. Epub 2015 May 13.

17. Zhang Y, Zhuang P, He W, et al. Association of fish and long-chain omega-3 fatty acids intakes with total and cause-specific mortality: prospective analysis of 421 309 individuals. *J Intern Med*. 2018;284(4):399-417. doi:10.1111/joim.12786. Epub 2018 July 17.

18. Orlich MJ, Fraser GE. Vegetarian diets in the Adventist Health Study 2: a review of initial published findings. *Am J Clin Nutr*. 2014;100 suppl 1(1):353S-358S. doi:10.3945/ajcn.113.071233.

19. Farvid M, Malekshah A, Pourshams A, et al. Dietary protein sources and all-cause and cause-specific mortality: the Golestan Cohort Study in Iran. *Am J Prev Med*. 2017;52(2):237-248. doi:10.1016/j.amepre.2016.10.041.

20. Nicholas RF, Sainsbury A, Caterson ID, Markovic TP. Egg consumption and human cardio-metabolic health in people with and without diabetes. *Nutrients*. 2015;7(9):7399-7420.

21. Sacks FM, Lichtenstein AH, Wu JHY, et al. Dietary fats and cardiovascular disease: a presidential advisory from the American Heart Association. *Circulation*. 2017;136:e1-e23.

22. Ismail SR, Maarof SK, Siedar Ali S, Ali A, Systematic review of palm oil consumption and the risk of cardiovascular disease. *PLoS One*. 2018;13(2):e0193533.

23. Eslamparast T, Sharafkhah M, Poustchi H, et al. Nut consumption and total and cause-specific mortality: results from the Golestan Cohort Study. *Int J Epidemiol*. 2017;46(1):75-85.

24. Luu HN, Blot WJ, Xiang YB, et al. Prospective evaluation of the association of nut/peanut consumption with total and cause-specific mortality. *JAMA Intern Med*. 2015;175(5):755-766.

25. Mackenbach JP. The origins of human disease: a short story on "where diseases come from", *J Epidemiol Community Health*. 2006. 60(1):81-86.

26. Tomljenović A. Effects of internal and external environment on health and well-being: from cell to society. *Coll Antropol*. 2014;38(1):367-372.

27. Jönsson T. *Healthy Satiety Effects of Paleolithic Diet on Satiety and Risk factors for Cardiovascular disease*. Sweden: Lund University; 2007.

28. O'Keefe JH, Vogel R, Lavie C, Cordain L. Exercise like a hunter-gatherer: a prescription for organic physical fitness. *Prog Cardiovasc Dis*. 2011;53(6):471-479.

29. Coker RH, Coker MS, Bartlett L, et al. The energy requirements and metabolic benefits of wilderness hunting in Alaska, *Physiol Rep*. 2018, 6(21):e13925.

30. Cheng E, Um CY, Prizment A, Lazovich D, Bostick RM. Associations of evolutionary-concordance diet, Mediterranean diet and evolutionary-concordance lifestyle pattern scores with all-cause and cause-specific mortality. *Br J Nutr*. 2018:1-10.

31. Draper HH. The aboriginal Eskimo diet in modern perspective. *Am Anthropol*. 1977;79(2):309-316.

32. Milton K. Hunter-gatherer diets—a different perspective. *Am J Clin Nutr*. 2000;71(3):665-667.

33. Walker AR, Walker BF, Adam F. Nutrition, diet, physical activity, smoking, and longevity: from primitive hunter-gatherer to present passive consumer–how far can we go? *Nutrition*. 2003;19(2):169-173.

34. O'Connor LE, Kim JE, Campbell WW. Total red meat intake of ≥0.5 servings/d does not negatively influence cardiovascular disease risk factors: a systemically searched meta-analysis of randomized controlled trials. *Am J Clin Nutr*. 2017;105(1):57-69.

35. Sharman MJ, Gómez AL, Kraemer WJ, Volek JS. Very low-carbohydrate and low-fat diets affect fasting lipids and postprandial lipemia differently in overweight men. *J Nutr*. 2004, 134(4):880-885.

36. Lanas F, Avezum A, Bautista LE, et al; INTERHEART Investigators in Latin America. Risk factors for acute myocardial infarction in Latin America: the INTERHEART Latin American study. *Circulation*. 2007;115(9):1067-1074.

37. Shai I, David Spence J, Schwarzfuchs D, et al. Dietary intervention to reverse carotid atherosclerosis. *Circulation*. 2010;121:1200-1208.

38. Newcombe CL. *The Nutritional Value of Sea Foods*. Richmond: William & Mary ScholarWorks; 1944.

39. Manninen SM, Lankinen MA, de Mello VD, Laaksonen DE, Schwab US, Erkkilä AT. Intake of fatty fish alters the size and the concentration of lipid components of HDL particles and camelina sativa oil decreases IDL particle concentration in subjects with impaired glucose metabolism. *Mol Nutr Food Res*. 2018;62(10):e1701042.

40. Erkkilä AT, Schwab US, Lehto S, et al. Effect of fatty and lean fish intake on lipoprotein subclasses in subjects with coronary heart disease: a controlled trial. *J Clin Lipidol*. 2014;8(1):126-133.

41. Prior IA, Davidson F, Salmond CE, Czochanska Z. Cholesterol, coconuts, and diet on Polynesian atolls: a natural experiment: the Pukapuka and Tokelau Island studies. *Am J Clin Nutr*. 1981;34(8):1552-1561.

42. Khaw KT, Sharp SJ, Finikarides L, et al. Randomised trial of coconut oil, olive oil or butter on blood lipids and other cardiovascular risk factors in healthy men and women. *BMJ Open*. 2018;8(3):e020167.

43. Chinwong S, Chinwong D, Mangklabruks A. Daily consumption of virgin coconut oil increases high-density lipoprotein cholesterol levels in healthy volunteers: a randomized crossover trial. *Evid Based Complement Alternat Med*. 2017;2017:7251562.

44. Harris M, Hutchins A, Fryda L. The impact of virgin coconut oil and high-oleic safflower oil on body composition, lipids, and inflammatory markers in postmenopausal women. *J Med Food*. 2017;20(4):345-351.

45. Dreon DM, Fernstrom HA, Campos H, Blanche P, Williams PT, Krauss RM. Change in dietary saturated fat intake is correlated with change in mass of large low-density-lipoprotein particles in men. *Am J Clin Nutr*. 1998;67(5):828-836.

46. Dreon DM, Fernstrom HA, Miller B, Krauss RM. Low-density lipoprotein subclass patterns and lipoprotein response to a reduced-fat diet in men. *FASEB J*. 1994;8(1):121-126.

47. Dreon DM, Fernstrom HA, Williams PT, Krauss RM. Reduced LDL particle size in children consuming a very-low-fat diet is related to parental LDL-subclass patterns. *Am J Clin Nutr*. 2000;71(6):1611-1616.

48. Dreon DM, Fernstrom HA, Williams PT, Krauss RM. A very low-fat diet is not associated with improved lipoprotein profiles in men with a predominance of large, low-density lipoproteins. *Am J Clin Nutr*. 1999;69(3):411-418.

49. Boers I, Muskiet AJ, Berkelaar E, et al. Favourable effects of consuming a Palaeolithic-type diet on characteristics of the metabolic syndrome: a randomized controlled pilot-study. *Lipids Health Dis*. 2014;13:160.

50. Masharani U, Sherchan P, Schloetter M, et al. Metabolic and physiologic effects from consuming a hunter-gatherer (Paleolithic)-type diet in type 2 diabetes. *Eur J Clin Nutr*. 2015;69:944-948.

51. Jönsson T, Granfeldt Y, Ahrén B, et al. Beneficial effects of a Paleolithic diet on cardiovascular risk factors in type 2 diabetes: a randomized cross-over pilot study. *Cardiovasc Diabetol*. 2009;8:35.

52. Blomquist C, Chorell E, Ryberg M, et al. Decreased lipogenesis-promoting factors in adipose tissue in postmenopausal women with overweight on a Paleolithic-type diet. *Eur J Nutr*, 2018;57(8):2877-2886.

53. Sebastian A, Cordain L, Frassetto L, Banerjee T, Morris RC. Postulating the major environmental condition resulting in the expression of essential hypertension and its associated cardiovascular diseases: dietary imprudence in daily selection of foods in respect of their potassium and sodium content resulting in oxidative stress-induced dysfunction of the vascular endothelium, vascular smooth muscle, and perivascular tissues. *Med Hypotheses*. 2018;119:110-119.

54. Denton D, Weisinger R, Mundy NI, et al. The effect of increased salt intake on blood pressure of chimpanzees. *Nat Med*. 1995;1(10):1009-1016.

55. Lee HA, Park H. Diet-related risk factors for incident hypertension during an 11-year follow-up: the Korean Genome Epidemiology Study. *Nutrients*. 2018;10(8). pii:E1077.

56. Chen X, Zou S, Wu X, et al. Dietary features and blood pressure among 18-88-year-old residents in an Island population in China. *J Nutr Health Aging*. 2016;20(2):107-113.

57. Yang B, Shi MQ, Li ZH, Yang JJ, Li D. Fish, long-chain n-3 PUFA and incidence of elevated blood pressure: a meta-analysis of prospective cohort studies. *Nutrients*. 2016;8(1). pii:E58.

58. Zurbau A, Jenkins AL, Jovanovski E, et al. Acute effect of equicaloric meals varying in glycemic index and glycemic load on arterial stiffness and glycemia in healthy adults: a randomized crossover trial. *Eur J Clin Nutr*. 2019;73(1):79-85.

59. Keogh JB, Brinkworth GD, Noakes M, et al. Effects of weight loss from a very-low-carbohydrate diet on endothelial function and markers of cardiovascular disease risk in subjects with abdominal obesity. *Am J Clin Nutr*. 2008;87(3):567-576.

60. O'Keefe JH, Gheewala NM, O'Keefe JO. Dietary strategies for improving post-prandial glucose, lipids, inflammation, and cardiovascular health. *J Am Coll Cardiol*. 2008;51(3):249-255.

61. Parr EB, Devlin BL, Callahan MJ, et al. Effects of providing high-fat versus high-carbohydrate meals on daily and postprandial physical activity and glucose patterns: a randomised controlled trial. *Nutrients*. 2018;10(5):557.

62. Klonoff DC. The beneficial effects of a Paleolithic diet on type 2 diabetes and other risk factors for cardiovascular disease. *J Diabetes Sci Technol*. 2009;3(6):1229-1232.

63. O'Dea K. Westernisation, insulin resistance and diabetes in Australian Aborigines. *Med J Aust*. 1991;155(4), 258-264.

64. O'Dea K, Spargo RM, Akerman K. The effect of transition from traditional to urban life-style on the insulin secretory response in Australian Aborigines. *Diabetes Care*. 1980;3(1):31-37.

65. O'Dea K, Spargo RM. Metabolic adaptation to a low carbohydrate-high protein ("traditional") diet in Australian Aborigines. *Diabetologia*. 1982;23(6):494-498.

66. Lindgärde F, Widén I, Gebb M, Ahrén B. Traditional versus agricultural lifestyle among Shuar women of the Ecuadorian Amazon: effects on leptin levels. *Metabolism*. 2004;53(10):1355-1358.

67. Jönsson T, Granfeldt Y, Erlanson-Albertsson C, Ahrén B, Lindeberg S. A Paleolithic diet is more satiating per calorie than a Mediterranean-like diet in individuals with ischemic heart disease. *Nutr Metab (Lond)*. 2010;7:85.

68. Katsiki N, Mikhailidis DP, Banach M. Leptin, cardiovascular diseases and type 2 diabetes mellitus. *Acta Pharmacol Sin*. 2018;39(7):1176-1188.

69. Manheimer EW, van Zuuren EJ, Fedorowicz Z, Pijl H. Paleolithic nutrition for metabolic syndrome: systematic review and meta-analysis. *Am J Clin Nutr*. 2015;102(4):922-932.

70. Melnik BC, John SM, Schmitz G. Over-stimulation of insulin/IGF-1 signaling by western diet may promote diseases of civilization: lessons learnt from laron syndrome. *Nutr Metab (Lond)*. 2011;8:41.

71. Stomby A, Otten J, Ryberg M, Nyberg L, Olsson T, Boraxbekk CJ. A Paleolithic diet with and without combined aerobic and resistance exercise increases functional brain responses and hippocampal volume in subjects with type 2 diabetes. *Front Aging Neurosci*. 2017;9:391.

72. Otten J, Stomby A, Waling M, et al. A heterogeneous response of liver and skeletal muscle fat to the combination of a Paleolithic diet and exercise in obese individuals with type 2 diabetes: a randomised controlled trial. *Diabetologia*. 2018;61(7):1548-1559.

73. Berrington de Gonzalez A, Hartge P, Cerhan JR, Flint AJ. Body-mass index and mortality among 1.46 million white adults. *N Engl J Med*. 2010;363(23):2211-2219.

74. Pontzer H, Wood BM, Raichlen DA. Hunter-gatherers as models in public health. *Obes Rev*. 2018;19, 24-35.

75. Colombo MG, Meisinger C, Amann U, et al. Association of obesity and long-term mortality in patients with acute myocardial infarction with and without diabetes mellitus: results from the MONICA/KORA myocardial infarction registry. *Cardiovasc Diabetol*. 2015;14:24.

76. Österdahl M, Kocturk T, Koochek A, Wändell PE. Effects of a short-term intervention with a Paleolithic diet in healthy volunteers. *Eur J Clin Nutr*. 2008;62:682-685.

77. Mellberg C, Sandberg S, Ryberg M, et al. Long-term effects of a Paleolithic-type diet in obese postmenopausal women: a 2-year randomized trial. *Eur J Clin Nutr*. 2014;68:350-357.

78. Martin SS, Qasim A, Reilly MP. Leptin resistance: a possible interface of inflammation and metabolism in obesity-related cardiovascular disease. *J Am Coll Cardiol*. 2008;52(15):1201-1210.

79. Fontes-Villalba M, Lindeberg S, Granfeldt Y, et al. Palaeolithic diet decreases fasting plasma leptin concentrations more than a diabetes diet in patients with type 2 diabetes: a randomised cross-over trial. *Cardiovasc Diabetol*. 2016;15:80.

80. O'Keefe JH Jr, Cordain L. Cardiovascular disease resulting from a diet and lifestyle at odds with our Paleolithic genome: how to become a 21st-century hunter-gatherer. *Mayo Clin Proc*. 2004;79(1):101-108.

81. Cordain L. The nutritional characteristics of a contemporary diet based upon paleolithic food groups. *JANA*. 2002;5(3).

82. Biolato M, Manca F, Marrone G, et al. Intestinal permeability after Mediterranean diet and low-fat diet in non-alcoholic fatty liver disease. *World J Gastroenterol*. 2019;25(4):509-520.

83. Porto F, Sakamoto YS, Salles C. Association between obstructive sleep apnea and myocardial infarction: a systematic review. *Arq Bras Cardiol*. 2017;108(4):361-369.

84. Varas-Lorenzo C, Rodriguez LA, Maguire A, et al. Use of oral corticosteroids and the risk of acute myocardial infarction. *Atherosclerosis*. 2007;192(2):376-383.

85. Whalen KA, McCullough ML, Flanders WD, et al. Paleolithic and Mediterranean diet pattern scores are inversely associated with biomarkers of inflammation and oxidative balance in adults. *J Nutr*. 2016;146(6):1217-1226.

86. de Punder K, Pruimboom L. The dietary intake of wheat and other cereal grains and their role in inflammation. *Nutrients*. 2013;5(3):771-787.

87. Irish AK, Erickson CM, Wahls TL, Snetselaar LG, Darling WG. Randomized control trial evaluation of a modified Paleolithic dietary intervention in the treatment of relapsing-remitting multiple sclerosis: a pilot study. *Degener Neurol Neuromuscul Dis*. 2017;7:1-18.

88. Jönsson T, Ahrén B, Pacini G, et al. A Paleolithic diet confers higher insulin sensitivity, lower C-reactive protein and lower blood pressure than a cereal-based diet in domestic pigs. *Nutr Metab (Lond)*. 2006;3:39.

89. Nam NH. Naturally occurring NF-kappaB inhibitors. *Mini Rev Med Chem*. 2006;6(8):945-951.

90. Kuipers RS, Luxwolda MF, Dijck-Brouwer DA, et al. Estimated macronutrient and fatty acid intakes from an East African Paleolithic diet. *Br J Nutr*. 2010;104(11):1666-1687.

91. Shelton RC, Miller AH. Eating ourselves to death (and despair): the contribution of adiposity and inflammation to depression. *Prog Neurobiol*. 2010;91(4):275-299.

92. Brown CM, Dulloo AG, Montani JP. Sugary drinks in the pathogenesis of obesity and cardiovascular diseases. *Int J Obes (Lond)*. 2008;32(suppl 6):S28-S34.

93. Statovci D, Aguilera M, MacSharry J, Melgar S. The impact of western diet and nutrients on the microbiota and immune response at mucosal interfaces. *Front Immunol.* 2017;8:838.

94. Jonasson L, Guldbrand H, Lundberg AK, Nystrom FH. Advice to follow a low-carbohydrate diet has a favourable impact on low-grade inflammation in type 2 diabetes compared with advice to follow a low-fat diet. *Ann Med.* 2014;46(3):182-187.

95. Afifi L, Danesh MJ, Lee KM, et al. Dietary behaviors in psoriasis: patient-reported outcomes from a U.S. National Survey. *Dermatol Ther (Heidelb).* 2017;7(2):227-242.

96. Wang C, Xiong B, Huang J. The role of omega-3 polyunsaturated fatty acids in heart failure: a meta-analysis of randomised controlled trials. *Nutrients.* 2017;9(1):18.

97. Konerman MC, Hummel SL. Sodium restriction in heart failure: benefit or harm? *Curr Treat Options Cardiovasc Med.* 2014;16(2):286.

98. González-Islas D, Orea-Tejeda A, Castillo-Martínez L, et al. The effects of a low-carbohydrate diet on oxygen saturation in heart failure patients: a randomized controlled clinical trial. *Nutr Hosp.* 2017;34(4):792-798.

99. Stanley WC, Dabkowski ER, Ribeiro RF, O'Connell KA. Dietary fat and heart failure: moving from lipotoxicity to lipoprotection. *Circ Res.* 2012;110(5):764-776.

100. Mozaffarian D, Bryson CL, Lemaitre RN, Burke GL, Siscovick DS. Fish intake and risk of incident heart failure. *J Am Coll Cardiol.* 2005;45(12):2015-2021.

101. Tavazzi L, Maggioni AP, Marchioli R, et al. Effect of n-3 polyunsaturated fatty acids in patients with chronic heart failure (the GISSI-HF trial): a randomised, double-blind, placebo-controlled trial. *Lancet.* 2008;372(9645):1223-1230.

102. Moertl D, Hammer A, Steiner S, et al. Dose-dependent effects of omega-3-polyunsaturated fatty acids on systolic left ventricular function, endothelial function, and markers of inflammation in chronic heart failure of nonischemic origin: a double-blind, placebo-controlled, 3-arm study. *Am Heart J.* 2011;161(5):915.e1-915.e9.

103. Chen J, Shearer GC, Chen Q, et al. Omega-3 fatty acids prevent pressure overload-induced cardiac fibrosis through activation of cyclic GMP/protein kinase G signaling in cardiac fibroblasts. *Circulation.* 2011;123(6):584-593.

104. Lepretti M, Martucciello S, Burgos Aceves MA, Putti R, Lionetti L. Omega-3 fatty acids and insulin resistance: focus on the regulation of mitochondria and endoplasmic reticulum stress. *Nutrients.* 2018;10(3). pii:E350.

105. Kaluza J, Åkesson A, Wolk A. Long-term processed and unprocessed red meat consumption and risk of heart failure: A prospective cohort study of women. *Int J Cardiol.* 2015;193:42-46.

106. Kaluza J, Akesson A, Wolk A. Processed and unprocessed red meat consumption and risk of heart failure: prospective study of men. *Circ Heart Fail.* 2014;7(4):552-557.

107. Koopman JJ, van Bodegom D, Westendorp RJ, Jukema JW. Scarcity of atrial fibrillation in a traditional African population: a community-based study. *BMC Cardiovasc Disord.* 2014;14:87.

108. Dewhurst MJ, Adams PC, Gray WK, et al. Strikingly low prevalence of atrial fibrillation in elderly Tanzanians. *J Am Geriatr Soc.* 2012;60(6):1135-1140.

109. Dinesen PT, Joensen AM, Rix TA, et al. Effect of dietary intake of saturated fatty acids on the development of atrial fibrillation and the effect of replacement of saturated with monounsaturated and polyunsaturated fatty acids. *Am J Cardiol.* 2017;120(7):1129-1132.

110. Wu JH, Lemaitre RN, King IB, et al. Association of plasma phospholipid long-chain omega-3 fatty acids with incident atrial fibrillation in older adults: the cardiovascular health study. *Circulation.* 2012;125(9):1084-1093.

111. Li FR, Chen GC, Qin J, Wu X. DietaryFish and long-chain n-3 polyunsaturated fatty acids intake and risk of atrial fibrillation: a meta-analysis. *Nutrients.* 2017;9(9), pii:E955.

112. Rix TA, Joensen AM, Riahi S, et al. A U-shaped association between consumption of marine n-3 fatty acids and development of atrial fibrillation/atrial flutter-a Danish cohort study. *Europace.* 2014;16(11):1554-1561.

113. Larsson SC, Drca N, Björck M, Bäck M, Wolk A. Nut consumption and incidence of seven cardiovascular diseases. *Heart.* 2018;104(19):1615-1620.

114. Djoussé L, Michael Gaziano J. Egg consumption and risk of heart failure in the physicians' health study. *Circulation.* 2008;117(4):512-516.

115. Iso H, Rexrode KM, Stampfer MJ, et al. Intake of fish and omega-3 fatty acids and risk of stroke in women. *JAMA.* 2001;285(3):304-312.

116. Qin ZZ, Xu JY, Chen GC, Ma YX, Qin LQ. Effects of fatty and lean fish intake on stroke risk: a meta-analysis of prospective cohort studies. *Lipids Health Dis.* 2018;17(1):264.

117. Kinoshita M, Yokote K, Arai H, et al. Japan Atherosclerosis Society (JAS) guidelines for prevention of atherosclerotic cardiovascular diseases 2017. *J Atheroscler Thromb.* 2018;25(9):846-984.

118. Kim K, Hyeon J, Lee SA, et al. Role of total, red, processed, and white meat consumption in stroke incidence and mortality: a systematic review and meta-analysis of prospective cohort studies. *J Am Heart Assoc.* 2017;6(9):e005983.

119. Cheng P, Pan J, Xia J, et al. Dietary cholesterol intake and stroke risk: a meta-analysis. *Oncotarget.* 2018;9(39):25698-25707.

120. Cheng P, Wang J, Shao W, Liu M, Zhang H. Can dietary saturated fat be beneficial in prevention of stroke risk? A meta-analysis. *Neurol Sci.* 2016;37(7):1089-1098.

121. Yamagishi K, Iso H, Yatsuya H, et al. Dietary intake of saturated fatty acids and mortality from cardiovascular disease in Japanese: the Japan Collaborative Cohort Study for Evaluation of Cancer Risk (JACC) Study. *Am J Clin Nutr.* 2010;92(4):759-765.

122. Hartman AL. Neuroprotection in metabolism-based therapy. *Epilepsy Res.* 2012;100(3):286-294.

123. Lee JE, Bisht B, Hall MJ, et al. A multimodal, nonpharmacologic intervention improves mood and cognitive function in people with multiple sclerosis. *J Am Coll Nutr.* 2017;36(3):150-168.

124. Lindeberg S, Lundh B. Apparent absence of stroke and ischaemic heart disease in a traditional Melanesian island: a clinical study in Kitava. *J Intern Med.* 1993;233(3):269-275.

125. Frassetto LA, Schloetter M, Mietus-Synder M, et al. Metabolic and physiologic improvements from consuming a paleolithic, hunter-gatherer type diet. *Eur J Clin Nutr.* 2009;63(8):947-955.

126. Kowalski LM, Bujko J. Evaluation of biological and clinical potential of paleolithic diet. *Rocz Panstw Zakl Hig.* 2012;63(1):9-15.

127. Otten J, Andersson J, Stahl J, et al. Exercise training adds cardiometabolic benefits of a paleolithic diet in type 2 diabetes mellitus. *J Am Heart Assoc.* 2019;8:e010634.

128. Severson T, Kris-Etherton PM, Robinson JG, Guyton JR. Roundtable discussion: dietary fats in prevention of atherosclerotic cardiovascular disease. *J Clin Lipidol,* 2018;12(3), 574-582.

129. Hu T, Jacobs DR, Bazzano LA, Bertoni AG. Low-carbohydrate diets and prevalence, incidence and progression of coronary artery calcium in the Multi-Ethnic Study of Atherosclerosis (MESA). *Br J Nutr.* 2019;121(4):461-468.

130. Pauletto P, Puato M, Caroli MG, et al. Blood pressure and atherogenic lipoprotein profiles of fish-diet and vegetarian villagers in Tanzania: the Lugalawa study. *Lancet.* 1996;348(9030):784-788.

131. Truswell AS, Hansen JDL. *Medical Research Among the !Kung.* Population and Health.

132. Truswell AS, Hansen JDL. *Medical Research Among the !Kung.* New Haven, CT: HRAF; 2005.

133. Cordain L, Eaton SB, Brand Miller J, Mann N, Hill K. The paradoxical nature of hunter-gatherer diets: meat-based, yet non-atherogenic. *Eur J Clin Nutr.* 2002;56:S42-S52.

134. Ander BP, Dupasquier CMC, Prociuk MA, Pierce GN. Polyunsaturated fatty acids and their effects on cardiovascular disease. *Exp Clin Cardiol.* 2003;8(4):164-172.

135. Simopoulos AP. Evolutionary aspects of diet, the omega-6/omega-3 ratio and genetic variation: nutritional implications for chronic diseases. *Biomed Pharmacother.* 2006;60(9):502-507.

136. Simopoulos AP. The importance of the omega-6/omega-3 fatty acid ratio in cardiovascular disease and other chronic diseases. *Exp Biol Med (Maywood).* 2008;233(6):674-688.

137. Metz J, Hart D, Harpending HC. Iron, folate, and vitamin B12 nutrition in a hunter-gatherer people: a study of the Kung Bushmen. *Am J Clin Nutr.* 1971;24(2):229-242.

138. Wood RJ, Volek JS, Davis SR, Dell'Ova C, Fernandez ML. Effects of a carbohydrate-restricted diet on emerging plasma markers for cardiovascular disease. *Nutr Metab (Lond).* 2006;3:19.

139. Krajčovičová-Kudláčková M, Blažíček P, Kopčová J, et al. Homocysteine levels in vegetarians versus omnivores. *Ann Nutr Metab.* 2000;44:135-138.

140. Li C, Gao M, Zhang W, et al. Zonulin regulates intestinal permeability and facilitates enteric bacteria permeation in coronary artery disease. *Sci Rep.* 2016;6:29142.

141. Carrera-Bastos P, Picazo Ó, Fontes-Villalba M, et al. Serum zonulin and endotoxin levels in exceptional longevity versus precocious myocardial infarction. *Aging Dis.* 2018;9(2):317-321.

142. Kaźmierski R, Baumann-Antczak A, Kozubski W. Serum autoantibodies to actin are associated with carotid artery wall adventitial thickness assessed using B-mode ultrasound. *Folia Neuropathol.* 2003;41(3):145-148.

143. Liljestrand JM, Paju S, Buhlin K, et al. Lipopolysaccharide, a possible molecular mediator between periodontitis and coronary artery disease. *J Clin Periodontol.* 2017;44(8):784-792.

144. Atarbashi-Moghadam F, Havaei SR, Havaei SA, et al. Periopathogens in atherosclerotic plaques of patients with both cardiovascular disease and chronic periodontitis. *ARYA Atheroscler.* 2018;14(2):53-57.

145. Ciaccio EJ, Lewis SK, Biviano AB, et al. Cardiovascular involvement in celiac disease. *World J Cardiol.* 2017;9(8):652-666.

146. Spreadbury I. Comparison with ancestral diets suggests dense acellular carbohydrates promote an inflammatory microbiota, and may be the primary dietary cause of leptin resistance and obesity. *Diabetes Metab Syndr Obes.* 2012;5:175-189.

147. Bischoff SC, Barbara G, Buurman W, et al. Intestinal permeability – a new target for disease prevention and therapy. *BMC Gastroenterol.* 2014;14:189.

148. Spruss A, Kanuri G, Stahl C, Bischoff SC, Bergheim I. Metformin protects against the development of fructose-induced steatosis in mice: role of the intestinal barrier function. *Lab Invest.* 2012;92(7):1020-1032.

149. Lerner A, Matthias T. Changes in intestinal tight junction permeability associated with industrial food additives explain the rising incidence of autoimmune disease. *Autoimmun Rev.* 2015;14(6):479-489.

150. Schnorr SL, Candela M, Rampelli S, et al. Gut microbiome of the Hadza hunter-gatherers. *Nat Commun.* 2014;5:3654.

151. Gomez A, Petrzelkova KJ, Burns MB, et al. Gut microbiome of coexisting BaAka pygmies and Bantu reflects gradients of traditional subsistence patterns. *Cell Rep.* 2016;14(9):2142-2153.

152. Segata N. Gut microbiome: westernization and the disappearance of intestinal diversity. *Curr Biol.* 2015;25(14):R611-R613.

153. De Filippo C, Cavalieri D, Di Paola M, et al. Impact of diet in shaping gut microbiota revealed by a comparative study in children from Europe and rural Africa. *Proc Natl Acad Sci USA.* 2010;107(33):14691-14696.

154. O'Keefe SJ, Li JV, Lahti L, et al. Fat, fibre and cancer risk in African Americans and rural Africans. *Nat Commun.* 2015;6:6342.

155. Tsai YL, Lin TL, Chang CJ, et al. Probiotics, prebiotics and amelioration of diseases. *J Biomed Sci.* 2019;26(1):3.

156. Zhang YG, Xia Y, Lu R, Sun J. Inflammation and intestinal leakiness in older HIV+ individuals with fish oil treatment. *Genes Dis.* 2018;5(3):220-225.

157. Koren O, Spor A, Felin J, et al. Human oral, gut, and plaque microbiota in patients with atherosclerosis. *Proc Natl Acad Sci USA.* 2011;108(suppl 1):4592-4598.

158. Lassalle F, Spagnoletti M, Fumagalli M, et al. Oral microbiomes from hunter-gatherers and traditional farmers reveal shifts in commensal balance and pathogen load linked to diet. *Mol Ecol.* 2018;27(1):182-195.

159. Dashti HM, Al-Zaid NS, Mathew TC, et al. Long term effects of ketogenic diet in obese subjects with high cholesterol level. *Mol Cell Biochem.* 2006;286(1-2):1-9.

160. Ness GC, Chambers CM. Feedback and hormonal regulation of hepatic 3-hydroxy-3-methylglutaryl coenzyme A reductase: the concept of cholesterol buffering capacity. *Proc Soc Exp Biol Med.* 2000;224(1):8-19.

161. Ducimetiere P, Eschwege E, Papoz L, et al. Relationship of plasma insulin levels to the incidence of myocardial infarction and coronary heart disease mortality in a middle-aged population. *Diabetologia.* 1980;19(3):205-210.

162. Mansoor N, Vinknes KJ, Veierød MB, Retterstøl K. Effects of low-carbohydrate diets v. low-fat diets on body weight and cardiovascular risk factors: a meta-analysis of randomised controlled trials. *Br J Nutr.* 2016;115(3):466-479.

163. Forsythe CE, Phinney SD, Fernandez ML, et al. Comparison of low fat and low carbohydrate diets on circulating fatty acid composition and markers of inflammation. *Lipids.* 2008;43(1):65-77.

164. Pinto A, Bonucci A, Maggi E, Corsi M, Businaro R. Anti-oxidant and anti-inflammatory activity of ketogenic diet: new perspectives for neuroprotection in Alzheimer's disease. *Antioxidants (Basel).* 2018;7(5):pii:E63.

165. Bueno NB, de Melo IS, de Oliveira SL, da Rocha Ataide T. Very-low-carbohydrate ketogenic diet v. low-fat diet for long-term weight loss: a meta-analysis of randomised controlled trials. *Br J Nutr.* 2013;110(7):1178-1187.

166. Cicero AF, Benelli M, Brancaleoni M, et al. Middle and long-term impact of a very low-carbohydrate ketogenic diet on cardiometabolic factors: a multi-center, cross-sectional, clinical study. *High Blood Press Cardiovasc Prev.* 2015;22(4):389-394.

167. Partsalaki I, Karvela A, Spiliotis BE. Metabolic impact of a ketogenic diet compared to a hypocaloric diet in obese children and adolescents. *J Pediatr Endocrinol Metab.* 2012;25(7–8):697-704.

168. Samaha FF, Iqbal N, Seshadri P, et al. A low-carbohydrate as compared with a low-fat diet in severe obesity. *N Engl J Med.* 2003;348(21):2074-2081.

169. Tay J, Luscombe-Marsh ND, Thompson CH, et al. A very low-carbohydrate, low-saturated fat diet for type 2 diabetes management: a randomized trial. *Diabetes Care.* 2014;37(11):2909-2918.

170. Krebs JD, Bell D, Hall R, et al. Improvements in glucose metabolism and insulin sensitivity with a low-carbohydrate diet in obese patients with type 2 diabetes. *J Am Coll Nutr.* 2013;32(1):11-17.

171. INTERMITTENT fasting and longevity in rats. *Nutr Rev.* 1946;4(7):218.

172. Tinsley GM, La Bounty PM. Effects of intermittent fasting on body composition and clinical health markers in humans. *Nutr Rev.* 2015;73(10):661-674.

173. Cherif A, Meeusen R, Farooq A, et al. Three days of intermittent fasting: repeated-sprint performance decreased by vertical-stiffness impairment. *Int J Sports Physiol Perform.* 2017;12(3):287-294.

174. Rahbar AR, Safavi E, Rooholamini M, et al. Effects of intermittent fasting during Ramadan on insulin-like growth factor-1, interleukin 2, and lipid profile in healthy Muslims. *Int J Prev Med.* 2019;10:7.

175. https://www.doh.wa.gov/CommunityandEnvironment/Food/Fish/FarmedSalmon.

176. https://www.ncbi.nlm.nih.gov/pubmed/17583796.

177. https://www.ncbi.nlm.nih.gov/pmc/articles/PMC6030944/.

178. https://www.ncbi.nlm.nih.gov/pmc/articles/PMC4937244/.

179. https://www.ncbi.nlm.nih.gov/pubmed/25550161.

180. https://www.ncbi.nlm.nih.gov/pubmed/30419974.

181. https://www.ncbi.nlm.nih.gov/pubmed/27993177.

182. https://www.ncbi.nlm.nih.gov/pmc/articles/PMC5532387/.

183. https://www.ncbi.nlm.nih.gov/pmc/articles/PMC4736892/.

184. https://www.ncbi.nlm.nih.gov/pubmed/18197175.

185. https://www.ncbi.nlm.nih.gov/pmc/articles/PMC3086762/.

186. https://pubs.rsc.org/en/content/articlelanding/2017/ra/c7ra10248h#!divAbstract.

187. http://www.scielo.br/scielo.php?script=sci_arttext&pid=S0102-311X2009000100004&lng=en&nrm=iso&tlng=en.

6

Food Sensitivities, Wheat-Related Disorders, and Cardiovascular Disease

Tom O'Bryan, DC, CCN, DACBN

Atherosclerosis is the most life-threatening pathology worldwide. Its major clinical complications, stroke, myocardial infarction, and heart failure, are on the rise in many regions of the world—despite considerable progress in understanding cause, progression, and consequences of atherosclerosis. Originally perceived as a lipid-storage disease of the arterial wall,[1] atherosclerosis was recognized as a chronic inflammatory disease in 1986.[2] From a clinician's point of view, there is great value in asking "*where is the chronic inflammation coming from?*"

The presence of lymphocytes in atherosclerotic lesions suggested an autoimmune process in the vessel wall. A substantial body of evidence identifies inflammatory and immunologic mechanisms as a driving force behind atherosclerosis and its clinical sequelae.

The origin, lineage, phenotype, and function of distinct inflammatory cells that trigger or inhibit the inflammatory response in the atherosclerotic plaque have been studied. Multiphoton microscopy recently enabled direct visualization of antigen-specific interactions between T cells and antigen-presenting cells in the vessel wall.[3] Vascular Immunology is now emerging as a new field, providing evidence for protective as well as damaging autoimmune responses.[4,5]

Arguably, the primary initiator of an inflammatory response in the human body is the choice of foods consumed habitually. For the last two decades, we have known a diet including chocolate, wine, fish, nuts, garlic, fruit, and vegetables represented a reduction in cardiovascular disease events by 76%, an increase in total life expectancy of 6.6 years, an increase in life expectancy free from cardiovascular disease of 9.0 years, and a decrease in life expectancy with cardiovascular disease of 2.4 years. The corresponding differences for women were 4.8, 8.1, and 3.3 years[6] (Table 6.1).

Food selections can have a profound positive or negative impact on the development of cardiovascular disease (Table 6.2).[7-15] This Chapter looks at the association of wheat-related disorders (WRDs) with cardiovascular disease (CVD).

Table 6.1

A DIET INCLUDING CHOCOLATE, WINE, FISH, NUTS, GARLIC, FRUIT, AND VEGETABLES REPRESENTED A REDUCTION IN CARDIOVASCULAR DISEASE EVENTS BY 76%

Men	Women
An increase in total life expectancy of 6.6 y	An increase in total life expectancy of 4.8 y
An increase in life expectancy free from cardiovascular disease of 9.0 y	An increase in life expectancy free from cardiovascular disease of 8.1 y
A decrease in life expectancy with cardiovascular disease of 2.4 y	A decrease in life expectancy with cardiovascular disease of 3.3 y

In industrialized nations such as the United States, the United Kingdom, and Germany, approximately 20% of the population has been reported to experience adverse reactions to food (ARF) with wheat, nuts, fruits, and cow's milk products among the most common triggers.[16]

Wheat Allergy

The most dangerous and life-threatening manifestation of allergic diseases is anaphylaxis, a condition in which the cardiovascular system is responsible for the majority of clinical symptoms and for potentially fatal outcome. The heart is both a source and a target of chemical mediators released during allergic reactions. Mast cells are abundant in the human heart, where they are located predominantly around the adventitia of large coronary arteries and in close contact with the small intramural vessels. Cardiac mast cells can be activated by a

Table 6.2

EFFECT OF INGREDIENTS OF POLYMEAL IN REDUCING RISK OF CARDIOVASCULAR DISEASE

Ingredients	Percentage Reduction (95% CI) in Risk of CVD
Wine (150 mL/d)	32 (23%-41%) (MA)
Fish (114 g four times/wk)	14 (8-19) (MA)
Dark chocolate (100 g/d)	21 (14%-27%) (RCT)
Fruit and vegetables (400 g/d)	21 (14%-27%) (RCT)
Garlic (2.7 g/d)	25 (21%-27%) (MA)
Almonds (68 g/d)	12.5 (10.5%-13.5%) (RCT)
Combined effect	76 (63-84)

CVD, cardiovascular disease; MA, meta-analysis; RCT, randomized controlled trial.

variety of stimuli including allergens, complement factors, general anesthetics, and muscle relaxants. Mediators released from immunologically activated human heart mast cells strongly influence ventricular function, cardiac rhythm, and coronary artery tone. The number and density of cardiac mast cells is increased in patients with ischemic heart disease and dilated cardiomyopathies. This observation may help explain why these conditions are major risk factors for fatal anaphylaxis. Although the skin (urticaria and angioedema) and the respiratory tract (laryngeal edema and bronchospasm) are the main organs involved in the early stages of anaphylaxis, dysfunction of the central and peripheral cardiovascular systems usually dictates the outcome of anaphylactic events.[17]

Gastrointestinal food allergies (an IgE immune response) do exist in both children and adults, but the majority of symptoms from ARF are due to either nonallergenic immune reactions to foods (IgG, IgA, or IgM mediated), or nonimmune reactions. Thus, although IgE immunoglobulin testing of food proteins is of clinical value in identifying an adverse reaction, exclusive use of such testing may be limiting.

Wheat allergy manifestations (an IgE-mediated response) affect the GI tract (vomiting, colic, diarrhea), skin (urticaria, eczema), respiratory tract (upper respiratory, asthma), or multiple systems (anaphylaxis). Sensitization is primarily through ingestion, but can be by inhalation or skin contact—even by wheat-containing cosmetics.[18] Wheat, specifically its omega-5 gliadin fraction, is the most common allergen implicated in food-dependent, exercise-induced anaphylaxis (FDEIA), being positive in 53% of provocation tests. However the importance of more comprehensive testing parameters (including oral challenge) cannot be overemphasized. Skin testing demonstrated a 29% positive predictive value (PPV), and serum IgE a 9% PPV.[19]

The most allergenic foods (determined by IgE positivity) change according to the age group: egg being the most

frequent in children under 5 years, and fresh fruits in children older than 5 years.

The most Common Clinical Manifestations of Food Allergy include:

- Digestive (25%-30%)—nausea/vomiting, abdominal pain, bloating, dizziness, diarrhea
- Respiratory (40%-60%)—conjunctival or nasal congestion and pruritus, laryngospasm, bronchospasm/asthma
- Cutaneous/mucous membranes (80%-90%)—atopic dermatitis, urticaria, angioedema, prurigo, pityriasis alba, cutaneous xerosis
- Cardiovascular (30%-35%)—hypotension/shock, cardiac arrest[20]

The global population has more than doubled in the last 40 years supported by the "green revolution" in agriculture producing high-yield grain varieties, including semidwarf, high-yield, disease-resistant varieties of wheat, that are central to the modern diet.[21] Awarding the Nobel Peace Prize in 1970 to Norman Ernest Borlaug recognized the value of dwarf wheat to humanity.

Arguably, one of the most researched conditions diagnosed from an ARF is celiac disease—an autoimmune reaction to wheat. Celiac disease has traditionally been clinically considered and then investigated with patients presenting with gastrointestinal (GI) symptoms. However, for every adverse reaction to wheat presenting with GI symptoms, there are eight presenting without GI symptoms.[22] Thus, dependence on GI complaints as a prerequisite in considering an adverse reaction to wheat will allow a majority to escape diagnosis. This is a critical point of recognition for the clinician when considering an association of WRDs and cardiovascular health.

Celiac disease is an autoimmune inflammatory disease in response to exposure to the environmental antigen, wheat. It is characterized by autoantibody production (tissue transglutaminase and/or endomysium), autoimmune enteropathy, and autoimmune comorbidities up to 30 times more prevalent than in the general population.[23] This overly active immune reactivity is evident in untreated adults with CD being at increased risk of early atherosclerosis, as suggested by the presence of chronic inflammation, vascular impairment, unfavorable biochemical patterns, and relative lack of the classical risk factors. Certain cardiovascular maladies, including cardiomyopathy, myocarditis, arrhythmias, and premature atherosclerosis, are substantially more prevalent in individuals with CD as compared to individuals without the disease.[24,25]

There has been a dramatic increase in the number of articles on CD and cardiovascular function in the last 15 years with the largest number of documents published concerned CD in conjunction with cardiomyopathy (33 studies) (**Figure 6.1**), and there have also been substantial numbers of studies published on CD and thrombosis (27), cardiovascular risk (17), atherosclerosis (13), stroke (12), arterial function (11), and ischemic heart disease (11).[26]

The 8:1 ratio of extraintestinal versus intestinal symptoms is not limited to celiac disease. In a prospective 1-year study of suspected nonceliac gluten sensitivity (NCGS)–related disorders from 38 Italian centers (27 centers of adult

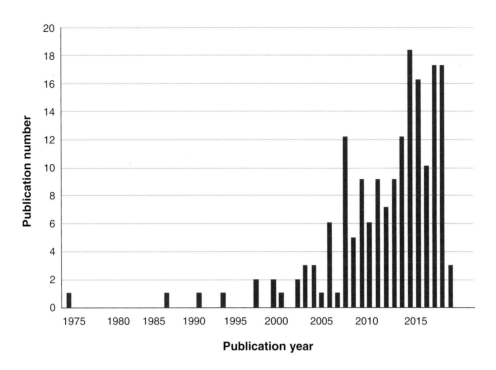

Figure 6.1 *Published studies on the association of celiac disease and cardiovascular function. (From Ciaccio EJ, Lewis SK, Biviano AB, Iyer V, Garan H, Green PH. Cardiovascular involvement in celiac disease.* World J Cardiol. *2017;9(8):652-666.)*

gastroenterology, 5 of internal medicine, 4 of pediatrics, and 2 of allergy)—all recognized as referral centers of excellence and included in the register of the Italian Health Ministry for the diagnosis of gluten-related disorders), 53% of patients presented with nonabdominal complaints. The most frequent extraintestinal manifestations were fatigue and lack of well-being, reported by 64% and 68%, respectively, of the enrolled subjects. In addition, a high prevalence of neuropsychiatric symptoms including headache (54%), anxiety (39%), "*foggy mind*" (38%), and arm/leg numbness (32%) were recorded. Other extraintestinal manifestations emerging from the analysis of the survey responses were joint/muscle pain often misdiagnosed as fibromyalgia (31%), weight loss (25%), anemia (22%), due both to iron deficiency and low folic acid, depression (18%), dermatitis (18%), and skin rash (29%).[27] With its global impact in the body and lack of isolated tissue vulnerability, a high degree of suspicion is required for a clinician to investigate a presenting patient for a WRD.

A gluten-free diet (GFD), the mainstay of treatment for CD, is increasingly being adopted by people without a diagnosis of celiac disease. Gluten-free (GF) eating patterns have become a mainstream phenomenon during recent years, and nearly one-third of Americans report having attempted to eliminate or reduce the amount of dietary gluten they consume.[28]

Intrauterine Growth Retardation and Failure to Thrive

Birthweight has been directly associated with later-in-life cardiovascular disease. Ascertained deaths from stroke and coronary heart disease in 13,249 men revealed standardized mortality ratios (SMRs) for stroke fell by 12% (95% CI 1-22) and for coronary heart disease by 10% (6-14) between each of five groupings of increasing birthweight (<or = 5.5 lb, 5.6-6.5 lb, 6.6-7.5 lb, 7.6-8.5 lb, and > 8.5 lb).[29] In an observational study, those who had had low birthweights had relatively high death rates from coronary heart disease in adult life.[30] It has been demonstrated that people who were small at birth as a result of growth retardation, rather than those born prematurely, were at increased risk of mortality from CVD.[31] Similarly, a systematic review of 34 studies examining the relation between birthweight and blood pressure in different populations around the world found strong support for an association between low birthweight and high blood pressure in prepubertal children and adults.[32]

Although the fetal genome determines growth potential in utero, the weight of evidence suggests that it plays a subordinate role in determining the growth that is actually achieved. Rather, it seems that the dominant determinant of fetal growth is the environmental milieu (nutrition, hormonal, microbial) in which the fetus develops, and in particular, the microbiome, nutrient and oxygen supply.[33,34]

One in every 70 pregnant women admitted to a major city hospital in Italy suffered from untreated celiac disease; 70% had a poor outcome of pregnancy, and 8/9 women had a second healthy baby after 1 year on a GFD.[35] An unfavorable neonatal outcome was not only associated with maternal celiac disease but also with paternal celiac disease. Infants of celiac mothers weighed 222 g less than the population average, and infants of celiac fathers weighed 266 g less than the population average. The risk of a low birthweight baby to celiac fathers was fivefold higher than that in the general population (11% versus 2.5%).[36]

Intrauterine growth retardation (IUGR) is defined as a poorly growing fetus whose weight is less than the tenth percentile for its gestational age based on a standard curve for the general population. In addition to common causes such as smoking and alcohol abuse, numerous studies have linked celiac disease and IUGR. Rates for IUGR are significantly higher (threefold) in celiac patients, 6.3% versus 2.1%.[37] In a study of 211 infants and 127 mothers with celiac disease and 1260 control deliveries, there was a 3.4-fold increased risk of IUGR in infants whose mothers had untreated celiac disease.[38] This study also found that women with celiac disease gave birth to infants with a mean birthweight that was 238 g lower than observed in the control deliveries. However, the women with celiac disease who were on GFDs gave birth to babies 67 g heavier than the controls. Investigating the correlation from a reverse perspective, patients with both repeated spontaneous abortions (RSA) and IUGR showed a statistically significant higher frequency of celiac disease when tested serologically than did the controls (with no RSA or IUGR). Specifically, 8 % of RSA patients and 15% of IUGR patients were positive for celiac antibodies, whereas all controls were negative.[39]

Wheat-Related Disorders and Increased Cardiac Risk

The frequency of vascular thrombotic events associated with CD are increased,[40] can be recurrent,[41] and may be present at multiple locations.[42] Endothelial dysfunction is the earliest sign of atherosclerosis and associated with cardiovascular events.[43,44] The detection of endothelial dysfunction in healthy subjects may indicate an increased risk for cardiovascular events (heart failure, stroke, erectile dysfunction, peripheral artery disease) and can be used as a predictor of clinical prognosis (morbidity/mortality) in patients with coronary artery disease. In the first functional challenge study of the brachial artery in individuals with CD, response to a hyperemic challenge revealed a significant reduced response of celiac patients versus controls.

Endothelial dysfunction at the macrovascular level was found in celiac patients and is one of the earliest signs of atherosclerosis.[45] Areas with improved markers on a GFD include the common carotid arteries for intima-media thickness and the humeral artery for endothelium-dependent dilatation.[46]

In an age- and sex-matched control study of 65 patients with CD (mean age 6.74 ± 4.6 years) and 51 controls, serum levels of vascular adhesion molecule-1, intercellular adhesion molecule-1, endothelial selectin, vascular endothelial cadherin, high-sensitivity C-reactive protein, and homocysteine levels were measured. The average soluble vascular adhesion molecule-1 (CD versus control group: 1320 ± 308 versus 1120 ± 406 ng/mL, $P = .006$), soluble intercellular adhesion molecule-1 (336 ± 99 versus 263 ± 67 ng/mL, $P = .025$), and soluble endothelial selectin (113.9 ± 70 versus 76.9 ± 32 ng/mL, $P = .007$) levels were significantly higher

in cases of newly diagnosed CD than in the control group. Soluble vascular adhesion molecule-1 (1050 ± 190 ng/mL) and soluble endothelial selectin (68.7 ± 45 ng/mL) levels in patients with CD, who were fully compliant with a GFD, were significantly lower than that in those newly diagnosed as having CD ($P = .003$ and $P = .0012$, respectively). These results show that serum adhesion molecule levels are higher in patients with CD and may explain some of the risks associated with endothelial dysfunction seen in CD.[47]

CD youth have also been associated with increased risk of developing early atherosclerosis. They are also more likely to have greater mean low-density lipoprotein (LDL) cholesterol and have thicker carotid intima-media as compared with controls, and their endothelium-dependent dilatation is decreased, all of which negatively affect vascular function.[48,49]

A relationship with increased carotid intima-media thickness (CIMT) and decreased flow-mediated dilatation (FMD) in addition to elevated CRP and homocysteine levels in recently diagnosed young CD patients has been identified. The GFD improved CIMT, FMD, and CRP levels.[50] These findings support the theory that chronic inflammation in CD patients increases the risk of premature atherosclerosis. CIMT values are significantly higher in patients with coexisting diabetes and CD as compared to those patients with diabetes or CD alone.[51]

In adult CD patients lacking cardiovascular risk factors, abnormal homocysteine, erythrocyte sedimentation rate, C-reactive protein, and insulin levels, along with inflammation, may be contributing to arterial stiffening.[52] Correlation has been shown between restoration of the small intestinal villous atrophy and normalization of vascular parameters in gluten-abstinent CD patients.[53,54]

Folic acid and vitamin B_{12}, along with vitamin B_6 and riboflavin, are needed for the metabolism of homocysteine, which is widely considered to be a risk factor for heart disease and stroke. Higher levels of homocysteine have been found in untreated patients with CD compared with healthy controls, with normalization after recovery from villous atrophy. The B-complex of vitamins are principally absorbed in the proximal part of the small intestine, which is the primary site of the inflammatory cascade in CD and NCWS (nonceliac wheat sensitivity). With associated deficiencies of the B-complex and protein S from malabsorption, a thrombophilia may result from hyperhomocysteinemia.[55-57] The thrombotic events in CD may also result from dehydration due to diarrhea.[58] Cerebral venous sinus thrombosis can occur in CD patients[55,59-61] even in absence of gastrointestinal symptoms,[60] but can resolve with symptomatic treatment.[55] Venous thrombosis can be a sequela of undetected CD[57,62-69] and may result in thromboembolic events.[63,70] CD may be accompanied by portal vein thrombosis,[71,72] and mesenteric[73] or splenic[74] vein thrombosis may present in occult or subclinical celiac disease.[73] There is an increased risk of developing venous thromboembolism from chronic inflammation and vitamin deficiency in CD.[59,75,76]

Wheat-Related Disorders and Strokes

Patients with CD have been found to be at an increased risk for stroke, and recurrent stroke, which can persist after onset of the GFD.[77-79] CD should be considered as a possible etiology for stroke cases of unknown cause, particularly in youth, whether gastrointestinal manifestations are evident or not.[80] The pathogenesis of stroke in CD youth may involve vitamin B_{12} deficiency[81] and possibly hyperhomocysteinemia, which may be secondary to folic acid deficiency,[82] cerebral arterial vasculopathy, and antiphospholipid syndrome, a secondary autoimmune disorder which also carries a higher prevalence in celiac disease.[83-85] Because CD is a potentially treatable cause of cerebral vasculopathy and stroke,[86] serology, specifically TG2 antibodies, should be included in the evaluation for cryptogenic stroke in childhood, even in the absence of typical gastrointestinal symptoms.[85,87]

Dramatically reduced cholecystokinin secretion, a common finding in CD,[88] is responsible for the reduced absorptive mechanism of fat-soluble vitamins, thus may result in coagulopathy attributable to vitamin K deficiency.[89,90]

In untreated CD, continual systemic inflammation can deteriorate aortic function, and this deterioration is predictive of subclinical atherosclerosis and future cardiovascular events.[91] Aortic strain and distensibility tend to be significantly lower, and the aortic stiffness index significantly higher, in untreated CD patients versus controls.[92] Owing to the continual systemic inflammation seen in CD (and NCWS), patients are at increased risk for coronary artery disease.[52]

The symptoms of malabsorption are alleviated with GFD. However, given the poor compliance to a recommended GFD (see below), vitamin B_6, B_{12}, and folate deficiencies might still be observed in patients with malabsorption. This may cause hyperhomocysteinemia, which may increase the risk of vascular diseases. Hyperhomocysteinemia may cause endothelial dysfunction including arterial vasospasm, activation of tissue-type plasminogen activator and factor V, increased platelet aggregation, and inhibition of protein C, all of which can result in plaque rupture, vascular damage, and vasoconstriction.[93] Elevated homocysteine levels are associated with spontaneous coronary artery dissection.[94]

Diastolic dysfunction is an important early finding in children with CD and postulated to be the earliest cardiac complication of pediatric CD. Examining cardiac function in pediatric controls, recently diagnosed pediatric CD (Group 1) and CD children 10+ months on a GFD (Group 2) revealed significantly shorter deceleration time (DT) and left ventricle (LV) isovolumetric relaxation time (IVRT) in Group 1 compared to Group 2 and the control group ($P = .002$, $P = .015$).[95] Suggested theories explaining cardiac dysfunction include nutritional deficiency triggered by intestinal malabsorption and an autoimmune inflammatory response in myocardial tissue via molecular mimicry caused by immune system activation from increased macromolecular absorption of numerous antigens following increased intestinal permeability.[96,97]

Adult patients with CD and diabetes demonstrate the microvascular complications in both conditions. At diagnosis of CD, adult type 1 diabetic patients had worse glycemic control (8.2 versus 7.5%, $P = .05$), lower total cholesterol (4.1 versus 4.9, $P = .014$), lower HDL cholesterol (1.1 versus 1.6, $P = .017$), and significantly higher prevalence of retinopathy (58.3% versus 25%, $P = .02$), nephropathy (41.6% versus 4.2%, $P = .009$), and peripheral neuropathy (41.6% versus 16.6%, $P = .11$) than adult type 1 diabetic patients without CD. After 1 year on a GFD, only the lipid profile improved overall, but in adherent individuals HbA1c and markers for nephropathy improved.[98] The potential role of altered apolipoprotein A-I (Apo A-I) secretion in newly diagnosed CD patients offers an explanation for the different results observed between diabetic nephropathy (DN) and diabetic retinopathy (DR). Apo A-I is the major HDL structural protein, essential for reverse transport of cholesterol from peripheral tissue to the liver. It is also characterized by antioxidant and anti-inflammatory effects. Apo A-I has been reported as being synthesized by the liver and the intestine and, more recently, by the vitreous fluid and retinal pigment epithelium. Serum levels of HDL and Apo A-I are decreased in individuals with CD, and subsequent restoration of blood lipid profile is observed after GFD.[99] The reduced intestinal secretion of Apo A-I in individuals with type 1 diabetes affected by CD could contribute to the increased prevalence of DN in these subjects compared with individuals with type 1 diabetes alone and would also be of relevance in the assessment of macrovascular complications in these patients. Also, the restoration of Apo A-I and HDL levels due to the normalization of the intestinal villi after GFD could be responsible, at least partially, for the improvement of DN.[100]

Wheat-Related Disorders and Ischemic Heart Disease

Ischemic heart disease (IHD, defined as death or incident disease in myocardial infarction or angina pectoris) is one of the main causes of death. The underlying pathology in IHD is atherosclerosis, and it seems that chronic inflammation plays an important role in the development of atherosclerosis. A population-based study of 28,190 unique individuals diagnosed with Marsh 3 CD, and 12,598 unique individuals diagnosed with inflammation without villous atrophy (Marsh 1-2), found a 19% increased risk of IHD in individuals with CD. This study also found a 28% increased risk of IHD in individuals with small intestinal inflammation but no villous atrophy and a 14% increase in individuals with normal mucosa but positive CD serology (latent CD).[101] The discovery of a suspected WRD demonstrating significant increased mortality independent of small intestinal histopathology is of critical importance to clinicians and reinforces the necessity of an understanding of WRD outside of total villous atrophy CD. These risks were found to persist for years after commencing the GFD.[102] Persistent inflammation maintaining increased intestinal permeability even in the presence of villous regeneration is suspect.

Wheat-Related Disorders, Molecular Mimicry, and Cross-reactivity

Autoimmune diseases tend to have long, asymptomatic prodromal periods and the initiating events leading to loss of self-tolerance occurring long before the disease becomes clinically manifest. Several different pathological processes have the potential to break tolerance and contribute to the development of autoimmune disease. The mechanism of molecular mimicry (antigenic similarity between pathogenic organisms or foreign proteins and self-proteins) is one of them.

Primary mechanisms involved in food protein–induced autoimmunity are antibody molecular mimicry, cross-reactivity, and covalent binding of food and human tissue proteins creating neoepitopes. Shared amino acid homology between multiple peptides of wheat and human tissues as well as dairy proteins and human tissues has been illustrated.[103-105]

The molecular mimicry or cross-reactivity hypothesis proposes that an exogenous substance, mostly produced or possessed by infectious agents or foods, may trigger an immune response against self-antigens. Susceptible individuals consume a food or have a bacterial exposure, and initiate an inflammatory immune response that has antigenic similarity to self-antigens. As the result, these food or pathogen-specific antibodies bind to the host structures possessing cross-reactive self-antigens and cause tissue damage and disease. The most familiar of these mechanisms occur in celiac disease with the antigen gluten. As an example, arguably, the most recognized preventive measure in health care to this mimicry mechanism is the use of antibiotics prior to dental visits. In rheumatic fever carditis, for example, the basic pathogenic process involves production of antibodies against *Streptococcus* which express high levels of M protein antigens, a molecule that shares structural similarities with those found in the heart valves and endocardial membrane. With standard dental care, perforation of the epithelial lining of the gums occurs creating potentially pathogenic gum permeability, allowing macromolecules of oral bacteria to migrate through the normally restrictive membrane barrier. The use of antibiotics in dental care is designed to mitigate the initial immune protective response against the invading pathogen (streptococcus), thus reducing the risk of a cross-reactivity to cardiac tissue.

If antibodies to these bacterial proteins reach high levels, there may be sufficient binding to the host cells possessing these cross-reactive antigens with activation of the complement system, production of neoepitopes, and induction of the autoimmune cascade creating pathological damages at these sites.

Known environmental triggers of autoimmune cross reactivity include:

- food proteins, for example, gluten instigates celiac disease, casein from dairy may instigate type 1 diabetes;
- chemicals, for example, bisphenol A[106-108] plays a role in thyroid disorders; and

- pathogens:
  - *Klebsiella pneumoniae* contributes to ankylosing spondylitis and Crohn disease,[109]
  - *Proteus* from asymptomatic urinary tract infections and *Porphyromonas gingivalis* contribute to rheumatoid arthritis,[110-112] and
  - *Chlamydia pneumoniae* contributes to multiple sclerosis.[113]

Several pathogens share antigenic determinants with host proteins. Often, these are used to gain entry into the cell; rhinovirus binds to an adhesion molecule (ICAM-1) on epithelial cells, and human immunodeficiency virus (HIV) binds to CD4, and enters the cell using a chemokine receptor. Eighty-nine (89%) of untreated celiac patients had antibodies to adenovirus 12, and these antibodies were also raised in treated children with celiac disease (31%) compared with controls (0%-13%). Antibodies to adenovirus 18 or echovirus 11 were not raised. A similar amino acid sequence between alpha-gliadin and the E1b protein of adenovirus 12 was reported, and this sequence was found to be an antigenic determinant in active celiac disease. This suggested that the viral protein might play a role in the pathogenesis of celiac disease by virtue of immune cross reactivity. It is possible that infection with adenovirus sensitizes the genetically predisposed host to A-gliadin by molecular mimicry, with resultant gluten-sensitive enteropathy, using a "hit and run" mechanism.[114]

Anti-ganglioside antibodies might arise through antigenic molecular mimicry and antibody cross-reactivity with foreign glycolipids or glycoproteins. In Guillain-Barre syndrome, for example, IgG anti-ganglioside antibodies appear to be induced by infection with bacteria such as *Campylobacter jejuni* or *Haemophilus influenzae*. These bacteria bear lipopolysaccharide (LPS) molecules that cross-react with gangliosides. In one review, every celiac patient suffering with peripheral neuropathies was positive to ganglioside antibodies.[115]

Although the avidity of the interactions between antigenic determinants and specific antibodies is considerably high, these antigen-binding sites can allow epitopes of similar shapes expressed on completely different microbial or animal cells to bind these antibodies, albeit with a lower binding avidity. These so-called cross-reactive epitopes are made up of essentially similar amino acid and carbohydrate molecules, and such cross-reactions are in fact common and may account for the undesirable production of antibodies against self-molecules, which occurs in some autoimmune diseases.

Gliadin antibodies can cross-react with multiple tissues in the body, which may result in autoantibody formation. When a WRD was identified by positive serology (IgG) to a family of peptides of incompletely digested wheat (native + deamidated β-gliadin-33 mer, β-gliadin-17 mer, β-gliadin-15 mer, β-gliadin-17 mer, glutenin-21 mer), 64% also had a positive reaction to self including 40% to myocardial peptide. To focus on WRD and avoid CD, IgA positive specimens were excluded so as to prevent using possible celiac patients. Yet 40% of positive specimens demonstrate cross-reactivity with myocardial peptides, an autoimmune reaction initiating myocardial inflammation.[116]

Wheat-Related Disorders and Myocarditis

Myocarditis, particularly the giant cell type, can be associated with systemic autoimmune disorders that if unrecognized and untreated can prevent the recovery of, or even worsen myocardial function.[117] A WRD is often uncovered while exploring the cause of a recognized anemia in cardiovascular patients.[118]

In a study of 187 patients diagnosed with myocarditis:
- Positivity for organ-specific anti-heart autoantibodies was evident in 53 (28%) of the patients.
- Thirteen (14%) were positive for IgA-tissue transglutaminase (tTG) antibodies, of which all showed iron deficiency anemia refractory to oral iron replacement suggesting a GI inflammatory malabsorption syndrome.
- Nine (4.4%) were found to have CD. In the 5 patients with CD and autoimmune myocarditis presenting with heart failure, all were unresponsive to full conventional therapy. However, when immunosuppressive treatment was administered together with a GFD, recovery of cardiac volumes and function was elicited in all.
- Fifty (50%) of patients with autoimmune myocarditis and CD had significant cardiac improvement with GFD. The remaining 50% experienced significant improvement with a combination of the GFD and immune suppression versus immune suppression alone.[119]

With a frequency of 4.4% of myocarditis patients presenting with an underlying WRD, the dramatic and significant improvement in LVEF (left ventricular ejection fraction) achievable in the majority of patients with autoimmune myocarditis and celiac disease warrants investigation of a WRD in all patients presenting with myocarditis (Table 6.3).

However, unless strict, complete GFD is implemented in these cases, progression to chronic dilated cardiomyopathy likely will occur.[96,120]

Wheat-Related Disorders and Atrial Fibrillation

Atrial fibrillation, a common cardiac arrhythmia, is a kind of supraventricular tachyarrhythmia, associated with substantial morbidity and mortality. Atrial fibrillation is associated with heart failure, increased hospitalization, decreased quality of life, decreased exercise capacity, a fivefold increased risk of stroke, and twofold increased risk of mortality.[121] Systemic inflammation plays a significant role in AF pathogenesis, and AF risk factors have been found to be linked to oxidative stress.[122,123] Inflammation causes formation of arrhythmogenic substrates by stimulating fibrosis and structural changes.[124] Inflammation and oxidative stress have been found to be the primary responsible molecular mechanisms of damage in CD.[125] Individuals with CD have been found to be more likely to have AF with an increased risk of 26%.[126] Eliminating wheat reduces the inflammatory "fuel on the fire" in WRD with associated reductions in inflammatory cytokine and chemokine levels, and a lowered number of adhered leukocytes in tissue vasculature.[127]

In a Swedish nationwide cohort study of more than 28,637 patients with biopsy-verified CD, a 36% increased risk of atrial fibrillation was identified. This association was seen both before and after diagnosis with CD and strongest around the time of diagnosis.[128]

The delays in interatrial and intra-atrial conduction time and increased electro-mechanical coupling have been shown to be related to the development and recurrence of AF in patients with or without apparent heart disease. Clinicians need to be aware that both left and right intra-atrial and interatrial electro-mechanic delay were found significantly prolonged in patients with anti-endomysium antibodies and in patients with anti-gliadin IgG positive antibodies (serology markers of CD and WRD) ($P = .07$, $P = .043$, respectively). The measurement of atrial interatrial electro-mechanic delay (EMD) may be used to determine who is prone to AF in CD patients, and impaired EMD parameters may be early and the only clinical clues of subclinical heart disease. In this regard, AF may be of concern to the CD patients and trans-thoracic echocardiography can easily be used in these patients to evaluate atrial electromechanic properties.[129]

Wheat-Related Disorders and Cardiomyopathy

Dilated cardiomyopathy (DCM) is defined by the presence of left ventricular dysfunction associated with chamber dilatation. The differentials are broad, but may include alcohol excess, chemotherapeutic agents, and myocarditis. A small cohort of patients has true idiopathic DCM where the etiology is unknown, although potentially related to an autoimmune pathogenesis.

An autoimmune response directed at antigenic components of both myocardium, peptides of wheat, and/or small bowel has been postulated to play a key role in the pathogenesis of inflammatory heart damage and cardiomyopathy. One mechanism contributing to this is molecular mimicry. Indeed, autoantibodies may have shared affinity to antigen epitopes in different tissues or, alternatively, different antigens could mimic tTG epitopes. The family of 9 transglutaminases (TGases) in the human body are enzymes normally expressed at low levels in many different tissues and are widely used in numerous biological systems for generic tissue stabilization purposes. TGases are particularly interesting enzymes to consider in the context of pathology because their many functions generally involve either protection and prevention of bodily injury, or tissue assembly and repair. TGases can be thought of as mediators of biological glues. Widely distributed in human organs, TTG is a multifunctional enzyme involved in the cross-linking of extracellular matrix proteins, fibrogenesis, and wound healing.[130]

Altered TTG expression is associated with the development of numerous inflammatory diseases, including cardiomyopathies. TTG is also the primary serology marker of CD.

Table 6.3

CHARACTERISTICS, TREATMENT, AND FOLLOW-UP OF PATIENTS WITH AUTOIMMUNE MYOCARDITIS AND CELIAC DISEASE

No.	Age/Sex	Clinical Presentation	Myocardial Histology	Duodenal Endoscopy	Duodenal Histology	Treatment	Follow-Up (Overall 12 mo)	IDA	LVEF Improvement
1	24/F	CHF (NYHA III; LVEF 32%) + IDA	ALM	Scalloped valvulae	SVA/CH	GFD+I	Improved (NYHA I; LVEF 54%)	Eliminated	1.68-fold
2	22/F	CHF (NYHA IV; LVEF 21%) + IDA	GCM	Reduction of duodenal folds	TVA/CH	GFD+I	Improved (NYHA I; LVEF 56%)	Eliminated	2.66-fold
3	35/F	VEB (Lown Class IVa) + IDA	ALM	Loss of duodenal folds	TVA/CH	GFD	Improved (Lown Class I)	Eliminated	Lown Class IVa-Lown Class I
4	16/F	VEB (Lown Class III) + IDA	ALM	Reduction of duodenal folds	SVA/CH	GFD	Improved (Lown Class I)	Eliminated	Lown Class III-Lown Class I
5	32/M	CHF (NYHA IV; LVEF 17%) + IDA	ALM	Scalloped valvulae	SVA/CH	GFD+I	Improved (NYHA II; LVEF 46%)	Eliminated	2.7-fold
6	38/F	VEB (Lown Class IVa) + IDA	ALM	Loss of duodenal folds	TVA/CH	GFD	Improved (Lown Class I)	Eliminated	Lown Class IVa-Lown Class I
7	16/F	CHF (NYHA II; LVEF 36%) + IDA	ALM	Loss of duodenal folds	SVA/CH	GFD+I	Improved (NYHA I; LVEF 54%)	Eliminated	1.5-fold
8	36/M	CHF (NYHA III; LVEF 27%) + IDA	ALM	Loss of duodenal folds	TVA/CH	GFD+I	Improved (NYHA I; LVEF 48%)	Eliminated	1.72-fold
9	14/F	VEB (Lown Class III) + IDA	ALM	Reduction of duodenal folds	SVA/CH	GFD	Improved (Lown Class I)	Eliminated	Lown Class III-Lown Class I

ALM, active lymphocytic myocarditis; CH, crypt hyperplasia; CHF, congestive heart failure; GCM, giant-cell myocarditis; GFD, gluten-free diet; I, immunosuppression; IDA, iron deficiency anemia; LVEF, left ventricular ejection fraction; NYHA, New York Heart Association class; SVA, subtotal villous atrophy; TVA, total villous atrophy; VEB, ventricular ectopic beats.

During an infectious disease, anti-transglutaminase antibodies can be produced temporarily and independently of gluten. The protein Hyphal Wall protein 1 (HWP1), expressed in the pathogenic phase of *Candida albicans*, presents sequence analogy with the gluten protein gliadin and is also a substrate for TTG.[131] HWP1 is a protein found on the germ tube cell wall of *C. albicans* which represents the potentially invasive, saprophytic-pathogenic stage of the fungus.

C. albicans might function as an adjuvant that stimulates antibody formation against HWP1 and gluten, and formation of autoreactive antibodies against tissue transglutaminase and endomysium.[132]

Infection-triggered anti-transglutaminase antibodies have the same biological properties as that of the celiac patient, with the same *in-vivo potential* for damage. The evidence that improvement of cardiac function and of ventricular arrhythmias was paralleled by the disappearance of CD antibodies in the serum supports this hypothesis.

A positive correlation between 13,358 CD patients and an increased risk to myocardial infarction, angina pectoris, congestive heart failure, intracranial bleeding, and ischemic stroke has been identified (**Figure 6.2**).

The risk of idiopathic DCM was found to be 73% greater in patients with celiac disease. Indeed, this risk was maintained in subanalyses after adjustment for confounders.[133] Patients diagnosed with celiac disease that adhere to gluten abstinence have been shown to demonstrate significant recovery of ventricular volumes and function, with adjunct suppression of dysrhythmic potential, and a reduction in cardiac inflammation.[134] Cardiomyopathy associated with celiac disease is a serious and potentially lethal condition. However, if diagnosed early, cardiomyopathy may be completely reversible with initiation of a GFD.[135]

Wheat-Related Disorders

The most researched WRDs have been identified as celiac disease (affecting approximately 1 in 100 in the general population) and wheat allergy (affecting approximately 1 in 1000 in the general population).[136] After celiac disease and wheat allergy have been (largely) excluded, numerous NCWS disorders may be considered. Recent studies and experimental data strongly indicate that NCWS exists in a substantial proportion of the population, and that it begins initially as an innate immune response to wheat exposure, which may progress to an adaptive immune response. Patients often present with extraintestinal symptoms, such as worsening of an underlying inflammatory disease in clear association with wheat consumption.[137]

There is indisputable evidence from the scientific community, supported by numerous studies recognizing the glutens, gliadins, and glutenin families of proteins in wheat, rye, and barley as primary, but not exclusive antigenic triggers of WRD.[138-143] The value for clinicians in understanding this diversity of antigens in wheat is the immediate recognition of the need for more comprehensive testing in identifying a WRD beyond an immune reaction to gluten.[144]

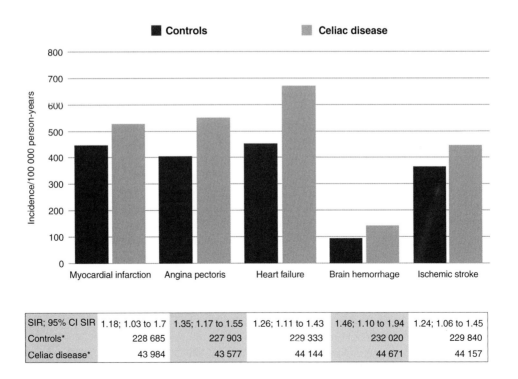

Figure 6.2 *Celiac disease and cardiovascular disease. (Modified from Ludvigsson et al. Vascular disease in a population-based cohort of individuals hospitalised with coeliac disease.* Heart. *2007;93:1111-1115.)*

A breakdown of sensitivities included within the category NCWS may include:

- Nonceliac gluten sensitivity (NCGS), whose published prevalence varies widely (0.5%-13%) in western populations.[145,146] In secondary care, 200 suspected gluten-sensitive patients referred to a secondary gastroenterologist (female 84%, mean age 39.6 years) were investigated. Seven (7%) were found to have CD and 93% to have NCGS.[147]

- Wheat germ agglutinin (WGA) sensitivity: a carbohydrate-binding protein that also functions as a natural pesticide. WGA initiates an immune response which has been associated with inhibition of gut epithelial cell repair and stimulating synthesis of proinflammatory cytokines and may have an antigenic impact on the intestinal epithelium at nanomolar concentrations.[148,149] WGA induces platelet activation and aggregation.[150] WGA has a potent, disruptive effect on platelet endothelial cell adhesion molecule-1, which plays a key role in tissue regeneration and safely removes neutrophils from our blood vessels.[151] Molecular cross-reactivity has been identified between wheat germ agglutinins and soybean agglutinins with cardiac muscle.[152]

- Wheat amylase trypsin inhibitors (ATIs), representing 2% to 4% of total wheat proteins, are primary activators of an innate immune response via activation of Toll-like receptor 4 (TLR4). They are a major stimulator of innate immune cells (dendritic cells > macrophages > monocytes) while intestinal epithelial cells were nonresponsive. ATIs lead to release of proinflammatory cytokines within 2 to 12 hours of ingestion, a time frame which is too short to induce adaptive immune response.[153] Wheat ATIs are a family of up to 17 similar proteins of molecular weights around 15 kDa which have been identified as the most likely triggers of NCWS. Acting as an adjuvant, they costimulate antigen-presenting cells, especially dendritic cells, and thus fuel an ongoing T-cell response as seen in celiac disease and chronic and inflammatory diseases of the gut, liver, heart, kidneys, brain, reproductive tract, blood vessels, and fat cells.[137,154]

- FODMAPs (fermentable oligo-, di-, monosaccharides and polyols) which may primarily cause gastrointestinal symptoms through gaseous production and osmotic diarrhea and are present in many food products, with fructans (arabinoxylans) commonly present in wheat.[139,155-157]

- Gluteomorphins: Gluten proteins can be degraded in the human digestive tract into several morphine-like substances named exorphins.[158] These compounds mimic endogenous opioid and could mask the deleterious effects of gluten protein on intestinal lining and function.[159] Gluten is not the only source of exorphins. Dairy products and certain vegetables such as soy and spinach also contain proteins, which can be converted into bioactive exorphins.[160] A recent review of the literature concluded that food-derived exorphins are bioactive and affect behavioral traits such as spontaneous behavior, memory, and pain perception. The highest behavioral influence was measured for casein and spinach-derived exorphins (respectively, B-casomorphin and rubiscolin).[161] Exorphins inhibit DPP IV activity and are known to increase the possibility of developing angioedema. CD produces the same symptoms as angioedema,[162] and both disorders are so similar that, in general, it is advised to screen people with hereditary angioedema for CD.[163]

Besides the multiple peptides of wheat that may be immunogenic and activate an immune response, the harvesting and storage of wheat may impact on its antigenicity. If not properly harvested and stored, wheat may also be infested with fungi such as aspergillus and fusarium, leading to consumption of harmful mycotoxins.[137] Fungal endocarditis is an uncommon form of infective endocarditis accounting for 1.3% to 6% of all cases and is often a lethal cardiac infection.[164] The *Candida* and *Aspergillus* species are the two most common etiologic fungi found responsible for fungal endocarditis. Treating *Candida* endocarditis can be difficult because the *Candida* species can form biofilms on native and prosthetic heart valves. *Aspergillus* species account for 20% to 30% of cases. Cardiac involvement (endocarditis, pancarditis, or pericarditis) accounts for 0.7% to 6% of cases of invasive aspergillosis.[165]

With clear evidence of an immune reaction to multiple peptides of incompletely digested wheat, and an immune reaction to mold infestations, in looking for evidence of an adverse reaction to wheat, if one is looking exclusively for celiac disease or an IgE allergy to wheat, it is likely for a clinician to arrive at a false conclusion of safety with wheat consumption.

Wheat and Cross-Reactivity

The main mechanisms involved in food protein–induced autoimmunity are antibody cross-reactivity and covalent binding of food and human tissue proteins producing neoepitopes. Shared amino acid homology between multiple peptides of wheat and human tissues as well as dairy proteins and human tissues has been illustrated.[103-105]

In a cohort of 118 patients suspected and checked for an immune reaction to wheat, of the 45 patients negative for IgG against alpha-gliadin protein, 16 (35%) were reactive against one or more tissues of self, while of 45 positive for IgG against alpha-gliadin proteins, 29 (64%) were reactive against tissues of self with 40% demonstrating a cross-reactivity to cardiac muscle and/or α-myosin.

Looking at other peptides of wheat and their immune cross-reactivity, of 25 patients negative for IgG against wheat germ agglutinin (WGA) (a lectin of wheat), 8 (22%) were reactive against one or more tissues of self, while of 25 patients positive for IgG against WGA, 19 (76%) were reactive against tissues of self. Forty (40) percent of gluten-positive serology demonstrated elevated antibodies to myocardial tissue versus 13% of gluten negative serology[116] (**Figures 6.3-6.5**).

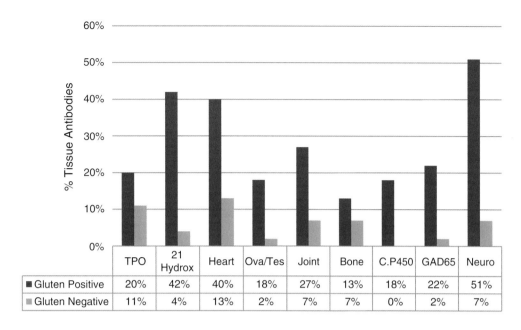

Figure 6.3 *Comparison of gluten family positive and negative tissue reactivity. A significant elevation of tissue antibodies in patients with gluten family protein IgG versus patients IgG negative for gluten family proteins is shown. TPO = thyroid peroxidase, 21 Hydrox = 21 hydroxylase (adrenal cortex), Heart = myocardial peptide and/or α-myosin, Ova/Tes = ovary/testis, Joint = fibulin, collagen and/or arthritic peptide, Bone = osteocyte, C.P450 = cytochrome P450 (hepatocyte), GAD65 = glutamic acid decarboxylase-65, Neuro = myelin basic protein, asialoganglioside, α+β-tubulin, cerebellar and/or synapsin. (From Lambert J, Vojdani A. Correlation of tissue antibodies and food immune reactivity in randomly selected patient specimens.* J Clin Cell Immunol. *2017;8(5):521.)*

Identifying a Wheat-Related Disorder

The first and most important aspect of identifying a WRD is for the clinician to suspect a WRD. With an extraintestinal to intestinal symptom ratio of 8:1, familiarity with its multiple cardiovascular manifestations is required. Historically, CD was defined as total villous atrophy and therefore small intestinal biopsy has been acknowledged as the "gold standard" for diagnosis.[166] However, celiac disease, as is true of all autoimmune diseases, develops on a spectrum.[167] Total villous atrophy can

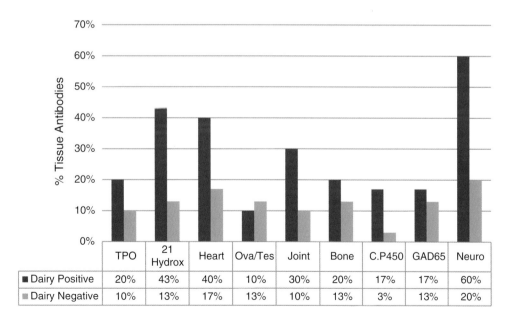

Figure 6.4 *Comparison of Dairy Family Positive and Negative Tissue Reactivity. A significant elevation of antibodies to most tissues in patients with Dairy family protein IgG + IgA versus patients IgG + IgA negative for Dairy family proteins is shown. Ovary/Testis is the one tissue that resulted with four dairy negative patient reacting, and only three dairy positive patients reacting. In this instance, each of the four dairy negative patients was positive for gluten family proteins. TPO = thyroid peroxidase, 21 Hydrox = 21 hydroxylase (adrenal cortex), Heart = myocardial peptide and/ or α-myosin, Ova/Tes = ovary/testis, Joint = fibulin, collagen and/or arthritic peptide, Bone = osteocyte, C.P450 = cytochrome P450 (hepatocyte), GAD65 = glutamic acid decarboxylase-65, Neuro = myelin basic protein, asialoganglioside, α+β-tubulin, cerebellar and/or synapsin. (From Lambert J, Vojdani A. Correlation of Tissue Antibodies and Food Immune Reactivity in Randomly Selected Patient Specimens.* Journal of Clinical & Cellular Immunology. *2017;8(5):521.)*

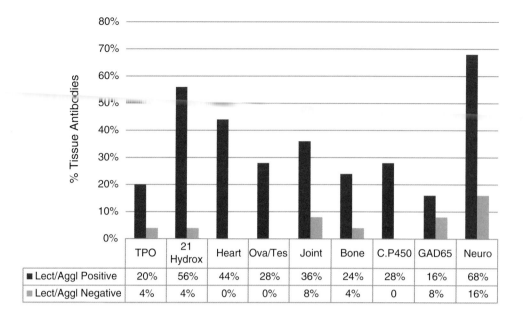

Figure 6.5 *Comparison of Lectin/Agglutinin Family Positive and Negative Tissue Reactivity. A significant elevation of antibodies to most tissues in patients with lectin/agglutinin family protein IgG or IgG + IgA versus patients IgG/IgA or IgG + IgA negative for lectin/agglutinin family proteins is shown. TPO = thyroid peroxidase, 21 Hydrox = 21 hydroxylase (adrenal cortex), heart = myocardial peptide and/or α-myosin, Ova/Tes = ovary/testis, Joint = fibulin, collagen and/or arthritic peptide, Bone = osteocyte, C.P450 = cytochrome P450 (hepatocyte), GAD65 = glutamic acid decarboxylase-65, Neuro = myelin basic protein, asialoganglioside, α+β-tubulin, cerebellar and/or synapsin. (From Lambert J, Vojdani A. Correlation of tissue antibodies and food immune reactivity in randomly selected patient specimens.* J Clin Cell Immunol. *2017;8(5):521.)*

be viewed as the "end stage" of an extended, activated immune response in the small intestine.

Tissue transglutaminase (tTG), also known as transglutaminase 2 (tTG or TG2), is an ubiquitous protein involved in a wide variety of cell processes and therefore has a role in wound healing, inflammation, autoimmunity, and others.[168] tTG is central to the pathogenesis of celiac disease. It potentiates the immunogenicity of gluten peptides in the small bowel through primarily deamidation. TG2 is the main target antigen for endomysial antibodies (EM) and TG2 is therefore recommended as a primary screening test for CD.[169] In celiac disease, antibodies are often also produced against endomysium, a structure of the smooth muscle connective tissue. Depending on the study, tTG and anti-endomysial antibodies both show a sensitivity and specificity > 95% for detecting total villous atrophy CD; however, both demonstrate a sensitivity as low as 27% to 31% with partial villous atrophy.[136,170,171] Thus, the serology "gold standard" of diagnosing CD, tTG, is in reality the "gold standard" for the *end stage* of the celiac spectrum—total villous atrophy. It is not the preferred screen for identifying the earlier stages of CD or of a WRD.[172]

Compelling evidence identifies a useful clinical role for immunoglobulin testing (IgG, IgA, IgM) to multiple peptides of gluten.[173] Clinically available for the last 8 years, screening for an immune response to multiple peptides of wheat has proven to be an extremely useful biomarker in reducing the false negative results of only checking tTG or one peptide of wheat, alpha-gliadin. And one of the earliest serology markers of being on the celiac spectrum that a clinician can identify, years before the end stage of villous atrophy has occurred, is an immune response to the neoepitope of Transglutaminase-Deamidated Gliadin

Complex.[174-176] These panel-of-peptide tests allowing for biomarkers of the earlier stages of WRD before the progression to end-stage disease have proven to be effective in identifying WRD and following progress on a GFD.[177]

Recently, novel sets of epitopes derived from gliadin which have a high degree of accuracy (99% sensitivity and 100% specificity, $P < .001$) in differentiating CD from controls, compared with standard serologic tests, have been identified.[178] This method of ultra-high-density peptide microarray is proving broadly useful in identifying an immune reaction to wheat outside of the standard anti-gliadin screen of a WRD. The relative noninvasiveness, broad availability, economic accessibility, and versatility of the high-throughput peptide microarrays make this technology well suited for incorporation into routine health care and also provide a promising new tool for biomarker discovery. And the latest, and now referred to as an even earlier marker of being on the celiac spectrum, is an immune response to any of 172 immunogenic epitopes of the tissue transglutaminase-deamidated gliadin complex (tTG-DGP). This screen, with 99% sensitivity and 100% specificity ($P < .001$) allows for identifying earlier stages of WRD and accurate follow-up of the GFD.[179]

Implementing the GFD

The GFD can be restrictive in social situations, leading to poor quality of life significantly correlated with anxiety and, ultimately, nonadherence. Twenty-eight (28%) of CD patients showed obsessive-compulsive behavior disorders. The percentages of CD patients with high levels of both state anxiety and trait anxiety were 27% and 24%, with mean scores of 56.26 and 54.17, respectively. A value of 45 indicates existing anxiety in both "state" and "trait" scales. For comparison purposes, in diabetic patients, these figures were 13% and 19%, with mean values of 55.72 and 51.75, respectively. The foremost pathogenetic mechanisms underlying psychiatric disorders in CD patients favor the role of malabsorption or poor vitamin status, endorphin and opioid antagonist activity in gluten-derived polypeptides and their possible role in schizophrenia, or an immune involvement of the central nervous system.[180]

In CD patients, the relationship between depression and duration of diet restriction may be explained by a progressively increased awareness of the effects of a chronic disease. Social phobia is a condition characterized by fear and/or avoidance of situations that involve possible scrutiny by others.[181] This is a primary contributor to the terrible statistic of a 55% overall increased suicide risk being seen in all celiac disease age groups, with CD diagnosed in childhood being associated with a 40% increase in suicide risk.[182]

Thus, successful transitioning to a GFD involves a gradual change in coping strategies, from avoidance to acceptance/resignation, and many years are needed to reach this goal. Thus, in the early phases, patients are angry, frustrated, and contentious about having a previously unknown disease (although CD is one of the most common genetically based diseases). Furthermore, a medical team willing to inform adequately and reassure patients, a strict follow-up in the early phases after diagnosis, and, last but not least, contact with other patients and patient associations are indispensable features.

All patients with a WRD should seek out community support because support groups can have varied roles: social and emotional support or empathy; adjustment; awareness of local and national sources of gluten-free foods; product sampling; practical advice for gluten-free food preparation; advocacy or representation; dissemination of up-to-date information; travel information ;and/or experience. Membership in celiac disease support groups has been associated with improved dietary adherence.[183]

Valid concerns exist that implementation of a nonguided GFD may result in micro and macro nutrient deficiencies, increased exposure to toxins such as arsenic and other heavy metals, and an increased cardiovascular risk.[184] The wide-ranging long-term health effects of a GFD, apart from its beneficial effect on enteropathy in celiac disease, have been reported. However, rates of strict adherence to a GFD in adults have been found to vary between 17% and 45%.[183]

The complex manufacture of modern processed food, the recognized inadequacies of the common GFD referenced below, and the required paradigm shift commonly referred to in the common press as the "dangers" of a GFD are easily remedied with structured guidance from specialty-trained professionals. The ongoing advice of a specialty-trained Dietician, Nutritionist, or Health Coach is required.[185]

Recognizing that dietary changes alter the gut microbiome in humans within 24 to 48 hours,[186] a 2011 study demonstrated that for celiac children following a GFD for 2 years, the GFD did not completely restore the microbiota and, consequently, the metabolome of CD children.[187] In another study, 10 healthy participants who did not have celiac disease or a recognized gluten sensitivity, following a GFD, found that their diet alone created a proinflammatory environment 100% of the time. Researchers concluded that when individuals discontinue eating wheat, the reduced polysaccharide intake (prebiotics) creates a shift in the diversity of the intestinal microbiome, with lowered bifidobacterium and lactobacillus and a concomitant increase in enterobacteriaceae, diminishing short chain fatty and organic acids and thus reducing competence of the immunomodulatory role of the microbiome with lowered TNFa, IFN gamma, IL-8, and IL-10. This outcome creates a proinflammatory environment.[188] The Reader is advised to review the Chapter 27 on the Microbiome with an understanding of the role that food sensitivities, and their treatment, may contribute to dysbiosis.

Numerous factors have been associated with this dysbiosis of the microbiome including:

- Wheat (78%) and barley (3%) together provide 81% of oligofructose and inulin for average North Americans, with onions giving 10%.[189] On a GFD, the prebiotic value of wheat is unavailable and is not consciously replaced with GF prebiotic foods. Without these fructan prebiotics in wheat called arabinoxylose, the microbiota which was accustomed to this family of prebiotics die off, creating a proinflammatory environment.[190]
- Thus, it appears that a GFD in both CD and WRD subjects could produce similar, potentially adverse, changes in the microbiota solely on the basis of a marked reduction in intake of naturally occurring fructans which have prebiotic action.[190]

A common misnomer is that GF foods are healthy. There is no evidence to support such a claim. While it is true that GF foods will eliminate a primary antigenic component of the diet, GF foods are calorie rich and nutrient poor. Restricting the intake of wheat in the diet can have serious consequences for the intake of essential nutrients and other beneficial components unless equivalent sources of these are provided.[191] It is generally considered that GF foods are less nutritionally adequate than standard products. GF bread products were significantly higher in fat and fiber. All GF products were lower in protein than standard products. Only 5% of GF breads were fortified with all four mandatory fortification nutrients (calcium, iron, niacin, and thiamin), only 9% of GF bread products were fortified with thiamine, riboflavin, and niacin, and 28% of GF breads were fortified with calcium and iron only. This lack of fortification may increase the risk of micronutrient deficiency in celiac sufferers.

Insulin resistance, a primary contributor to cardiovascular dysfunction, is enhanced with GF products. The incorporation of a commercial GF pasta composed of rice and corn flours into a common recipe, macaroni and cheese, increased the peak postprandial glycemic response by 57% compared to conventional wheat pasta.[192] GF foods have demonstrated a lower allergenic potential but are not considered "healthy." Consumption of GF products in moderation is highly recommended. The advice and guidance from a trained professional focusing on a variety of prebiotic and fermented foods is highly recommended to ensure lowering the antigenic load, reducing the inflammatory cascade, replacing the lost oligofructose and inulin, reinoculating, maintaining, and propagating a diverse microbiome.

Higher levels of fat, sugar, and salt are observed in GF foods compared with standard foods. Iron fortification is present in only 23% of GF breads and no fortification in GF pasta products. CD patients following a GFD consume inadequate fiber levels, especially women, with intakes of 13.7 g per day (RDA 30 g/d). There is no apparent reason GF products are not included in fortification legislation. This lack of fortification of GF foods may increase the risk of micronutrient deficiency and have severe health consequences for CD patients and consumers who choose to avoid gluten.[193] A medical team willing to inform adequately and reassure patients, a strict follow-up in the early phases after diagnosis, and, last but not least, contact with other patients and patient associations are indispensable features.[180]

With the increased dependence on processed foods, increased levels of toxin exposures from our foods impacting on the microbiome and triggering inflammatory responses, and the concomitant rise in adverse reactions to foods in the last few years, the necessity of screening for an immune reaction to foods is more essential than at any time in our human history. Once the ARF has been identified, complete elimination is essential to calm the inflammatory immune response. It is this author's opinion the missing link in successfully transitioning a patient onto a healthy, balanced GFD, is the absence of trained support personnel focusing on guiding the patient through the trials and errors of modifying lifetime habits. The GFD can be restrictive in social situations, leading to poor quality of life and, ultimately, nonadherence. As the number of patients with WRDs increases worldwide, clinicians need to be aware of the challenges patients face. Heightened awareness by physicians, dietitians, and other health providers can help maximize successful treatment, improve outcomes, and reduce health-care costs and disease burden.[194]

References

1. Virchow R. *Die cellularpathologie in ihrer begründung auf physiologische und pathologische gewebelehre.* Berlin: August Hirschwald Verlag; 1871.
2. Ross R. The pathogenesis of atherosclerosis–an update. *New Engl J Med.* 1986;314:488-500.
3. Koltsova EK, Garcia Z, Chodaczek G, et al. Dynamic t cell-apc interactions sustain chronic inflammation in atherosclerosis. *J Clin Invest.* 2012;122:3114-3126.
4. Tse K, Tse H, Sidney J, Sette A, Ley K. T cells in atherosclerosis. *Int Immunol.* 2013;25:615-622.
5. Lichtman AH, Binder CJ, Tsimikas S, Witztum JL. Adaptive immunity in atherogenesis: new insights and therapeutic approaches. *J Clin Invest.* 2013;123:27-36.
6. Franco OH, Bonneux L, de Laet C, Peeters A, Steyerberg EW, Mackenbach JP. The Polymeal: a more natural, safer, and probably tastier (than the Polypill) strategy to reduce cardiovascular disease by more than 75%. *BMJ.* 2004;329(7480):1447-1450.
7. Di Castelnuovo A, Rotondo S, Iacoviello L, Donati MB, De Gaetano G. Meta-analysis of wine and beer consumption in relation to vascular risk. *Circulation.* 2002;105:2836-2844.
8. Whelton SP, He J, Whelton PK, Muntner P. Meta-analysis of observational studies on fish intake and coronary heart disease. *Am J Cardiol.* 2004;93:1119-1123.
9. Taubert D, Berkels R, Roesen R, Klaus W. Chocolate and blood pressure in elderly individuals with isolated systolic hypertension. *JAMA.* 2003;290:1029-1030.
10. John JH, Ziebland S, Yudkin P, Roe LS, Neil HA. Effects of fruit and vegetable consumption on plasma antioxidant concentrations and blood pressure: a randomised controlled trial. *Lancet.* 2002;359:1969-1974.
11. Ackermann RT, Mulrow CD, Ramirez G, Gardner CD, Morbidoni L, Lawrence VA. Garlic shows promise for improving some cardiovascular risk factors. *Arch Intern Med.* 2001;161:813-824.
12. Silagy C, Neil A. Garlic as a lipid lowering agent—a meta-analysis. *J R Coll Physicians Lond.* 1994;28:39-45.
13. Berthold HK, Sudhop T, von Bergmann K. Effect of a garlic oil preparation on serum lipoproteins and cholesterol metabolism: a randomized controlled trial. *JAMA.* 1998;279:1900-1902.
14. Sabate J, Haddad E, Tanzman JS, Jambazian P, Rajaram S. Serum lipid response to the graduated enrichment of a step I

15. Jenkins DJ, Kendall CW, Marchie A, et al. Dose response of almonds on coronary heart disease risk factors: blood lipids, oxidized low-density lipoproteins, lipoprotein(a), homo- cysteine, and pulmonary nitric oxide: a randomized, controlled, crossover trial. *Circulation.* 2002;106:1327-1332.
16. Bischoff S, Crowe SE. Gastrointestinal food allergy: new insights into pathophysiology and clinical perspectives. *Gastroenterology.* 2005;128(4):1089-1113.
17. Triggiani M, Montagni M, Parente R, Ridolo E. Anaphylaxis and cardiovascular diseases: a dangerous liaison. *Curr Opin Allergy Clin Immunol.* 2014;14(4):309-315.
18. Kobayashi T, Ito T, Kawakami H, et al. Eighteen cases of wheat allergy and wheat-dependent exercise-induced urticaria/anaphylaxis sensitized by hydrolyzed wheat protein in soap. *Int J Dermatol.* 2015;54:302-305.
19. Asaumi T, Yanagida N, Sato S, Shukuya A, Nishino M, Ebisawa M., Provocation tests for the diagnosis of food-dependent exercise-induced anaphylaxis. *Pediatr Allergy Immunol.* 2016;27:44-49.
20. Ruiz Sánchez JG, Palma Milla S, Pelegrina Cortés B, López Plaza B, Bermejo López LM, Gómez-Candela C. A global vision of adverse reactions to foods: food allergy and food intolerance. *Nutr Hosp.* 2018;35(Spec No4):102-108.
21. Hedden P. The genes of the green revolution. *Trends Genet.* 2003;19:5-9.
22. Fasano A, Catassi C. Current approaches to diagnosis and treatment of celiac disease: an evolving spectrum. *Gastroenterology.* 2001;120:636-651.
23. Nass FR, Kotze LM, Nisihara RM, Messias-Reason IT, Utiyama SR. Autoantibodies in relatives of celiac disease patients: a follow-up of 6-10 years. *Arq Gastroenterol.* 2012;49(3):199-203.
24. Bayar N, Çağırcı G, Üreyen ÇM, Kuş G, Küçükseymen S, Arslan Ş. The relationship between spontaneous multi-vessel coronary artery dissection and celiac disease. *Korean Circ J.* 2015;45:242-244.
25. Wang I, Hopper I. Celiac disease and drug absorption: implications for cardiovascular therapeutics. *Cardiovasc Ther.* 2014;32:253-256.
26. Ciaccio EJ, Lewis SK, Biviano AB, Iyer V, Garan H, Green PH. Cardiovascular involvement in celiac disease. *World J Cardiol.* 2017;9(8):652-666.

27. Volta U, Bardella MT, Calabrò A, Troncone R, Corazza GR; The Study Group for Non-Celiac Gluten Sensitivity. An Italian prospective multicenter survey on patients suspected of having non-celiac gluten sensitivity. *BMC Med*. 2014;12:85.

28. Taetzsch A, Das SK, Brown C, Krauss A, Silver RE, Roberts SB. Are gluten-free diets more nutritious? An evaluation of self-selected and recommended gluten-free and gluten-containing dietary patterns. *Nutrients*. 2018;10(12):1-8.

29. Martyn CN, Barker DJP, Osmond C. Mothers pelvic size, fetal growth and death from stroke in men. *Lancet*. 1996;348:1264-1268.

30. Osmond C, Barker DJP, Winter PD, Fall CHD, Simmonds SJ. Early growth and death from cardiovascular disease in women. *BMJ*. 1993;307:1519-1524.

31. Barker DJP, Osmond C, Simmonds SJ, Wield GA. The relation of small head circumference and thinness at birth to death from cardiovascular disease in adult life. *BMJ*. 1993;306:422-426.

32. Law CM, Shiell AW. Is blood pressure inversely related to birthweight? The strength of evidence from a systematic review of the literature. *J Hypertens*. 1996;14:935-941.

33. Ounsted M, Ounsted C. Maternal regulation of intrauterine growth. *Nature*. 1966;212:687-689.

34. Barker DJP, Gluckman PD, Godfrey KM, Harding J, Owens JA, Robinson JS. Fetal nutrition and adult disease. *Lancet*. 1993;341:938-941.

35. Greco L, Veneziano A, Di Donato L, et al. Undiagnosed coeliac disease does not appear to be associated with unfavourable outcome of pregnancy. *Gut*. 2004;53:149-151.

36. Greco L. The father figure in celiac disease. *Gut*. 2001;49:163-166.

37. Sheiner E, Peleg R, Levy A. Pregnancy outcome of patients with known celiac disease. *Eur J Obstet Gynecol Reprod Biol*. 2006;129(1):41-45.

38. Norgard S, Fonager K, Sorensen HT, Olsen J. Birth outcomes of women with celiac disease: a nationwide historical cohort study. *Am J Gastroenterol*. 1999;94:2435-2440.

39. Gasbarrini A, Torre ES, Trivellini C, Carolis SD, Caruso A, Gasbarrini G. Recurrent spontaneous abortion and intrauterine growth restriction as symptoms of celiac disease. *Lancet*. 2000;356:399.

40. Boucelma M, Saadi M, Boukrara H, Benaalah D, Hakem D, Berrah A. Association of celiac disease and cerebral venous thrombosis: report of two cases. *J Mal Vasc*. 2013;38:47-51.

41. Beyrouti R, Mansour M, Kacem A, Derbali H, Mrissa R. Recurrent ccrebral venous thrombosis revealing celiac disease: an exceptional case report. *Acta Neurol Belg*. 2017;117:341-343.

42. Poulin W, Gaertner S, Cordeanu EM, Mirea C, Andrès E, Stephan D. Stroke revealing celiac disease associated with multiple arterial thrombotic locations. *Presse Med*. 2015;44:537-538.

43. Vita JA, Keaney JF Jr. Endothelial function: a barometer for cardiovascular risk? *Circulation*. 2002;106:640-642.

44. Celermajer DS, Sorensen KE, Bull C, et al. Endothelium-dependent dilation in the systemic arteries of asymptomatic subjects relates to coronary risk factors and their interaction. *J Am Coll Cardiol*. 1994;24:1468-1474.

45. Sari C, Bayram NA, Doğan FE, et al. The evaluation of endothelial functions in patients with celiac disease,. *Echocardiography*. 2012;29(4):471-477.

46. Demir AM, Kuloğlu Z, Yaman A, Fitöz S, Nergizoğlu G, Kansu A. Carotid intima-media thickness and arterial stiffness as early markers of atherosclerosis in pediatric celiac disease. *Turk J Pediatr*. 2016;58:172-179.

47. Comba A, Çaltepe G, Yank K, Gör U, Yüce Ö, Kalayc AG. Assessment of endothelial dysfunction with adhesion molecules in patients with celiac disease. *J Pediatr Gastroenterol Nutr*. 2016;63(2):247-252.

48. Valitutti F, Trovato CM, Barbato M, Cucchiara S. Letter: atherosclerosis and coeliac disease – another feature of the changing paradigm?. *Aliment Pharmacol Therap*. 2013;38:559.

49. Emilsson L, Carlsson R, James S, Ludvigsson JF. Letter: coeliac disease and ischaemic heart disease – a true additional risk factor? Authors' reply. *Aliment Pharmacol Therap*. 2013;37:1118.

50. De Marchi S, Chiarioni G, Prior M, Arosio E. Young adults with coeliac disease may be at increased risk of early atherosclerosis. *Aliment Pharmacol Ther*. 2013;38:162-169.

51. Pitocco D, Giubilato S, Martini F, et al. Combined atherogenic effects of celiac disease and type 1 diabetes mellitus. *Atherosclerosis*. 2011;217(2):531-535.

52. Korkmaz H, Sozen M, Kebapcilar L. Increased arterial stiffness and its relationship with inflammation, insulin, and insulin resistance in celiac disease. *Eur J Gastroenterol Hepatol*. 2015;27:1193-1199.

53. De Marchi S, Chiarioni G, Prior M, Arosio E. Commentary: coeliac disease and atherosclerosis–hand in hand? Authors' reply. *Aliment Pharmacol Ther*. 2013;38:550-551. PMID:23937458. doi:10.1111/apt.12405.

54. Martini F, Pitocco D, Zaccardi F, et al. Early detection of cardiovascular disease in patients with associated type 1 diabetes mellitus and celiac disease.

55. Bahloul M, Chaari A, Khlaf-Bouaziz N, et al. Celiac disease, cerebral venous thrombosis and protein S deficiency, a fortuitous association? *J Mal Vasc*. 2005;30:228-230.

56. Kallel L, Matri S, Karoui S, Fekih M, Boubaker J, Filali A. Deep venous thrombosis related to protein S deficiency revealing celiac disease. *Am J Gastroenterol*. 2009;104:256-257. PMID:19098891. doi:10.1038/ajg.2008.48.

57. Baryshnikov EN, Krums LM, Vorob'eva NN, Parfenov AI. Lower extremity deep vein thrombosis associated with gluten-sensitivity celiac disease. *Ter Arkh*. 2010;82:52-54.

58. Lee ES, Pulido JS. Nonischemic central retinal vein occlusion associated with celiac disease. *Mayo Clin Proc*. 2005;80:157.

59. Johannesdottir SA, Erichsen R, Horváth-Puhó E, Schmidt M, Sørensen HT. Coeliac disease and risk of venous thromboembolism: a nationwide population-based case control study. *Br J Haematol*. 2012;157:499-501. PMID:22296563. doi:10.1111/j.1365-2141.2012.09030.x.

60. Doğan M, Peker E, Akbayram S, et al. Cerebral venous sinus thrombosis in 2 children with celiac disease. *Clin Appl Thromb Hemost*. 2011;17:466-469.

61. Grover PJ, Jayaram R, Madder H. Management of cerebral venous thrombosis in a patient with Lane-Hamilton syndrome and coeliac disease, epilepsy and cerebral calcification syndrome. *Br J Neurosurg*. 2010;24:684-685.

62. Ghoshal UC, Saraswat VA, Yachha SK. Association of splenic vein obstruction and coeliac disease in an Indian patient. *J Hepatol*. 1995;23:358. PMID:8551004. doi:10.1016/S0168-8278(95)80019-0.

63. Beyan E, Pamukcuoglu M, Beyan C. Deep vein thrombosis associated with celiac disease. *Bratisl Lek Listy*. 2009;110:263-264.

64. Grigg AP. Deep venous thrombosis as the presenting feature in a patient with coeliac disease and homocysteinaemia. *Aust N Z J Med*. 1999;29:566-567. PMID:10868541. doi:10.1111/j.1445-5994.1999.

65. Casella G, Baldini V, Perego D, Brambilla M, Fraterrigo RT. A rare association between inflammatory bowel disease (IBD), coeliac disease, membranous glomerulonephritis and leg venous thrombosis associated to heterozygosis of V Leiden factor. *Dig Liver Dis*. 2000;32:A44.

66. Casella G, Perego D, Baldini V, Monti C, Crippa S, Buda CA. A rare association between ulcerative colitis (UC), celiac disease (CD), membranous glomerulonephritis, leg venous thrombosis, and heterozygosity for factor V Leiden. *J Gastroenterol*. 2002;37:761-762.

67. Hida M, Erreimi N, Ettair S, Mouane N, Bouchta F. Associated celiac disease and venous thrombosis. *Arch Pediatr*. 2000;7:215-216.

68. Mezalek ZT, Habiba BA, Hicham H, et al. C0396 Venous thrombosis revealing celiac disease. Three cases. *Throm Res*. 2012;130:S154-S155.

69. Kremer Hovinga JA, Baerlocher G, Wuillemin WA, Solenthaler M. Deep venous thrombosis of the leg in acquired thrombophilia – hyperhomocysteinemia as a sequela of undetected celiac disease. *Ther Umsch*. 1999;56:519-522.

70. Ludvigsson JF, Welander A, Lassila R, Ekbom A, Montgomery SM. Risk of thromboembolism in 14,000 individuals with coeliac disease. *Br J Haematol*. 2007;139:121-127 cx.

71. Karoui S, Sfar S, Kallel M, Boubaker J, Makni S, Filali A. Antiphospholipid syndrome revealed by portal vein thrombosis in a patient with celiac disease. *Rev Med Interne*. 2004;25:471-473

72. Zenjari T, Boruchowicz A, Desreumaux P, Laberenne E, Cortot A, Colombel JF. Association of coeliac disease and portal venous thrombosis. *Gastroenterol Clin Biol*. 1995;19:953-954.

73. Azzam NA, Al Ashgar H, Dababo M, Al Kahtani N, Shahid M. Mesentric vein thrombosis as a presentation of subclinical celiac disease. *Ann Saudi Med.* 2006;26:471-473.

74. Khanna S, Chaudhary D, Kumar P, Mazumdar S. Occult celiac disease presenting as splenic vein thrombosis. *Indian J Gastroenterol.* 2008;27:38-39.

75. Ungprasert P, Wijarnpreecha K, Tanratana P. Risk of venous thromboembolism in patients with celiac disease: a systematic review and meta-analysis. *J Gastroenterol Hepatol.* 2016;31:1240-1245.

76. Gabrielli M, Santoliquido A, Santarelli L, et al. 6 P Venous thromboembolism, hyperhomocysteinemia and silent coeliac disease: a case report. *Dig Liver Dis.* 2002;34:A27.

77. Emilsson L, Lebwohl B, Sundström J, Ludvigsson JF. Cardiovascular disease in patients with coeliac disease: a systematic review and meta-analysis. *Dig Liver Dis.* 2015;47:847-852.

78. Ludvigsson JF, West J, Card T, Appelros P. Risk of stroke in 28,000 patients with celiac disease: a nationwide cohort study in Sweden. *J Stroke Cerebrovasc Dis.* 2012;21:860-867.

79. Ozge A, Karakelle A, Kaleağasi H. Celiac disease associated with recurrent stroke: a coincidence or cerebral vasculitis?. *Eur J Neurol.* 2001;8:373-374.

80. El Moutawakil B, Chourkani N, Sibai M, et al. Celiac disease and ischemic stroke. *Rev Neurol (Paris).* 2009;165:962-966.

81. Rachid B, Zouhayr S, Chtaou N, Messouak O, Belahsen F. Ischemic stroke revealing celiac disease. *Pan Afr Med J.* 2010;5:2.

82. Gefel D, Doncheva M, Ben-Valid E, el Wahab-Daraushe A, Lugassy G, Sela BA. Recurrent stroke in a young patient with celiac disease and hyperhomocysteinemia. *Isr Med Assoc J.* 2002;4:222-223.

83. Ajello A, Vitullo G. Stroke and coeliac disease: a new face for an old lady. *Ital J Pediatr.* 2006;32:259.

84. Audia S, Duchêne C, Samson M, et al. Stroke in young adults with celiac disease. *Rev Med Interne.* 2008;29:228-231. PMID:17976872. doi:10.1016/j.revmed.2007.08.013.

85. Goodwin FC, Beattie RM, Millar J, Kirkham FJ. Celiac disease and childhood stroke. *Pediatr Neurol.* 2004;31:139-142. PMID:15301836. doi:10.1016/j.pediatrneurol.2004.02.014.

86. Slimani N, Hakem D, Mansouri B, Berrah A. Ischemic stroke revealing a celiac disease: a case report and review of the literature. *J Neurol Sci.* 2013;333:e248.

87. Balci O, Sezer T. The prevalence of celiac disease in children with arterial ischemic stroke. *J Pediatr Hematol Oncol.* 2017;39:46-49.

88. Rubio-Tapia A, Murray J. The liver in celiac disease. *Hepatology.* 2007;46:1650-1658.

89. Chen CS, Cumbler EU, Triebling AT. Coagulopathy due to celiac disease presenting as intramuscular hemorrhage. *J Gen Intern Med.* 2007;22:1608-1612.

90. Abenavoli L, Delibasic M, Peta V, Turkulov V, De Lorenzo A, Medić-Stojanoska M. Nutritional profile of adult patients with celiac disease. *Eur Rev Med Pharmacol Sci.* 2015;19(22):4285-4292.

91. Sari C, Ertem AG, Sari S, et al. Impaired aortic function in patients with coeliac disease. *Kardiol Pol.* 2015;73:1108-1113.

92. Bayar N, Çekin AH, Arslan Ş, et al. Assessment of aortic elasticity in in patients with celiac disease. *Korean Circ J.* 2016;46:239-245.

93. Welch GN, Loscalzo J. Homocysteine and atherothrombosis. *N Engl J Med.* 1998;338:1042-1050.

94. Najaf SM, Quraishi AR, Kazmi KA. Spontaneous multivessel coronary artery dissection associated with elevated homocysteine levels. *J Coll Physicians Surg Pak.* 2005;15:108-109.

95. Karadaş U, Eliaçık K, Baran M, et al. The subclinical effect of celiac disease on the heart and the effect of gluten-free diet on cardiac functions. *Turk J Pediatr.* 2016;58(3):241-245.

96. Curione M, Barbato M, Viola F, Francia P, De Biase L, Cuchiara S. Idiopathic dilated cardiomyopathy associated with coeliac disease: the effect of a gluten- free diet on cardiac performance. *Dig Liver Dis.* 2002;34:866-869.

97. Bardella MT, Fraquelli M, Quatrini M, Molteni N, Bianchi P, Conte D. Prevalence of hypertransaminasemia in adult patients an effect of gluten-free diet. *Hepatology.* 1995;22:833-836.

98. Leeds JS, Hopper AD, Hadjivassiliou M, Tesfaye S, Sanders DS. High prevalence of microvascular complications in adults with

99. type 1 diabetes and newly diagnosed celiac disease. *Diabetes Care.* 2011;34:2158-2163.

99. Capristo E, Malandrino N, Farnetti S, et al. Increased serum high-density lipoprotein- cholesterol concentration in celiac disease after gluten-free diet treatment correlates with body fat stores. *J Clin Gastroenterol.* 2009;43:946-949.

100. Malandrino N, Capristo E. Comment on: Leeds et.al. High prevalence of microvascular complications in adults with type 1 diabetes and newly diagnosed celiac disease. Diabetes Care 2011;34:2158-2163. *Diabetes Care.* 2012;35(6):e44.

101. Ludvigsson JF, James S, Askling J, Stenestrand U, Ingelsson E. Nationwide cohort study of risk of ischemic heart disease in patients with celiac disease. *Circulation.* 2011;123(5):483-490.

102. Lebwohl B, Emilsson L, Fröbert O, Einstein AJ, Green PH, Ludvigsson JF. Mucosal healing and the risk of ischemic heart disease or atrial fibrillation in patients with celiac disease; a population-based study. *PLoS One.* 2015;10(1):e0117529.

103. Carter C. Evidence for gliadin antibodies as causative agents in schizophrenia. *Nature Precedings.* 2010. doi:10.1038/npre.2010.5351.1. Accessed December 22, 2018.

104. Riemekasten G, Marell J, Hentschel C, et al. Casein is an essential cofactor in autoantibody reactivity directed against the C-terminal SmD1 peptide AA 83-119 in systemic lupus erythematosus. *Immunobiology.* 2002;206:537-545.

105. Vojdani A, Kharrazian D, Mukherjee PS. The prevalence of antibodies against wheat and milk proteins in blood donors and their contribution to neuroimmune reactivities. *Nutrients.* 2014;6:15-36.

106. Kharrazian D. The potential roles of bisphenol A (BPA) pathogenesis in autoimmunity. *Autoimmune Dis.* 2014;2014:743616.

107. Moriyama K, Tagami T, Akamizu T, et al. Thyroid hormone action is disrupted by bisphenol A as an antagonist. *J Clin Endocrinol Metab.* 2002;87:5185-5190.

108. Lang IA, Galloway TS, Scarlett A, et al. Association of urinary bisphenol A concentration with medical disorders and laboratory abnormalities in adults. *JAMA.* 2008;300:1303-1310.

109. Rashid T, Ebringer A. Autoimmunity in rheumatic diseases is induced by microbial infections via crossreactivity or molecular mimicry. *Autoimmune Dis.* 2012;2012:539282.

110. Routsias JG, Goules JD, Goules A, et al. Autopathogenic correlation of periodontitis and rheumatoid arthritis. *Rheumatology.* 2011;50:1189-1193.

111. Mikuls TR, Thiele GM, Deane KD, et al. Porphyromonas gingivalis and disease-related autoantibodies in individuals at increased risk of rheumatoid arthritis. *Arthritis Rheum.* 2012;64:3522-3530.

112. Nielen MM, van Schaardenburg D, Reesink HW, et al. Speci c autoantibodies precede the symptoms of rheumatoid arthritis: a study of serial measurements in blood donors. *Arthritis Rheum.* 2004;50:380-386.

113. Libbey JE, McCoy LL, Fujinami RS. Molecular mimicry in multiple sclerosis. *Int Rev Neurobiol.* 2007;79:127-147.

114. Leech S. Molecular mimicry in autoimmune disease. *Arch Dis Child.* 1998;79:448-451.

115. Alaedini A, Green PH, Sander HW, et al. Ganglioside reactive antibodies in the neuropathy associated with celiac disease. *J Neuroimmunol.* 2002;127(1-2):145-148.

116. Lambert JJ, Vojdani A. Correlation of tissue antibodies and food immune reactivity in randomly selected patient specimens. *J Clin Cel Immunol.* 2017;8:5-21.

117. Cooper LT Jr, Berry GJ, Shabetai R. Idiopathic giant-cell myocarditis natural history and treatment: Multicenter Giant Cell Myocarditis Study Group Investigators. *N Engl J Med.* 1997;336:1860-1866.

118. Patel P, Smith F, Kilcullen N, Artis N. Dilated cardiomyopathy as the first presentation of coeliac disease: association or causation? *Clin Med (Lond).* 2018;18(2):177-179.

119. Frustaci A, Cuoco L, Chimenti C, et al. Celiac disease associated with autoimmune myocarditis. *Circulation.* 2002;105(22):2611-2618.

120. Milisavljević N, Cvetković M, Nikolić G, Filipović B, Milinić N. Dilated cardiomyopathy associated with celiac disease: case report and literature review. *Srp Arh Celok Lek.* 2012;140(9-10):641-643.

121. Kannel WB, Wolf PA, Benjamin EJ, Levy D. Prevalence, incidence, prog- nosis, and predisposing conditions for atrial fibrillation: popula- tion- based estimates. *Am J Cardiol.* 1998;82:2N-9N.

122. Boos CJ, Anderson RA, Lip GY. Is atrial fibrillation an inflammatory disorder? *Eur Heart J.* 2006;27:136-149.

123. Youn JY, Zhang J, Zhang Y, et al. Oxidative stress in atrial fibril- lation: an emerging role of NADPH oxidase. *J Mol Cel Cardiol.* 2013;62:72-79.

124. Kirchhof P, Bax J, Blomstrom-Lundquist C, et al. Early and com- prehensive management of atrial fibrillation: proceedings from the 2nd AFNET/EHRA consensus conference on atrial fibrillation entitled "research perspectives in atrial fibrillation". *Europace.* 2009;11:860-885.

125. Ferretti G, Bacchetti T, Masciangelo S, Saturni L. Celiac disease, inflammation and oxidative damage: a nutrigenetic approach. *Nutrients.* 2012;4:243-257.

126. West J, Logan RF, Card TR, Smith C, Hubbard R. Risk of vascular disease in adults with diagnosed coeliac disease: a population-based study. *Aliment Pharmacol Ther.* 2004;20:73-79.

127. Soares FL, de Oliveira Matoso R, Teixeira LG, et al. Gluten-free diet reduces adiposity, inflammation and insulin resistance associated with the induction of PPAR-alpha and PPAR-gamma expression. *J Nutr Biochem.* 2013;24(6):1105-1111.

128. Emilsson L, Smith J, West J, Melander O, Ludvigsson J. Increased risk of atrial fibrillation in patients with coeliac disease: a nationwide cohort study. *Eur Heart J.* 2011;32:2430-2437.

129. Efe TH, Ertem AG, Coskun Y, et al. Atrial electromechanical proper- ties in coeliac disease. *Heart Lung Circ.* 2016;25(2):160-165.

130. Picarelli A, Di Tola M, Sabbatella L, et al. Anti-tissue transglutami- nase antibodies in arthritic patients: a disease specific finding? *Clin Chem.* 2003;49(12):2091-2094.

131. Corouge M, Loridant S, Fradin C, et al. Humoral immunity links Candida albicans infection and celiac disease. *PLoS One.* 2015;10(3):e0121776.

132. Nieuwenhuizen WF, Pieters RH, Knippels LM, Jansen MC, Koppelman SJ. Is Candida albicans a trigger in the onset of coeliac disease? *Lancet.* 2003;361(9375):2152-2154.

133. Emilsson L, Andersson B, Elfström P, Green PH, Ludvigsson JF. Risk of idiopathic dilated cardiomyopathy in 29,000 patients with celiac disease. *J Am Heart Assoc.* 2012;1:e001594.

134. Ludvigsson JF, de Faire U, Ekbom A, Montgomery SM. Vascular disease in a population-based cohort of individuals hospitalised with coeliac disease. *Heart.* 2007;93:1111-1115.

135. Goel NK, McBane RD, Kamath PS. Cardiomyopathy associated with celiac disease. *Mayo Clin Proc.* 2005;80(5):674-676.

136. Lebwohl B, Murray JA, Verdú EF, et al. Gluten introduction, breastfeeding, and celiac disease: back to the drawing board. *Am J Gastroenterol.* 2016;111:12-14.

137. Schuppan D, Pickert G, Ashfaq-Khan M, Zevallos V. Non-celiac wheat sensitivity: differential diagnosis, triggers and implications. *Best Pract Res Clin Gastroenterol.* 2015;29:469-476.

138. Molina-Infante J, Carroccio A. Suspected non-celiac gluten sensi- tivity confirmed in few patients after gluten challenge in double- blind, placebo-controlled trials. *Clin Gastroenterol Hepatol.* 2017;15:339-348.

139. Biesiekierski JR, Peters SL, Newnham ED, Rosella O, Muir JG, Gibson PR. No effects of gluten in patients with self-reported non- celiac gluten sensitivity after dietary reduction of fermentable, poorly absorbed, short-chain carbohydrates. *Gastroenterology.* 2013;145:320-328.

140. Zevallos VF, Raker V, Tenzer S, et al. Nutritional wheat amylase- trypsin inhibitors promote intestinal inflammation via activation of myeloid cells. *Gastroenterology.* 2017;152:1100-1113.

141. Zanini B, Baschè R, Ferraresi A, et al. Randomised clinical study: gluten challenge induces symptom recurrence in only a minority of patients who meet clinical criteria for non-coeliac gluten sensitivity. *Aliment Pharmacol Ther.* 2015;42:968-976.

142. Bucci C, Zingone F, Russo I, et al. Gliadin does not induce mucosal inflammation or basophil activation in patiens with nonceliac gluten sensitivity. *Clin Gastroenterol Hepatol.* 2013;11:1294-1299.

143. Rosinach M, Fernández-Bañares F, Carrasco A, et al. Double-blind randomized clinical trial: gluten versus placebo rechallange in patiens with lymphocytic enteritis and suspected celiac disease. *PLoS One.* 2016;11:e0157879.

144. Vojdani A, Vojjdani E. Gluten and non-gluten proteins of wheat as target antigens in autism, Crohn's and celiac disease. *J Cereal Sci.* 2017;75:252:e260.

145. Fasano A, Sapone A, Zevallos V, Schuppan D. Nonceliac gluten sensitivity. *Gastroenterology.* 2015;148:1195-1204.

146. Molina-Infante J, Santolaria S, Sanders DS, Fernández-Bañares F. Systematic review: noncoeliac gluten sensitivity. *Aliment Pharmacol Ther.* 2015;41:807-820.

147. Aziz I, Lewis N, Hadjivassiliou M, et al. A UK study assessing the population prevalence of self-reported gluten sensitivity and referral characteristics to Secondary Care. *Eur J Gastroenterol Hepatol.* 2014;26(1):33-39.

148. Pellegrina CD, Perbellini O, Scupoli MT, et al. Effects of wheat germ agglutinin on human gastrointestinal epithelium: insights from an experimental model of immune/epithelial cell interaction. *Toxicol Appl Pharmacol.* 2009;237:146-153.

149. Miyake K, Tanaka T, McNeil PL. Lectin-based food poisoning: a new mechanism of protein toxicity. *PLoS One.* 2007;2:687.

150. Lebret M, Rendu F. Further characterization of wheat germ agglutinin interaction with human platelets: exposure of fibrinogen receptors. *J Thromb Haemost.* 1986;56(3):323-327.

151. Ohmori T, Yatomi Y, Wu Y, Osada M, Satoh K, Ozaki Y. Wheat germ agglutinin-induced platelet activation via platelet endothelial cell adhesion molecule-1: involvement of rapid phospholipase C gamma 2 activation by Src family kinases. *Biochemistry.* New York: Bedford, Freeman & Worth. 2001.

152. Lambert J, Vojdani A, Correlation of tissue antibodies and food immune reactivity in randomly selected patient specimens, *J Clin Cell Imm Sept.* 2017;8:5.

153. Junker Y, Zeissig S, Kim SJ, et al. Wheat amylase trypsin inhibitors drive intestinal inflammation via activation of toll-like receptor 4. *J Exp Med.* 2012;209:2395-2408.

154. Schuppan D, Zevallos V. Wheat amylase trypsin inhibitors as nutritional activators of innate immunity. *Dig Dis.* 2015;33: 260-263.

155. Shepherd SJ, Parker FC, Muir JG, Gibson PR. Dietary triggers of abdominal symptoms in patients with irritable bowel syndrome: randomized placebo-controlled evidence. *Clin Gastroenterol Hepatol.* 2008;6:765-771.

156. Murray K, Wilkinson-Smith V, Hoad C, et al. Differential effects of FODMAPs (fermentable oligo-, di-, mono-saccharides and polyols) on small and large intestinal contents in healthy subjects shown by MRI. *Am J Gastroenterol.* 2014;109:110-119.

157. Halmos EP, Power VA, Shepherd SJ, Gibson PR, Muir JG. A diet low in FODMAPs reduces symptoms of irritable bowel syndrome. *Gastroenterology.* 2014;146:67-75.

158. Vojdani A, O'Bryan T, Green JA, et al. Immune response to dietary proteins, gliadin and cerebellar peptides in children with autism. *Nutr Neurosci.* 2004;7:151-161.

159. Pruimboom L, de Punder K. The opioid effects of gluten exorphins: asymptomatic celiac disease. *J Health Popul Nutr.* 2015;33:24.

160. Teschemacher H. Opioid receptor ligands derived from food proteins. *Curr Pharm Des.* 2003;9(16):1331-1344.

161. Lister J, Fletcher PJ, Nobrega JN, Remington G. Behavioral effects of food- derived opioid-like peptides in rodents: Implications for schizo- phrenia? *Pharmacol Biochem Behav.* 2015;134:70-78. doi:10.1016/j. pbb.2015.01.020.

162. Gosmanov AR, Fontenot EC. Sitagliptin-associated angioedema. *Diabetes Care.* 2012;35(8):e60. doi:10.2337/dc12-0574.

163. Csuka D, Kelemen Z, Czaller I, et al. Association of celiac disease and hereditary angioedema due to C1-inhibitor deficiency. Screening patients with hereditary angioedema for celiac disease: is it worth the effort? *Eur J Gastroenterol Hepatol.* 2011;23(3):238-244. doi:10. 1097/MEG.0b013e328343d3b2.

164. Jain AG, Guan J, D'Souza J. Candida parapsilosis: an unusual cause of infective endocarditis. *Cureus.* 2018;10(11):e3553.

165. Pavlina AA, Peacock JW, Ranginwala SA, Pavlina PM, Ahier J, Hanak CR. Aspergillus mural endocarditis presenting with multiple cerebral abscesses. *J Cardiothorac Surg*. 2018;13(1):107.

166. DeMelo EN, McDonald C, Saibil F, Marcon MA, Mahmud FH. Celiac disease and type 1 diabetes in adults: is this a high-risk group for screening? *Can J Diabetes*. 2015;39:513-519.

167. Arbuckle MR, McClain MT, Rubertone MV, et al. Development of autoantibodies before the clinical onset of systemic lupus erythematosus. *N Engl J Med*. 2003;349:1526-1533.

168. Nurminskaya MV, Belkin AM. Cellular functions of tissue transglutaminase. *Int Rev Cel Mol Biol*. 2012;294:1-97.

169. Schuppan D, Zimmer K-P. The diagnosis and treatment of celiac disease. *Dtsch Arztebl Int*. 2013;110:835-846.

170. Kaswala DH, Veeraraghavan G, Kelly CP, Leffer DA. Celiac disease: diagnostic standards and dilemmas. *Diseases*. 2015;3:86-101.

171. Rostami K, Kerckhaert J, Tiemessen R, von Blomberg BM, Meijer JW. Sensitivity of antiendomysium and antigliadin antibodies in untreated celiac disease: disappointing in clinical practice. *Am J Gastroenterol*. 1999;94:888-894.

172. O'Bryan T. Review of three pediatric wheat-related disorder cases with disparate clinical manifestations. *J Gastroenterol Hepatol Res*. 2018;3:020.

173. Vojdani A, Perlmutter D. Differentiation between celiac disease, non-celiac gluten sensitivity, and their overlapping with crohn's disease: a case series. *Case Rep Immunol*. 2013;2013:248482.

174. Lerner A. Comparison of the reliability of 17 Celiac disease associated biomarkers to reflect intestinal damage. *J Clin Cel Immunol*. 2017;8:1.

175. Di Pisa M, Pascarella S, Scrima M, et al. Synthetic peptides reproducing tissue transglutaminase-gliadin complex neo-epitopes as probes for antibody detection in celiac disease patients' sera. *J Med Chem*. 2015;58:1390-1399.

176. Porcelli B, Ferretti F, Vindigni C, et al. Assessment of a test for the screening and diagnosis of celiac disease. *J Clin Lab Anal*. 2016;30:65-70.

177. Perlmutter D, Vojdani A. Association between headache and sensitivities to gluten and dairy. *Integr Med*. 2013;12(2).

178. Choung RS, Marietta EV, Van Dyke CT, et al. Determination of B-cell epitopes in patients with celiac disease: peptide microarrays. *PLoS One*. 2016;11:0147777.

179. Choung R, Rostamkolaei S, Ju J, et al. Synthetic neoepitopes of the transglutaminase–deamidated gliadin complex as biomarkers for diagnosing and monitoring celiac disease. *Gastroenterology*. 2018. S0016-5085(18)35156-4.

180. Fera T, Cascio B, Angelini G, Martini S, Guidetti CS. Affective disorders and quality of life in adult coeliac disease patients on a gluten-free diet. *Eur J Gastroenterol Hepatol*. 2003;15(12):1287-1292.

181. Addolorato G, Mirijello A, D'Angelo C, et al. Social phobia in coeliac disease. *Scand J Gastroenterol*. 2008;43(4):410-415.

182. Ludvigsson JF, Sellgren C, Runeson B, Långström N, Lichtenstein P. Increased suicide risk in coeliac disease–a Swedish nationwide cohort study. *Dig Liver Dis*. 2011;43(8):616-622.

183. Leffler DA, Edwards-George J, Dennis M, et al. Factors that influence adherence to a gluten-free diet in adults with celiac disease. *Dig Dis Sci*. 2008;53:1573-1581.

184. Potter MDE, Brienesse SC, Walker MM, Boyle A, Talley NJ. Effect of the gluten-free diet on cardiovascular risk factors in patients with celiac disease: a systematic review. *J Gastroenterol Hepatol*. 2018;33(4):781-791.

185. See JJ, Murray J. Gluten-free diets: the medical and nutritional management of celiac disease. *Nutr Clin Pract*. 2006;21:1.

186. David L, Maurice C, Carmody R, et al. Diet rapidly and reproducibly alters the human gut microbiome. *Nature*. 2014;505(7484):559-563.

187. Di Cagno R, De Angelis M, De Pasquale I, et al. Duodenal and faecal microbiota of celiac children: molecular, phenotype and metabolome characterization. *BMC Microbiol*. 2011;11:219.

188. Sanz Y. Effects of a gluten-free diet on gut microbiota and immune function in healthy adult humans. *Gut Microbes*. 2010;1(3):135-137.

189. Moshfegh AJ, Friday JE, Goldman JP, et al. Presence of inulin and oligofructose in the diets of Americans. *J Nutr*. 1999;129:1407S-1411S.

190. Jackson FW. Effects of a gluten-free diet on gut microbiota and immune function in healthy adult human subjects - comment by Jackson. *Br J Nutr*. 2010;104(5):773.

191. Shewry PR, Tatham AS. Improving wheat to remove coeliac epitopes but retain functionality. *J Cereal Sci*. 2016;67:12-21.

192. Johnston CS, Snyder D, Smith C. Commercially available gluten-free pastas elevate postprandial glycemia in comparison to conventional wheat pasta in healthy adults: a double-blind randomized crossover trial. *Food Funct*. 2017;8(9):3139-3144.

193. Allen B, Orfila C. The availability and nutritional adequacy of gluten-free bread and pasta. *Nutrients*. 2018;10(10).

194. See JA, Kaukinen K, Makharia GK, Gibson PR, Murray JA. Practical insights into gluten-free diets. *Nat Rev Gastroenterol Hepatol*. 2015;12(10):580-591.

7

Marine-Derived Omega-3 Fatty Acids and Cardiovascular Disease

Thomas G. Guilliams, PhD and Jørn Dyerberg, MD, DMSc, DHC

Omega-3 Fatty Acids and Cardiovascular Disease

One of the most complex (and controversial) associations between food intake and cardiovascular disease (CVD) risk involves the dietary intake of fatty acids. Epidemiological and animal model data from the early 20th century linked the dietary intake of fat (primarily saturated) and cholesterol with increased risk for cardiovascular events in Western countries, which was followed by decades of recommendations for a low-fat/low-cholesterol diet to prevent CVD.[1-3] Today, there is a much more nuanced understanding of the complex relationship between fats and CVD risk, including their types (eg, saturated, unsaturated, omega-3, omega-6, omega-9), molecular structures (eg, trans versus cis bonds, triglycerides, phospholipids [PLs], free fatty acids, ethyl esters [EEs]), sources (eg, plant, animal, marine), and the doses and ratios of each. Among other discoveries, a significant shift in our understanding of the association between fatty acid intake and CVD occurred 50 years ago when Hans Olaf Bang and Jørn Dyerberg discovered that the Inuit populations of Greenland, eating a traditional diet with an extremely high intake of dietary fat, had a lower risk for cardiovascular events than Western populations consuming less fat. This discovery, and the subsequent publication of these findings by Bang and Dyerberg, initiated a revolution in both nutritional research and cardiovascular intervention.[4-6] Since then, the long-chain marine omega-3 fatty acids discovered in the Inuit diet and blood samples have been investigated for nearly every disease outcome and biomarker, including hundreds of clinical trials in healthy and at-risk populations. In that time, omega-3 fatty acid supplementation (primarily eicosapentaenoic acid [EPA] and/or docosahexaenoic acid [DHA] from fish) has become increasingly popular as a means for reducing CVD risk, as illustrated by the inclusion of omega-3 fatty acids in the American Heart Association dietary recommendations for the prevention of heart disease and the US Food and Drug Administration (FDA) approval of several omega-3 pharmaceutical products for a CVD-related biomarker.

However, the increased popularity of omega-3 fatty acid supplementation is not without controversy or confusion. Recent reevaluation of clinical trials performed years ago, through meta-analytical methodology, has led to several publications suggesting there is limited cardiovascular risk reduction associated with EPA and DHA supplementation, whereas epidemiological studies on the effect of a high fish intake continue to show a positive association with reduced CVD risk. These controversies are further mixed with numerous other debates surrounding the design of clinical trials testing omega-3 fatty acids for CVD outcomes, including how CVD risk should be measured (ie, biomarker versus end points), whether primary or secondary prevention studies are more appropriate to measure risk, bioavailability issues of omega-3 fatty acid supplements, the baseline omega-3 status of trial participants, and the concomitant use of other risk-reducing agents (ie, statin drugs) in these trials. At nearly the same time, the results of large and well-designed intervention trials have been recently published demonstrating significant CVD risk reduction after consuming n-3 fatty acid supplements. It is not surprising, then, that there is still much confusion as to the utility of supplementing omega-3 fatty acids for cardiovascular event risk reduction.

In this chapter, we will review these recent studies, as well as several seminal clinical trials from the recent past. In addition, we will discuss the mechanisms underlying the association between omega-3 fatty acid intake and the pathophysiology and biomarkers known to influence the risk for CVD. Included in this chapter is a discussion of various products (eg, dietary supplements, pharmaceuticals) designed to deliver omega-3 fatty acids for therapeutic use and important distinctions between these products.

Omega-3 Fatty Acids

Omega-3 (n-3) fatty acids are a class of polyunsaturated fatty acids derived from the 18-carbon essential fatty acid alpha-linolenic acid (ALA, 18:3 (n-3)). Although ALA is only synthesized in plants, some plants (eg, algae) and animals consuming ALA can elongate and desaturate this molecule to produce several different long-chain polyunsaturated fatty acids (LCPUFAs) such as stearidonic acid (18:4 (n-3)), eicosatetrae-noic acid (ETA, 20:4 (n-3)), EPA (20:5 (n-3)), docosapentae-noic acid (DPA, 22:5 (n-3)), and DHA (22:6 (n-3)). Although each of these fatty acids have been associated with health benefits in humans and garnered research attention, the two fatty acids that have gained the most attention and research focus are EPA and DHA. In fact, the vast majority of epidemiological studies connecting n-3 fatty acids and cardiovascular risk often only measure dietary intake of, or biomarkers for, EPA and DHA; furthermore, intervention trials using supplemental n-3 fatty acids are often described solely by their EPA and/or DHA content (even though they may contain other n-3 intermediates). Therefore, before diving into the epidemiological, interventional, and mechanistic studies of EPA and DHA, it is important to briefly describe the sources and molecular structures of these compounds as they are found in foods, supplements, and pharmaceuticals—because these factors can greatly influence their bioavailability, efficacy, and cost.

Sources of Marine Omega-3 Ingredients

For the most part, the marine n-3 fatty acid category is dominated by products best described as "fish oil"—that is, although there are products available that deliver n-3 fatty acids from other marine sources, nearly all the available research has been done with fish oil–derived fatty acids. These data using fish oil have become the benchmark for efficacy and safety and are the standard to which we compare other sources. Although pharmaceutical products often avoid the use of the term "fish oil," these products are currently all made from fish-derived fatty acids.

The following are the main sources of marine omega-3 fatty acids.

- **Fish Body Oil:** The largest biomass used to create marine-derived n-3 fatty acids are small oily fish caught in the cold waters off the coast of Chile and Peru. The fish species most commonly used are anchovies and sardines, with some mackerel. Concentrations of these purified oils are the most common therapeutic ingredient used in dietary supplements and pharmaceutical products throughout the world. Other species used to produce fish oil may include salmon, tuna, menhaden, herring, and other minor species. The EPA and DHA (and other fatty acids) content, which is predominantly in the triglyceride form, is dependent on the species of fish, the water temperature, and other variables on a seasonal basis.
- **Cod Liver:** As a by-product of the cod meat market, cod livers are used to provide a blend of fatty acids similar to unconcentrated fish body oil.

- **Krill:** These small crustaceans feed on plankton and are subsequently eaten by many marine mammals, especially penguins and whales. Factory ships process krill immediately upon capture off the coast of Antarctica. Krill oil, in which the n-3 LCPUFAs are predominantly in a free fatty acid and PL form, is relatively low in EPA and DHA but contains small amount of the carotenoid astaxanthin.
- **Calamari:** A more recent, but small, player in the n-3 fatty acid industry is calamari or squid oil. This oil, which is predominantly in the triglyceride form, has a higher ratio of DHA over EPA than is typical of fish oil. This material is a by-product of the calamari food industry.
- **Mussels:** Shellfish are only a minor source of commercially available n-3 fatty acids. Nonetheless, several products are currently available from the fatty acids derived from green-lipped mussels (*Perna canaliculus*). These ingredients are not typically marketed for cardiovascular benefits.
- **Algae:** Various species of algae are commercial sources for n-3 fatty acids. Algae can be grown in large inland production sites where access to sunlight is plentiful. These products are very high in DHA, with only small amounts of EPA, predominantly in the triglyceride form. Most of the pure DHA raw materials, especially pure DHA used for the fortification of infant formula, is sourced from algae. In addition, algae are currently the only vegan source of DHA available.
- **EPA and DHA from genetically modified plants:** Various algae, plants, and fungi have been genetically modified to produce various fatty acids, including both EPA and DHA. These ingredients are designed to help increase the global supply of these fatty acids, while limiting the harvesting burden on marine animals. As of 2018, these ingredients were only being produced for the supplementation of farm-raised fish (not directly used in dietary supplement ingredients).[7,8] It is possible these plant-derived EPA and DHA fatty acids may be approved for direct human consumption in the future.

Delivery Forms for Supplementation

When fatty acids are harvested from their source, they are typically in the form of triglycerides (TGs), PLs, or free fatty acids (FFAs) and are relatively low in total EPA and DHA (<30%). When consuming fish or unconcentrated fish oil (ie, fish body oil or cod liver oil), these fatty acids are in the TG form, as they are in most plant and animal sources of fat. However, because the recommended doses of EPA and DHA are often difficult to consume using unconcentrated oils, several steps can be used to increase the EPA and DHA concentration of the product while increasing the purity of the fatty acids delivered. The EPA and DHA fatty acids can be removed from their glycerol backbone and separated from other fatty acids (via hydrolysis and distillation). These fatty acids are then concentrated as EEs of EPA and DHA. These concentrated fatty acids can be reattached to a glycerol backbone to form re-esterified TG (rTG) molecules that contain a much higher concentration of EPA and DHA compared with the original TG molecule. These two forms of concentrated fish oil (EE and rTG) are the most common sources used in clinical trials and often recommended by physicians (as dietary supplements or pharmaceuticals). It is important to note the distinctions between the various delivery forms of these fatty acids, as this often impacts their bioavailability and efficacy. The use of FFAs and PLs (primarily from krill), as well as other factors affecting the quality, safety, and bioavailability of n-3 products (eg, heavy metals, pesticides, oxidation), will be discussed further.

The Epidemiology of Omega-3 FA and CVD

Epidemiological and cohort studies have repeatedly shown that higher dietary intake of fatty fish and/or a person's n-3 status (as measured by EPA and DHA in serum, plasma, or red blood cell [RBC] membranes) is inversely associated with cardiovascular events and/or cardiovascular mortality.[9-12] For instance, in a cohort of 20,551 men from the Physician's Health Study, the multivariate relative risk (RR) for sudden cardiac death in those consuming one fish meal per week was 0.48 ($P = .04$), compared with men who consumed fish less than once per month.[13] The adjusted RR in the highest quartile of RBC n-3 levels (compared with the lowest quartile) in this population was just 0.19 ($P = .007$).[9] The Honolulu Heart Program followed Japanese-Americans living in Hawaii and found the RR for coronary heart disease (CHD) mortality was cut in half for heavy smokers (>30 cigarettes/d) if they consumed more than two fish meals per week.[14] Several recent meta-analyses of prospective cohort studies have confirmed these overall results. Chowdhury et al. (2014) analyzed 16 studies exploring the relationship between long-chain n-3 dietary intake (lowest versus highest tertile) and coronary outcomes and reported an RR of 0.87 (95% confidence interval [CI], 0.78-0.97).[15] By comparison, ALA intake had no statistical relation to coronary outcomes (RR = 0.99, N = 7 studies), whereas total trans fatty acid intake contributed to a significant increase in coronary outcomes (RR = 1.16, N = 5). Furthermore, their analysis of studies comparing coronary outcomes based on circulating fatty acids (top versus lowest tertile, N = 13) revealed statistically significant risk reduction for EPA (RR = 0.78), DHA (RR = 0.79), and EPA + DHA (RR = 0.75). In a more recent meta-analysis, Alexander et al. (2017) analyzed 17 prospective cohort studies and found a significant reduction in CHD events (RR = 0.82), coronary deaths (RR = 0.82), and sudden cardiac deaths (RR = 0.53) comparing subjects consuming the highest versus lowest intake of n-3 fatty acids.[16] Notably, an analysis of data generated through the National Health and Nutrition Examination Survey (NHANES-2012) estimated that insufficient intake of marine n-3 fatty acids was the "cause" of over 54,000 CVD-related deaths annually.[17]

Omega-3 Index and CVD Risk

Because the dietary intake of omega-3 fatty acids from foods or supplements may not always correlate with biomarkers of omega-3 status, several investigators have focused on the incorporation of long-chain n-3 fatty acids (primarily EPA and DHA) within RBC membrane fatty acids as a way to measure the long-term absorption and tissue deposition of n-3 fatty acids.[18] In fact, the percentage of EPA and DHA within RBC membranes, known generally as the "Omega-3 Index" or O-3I, is inversely related to cardiovascular events and mortality, whereby the highest risk is associated with subjects with an omega-3 index less than 4% and the lowest risk is in subjects with an omega-3 index greater than 8%.[19] A recent meta-analysis of 10 cohort studies measuring risk in subjects based on their estimated omega-3 index predicted that subjects with an omega-3 index of 8% had a 30% lower risk for fatal CHD compared with those with an omega-3 index of 4%.[20] Therefore, because the risk reduction potential of supplemental EPA and/or DHA is likely dependent on dose, absorption, and tissue incorporation, determining a subject's baseline and postsupplemental omega-3 index may be necessary to optimize risk reduction–related n-3 supplementation.

Testing a patient's omega-3 index may be especially important to ensure that they are being recommended the correct dose to optimize their CVD risk reduction. Flock et al. have convincingly shown that the treatment dose of EPA and DHA (TG from fish) has a predictable effect on the change in omega-3 index, but they also discovered interindividual differences (especially based on a person's body weight) account for a high degree of variability in the omega-3 index changes seen after consuming EPA and DHA (**Figure 7.1**).[21] Therefore, based on this study, it is essential for the clinician to understand that, without testing a person's omega-3 index, it is not possible to predict the patient's current (or change in) omega-3 index, based simply on the n-3 fatty acid dose given (an important factor in interpreting clinical trials where all subjects are given the same dose of n-3). The omega-3 index is readily available through numerous laboratories and can easily be incorporated into a clinician's CVD risk assessment.

CVD Intervention Studies Using Omega-3 Fatty Acid

Although epidemiological and cohort studies have consistently shown substantial risk reduction in subjects consuming higher amounts of long-chain n-3 fatty acids, primary and secondary prevention trials have resulted in much more heterogeneity. One of the first studies assessing the secondary prevention potential of n-3 fatty acids from fish was the Diet And Reinfarction Trial (DART).[22] Men (N = 2033) recovering from a myocardial infarction (MI) were randomized to receive one of three different dietary recommendations: to increase fatty fish consumption, to increase fiber, or to reduce fat intake. Those advised to increase fatty fish

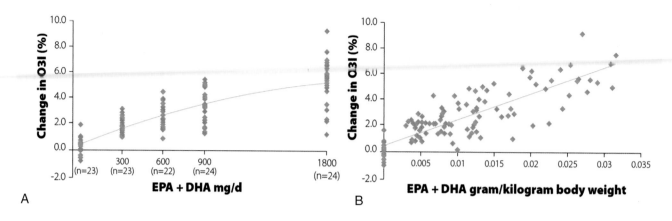

Figure 7.1 *Change in omega-3 index after 5 months of different doses of EPA + DHA in healthy subjects. A, Treatment dose significantly predicted changes in omega-3 index. Baseline omega-3 index for groups was 4.3%. Note that, although the average increases as the dose increases, there are many individuals with much higher (or lower) than average changes with each dose. B, Body weight effects on omega-3 index changes. The amount of EPA + DHA in grams consumed per kilogram of body weight significantly predicted changes in the omega-3 index. (From Flock MR, Skulas-Ray AC, Harris WS, et al. Determinants of erythrocyte omega-3 fatty acid content in response to fish oil supplementation: a dose-response randomized controlled trial.* J Am Heart Assoc. 2013;2:e000513.)

consumption had a 29% reduction in 2-year all-cause mortality, whereas neither the low-fat or fiber recommendation groups had a meaningful risk reduction. Unfortunately, like many lifestyle changes, this advice was difficult to maintain over many years and both compliance and benefits diminished after a decade.[23]

Until recently, the largest and most cited secondary prevention trial investigating the supplementation of EPA and DHA was the GISSI-prevention trial.[24] In this study, over 11,000 patients (surviving a recent MI) were randomized to one of three supplement groups: those given one gelatin capsule containing 850 to 882 mg of EPA and DHA (as EEs in the average ratio of EPA:DHA, 1:2), those given 300 mg of vitamin E (as acetyl alpha tocopherol, synthetic *all racemic*), or those give both n-3 fatty acids and vitamin E. Most of these patients were concomitantly taking nonstatin cardiovascular pharmaceuticals of various kinds, as well as advised about diet and lifestyle changes. Total (RR = 0.59) and cardiovascular mortality (RR = 0.66) were significantly reduced in the fish oil groups as early as 3 and 4 months into the study, respectively. The most dramatic reduction was in sudden deaths, for which RRs of 0.37 (after 9 months) and 0.55 (42 months) were reported.[25] Among the lipids measured, only triglyceride levels showed significant improvements. The results of the GISSI-prevention trial initiated the widespread use of concentrated EPA and DHA products around the world and justified numerous official recommendations for the use of EPA and DHA for CVD prevention and management (eg, American Heart Association's recommendation to consume 1 g/d of EPA and DHA from fatty fish or supplements).[26]

In the years between the publication of the DART and GISSI trials (1988-1999) there were over 20 randomized clinical trials evaluating the role of n-3 supplementation or increased fatty fish consumption on CVD, 10 of which met the criteria for a meta-analytical study.[27] Although many of these trials were of suboptimal quality, these data showed that the daily intake of long-chain n-3 fatty acids from fish for an average of 3 years resulted in a 16% decrease in all-cause mortality and a 24% decrease in the incidence of death from MI. We should note that none of the subjects in these 10 trials were taking statin drugs and, with the exception of the GISSI-prevention trial, the n-3 fatty acid doses given were all > 1.5 g of EPA and DHA per day. Both are important factors in comparing these data with more recent clinical trials, which are almost universally performed in statin-treated individuals (for secondary prevention) and often use n-3 fatty acid doses below 1 g/d.

In the past two decades, hundreds of clinical trials have been performed using a variety of doses, combinations, and types of EPA and DHA with respect to nearly every CVD-related end point. Although many of these were trials exploring the effects of n-3 FA on a variety of biomarkers (eg, TG, C-reactive protein [CRP], low-density lipoprotein-cholesterol [LDL-C], lipoprotein number and size, blood pressure), several of these studies were designed as primary and secondary prevention trials, measuring MACE (major adverse cardiac events; nonfatal MI/strokes, CVD deaths) and/or all-cause mortality. In 2017 and 2018, several well-publicized meta-analyses examined and compared these latter trials with some of the earlier trials mentioned before, determining there was no significant reduction in fatal or nonfatal CVD events in subjects randomized to n-3 FA therapies in these trials.[16,28,29] Of these, Aung et al., published in *JAMA Cardiology*, has had a significant negative impact on cardiologists' view of n-3 supplementation.[28]

However, as with many large intervention trials evaluating nutrients for drug-like outcomes, this meta-analysis, and the studies upon which it was based, has significant limitations. First, the analysis included only studies with greater than 500 participants treated for more than 1 year, which restricted their analysis to only 10 trials. Furthermore, 83.4% of the nearly 78,0000 subjects included in the analysis were concurrently using statin therapy, which reflects the changes in cardiovascular therapy from the previously mentioned cohort of n-3 studies. Perhaps more problematic was the fact that the omega-3 status was not used as an inclusion/exclusion criterion for any of these trials nor reported as a biomarker in these studies. This is important because, unlike drugs, participants would have started each trial with varying levels of EPA and DHA, greatly influencing their ability to achieve risk reduction through n-3 supplementation. In addition, as pointed out by von Schacky, these trials used a fixed dose of EPA and DHA, most often below 1 g (usually during a low-fat breakfast), which was likely to result in poor bioavailability (overall) and a large interindividual dose-response on improved omega-3 index.[30] Although some of the same limitations apply to the meta-analysis performed by Alexander et al., published in *Mayo Clinic Proceedings*, subgroup analysis of their 17 included trials revealed statistically significant benefits in subjects with elevated baseline TG > 150 mg/dL (RR = 0.84; 95% CI, 0.72-0.98) or baseline LDL-C >130 mg/dL (RR = 0.86; 95% CI, 0.76-0.98). Importantly, in this study, the strongest benefit was seen in subjects with elevated baseline TG given an n-3 fatty acid dose greater than 1 g/d of EPA and DHA (RR = 0.75; 95% CI, 0.64-0.89). This magnitude of risk reduction aligns with the prospective cohort data mentioned previously, suggesting that higher doses of n-3 fatty acids over a short-term period (ie, less than 5 years) may be needed to realize benefits that are typically achieved by extended periods of low to moderate n-3 intake. Data from recent large clinical trials may confirm this notion.

REDUCE-IT (2018)

One of these large clinical trials, the Reduction of Cardiovascular Events with Icosapent Ethyl-Intervention Trial (REDUCE-IT), has garnered much attention.[31] Like the successful Japan EPA Lipid Intervention Study (JELIS), the REDUCE-IT trial employed the use of the approved drug Vascepa, which is an EPA-only, EE product.[32] In this secondary prevention study, 8179 subjects with elevated fasting TG (between 150 and 499 mg/dL) and LDL-C of 41 to 100 mg/dL (all subjects were concurrently medicated with a stable dose of statin therapy) were randomized to receive placebo (mineral oil) or 4 g daily (2 g twice daily, with food) of EPA-EEs and followed for nearly 5 years. The major clinical end point was the cumulative incidence of cardiovascular events (CVD deaths, nonfatal MI, nonfatal stroke, coronary revascularization or unstable angina), which was 25% lower in the fish oil therapy group compared with placebo (hazard ratio 0.75, P < .001). As anticipated, TG levels in these subjects, which averaged 216.5 mg/dL at baseline, were significantly reduced (18.3%-21.7%) during the trial. Although the company producing Vascepa (Amarin) often remarks that EPA therapy (as opposed to DHA therapy) does not raise

LDL-C, these subjects realized a small but statistically significant increase in LDL-C from baseline (3.1%, P < .001). Because the LDL-C increase was coincident with an increase in HDL-C and a decrease in ApoB of similar magnitudes, these changes likely reflect a beneficial shift in LDL particle size and number (not reported). The lowest statistically significant hazard ratio (HR) following n-3 therapy was for subjects having baseline TG > 200 mg/dL and HDL <35 mg/dL (HR = 0.62). There is significant debate (both scientifically and commercially) as to the applicability of these data to other (similar) available products (ie, dietary supplements) that provide concentrated EPA or EPA/DHA in either the EE or rTG form. For a discussion of the potential differences between EPA and DHA and the bioavailability differences between EE and rTG see subsequent text.

VITAL (2018)

Published in the same November 2018 issue of the *New England Journal of Medicine* as the REDUCE-IT trial, the Vitamin D and Omega-3 Trial (VITAL) evaluated a more traditional n-3 dose and product in a large primary prevention study.[33] Participants (N = 25,871) were randomized to one of four groups: (1) n-3 fatty acids (1 g fish oil capsule/day [Omacor/Lovaza] providing EE forms of EPA [460 mg] and DHA [380 mg]), (2) vitamin D_3 (2000 IU/d), (3) both n-3 and vitamin D_3, or (4) both placebos (olive oil used for fish oil placebo). This dose and n-3 form was based on the recommendation of the American Heart Association (for cardioprotection) and the late-1990s GISSI-prevention trial. As a primary prevention trial in subjects over the age of 50 years (mean 67.1 years), only 4.2% of the subjects in VITAL experienced a cardiovascular event (defined in the composite end points: MI, stroke, cardiovascular deaths, or coronary revascularization) during the 5 years of the trial compared with greater than 19% of subjects in the REDUCE-IT trial. However, when subjects taking the n-3 supplements were compared with those taking olive oil, there was only a non-statistical trend in the reduction of major cardiovascular events (HR = 0.93; 95% CI, 0.80-1.04). Secondary end-point analysis suggested some benefits with n-3 supplementation, such as total MI (HR = 0.72; 95% CI, 0.59-0.90), deaths from MI (HR = 0.50; 95% CI, 0.26-0.97), and events in subjects with fish consumption <1.5 servings per week (HR = 0.81; 95% CI, 0.67-0.98).

Overall, these data are not unexpected, based on the shortcomings of the trial design: primarily the low number of events in this populations, the comparatively low n-3 dose to achieve meaningful event reduction (evidenced by achieving an omega-3 index of only 4.1% [from 2.7%] after 1 year of n-3 supplementation), and the use of olive oil (known to reduce CVD events at higher doses) as a placebo.[34] These shortcomings should be considered when evaluating the (mostly) negative results of VITAL, one of the largest clinical trials performed using EPA and DHA for the primary prevention of CVD. Unfortunately, some of these same shortcomings exist in a similar trial published earlier in 2018, ASCEND.

ASCEND (2018)

A Study of Cardiovascular Events in Diabetes (ASCEND) was also a primary prevention trial including only diabetic subjects (N = 15,480) with no evidence of CVD.[35] Subjects were randomized to receive a 1-g fish oil capsule per day (Omacor/Lovaza, providing EE forms of EPA [460 mg] and DHA [380 mg]) or placebo (olive oil) and followed for an average of 7.4 years. The primary outcome was a composite of nonfatal MI, stroke, or vascular deaths, whereas secondary end points included other serious vascular events or any arterial revascularization. Over the length of the trial, the group randomized to fish oil had 689 events (8.9%), whereas the olive oil group had 712 events (9.2%); this difference was not statistically significant (RR = 0.97; 95% CI, 0.87-1.08). In fact, with the exception of vascular deaths (RR = 0.81; 95% CI, 0.67-0.99), there were no beneficial differences in events reported between the n-3 and olive oil groups.

Again, these data are not surprising for some of the same reasons discussed previously in the VITAL study (eg, low n-3 dose, olive oil placebo), with two important differences. Because this group included only diabetic subjects (all types), these subjects had a higher CVD risk, which was evidenced by the higher number of events recorded in ASCEND (9.0%) compared with VITAL (4.2%), although still much fewer than the secondary prevention REDUCE-IT trial (19%). However, unlike the American subjects recruited for VITAL who had a mean baseline omega-3 index of just 2.7% (high risk), the UK subjects recruited for ASCEND had a mean baseline omega-3 index of 7.1% (which increased to 9.1% after supplementation). This suggests that the ASCEND subjects were already at low risk based on their baseline n-3 levels, limiting the ability of n-3 supplementation to alter that risk. On the other hand, because the VITAL group was only able to achieve an omega-3 index of 4.1% after supplementation, these subjects never achieved an omega-3 status associated with lower risk. Because neither trial reported TG levels of the participants, it is difficult to know whether either group included subjects with TG-associated risk and whether n-3 supplementation altered subjects' TG levels. Overall, these data suggest that routine n-3 supplementation of less than 1 g/d is unlikely to reduce measures of CVD events in populations with an average baseline omega-3 index of less than 4% or greater than 7%, at least when compared with subjects given olive oil placebos, over a span of less than 7 years.[36] However, several large clinical trials are currently underway that are soon likely to influence our understanding of the role of n-3 fatty acid supplementation in CVD primary and secondary prevention.[37-39]

Cardiometabolic Mechanisms and Biomarkers Related to EPA and/or DHA

Although the use of large clinical trials using major cardiovascular events as primary end points is viewed as the standard for measuring effects in drug trials, there are many studies linking the intake of EPA and/or DHA to a range of well-established CVD risk biomarkers.[40] For the most part, EPA and DHA are considered to have similar health benefits because they are most often delivered together, at various ratios, in fish food and in clinical trials; hence recommendations usually describe a combination of the two (EPA plus DHA), without differentiation. However, over the past decade a number of studies have hinted at both mechanistic and clinically relevant differences between these two similar fatty acids, potentially leading to subtle therapeutic differences for each. In some cases, there are head-to-head comparisons between the two fatty acids in clinical trials; in other cases, there are epidemiological or basic science discoveries that are driving clinical focus on one fatty acid over the other for specific health outcomes (eg, eye health, depression). Here we will briefly overview some of these discoveries as they relate to CVD biomarkers and outcomes, outlining where these differences between EPA and DHA may be clinically relevant.

Although it is generally assumed that EPA and DHA have identical benefits in preventing cardiovascular risk, and there is some limited evidence that the two molecules can be converted back and forth in humans,[41] there is accumulating evidence that DHA may be more favorable (overall) in cardiovascular-related outcomes. Mori and Woodman concluded in a review published in 2006 that "The data in humans suggest that DHA may be more favorable in lowering blood pressure and improving vascular function, raising HDL cholesterol and attenuating platelet function. Future studies will need to carefully assess the independent effects of EPA and DHA on other clinical and biochemical measures before decisions can be made with respect to dietary supplements and the fortification of foods with either EPA or DHA."[42] Others have published similar observations.[43,44] Since then, many advances, including the introduction and approval of an EPA-only EE pharmaceutical n-3 product, have been added to these early findings. Nonetheless, a systematic review published in 2018 came to a similar conclusion: "*Both EPA and DHA lowered triglyceride concentration, with DHA having a greater triglyceride-lowering effect. Whilst total cholesterol levels were largely unchanged by EPA and DHA, DHA increased high-density lipoprotein (HDL) cholesterol concentration, particularly HDL$_2$, and increased low-density lipoprotein (LDL) cholesterol concentration and LDL particle size. Both EPA and DHA inhibited platelet activity, whilst DHA improved vascular function and lowered heart rate and blood pressure to a greater extent than EPA.*"[45] Perhaps the ability of high-dose DHA to increase the omega-3 index to a greater extent than high-dose EPA helps explain some of these differences.[46] Below we will explore the data behind these statements further.

Triglyceride Reduction

One of the most consistent CVD-related biomarker changes resulting from supplementation with EPA and/or DHA preparations is the reduction in fasting and nonfasting serum TG.[47] These results have been consistently reported for decades, where the magnitude of reduction is often related to the dose of EPA and/or DHA, as well as the subject's baseline TG levels.[48-50] The TG-lowering effects of EPA and DHA are so well established that, currently, each of the omega-3 pharmaceutical products approved by the FDA are indicated specifically for severe hypertriglyceridemia (TG >500 mg/dL).

In many cases, the magnitude of the TG-lowering effect following EPA and/or DHA supplementation influences changes in other lipoprotein biomarkers, such as very low-density lipoprotein (VLDL) number and size, LDL number and size, LDL-C and HDL-C. These effects are thought to be mostly driven by the effects of these fatty acids on lipid-modulating transcription factors in hepatocytes and adipocytes (eg, PPAR family, RXR, SREBP1), and lipoprotein enzymes such as cholesterol ester transfer protein (CETP) and apoCIII.[51] Ultimately, these effects result in reduced hepatic synthesis of VLDL-TG, an increased clearance of TG, reduced levels of ApoB100, and a shift in cholesterol from VLDL particles to HDL and LDL particles. When compared head-to-head, DHA is often reported to have a slightly greater ability to lower TG levels versus EPA.[44,52,53]

LDL, HDL, and Non-HDL Cholesterol

There is much controversy surrounding the ability of fish oil supplementation to affect LDL-C and HDL-C levels, especially related to fish oil's ability to *raise* LDL-C. Research shows that long-chain n-3 fatty acid supplementation, and particularly DHA supplementation, raises both HDL-C and LDL-C, although it does not increase non-HDL-C. These increases in both HDL-C and LDL-C appear to be greater where TG-lowering is greatest.[54] As the triglyceride-rich lipoprotein VLDL is metabolized to LDL, a concomitant rise in LDL particles is, therefore, a natural consequence of triglyceride lowering (ie, VLDL lowering). Because the increase in LDL-C does not translate to higher non-HDL-C, this effect is likely the result of shifting cholesterol from VLDL particles to LDL and HDL particles, which then shifts LDL particles toward a larger and less atherogenic phenotype (see later discussion on particle size changes). The increase in LDL-C (and HDL-C) after DHA supplementation should therefore be viewed as metabolically favorable and indicative of shifting of lipids away from the triglyceride-rich VLDL particles, effects associated with reduced CVD risk.

Lipoprotein Particle Size

Combinations of EPA and DHA have been shown to favorably alter lipoprotein particle size: increasing both LDL and HDL particle sizes, as well as decreasing VLDL particle size. When EPA and DHA are compared with respect to their ability to improve HDL particle size, DHA-rich oils show more consistent improvements.[55,56] This may be because DHA has a greater inhibition of CETP activity, one of the enzymes responsible for altering lipoprotein particle size.[57] DHA, but not EPA, was capable of increasing LDL particle size in treated hypertensive patients with type 2 diabetes, as well as overweight hypercholesterolemic subjects.[54,58]

Blood Pressure

Omega-3 fatty acid therapy has shown modest improvements in both systolic and diastolic blood pressure and endothelial function, particularly in hypertensive patients.[59-61] In animal and human studies, DHA supplementation has a more significant impact on reducing both systolic and diastolic blood pressure than EPA supplementation.[62] DHA also showed greater improvement in endothelial function in these patients.[63] Both EPA and DHA improve arterial compliance.[64]

Heart Rate: An increased heart rate is an independent risk factor for CVD mortality. A meta-analysis of 30 studies investigating the role of fish oil supplements on heart rate showed a modest, statistically significant improvement in subjects consuming fish oil, compared with placebo (1.6 bpm; $P = .002$).[65] Heart rate was reduced by 2.6 bpm ($P < .001$) in studies lasting longer than 12 weeks or in studies in which the baseline median heart rate was above 69 bpm. In a study comparing DHA with EPA in their ability to affect heart rate, DHA was able to lower heart rate in overweight hyperlipidemic men, whereas EPA was not.[54] Other studies have shown similar superiority of heart rate lowering using DHA as compared with EPA.[52,66]

Inflammatory Biomarkers and Proresolving Mediators

Inflammation is a critical initiator and mediator of atherosclerosis and CVD events. Therefore, agents that reduce inflammatory biomarkers in at-risk subjects are considered to be helpful in risk reduction. CRP has been recognized as a universal biomarker of systemic and cardiovascular inflammation and has been used as a biomarker of CVD risk for many years.[67] Numerous studies have investigated the ability of n-3 supplements (primarily EPA and DHA) to improve biomarkers of inflammation (eg, CRP, tumor necrosis factor [TNF]-α, interleukin [IL]-6, eicosanoids) in human clinical trials, animal studies, and cell culture experiments, although many of these are in non-CVD-related experimental designs. A meta-analysis of 68 clinical trials evaluating the effects of marine-derived n-3 fatty acids on CRP, IL-6, and TNF-α have been performed.[68] This included studies performed in healthy subjects, as well as in patients with chronic autoimmune and nonautoimmune diseases. Overall, subjects given n-3 supplements had clinically meaningful, statistically significant reduction in fasting blood CRP, IL-6, and TNF-α, when compared with subjects given placebo. The cohort of studies that included those with CVD (chronic nonautoimmune diseases) had reductions of −18% for CRP and −20% for IL-6; the reduction in TNF-α was not statistically significant. Of the three biomarkers measured, only IL-6 lowering (−7.7%) reached statistically significance when these biomarkers were assessed based on n-3 from dietary intake (rather than supplementation). In subgroup analysis, significant lowering of CRP was observed only when n-3 supplementation was paired with a placebo that contained the n-6 fatty acid linolenic acid (primarily corn, sunflower, or soybean-containing oils), whereas this difference was not statistically significant in trials in which olive oil was used as the placebo. As noted earlier in our discussion of the VITAL and ASCEND clinical trials, olive oil has known benefits in CVD subjects, including documented anti-inflammatory activity.[69] In a meta-analysis of eight studies evaluating the effects of n-3 supplementation in type 2 diabetic subjects, there was a modest but statistical mean reduction of CRP.[70]

There are numerous mechanisms that have been postulated to account for the anti-inflammatory activities of EPA and DHA including the downregulation of various eicosanoids (prostaglandins, thromboxanes, and leukotrienes), PPAR-mediated modulation of NFκB pathways, and as precursors for specialized proresolving mediators (SPMs).[71] This latter mechanism has recently gained much attention, especially as it pertains to n-3 supplementation. SPMs are cell-signaling molecules derived from LCPUFA that function primarily to resolve (rather than inhibit) inflammatory processes.[72] Categories of SPMs include lipoxins (derived from arachidonic acid), resolvins (from EPA and DHA), protectins/neuroprotectins (from DPA and DHA), and maresins (from DPA and DHA).

Currently, there are several studies that associate biomarkers of SPMs with n-3 intake in human subjects. A secondary analysis of subjects with peripheral arterial disease given high doses of fish oil n-3 fatty acids (4.4 g of EPA and DHA per day) showed a significant 1-month increase in their omega-3 index (from 5% to 9%), which corresponded to significant increases in four different SPM precursors. Similarly, subjects with chronic kidney disease given 4 g per day of n-3 fatty acids (Omacor) saw significant increases in E and D-series resolvins after 8 weeks of supplementation. These studies, along with other similar findings, suggest that the intake of n-3 fatty acids (particularly EPA, DPA, and DHA) may augment the fatty acid reserve needed for the local production of SPMs to allow for appropriate resolution of local inflammatory processes.[73-75]

Bioavailability of n-3 Supplements

The efficacy of omega-3 fatty acid therapy is significantly affected by tissue availability, particularly its ability to increase a person's omega-3 index, which is affected by its initial bioavailability.[76] Therefore, numerous studies have been performed to compare short- and long-term bioavailability in human subjects using omega-3 fatty acids from different sources and in different molecular forms. We will first discuss studies using fish oil preparations and subsequently address the question of krill versus fish oil.[77]

Ethyl Esters Versus Triglycerides

Since the initial production and use of EE forms of omega-3 fatty acids, many have questioned the potential difference in bioavailability of these forms compared with other natural fatty acid forms. The early studies were small, but these data revealed either a slightly reduced bioavailability of the EE

forms (compared with TG forms) in the absence of additional dietary fat or a statistically similar bioavailability between EE and TG forms. More recently, several larger and better-designed studies have shown a superior bioavailability of rTG forms over EE forms.

One of the largest studies performed to date compared similar doses of EPA and DHA using five different forms: unconcentrated triglycerides (which the researchers called fish body oil [FBO]), cod liver oil (CLO, similar TG form as FBO), rTG, EE, or FFA, along with a "placebo" of corn oil (CO). In this study, 72 subjects were randomly assigned 3.3 g/d of an EPA + DHA blend as capsules for 2 weeks.[78] Serum fatty acids (combined serum TG, PL, and cholesterol esters) were analyzed at baseline and after 2 weeks. In these subjects, the bioavailability of EPA + DHA from re-esterified triglycerides (rTG) was superior (+24%) when compared with natural fish oil (FBO or CLO), whereas the bioavailability from EEs was inferior (−27%) to natural TG and nearly 70% less bioavailable than rTG. The authors suggest that the increased bioavailability of rTG over the unconcentrated TG form may be due to diglycerides contained in the rTG products, along with a small amount of monoglycerides, which act as "partially digested forms" of the natural triglyceride, potentially enhancing bioavailability over the natural fish body oil. Concerning the EE form, studies have shown a decreased lipase enzymatic activity when EE substrates are used, perhaps accounting for their decreased absorption when consumed away from a meal containing fat.[79]

Ultimately, it is critical to know whether these differences in bioavailability over 2 weeks might translate into long-term differences in fatty acid incorporation into important tissues (eg, RBC or cardiovascular tissues) and whether these differences can be measured in a clinically meaningful outcome (eg, reductions in TG). These sorts of studies have been carried out by researchers in Germany, who analyzed the incorporation of EPA and DHA into red blood cell membranes, commonly referred to as the omega-3 index, when individuals consumed either EE or rTG forms of fish oil.[80] One particular study included 150 hyperlipidemic subjects who were also taking statin drugs. Subjects were given soft gelatin capsules containing EPA (1008 mg) and DHA (672 mg) daily as either rTG or EE forms (corn oil used in placebo group) and were followed for 6 months. Subjects consuming the rTG form had, on average, a statistically higher omega-3 index than those consuming the EE form after 3 months, which was maintained after 6 months of daily intake. In a separate publication, the lipid-lowering effects of these two therapies were also reported.[81] Although both the EE and rTG reduced serum TG levels in these patients compared with placebo, the change resulting from rTG was nearly double that of the EE form (−18.7% versus −9.4%). The only therapy to reach a statistically significant decrease from baseline was rTG therapy.

These differences between rTG and EE have become hotly debated, because pharmaceutical products are primarily delivered as EE, whereas dietary supplement forms are available as both EE and rTG. Therefore, in a more recent trial, researchers performed a head-to-head trial comparing the TG-lowering effects of one of the popular EE pharmaceutical products (Lovaza) and an rTG fish oil product.[82] In this randomized, double-blind placebo-controlled trial, 120 subjects with nonfasting plasma TG levels of 150 to 500 mg/dL were given 3 g/d EPA and DHA as either an EE or rTG (or placebo) for 8 weeks. After supplementation, nonfasting plasma TG decreased 28% in the rTG group and 22% in the EE group (both $P < .001$ versus placebo), with no statistically significant difference between the two groups. The TG-lowering effect was seen after 4 weeks and was inversely correlated with the omega-3 index, which increased 63.2% in the rTG group and 58.5% in the EE group. In addition, heart rate decreased by three beats per minute ($P = .045$) and HDL-C increased only in the rTG group ($P < .001$). These data confirm that rTG products delivering similar amounts of total EPA and DHA as pharmaceutical EE products are at least as effective for lowering TG and may provide other cardioprotective benefits beyond the EE forms.[a]

Krill Oil Versus Fish Oil

In the past decade, the market has been flooded with information about the use of, and purported superiority of, omega-3 fatty acids from krill.[83] These claims have primarily come from two properties of krill oil: that it is composed mostly of PLs (as opposed to TG) and that it contains trace levels of astaxanthin, a bioactive carotenoid. Additionally, some studies have suggested these properties, particularly the PL nature of the fatty acids, account for superior bioavailability compared with fish oil. We will examine this claim first.

In general, only short-term and limited comparisons are available to ascertain the relative bioavailability of krill oil versus fish oil, a research question complicated by krill oil's very low concentration of EPA and DHA. One group studied the difference between the use of krill oil and menhaden oil (fish body oil, natural TG) or placebo (olive oil) in their ability to alter plasma fatty acids when consumed by overweight and obese subjects (N = 76).[84] Each subject was to consume 2 g/d of each oil for 4 weeks before being tested for changes in plasma fatty acid levels. The 2 g of menhaden oil contained 212 mg of EPA and 178 mg of DHA (390 mg total), whereas the krill oil preparation contained 216 mg EPA and 90 mg of DHA (306 mg total). Compared with olive oil, both the krill and menhaden oil significantly increased the EPA and DHA levels of the subjects: krill increased EPA by 89% and DHA by 23%; menhaden increased EPA by 81% and DHA by 45%. These data suggest that the bioavailability of EPA and DHA from krill and unconcentrated menhaden oil are similar.

The second study often cited was a 7-week study comparing the change in plasma fatty acids in subjects with "normal or slightly elevated" lipids when given either krill or fish oil.[85] This study compared six capsules of krill oil, providing 543 mg of EPA + DHA, and three capsules of fish oil (unspecified form), providing 864 mg of EPA + DHA. Compared with control subjects (unsupplemented subjects), both krill and fish oil were able to statistically increase EPA and DHA in those consuming each. However, although the average increase in EPA and DHA was slightly higher in the fish oil group, the difference between the groups was not statistically significant.

Unfortunately, trials using equal amounts of EPA/DHA from fish and krill are limited or severely flawed. One recent study compared equivalent doses of EPA + DHA from krill, rTG, and EE fish oils.[86] This was a single-dose, 72-hour study that measured changes in plasma PLs only, unlike the previous krill studies (measuring plasma fatty acids) or the long-term fish oil study (omega-3 index/RBC FA). Here, 12 healthy males were recruited to consume each of the three omega-3 preparations (crossover design, 14 days apart) containing a total of 1680 mg of EPA + DHA. The particular products used required 4 capsules of fish oil (rTG or EE) or 14 krill oil capsules to obtain the necessary EPA + DHA. Blood samples were taken before dosing (7 AM) and at 2, 4, 6, 8, 24, 48, and 72 hours after capsule intake. Like previous studies, there were no significant differences in the changes in plasma PL levels of EPA, DHA, or the sum of EPA + DHA between the three treatments. The authors did note nonstatistical "trends" of higher levels of plasma PL-EPA when subjects consumed krill. When one examines the data closely, it does appear that a higher plasma PL level did indeed occur in individuals consuming equal levels of EPA + DHA from krill versus fish. However, because the authors measured plasma PLs only, and krill oil is enriched with the PL form of the fatty acids, this trend may have been an artifact of fatty acid metabolism. Lastly, and perhaps most important for practical clinical consideration, it took 14 krill oil capsules to provide 1680 mg of EPA + DHA, something now provided easily in two concentrated fish oil capsules (they used four in this study). We conclude, as others have, that the bioavailability of EPA and DHA from krill is not superior to that of fish oil TG or rTG forms and the low concentration of EPA and DHA from krill make it an especially uneconomical way to deliver these compounds.[87]

Astaxanthin From Krill

Astaxanthin is a reddish-colored xanthophyll (carotenoid, similar to the compound zeaxanthin) found in a variety of marine organisms, from algae to salmon. Krill biomass contains about 120 ppm astaxanthin, and most krill oil preparations claim a small amount of it on their label. To date, no human studies have been performed using krill oil–derived astaxanthin, making the various marketing claims difficult to evaluate. Microalgae sources, and some synthetic sources, are the commercially available forms used in the limited

---

[a]It may be important to note that the rTG fish oil product had a higher content of DHA than the pharmaceutical EE product (1930 mg versus 1382 mg), although the rTG product had a lower level of total EPA and DHA (2885 mg versus 3306 mg). Even though the rTG dose was lower, the higher level of DHA may have accounted for some of these differences.

clinical studies that have evaluated astaxanthin. For context, the few studies available for astaxanthin supplementation in humans used doses ranging from 4 to 20 mg/d, and the average krill oil capsule claims to have 0.5 to 0.8 mg of astaxanthin per capsule.[88,89] Additional studies must be performed to understand the role and benefits of delivering astaxanthin from krill oil.

Additional Considerations on Marine Omega-3 Sourcing

Kosher

Only products derived from fish or algae sources can be deemed truly "kosher"; however, additional manufacturing processes may influence the ability to officially label a finished product (eg, soft gelatin capsules) with a particular kosher certificate.

Vegetarian/Vegan

Although many vegetarians choose to consume fish oil products even if they avoid consuming fish, strict vegans will avoid all marine lipids with the exception of algae-sourced products. Because EPA can be formed by consuming either DHA from algae or alpha-linolenic acid from flaxseed oil, these may be suitable options for strict vegan individuals. It should be noted that, although these vegan omega-3 sources are likely to increase blood levels of EPA and DHA, there are limited data to suggest that these alternatives will have the same risk-lowering benefits as EPA and DHA from fish.

Gluten

Marine fatty acids are gluten-free, and softgel manufacturing typically does not introduce gluten to finished products.

Sustainability Issues

One of the concerns with using large quantities of marine omega-3 fatty acids for therapeutic use is the long-term sustainability of harvesting the needed biomass. The debate over which source(s) might be in danger of overharvesting or are being harvested in an ecologically sound manner is controversial and made more difficult by the fact that no single final authority defines "sustainability" for the global community. Fisheries that supply both fish meal and fish oil are managed by a number of regulatory bodies around the world, and harvest limits are set for certain fish species, fishing seasons, and fishery zones. There is a seasonal variability in biomass, which is controlled by both local and global ocean conditions, affecting the year-to-year availability of EPA and DHA.[b]

Controversy over krill sustainability is especially keen. Most notably, in 2010 the retailer Whole Foods declared they would not sell krill products because of data they believed linked krill harvesting with reduced levels of animals that depend on krill for food. Since that time, the Marine Stewardship Council and other organizations have approved several of the largest krill harvesting companies as being "sustainable." The future of the sustainability of marine biomass is influenced by global ocean fluctuations and the growing need for EPA and DHA. Tension between marine-derived EPA and DHA sustainability and the development of more sustainable genetically modified organism-produced EPA and DHA from plants will no doubt heighten the controversy.

Allergies to Fish and Shellfish Related to Omega-3 Products

Since the changes required for food allergen labeling went into effect in the United States in 2006, there is confusion as to how fish oil products should be labeled and whether individuals allergic to fish can safely consume fish oil. The eight allergens requiring mandatory labeling include both fish and shellfish (also soy, wheat, eggs, peanuts, tree nuts, and milk). However, the labeling requirements exempt the need to label ingredients that are highly refined oils containing no allergenic proteins specifically as allergens. Therefore, highly refined fish oils, like certain soybean oils, do not need to be listed in a separate "contains the following allergens" statement on the label, although most companies using highly refined fish oils still choose to include "fish" in a list of allergens, primarily from a product liability standpoint. Nonetheless, the supplement facts box or front panel of a fish oil product must still declare that the ingredient itself is concentrated fish oil, thereby notifying users that the content contains fish-derived oils, even if no official declaration is made pertaining to fish-derived allergens.

Labeling issues aside, what is the likelihood that individuals who have known allergies to finned fish might also have an allergic reaction to a fish oil product? The answer appears to be: *extremely unlikely*. First, allergic reactions to fish are well understood and linked to specific proteins. Highly refined fish oil products are virtually free from any detectable protein, and there are no known allergens in fish-derived fatty acids. This notion was actually tested in a small-scale study where individuals with known allergies to finned fish were given fish oil supplements to evaluate their reaction.[90] Two different fish oil supplements were tested in six subjects with known fish allergies by both skin and oral challenges. None of the subjects reacted in any way to either product.

These data, although limited, agree with the notion that highly refined fish oil products contain no reactive allergens and should be safe to consume by individuals with mild to moderate fish allergies, although published case reports suggest it may occur rarely.[91] Ironically, delivering fish oil using fish gelatin capsules (to avoid animal versions of gelatin)

---

[b]For detailed information about the status and environmental performance of fisheries worldwide (eg, fish species, harvest statistics, regulations, and sustainability), see www.fishsource.com.

may inadvertently increase the likelihood of an allergic reaction in sensitive individuals.[92] Highly sensitive individuals and those with life-threatening fish allergies should probably avoid the use of fish oil products as a precaution and look to obtain omega-3 fatty acids from plant sources such as algae (DHA) or flax (ALA). Likewise, subjects with shellfish allergies should avoid krill and mussel-derived oils.[93]

Quality Control Issues of Fish Oil and Related Products

Fish oil–derived omega-3 fatty acids have been used as dietary supplements and pharmaceutical products for several decades. The quality control issues that plagued the first few years of fish oil availability, such as heavy metal contamination, pesticide residues, and oxidation, rarely occur in today's products. Several highly reputable organizations (eg, Global Organization for EPA and DHA [GOED], The Council of Responsible Nutrition [CRN]) have developed quality and regulatory standards for fish oil and related omega-3 products that set specific limits for heavy metal contamination, a wide variety of organic pollutants, and oxidation.[94] Because of these standards, most global fish oil providers maintain their products to these high standards—this is especially true of the concentrated products (ie, rTG and EE forms). Because heavy metal and pesticide residues are virtually impossible to be added during the manufacturing process, monitoring oxidation of the fatty acids is one of the critical steps in producing a high-quality product.

Fish oil oxidation is measured using two methods. The first measures oxidized fatty acids directly as a peroxide value (PV or POV). Because these peroxides are transient and can form secondary oxidized molecules, such as aldehydes, a second test is used to detect these oxidized compounds: the anisidine (or p-anisidine) test. By adding the anisidine value to twice the peroxide value (AV+2PV), we get the TOTOX value, which allows for evaluating an oil's rancidity.[95] To control the oxidation of the oil raw material

and finished product, most manufacturers add a variety of antioxidant compounds. The most popular are vitamin E, vitamin A, flavonoids, and rosemary or other spice extracts; synthetic antioxidants are rarely used. Most commercially available products contain one or more of these antioxidants, at very low doses, in the finished product. Manufacturers of liquid-filled bottles or softgel capsules also utilize nitrogen (to purge available oxygen), low light, and cold temperatures in the manufacturing process to reduce oxidation and extend shelf life. Products that have passed their expiration date should be thrown away, as oxidized fish oil can act as a pro-oxidant and limit the benefits realized if consumed.[96,97]

Conclusion and Recommendation

Based on the current available evidence, there is a significant inverse relationship between a person's omega-3 status (as measured by their omega-3 index) and their risk for CVD. In addition, there is a strong correlation between their dietary intake and/or supplementation with EPA and DHA and their omega-3 index. Therefore, clinicians should routinely measure the n-3 status of their patients and make dietary and supplemental recommendations according to their results. Although many forms of n-3 supplements have been shown to improve a subject's n-3 status and reduce CVD risk, evidence suggests that rTG forms may increase a patient's omega-3 index greater than EE forms, although individual variability (and subject body mass index) can affect this relationship. Also, although most studies are performed on products providing both EPA and DHA (some with only EPA), head-to-head studies often favor DHA for CVD-related outcomes. Therefore, some subjects may benefit from rTG products providing more DHA than EPA for CVD-related outcomes. Subjects should be monitored to achieve an omega-3 index of greater than 8%, which will often require doses greater than 1.5 g of EPA/DHA per day. These doses are easy to achieve using rTG or EE forms of fish oil, although they are difficult to achieve using low-dose fish or krill oil products.

References

1. Buja LM. Nikolai N. Anitschkow and the lipid hypothesis of atherosclerosis. *Cardiovasc Pathol.* 2014;23:183-184.
2. Mahmood SS, Levy D, Vasan RS, et al. The Framingham Heart Study and the epidemiology of cardiovascular disease: a historical perspective. *Lancet.* 2014;383:999-1008.
3. Andrade J, Mohamed A, Frohlich J, et al. Ancel Keys and the lipid hypothesis: from early breakthroughs to current management of dyslipidemia. *Br Columbia Med J.* 2009;51:66-72.
4. Bang HO, Dyerberg J. Plasma lipids and lipoproteins in Greenlandic west coast Eskimos. *Acta Med Scand.* 1972;192:85-94.
5. Dyerberg J, Bang HO, Hjorne N. Fatty acid composition of the plasma lipids in Greenland Eskimos. *Am J Clin Nutr.* 1975;28:958-966.
6. Dyerberg J. Coronary heart disease in Greenland Inuit: a paradox. Implications for western diet patterns. *Arctic Med Res.* 1989;48:47-54.
7. Sprague M, Betancor MB, Tocher DR. Microbial and genetically engineered oils as replacements for fish oil in aquaculture feeds. *Biotechnol Lett.* 2017;39:1599-1609.
8. Betancor MB, Li K, Sprague M, et al. An oil containing EPA and DHA from transgenic Camelina sativa to replace marine fish oil in feeds for Atlantic salmon (Salmo salar L.): effects on intestinal transcriptome, histology, tissue fatty acid profiles and plasma biochemistry. *PLoS One.* 2017;12:e0175415.
9. Albert CM, Campos H, Stampfer MJ, et al. Blood levels of long-chain n-3 fatty acids and the risk of sudden death. *N Engl J Med.* 2002;346:1113-1118.
10. Hu FB, Bronner L, Willett WC, et al. Fish and omega-3 fatty acid intake and risk of coronary heart disease in women. *JAMA.* 2002;287:1815-1821.
11. Gammelmark A, Nielsen MS, Bork CS, et al. Association of fish consumption and dietary intake of marine n-3 PUFA with myocardial infarction in a prospective Danish cohort study. *Br J Nutr.* 2016;116:167-177.
12. Miyagawa N, Miura K, Okuda N, et al. Long-chain n-3 polyunsaturated fatty acids intake and cardiovascular disease mortality risk in Japanese: a 24-year follow-up of NIPPON DATA80. *Atherosclerosis.* 2014;232:384-389.

13. Albert CM, Hennekens CH, O'Donnell CJ, et al. Fish consumption and risk of sudden cardiac death. *JAMA*. 1998;279:23-28.

14. Rodriguez BL, Sharp DS, Abbott RD, et al. Fish intake may limit the increase in risk of coronary heart disease morbidity and mortality among heavy smokers. The Honolulu Heart Program. *Circulation*. 1996;94:952-956.

15. Chowdhury R, Warnakula S, Kunutsor S, et al. Association of dietary, circulating, and supplement fatty acids with coronary risk: a systematic review and meta-analysis. *Ann Intern Med*. 2014;160:398-406.

16. Alexander DD, Miller PE, Van Elswyk ME, et al. A meta-analysis of randomized controlled trials and prospective cohort studies of eicosapentaenoic and docosahexaenoic long-chain omega-3 fatty acids and coronary heart disease risk. *Mayo Clin Proc*. 2017;92:15-29.

17. Micha R, Penalvo JL, Cudhea F, et al. Association between dietary factors and mortality from heart disease, stroke, and type 2 diabetes in the United States. *JAMA*. 2017;317:912-924.

18. Harris WS, Von Schacky C. The Omega-3 Index: a new risk factor for death from coronary heart disease?. *Prev Med*. 2004;39:212-220.

19. Harris WS. The omega-3 index: clinical utility for therapeutic intervention. *Curr Cardiol Rep*. 2010;12:503-508.

20. Harris WS, Del Gobbo L, Tintle NL. The Omega-3 Index and relative risk for coronary heart disease mortality: estimation from 10 cohort studies. *Atherosclerosis*. 2017;262:51-54.

21. Flock MR, Skulas-Ray AC, Harris WS, et al. Determinants of erythrocyte omega-3 fatty acid content in response to fish oil supplementation: a dose-response randomized controlled trial. *J Am Heart Assoc*. 2013;2:e000513.

22. Burr ML, Fehily AM, Gilbert JF, et al. Effects of changes in fat, fish, and fibre intakes on death and myocardial reinfarction: diet and reinfarction trial (DART). *Lancet*. 1989;2:757-761.

23. Ness AR, Hughes J, Elwood PC, et al. The long-term effect of dietary advice in men with coronary disease: follow-up of the Diet and Reinfarction trial (DART). *Eur J Clin Nutr*. 2002;56:512-518.

24. Gruppo Italiano per lo Studio della Sopravvivenza nell'Infarto miocardico. Dietary supplementation with n-3 polyunsaturated fatty acids and vitamin E after myocardial infarction: results of the GISSI-Prevenzione trial. *Lancet*. 1999;354:447-455.

25. Marchioli R, Barzi F, Bomba E, et al. Early protection against sudden death by n-3 polyunsaturated fatty acids after myocardial infarction: time-course analysis of the results of the Gruppo Italiano per lo Studio della Sopravvivenza nell'Infarto Miocardico (GISSI)-Prevenzione. *Circulation*. 2002;105:1897-1903.

26. Kris-Etherton PM, Harris WS, Appel LJ. Fish consumption, fish oil, omega-3 fatty acids, and cardiovascular disease. *Circulation*. 2002;106:2747-2757.

27. Yzebe D, Lievre M. Fish oils in the care of coronary heart disease patients: a meta-analysis of randomized controlled trials. *Fundam Clin Pharmacol*. 2004;18:581-592.

28. Aung T, Halsey J, Kromhout D, et al. Associations of omega-3 fatty acid supplement use with cardiovascular disease risks: meta-analysis of 10 trials involving 77917 individuals. *JAMA Cardiol*. 2018;3:225-234.

29. Abdelhamid AS, Brown TJ, Brainard JS, et al. Omega-3 fatty acids for the primary and secondary prevention of cardiovascular disease. *Cochrane Database Syst Rev*. 2018;11:Cd003177.

30. von Schacky C. Rebuttal to Aung et al, "Associations of omega-3 fatty acid supplement use with cardiovascular disease risks: meta-analysis of 10 trials involving 77 917 individuals". *Altern Ther Health Med*. 2018;24:8-9.

31. Bhatt DL, Steg PG, Miller M, et al. Cardiovascular risk reduction with icosapent ethyl for hypertriglyceridemia. *N Engl J Med*. 2019;380:11-22.

32. Yokoyama M, Origasa H, Matsuzaki M, et al. Effects of eicosapentaenoic acid on major coronary events in hypercholesterolaemic patients (JELIS): a randomised open-label, blinded endpoint analysis. *Lancet*. 2007;369:1090-1098.

33. Manson JE, Cook NR, Lee IM, et al. Marine n-3 fatty acids and prevention of cardiovascular disease and cancer. *N Engl J Med*. 2019;380:23-32.

34. Guasch-Ferre M, Hu FB, Martinez-Gonzalez MA, et al. Olive oil intake and risk of cardiovascular disease and mortality in the PREDIMED Study. *BMC Med*. 2014;12:78.

35. Bowman L, Mafham M, Wallendszus K, et al. Effects of n-3 fatty acid supplements in diabetes mellitus. *N Engl J Med*. 2018;379:1540-1550.

36. Maki KC, Dicklin MR. Omega-3 fatty acid supplementation and cardiovascular disease risk: glass half full or time to nail the coffin shut? *Nutrients*. 2018;10:864.

37. Daida H. *Randomized trial for Evaluation in Secondary Prevention Efficacy of Combination Therapy – Statin and Eicosapentaenoic Acid*; 2018. https://upload.umin.ac.jp/cgi-open-bin/ctr_e/ctr_view.cgi?recptno=R000014051.

38. Budoff M, Brent Muhlestein J, Le VT, et al. Effect of Vascepa (icosapent ethyl) on progression of coronary atherosclerosis in patients with elevated triglycerides (200-499 mg/dL) on statin therapy: rationale and design of the EVAPORATE study. *Clin Cardiol*. 2018;41:13-19.

39. Nicholls SJ, Lincoff AM, Bash D, et al. Assessment of omega-3 carboxylic acids in statin-treated patients with high levels of triglycerides and low levels of high-density lipoprotein cholesterol: rationale and design of the STRENGTH trial. *Clin Cardiol*. 2018;41:1281-1288.

40. Thota RN, Ferguson JJA, Abbott KA, et al. Science behind the cardiometabolic benefits of omega-3 polyunsaturated fatty acids: biochemical effects vs. clinical outcomes. *Food Funct*. 2018;9:3576-3596.

41. Arterburn LM, Hall EB, Oken H. Distribution, interconversion, and dose response of n-3 fatty acids in humans. *Am J Clin Nutr*. 2006;83:1467s-1476s.

42. Mori TA, Woodman RJ. The independent effects of eicosapentaenoic acid and docosahexaenoic acid on cardiovascular risk factors in humans. *Curr Opin Clin Nutr Metab Care*. 2006;9:95-104.

43. Cottin SC, Sanders TA, Hall WL. The differential effects of EPA and DHA on cardiovascular risk factors. *Proc Nutr Soc*. 2011;70:215-231.

44. Wei MY, Jacobson TA. Effects of eicosapentaenoic acid versus docosahexaenoic acid on serum lipids: a systematic review and meta-analysis. *Curr Atheroscler Rep*. 2011;13:474-483.

45. Innes JK, Calder PC. The differential effects of eicosapentaenoic acid and docosahexaenoic acid on cardiometabolic risk factors: a systematic review. *Int J Mol Sci*. 2018;19(2):532.

46. Allaire J, Harris WS, Vors C, et al. Supplementation with high-dose docosahexaenoic acid increases the Omega-3 Index more than high-dose eicosapentaenoic acid. *Prostaglandins Leukot Essent Fatty Acids*. 2017;120:8-14.

47. Pirillo A, Catapano AL. Omega-3 polyunsaturated fatty acids in the treatment of atherogenic dyslipidemia. *Atheroscler Suppl*. 2013;14:237-242.

48. Skulas-Ray AC, Alaupovic P, Kris-Etherton PM, et al. Dose-response effects of marine omega-3 fatty acids on apolipoproteins, apolipoprotein-defined lipoprotein subclasses, and Lp-PLA2 in individuals with moderate hypertriglyceridemia. *J Clin Lipidol*. 2015;9:360-367.

49. Balk EM, Lichtenstein AH, Chung M, et al. Effects of omega-3 fatty acids on serum markers of cardiovascular disease risk: a systematic review. *Atherosclerosis*. 2006;189:19-30.

50. Backes J, Anzalone D, Hilleman D, et al. The clinical relevance of omega-3 fatty acids in the management of hypertriglyceridemia. *Lipids Health Dis*. 2016;15:118.

51. Martinez-Fernandez L, Laiglesia LM, Huerta AE, et al. Omega-3 fatty acids and adipose tissue function in obesity and metabolic syndrome. *Prostaglandins Other Lipid Mediat*. 2015;121:24-41.

52. Grimsgaard S, Bonaa KH, Hansen JB, et al. Effects of highly purified eicosapentaenoic acid and docosahexaenoic acid on hemodynamics in humans. *Am J Clin Nutr*. 1998;68:52-59.

53. Allaire J, Couture P, Leclerc M, et al. A randomized, crossover, head-to-head comparison of eicosapentaenoic acid and docosahexaenoic acid supplementation to reduce inflammation markers in men and women: the Comparing EPA to DHA (ComparED) Study. *Am J Clin Nutr*. 2016;104:280-287.

54. Mori TA, Burke V, Puddey IB, et al. Purified eicosapentaenoic and docosahexaenoic acids have differential effects on serum lipids and lipoproteins, LDL particle size, glucose, and insulin in mildly hyperlipidemic men. *Am J Clin Nutr*. 2000;71:1085-1094.

55. Buckley R, Shewring B, Turner R, et al. Circulating triacylglycerol and apoE levels in response to EPA and docosahexaenoic acid supplementation in adult human subjects. *Br J Nutr.* 2004;92:477-483.

56. Allaire J, Vors C, Tremblay AJ, et al. High-dose DHA has more profound effects on LDL-related features than high-dose EPA: the ComparED study. *J Clin Endocrinol Metab.* 2018;103:2909-2917.

57. Hirano R, Igarashi O, Kondo K, et al. Regulation by long-chain fatty acids of the expression of cholesteryl ester transfer protein in HepG2 cells. *Lipids.* 2001;36:401-406.

58. Woodman RJ, Mori TA, Burke V, et al. Docosahexaenoic acid but not eicosapentaenoic acid increases LDL particle size in treated hypertensive type 2 diabetic patients. *Diabetes Care.* 2003;26:253.

59. Zehr KR, Walker MK. Omega-3 polyunsaturated fatty acids improve endothelial function in humans at risk for atherosclerosis: a review. *Prostaglandins Other Lipid Mediat.* 2018;134:131-140.

60. Balakumar P, Taneja G. Fish oil and vascular endothelial protection: bench to bedside. *Free Radic Biol Med.* 2012;53:271-279.

61. Cicero AF, Ertek S, Borghi C. Omega-3 polyunsaturated fatty acids: their potential role in blood pressure prevention and management. *Curr Vasc Pharmacol.* 2009;7:330-337.

62. Mori TA, Bao DQ, Burke V, et al. Docosahexaenoic acid but not eicosapentaenoic acid lowers ambulatory blood pressure and heart rate in humans. *Hypertension.* 1999;34:253-260.

63. Mori TA, Watts GF, Burke V, et al. Differential effects of eicosapentaenoic acid and docosahexaenoic acid on vascular reactivity of the forearm microcirculation in hyperlipidemic, overweight men. *Circulation.* 2000;102:1264-1269.

64. Nestel P, Shige H, Pomeroy S, et al. The n-3 fatty acids eicosapentaenoic acid and docosahexaenoic acid increase systemic arterial compliance in humans. *Am J Clin Nutr.* 2002;76:326-330.

65. Mozaffarian D, Geelen A, Brouwer IA, et al. Effect of fish oil on heart rate in humans: a meta-analysis of randomized controlled trials. *Circulation.* 2005;112:1945-1952.

66. Hidayat K, Yang J, Zhang Z, et al. Effect of omega-3 long-chain polyunsaturated fatty acid supplementation on heart rate: a meta-analysis of randomized controlled trials. *Eur J Clin Nutr.* 2018;72:805-817.

67. Avan A, Tavakoly Sany SB, Ghayour-Mobarhan M, et al. Serum C-reactive protein in the prediction of cardiovascular diseases: overview of the latest clinical studies and public health practice. *J Cell Physiol.* 2018;233:8508-8525.

68. Li K, Huang T, Zheng J, et al. Effect of marine-derived n-3 polyunsaturated fatty acids on C-reactive protein, interleukin 6 and tumor necrosis factor alpha: a meta-analysis. *PLoS One.* 2014;9:e88103.

69. Schwingshackl L, Christoph M, Hoffmann G. Effects of olive oil on markers of inflammation and endothelial function-a systematic review and meta-analysis. *Nutrients.* 2015;7:7651-7675.

70. Lin N, Shi JJ, Li YM, et al. What is the impact of n-3 PUFAs on inflammation markers in Type 2 diabetic mellitus populations?: a systematic review and meta-analysis of randomized controlled trials. *Lipids Health Dis.* 2016;15:133.

71. Calder PC. Omega-3 fatty acids and inflammatory processes: from molecules to man. *Biochem Soc Trans.* 2017;45:1105-1115.

72. Conte MS, Desai TA, Wu B, et al. Pro-resolving lipid mediators in vascular disease. *J Clin Invest.* 2018;128:3727-3735.

73. Barden AE, Mas E, Mori TA. n-3 Fatty acid supplementation and proresolving mediators of inflammation. *Curr Opin Lipidol.* 2016;27:26-32.

74. Barden AE, Mas E, Croft KD, et al. Specialized proresolving lipid mediators in humans with the metabolic syndrome after n-3 fatty acids and aspirin. *Am J Clin Nutr.* 2015;102:1357-1364.

75. Mas E, Croft KD, Zahra P, et al. Resolvins D1, D2, and other mediators of self-limited resolution of inflammation in human blood following n-3 fatty acid supplementation. *Clin Chem.* 2012;58:1476-1484.

76. von Schacky C. Omega-3 fatty acids in cardiovascular disease–an uphill battle. *Prostaglandins Leukot Essent Fatty Acids.* 2015;92:41-47.

77. Schuchardt JP, Hahn A. Bioavailability of long-chain omega-3 fatty acids. *Prostaglandins Leukot Essent Fatty Acids.* 2013;89:1-8.

78. Dyerberg J, Madsen P, Moller JM, et al. Bioavailability of marine n-3 fatty acid formulations. *Prostaglandins Leukot Essent Fatty Acids.* 2010;83:137-141.

79. Krokan HE, Bjerve KS, Mork E. The enteral bioavailability of eicosapentaenoic acid and docosahexaenoic acid is as good from ethyl esters as from glyceryl esters in spite of lower hydrolytic rates by pancreatic lipase in vitro. *Biochim Biophys Acta.* 1993;1168:59-67.

80. Neubronner J, Schuchardt JP, Kressel G, et al. Enhanced increase of omega-3 index in response to long-term n-3 fatty acid supplementation from triacylglycerides versus ethyl esters. *Eur J Clin Nutr.* 2011;65:247-254.

81. Schuchardt JP, Neubronner J, Kressel G, et al. Moderate doses of EPA and DHA from re-esterified triacylglycerols but not from ethyl-esters lower fasting serum triacylglycerols in statin-treated dyslipidemic subjects: results from a six month randomized controlled trial. *Prostaglandins Leukot Essent Fatty Acids.* 2011;85:381-386.

82. Hedengran A, Szecsi PB, Dyerberg J, et al. n-3 PUFA esterified to glycerol or as ethyl esters reduce non-fasting plasma triacylglycerol in subjects with hypertriglyceridemia: a randomized trial. *Lipids.* 2015;50:165-175.

83. Kwantes JM, Grundmann O. A brief review of krill oil history, research, and the commercial market. *J Diet Suppl.* 2015;12:23-35.

84. Maki KC, Reeves MS, Farmer M, et al. Krill oil supplementation increases plasma concentrations of eicosapentaenoic and docosahexaenoic acids in overweight and obese men and women. *Nutr Res.* 2009;29:609-615.

85. Ulven SM, Kirkhus B, Lamglait A, et al. Metabolic effects of krill oil are essentially similar to those of fish oil but at lower dose of EPA and DHA, in healthy volunteers. *Lipids.* 2011;46:37-46.

86. Schuchardt JP, Schneider I, Meyer H, et al. Incorporation of EPA and DHA into plasma phospholipids in response to different omega-3 fatty acid formulations–a comparative bioavailability study of fish oil vs. krill oil. *Lipids Health Dis.* 2011;10:145.

87. Salem N Jr, Kuratko CN. A reexamination of krill oil bioavailability studies. *Lipids Health Dis.* 2014;13:137.

88. Earnest CP, Lupo M, White KM, et al. Effect of astaxanthin on cycling time trial performance. *Int J Sports Med.* 2011;32:882-888.

89. Choi HD, Kim JH, Chang MJ, et al. Effects of astaxanthin on oxidative stress in overweight and obese adults. *Phytother Res.* 2011;25:1813-1818.

90. Mark BJ, Beaty AD, Slavin RG. Are fish oil supplements safe in finned fish-allergic patients? *Allergy Asthma Proc.* 2008;29:528-529.

91. Howard Thompson A, Dutton A, Hoover R, et al. Flushing and pruritus secondary to prescription fish oil ingestion in a patient with allergy to fish. *Int J Clin Pharm.* 2014;36:1126-1129.

92. Sakaguchi M, Toda M, Ebihara T, et al. IgE antibody to fish gelatin (type I collagen) in patients with fish allergy. *J Allergy Clin Immunol.* 2000;106:579-584.

93. Motoyama K, Suma Y, Ishizaki S, et al. Identification of tropomyosins as major allergens in Antarctic krill and mantis shrimp and their amino acid sequence characteristics. *Mar Biotechnol (NY).* 2008;10:709-718.

94. Global Organization for EPA and DHA Omega-3. *GOED Voluntary Monograph*; 2018. http://goedomega3.com/index.php/goed-monograph.

95. Miller M. *Oxidation of Food Grade Oils*; n/a. https://www.oilsfats.org.nz/documents/Oxidation%20101.pdf.

96. Jackowski SA, Alvi AZ, Mirajkar A, et al. Oxidation levels of North American over-the-counter n-3 (omega-3) supplements and the influence of supplement formulation and delivery form on evaluating oxidative safety. *J Nutr Sci.* 2015;4:e30.

97. Rundblad A, Holven KB, Ottestad I, et al. High-quality fish oil has a more favourable effect than oxidised fish oil on intermediate-density lipoprotein and LDL subclasses: a randomised controlled trial. *Br J Nutr.* 2017;117:1291-1298.

Section 4

The Role of Exercise

Chapter 8   **The Role of Exercise in Hypertension, Dyslipidemia, Insulin Resistance, Metabolic Syndrome, Obesity, CHD, and CHF**
Mark C. Houston, MD, MS, MSc, FACP, FAHA, FASH, FACN, FAARM, ABAARM, DABC

8

The Role of Exercise in Hypertension, Dyslipidemia, Insulin Resistance, Metabolic Syndrome, Obesity, CHD, and CHF

Mark C. Houston, MD, MS, MSc, FACP, FAHA, FASH, FACN, FAARM, ABAARM, DABC

The Health Benefits of Exercise

The health benefits of exercise are many (Table 8.1) and include improvements in virtually every organ system in the body. Some of these benefits are increased longevity and reductions in cardiovascular disease, myocardial infarction, congestive heart failure (CHF), stroke, hypertension, dyslipidemia, dysglycemia, obesity, thrombosis, cancer, immune function, infections, and gastrointestinal illness. Memory and central nervous system function improve with reductions in anxiety, stress, depression, disturbances in sleep, and more.[1,2] Whether exercise is dynamic/isotonic, isometric, aerobic, anaerobic, based on oxygen utilization, there are specific benefits.[1-5] Aerobic or endurance exercise (AE) imposes a volume overload on the cardiovascular system with increased VO2, heart rate, cardiac output, and stroke volume; reduced systemic vascular resistance; decreased diastolic blood pressure (BP); and increased A-VO2. Resistance training (RT) exerts both a volume and a pressure overload state with little change in heart rate, cardiac output, stroke volume, systolic or diastolic BP; it increases or does not change VO2.[3] The relative merits and specific combinations of interval and endurance aerobics and RT will be discussed in more detail later in this chapter.

Exercise Physiology and Theory

Skeletal muscle is a secretory (endocrine) organ, and exercise increases the metabolic and secretory/endocrine capacity of muscle.[1] Specific kinds of exercise can alter the ways genes function and interact with cells.[1] By triggering the right exercise-gene interactions, inflammation, oxidative stress, and immune dysfunction are improved.[1]

The slow physical deterioration of the cardiovascular system and body in general that is seen with age is not inevitable. It is largely the result of diet and movement—or the lack thereof. Movement is one of the primary keys to overall health and especially cardiovascular health. The movement required is the same kind of natural movement that kept humans in robust physical health for millennia. This is not the kind of exercise that most personal trainers, fitness enthusiasts, or doctors recommend. As a matter of fact, most doctors and trainers recommend the exact opposite approach to movement and exercise, one that may actually accelerate the deterioration of health, cardiovascular benefits, and overall aging. In this chapter, we will discuss the optimal type and duration of exercise required to improve health. It is important to avoid the overtraining syndrome that actually increases muscle breakdown, elevates cortisol levels and sympathetic tone, increases oxidative stress and inflammation, and results in the opposite effects of those noted in Table 8.1.

The power of exercise is a function of the numerous hormones, cytokines, chemokines, interleukins, and other signaling molecules and mediators that are released with the proper type of exercise; these substances influence genes, inflammation, oxidative stress, and immune function. The effects of exercise on human genetics are shown in Table 8.2.[1,5,6] Exercise modifies the expression of at least 397 of 14,500 genes tested linked to energy metabolism upregulation, protein and amino acid dephosphorylation, heme biosynthesis, downregulation of protein catabolism, and the other effects shown in Table 8.2.[6] Skeletal muscle has the ability to alter the type and amount of protein depending on the disruptions that occur in cellular homeostasis.[5] The exercise adaptation of skeletal muscle involves numerous signaling mechanisms that initiate replication of DNA genetic sequences that signal

129

Table 8.1

CARDIOVASCULAR AND OVERALL HEALTH: BENEFITS OF EXERCISE

- Reduces risk of MI, recurrent MI, angina, CHD arrhythmias, and recurrent MI
- Improves heart function, ejection fraction, cardiac output, coronary blood flow and reserve, oxygen consumption, aerobic capacity, LVEDV, and CHF
- Lowers blood pressure (average reduction is 11/7.5 mm Hg with optimal training), reduces risk of developing hypertension, decreases heart rate, improves heart rate variability and heart rate recovery time, lowers SVR, and increases eNOS and NO
- Reduces total cholesterol, triglycerides, and LDL; increases HDL
- Reduces body weight and body fat and increases lean muscle mass
- Reduces clotting tendencies and blood viscosity
- Lowers blood sugar, decreases risk of diabetes, and improves insulin sensitivity
- Improves all abnormalities of metabolic syndrome
- Improves immune function and decreases infections
- Reduces risk of stroke
- Increases muscle mass and decreases sarcopenia (resistance exercise)
- Improves memory and focus and reduces risk of Alzheimer disease and dementia
- Improves skin tone and elasticity and decreases wrinkles
- Improves depression, stress, anxiety, and overall psychological well-being
- Improves quality of life
- Improves sleep and sleep quality
- Reduces risk of certain cancers, such as colon, breast, and prostate
- Decreases risk of gallstones and peptic ulcer disease
- Increases telomerase and slows telomere attrition rate and aging
- Decreases sympathetic nervous system activity, cortisol, and catecholamines; increases parasympathetic activity
- Reduces inflammation
- Decreases fatigue
- Decreases osteoporosis

CHD, coronary heart disease; eNOS, endothelial nitric oxide synthase; HDL, high-density lipoprotein; LDL, low-density lipoprotein; LVEDV, left ventricular end-diastolic volume; MI, myocardial infarction; NO, nitric oxide; SVR, systemic vascular resistance.

RNA production of amino acids and proteins that peak about 3 to 12 hours post exercise.[5] Training volume, intensity, and frequency as well as the half-life of the proteins will determine the final functional outcomes of exercise.[5] Endurance training increases mitochondrial biogenesis, fast to slow fiber type transformation, and substrate metabolism, whereas heavy resistance exercise stimulates synthesis of contractile proteins to induce muscle hypertrophy and increase maximal contractile force.[5] Increased muscle cross-sectional area and altered neural recruitment patterns are the principal adaptations to repeated bouts of heavy resistance exercise. A balance of protein synthesis, protein degradation, and muscle remodeling also reduces atrophy pathways with a result net increase in protein synthesis and muscle hypertrophy with RT.

Signal Transduction Pathways in Skeletal Muscle: Muscle Molecules, Hormones, Other Mediators, and Myokines

Many of the health benefits of exercise are partly linked to reduced levels of inflammation and oxidative stress with chronic adaptive mechanisms. Optimal exercise regimens release numerous signaling molecules that stimulate healthy responses that include inflammation, anti-inflammation, oxidative stress, oxidative defense, proimmune and anti-immune mechanisms for muscle, and other organ repair, regeneration, and growth. Exercise, when performed properly, is the ultimate metabolomic and proteomic prescription to connect the internal weblike signaling within the human body. Hormones, myokines (cytokines specific to skeletal muscle), cytokines, nitric oxide, and other mediators of muscle have numerous functions in the body, including control of fuel mechanisms, reproduction, hunger, immune function, gene expression, and every other metabolic process in the body. Human physiology is designed around movement, with a variety of hormones being released by body movement that produce intracellular signaling. But not all exercise has the same effect on genetic signaling.[1]

The muscular Olympic sprinters and wiry and gaunt Olympic marathon runners are extremes of the exercise regimen. Both have low percentages of body fat, but the sprinters have even less. The key difference is that sprinters exercise in very short, all-out bursts of energy, whereas marathon runners exercise for hours at a slower, steadier pace.

Caloric expenditure is really just a side effect of exercise, inconsequential compared with the enormous release of hormones and other signaling substances that determine cell function. Although the short, intense activity of sprinting does not burn many calories, it triggers the release of anabolic hormones such as human growth hormone and testosterone. This hormonal mix elevates caloric consumption for hours and even days after the sprinter has stopped running. Long-distance running does not elicit the same effect. Instead, it leads to the production of a catabolic hormonal mix (such as cortisol elevations) that causes muscle wasting, inefficient metabolic processing, and physical decay. Higher-intensity exercise produces the most muscle signaling. Exercise using full body movements, incorporating great amounts of muscle, requiring a combination of strength and endurance and forcing the muscle to do a lot of work in a short amount of time results in powerful muscle-building, fat-burning, anti-inflammatory, and brain-stimulating effects.

Table 8.2

METABOLIC GENE EXPRESSION: HUMAN GENES AFFECTED BY EXERCISE

- Genes that regulate energy metabolism, control weight, and improve energy levels. Metabolic gene expression affects enzymes in carbohydrate and fat metabolism, such as hexokinase, lipoprotein lipase, and carnitine palmitoyltransferase, which peak within a few hours and return to resting state in 24 h
- Genes that improve protein synthesis and decrease protein degradation. This especially involves IGF-1 and IGF-BP and the PI3-k-Akt-mTOR signaling pathways
- Genes that improve production of hemoglobin and reduce anemia
- Genes that improve mitochondrial biogenesis. Exercise can increase the steady state mitochondrial protein content by 50%-100% within 6 wk, but a protein turnover half-life of 1 wk means a continuous training stimulus is required to maintain elevated mitochondrial content. Exercise increases mitochondrial TFAM, NRF-2, and PGC1–alpha, which increases mitofusin and protein assembly
- Nitric oxide (NO) genes that reduce aging, improve mitochondrial function, improve vascular health, reduce inflammation, reduce oxidative stress, slow atherosclerosis, and lower blood pressure
- Interleukin (IL) genes for IL-10, IL-8, which reduce inflammation and increase growth hormone and testosterone
- Genes for heme-oxygenase I (HO-1), which removes toxic heme and protects cells from various insults such as low oxygen, heavy metals, oxidative stress, and inflammation and helps to regulate vascular tone and the transmission of nerve impulses
- Genes for heat shock proteins, such as numbers 70 and 72 (HSP-70 and 72) (stress proteins), which are chaperones for proteins in cells and protect cells from low oxygen and other stress to reduce the risk of cardiovascular disease, myocardial infarction, and cancer and to improve immune function
- Genes that increase muscle proteins to increase lean muscle mass, such as HIF-1 and 2 (hypoxic inducible factor), P21, Myo D, muscle ring finger (MURF-1) and decrease myostatin and REDDI
- Genes that improve cholesterol and other blood lipids, such as PPAR gamma (increases removal of the toxic oxidized LDL cholesterol and stimulates the removal of LDL cholesterol from the cells)
- Genes that improve blood sugar levels and insulin resistance, such as PPAR gamma, PGC-1 alpha, GLUT 4 (glucose uptake transporter 4), and other nuclear-coded mitochondrial genes
- Genes that protect from cancers, such as BHMT 2 (betaine homocysteine methyltransferase), VEGF (vascular endothelial growth factor), ANG 2 (angiopoietin 2), and IPL-A2 (phospholipase A2), for colon cancer prevention and calprotectin for antibacterial activity
- Genes that cause inflammation are decreased, such as NF-Kappa B (nuclear factor kappa beta), iNOS (inducible nitric oxide synthase), TNF-alpha, and COX 2 (cyclooxygenase 2)
- Genes involved in stress management, anxiety, and depression, such as VGF nerve factor, opioids, and opioid receptors
- Antioxidant genes such as superoxide dismutase (SOD), endothelial nitric oxide synthase (eNOS), and NF-Kappa B.
- Genes that slow aging in muscle, slow telomere attrition rate, and reduce sarcopenia, such as MURF protein, atrogin, FOXO 3A, TNF-alpha, ILGF-1, AMPK, IGFBPS, CNF (ciliary neurotrophic factor), and MMP 2
- Genes that regulate the growth of new blood vessels (angiogenesis) and improve remodeling and structure of blood vessel cells
- Genes that reduce heart disease, stroke, and other cardiovascular diseases, such as prostaglandins, CNP (c-type natriuretic peptide), nitric oxide, HO-1, COX 2, and HSPs

The conversion of mechanical signals during muscular contraction into a molecular event involves primary and secondary messengers to activate or repress specific signaling pathways to regulate exercise-induced gene expression and protein synthesis and degradation.[5] The mechanisms include[1,5-13]:

1. Interleukins, tumor necrosis factor (TNF)-alpha, nuclear factor (NF)-KB, and other cytokines (discussed in detail later).
2. Mechanical stretch: This activates calcineurin, MAPK, and IFG signaling pathways.
3. Calcium flux: Neural activation of skeletal muscle generates an action potential that releases calcium from the sarcoplasmic reticulum. The amplitude and duration of calcium flux is regulated by the duration and frequency of the contractile stimulus.
4. Redox state: The NAD/NADH ratio is the primary redox mechanism in skeletal muscle that results from glycolysis and lipolysis in the mitochondria. The high production of reactive oxygen species (ROS) with exercise is buffered by Gpx, Mn, SOD, and catalase. Oxidative stress helps modulate exercise-induced adaptive signaling by serving as a primary messenger on transcriptional regulation and DNA binding with NF-KB and AP-1, direct effects on mitochondrial metabolism, decrease in myofilament calcium sensitivity, and hormetic effects to increase oxidative defense.
5. Phosphorylation status: Changes in the AMP/ATP ratio initiate numerous downstream molecular events in muscle such as activation of AMPK.

6. AMPK serves a primary role as the energy sensing kinase in both RT and AE related to cellular AMP/ATP ratios. AMPK stimulates insulin-independent glucose uptake and fat oxidation and regulates protein synthesis and gene expression via insulin IGF pathways.

7. Calmodulin and calcineurin regulate gene expression of contractile and mitochondrial proteins, fiber type plasticity, fast-to-slow phenotype transformation and fiber growth, hypertrophy, and regeneration.

8. IGF is stimulated during exercise and relates to glucose uptake, glycogen synthesis, and cell growth and differentiation through TOR, FoxO-1, and Akt pathways.

Interleukin-10—Fat Burning and Anti-inflammatory

Interleukin (IL)-10 regulates the muscle's current and future energy needs. It is the most powerful metabolic signaling agent released from muscle as soon as the muscle starts to contract and move. It is released in even greater amounts as the activity becomes more intense. IL-10's actions decrease inflammation; increase serum testosterone, growth hormone, and fat metabolism; regulate glucose; reduce weight; increase lean muscle mass; optimize fuel metabolism; and reduce the risk of myocardial infarction and stroke.

Interleukin-15—Muscle Sparing and Fat Burning

The major task of IL-15, which is released primarily through weight training, is to regulate the breakdown of muscle tissue. It is a major factor in determining the body's muscle-to-fat ratio, which is an important contributor to coronary heart disease (CHD). Unfortunately, most modern exercise regimens do not trigger the release of adequate amounts of IL-15, for they avoid the short bursts of intense energy expenditure needed to produce it in sufficient amounts.

Interleukin-8—Muscle Angiogenesis

IL-8 is synthesized in muscle whenever the muscle is forced to produce energy anaerobically. When this happens, the muscle releases IL-8, which results in angiogenesis in skeletal and cardiac muscle that improves muscles oxygenation. This is a remarkable example of exercise's ability to mold metabolism.

Interleukin-6—Inflammatory or Anti-inflammatory Myokine?[5-13]

IL-6 is generally an inflammatory cytokine when released from nonskeletal muscle cells.[5-13] However, when released in high concentrations from skeletal muscle in the absence of TNF-alpha and IL-1, it is anti-inflammatory by actually blocking both via IL-1ra (receptor to IL-1) and soluble TNFR (TNF-alpha receptors) and stimulating the release of IL-10. The amount of IL-6 released during exercise far exceeds the level of TNF-alpha.[5-13] This low ratio may account for the anti-inflammatory effects. The amount of IL-6 released is dependent on the intensity of the exercise, amount of muscle being used, and liver and skeletal muscle glycogen, with 20- to 100-fold increases over rest. IL-6 circulates as a myokine to all organs such as brain, liver, adipose tissue, heart, and blood vessels to control fat and glucose metabolism with adipose tissue fatty acid oxidation and liver glycogenolysis. There is also a reduction in inflammation and immune function with a shift to TH2 dominance. Finally, there are alterations in cortisol and leukocyte levels, central nervous system function (appetite regulation, fuel regulation, and body composition), BP, cardiovascular disease (CVD), and cancer risk, as well as promotion of many other health benefits.[5-13]

TNF-Alpha

This is suppressed in both RT and AE programs, which improves insulin sensitivity, reduces inflammation, and improves anabolic effects as long as muscle has time to recover during exercise regimens and there is no overtraining, which could actually increase TNF-alpha.

Lactic Acid—Growth Promoter, Energy Enhancer

Lactic acid, also known as lactate, is not just a waste product but actually has several beneficial effects. One of the immediate effects of lactic acid is to balance the acid pH that accumulates as a result of intense movement. The burn during intense exercise, usually blamed on lactic acid, is really caused by the accumulation of toxic metabolic waste products, such as ammonia and hydrogen. Lactic acid buffers their effects and improves exercise performance.

Lactic acid functions like a hormone by stimulating the release of testosterone and growth hormone that induce anabolic effects for increased lean muscle mass and better strength and function. In addition, lactic acid signals the muscle cells to increase both the number and efficiency of mitochondria to increase ATP, reduce production of radical oxygen species, and increase burning of body fat.

Nitric Oxide

Nitric oxide (NO) has numerous beneficial effects, including reducing arterial inflammation and oxidative stress, vasodilation, lowering systemic vascular resistance (SVR) and BP, decreasing atherosclerosis and CHD, improving mitochondrial biogenesis, and inhibiting thrombosis, permeability, and abnormal growth of vascular tissue. NO production is largely controlled by the endothelial cells, but activated muscles also release NO, allowing blood vessels supplying the muscle to remain open to maintain blood flow.

Effects of Exercise on Cardiovascular Disease and Metabolic Parameters

Combined aerobic and resistance exercise have numerous beneficial effects on CHD, CVD, cardiac arrhythmias, stroke, and CHD risk factors such a serum glucose, lipids, BP, body composition, and obesity[1-5] (Table 8.3).

Table 8.3

EFFECTS OF EXERCISE ON CARDIOVASCULAR DISEASE

1. Reduces resting and exercise systolic and diastolic blood pressure
2. Reduces rest and exercise heart rate
3. Improves heart rate variability and heart rate recovery time
4. Helps to balance the SNS and PNS
5. Lowers fasting and postprandial glucose
6. Improves diabetes mellitus and insulin sensitivity
7. Increases adiponectin
8. Improves metabolic syndrome
9. Improves lipid profile: Reduces TC, LDL-C, TG, VLDL, LDL-P, and Lp(a); increases HDL, HDL particle size and HDL functionality, and LDL particle size
10. Lowers total and visceral body fat and increases lean muscle mass
11. Improves CHF symptoms, exercise tolerance, ejection fraction, CO, CI, SV, MVO2, quality of life, and survival
12. Improves CHD symptoms and progression of CHD plaque progressions, angina and future MI
13. Improves coronary artery blood flow and coronary reserve
14. Reduces PACs, PJCs, and PVCs and sudden death from cardiac arrhythmias
15. Reduces stroke
16. Improves PAD
17. Improves endothelial dysfunction and arterial compliance

CHD, coronary heart disease; CI, cardiac index; CO cardiac output; HDL, high-density lipoprotein; LDL, low-density lipoprotein; LDL-C, low-density lipoprotein-cholesterol; LDL-P, low density lipoprotein particle number; MI, myocardial infarction; MVO2, myocardial volume oxygen consumption; PNS, parasympathetic nervous system; SI, stroke volume; SNS, sympathetic nervous system; TC, total cholesterol; TG, triglyceride; VLDL, very low-density lipoprotein.

Aerobic Exercise and Resistance Training

RT improves cardiovascular conditioning; increases basal femoral blood flow and vascular conductance, basal metabolic rate (BMR), quality of life, muscle strength, endurance, lean muscle mass, and insulin sensitivity; decreases the risk of metabolic syndrome; and reduces sarcopenia, body fat, and risk of osteoporosis.[1,3-5,14,15] The increase in strength and endurance varies from 25% to 100%. The BMR increases 7.7% in both genders within 3 to 6 months following moderate- to high-intensity training.[2,5,14] AE after RT rather than before RT can prevent deterioration of vascular function such as reduction in pulse wave velocity, brachial artery diameter, mean blood velocity, and blood flow.[15,16] BP remains in an acceptable range as long as the one RM (repetition maximum) stays between 40% and 60%, but significant BP elevations occur at over 80% of one RM.[3,17] As will be discussed later, this is the reason for the recommendation of RT before AE with a specific time relationship of two to one ratio of RT to AE.

The cardiovascular responses to exercise differ between RT and AE.[3] AE imposes a volume-overload state on the cardiovascular system with increased VO2, heart rate cardiac output, and stroke volume and acute increases in systolic BP (SBP) but no change or decrease in diastolic BP (DBP).[3] With prolonged AE, both SBP and DBP fall as there is decrease in SVR.[3] There is asymmetric left ventricular (LV) hypertrophy with AE.[3]

In contrast, RT is a pressure-overload state on the cardiovascular system with little increase in VO2, mild increase in cardiac output, increased heart rate, and acute increase in SBP and DBP, but SBP and DBP decrease with chronic RT.[3] There is symmetric LV hypertrophy with a change in the ventricular diameter.[3] RT improves cardiovascular function, overall metabolic state, and general quality of life. An increase in strength and endurance of 25% to 100% in both genders occurs in 3 to 6 months.[3] There is decreased adipose tissue; increased lean muscle mass, BMR, and bone mass; reduced oxidative stress with increased muscle antioxidants; reduced risk of metabolic syndrome and osteoporosis; and improvement in peripheral arterial disease (PAD).[3] RT also improves clinical symptoms in patients with CHF.[3,18]

Both RT and AE prevent and treat hypertension; improve dyslipidemia, insulin resistance, metabolic syndrome, diabetes mellitus, and body composition problems; and reduce cardiovascular morbidity and mortality.[1,3,19-22] In type 2 diabetes mellitus, the combined RT and AE reduced hemoglobin A1C by 0.34% compared with control or RT or AE alone.[19] In a controlled study, 357 males with essential hypertension were grouped into control, interval training (IT), or continuous training (CT) programs at 60% to 79% maximum heart rate (MHR) for 45 to 60 minutes three times per week over 8 weeks. Both the IT and CT resulted in significant reductions in SBP, DBP, heart rate (HR), pulse pressure (PP), and mean arterial pressure (MAP) and improved VO2 (P < .05) compared with the control group.[21] BP was reduced by 16,4/4.01 mm Hg in the IT group and 13.94/7.41 mm Hg in the CT group, and HR fell 8 and 12 b/min, respectively. VO2 was significantly improved in the IT group by 13.85 mL/kg/min versus 7.99 in the CT group, which is consistent with other studies. The combination of AE and RT at an energy expenditure of 4200 kcal per week is superior to either AE or RT alone in reducing BP, achieving weight loss, improving body composition, increasing upper and lower body strength, and improving cardiovascular fitness (VO2 max), CVD, and CHD.[23-25] Increasing energy expenditure over 4200 kcal per week did not result in any additional benefit in reducing the relative CHD risk and may actually increase the risk.[25]

ABCT Exercise

The ABCT exercise program has numerous positive effects on body and mind, much more than the typical aerobic-based programs (see Table 8.1). The ABCT exercise program is a modern way of exercising the way our ancestors did. The program is specifically designed to get the muscles and body moving in short burns of intense activity and to mix anaerobic with just enough AE to improve cardiovascular health, overall health, and conditioning.[1] In addition, proper nutrition is emphasized before, during, and after exercise training.[26-53]

Nutrition and nutritional supplements may help to dampen some of the oxidative stress, inflammation, muscle damage, muscle fatigue, lipid peroxidation, and damage to cellular proteins and DNA that occur with exercise.[30] Cytokine production increases ROS, reactive nitrogen species (RNS), and oxidative stress. Cytokine production is regulated by calcium, muscle glycogen breakdown, mobilization of immune cells, catecholamines, growth hormone, cortisol, increased core temperature, increased intestinal permeability to lipopolysaccharides and endotoxins, and oxidative stress.[30]

The ABCT exercise program is simple, effective, scientifically sound, and adaptable to everyone's exercise needs. It allows for optimal training benefits in a shorter period of time to build and tone muscle, reduce body fat, lose weight, improve hormone levels, lower inflammation and oxidation, decrease blood sugar, reduce BP, improve the lipid profile and quality of life, increase life expectancy, and slow the aging process. In addition, this type of exercise avoids overtraining associated with increased cortisol levels, catabolic effects on muscle, or chronic fatigue. Finally, the **EPOC** (post-exercise oxygen consumption) is optimized. This means that the postexercise hormonal effects continue to increase calorie expenditure and provide other health-promoting benefits, long after the exercise is completed.[54]

The ABCs of Exercise With a Twist

The most efficient and effective means of achieving all the health benefits of exercise is to combine interval aerobic with anaerobic or resistance exercise in a way that causes body restoration and proper muscle growth and efficiency. ABCT exercise program represents **A**erobics, **B**uild, **C**ontour, and **T**one. It has additional meanings that help define its goals.

- **A** = **A**erobics plus action and adaptation: The program focuses on the types of action best suited for muscle and cardiovascular conditioning to adapt to new exercises so muscles do not accommodate to the same daily training.
- **B** = **B**uild plus bulk, burn, and breathe: The program builds and increases muscle strength more than any other exercise regimen while learning to use muscle burn to the best advantage with proper breathing to increase oxygen consumption and to eliminate carbon dioxide to improve cardiovascular and muscle conditioning and function while reducing fatigue.
- **C** = **C**ontour plus core and controlling your genes: Muscular exercise regulates the expression of more than 400 genes that mediate the beneficial effects of physical activity. In addition to aerobics and resistance exercise this program will combine core exercises that improve abdominal and back muscle strength as well as exercises for flexibility and balance.
- **T** = **T**one plus trim and tight: Total body fat, visceral body fat, and body weight are decreased while lean muscle mass increases.

The ABCT exercise program emphasizes interval aerobic and anaerobic resistance movements. Proper warm-up and stretching before beginning every exercise session and cooling down and stretching again when finished are mandatory to avoid muscle, tendon, and ligament injuries while promoting the flexibility that is necessary for exercising.

Before embarking on an exercise program of any kind or changing the exercise regimen you already have, a complete history, physical examination, laboratory tests, cardiovascular risk factor analysis, and stress test are suggested. Interval training with rapid bursts of activity may precipitate plaque rupture in a coronary artery in some predisposed individuals and result in a myocardial infarction.

The Elements of ABCT

Here are the main elements of ABCT, each of which will be discussed in more detail later.

- **Resistance Training**—Weight lifting modified properly will encourage optimal muscle physiology and release of hormones, mediators, and interleukins. ABCT uses graduated weights and variable repetitions. In brief, initially lift the heaviest weight possible 12 times to get the muscle burn, then decrease the weight with each subsequent set, but keep increasing the number of times the weight is lifted. This maximizes postexercise oxygen consumption, depletes glycogen, and increases the production of lactic acid to achieve all the muscle-, hormone-, cytokine-, and interleukin-stimulating effects that lead to the health benefits of exercise.
- **Aerobic Training in Intervals**—Jogging, swimming, biking, and other forms of continual movement should be done at specific levels of submaximal and maximal aerobic capacity (MAC) or estimated heart rate for age and level of exercise (MHR). The best technique is aerobic interval training, which consists of short periods ranging from 20 seconds to 2 minutes of "burst" aerobic training of varying intensities, depending on one's present level of exercise conditioning. This more closely mimics the natural activities we evolved to perform and benefit from and strings together several periods of intense and semi-intense activity into a single, longer exercise period that still burns calories and builds endurance.
- **Proper Ratio of Aerobic Training to Resistance Training**—The optimal ratio of resistance to interval aerobic training should be 2:1. For example, during a 60-minute workout, you would perform 40 minutes of RT and 20 minutes of interval aerobics, with the aerobics coming after the RT.
- **Core Exercises**—Exercises designed to improve abdominal and back strength while increasing flexibility. These exercises are important for the core (abdomen and lower back), which is often neglected.
- **Time-Intense Exercise**—Rather than methodically working one muscle or muscle group after another, then doing the AEs—or even saving the aerobics for the next

day—ABCT challenges the body by combining exercises as much as possible. For example, instead of doing leg squats followed by shoulder presses, with ABCT they are done at the same time, mimicking the real-life movements.

- **Busy Rest Periods**—These are used to insert small bursts of AE into the RT period.
- **Water and the ABCT Energy Shake**—Drinking plenty of water while working out is vital. (If you get thirsty during the workout, you have waited too long to drink.) You must drink water before beginning to exercise, at set intervals during exercise, and afterward. Your water should be of high quality and not from plastic containers, due to the risk of ingesting chemical compounds like polychlorinated biphenyls (PCBs) that get into the water from the plastic. In addition, about 10 minutes after starting your workout, you begin consuming an energy drink consisting of fresh orange juice and water, raw honey, D-ribose, carnitine, glutamine, vitamin C, whey protein, and other supplements to provide ATP and energy as well as nutritional substrates to maximize exercise performance and increase muscle strength and performance as well as lean muscle mass.[1,26-36]
- **Exercise in the Morning**—Exercising in the morning after a 12-hour fast is best for numerous reasons, including the fact that an empty stomach optimizes fat burning, IL-10 and myokine surges, and the resulting increase in muscle strength, bulk, tone, and contour, as well as weight loss and improved energy level, focus, and concentration during the day.
- **Exercise on an Empty Stomach**—Begin exercising on an empty stomach after a 12-hour fast, except for water and whey protein consumed about 10 minutes before exercise, and have nothing but more water and the energy drink while exercising. This allows for depletion of liver and muscle glycogen while generating maximal surges of IL-10. It also increases fat burning and accelerates weight and fat loss from both inside and outside the skeletal muscle.
- **Push and Rest**—Exercise to maximal effort during each set until the burn is significant. The burn should be severe and last for about 4 to 5 seconds after you stop the exercise. Then rest for 60 seconds before beginning the next set or exercise but you may take 3-second rest periods between repetitions, if necessary. Also, performing supersets with minimal rest between sets of exercises or using the rest period for core exercises or alternative upper or lower body exercises will improve the time intensity of the exercise session.
- **Exercise Daily, Utilizing Cross-Training**—To achieve the best results, perform interval aerobic and resistance training at least 4 days per week or if desired every day, but alternate the muscle groups for upper and lower body as well as the type of AE performed. It is important to change the exercise routine every few weeks to avoid muscle accommodation to the exercise regimen.
- **Breathe**—Mastering proper breathing techniques will ensure ample oxygenation for the muscle performance, as well as prompt the removal of carbon dioxide.

The ABCT Elements in Detail

RESISTANCE TRAINING

ABCT RT takes a radically different approach, mixing heavier weights and lower repetitions with lower weights and greater repetitions to increase the lactic acid burn as well as to maximize muscle contractions and the release of myokines. With ABCT, the real goal is neither to bulk nor to contour the muscles but to use muscle movements to improve body biochemistry and improve cardiovascular and overall health.

ABCT RT is based on five sets, each with a different number of repetitions. Here is the **ABCT Five-Set Schedule** that starts with the heaviest weight with low repetitions and advances to lighter weight with increasing repetitions:

- ABCT Set 1: 12 repetitions at maximum weight
- ABCT Set 2: 18 repetitions at 75% of maximum weight
- ABCT Set 3: 24 repetitions at 50% of maximum weight
- ABCT Set 4: 50 repetitions at 25% of maximum weight
- ABCT Set 5: 12 repetitions at maximum weight

ABCT Five-Set schedule should be phased in slowly to avoid injury or excessive fatigue, depending on one's present level of physical conditioning:

- Beginners: ABCT 1, or ABCT 1 and 2
- Intermediate: ABCT 1, 2, and 3
- Advanced: ABCT 1, 2, 3, and 4
- Professional: ABCT 1, 2, 3, 4, and 5

This burn scale can be used as a guide to the exercise level. The idea is to attempt to score a five multiple times during your workouts, stopping only briefly (3 seconds) to clear the burn before continuing again.

1—No burn in the muscle
2—Light burn
3—Moderate burn
4—Strong burn
5—Intense burn; must rest

WHAT, HOW, AND WHEN TO LIFT

Descriptions of the key ABCT resistance exercises are found at the end of the chapter under the heading "Getting Started with ABCT: Training Session Schedules and Descriptions of the Lifts."

UPPING THE INTENSITY WITH SUPERSETS, HYBRIDS, AND RAPID SETS

Simply following the ABCT 5-Set Schedule will improve cardiovascular and general health. Incorporating hybrids, supersets, and rapid sets as one gains strength and endurance will improve exercise outcomes.

- *Hybrids* are two exercises performed at once, ie, do a full leg squat while also performing an overhead press. Using more muscles simultaneously increases the burn, lactic acid, release of IL-10, and postexercise oxygen consumption.

- *Supersets* are exercises done back to back, with almost no rest period between (15 seconds maximum). These can be the same exercise, such as biceps curls back to back, or different exercises, such as a biceps curl followed immediately by a tricep lift. Supersets dramatically increase the burn and other beneficial effects of exercise. Supersets should be done only after one has trained for some time to avoid overuse injury or excessive heart rate.
- *Rapid sets* are sets performed faster than normal to compress the workout time, enhance mechanical and metabolic burnout, and improve both resistance and aerobic conditioning. For example, with a biceps curl, increase the speed from one every second to two every 3 seconds.

ABCT RESISTANCE TRAINING HINTS

1. Take 3-second breaks along the way, if necessary.
2. Drink water and the ABCT energy drink after each set of exercises.
3. Even if the number of repetitions cannot be done in each set, attempt to push to the limit until the maximum burn occurs.
4. If the percentage reduction in weight is a fraction of a number, round up to the next highest whole number on the weight system you are using. This may be 1 pound or 5 pounds in most systems.

Aerobic Training in Intervals

Aerobic means "with oxygen" and refers to the use of oxygen in the body's metabolic processes. Aerobic training consists of continuous movements that demand more oxygen consumption and ultimately improve the body's oxygen use. Rapid walking, jogging, running, swimming, bicycling, dancing, and aerobics classes can all be aerobic exercises if they keep the body in moderate to intense motion for a moderately long period of time, with an elevated heart rate representing the body's heightened level of activity.

For best results, aerobic training should be broken up into periods of differing intensities or interval training with differing lengths and intensities. In general, the interval would be at 90% MHR for a period of time followed by 50% of MHR for one to three times that period, depending on conditioning. For example, a 30-second sprint would be followed by a 30- to 90-second slow jog.

The ideal ratio for aerobic interval training is 1:3. This means for every unit of time spent exercising at 90% of your maximal heart rate, spend an additional three units of time exercising at 50% of maximal heart rate (MHR). Then you repeat this 1:3 sequence about six times over about 20 minutes. The MHR calculation is shown in the subsequent text.

For best results, an interval AE program should consist of a 5-minute warm-up period, followed by moderate to intense interval training involving large and multiple muscle groups lasting about 20 minutes, followed by a cooling-down period of about 5 minutes at the end.

Aerobic sessions should utilize cross-training by rotating through different aerobic activities to improve cardiovascular and muscle performance. For example, jog or run on Monday, Wednesday, and Friday; swim on Tuesday and Thursday; bike on Saturday and Sunday.

MAXIMUM HEART RATE AND MAXIMUM AEROBIC CAPACITY

MAC = 220 minus age. Then, to get the MHR, multiply by the desired heart rate, which should range between 50% and 90% depending on level of exercise and age.

For example, if you are age 40 years, the MAC would be $220 - 40$, or 180. If you wanted to push to 80% of MAC, then multiply $180 \times 0.80 = 144$ beats/min as MHR.

Always combine resistance and aerobic exercises. The optimal ratio is two parts RT to one part interval aerobic training, with the RT first. Here is how the ratio works out with differing total exercise time frames.

- 15 minutes total = 10 minutes of RT, 5 minutes of aerobic training
- 30 minutes total = 20 minutes of RT, 10 minutes of aerobic training
- 45 minutes total = 30 minutes of RT, 15 minutes of aerobic training
- 60 minutes total = 40 minutes of RT, 20 minutes of aerobic training

Core Exercises

Exercising body core, such as the belly and lower back, increases abdominal and back strength while improving flexibility and balance. These can be done in sets of one to four per exercise, with the number of repetitions necessary to create the same burn that one gets with the resistance weight training program. Doing the core exercises during the 60-second break periods while the upper or lower body muscles are resting will improve the time efficiency of the workout. Core exercises include sit-ups, abdominal crunches, leg lifts, leg scissor crosses, etc.

Time-Intensive Exercise

Two additional steps are required to efficiently and effectively build muscle strength, tone, and contour while simultaneously improving cardiovascular conditioning and cardiovascular health: time-intensive resistance exercises and combined aerobic and RT.

1. **Time-Intensive Resistance Exercises**—Performing time-intense exercises requires using multiple and large muscle groups simultaneously, with minimal rest periods, for example, lifting light weights over the head while doing deep knee bends. This increases the release of IL-10 and other muscle cytokines, reduces inflammation, increases lactic acid burn, enhances postexercise oxygen consumption, builds muscle, optimizes metabolic and hormonal responses, and increases fat metabolism and fat and weight loss.

2. **Combined Aerobic and Resistance Training**—Instead of standing or sitting during the 60-second between-set rest periods, another resistance or aerobic exercise should be done to maintain heart rate and respiratory rate. For example, on completing an upper body exercise, immediately start doing a lower body exercise or a core exercise that engages large muscle groups and requires big action. This technique maintains heart rate and provides more cardiovascular and muscular conditioning.

NUTRITION, NUTRITIONAL SUPPLEMENTS, WATER, AND ABCT ENERGY DRINK[1,26-53]

Nutritional macronutrient and micronutrient intake relative to exercise can optimize recovery, enhance subsequent performance, synthesize muscle (anabolism > catabolism), and provide optimal metabolic and nutrient-genetic interaction for muscle signaling.[29] During exercise, inflammation and oxidative stress are linked via muscle metabolism and muscle damage.[30] The role of antioxidant supplements around the exercise time may have beneficial effects on muscle damage, ROS, RNS, inflammation, recovery, and fatigue.[30] Consumption of a carbohydrate supplement immediately after exercise will improve insulin action and synthesize muscle glycogen significantly faster than when the same amount of carbohydrate is consumed 2 hours post exercise.[29] However, the type and amount of carbohydrate determine the muscle response.[28] Fructose and glucose co-ingestion during prolonged exercise increase lactate and glucose fluxes and oxidation more, compared with an equimolar intake of glucose.[28] Regardless of the amount of exogenous glucose intake during exercise, there is a maximal exogenous oxidation rate of 1 g/min[28] However, adding fructose to glucose during exercise increases exogenous carbohydrate oxidation rate up to 1.75 g/min[28]

Fructose metabolism is different from glucose metabolism for many reasons.[28] Fructose is absorbed by intestinal and liver cells rapidly and converted into triose-phosphates, so serum fructose levels are usually not elevated.[28] Fructose is not metabolized in skeletal muscle owing to lack of fructokinase and the low affinity of hexokinase for fructose. Most of the fructose is converted to glucose and lactate in the liver.[28] Lactate is efficiently oxidized during exercise by skeletal muscle as well as cardiomyocytes.[28] Thus, ingestion of the combination of glucose and fructose during exercise provides an additional oxidative fuel to active skeletal muscles that improves exercise performance and reduces muscle fatigue.[28]

Protein intake and exercise have synergistic effects on increasing the rate of muscle protein synthesis, leading to a more positive protein balance, but effects vary depending on the timing of the protein intake and the exercise session.[29] The timing of whole protein may not be as crucial as the timing of specific amino acid supplements and anabolism.[29] Most studies suggest that consuming free amino acids immediately before exercise or within 10 minutes of the initiation of exercise is more effective to increase muscle protein accretion compared with consumption after exercise.[27,29] In contrast, whey protein may be consumed before, during, or after exercise. The effects on muscle anabolism are enhanced with immediate and simultaneous consumption post exercise of carbohydrates and fats as long as this occurs within less than 2 hours post exercise.[29] The timing of a fat meal and exercise will alter the postprandial hypertriglyceridemia because exercise stimulates lipoprotein lipase for several hours post exercise.[29] Studies suggest that chronic exercise may reduce postprandial hypertriglyceridemia throughout a 24-hour day, but it may be optimal within 12 hours of exercise.[29]

Hydration before, during, and after the exercise program is vital. Two types of hydration are necessary: plain water and the ABCT energy drink. Begin the exercise program well hydrated, drinking about 6 ounces of water mixed with 20 g whey protein and an amino acid mixture before starting the exercise. The amount of fluids and water consumed depends on body size, the ambient temperature, and the length and intensity of the workout. As a rule of thumb, 24 to 32 ounces or more of fluid and water are needed during the typical 60-minute workout, with consumption of about 4 ounces of water between each exercise set.

Whey protein supplies glutathione precursors (cysteine, glutamine), is anabolic with an increase in muscle mass, and reduces oxidative stress and inflammation.[1,29] The ingredients in whey help maximize ATP (adenosine triphosphate) production, improve muscle performance, increase muscle mass, and reduce muscle fatigue.[1,29]

Numerous other nutritional supplements will improve exercise performance and/or increase skeletal muscle mass, including creatine, caffeine, carnitine, D-ribose, glutamine, vitamin C, mixed tocopherols, arginine, citrulline, taurine, and branched-chain amino acids (BCAAs), especially leucine, mixed amino acid blends, whey protein, Cordyceps, and Rhodiola.[1,30-53]

The recommended combination is water, whey protein, fresh orange juice, organic raw honey, carnitine, vitamin C, glutamine, taurine, arginine, and D-ribose throughout the workout. Consumption of some type of carbohydrates (glucose) during, rather than before, exercise has only a minor impact on fat oxidation when starting exercise in the fasting state. Into a 24- to 32-ounce bottle, add the following:

- 4 to 6 ounces of fresh orange juice diluted with 12 ounces of water
- One tablespoon of organic raw honey
- 20 g whey protein powder
- Amino acid blend—6.6 g DaxibeQol
- 10 g D-ribose powder
- 2 g carnitine tartrate powder
- 2 g of glutamine powder
- 2 g buffered vitamin C
- 2 g taurine powder
- 2 g arginine powder
- Cordyceps 3000 mg standardized
- Rhodiola 300 mg standardized

Between each set, drink 2 to 4 ounces of the energy drink. Also take 5 g BCAAs, with at least 3 g leucine, at the completion of the exercise. The BCAAs include leucine, isoleucine, and valine. The benefits of each ingredient in the energy drink are as follows:

- **Orange juice and organic raw honey**—provides carbohydrates in the form of glucose and fructose, as well as lactate for cardiac and skeletal muscle oxidation.[1,28] Expending energy while exercising ensures the maintenance of normal blood sugar, despite the glucose and fructose in the juice and honey.
- **Whey protein** contains amino acids and protein for muscle anabolism, plus precursors such as cysteine and glutamine for the production of glutathione to help reduce excessive oxidative stress and inflammation and to provide additional immune support.[1,27-29]
- **D-Ribose** provides immediate ATP production for energy, improved mitochondrial function, cardiovascular support, reduction in ROS, inhibition of the breakdown of adenine nucleotides during hypoxia/ischemia, and cellular protection, with increased glutathione levels.[1,37-39]
- **Carnitine** improves beta oxidation in skeletal and cardiac muscle by transport of fatty acids longer than C-12, which provides energy to all muscles. Carnitine is also an excellent antioxidant and reduces exercise-induced oxidative stress, decreases fatigue, and enhances muscle performance and endurance.[34-36]
- **Glutamine** increases muscle growth, and glutathione induces gastrointestinal repair and improves immune function and exercise performance.[1,40]
- **L-Arginine** increases NO, increases exogenous carbohydrate oxidation, and decreases the oxygen cost of exercise.[1,41]
- **Taurine** decreases muscle soreness and muscle damage during and following high-intensity exercise that is additive to BCCA.[42]
- **Vitamin C** reduces cortisol levels during exercise, provides antioxidant protection, and inhibits NF-KB.[30] Vitamin C given with the carbohydrates and tocopherol reduces IL-6 and high-sensitivity CRP.[30] Some studies show mixed results.[30,32] If epigallocatechin gallate (EGCG) is added to the regimen, oxidative stress is reduced more.[33]
- **BCAA (valine, leucine, and isoleucine)** increases muscle mass, muscle protein synthesis, and anabolism via mRNA translation; reduces muscle damage; accelerates recovery; and provides important amino acids, especially leucine.[1,44-46]
- **Cordyceps** is an adaptogen that increases MVO2, red blood cell delivery, coronary vasodilation, ATP, and O2 utilization by 15% and improves stamina and metabolic and ventilator threshold and performance.[47,48] Cordyceps activates skeletal muscle metabolic regulators and angiogenesis, improves glucose and lactate uptake, and coordinates antioxidant responses via AMPK, PGC1alpha, PPAR gamma, GLUT 4, VEGF, MCT 1, MCT 4, NRF-2, SOD1, and TRX.[47,48]
- **Rhodiola** is an adaptogen that decreases exercise-induced HR, reduces norepinephrine and epinephrine, increases serotonin and beta endorphins, reduces arrhythmias, improves performance and exercise efficiency (mental and physical), decreases the perception of effort, decreases fatigue, reduces lactate levels, decreases parameters of skeletal muscle damage, ameliorates fatty acid consumption, and increases liver glycogen.[49-53] Rhodiola reduces oxidative stress and malondialdehyde (MDA) and increases oxidative defense by upregulating catalase, SOD, and glutathione peroxidase (GSH-Px).[49-53]

EXERCISE ON AN EMPTY STOMACH (EXCEPT FOR WATER-WHEY MIX)

The exercising program should begin in the morning on an empty stomach, following an 8- to 12-hour fast, with the exception of drinking water and whey protein. That is followed during exercise with the ABCT Energy Drink. Consumption of carbohydrates before exercise decreases fat burning and weight loss. Exercising on an empty stomach burns more than twice as much fat as does exercising after consuming carbohydrates. Exercising in a fasting state may increase the utilization of muscle protein for energy slightly, but this effect is relatively small and is minimized when whey protein is consumed.

Optimal exercise benefits occur when skeletal muscle and liver glycogen are depleted. Glycogen depletion triggers the maximal release of IL-10 from muscle, increases muscle growth and fat burning for energy, accelerates fat loss from inside and outside muscle, and improves weight loss. All of this, in turn, reduces inflammation by increasing the levels of IL-10 while lowering IL-1, IL-6, and TNF-alpha, increasing the production of testosterone and growth hormone, improving insulin sensitivity, and lowering insulin and glucose levels.

The intramuscular triglycerides are metabolized better during glycogen-depleted exercise. The intramuscular triglycerides are far less responsive to insulin, which slows the breakdown of stored fat. Exercising while fasting suppresses insulin levels and maximizes the hormonal and cytokine effects of the exercise program.

HORMONAL CHANGES

Performing ABCT exercises on an empty stomach, after consuming only water and whey, generates the following results:

- Testosterone levels increase, enhancing muscle growth, mass, tone, and contour; improving insulin sensitivity, which lowers blood sugar and reduces the risk of diabetes and heart disease; elevating the energy level and libido; and slowing aging.
- Growth hormone levels increase, improving muscle growth, mass, tone, and contour; improving energy; increasing the sense of well-being; and slowing aging.
- Insulin levels decrease as a result of the improved insulin sensitivity that develops as lean muscle mass increases. (Lean muscle accounts for about 80% of

insulin sensitivity or resistance in humans.) These changes help reduce intramuscular triglycerides and extramuscular fat tissue while reducing the risk of heart disease and inflammation.

- Cortisol levels drop, improving muscle growth, lowering cholesterol and triglyceride, reducing blood sugar, and decreasing visceral fat, which is associated with inflammation, diabetes, metabolic syndrome, insulin resistance, high BP, elevated cholesterol, cancer, heart disease, and stroke.

NUTRITION BEFORE, DURING, AND AFTER THE EXERCISE SESSION

Nutrient availability serves as a potent modulator of many acute responses and chronic adaptations to both RT and AE. Changes in the macronutrient intake quickly change the concentration of substrates and hormones with alterations in the storage profile of skeletal muscle and other insulin-sensitive organs. This, in turn, regulates gene expression and cell signaling. Nutrient-exercise interactions activate or inhibit biochemical pathways during training. Proper nutrition after exercise (eg, a breakfast containing fluids, high-quality protein, complex carbohydrates, omega-3 fatty acids, and monounsaturated fatty acids) is essential to increase muscle mass and overall muscle performance and cardiovascular conditioning for each subsequent exercise session. Some food options include:

- whole-grain cereal with whole milk, rice milk, or almond milk; raw oats; and wheat germ
- ½ cup of each of the following: fresh blueberries, raspberries, blackberries, and strawberries
- 6 ounces fresh orange or vegetable juice or another fresh juice, such as pomegranate, grape, or grapefruit, or have an orange, grapefruit, grapes, or green vegetable like kale, spinach, or broccoli
- 4 to 6 oz smoked salmon spiced with lemon juice, capers, hot sauce, and jalapeño peppers
- tuna or other cold-water fish, lean organic meat (buffalo, elk, venison, beef), organic chicken, or organic turkey
- whole-wheat toast with omega-3 margarine and raw honey
- one or two eggs
- low-fat and low-sugar yogurt with mixed nuts

Getting Started With ABCT: Training Schedules and Descriptions of the Lifts

This section contains different training schedules, ranging from beginner to professional levels. General guidelines include:

- Alternate days with the various resistance programs (numbers 1-4) listed below for each of the week's sessions.
- Vary the type of AE, for example, running 1 day, swimming the next, and bicycling the third.

- Do the AE after the resistance exercises.
- Always do the correct number of sets with each type of ABCT session for the upper body, lower body, core, flexibility, and balance exercises. For example, if you are doing ABCT 1, do only one set for each exercise. With ABCT 2, do two sets for each exercise, with ABCT 3, do three sets for each exercise, and so on.
- Customize the exercise program depending on your goals and time commitment. If you wish to build more muscle, do ABCT 1, 2, and 5; or ABCT 1, 2, 3, and 5. If your goal is to contour and tone, do ABCT 2, 3, and 4. If you wish to have bulk, contour, and tone, then do ABCT 1 to 5.

The ABCT Training Schedules

WEEK ONE: BEGINNING SESSION #1, WITH ABCT 1

1. Resistance training for 10 minutes: Pick the maximum weight you can do for 12 repetitions, and do one set for each exercise.
   a. Two upper body exercises: 1 biceps, 1 triceps
   b. Two lower body exercises: squat, lunges
   c. One core: 25 to 50 or more sit-ups until maximum burn
2. Aerobic exercise for 5 minutes

WEEK ONE: BEGINNING SESSION #2, WITH ABCT 1

3. Resistance training for 10 minutes: Pick the maximum weight you can do for 12 repetitions, and do one set for each exercise.
   a. Two upper body exercises: one chest, one deltoid
   b. Two lower body exercises: leg press, hamstring press
   c. One core: abdominal crunches until maximum burn
4. Aerobic exercise for 5 minutes

WEEK ONE: BEGINNING SESSION #3, WITH ABCT 1

5. Resistance training for 10 minutes: Pick the maximum weight you can do for 12 repetitions, and do one set for each exercise.
   a. Two upper body exercises: 1 shoulder, 1 forearm
   b. Two lower body exercises: squat with weights, lunges
   c. One core: leg lift
6. Aerobic exercise for 5 minutes

WEEK ONE: BEGINNING SESSION #4, WITH ABCT 1

7. Resistance training for 10 minutes: Pick the maximum weight you can do for 12 repetitions, and do one set for each exercise.
   a. Two upper body exercises: one reverse biceps curl, one pull-down back exercise
   b. Two lower body exercises: leg press, hamstring press
   c. One core: leg scissor crosses
8. Aerobic exercise for 5 minutes

9. Resistance training for 20 minutes: Do 12 repetitions at the maximum weight you can do, then 18 repetitions at 75% of original weight.
   a. Three upper body exercises: one chest press, one biceps, one triceps
   b. Two lower body exercises: squats, lunges
   c. One core exercise: sit-ups
10. Aerobic exercise for 10 minutes

11. Resistance training for 20 minutes: Do 12 repetitions at the maximum weight you can do, then 18 repetitions at 75% of original weight.
   a. Three upper body exercises: one chest press, one biceps, one deltoid
   b. Two lower body exercise: lunges, hamstring leg press
   c. One core exercise: abdominal crunches
12. Aerobic exercise for 10 minutes

13. Resistance training for 20 minutes: Do 12 repetitions at the maximum weight you can do, then 18 repetitions at 75% of weight.
   a. Three upper body exercises: one upper shoulder and trapezius, one biceps with reverse curl, one forearm
   b. Two lower body exercises: squat with overhead press, quadriceps leg press
   c. One core: leg lifts at variable heights
14. Aerobic exercise for 10 minutes

15. Resistance training for 20 minutes: Do 12 repetitions at the maximum weight you can do, then 18 repetitions at 75% of weight.
   a. Three upper body exercises: one reverse bicep, one pull-down back exercise, one chest
   b. Two lower body exercises: lunges with weights, squats
   c. One core: leg scissor crosses
16. Aerobic exercise for 10 minutes

17. Resistance exercise for 30 minutes with ABCT 1 to 3: Use maximum weight for 12 repetitions, 75% weight for 18 repetitions, and 50% weight for 24 repetitions.
   a. Three upper body exercises: one biceps, one chest, one triceps
   b. Three lower body exercises: squat, lunges, quadriceps leg press
   c. Two core exercises: sit-ups, leg lifts
18. Aerobic exercise for 15 minutes

19. Resistance exercise for 30 minutes with ABCT 1 to 3; Use maximum weight for 12 repetitions, 75% weight for 18 repetitions, and 50% weight for 24 repetitions.
   a. Three upper body exercises: one deltoid, one reverse biceps curl, one pull-down back exercise
   b. Three lower body exercises: squats with weights, lunges, hamstring press
   c. Two core exercises: leg scissor crosses, abdominal crunches
20. Aerobic exercise for 15 minutes

21. Resistance exercise for 30 minutes with ABCT 1 to 3: Use maximum weight for 12 repetitions, 75% weight for 18 repetitions, and 50% weight for 24 repetitions.
   a. Three upper body exercises: one forearm, one upper shoulder and trapezius, one chest
   b. Three lower body exercises: lunges with weights, quadriceps leg press, hamstring press
   c. Two core exercises: leg lifts to chest with floor extension, supine "bicycle" movement with elbows to opposite knees
22. Aerobic exercise for 15 minutes

23. Resistance exercise for 30 minutes with ABCT 1 to 3: Use maximum weight for 12 repetitions, 75% weight for 18 repetitions, and 50% weight for 24 repetitions.
   a. Three upper body exercises: one biceps, one triceps, one forearm
   b. Three lower body exercises: leg quadriceps press, squats, hamstring press
   c. Two core exercises: leg lifts, sit-ups
24. Aerobic exercise for 15 minutes

25. Resistance exercise for 40 minutes with ABCT 1 to 4: Use maximum weight for 12 repetitions, 75% weight for 18 repetitions, 50% weight for 24 repetitions, and 25% weight for 50 repetitions.
   a. Four upper body exercises: one biceps, one triceps, one shoulder and trapezius, one deltoid
   b. Three lower body exercises: leg quadriceps press, leg hamstring press, squats
   c. Two core exercises: sit-ups, leg lifts
26. Aerobic exercise for 20 minutes

27. Resistance exercise for 40 minutes with ABCT 1 to 4: Use maximum weight for 12 repetitions, 75% weight for 18 repetitions, 50% weight for 24 repetitions, and 25% weight for 50 repetitions.

a. Four upper body exercises: one pull-down back exercise, one reverse curl, one forearm, one chest
b. Three lower body exercises: lunges, leg quadriceps press, squats
c. Two core: abdominal crunches, leg scissor crosses

28. Aerobic exercise for 20 minutes

WEEK FOUR: ADVANCED SESSION #3 WITH ABCT 1 TO 4

29. Resistance exercise for 40 minutes with ABCT 1 to 4: Use maximum weight for 12 repetitions, 75% weight for 18 repetitions, 50% weight for 24 repetitions, and 25% weight for 50 repetitions.
    a. Four upper body exercises: one biceps front curl with reverse curl, one chest, one deltoid, one triceps
    b. Three lower body exercises: hamstring press, lunges with weights, squats with weights
    c. Two core: Lie on back and do leg extensions from chest, supine "bicycle" touching opposite elbow to knee

30. Aerobic exercise for 20 minutes

WEEK FOUR: ADVANCED SESSION #4 WITH ABCT 1 TO 4

31. Resistance exercise for 40 minutes with ABCT 1 to 4: Use maximum weight for 12 repetitions, 75% weight for 18 repetitions, 50% weight for 24 repetitions, and 25% weight for 50 repetitions.
    a. Four upper body exercises: one forearm, one biceps, one upper shoulder trapezius, one pull-down back exercise
    b. Three lower body exercises: lunges with weights, squats with weights, quadriceps leg press
    c. Two core exercises: leg lifts, sit-ups

32. Aerobic exercise for 20 minutes

WEEK FIVE AND BEYOND: PROFESSIONAL SESSIONS WITH ABCT 1 TO 5

33. Resistance exercise for 40 minutes with ABCT 1 to 5: Use maximum weight for 12 repetitions, 75% for 18 repetitions, 50% weight for 24 repetitions, 25% weight for 50 repetitions, and maximum weight for an additional 12 repetitions
    a. Five upper body exercises with selection from the following: one biceps curl, one upper shoulder pull-up, one triceps, one forward with reverse biceps curl, one deltoid, one forearm/wrist curl/extension, one back pull-down exercise, one forearm reverse curl, one neck flexion and extension
    b. Four lower body exercises with selection from the following: squats, lunges, quadriceps press, hamstring press.
    c. Two to three core exercises with selection from the following: sit-ups, crunches, leg lifts, leg scissor crosses, leg extensions to chest

34. Aerobic exercise for 20 minutes

CHEST EXERCISES

Push-up—Position yourself like a plank, on your hands and toes. The hands should be in alignment with the chest, fingers pointing straight forward, with the hands spaced a little wider than shoulder-width apart. The tummy is tucked in, and the butt muscle is down and straight, in alignment with the back. To work different areas of the muscles, the hands can be moved further apart (more chest) or closer together (more triceps).
→ Primary areas worked: chest
→ Secondary areas worked: triceps, shoulders

Bench Press—This uses the same movement as a push-up, except you lie on your back and push a weight up instead of raising the body. It can be done with dumbbells, a barbell, or on a machine. It can also be done in an incline or decline position.
→ Primary areas worked: chest
→ Secondary areas worked: triceps, shoulders

Dip—Best done on a "dipping bar," where the body is suspended and supported only by the arms. In the beginning position, the legs hang down, the body leans slightly forward, and the arms are fully extended. The elbows bend, and the arms lower the body down, then straighten to raise the body back to the starting position.
→ Primary areas worked: chest
→ Secondary areas worked: triceps, shoulders

Chest Fly—Can be performed using either dumbbells or a fly machine. Lie on your back on a bench with your arms out to the sides holding weights (or gripping the machine bars). Arc your arms up and in from the outstretched position until they are pressed together above the chest, with arms straight out and up. Keep a slight bend in the elbows the entire time. Get a good stretch at the bottom of the movement and a good squeeze at the top.
→ Primary areas worked: chest
→ Secondary areas worked: front deltoid

Cable Chest Fly—Done on a cable machine, standing, with each hand gripping a handle. Stand with one leg in front of the other, leaning slightly forward, the arms outstretched and back, with elbows slightly bent. The arms are then pulled forward until they are aligned directly in front of the chest.
→ Primary areas worked: chest
→ Secondary areas worked: front deltoid

BACK EXERCISES

Back Row—Done with dumbbells (one or two), a barbell, or machines. Start lying face down on a bench, with the arms hanging down straight and gripping the weights or the machine bars. The goal is to pull weight up toward the body. There are many variations, including close-grip rows performed on a pulley machine and the one-arm version done while leaning over a bench.
→ Primary areas worked: latissimi, rhomboids, trapezii
→ Secondary areas worked: biceps, rear deltoid

Pullover—Begin lying face up on a bench, with the arms extended beyond the head and down, holding the weight. Keeping the arms close together and elbows slightly bent, bring them up over the head in an arcing motion, then lower them back to the starting position. This is usually done with one dumbbell, although there are variations using a barbell, two dumbbells, or a pullover machine.
→ Primary areas worked: latissimi
→ Secondary areas worked: triceps, chest

Lat Pull-Down—Done using a weight machine. While sitting on the bench, reach up to grasp the bar and pull it down the top of the upper chest or upper back.
→ Primary areas worked: latissimi
→ Secondary areas worked: biceps

Dickerson—Done using either a lat pull-down machine or a pulley system. Begin with the arms straight out in front of the body, slightly elevated to forehead level. Grasp the vertical bar. Keeping the arms stiff, elbows slightly bent and shoulder width (or a little wider apart), pull the bar down to just above the hips.
→ Primary areas worked: latissimi
→ Secondary areas worked: triceps

Pull-Up—This exercise uses body weight only. It is done hanging from a bar and pulling yourself up, or using a machine with a counterbalanced weight bar you stand on for a little help. This is ideal for those not yet strong enough to lift their own body weight.
→ Primary areas worked: latissimi
→ Secondary areas worked: biceps

Shrug—Standing and holding on to barbells or dumbbells, "shrug" your shoulders up toward your ears to pull the weight up. Arms remain straight the whole time.
→ Primary areas worked: trapezii
→ Secondary areas worked: none, or very minor shoulder action

Shoulder Exercises

Shoulder Press—The goal of this exercise is to push a weight up over the head. It can be done with dumbbells or barbells, or using a weight machine. Hand position can be varied. If a barbell or machine is used, the hands can be placed closer or farther apart on the bar. If dumbbells are used, the palms can be facing out (forward) or each other, or changed from one position to the other as the arms are raised.
→ Primary areas worked: deltoids
→ Secondary areas worked: triceps

Lateral Raise—Done with dumbbells, one held in each hand, arms hanging down to the sides, with the weights slightly in front of the body. The arms are raised to the side until the elbows reach just above the shoulder level, then are lowered back down. This exercise can be varied by keeping the elbows slightly bent, which makes it a bit harder, or completely bent, which is easier and safer for the shoulder joint.
→ Primary areas worked: side deltoids
→ Secondary areas worked: trapezii

Front Raise—Similar to the lateral raise, performed with dumbbells or a barbell. Begin with the weight(s) held in the hands, arms straight down in front of body. The arms are lifted straight out and up in front of the body in an arcing movement, stopping just above shoulder level.
→ Primary areas worked: front deltoids
→ Secondary areas worked: trapezii, chest

Rear Fly—Performed with dumbbells, with the body leaning over the legs. It can be done either seated or standing with knees bent and leaning over. Start with weights hanging straight down from the body, level with the abdominal muscles. The weight is then lifted out to the side of the body, keeping a slight bend in the elbows.
→ Primary areas worked: rear deltoids
→ Secondary areas worked: rhomboids

Upright Row—Done with a barbell or two dumbbells. Begin standing, with the arms hanging down and weights in front of the body, palms facing in toward the body. The weight is lifted up to just below chin level, with the elbows kept high through the motion.
→ Primary areas worked: front deltoids
→ Secondary areas worked: trapezii

ARM EXERCISES

Biceps Curl—This exercise involves lifting a weight held in the hand by bending the elbow to bring the hands up toward the shoulders. There are many variations, including using dumbbells, a barbell, or a machine; you can stand or be seated; and the palms may be facing out, in, or rotating through the movement.
→ Primary areas worked: biceps
→ Secondary areas worked: front deltoid

Triceps Extension—The "reverse" of the biceps curl, with the goal being to straighten a bent arm while holding a weight, then releasing it back into the starting position. If you are using a dumbbell, begin leaning over a bench, supporting yourself with one hand, holding a dumbbell in the other, with the dumbbell arm pulled back and its elbow bent at a 90-degree angle. Keeping the upper arm stationary, extend the arm straight out so that the dumbbell moves backward and up. This can also be done using a pulley.
→ Primary areas worked: triceps
→ Secondary areas worked: shoulder, latissimi

Bench Dip—Similar to the dip but performed using a weight bench to support the upper body and with the feet on the ground. Begin with your hands on the edge of the bench, palms down and supporting your weight, with your rear end hanging just off the bench and your legs straight out in front, angling down to the floor so that your heels are resting on the floor. The fingers should be facing the body and the elbows close together. The arms are then bent, lowering the body toward the floor, then straightened so the body is raised.
→ Primary areas worked: triceps
→ Secondary areas worked: shoulders, chest

LEG EXERCISES

Squat—The goal of this exercise is to "sit" and stand back up while holding a weight. Starting in a standing position, push the gluteus muscles backward and lower yourself as if you are going to sit in a chair until you are in a squatting position. The upper body leans slightly forward, toes are pointed straight out in front, feet are slightly wider than shoulder-width apart. This exercise can be done with a barbell held across the back, or using a squat machine, a Smith machine, a hack squat machine, or a Smith ball on the wall.
→ Primary areas worked: quadriceps, gluteals, hamstrings
→ Secondary areas worked: back

Leg Press—Similar to a bench press, but it works the leg rather than the chest muscles. Sit or lie down in a leg press machine, with knees bent toward the chest and feet against the weight platform. Push hard with the legs against the platform until the legs straighten but not entirely; the knees should be slightly bent.
→ Primary areas worked: quadriceps, gluteals, hamstrings
→ Secondary areas worked: back

Leg Extension—Done on a machine while sitting up, with the legs down and the ankles pressing up against a padded bar. The legs are lifted with the feet rising up in an arc, pushing the bar up, until the legs are straight out in front of the body.
→ Primary areas worked: quadriceps
→ Secondary areas worked: none, or minor hip flexor action

Leg Curl—The "reverse" of the leg extension, performed lying face down on a bench with the Achilles tendons pressed up into a padded bar or sitting up, legs straight out in front, with the Achilles tendons resting on a padded bar. The legs are flexed, pushing against the bar until the knees are bent, with the heel toward the gluteals.
→ Primary areas worked: hamstrings
→ Secondary areas worked: none, or slight lower back action

Calf Raise—The goal is to stand up on tiptoes against resistance. This can be done various ways. The simplest is to stand straight up, feet flat on the ground, holding dumbbells by the sides. Stand up on tiptoes, then descend back to feet flat on the ground.
→ Primary areas worked: calves
→ Other benefit: full body stabilization

Lunge—The idea is to "dip" one leg, knee bent, similar to the way a fencer does when lunging with the foil. Begin standing. Keeping the upper body erect, step forward so that one leg is in front of the body and one is behind. Lower the back knee toward the ground, bending the front leg as well, until the front leg is bent in a perfect 90-degree angle at the knee. The upper body is kept erect. There are many variations of this exercise, including holding the lunge while moving up and down, stepping out and pushing back, and walking. It can be done with dumbbells, barbells, and using a machine such as the Smith machine.
→ Primary areas worked: gluteals, quadriceps, hamstrings
→ Secondary areas worked: low back, abductors, adductors

Step-up—Holding dumbbells at the sides or a barbell across the back, step up onto a step or low bench (as long as it is very secure and safe) and then back down. It can be done working one leg at a time and then the other, or with alternating legs.
→ Primary areas worked: gluteals, hamstrings, quadriceps
→ Secondary areas worked: low back, abductors, and adductors

Abductor and Adductor Toners—Performed with machines, these exercises work the "outside" and "inside" of the thighs. To work the muscles on the outsides of your thighs (abductors), you sit in the machine, legs straight forward and resting on pads attached to weights, then spread them out to the sides. To work the muscles on the insides of your thighs (adductors), you do the reverse, beginning in a seated position, legs straight out in front but spread, then squeeze them together.
→ Primary areas worked: abductors, adductors
→ Secondary areas worked: none

Dead Lift—Performed with dumbbells or barbells. Begin in a kneeling position, with the butt pushed back, upper body leaning forward, and the toes pointed straight out. The back is kept in alignment, without rounding. Hands grip the weights, which rest on the floor. Stand up, using only the legs, with the arms and hands acting only as hooking and carrying mechanisms. After reaching the standing position, lower the weight in the same fashion.
→ Primary areas worked: trapezius, latissimi, erector spinae, gluteals, hamstrings, quadriceps, and psoas

ABCT Summary (Table 8.4)

- Exercise in the morning on an empty stomach after an 8- to 12-hour fast.
- Drink 6 ounces of water mixed with 10 g whey protein before starting warm-up or doing any exercise.
- Warm up for 5 minutes with stretching, flexing, and extension exercises of the upper and lower body.
- Start the resistance portion of ABCT based on one's present exercise level, time commitment, and desired intensity of workout. Pick ABCT 1, 2, 3, 4, or 5, with varied mixing and matching to accomplish the goals of bulk, contour, and tone. Do the intense exercise to the muscle burn. Alternate muscle groups each day for both upper and lower body, and do core exercises.
- Exercise two or three upper body and two or three lower body muscle groups per session, and increase the number of muscle groups exercised with your desired intensity and training time. Do two or three core exercises with some flexibility and balance work as well.

Table 8.4

RECOMMENDED EXERCISES FOR ABCT FITNESS WITH AEROBIC INTERVALS AND RESISTANCE TRAINING BASED ON TIME SCHEDULE

15 min: Aerobic intervals for 5 min
    Resistance training for 10 min
        Two upper body exercises with ABCT 1
        Two lower body exercises
        One core exercise
30 min: Aerobic intervals for 10 min
    Resistance training for 20 min
        Three upper body exercises with ABCT 1 and 2
        Two lower body exercises
        One core exercise
        One flexibility exercise
45 min: Aerobic intervals for 15 min
    Resistance training for 30 min
        Three upper body exercises with ABCT 1, 2, and 3
        Three lower body exercises
        Two core exercises
        One flexibility exercise
60 min: Aerobic intervals for 20 min
    Resistance training for 40 min
        Four upper body exercises with ABCT 1, 2, 3, and 4
        Three lower body exercises
        Two core exercises
        One flexibility exercise
90 min: Aerobic intervals for 30 min
    Resistance training for 60 min
        Five upper body exercises with ABCT 1, 2 3, 4, and 5
        Three lower body exercises
        Two core exercises
        One flexibility exercise
120 min: Aerobic intervals for 40 min
    Resistance training for 80 min
        Six upper body exercises with ABCT 1, 2, 3, 4, and 5
        Four lower body exercises
        Three core exercises
        Two flexibility exercises

- Ten minutes into the resistance workout, start drinking 4 ounces of the ABCT Energy Shake at intervals after each exercise set.
- Rest 60 seconds between each repetition unless doing supersets or taking minimal rest periods.
- Take 3-second rests as needed to combat muscle fatigue.
- After completing the resistance exercises, start the aerobic program, utilizing cross-training.
- Keep the ratio of resistance training to aerobic exercise at 2:1.
- Exercise at least four times per week, but daily is best with 1 day off every week if necessary.
- Compress the exercise time and increase training intensity by doing core exercises or other lower-intensity exercises during the 60-second rest periods. Alternatively, you can do the core exercises as part of the resistance exercise session.
- Eat the recommended postexercise breakfast.

Conclusion

Optimal exercise with the ABCT program, combining AE and RT and taking proper nutrition and nutraceutical supplements, results in numerous cardiovascular and overall health benefits and slows aging. Skeletal muscle is an endocrine organ that secretes over 400 myokines, hormones, and mediators that result in gene expression patterns and intracellular and extracellular signaling to reduce inflammation and oxidative stress and modulate immune function during chronic adaptive training. An understanding of the nutrient-gene-muscle interconnections related to proteomics and metabolomics will allow for a more scientific recommendation for the types and duration of exercise coupled with nutritional support to enhance good health outcomes and reduce morbidity and mortality.

References

1. Houston MC. *What Your Doctor May Not Tell You About Heart Disease. The Revolutionary Book that Reveals the Truth Behind Coronary Illnesses—and How You Can Fight Them.* New York, NY: Grand Central Life and Style, Hachette Book Group; 2012.
2. Vina J, Sanchis-Gomar F, Martinez-Bello V, Gomez-Cabrera MC. Exercise acts a drug; the pharmacological benefits of exercise. *Br J Pharmacol.* 2012;167(1):1-12.
3. Meka N, Katragadda S, Cherian B, Arora RR. Endurance exercise and resistance training in cardiovascular disease. *Ther Adv Cardiovasc Dis.* 2008;2(2):115-121.
4. Coffey VG, Hawley JA. The molecular bases of training adaptation. *Sports Med.* 2007;37(9):737-763.
5. McCall GE, Byrnes WC, Dickinson A, Pattany PM, Fleck SJ. Muscle fiber hypertrophy, hyperplasia, and capillary density in college men after resistance training. *J Appl Physiol.* 1996;81(5):2004-2012.
6. Radom-Aizik S, Hayek S, Shahar I, Rechavi G, Kaminski N, Ben-Dov I. Effects of aerobic training on gene expression in skeletal muscle of elderly men *Med Sci Sports Exerc.* 2005;37(10):1680-1696.
7. Ostrowski K, Schjerling P, Pedersen BK. Physical activity and plasma interleukin-6 in humans–effect of intensity of exercise *Eur J Appl Physiol.* 2000;83(6):512-515.
8. Pedersen BK, Ostrowski K, Rohde T, Bruunsgaard H, Can J. The cytokine response to strenuous exercise. *Physiol Pharmacol.* 1998;76(5):505-511.
9. Steensberg A. The role of IL-6 in exercise-induced immune changes and metabolism. *Exerc Immunol Rev.* 2003;9:40-47.

10. Petersen AM, Pedersen BK. The anti-inflammatory effect of exercise. *J Appl Physiol.* 2005;98(4):1154-1162.

11. Bruunsgaard H. Physical activity and modulation of systemic low-level inflammation. *J Leukoc Biol.* 2005;78(4):819-835.

12. Scott JP, Sale C, Greeves JP, Casey A, Dutton J, Fraser WD. Cytokine response to acute running in recreationally active and endurance-trained men. *Eur J Appl Physiol.* March 6, 2013. [Epub ahead of print].

13. Welc SS, Clanton TL. The regulation of interleukin-6 implicates skeletal muscle as an integrative stress sensor and endocrine organ. *Exp Physiol.* 2013;98(2):359-371.

14. Pratley R, Nicklas B, Rubin M, et al. Strength training increases resting metabolic rate and norepinephrine levels in healthy 50- to 65-yr-old men. *J Appl Physiol.* 1994;76(1):133-137.

15. Anton MM, Cortez-Cooper MY, DeVan AE, Neidre DB, Cook JN, Tanaka H. Resistance training increases basal limb blood flow and vascular conductance in aging humans. *J Appl Physiol.* 2006;101(5):1351-1355.

16. Okamoto T, Masuhara M, Ikuta M. Combined aerobic and resistance training and vascular function: effect of aerobic exercise before and after resistance training *J Appl Physiol.* 2007;103(5):1655-1661.

17. McCartney N, McKelvie RS, Haslam DR, Jones NL. Usefulness of weightlifting training in improving strength and maximal power output in coronary artery disease. *Am J Cardiol.* 1991;67(11):939-945.

18. Pu CT, Johnson MT, Forman DE, et al. Randomized trial of progressive resistance training to counteract the myopathy of chronic heart failure. *J Appl Physiol.* 2001;90(6):2341-2350.

19. Church TS, Blair SN, Cocreham S, et al. Effects of aerobic and resistance training on hemoglobin A1c levels in patients with type 2 diabetes: a randomized controlled trial. *JAMA.* 2010;304(20):2253-2262.

20. Mujica V, Urzúa A, Leiva E, et al. Intervention with education and exercise reverses the metabolic syndrome in adults. *J Am Soc Hypertens.* 2010;4(3):148-153.

21. Warner SO, Linden MA, Liu Y, et al. The effects of resistance training on metabolic health with weight regain *J Clin Hypertens (Greenwich).* 2010;12(1):64-72.

22. Lamina S. Effects of continuous and interval training programs in the management of hypertension: a randomized controlled trial. *J Clin Hypertens (Greenwich).* 2010;12(11):841-849.

23. Marzolini S, Oh PI, Brooks D. Effect of combined aerobic and resistance training versus aerobic training alone in individuals with coronary artery disease: a meta-analysis. *Eur J Prev Cardiol.* 2012;19(1):81-94.

24. Rossi A, Dikareva A, Bacon SL, Daskalopoulou SS. The impact of physical activity on mortality in patients with high blood pressure: a systematic review. *J Hypertens.* 2012;30(7):1277-1288.

25. Sesso HD, Paffenbarger RS Jr, Lee IM. Physical activity and coronary heart disease in men: The Harvard Alumni Health Study. *Circulation.* 2000;102(9):975-980.

26. Hawley JA, Burke LM, Phillips SM, Spriet LL. Nutritional modulation of training-induced skeletal muscle adaptations. *J Appl Physiol.* 2011;110(3):834-845.

27. Pennings B, Koopman R, Beelen M, Senden JM, Saris WH, van Loon LJ. Exercising before protein intake allows for greater use of dietary protein-derived amino acids for de novo muscle protein synthesis in both young and elderly men. *Am J Clin Nutr.* 2011;93(2):322-331.

28. Lecoultre V, Benoit R, Carrel G, et al. Fructose and glucose co-ingestion during prolonged exercise increases lactate and glucose fluxes and oxidation compared with an equimolar intake of glucose. *Am J Clin Nutr.* 2010;92(5):1071-1079.

29. Stephens BR, Braun B. Impact of nutrient intake timing on the metabolic response to exercise. *Nutr Rev.* 2008;66(8):473-476.

30. Peake JM, Suzuki K, Coombes JS. The influence of antioxidant supplementation on markers of inflammation and the relationship to oxidative stress after exercise. *J Nutr Biochem.* 2007;18(6):357-371.

31. Fukuda DH, Smith AE, Kendall KL, Stout JR. The possible combinatory effects of acute consumption of caffeine, creatine, and amino acids on the improvement of anaerobic running performance in humans. *Nutr Res.* 2010;30(9):607-614.

32. Wray DW, Uberoi A, Lawrenson L, Bailey DM, Richardson RS. Oral antioxidants and cardiovascular health in the exercise-trained and untrained elderly: a radically different outcome. *Clin Sci (Lond).* 2009;116(5):433-441.

33. Panza VS, Wazlawik E, Ricardo Schütz G, Comin L, Hecht KC, da Silva EL. Consumption of green tea favorably affects oxidative stress markers in weight-trained men. *Nutrition.* 2008;24(5):433-442.

34. Karanth J, Jeevaratnam K. Effect of carnitine supplementation on mitochondrial enzymes in liver and skeletal muscle of rat after dietary lipid manipulation and physical activity. *Indian J Exp Biol.* 2010;48(5):503-510.

35. Huang A, Owen K. Role of supplementary L carnitine in exercise and exercise recovery. *Med Sport Sci.* 2012;59:135-142.

36. Broad EM, Maughan RJ, Galloway SDR. Effects of exercise intensity and altered substrate availability on cardiovascular and metabolic responses to exercise after oral carnitine supplementation in athletes. *Int J Sport Nutr Exerc Metab.* 2011;21(5):385-397.

37. Addis P, Shecterle LM, St Cyr JA. Cellular protection during oxidative stress: a potential role for D-ribose and antioxidants. *J Diet Suppl.* 2012;9(3):178-182.

38. Cramer JT, Housh TJ, Johnson GO, Coburn JW, Stout JR. Effects of a carbohydrate-, protein-, and ribose- containing repletion drink during 8 weeks of endurance training on aerobic capacity, endurance performance, and body composition. *J Strength Cond Res.* 2012;26(8):2234-2242.

39. Seifert JG, Subudhi AW, Fu MX, et al. The role of ribose on oxidative stress during hypoxic exercise: a pilot study. *J Med Food.* 2009;12(3):690-693.

40. Hoffman JR, Williams DR, Emerson NS, et al. L-alanyl-L-glutamine ingestion maintains performance during a competitive basketball game. *J Int Soc Sports Nutr.* 2012;9(1):4.

41. Rowlands DS, Clarke J, Green JG, Shi X. L-Arginine but not L-glutamine likely increases exogenous carbohydrate oxidation during endurance exercise. *Eur J Appl Physiol.* 2012;112(7):2443-2453.

42. Ra SG, Miyazaki T, Ishikura K, et al. Additional effects of taurine on the benefits of BCAA intake for the delayed-onset muscle soreness and muscle damage induced by high-intensity eccentric exercise. *Adv Exp Med Biol.* 2013;776:179-187.

43. Tang FC, Chan CC, Kuo PL. Contribution of creatine to protein homeostasis in athletes after endurance and sprint running. *Eur J Nutr.* February 8, 2013. [Epub ahead of print].

44. Howatson G, Hoad M, Goodall S, Tallent J, Bell PG, French DN. Exercise-induced muscle damage is reduced in resistance-trained males by branched chain amino acids: a randomized, double-blind, placebo controlled study. *J Int Soc Sports Nutr.* 2012;9(1):20. [Epub ahead of print].

45. Breen L, Phillips SM. Nutrient interaction for optimal protein anabolism in resistance exercise. *Curr Opin Clin Nutr Metab Care.* 2012;15(3):226-232.

46. Pasiakos SM, McClung HL, McClung JP, et al. Leucine-enriched essential amino acid supplementation during moderate steady state exercise enhances postexercise muscle protein synthesis. *Am J Clin Nutr.* 2011;94(3):809-818.

47. Chen S, Li Z, Krochmal R, Abrazado M, Kim W, Cooper CBJ. Effect of Cs-4 (Cordyceps sinensis) on exercise performance in healthy older subjects: a double-blind, placebo-controlled trial. *Altern Complement Med.* 2010;16(5):585-590.

48. Kumar R, Negi PS, Singh B, Ilavazhagan G, Bhargava K, Sethy NK. Cordyceps sinensis promotes exercise endurance capacity of rats by activating skeletal muscle metabolic regulators. *J Ethnopharmacol.* 2011;136(1):260-266.

49. Noreen EE, Buckley JG, Lewis SL, Brandauer J, Stuempfle KJ. The effects of an acute dose of *Rhodiola rosea* on endurance exercise performance. *J Strength Cond Res.* 2013;27(3):839-847.

50. Xu J, Li Y. Effects of salidroside on exhaustive exercise-induced oxidative stress in rats. *Mol Med Rep.* 2012;6(5):1195-1198.

51. Noreen EE, Buckley JG, Lewis SL, Brandauer J, Stuempfle KJ. The effects of an acute dose of *Rhodiola rosea* on endurance exercise performance. *J Strength Cond Res.* May 24, 2012. [Epub ahead of print].

52. Parisi A, Tranchita E, Duranti G, et al. Effects of chronic Rhodiola rosea supplementation on sport performance and antioxidant capacity in trained male: preliminary results. *J Sports Med Phys Fitness.* 2010;50(1):57-63.

53. Evdokimov VG. Effect of cryopowder *Rhodiola rosae* L. on cardiorespiratory parameters and physical performance of humans. *Aviakosm Ekolog Med.* 2009;43(6):52-56.

54. Osterberg KL, Melby CL. Effect of acute resistance exercise on postexercise oxygen consumption and resting metabolic rate in young women. *Int J Sport Nutr Exerc Metab.* 2000;10(1):71-81.

Section 5

Cardiovascular Genomics

Chapter 9   **Cardiogenomics in the Age of Personalized Lifestyle Medicine**
Jeffrey S. Bland, PhD, FACN, FACB

9

Cardiogenomics in the Age of Personalized Lifestyle Medicine

Jeffrey S. Bland, PhD, FACN, FACB

In 2019, the American Heart Association published an update of heart disease and stroke statistics for the United States. This report was compiled using data collected between 2013 and 2016 for the National Health and Nutrition Examination Survey. The prevalence of cardiovascular disease (CVD)—coronary heart disease, heart failure, stroke, and hypertension—in adults greater than 20 years of age is 48% overall (121.5 million in 2016) and increases with advancing age in both men and women. Globally, CVD is the number one cause of death and in fact has increased by 14.5% since 2006.[1] Evidence has clearly demonstrated the importance of lifestyle factors in the development of CVDs.[2] Even so, population-based public health criteria for lifestyle interventions have had mixed success in reducing CVD incidence.[3] Personalized lifestyle medicine—a concept that takes into account an individual's unique response to lifestyle, diet, physical activity, stress, environmental exposures, and medications—may represent a more effective approach to the management of CVDs.[4] On a global scale, the prevalence of many noncommunicable diseases are on the rise, and this trend has led researchers to focus on the interaction between genetics and lifestyle, diet, social, and environmental factors.[5]

There is emerging evidence that implementation of individualized preventive health care could help bend the curve of health care costs downward.[6] In preventive cardiology, advancements would include integration of genomic, biometric, dietary, and lifestyle data to improve precision in both diagnosis and therapy. In an editorial titled "Introducing 'Genomics and Precision Health'," which was published in the *Journal of the American Medical Association* in May 2017, Dr William Feero asserted: "This shift is inexorably moving medicine from an endeavor in which care for individual patients is driven by trial and error informed by studies designed to measure populations outcomes to one in which care is selected based on a deep understanding of health and disease attributes unique to each individual."[7] What

forces are driving this shift in perspective? The Framingham Cardiovascular Risk Score is one of the best known and most widely used tools to emerge from a population-based study. It is calculated using data related to smoking history, elevated serum cholesterol (and specifically elevated low-density lipoprotein [LDL] cholesterol), obesity, hypertension, maleness, and age. Yet despite its iconic standing and its deep roots in clinical care, it has been reported that the Framingham Risk Score has less than a 50% probability of predicting CVD within 10 years in men 30 to 39 years of age.[8]

To better appreciate how the concept of personalization is shaping the future of cardiology, we can look to a well-known and significant study from the recent past: the JUPITER primary prevention trial (Justification for the Use of Statins in Prevention: an Intervention Trial Evaluating Rosuvastatin). When the results of this study were published in 2008, a key finding was the demonstration that CVD risk is linked to more factors than just elevated serum lipids. The JUPITER researchers found that people with low serum LDL cholesterol and elevated serum high-sensitivity C-reactive protein (hsCRP), which is an inflammatory biomarker, had a reduction in both hsCRP and cardiovascular events when treated with the statin rosuvastatin.[9] This observation contributed to the increased recognition that CVD results from the interaction of many variables and some of these variables are controlled by numerous genes.[10] Cardiology is now moving toward new therapeutic frontiers based on an expanded understanding of the complexities of gene-environment interaction and its connection to health and disease.[11]

"Polygenic" is a word used to describe the interaction of multiple genes in a network for the regulation of physiological function.[12] According to Boyle et al, authors of an important 2017 publication called "An Expanded View of Complex Traits: From Polygenic to Omnigenic," this definition may be too limited; they write: "A central role of genetics is to understand the links between genetic variation and disease.... But for complex traits, association signals tend to be spread across most of the genome-including many genes without an obvious connection to disease."[13] These authors suggest that these gene regulatory networks are so interconnected to the etiology of complex diseases that a more appropriate characterization would be to refer to them as "omnigenic." The functional expression of omnigenic networks that are involved in the etiology of complex chronic diseases such as CVD are influenced by signals derived from lifestyle, diet, and environmental exposures, including pharmaceutical drugs that are used for treatment.

How do we develop a unified conceptual approach to managing the complex interaction of gene networks and lifestyle variables? In cardiac care, a systems biology approach to precision personalized cardiology must be developed, and we are now starting to witness translation of this emerging scientific understanding. In a 2017 article, Bland, Minich, and Eck assert the following: "Emerging groundbreaking research projects have given us a glimpse of how systems thinking and computational methods may lead to personalized health advice. It is important that all stakeholders work together to create the needed paradigm shift in healthcare before the rising epidemic of NCDs [non-communicable diseases] overwhelm the society, the economy, and the dated health system."[14]

Genetic Regulation of Cardiovascular Function: An Omnigenic Network

Cardiogenomics is a relatively new term that is being used to describe the use of genomic profiling to assess risk for CVD. An example of the advancement in this field is the recognition that polymorphisms of specific genes such as LDLR, APOB, and PCSK9 have been found to be important in establishing individual risk to CVD.[15] The functional impact of these genes is known to be influenced by lifestyle, dietary, and environmental factors. For example, PCSK9 was discovered through genetic studies documenting familial hypercholesterolemia, and PCSK9 protein, which is secreted by the liver, binds to the LDL receptor and targets it for degradation; this results in alteration in LDL signaling and ApoB degradation that contributes to CVD risk.[16] Additional research has demonstrated that variations in both the PCSK9 and hydroxymethylglutaryl CoA Reductase (HMGCR) genes contribute to CVD risk.[17] Multiple single nucleotide polymorphisms (SNPs) exist for these genes and impart varying degrees of individual risk to CVD; it is becoming recognized that SNPs with a more mild influence on the disease phenotype are more significantly influenced by lifestyle, diet, and environmental factors.[18] Clinical intervention trials in patients with existing atherosclerotic CVD who were administered a biological drug that blocks the binding of PCSK9 with the LDL receptor when administered along with statins demonstrated significant reduction in LDL cholesterol—beyond results that high-dose statins alone can produce—and also a reduction in the risk of subsequent cardiovascular events.[19]

These trials support the important understanding that variations in the PCSK9 gene can impact vascular biology and cardiovascular risk. A complete understanding of how PCSK9 fits into the omnigenic cardiovascular risk story is yet to be developed, but this work clearly indicates that multiple genes influence cardiovascular function and that single nucleotide variations in these genes can result in risk that is highly personalized to the individual. Recently, a controlled animal trial demonstrated that PCSK9 activity can be inhibited by the alkaloid berberine.[20] Berberine is found in a variety of traditional medicinal plants historically used by a number of cultures, including barberry, tree turmeric, Oregon grape, goldenseal, yellow root, and California poppy. The results of this study indicated that, with pharmacological doses of berberine (200 mg/kg by gavage in mice), the hepatocyte nuclear factor 1alpha, which is known to be an obligate transactivator for PCSK9 gene expression, was inhibited, thereby reducing the genetic expression of PCSK9 and improving LDL metabolism. This is an interesting study in that it suggests that there are multiple ways in which a risk gene can be modulated in its expression through different environmental exposures. It is often thought that to block the effects of a risk gene you have to directly inhibit its expression, but in fact there are many upstream and downstream events linked to lifestyle, diet, and environmental factors that can modify the expression of the genetic risk factor. This demonstrates the concept that regulatory functions can be connected to the uniqueness of an individual's gene-environment status.

Within cardiology, there has been a long-standing belief that elevated serum LDL cholesterol is always a risk factor for CVD, but recent cardiogenomic studies have found that, when serum LDL is elevated but apoB is low, cardiovascular risk is low.[21] This suggests that omnigenic regulation of cardiovascular signaling processes—as reflected in the level of apoB—is more important than a single surrogate marker for CVD, such as serum LDL.[22] Infiltration of an apoB particle into the arterial wall is the first step in initiating the atherosclerotic process. We are now learning that this process is the result of many genetically controlled functions that relate to lipid metabolism, immune function, inflammation, coagulation factors, and vascular smooth muscle cell proliferation, all of which can be influenced by lifestyle, dietary, and environmental factors.

Ference et al have found that genetic variants that regulate cholesterol transport through the cholesterol ester transport protein system (CETP) and its impact on apoB structure and function impart varying degrees of CVD risk. This team conducted a retrospective analysis of 14 cohort or case-controlled studies conducted in North America or the United Kingdom between 1948 and 2012. When the results of this effort were published in the *Journal of the American Medical Association* in 2017, the following conclusion was reached: "Combined exposure to variants in the genes that encode the targets of CETP inhibitors and statins was associated with discordant reductions in LDL-C and apoB levels and a corresponding risk of cardiovascular events that was proportional to the attenuated reduction in apoB but significantly less than expected per unit change in LDL-C."[21]

Specific genes have also been linked to diet-related CVD risk; for example, the cardiometabolic effects of omega-3 long-chain fatty acids, such as eicosapentaenoic acid (EPA) and docasahexaenoic acid (DHA).[23] In a recent study of the relationship between PCSK9 genetic variants and the risk of nonfatal myocardial infarction, it was found that increased consumption of omega-3 polyunsaturated fatty acids was associated with a lower risk in C-allele carriers of PCSK9 rs11206510 but not in the non-C allele carriers.[24] One important implication of this study is that, in designing future clinical studies to evaluate the health benefits of omega-3 fatty acid supplementation, stratification for specific genetic responders versus nonresponders might be significant.

Agents that have weaker interaction with genomic signaling processes (which is often the case with lifestyle, diet, and environmental factors) may have more sensitivity to genetic variants than therapeutic agents that are designed to have a strong target affinity for a specific gene product. Because these factors can impact complex cellular interactions, the relationship between lifestyle, diet, environment, and the network biology associated with altered genomic signaling may be much more important in determining long-term cardiovascular risk than previously recognized. As greater insight and understanding emerges, the future points toward applying cardiogenomics to the design of personalized lifestyle approaches for the primary prevention of vascular disease.

Genetic Risk, Adherence to a Healthy Lifestyle, and Cardiovascular Disease

Data compiled from the Nurses' Health Study between 1976 and 2016 demonstrated that women who ate a diet that was low in transfat, saturated fat, refined carbohydrates, and sugar-sweetened beverages and rich in fruits and vegetables, whole grains, and sources of unsaturated fats had a reduced risk of CVD. This reduced risk was further amplified if their lifestyle incorporated regular physical activity, maintenance of a normal body mass index, moderate alcohol intake, and no smoking. Researchers who recently reviewed these data concluded the following: "Adherence to a combination of a healthy diet and lifestyle behaviors may prevent most vascular events."[25]

Recommendations that result from large-scale, longitudinal studies are important public health messages, but it has been reported that at least one of every six people who sustain a myocardial infarction have no significant risk based on traditional cardiovascular risk factors and those with the lowest risk factors have the highest death rate after a myocardial infarction.[26] These data suggest that we have much yet to learn about the etiology of CVD and its complex relationship to individual genetics lifestyle, diet, and environment.

A recent study that shines a particularly bright light on the future of precision cardiology framed within a personalized lifestyle medicine context is the work of Dr Sekar Kathiresan at the Center for Human Genetic Research and Cardiology, Massachusetts General Hospital, and his collaborators at Massachusetts General Hospital, Brigham and Women's Hospital, the Broad Institute, Mount Sinai Medical Center, Lund University Department of Clinical Sciences, Perelman School of Medicine, and the University of Texas Health Sciences Center. This study, which was published in the *New England Journal of Medicine* in 2016, used a polygenic score of DNA sequence polymorphisms of 50 genes identified from genome-wide association studies (GWASs) in three prospective studies: 7814 participants in the Atherosclerosis Risk in Communities Study, 21,222 in the Women's Genome Health Study, and 22,389 in the Malmo Diet and Cancer Study, and also in 4260 participants in the cross-sectional BioImage Study for whom genotype and covariate data were available. All of the participants in these studies also had the quality of their lifestyle evaluated using a scoring system consisting of four factors: smoking status, physical activity index, body mass index, and diet.[27]

The objective of the study, which included data collected since 1987, was to determine if there was a correlation between the polygenic cardiovascular risk score and the aggregate lifestyle score in CVD outcome in people enrolled in the studies. The results were instructive about the nature of the interaction between various risk genotypes and modifiable lifestyle factors. The relative risk of incident cardiovascular events was 91% higher in the participants in the highest genetic risk group than in those of the lowest genetic risk, indicating that genetics does play a role in CVD. This research team also found that a favorable lifestyle was associated with a substantially lower risk of cardiovascular events than an unfavorable lifestyle, regardless of the genetic risk category. Most importantly, among participants at the highest genetic risk, a favorable lifestyle was associated with a 46% lower risk of cardiovascular events than in those with an unfavorable lifestyle. The authors suggest that this finding translates to a reduction in the standardized 10-year incidence of coronary events from approximately 10% for an unfavorable lifestyle to 5% risk for a favorable lifestyle in the high-genetic-risk category. They also reported that in the BioImage Study participants, a favorable lifestyle score was associated with a significant reduction in coronary artery calcification in each genetic risk category.

The conclusions of this study were truly frameshifting in terms of increasing the understanding of the nature of the interaction of genes with lifestyle in the etiology of CVD. The findings were summarized with the following statement: "Across four studies involving 55,685 participants, genetic and lifestyle factors were independently associated with susceptibility to coronary artery disease. Among participants at high genetic risk, a favorable lifestyle was associated with a nearly 50% lower relative risk of coronary artery disease than was an unfavorable lifestyle."

Review and analysis indicate that 29 of the 50 genes identified by GWAS to be associated with CVD risk can be linked to five different physiological processes and grouped into the following functional states:

Inflammation-related genes

- **MRAS**
- **SCL22A4**
- **TRB1B1**
- **ADAMT**
- **BCAP29**
- **GGCX**

Lipid metabolism–related genes

- **LIPA**
- **SH2B3**
- **HHIPL1**
- **UBE2Z**
- **SMG6**

Vascular endothelial biology–related genes

- **SORT1**
- **MIA3**
- **EDNRA**
- **GUCY1A3**
- **PDGFD**
- **FLT1**
- **COL4A1**
- **KCNK5**

Vascular smooth muscle proliferation–related genes

- **RASD1**
- **CYP17A1**
- **ZC3HC1**
- **TCF21**
- **ANKS1A**
- **WOR12**

Coagulation-related genes

- **ZEB2**
- **PLG**
- **ABO**
- **DHACTR1**

This approach of grouping individual risk genes into five functional polygenic assessment areas provides a model for personalizing recommendations regarding lifestyle, diet, and environment and allows for the development of medical therapy based on the identified function and specific gene network. Many studies have been published in the medical literature about these five different functional areas, some of which demonstrate clear links to lifestyle factors such as diet and nutrients, botanical medicine, physical activity, stress, sleep, environmental exposures, and medication. Consolidation of this information could serve as a framework for a new personalized lifestyle medicine approach to precision preventive cardiology. By pairing information obtained through whole genome sequencing with a polygenic portfolio of specific single nucleotide polymorphisms (SNPs) related to cardiovascular function, a clinician would have powerful new tools for applying a systems biology approach to clinical decision-making.

Polygenic Analysis and Cardiogenomics

Cardiogenomic analysis is going to become increasingly important in vascular care. Recent studies can serve as examples of GWAS/SNP approaches to cardiogenomics. The results of a study of 61,079 individuals who were part of a genome-wide association meta-analysis correlating specific SNPs with serum calcium and cardiovascular outcomes were published in the *Journal of the American Medical Association* in 2017; this work demonstrated that a genetic predisposition to higher serum calcium is associated with an increased risk of coronary artery disease and myocardial infarction.[28] In 2018, an important report appeared in that same journal about the association of specific genetic variants related to gluteofemoral versus abdominal fat distribution with coronary disease risk.[29] Genetic variants of genes that control the metabolism of homocysteine that have been linked to increased CVD include methylenetetrahydrofolate reductase, betaine-homocysteine methyltransferase, 5-methyltetrahydrofolate-homocysteine methyltransferase, and cystathionine beta synthase. Controlling the metabolism of homocysteine has been linked to increased CVD risk.[30] Historically, this area of study is closely associated with early work on the genetics of hyperhomocysteinemia and its relationship to coronary artery disease risk.[31]

Recently, it has become well recognized that analysis of multiple SNPs using polygenic algorithms has great predictive power for determining CVD risk. In a GWAS analysis of 1 million genotyped individuals, a specific family of genetic polymorphisms associated with risk was identified.[32] In 2018, a research group at the Center for Genomic Medicine at the Massachusetts General Hospital led by Khera and Kathiresan established a polygenic risk score from GWAS data for five common diseases: coronary heart disease, atrial fibrillation, type 2 diabetes, inflammatory bowel disease, and breast cancer. For coronary artery disease, the prevalence is 20-fold higher than the carrier frequency of rare monogenic mutations conferring comparable risk. When these findings were published in *Nature Genetics*, the authors wrote the following: "We propose that it is time to contemplate the inclusion of polygenic risk prediction in clinical care, and discuss relevant issues."[33]

In 2019, an article titled "The Evolution of Genetic-Based Risk Scores for Lipids and Cardiovascular Disease" was published in *Current Opinion in Lipidology*. The authors, Dron and Hegele, write about entering a new era of risk assessment, and they state: "We are on the verge of clinical applications of GRSs [genetic risk scores] to provide incremental information on dyslipidemia and CVD risk above and beyond traditional clinical variables."[34] A research team known as the UK Biobank CardioMetabolic Consortium CHD Working Group applied this concept to genomic risk prediction for coronary artery disease in 480,000 adults and found that a genetic risk score was more predictive than any previous risk assessment tool. These investigators concluded that the polygenomic risk score substantially advances the concept of using genomic information to stratify individuals with different trajectories of coronary artery disease risk.[35]

Use of genetic risk evaluation may potentially provide clinical guidance on how to personalize diet and lifestyle intervention programs. It has recently been reported that nutritional genomics can be applied to cardiogenomic profiling to improve diet and lifestyle recommendations.[36] Evidence from recent studies demonstrates important clinical relationships between specific diet and gene interactions related to CVD risk. The cardiovascular relationships to diet-related genes such as FTO, ACE, PPARs, TCF7L2, BDNF, MC4R, APOAs, ANGPTL3, and FADS consistently demonstrate predictive ability across age groups and populations.

Additionally, specific mutations that result in clonal hematopoiesis of indeterminate potential are associated with CVD risk.[37] Of all the Framingham risk factors, age is known to be the strongest predictor of CVD risk. There is strong evidence that age is also an independent risk factor to hypertension and elevated LDL cholesterol. Modifiable risk factors derived from the Framingham Risk Score only account for 12% of age effect in men and 40% in women. It appears as if a collection of specific clonal mutations in immune cells, such as TET2, DNMT3A, and ASXL1, which control epigenetic regulation of inflammatory gene expression through the process of genomic methylation, may account for an increase in cardiovascular risk with age beyond that of the traditional Framingham risk factors.[38,39]

The role of the epigenetic DNA methylation process in CVD risk is another innovative and important area of investigation. It is now known that a polygenic risk score comprising specific genetic polymorphisms provides more precise cardiovascular risk evaluation but still accounts for a relatively small incremental risk. The SNPs alone do not predict the full impact of the gene-environment interaction that influences the expression of genes that establish CVD risk. Accumulating evidence suggests that epigenetic modifications of the genome in specific cells that occur as a result of environmental, dietary, and lifestyle factors are important as determining processes for establishing a more clinically precise understanding of the genetic regulation of cardiovascular function.[40] Considerable progress is being made in assessing the methylome as an approach toward early evaluation of cardiovascular risk associated with epigenomic effects. This research may increase our understanding of the role and influence of epigenetics in cardiovascular function, which in turn may increase the specificity of personalized genomic risk profiling.

Summary

This is an exciting time for cardiovascular medicine. We are witnessing the creation of a new approach to the prevention and treatment of CVD. It is an omnigenic approach—powered by systems biology—to assembling patient-specific information about how genes, environment, diet, and lifestyle interact. When combined with other new technologies such as artificial intelligence and machine learning informatics, the result will be the development of a precision approach to CVD risk assessment and management through the application of personalized medicine. Advancements in cardiogenomics will open a gateway for change throughout the entire segment of the health care system that is focused on the risk assessment for many complex, chronic, noncommunicable diseases affecting our world population.

References

1. Benjamin EJ, Munter P, Alonso A, et al. Heart disease and stroke statistics-2019 update: a report from the American Heart Association. *Circulation*. 2019:139(10):e56-e528. doi:10.1161/CIR.0000000000000659.

2. Doughty KN, Del Pilar NX, Audette A, Katz DL. Lifestyle medicine and the management of cardiovascular disease. *Curr Cardiol Rep*. 2017;19(11):116.

3. Gaziano TA. Lifestyle and cardiovascular disease: more work to do. *J Am Coll Cardiol*. 2017;69(9):1126-1128.

4. Minich DM, Bland JS. Personalized lifestyle medicine: relevance for nutrition and lifestyle recommendations. *ScientificWorldJournal*. 2013;2013:129841.

5. GBD 2016 DALYs and HALE Collaborators. Global, regional, and national disability-adjusted life-years (DALYs) for 333 diseases and injuries and healthy life expectancy (HALE) for 195 countries and territories, 1990-2016: a systematic analysis for the Global Burden of Disease Study 2016. *Lancet*. 2017;390(10100):1260-1344.

6. Mehrian-Shai R, Reichardt JK. Genomics is changing personal healthcare and medicine: the dawn of iPH (individualized preventive healthcare). *Hum Genomics*. 2015;9:29.

7. Feero WG. Introducing "Genomics Precision Health". *JAMA*. 2017;317(18):1842-1843.

8. Berry TD, Lloyd-Jones DM, Garside DB, Greenland P. Framingham risk score and prediction of coronary heart disease death in young men. *Am Heart J*. 2007;154(1):80-86.

9. Ridker PM, Danielson E, Fonseca FA, et al. Rosuvastatin to prevent vascular events in men and women with elevated C-reactive protein. *N Engl J Med*. 2008;359(21):2195-2207.

10. Hlatky MA. Expanding the orbit of primary prevention—moving beyond JUPITER. *N Engl J Med*. 2008;359(21):2280-2282.

11. Narasimhan SD. Beyond statins: new therapeutic frontiers for cardiovascular disease. *Cell*. 2017;169(6):971-973.

12. Gustafsson M, Nestor CE, Zhang H, et al. Modules, networks and systems medicine for understanding disease and aiding diagnosis. *Genome Med*. 2014;6(10):82.

13. Boyle EA, Li YI, Pritchard JK. An expanded view of complex traits: from polygenic to omnigenic. *Cell*. 2017;169(7):1177-1186.

14. Bland JS, Minich DM, Eck BM. A systems medicine approach: translating emerging science into individualized wellness. *Adv Med*. 2017;2017:1718957.

15. O'Donnell CJ, Nabel EG. Genomics of cardiovascular disease. *N Engl J Med*. 2011;365(22):2098-2109.

16. Dullaart RPF. PCSK9 inhibition to reduce cardiovascular events. *N Engl J Med*. 2017;376(18):1790-1791.

17. Ference BA, Robinson JG, Brook RD, et al. Variation in PCSK9 and HMGCR and risk of cardiovascular disease and diabetes. *N Engl J Med*. 2016;375(22):2144-2153.

18. Gorlov IP, Gorlova OY, Amos CI. Allelic spectra of risk SNPs are different for environment/lifestyle dependent versus independent diseases. *PLoS Genet*. 2015;11(7):e1005371.

19. Sabatine MS, Giugliano RP, Keech AC, et al. Evolocumab and clinical outcomes in patients with cardiovascular disease. *N Engl J Med.* 2017;376(18):1713-1722.

20. Dong B, Li H, Singh AB, et al. Inhibition of PCSK9 transcription by berberine involves down-regulation of hepatic HNF1α protein expression through the ubiquitin-proteasome degradation pathway. *J Biol Chem.* 2015;290(7):4047-58.

21. Ference BA, Kastelein JJP, Ginsberg HN, et al. Association of genetic variants related to CETP inhibitors and statins with lipoprotein levels and cardiovascular risk. *JAMA.* 2017;318(10):947-956.

22. Sniderman AD, Peterson ED. Genetic studies help clarify the complexities of lipid biology and treatment. *JAMA.* 2017;318(10):915-917.

23. Muhlhausler BS. Variability in the cardiometabolic effects of ω-3 long-chain PUFAs: background diet, timing, and genetics. *Am J Clin Nutr.* 2017;105(5):1029-1030.

24. Yu Z, Huang T, Zheng Y, et al. PCSK9 variant, long-chain n-3 PUFAs, and risk of nonfatal myocardial infarction in Costa Rican Hispanics. *Am J Clin Nutr.* 2017;105(5):1198-1203.

25. Yu E, Rimm E, Qi L, et al. Diet, lifestyle, biomarkers, genetic factors, and risk of cardiovascular disease in the nurses' health studies. *Am J Public Health.* 2016;106(9):1616-23.

26. Canto JG, Kiefe CI, Rogers WJ, et al. Number of coronary heart disease risk factors and mortality in patients with first myocardial infarction. *JAMA.* 2011;306(19):2120-7.

27. Khera AV, Emdin CA, Drake I, et al. Genetic risk, adherence to a healthy lifestyle, and coronary disease. *N Engl J Med.* 2016;375(24):2349-2358.

28. Larsson SC, Burgess S, Michaëlsson K. Association of genetic variants related to serum calcium levels with coronary artery disease and myocardial infarction. *JAMA.* 2017;318(4):371-380.

29. Lotta LA, Wittemans LBL, Zubar V, et al. Association of genetic variants related to gluteofemoral vs abdominal fat distribution with type 2 diabetes, coronary disease, and cardiovascular risk factors. *JAMA.* 2018;320(24):2553-2563.

30. Fan AZ, Yesupriya A, Chang MH, et al. Gene polymorphisms in association with emerging cardiovascular risk markers in adult women. *BMC Med Genet.* 2010;11:6.

31. Wilcken DE, Wilcken B, Dudman NP, Tyrrell PA. Homocystinuria—the effects of betaine in the treatment of patients not responsive to pyridoxine. *N Engl J Med.* 1983;309(8):448-53.

32. Timmers PR, Mounier N, Lall K, et al. Genomics of 1 million parent lifespans implicates novel pathways and common diseases and distinguishes survival chances. *Elife.* 2019;8:e39856.

33. Khera AV, Chaffin M, Aragam KG, et al. Genome-wide polygenic scores for common diseases identify individuals with risk equivalent to monogenic mutations. *Nat Genet.* 2018;50(9):1219-1224.

34. Dron JS, Hegele RA. The evolution of genetic-based risk scores for lipids and cardiovascular disease. *Curr Opin Lipidol.* 2019;30(2):71-81.

35. Inouye M, Abraham G, Nelson CP, et al. Genomic risk prediction of coronary artery disease in 480,000 adults: implications for primary prevention. *J Am Coll Cardiol.* 2018;72(16):1883-1893.

36. Voruganti VS. Nutritional genomics of cardiovascular disease. *Curr Genet Med Rep.* 2018;6(2):98-106.

37. Keaney JF Jr. CHIP-ping away at atherosclerosis. *N Engl J Med.* 2017;377(2):184-185.

38. Jaiswal S, Natarajan P, Silver AJ, et al. Clonal hematopoiesis and risk of atherosclerotic cardiovascular disease. *N Engl J Med.* 2017;377(2):111-121.

39. Li F, Wu X, Zhou Q, Zhu DW. Clonal hematopoiesis of indeterminate potential (CHIP): a potential contributor to atherosclerotic cardio/cerebro-vascular diseases? *Genes Dis.* 2018;5(2):75-76.

40. Aavik E, Babu M, Ylä-Herttuala S. DNA methylation processes in atherosclerotic plaque. *Atherosclerosis.* 2018;281:168-179.

Section 6

Testing And Cardiovasular Disease

10

Introduction to Anatomic and Functional Testing in Patients With Known or Suspected Coronary Artery Disease

Bjarki J. Olafsson, MD, FACC

As physicians, we see patients on a daily basis who have complaints of chest discomfort, atypical and typical of myocardial ischemia. The burden is on us to assess not only if coronary artery disease (CAD) is responsible for the symptoms but also if present, how extensive it is and what the patient's prognosis is. Patients are not only asking us to diagnose the underlying condition but also tell them how the disease, if present, will affect their lifestyle and the prognostic implications of the diagnosis. The diagnostic modalities that are available can grossly be divided into anatomic testing and functional testing.

In terms of functional testing the standard treadmill testing (ETT or TMT) has been in use for over 70 years and is still the most frequently used test.[1] ETT is being used for not only diagnosis but also prognostic purposes in clinically stable patients.[1] ETT is generally a safe test and is cost-effective and free of radiation or contrast exposure. ETT has maximal diagnostic value in the patient population with intermediate (10%-90%) pretest probability of CAD.[2] ETT is of little diagnostic value in patients with either low or high pretest probability and is generally discouraged for asymptomatic individuals.[3] ETT is thought, based on meta-analysis, to have a sensitivity of 68% and a test specificity of 77%. Test accuracy (both sensitivity and accuracy) is lower in women than in men, and this is in part related to lower prevalence of CAD in women. Exercise capacity is the most important prognostic variable as patients with poor exercise capacity are at high risk for poor clinical outcome, often related to underlying left main or three-vessel CAD.[4]

The American College of Cardiology (ACC)/American Heart Association (AHA) 2002 Guideline Update for Exercise Testing identifies three CAD risk categories and allows the physician to classify the patient based on annual mortality rates: low <1%, intermediate 1% to 3%, or high >3% risk. The guidelines emphasize that low-risk patients do not need further cardiac testing and can be treated medically. The intermediate risk category may or may not require further testing, and the high risk is generally referred for coronary angiography.[1,3] Stress imaging (SPECT or ECHO) has higher sensitivity and similar specificity.[2,5,6] Despite advances in noninvasive testing over the last decades, there is still no consensus on which noninvasive test is preferable, and we continue to be faced with the dilemma of how to approach the patient in the best, safest, and most cost-effective way.[7] In part, this may also be related to which test the individual physician or institution has most experience and expertise in. Historically we have much evidence that traditional functional testing, exercise electrocardiography, exercise or dobutamine echocardiography, exercise or chemical myocardial perfusion imaging, and cardiac magnetic resonance imaging, provides excellent prognostic information. An abnormal functional test (FT) has been shown to be associated with a significantly increased (5- to 10-fold) risk of adverse cardiovascular events.

In terms of anatomical testing, invasive coronary angiography has been the gold standard for documenting obstructive coronary disease (usually defined as greater than 50%-70% luminal narrowing) but is expensive and has well-known shortcomings and potential complications. Coronary computed tomography angiography (CTA) is now widely available and gives noninvasive anatomic information, although it is also associated with radiation and risks associated with the use of iodinated contrast agent such as allergic reaction and reduced renal function. Noninvasive assessment of FFR (fractional flow reserve) is now becoming available, and CTA may therefore in the future play an increasingly important role as it may provide a combination of anatomic and functional data.

The PROMISE trial (Prospective Multicenter Imaging Study for Evaluation of Chest Pain) compared anatomic testing with functional testing among low- to intermediate-risk patients with chest pain suspicious for CAD. In this trial, 10,003 patients with stable chest pain and suspected CAD were randomized to initial strategy of CTA or functional stress testing (ETT), exercise or pharmacological nuclear testing, or stress echocardiography. The findings were that both approaches have similar prognostic value and CTA, as compared with the use of functional testing, did not reduce the incidence of events over a median follow-up of 25 months.[8] CTA, by visualizing nonobstructive (1%-69% luminal narrowing) CAD, identified additional at-risk patients, and CTA strategy was associated with a lower incidence of invasive cardiac catheterization probably due to lower false-positive rate with the CTA.[8] The PROMISE trial showed that coronary CTA was an alternative to stress testing among low- to intermediate-risk patients presenting with chest pain. Another finding in the study was that a normal CTA, in contrast to a completely normal functional test, is highly unlikely to be associated with a major adverse cardiac event (MACE) for at least 2 years.[9]

The 2012 ACC/AHA guidelines basically recommend ETT as a first step as supported by appropriate use criteria and emphasize that it is a process of shared decision making involving the patient and provider, taking into account risks, benefits, and costs to the patient.[7]

The European Society of Cardiology Guidelines make a class I recommendation for ETT in patients with an intermediate likelihood of CAD as long as they can exercise and do not have an abnormal EKG.[10]

Cardiac stress perfusion MRI (CMR) has been compared with SPECT imaging and both the CE-MARC (Clinical Evaluation of Magnetic Resonance Imaging in Coronary heart disease) and the MR-IMPACT (Magnetic Resonance Imaging for Myocardial Perfusion Assessment in Coronary artery disease Trial) studies found CMR to have superior sensitivity and preserved or improved specificity. Stress perfusion CMR is being used in some centers as the first-line test, but reimbursement may be an issue as the cost is universally higher.

In conclusion, although we have literally thousands of studies and papers on the diagnostic approach to the patient with possible CAD, the fact remains that no two patients are alike and the diagnostic path taken is a joint intellectual process between the patient and the physician.

References

1. Fraker TD Jr, Fihn SD; 2002 Chronic Stable Angina Writing Committee, et al. 2007 chronic angina focused update of the ACC/AHA 2002 guidelines for the management of patients with chronic stable angina: a report of the ACC/AHA Task Force on Practice Guidelines Writing Group to develop the focused update of the 2002 guidelines. *J Am Coll Cardiol.* 2007;50:2264-2274.
2. Gibbons RJ, Balady GJ, Bricker JT, et al; Task Force on Practice Guidelines, Committee to Update the 1997 Exercise Testing Guidelines. ACC/AHA 2002 guideline update. *J Am Coll Cardiol.* 2002;40:1431-1440.
3. Greenland P, Alpert JS, Beller GA, et al. 2010 ACCF/AHA guideline for assessment of cardiovascular risk in asymptomatic adults: a report of the ACC Foundation/AHA Task Force on Practice Guidelines. *J Am Coll Cardiol.* 2010;56:e50-e103.
4. Kligfield P, Lauer MS. Exercise electrocardiogram testing: beyond the ST segment. *Circulation.* 2006;114:2070-2082.
5. Klocke FJ, Baird MG, Lorell BH, et al. ACC/AHA/ASNC guidelines for the clinical use of cardiac radionuclide imaging-executive summary. *J Am Coll Cardiol.* 2003;42:1318-1333.
6. Cheitlin MD, Armstrong WF, Aurigemma GP, et al. ACC/AHA/ASE 2003 guideline update for the clinical application of echocardiography-summary article. *J Am Coll Cardiol.* 2003;42:954-970.
7. Fihn SD, Gardin JM, Abrams J, et al. 2012 ACCF/AHA/ACP/AATS/PCNA/SCAI/STS Guideline for the diagnosis and management of patients with stable ischemic heart disease. *J Am Coll Cardiol.* 2012;60:e44-e164.
8. Pamela S, Douglas MU. Outcomes of anatomical versus functional testing for coronary artery disease. *N Engl J Med.* 2015;372:1291-1300.
9. Hoffmann U, Ferencik M, Udelson JE, et al. Prognostic value of noninvasive cardiovascular testing in patients with stable chest pain. *Circulation.* 2017;135:2320-2332.
10. Montalescot G, Sechtem U, Achenbach S, et al. 2013 ECG guidelines on the management of stable coronary disease of the European Society of Cardiology. *Eur Heart J.* 2013;34:2949-3003.

11

Endothelial Dysfunction and Testing

Mark C. Houston, MD, MS, MSc, FACP, FAHA, FASH, FACN, FAARM, ABAARM, DABC

Fortunately, many noninvasive tests exist that will determine cardiovascular (CV) pathology before clinical coronary heart disease (CHD). One of the best validated early detection tests for functional abnormalities of the endothelium is the EndoPAT, which determines endothelial function and dysfunction[1-5] (Figure 11.1). The EndoPAT measures postocclusion brachial artery hyperemia, which is an excellent indirect measure of nitric oxide bioavailability and endothelial dysfunction in the coronary arteries The EndoPAT predicts accurately the future risk for hypertension, CHD, unstable angina, cardiovascular disease (CVD), congestive heart failure (CHF), myocardial infarction (MI), cardiac death, hospitalization, coronary artery bypass graft, stent restenosis, the presence of plaque in the coronary arteries that are rupture prone, peripheral arterial disease (PAD), and cerebrovascular accidents (CVAs) beyond the Framingham risk scoring (FRS).[1-5]

In a study of 528 patients with high risk for CV events over 5 years, the EndoPAT reactive hyperemia index (RHI) was measured before and after coronary angiogram.[4] The RHI, brain natriuretic peptide (BNP), and CV score by SYNTAX were independent risk predictors for all future CV events such as MI, CV death, unstable angina, ischemic CVA, coronary artery bypass graft, CHF, and PAD. When RHI was added to FRS, BNP, and SYNTAX, the net reclassification index was significantly improved by 27.5 % with a significant increase in the

EndoPAT Good and poor results

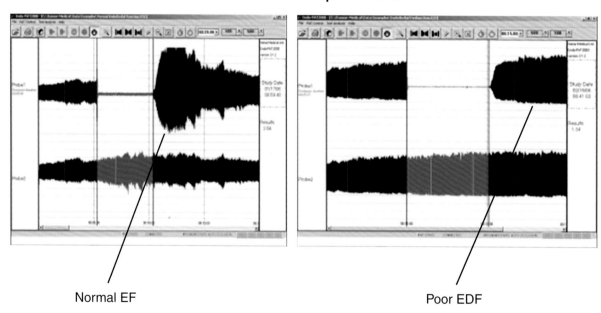

Normal EF

Poor EDF

Figure 11.1 *EndoPAT.*

C-statistic from 0.728 to 0.766. A normal RHI is over 1.67.[4,5] An index of 1.67 has sensitivity of 82% and specificity of 77% to diagnose coronary endothelial dysfunction and highly correlates to brachial artery flow mediated vasodilation (r = .0.33-0.55).

The endothelium is a very thin lining of vascular cells forming an interface between the arterial lumen and the vascular smooth muscle.[6-10] Endothelial dysfunction occurs when nitric oxide bioavailability is reduced, which leads to vascular inflammation, oxidative stress, immune dysfunction, abnormal vascular growth, vasoconstriction, increased permeability, thrombosis, and CHD.[6-10] Low-density lipoprotein (LDL)-cholesterol has a primary role in the development of atherosclerotic plaque formation starting at birth.[6,7] LDL-cholesterol migrates from the blood into the subendothelial layer, attaches to proteoglycans, and becomes modified, antigenic, and toxic primarily via oxidation of LDL (oxLDL) and glycation of LDL (glyLDL).[6,7] The modified LDLs produce numerous cytokines and chemokines that attract monocytes into the subendothelial layer, which transform into macrophages. The modified LDL is taken up by scavenger receptors on the macrophage cell membranes, which transform into foam cells, then form fatty streaks, and eventually form a coronary artery plaque (stable plaque or a soft rupture-prone plaque) that can result in an MI. Approximately 45 different steps exist in this process of dyslipidemia-induced vascular disease that can be interrupted with nutrition, nutritional supplements, and drugs.[6,7] Endothelial dysfunction, arterial pathology, cardiac dysfunction, and CHD represent a delicate balance of vascular injury (angiotensin II and endothelin), vascular protection with nitric oxide, and vascular repair from endothelial progenitor cells, produced by the bone marrow.[6-10]

References

1. Matsuzawa Y, Sugiyama S, Sugamura K, et al. Digital assessment of endothelial function and ischemic heart disease in women. *J Am Coll Cardiol.* 2010;55(16):1688-1696.
2. Bonetti PO, Pumper GM, Higano ST, Holmes DR Jr, Kuvin JT, Lerman A. Noninvasive identification of patients with early coronary atherosclerosis by assessment of digital reactive hyperemia. *J Am Coll Cardiol.* 2004;44(11):2137-2141.
3. Hamburg NM, Keyes MJ, Larson MG, et al. Cross-sectional relations of digital vascular function to cardiovascular risk factors in the Framingham Heart Study. *Circulation.* 2008;117(19):2467-2474.
4. Schoenenberger AW, Urbanek N, Bergner M, Toggweiler S, Resink TJ, Erne P. Associations of reactive hyperemia index and intravascular ultrasound-assessed coronary plaque morphology in patients with coronary artery disease. *Am J Cardiol.* 2012;109(12):1711-1716.
5. Matsuzawa Y, Sugiyama S, Sumida H, et al. Peripheral endothelial function and cardiovascular events in high-risk patients. *J Am Heart Assoc.* 2013;2(6);e000426.
6. Houston Mark C. *What Your Doctor May Not Tell You About Heart Disease. The Revolutionary Book that Reveals the Truth Behind Coronary Illnesses and How You Can Fight Them. Grand Central Life and Style.* New York, New York. Hachette Book Group. 237 Park Ave; 2012.
7. Houston MC. Nutrition and nutraceutical supplements in the treatment of hypertension. *Expert Rev Cardiovasc Ther.* 2010;8:821-833.
8. Duprez DA, Florea N, Zhong W, et al. Vascular and cardiac functional and structural screening to identify risk of future morbid events: preliminary observations. *J Am Soc Hypertens.* 2011;5(5):401-409.
9. Houston Mark C. *Handbook of Hypertension.* Oxford UK: Wiley – Blackwell; 2009.
10. Della Rocca DG, Pepine CJ. Endothelium as a predictor of adverse outcomes. *Clin Cardiol.* 2010;33(12):730-732.

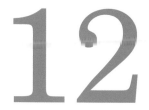

Multifunction Cardiogram, a.k.a. MCG

Raffi B. Shen, BA, Norbert W. Rainford, MD, FACC, FACP, and
Joseph T. Shen, MD

Introduction

Coronary artery heart disease (CAD) is a major cause of death and disability in developed countries. Although CAD mortality rates worldwide have decreased over the past four decades, CAD remains the cause of about one-third of all deaths among individuals over age 35 years.[1-3] About half of all middle-aged men and one-third of middle-aged women in the United States will develop some manifestation of CAD.[4] There are several unrecognized drivers or causes of the persistence of this morbidity despite our general knowledge of major risk factors based on population data such as the Framingham Heart Study. The lack of adaptable, inexpensive, noninvasive, and accurate modalities to detect CAD in its early stages as well as the lack of effective monitoring of the effects of diet and other lifestyle intervention has been a major factor.

Electrocardiogram (ECG) stress testing, nuclear scintigraphy, stress echocardiography, and other various types of cardiac stress imaging testing are considered the standard noninvasive techniques for evaluating cardiac ischemia. Although these are recognized as sensitive tests for the detection of CAD in two or more large epicardial vessels, it also has been widely acknowledged that they have poor specificity as shown by evidence of a high number of false-positive results. There is growing consensus that this lack of specificity results in a significant number of unnecessary coronary angiographies, thereby subjecting many patients to the potential risks involved with invasive procedures and radiation exposure without expected commensurate clinical benefit. For example, in 2010, Patel and colleagues published an analysis of the American College of Cardiology National Cardiovascular Data Registry, which included 397,954 patients without known CAD who were undergoing elective angiography.[5] At catheterization, 149,739 patients (37.6%) had obstructive coronary artery disease (70% obstruction or greater), requiring an interventional procedure. Stated bluntly, up to 62.4% of those patients could have avoided

coronary angiography if more accurate noninvasive testing modalities were available. Compounding the diagnostic inadequacy of conventional testing of obstructive CAD is the emerging consensus of the role of nonobstructive coronary disease and microvascular disease in the clinical manifestation of ischemic heart disease. A review in *Circulation* 1995 by Erlin Falk demonstrated that the progression to plaque rupture and myocardial infarction (MI) over time occurs most frequently in patients with obstruction of 50% or less.[6]

It is within this context of complex and evolving concepts that Premier Heart is proud to introduce the Multifunction Cardiogram (MCG), a noninvasive, physical-stress-free, and nonionizing diagnostic tool that can be used to quantitatively assess lesions across the very early nonobstructive to significantly obstructive spectrum and to monitor any form of therapeutic intervention.

The Purpose of This Chapter

This chapter provides an opportunity for the health professional to learn about a "new" diagnostic tool that has been more than 20 years in the making. It provides an outline as to why conventional cardiac testing is inadequate and why MCG is the ideal tool to fulfill this unmet need. There are several paradoxical or unexpected clinical developments in the management of CAD over the last several years. Although it is generally accepted that low-density lipoprotein (LDL) cholesterol plays a central role in the initiation of the coronary plaque, it is known that 50% of patients presenting with a MI have normal total cholesterol.[7] Additionally, the data from several primary and secondary prevention trials have shown that the majority of the risk of CAD still remains even after LDL reduction.[8] Perhaps the most glaring event of the inadequacy of conventional approach to the management of CAD is the 15-year outcome status report of the COURAGE trial (Clinical Outcomes Utilizing Revascularization and Aggressive Drug Evaluation).[9] The 15-year status of this study essentially demonstrated that percutaneous coronary intervention (stent placement) in patients with stable CAD did not improve in mortality outcome when compared with similar patients who were treated using only optimal medical management. Perhaps related is an older but interesting piece of data from the FAME (Fractional Flow Reserve versus Angiography for Multivessel Evaluation) study.[10] The FAME study looked at 1-year outcomes (death, MI, major adverse cardiovascular event) in one group of patients whose management was guided by angiographic results versus a similar group guided by the fractional flow reserve (FFR) data. The FFR-guided group had significantly better outcome in all categories. A systems approach to address the functional aspects of this complex biological conundrum, known as the cardiovascular system, is desperately required.

What Is MCG and What Does It Measure?

The MCG is the first embodiment of a mathematical application of systems theory to a dynamic biological (cardiovascular) environment, which expresses the physiologic state of the heart, with a primary focus on the level of its ischemic burden. In other words, the MCG describes the dynamic functional sate of the heart, beyond relying upon anatomical status. Premier Heart's greatest priority was always the measurement of the ischemic burden, but there were additional markers that needed to be recruited to describe the heart within a functional perspective. That expression was (is) the mathematical articulation of the communication between two standard ECG leads over multiple cycles, beginning with the conversion of the signals into a frequency domain via multiple nonlinear mathematical functions, thus the use of the term "multifunction cardiography." The adaptation of systems analysis principles, combined with Lagrangian mechanics, empirical data mining, deep machine learning, and neural network development, created, to our knowledge, the first example of a commercially available information technology solution in the discipline of "Clinical Computational Electrophysiology." Following decades of research and development, through the diligent work of two generations of dedicated scientists, clinicians, and engineers, MCG technology has evolved from conceptual mathematical designs to animal testing and finally to human application. Although x-ray, computed tomography,[11] magnetic resonance (MR), or ultrasound technologies describe **spatial** anatomic separation, MCG describes **frequency** separation, whereby specific mathematical elements from the multiple functions in frequency domains via power spectra are ascribed to specific anatomical or physiologic functions of the whole cardiovascular system.[12]

It is beyond the scope of this chapter to delve into full explanation of the applied Lagrangian mechanics used by this technology, but it is helpful to outline a few basic principles. Blood flow is a non-Newtonian fluid that is optimally assessed and reported with Euler coordinates. Cardiac tissue and brain tissue are viscoelastic solids, and they are assessed and reported with Lagrange coordinates. Among the infinitely possible mathematical expressions within this system, we have empirically selected six dynamic and integrative mathematical functions that act as the backbone of our mathematical analysis, namely, auto power spectrum, phase angle shift, impulse response, cross correlation, coherence function, and transfer function. The Euler and Lagrange coordinates are then linked by a Laplace transformation application (see **Figure 12.1**).

The deeper questions as to what these frequency interrogations represent are issues such as:
- Quantification of the abnormal electromechanical expression patterns of stress (physical) and strain and intracardiac blood flow.
- Integration of all myocardial electrical power required to function under normal and abnormal conditions delivered by sodium (Na^+), hydrogen (H^+), potassium (K^+), calcium (Ca^{2+}), and magnesium (Mg^{2+}) channels and ATPase activities of all myocardial cells through multiple cardiac cycles.
- Oxidative stress caused by supply and demand imbalances, free radical formation, and lactic acidosis leading to ion channelopathies, particularly gradient dependent H^+ channel (a subunit of F1-F0 ATPase) in addition to chronic damage/mutation of the mitochondrial gene transcription/translation mechanics, resulting in gradual myocardial power production.

All of this information and analyses are collected and collated by a bedside device within 10 minutes on the average patient, with the patient lying down (or sitting) quietly and remaining still for a few minutes. The device is the size of standard laptop. Electrocardiographic signals from two leads (II and V5) are recorded for 82 seconds per cycle and repeated for three to five times per session. Data are then uploaded and compared with the data patterns of hundreds of thousands of patients who have had the MCG test and who have had cardiac catheterization with angiogram. The database is equally male/female to eliminate gender bias, with an age range of 14 to 100 years. Every patient who has an MCG test in effect undergoes a virtual cardiac catheterization with an FFR assessment. How was this database built? The database is the end product of a laborious creation that is central to understanding MCG technology and may well be the most uniquely constructed database in all of medical data. The team, led by Dr Shen, embarked on a two-decade-long journey of research and development via digital signal processing, empirical clinical data collection, data mining, supervised machine learning, neural network development, artificial intelligence algorithm development, and countless iterations of optimization and improvement to create computer recognition of all forms of heart disease. In this endeavor, 2 million individuals were tested on MCG and more than 100,000 people with various heart diseases had their angiographic data strategically added to the system to build a production database for system software development. All the data sets used in analysis and the proposed statistical models had to satisfy the tests of

$$L_x(t,q(t),q'(t)) - \frac{a}{A+} \; L_y(t,q(t),q'(t)) = 0.$$

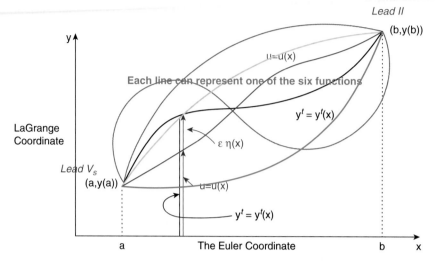

Euler-Lagrange equation in the Lagrangian Mechanics
Applied Computational Electrophysiology

Figure 12.1 *Graphic representation of the linkages between the Euler coordinate and Lagrange coordinate.*

both null hypothesis and alternative hypothesis. The extremely carefully verified and thoroughly validated data sets were used in the discovery of over 200 mathematical elements from the six nonlinear functions. We ensured that the development of the machine learning algorithms for the quantitative automatic heart disease pattern classification and differentiation were based purely on thoroughly vetted and trusted empirical evidence. Based on well-defined frequency and separation, the aim was to systematically explore, define, express, measure, quantify, and differentiate the hidden NORMAL and ABNORMAL electromechanical, electrostructural, electrobiochemical, electrohematologic, electroneuroendocrine, neurohormonal, and electroimmunological expressions, as well as the highly elusive, yet vitally important diverse expressions of electromyocardial perfusion pattern of the cardiovascular system. It is this kind of unique analysis, coupled with the 24/7 accessibility and reliability, that positions MCG well beyond more expensive and more cumbersome imaging and perfusion techniques.

The final report gives an overall functional severity score between 0 (totally normal) and 22 (the most severe) (see Table 12.1). The report also gives an assessment of secondary pathological and physiopathological conditions. These secondary conditions or markers include the following: cardiomyopathy (derangements in myocardial wall motion and/or structure), hypertrophy, arrhythmias or precipitating substrates, rheumatic pattern (LV, aortic/mitral valve derangements), pulmonary pattern (right heart, pulmonic/tricuspid valve derangements), myocardial damage (MI, contusion, etc.), congenital abnormalities, compliance changes, remodeling, energy output, ejection fraction, and angle phase shift. Although there is a generally good correlation between the severity score and the level of obstruction, there is no specific correlation between the numerical severity score and the percentage of blockage. This fact underscores the contribution of the secondary factors to the functional assessment of the heart and highlights the difference between conventional anatomical imaging and MCG's functional physiological assessment. It also underscores the importance of the FFR information alluded to earlier in the FAME study.

The validation of MCG in the detection of myocardial ischemia caused by obstructive coronary artery disease (CAD) has been demonstrated in multiple independently conducted clinical trials in eight countries[13-23] with high sensitivity (89%-100%), specificity (83%-94%), and negative predictive values over 95%. The accuracy can be improved when the results of MCG are corelated with serum biomarkers such as abnormal fasting glucose, hemoglobin A1c, LDL cholesterol, and the heart failure marker, pro-BNP. The details of each study will not be discussed here, but there are a few that should be highlighted. The landmark clinical validation of MCG was a study by Amano, Shinoda, Kunimura et al[20] (see Table 12.2). The study was done in Japan but published in the *Open Heart Journal* of the *British Medical Journal*. They combined angiographic and functional flow reserve (FFR) data and demonstrated that MCG has high specificity with high negative predictive value and concluded that MCG can be used not only to identify functionally significant ischemia but also to reduce unnecessary angiograms.

Another Japanese study by Takeshita and Shinoda[21] (see Table 12.3) compared classic syntax scores (SS) with functional syntax scores (FSS). The SS is derived purely from anatomical analysis of angiographic data. The FSS is derived from the addition of fractional flow reserve (FFR) information to the analysis. FFR is the percentage of reduction in pressure recordings across both obvious obstructive lesions

Table 12.1

8 CATEGORIES OF DISEASE SEVERITY

7	Extremely High Myocardial Dysfunction	Minimum MCG Severity Scores ≥ 15, *oscillating between 15 and ≤22*
6	Very High Myocardial Dysfunction	Maximum MCG Severity Score ≥ 15 and a minimum of 7.0 *oscillating between 7 and ≤15*
5	High Myocardial Dysfunction	Minimum MCG Severity Scores ≥ 3.5 and maximum score 7.0, and *oscillating between 3.5 and ≤7*
4	Intermediate Myocardial Dysfunction	All MCG Severity Scores fluctuating above or below 3.5, ie, any score lower or higher than 3.5 appearing in the same session; *oscillating between 0 and ≤X*
3	Collateral Circulation Group	Any MCG Severity Scores ≥ or ≤ 2.0 with or without significant pathological and physiopathological conditions
2	*Low Myocardial Dysfunction*	*Maximum MCG Severity Scores ≤ 3.5, or session scores oscillating between 0 and ≤3.5*
1	*Clinically normal*	*Maximum MCG Severity Scores ≤ 2.0 in a session, including 0, oscillating between 0 and ≤ 2.0;*
0	True Normal	MCG Score a "Zero"

and not-so-obvious nonobstructive lesions. They concluded that MCG showed high specificity and predictive accuracy especially for FSS, again supporting MCG's usefulness in identifying functionally significant ischemia and potentially its role in reducing unnecessary catheterizations.

A poster presentation at the Transcatheter Cardiovascular Therapeutics (TCT) 2015 meeting in San Francisco: TCT is a prestigious professional society that focuses on interventional cardiology. The poster by T. Amano et al[22] showed that MCG correctly identified all six restenosis and two new blockages among 45 patients who were followed 1 year post placement of coronary stents. With a sensitivity of 94.3% and a specificity of 97.3% among 720 epicardial coronary artery

segments, 16 per patient, MCG delivered a 0.94 (0.89-1.0) in the area under the receiver operating curve (ROC) analysis for the prediction of adverse events.

Finally, a word on the only outlier (negative) among these trials: Kawaji et al[23] published a study allegedly showing poor correlation between angiographic with FFR and MCG. However, there were several problems including a significant deviation from the original protocol.[24] They did not consider collateralization as a cause of false-negative results. Also, the decision not to perform FFRs on many diabetic patients with nonobstructive disease inserted a significant degree of bias. The authors, subsequently, reanalyzed the same data and retracted their initial position at a later date, in a Japanese language journal.

Table 12.2

MCG VERSUS CORONARY ANGIOGRAPHY (CAG)/FRACTIONAL FLOW RESERVE (FFR)

Predictive power of spectral ECG components stenosis through mathematical analysis of spectral ECG components

Conclusions: The MCG showed high specificity and predictive accuracy especially for the FRR + CAG, suggesting that it is useful not only in identifying functionally significant ischemia but also in reducing unnecessary CAGs.

- A high MCG score had a specificity of 90.4% (87.0%-93.9%) in model 1 adjusted by FFR≤0.8 threshold and of 87.0% (83.2%-90.8%) in model 2 adjusted by FFR ≤0.75 threshold, and a negative predictive value of 82.5% (78.3%-86.7%) in model 1 and of 83.8% (79.6%-87.9%) in model 2 for the prediction of severe ischemia.
- Conclusions: MCG showed high specificity with a high negative predictive value, suggesting that MCG could be used not only to identify functionally significant ischemia but to reduce unnecessary CAGs.
- Caveat—If the investigator had adopted the seven categories while also including the impact of collateral circulation on a patient's myocardial functionality and the presence of intermediate ischemic levels, MCG's would have reached an accuracy rating between 94% and 100% if a new model was adopted. The investigators are considering the possibility of reanalyzing the data using the seven categories we have developed.

Data from Amano T, Shinoda N, Kunimura A, et al. Non-invasive assessment of functionally significant coronary stenoses through mathematical analysis of spectral ECG components. *Open Heart*. 2014;1:e000144.

Table 12.3

PREDICTING ONE- YEAR OUTCOMES TARGETING MCG RESULTS VERSUS SS/FSS

Predicting one-year outcomes targeting MCG results versus SS/FSS
a.k.a. syntax score and functional syntax scores, the platinum standards for one-year mace outcome measures used by interventional cardiologists

Conclusions: The MCG showed high specificity and predictive accuracy especially for the FSS, suggesting that it is useful not only in identifying functionally significant ischemia but also in reducing unnecessary CAGs.
MCG was the only test significantly associated with the SS (odds ratio, 2.92 [1.60-5.31], P < .001) and FSS (odds ratio, 3.66 [1.95-6.87], P < .001). A high MCG score had a specificity of 92.6% (89.0%-96.2%) and 92.3% (89.0%-95.6%), and a predictive accuracy of 90% (89%-100%) and 94% (89%-100%) for the prediction of SS and FSS, respectively.

Data from Klein LW, et al. Occupational health hazards of interventional cardiologists in the current decade: Results of the 2014 SCAI membership survey. *Catheter Cardiovasc Interv*. 2015;86(5):913-924.

It is clearly evident that MCG's capabilities for the detection of early, intermediate-, and late-stage myocardial ischemia and natural recovery stages go far beyond conventional diagnostic stratagem and are of special value in women or individuals with microvascular or nonobstructive diseases, such as diabetes mellitus. MCG has also been demonstrated to have a direct and close correlation with the physiologic FFR measurement. MCG provides a uniquely positioned high-quality diagnostic tool to clinicians for making critical diagnostic and clinical management decisions in a timely, affordable, and dependable manner at the patient's bedside in real time.

Clinical Applications

MCG can be used in a number of clinically appropriate situations. It may be used in any situation wherein there is a clinical suspicion of CAD based on signs or symptoms. These signs or symptoms may be typical but may also be atypical, especially in women. Metabolic disorders such as diabetes mellitus, metabolic syndrome, and obesity have particularly striking features in MCG's capability of unmasking underlying CAD. The MCG may be used before or after conventional testing such as myocardial perfusion stress test. Although data have suggested that inappropriate coronary angiograms may be avoided by MCG testing, the reverse is also true—MCG may dictate coronary angiogram by uncovering severe CAD in unsuspecting patients. Then, as shown earlier, the technology can be used to assess the effectiveness of any form of intervention, conventional or lifestyle.

Case Studies

The following three case studies are illustrative of MCG's clinical utility.

SG is a 54-year-old woman with a history of dextrocardia who was concerned about a calcium score of 75 and a family history of CAD (her father died of an MI before age 60 years). She had atypical pains (neck, upper back). Her MCG scores were 4, 7, 7, 7, and 9 with indications of predominantly local (focal) ischemia. The secondary markers were positive for cardiomyopathy (wall motion dysfunction), atrial fibrillation, myocardial damage, and myocardial inflammation. Compliance abnormalities were absent. The study was interpreted as consistent with probably nonobstructive disease, predominantly in the left anterior descending (LAD)/circumflex (LCx) distribution (localization based on the dextrocardia) but could not exclude diffuse (global) disease. A cardiac magnetic resonance (MR) perfusion test was done as the next step. The cardiac MR report showed "decreased sub-endocardial signal in all three coronary territories. Differential diagnosis includes reversible ischemic disease versus 3-vessel obstructive disease." A cardiac angiogram was suggested. Subsequent catheterization report showed proximal LAD 30% to 40%, proximal LCx 30% to 40% lesion, and right coronary artery dominant, with luminal irregularities (small nonobstructive lesions). Intensive dietary and lifestyle intervention was begun. MCG correctly identified a pattern that more expensive and invasive techniques subsequently verified.

JR is 43-year-old man with a body mass index greater than 25 with poorly controlled type 2 diabetes, high cholesterol, recurrent chest pains, and a family history of early MI affecting his father, uncles, and brother. He presented to the emergency departments multiple times complaining of chest pains. His ECG readings, blood tests, and stress tests were all interpreted as "normal." However, MCG detected global ischemia with a severity score between 8.5 and 9.5. At one of his emergency room visits, a coronary angiogram was done and it showed no coronary obstruction but narrowed distal arteries showing TIMI II flow, indicating possible small vessel disease. He was subsequently managed with aggressive lifestyle changes and medication. In 60 days, he lost 35 pounds and was asymptomatic. His MCG severity scores fell to less than four, and the MCG functional expressions showed gradual normalization. At his request, he is now being monitored quarterly by MCG.

In another case, RR is a 77-year-old with known severe obstructive coronary artery disease and high MCG scores, with high cholesterol, LDL, and a history of prostate cancer with radical prostatectomy. He refused to undergo any revascularization procedure. He decided to try a ketogenic diet to lose weight and hopefully to improve his cardiovascular function. MCG overtime demonstrated steady improvement, as his scores fell from a range of 7.5 to 10 down to a range of 4 to 7. The elements of his mathematical matrix also showed functional improvements. This demonstrates that the metabolic component of a patient with severe ischemia can be reversed and that reversal can be measured and monitored by using MCG.

Summary

- The Multifunction Cardiogram (MCG) is the first purpose-built artificial intelligence cardiac disease diagnostic tool that utilizes systems theory within a biological context to give a functional analysis of the heart.
- It is a physiological test, not an anatomical imaging test, but the severity of ischemic score and the presence/absence of certain secondary factors (eg, phase shift) give its users actionable anatomical and functional information.
- MCG is capable of identifying CAD in its early stages long before it is demonstrable by more conventional testing. It is particularly powerful when combined with biomarkers such as B-type natriuretic peptide, myeloperoxidase, asymmetric dimethyl arginine or measures of oxidative stress. Thus early detection and primary prevention can be measured and monitored objectively and qualitatively based on functional outcome.
- It is an excellent tool for assesing subsets of patients whose anatomic features elude accurate diagnostic testing by conventional imaging methods. These include women (also men) with small vessel disease and patients with microvascular or non-obstructive disease seen in conditions such as diabetes and the metabolic syndrome.
- MCG is more accurate in the detection of myocardial ischemia caused by obstructive coronary artery disease than conventional tests, such as nuclear stress tests and echocardiography. Thus MCG should be provided BEFORE the stress imaging tests are used. This recommendation is consistent with the independent decision by Highmark Medicare contractor medical directors in a local coverage determination draft policy (LCD) in 2012-2013.
- MCG should be used as the first line tool for patients presenting to the emergency room for chest pain to reduce false negative discharges and false positive admissions, which would lead to effective resource allocations and value based care delivery.

- MCG is also an excellent tool for pre-surgical cardiac clearance, since it is more sensitive and specific for the detection of obstructive coronary artery disease.
- For patient safety, MCG should be utilized especially when the stress imaging tests are relatively contraindicated, eg, elderly patients who may be incapable of undergoing the demands of a stress imaging test session; and for patients with end stage renal diseases, since intravenous contrast agents applied in computed tomographic or magnetic resonance angiographic imaging may hasten the deterioration of renal function.
- MCG is the ideal, convenient, and flexible tool to measure the real-time outcome of lifestyle or other therapeutic interventions.

Future Challenges and Opportunities

- Medicare and commercial insurance coverage is needed for easier access to patients in the provider community. A forthcoming publication on MCG's utility as a triage tool in the assessment of emergency department patients with chest pain here in the United States will be extremely useful in the quest for insurance coverage.
- Premier Heart is actively working on developing a robust graphic interpretation report that captures and illustrates all the important variables that are measured in a study.
- One of the weaknesses of an MCG is its requirement for the patient to be still and for the environment to have minimum electrical interference. The technology is evolving so that devices will be wearable for remote personal use and can be adapted for a true exercise stress test.
- The technology and adaptability of MCG open paths for assessments in complex and difficult situations. The detection and monitoring of CAD in patients with the clonal hematopoiesis of indeterminate potential (CHIP) mutations and the monitoring of CAD in patients who are treated for elevated levels of trimethylamine-N-oxide are two areas of tremendous interest.
- Analysis of hundreds of MCG data has revealed a unique pattern of infiltrative disease correlating with possible chemotherapy induced cardiomyopathy and cardiac amyloidosis. These observations provide another opportunity for early recognition of two vexing clinical entities. Future studies need to be done to establish clinical utility.
- Since MCG represents an individual's phenotypic expressions, the information can be combined with genotypes to establish a unique MCG + Genomic database for studying clinical, pharmaceutical and medical/surgical treatments at an unprecedented depth to customize better personalized drugs and devices, and create outcome/evidence based management modalities.

References

1. Rosamond W, Flegal K, Furie K, et al. Heart disease and stroke statistics–2008 update: a report from the American Heart Association Statistics Committee and Stroke Statistics Subcommittee. *Circulation*. 2008;117:e25.

2. Nichols M, Townsend N, Scarborough P, Rayner M. Cardiovascular disease in Europe 2014: epidemiological update. *Eur Heart J*. 2014;35:2950.

3. Benjamin EJ, Virani SS, Callaway CW, et al. Heart disease and stroke statistics-2018 update: a report from the American Heart Association. *Circulation*. 2018;137:e67.

4. Lloyd-Jones DM, Larson MG, Beiser A, Levy D. Lifetime risk of developing coronary heart disease. *Lancet*. 1999;353:89.

5. Patel MR, Peterson ED, Dai D, et al. Low diagnostic yield of elective coronary angiography. *N Engl J Med*. 2010;362:886-895.

6. Falk E, Shah PK, Fuster V. Coronary plaque disruption. *Circulation*. 1995;92:657-671.

7. Sachdeva A, Cannon CP, Deedwania PC, et al. Lipid levels in patients hospitalized with coronary artery disease: an analysis of 136,905 hospitalizations in get with the guidelines. *Am Heart J*. 2009;157(1):111-117.e2.

8. Libby P. The forgotten majority: unfinished business in cardiovascular risk reduction. *J Am Coll Cardiol*. 2005;46(7):1225-1228.

9. Sedlis SP, Hartigan PM, Teo KK. Effect of PCI in long term survival in patients with stable ischemic heart disease. *N Engl J Med*. 2015;373:1937.

10. Tonino PA, De Bruyne B, Pijls NH, et al. Fractional flow reserve versus angiography for guiding percutaneous coronary intervention. *New Engl J Med*. 2009;360:213-224.

11. Sarno G, Decraemer I, Vanhoenacker PK, et al. On the appropriateness on noninvasive multidetector computed tomography coronary angiography to trigger coronary revascularization. *J Am Coll Cardiol Intervent*. 2009;2:550-557.

12. von Bertalanffy's L. *General System Theory: Foundations, Development, Applications* (Revised Edition) ISBN-10: 0807604534 | ISBN-13: 978-0807604533. New York, NY: George Braziller Inc.; March 17, 1969.

13. Weiss WB, Narasimhadevara SM, Feng GQ, Shen JT. Computer-enhanced frequency-domain and 12-lead electrocardiography accurate detect abnormalities consistent with obstructive and non-obstructive coronary artery disease. *Heart Dis*. 2002;4:2-12.

14. Grube E, Bootsveld A, Yuecel S, et al. Computerized two-lead resting electro-myocardium analysis for the detection of coronary artery stenosis. *Int J Med Sci*. 2007;4:249-263.

15. Grube E, Bootsveld A, Buellesfeld L, et al. Computerized two-lead resting electro-myocardium analysis for the detection of coronary artery stenosis after coronary revascularization. *Int J Med Sci*. 2008;5(2):50-61.

16. Hoshino J, Chou JT, Imhoff M. Computerized 2-lead resting ECG analysis for the detection of relevant coronary artery stenosis in comparison with angiographic findings. *Congest Heart Fail*. 2008;14:251-260.

17. Strobeck JE, Shen JT, Singh B, et al. Comparison of a two-lead, computerized, resting ECG signal analysis device, the MultiFunction-CardioGrams or MCG (a.k.a. 3DMP), to quantitative coronary angiography for the detection of relevant coronary artery stenosis (>70%) – a meta-analysis of all published trials performed and analyzed in the US. *Int J Med Sci*. 2009;6:143-155.

18. Strobeck JE, Mangieri A, Rainford N, et al. A paired-comparison of the MultiFunction Cardiogram (MCG) and sestamibi SPECT myocardial perfusion imaging (MPI) to quantitative coronary angiography for the detection of relevant coronary artery obstruction (≥70%) – a single-center study of 116 consecutive patients referred for coronary angiography. *Int J Med Sci*. 2011;8(8):717-724.

19. Strobeck JE, Rainford N, Arkus B, Imhoff M. Comparing Multifunction-Cardiogram and Coronary Angiography for Detection of Hemodynamically Relevant Coronary Artery Stenosis (>70%) in Women. *Treat Strateg*. 2010:83.

20. Amano T, Shinoda N, Kunimura A, et al. Non-invasive assessment of functionally significant coronary stenoses through mathematical analysis of spectral ECG components. *BMJ/Open Heart*. 2014;1:e000144. doi:10.1136/openhrt-2014-000144.

21. Takeshita M, Shinoda N, Takashima H, et al. Noninvasive mathematical analysis of spectral electrocardiographic components for coronary lesions of intermediate to obstructive stenosis severity–relationship with classic and functional SYNTAX score. *Catheter Cardiovasc Interv*. 2015;86(1):21-29. doi:10.1002/ccd.25924.

22. Tetsuya A, Norihiro S, Hiroaki T, et al. Impact of noninvasive mathematical analysis of spectral electrocardiographic components on the prediction of recurrent cardiac ischemic events after coronary intervention, An Abstract submitted for 2015 PCI TCT San Francisco.

23. Kawaji T, Shiomi H, Morimoto T, et al. Noninvasive detection of functional myocardial ischemia: multifunction cardiogram evaluation in diagnosis of functional coronary ischemia study. *Ann Noninvasive Electrocardiol*. 2015;20(5):446-453.

24. Imhoff M, Rainford N. It all depends on your references: electrophysiology compared to angiography. *Ann Noninvasive Electrocardiol*. 2015;20(5):506-507.

13

CAPWA: Computerized Arterial Pulse Wave Analysis

Daniel Duprez, MD, PhD and Jay N. Cohn, MD

Arterial Elasticity (1/Arterial Stiffness) and Blood Pressure

The clinical assessment of the arterial pressure wave, which is a powerful marker for cardiovascular disease, has for more than a century been dependent on sounds or arterial wall motion depicting the peak (systolic) and trough (diastolic) pressure.[1] The guidelines for the diagnosis of arterial hypertension have changed over time, but they are still based on the two extreme points of the arterial blood pressure waveform.[1] During the last decade, more emphasis has been placed on the systolic hypertension because of the growing elderly population with elevated systolic blood pressure.[2] The recent blood pressure guidelines have targeted a lower pressure, such as 120/80 mm Hg, as an ideal goal of management.[3]

This emphasis on pressure rather than vascular health has deprived the care givers from access to information that can provide far more insight into the health of the vasculature. It is known that arterial hypertension is associated with endothelial dysfunction, one of the most powerful regulators of vascular tone, especially in the small arteries[4] (**Figure 13.1**). Therefore, assessment of endothelial dysfunction and microvascular functional and structural abnormalities is important in the early detection of vascular changes that raise blood pressure in asymptomatic people at risk for cardiovascular disease. This diagnostic approach may be based on the morphology of the arterial pulse waveform.

Arterial stiffness and arterial elasticity (1/arterial stiffness) are important markers for vascular health and disease.[4] These parameters can be obtained noninvasively using different techniques such as the measurement of the difference in arrival time of the pulse at the carotid and femoral artery (carotid-femoral pulse wave velocity) or radial artery pulse wave analysis (systolic or diastolic part). To implement one of these techniques in daily practice the following criteria need to be addressed: (1) Proof of concept—does the novel marker level differ between subjects with and without adverse outcomes? (2) Prospective validation—does the novel marker predict development of future outcomes in a prospective cohort study? (3) Incremental value—does the novel risk marker change predictive information from established, standard risk markers? (4) Clinical utility—does the novel marker change predicted risk sufficiently to change recommended therapy? (5) Clinical outcome prediction—does use of the novel marker for therapeutic guidance improve clinical outcomes, especially when tested in a randomized trial? (6) Cost-effectiveness—does use of the marker improve clinical outcomes sufficiently to justify additional costs of testing or treatment?

Although some data are available to support wider use of measures of arterial stiffness or elasticity in both the small and large arteries, critical documentation of its incremental value still requires further validation.

Radial artery pulse contour analysis is the continuous analysis of either the systolic part or the diastolic part of the radial artery and is convenient for patient and technician. In this chapter, we describe specifically the diastolic pulse contour analysis methodology.

Technique Diastolic Radial Artery Pulse Contour Analysis

Radial artery waveforms are recorded using the Hypertension Diagnostics PulseWave CR-2000 instrument. A solid-state pressure transducer array (tonometer) is placed over the radial artery of the dominant arm to record the pulse contour. Once a stable measurement is achieved, a 30-second analog tracing of the radial waveform, excluding the dicrotic notch, is digitized at 200 samples per second, with accompanying automated, oscillatory blood pressure measurement. Measures of small artery elasticity (SAE) and large artery elasticity (LAE) (change in arterial volume per change in

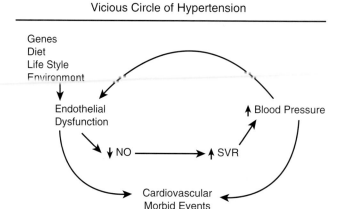

Vicious Circle of Hypertension

Figure 13.1 *Endothelial dysfunction results from genetic factors and environmental exposure. The resultant decrease in nitric oxide (NO) produces small artery narrowing and remodeling that raises systemic vascular resistance (SVR) and blood pressure. Morbid events result from the vasoconstriction and the rise in blood pressure.*

arterial pressure) are produced by the device. C1 (defined as LAE or capacitive compliance or proximal arterial compliance) and C2 (defined as SAE or oscillatory compliance or distal compliance) are estimated by the device from the waveform modeled as a sinusoidal function dampened by a decaying exponential.[5]

C2 is also an indicator for endothelial function. Gilani et al studied the effect of the inhibitor of nitric oxide release arginine NG-nitro-L-arginine-methyl ester (L-NAME).[6] The magnitude of effect of L-NAME on SAE (−31.2% ± 18.4%) was significantly greater and more consistent than its effect on other vascular measurements. LAE index, brachial artery caliber, and brachial artery compliance were unchanged. Flow-mediated brachial artery dilation was blunted slightly, and aortic pulse wave velocity increased slightly but significantly because of the rise in pressure. Reduction in SAE is a sensitive marker for endothelial dysfunction and may serve as a useful marker for prehypertensive patients at risk for cardiovascular morbid events.

Validation Small Artery Elasticity and Large Artery Elasticity

A diagnostic challenge is to detect abnormal function in the vascular system before the development of symptoms or signs of cardiovascular disease. Variability in arterial elasticity may help account for race/ethnic and sex differences in cardiovascular (CVD) risk, and knowledge of arterial elasticity might improve risk stratification and help identify individuals with early vascular damage who are predisposed to future vascular events. The SAE and LAE have been studied and validated in the multiethnic study of atherosclerosis (MESA).[7,8] The MESA study cohort consists of 6814 men and women who were recruited between 2000 and 2002 from six US communities and identified themselves as white, African American, Hispanic, or Chinese and were aged 45 to 84 years, free of clinically apparent CVD and never treated for cancer. The results of this multiethnic study at baseline

showed that African Americans had the lowest SAE, with somewhat higher values in Hispanics. SAE values were higher in Whites and Chinese. Women in general had lower SAE than men, which was mainly because of the difference in height. LAE did not differ by race/ethnicity.

Predictive Value of SAE and LAE

Hypertension

Hypertension is characterized by increased arterial stiffness and endothelial dysfunction. We studied the MESA study participants, who had their blood pressure measured at baseline and were not hypertensive at the baseline visit, which was defined as having a systolic blood pressure of <130 mm Hg and a diastolic blood pressure of <80 mm Hg and not taking any antihypertensive medication, and reported no history of hypertension.[9] We chose the cut point 130/80 mm Hg to increase the likelihood that participants were free of the outcome at the beginning of the study. New development of arterial hypertension was defined as a systolic blood pressure of ≥140 mm Hg, a diastolic blood pressure of ≥90 mm Hg, or the use of medication for hypertension during a mean follow-up at 4.3 years. Lower SAE is independently associated with new onset of hypertension, whereas LAE is also associated with development of hypertension but to a lesser extent than SAE.[9] It is possible that the small arteries, which represent the oscillatory compliance of the vascular tree, are uniquely important in the development and initiation of hypertension, relative to the vascular stiffness and atherosclerotic plaque deposition of the larger vessels.

Cardiovascular Disease Morbidity and Mortality

In contrast to several structural markers for vascular disease, such as carotid intima-media thickness and coronary calcium score[10,11] that have been studied in relation to CVD risk factors and coronary heart disease events, the functional vascular stiffness markers probably capture an earlier phase of cardiovascular disease development. In the MESA study cohort, we studied the predictive value of SAE and LAE for any CVD event and for each of its different components: myocardial infarction and coronary heart disease, death, angina, heart failure, stroke, and peripheral vascular disease during median 5.8 years of follow-up.[12] The predictive value of SAE was statistically significant not only after adjustment for demographic and anthropometric characteristics but also with further adjustment for CVD risk factors. In contrast to SAE, LAE was also predictive of CVD events in models adjusted for demographic factors, but after adjustment, LAE is predictive only for heart failure. This study therefore supports the concept that vascular disease originates with endothelial dysfunction, which has a profound influence on the microvasculature. In this view, evaluation of the smaller arteries and other microvasculature, assessed by SAE, is helpful in predicting early clinical CVD events. The findings have now been extended for more than a decade that the MESA study cohort has been followed for CVD events.[13]

Renal Function Decline

Decline in renal function is an independent risk factor for CVD. We addressed the question that subclinical vascular dysfunction may also contribute to the initiation and progression of kidney disease.[14] In the MESA study cohort, we studied the predictive value of SAE and LAE on early decline of renal function in study participants who had an estimated glomerular filtration rate (eGFR) of $\geq$60 mL/min/1.73 m^2. We found that decreased SAE and LAE were significantly and linearly associated with faster decline in kidney function among persons with eGFR >60 mL/min/1.73 m^2 during 5 years follow-up. Future studies with pharmacological interventions, which improve SAE and/or LAE, are warranted.

Medical Therapy

Cardiovascular disease appears to begin in the endothelium where it leads to functional changes in the vasculature. These changes can be detected by assessment mainly of SAE and to a lesser extent by LAE. SAE provides extra prognostic information beyond arterial blood pressure measurement. SAE and LAE may be used as a tool in the selection and

follow-up monitoring of therapeutic strategies aimed at preventing or delaying progression of vascular disease.[15] During the last decade, we have studied several antihypertensive agents in placebo-controlled trials in patients with either borderline hypertension or prehypertension with decreased SAE. In the DETECTIV (DEtection and Treatment of Early Cardiovascular disease Trial: Intervention with Valsartan) study, a double-blind study where valsartan was compared with placebo to slow the progression of early CVD in asymptomatic high-risk patients with prehypertension or hypertensive patients, valsartan treatment results in a significant improvement of SAE.[16] In the DETECT (DEtection and Treatment of Early Cardiovasular disease Trial) study, we showed in a group of prehypertensive subjects that 9 months of double-blind therapy with carvedilol, lisinopril, or their combination versus placebo resulted in a significantly sustained and well-tolerated functional improvement in SAE and to a lesser extent of LAE.[17] The EVIDENCE (Early Vascular Intervention—Determine Efficacy of Nebivolol, Comparator Examination) study was a double-blind study in which nebivolol was compared with atenolol in prehypertensive or borderline blood pressure and abnormal SAE. Nebivolol increased SAE, whereas there was no significant change in the atenolol and placebo groups.[18] In a nested substudy of the AVALON trial, which assessed the effects of coadministered amlodipine and atorvastatin versus either therapy alone or placebo on SAE and LAE, to evaluate the vascular benefits of coadministered therapy, early and sustained improvement in SAE was observed following coadministration of amlodipine and atorvastatin, thus demonstrating a vascular benefit with simultaneous treatment of hypertension and dyslipidemia.[19]

Conclusion

Noninvasive analysis of small artery function (SAE) through pulse contour analysis of radial artery waveforms provides an independent predictor of arterial hypertension and CVD morbid events, including coronary heart disease, angina, myocardial infarction, heart failure, stroke, and also a decline in renal function. LAE is to a lesser extent associated with CVD. These parameters can be used as phenotype for early detection of asymptomatic CVD. Moreover, SAE may serve as a guide to follow-up of vascular preventive therapy to reduce CVD events. Pulse contour analysis therefore provides diagnostic information well beyond the pressure itself in identifying and monitoring individuals in need of antihypertensive therapy to protect them from cardiovascular morbid events.

References

1. Stolarz-Skrzypek K, Thijs L, Wizner B, et al. From pioneering to implementing automated blood pressure measurement in clinical practice: Thomas Pickering's legacy. *Blood Press Monit*. 2010;15: 72-81.
2. Duprez DA. Systolic hypertension in the elderly: addressing an unmet need. *Am J Med*. 2008;121:179-184.
3. Whelton PK, Carey RM, Aronow WS, et al. 2017 ACC/AHA/AAPA/ABC/ACPM/AGS/APhA/ASH/ASPC/NMA/PCNA Guideline for the prevention, detection, evaluation, and management of high blood pressure in adults: executive summary: a report of the American College of Cardiology/American Heart Association Task Force on Clinical Practice Guidelines. *Hypertension*. 2018;71:1269-1324.

4. Duprez DA, Cohn JN. Monitoring vascular health beyond blood pressure. *Curr Hypertens Rep*. 2006;8:287-291.

5. Finkelstein SM, Cohn JN. First- and third-order models for determining arterial compliance. *J Hypertens Suppl*. 1992;10(6):S11-S14.

6. Gilani M, Kaiser DR, Bratteli CW, et al. Role of nitric oxide deficiency and its detection as a risk factor in pre-hypertension. *J Am Soc Hypertens*. 2007;1(1):45-55.

7. Duprez DA, Jacobs DR Jr, Lutsey PL, et al. Race/ethnic and sex differences in large and small artery elasticity–results of the multi-ethnic study of atherosclerosis (MESA). *Ethn Dis*. 2009;19(3):243-250.

8. Bild DE, Bluemke DA, Burke GL, et al. Multi-Ethnic Study of Atherosclerosis: objectives and design. *Am J Epidemiol*. 2002;156(9):871-881.

9. Peralta CA, Adeney KL, Shlipak MG, et al. Structural and functional vascular alterations and incident hypertension in normotensive adults: the multi-ethnic study of atherosclerosis. *Am J Epidemiol*. 2010;171(1):63-71.

10. O'Leary DH, Polak JF, Kronmal RA, Manolio TA, Burke GL, Wolfson SK Jr. Carotid-artery intima and media thickness as a risk factor for myocardial infarction and stroke in older adults. Cardiovascular Health Study Collaborative Research Group. *N Engl J Med*. 1999;340(1):14-22.

11. Folsom AR, Kronmal RA, Detrano RC, et al. Coronary artery calcification compared with carotid intima-media thickness in the prediction of cardiovascular disease incidence: the Multi-Ethnic Study of Atherosclerosis (MESA). *Arch Intern Med*. 2008;168(12):1333-1339.

12. Duprez DA, Jacobs DR Jr, Lutsey PL, et al. Association of small artery elasticity with incident cardiovascular disease in older adults: the multi-ethnic study of atherosclerosis. *Am J Epidemiol*. 2011;174(5):528-536.

13. Hom EK, Duprez DA, Jacobs DR Jr, et al. Comparing arterial function parameters for the prediction of coronary heart disease events: the Multi-Ethnic Study of Atherosclerosis (MESA). *Am J Epidemiol*. 2016;184(12):894-901.

14. Peralta CA, Jacobs DR Jr, Katz R, et al. Association of pulse pressure, arterial elasticity, and endothelial function with kidney function decline among adults with estimated GFR >60 mL/min/1.73 m(2): the Multi-Ethnic Study of Atherosclerosis (MESA). *Am J Kidney Dis*. 2012;59(1):41-49.

15. Duprez DA. Is vascular stiffness a target for therapy? *Cardiovasc Drugs Ther*. 2010;24(4):305-310.

16. Duprez DA, Florea ND, Jones K, Cohn JN. Beneficial effects of valsartan in asymptomatic individuals with vascular or cardiac abnormalities: the DETECTIV Pilot Study. *J Am Coll Cardiol*. 2007;50(9):835-839.

17. Saul SM, Duprez DA, Zhong W, Grandits GA, Cohn JN. Effect of carvedilol, lisinopril and their combination on vascular and cardiac health in patients with borderline blood pressure: the DETECT Study. *J Hum Hypertens*. 2013;27(6):362-367.

18. Duprez DA, Florea N, Duval S, Koukol C, Cohn JN. Effect of nebivolol or atenolol vs. placebo on cardiovascular health in subjects with borderline blood pressure: the EVIDENCE study. *J Hum Hypertens*. 2017;32(1):20-25.

19. Cohn JN, Wilson DJ, Neutel J, et al. Coadministered amlodipine and atorvastatin produces early improvements in arterial wall compliance in hypertensive patients with dyslipidemia. *Am J Hypertens*. 2009;22(2):137-144.

14

Cardiopulmonary Exercise Testing

Don Chomsky, MD

Cardiopulmonary exercise testing (CPXT) was once primarily utilized as a research tool. It is now more widely available and has a substantial evidence base supporting its application in everyday care in the management of a wide array of clinical conditions and situations. Despite its widespread applicability, the actual utilization of this form of testing in clinical practice is woefully inadequate likely largely due to a lack of awareness. The goal of this chapter is to provide a basic overview of the general principles of CPXT, clinical indications, and key elements of interpretation.

CPXT is most commonly used to objectively and reproducibly establish the degree of exercise limitation, identify the underlying mechanism of this limitation, and specifically identify the relative contributions of cardiac and pulmonary impairment to a patient's exercise intolerance. There is an abundance of literature supporting the more widespread use of this form of testing in several clinical settings including the evaluation of unexplained dyspnea, perioperative risk assessment, functional significance of valvular disease, disability assessment, and, most notably, the prognostic assessment of patients with chronic systolic heart failure. In the latter case, CPXT is now considered a critical element in determining a patient's eligibility for advanced congestive heart failure (CHF) therapies such as cardiac transplantation and left ventricular assist device (LVAD) support. The key clinical applications and contraindications for CPXT are listed in Table 14.1.

CPXT Protocol

Pre-exercise assessment includes resting electrocardiogram (ECG), oxygen saturation, blood pressure (BP), and pulse, as well as resting spirometry including vital capacity, FEV1 (forced expiratory volume in 1 second), and MVV (maximum voluntary ventilation). During exercise, the patient remains connected to an ECG monitor as well as facemask or mouthpiece which is in turn connected to a gas analyzer. A pulse oximeter and sphygmomanometer are attached.

Incremental exercise is then performed to maximal effort either on a bicycle or treadmill utilizing any of several standard exercise protocols, such as a modified Bruce or Naughton protocol. It is important to note that high increments of workload, such as in the Bruce exercise protocol, are avoided to reliably measure steady state conditions within each stage of exercise. Table 14.2 demonstrates and defines the most common elements of respiratory gas analysis during exercise. The primary physiologic measures assessed include peak oxygen consumption (PvO_2), anaerobic threshold (AT), and respiratory exchange ratio (RER) or respiratory quotient (RQ).

The Normal Cardiopulmonary Response to Exercise

Under normal conditions, incremental exercise work is accomplished by physiologic changes including a reduction in systemic vascular resistance, augmentation of stroke volume, and a progressive rise in heart rate (HR) all leading to progressive rise in cardiac output. Maximal exercise is normally limited by heart rate reserve, with maximal predicted HR not exceeding 220−age. Beyond this limit, cardiac output can no longer be augmented further to sustain incremental physical workload. Normal individuals exhaust their cardiovascular reserve at peak exercise. In contrast, lung mechanics are not limiting in healthy individuals. A ventilatory reserve, or **breathing reserve (BR)**, of 30% to 50% would be considered normal for a healthy control exercising maximally. As a result, oxygen desaturation during exercise does not occur in a maximally exercising healthy individual and, additionally, does not occur during maximal exercise in those with significant circulatory dysfunction when there is no intrinsic pulmonary abnormality.

During exercise with incremental workload, oxygen consumption and carbon dioxide production rise in a parallel linear fashion. As an individual's exercise effort begins to exceed their ability to deliver blood flow and oxygen to working muscles, anaerobic metabolism begins. This is defined as the **anaerobic threshold (AT)**. Energy-starved muscle begins to produce lactic acid leading to a disproportionate

Table 14.1

CLINICAL INDICATIONS AND CONTRAINDICATIONS FOR CARDIOPULMONARY EXERCISE TESTING

Indications

Evaluation of breathlessness or fatigue of unknown cause

Cardiac ischemia

Risk stratification and assessment of prognosis in heart failure

Direct measurement of functional capacity

Disability determination

Assess functional significance of valvular heart disease

Perioperative risk assessment

Risk of lung resection surgery

Congenital heart disease: Assessment of functional capacity and prognosis

Absolute Contraindications

Acute myocardial infarction

Acute myocarditis

Critical symptomatic aortic stenosis

Severe uncontrolled heart failure

Uncontrolled arrhythmia

Severe resting hypoxia

Aortic dissection

rise in expired CO_2 relative to oxygen consumption (**Figure 14.1**). Identification of AT is an easily derived measurement during CPXT and should occur at approximately 40% to 65% of the VO_2 max in a healthy individual.

The **respiratory exchange ratio (RER)** is defined as the ratio of VCO_2 to VO_2 ($RER = VCO_2/VO_2$). As noted above, VO_2 and VCO_2 rise linearly in parallel during exercise until the AT is achieved and lactate is produced. At this point, VCO_2 rises more steeply and exceeds VO_2, resulting in an RER >1.0 (**Figure 14.2**). An RER <1.0 at maximal exercise would indicate that anaerobic metabolism has not yet occurred and is therefore an indication of submaximal effort by the individual being tested. This becomes a very useful tool for objectively assessing the adequacy of patient effort with RER >1.1, indicating good to excellent effort, and RER <1.0 indicate submaximal effort in a very reproducible fashion. There are a few important exceptions to this rule in that RER <1.0 can still be seen in situations of maximal effort if certain underlying neuromuscular limitations exist or in patients with severe ventilatory impairment, as well as in patients who experience cardiac or peripheral muscle ischemia at low levels of stress.

The **peak oxygen consumption (PvO_2)** is the amount of oxygen consumption achieved at peak exercise and represents the most objective measure of one's cardiopulmonary fitness or conversely the degree of one's cardiopulmonary limitation/impairment. It is related to the more popular, but less accurate, calculation of metabolic equivalents (METS) to describe an individual's maximal workload on standard stress testing by dividing the peak VO_2 by 3.5 (a peak VO_2 of 17.5 mL/kg/min is equivalent to 5 METS). It is important to realize that expected

Table 14.2

ABBREVIATIONS AND DEFINITIONS OF KEY COMPONENTS IN CPXT

VO_2 (oxygen uptake)	Amount of oxygen extracted from inspired gas per unit time—may be expressed as an absolute value (mL/min) or corrected for weight (mL/kg/min)
VCO_2	Amount of carbon dioxide exhaled from the body per unit time (usually, per minute)
VO_2 max	Maximum oxygen uptake achievable (confirmed by repeated tests), despite further work rate increases
Peak VO_2	Highest VO_2 achieved during presumed maximal effort (as indicated by RER >1.15), for that test
R (or respiratory exchange ratio, RER)	Ratio of carbon dioxide output to oxygen uptake (VCO_2/VO_2)
VE	Volume of air inhaled or exhaled by the body in 1 min
MVV (maximum voluntary ventilation)	The maximum potential ventilation achievable (estimated as forced expiratory volume in 1 s [FEV_1] × 40)
Anaerobic threshold (AT)	Exercise limit above which the subject's anaerobic high-energy phosphate production supplements aerobic metabolism
Breathing reserve	The difference between maximum voluntary ventilation and the achieved maximum exercise minute ventilation

CPXT, cardiopulmonary exercise testing.

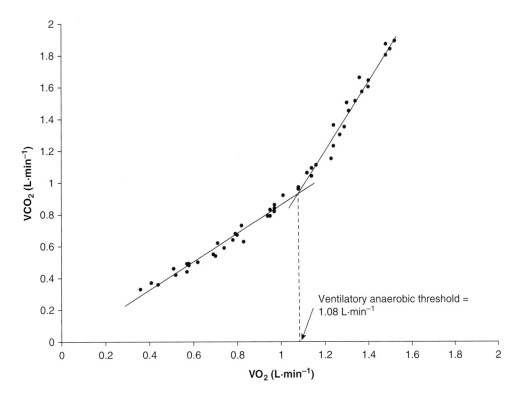

Figure 14.1 *Determination of anaerobic threshold.*

Interpretation of CPXT Results

peak VO_2 will be lower in women than in men and decreases with age, when interpreting the results of CPXT and results should be compared with predicted values for age and sex.

CPXT allows for precise measurement of an individual's cardiopulmonary capacity in a reproducible manner. In addition, as previously noted, it allows the interpreter to easily gauge the adequacy of patient effort by evaluating the RER, thus eliminating the subjective nature of standard exercise testing. In individuals who do demonstrate exercise impairment, analysis of gas exchange data allows for assessment of the relative contributions of cardiac and/or pulmonary derangement. CPXT can thereby provide invaluable information in assessing the patient who presents with unexplained exertional dyspnea or fatigue. It can also provide accurate assessment of the functional significance and severity of certain disease states both at a static point in time and longitudinally as the disease state potentially progresses. The evidence base for this latter utility of CPXT is most notable in the case of chronic systolic heart failure where it has become a mainstay of assessment in advanced disease and, at all stages of this disease, can provide powerful prognostic information.

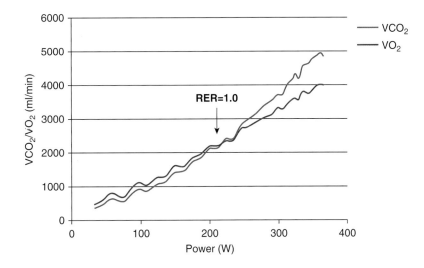

Figure 14.2 *Relationship of VO_2 to VCO_2 during cardiopulmonary exercise testing (CPXT), identification of respiratory exchange ratio (RER).*

Practical Application in the Patient With Systolic Heart Failure

CPXT has gained widespread acceptance as a critical part of the prognostic evaluation of individuals with systolic heart failure. As such, this testing deserves more broad utilization in this patient population and is generally greatly underutilized. Numerous studies have demonstrated that as peak VO_2 falls so too does life expectancy with this disorder. Interestingly, left ventricular ejection fraction does not correlate with peak VO_2 yet reproducibly peak VO_2 has been found to be a better predictor of death. In fact, multivariate analyses have demonstrated that peak VO_2 is a more powerful predictor of 1-year prognosis than all other prognostic markers including, left ventricular ejection fraction (LVEF), left ventricular end-diastolic diameter (LVEDD), New York Heart Association (NYHA), hemodynamic parameters such as cardiac output and pulmonary capillary wedge pressure, etc.

Because of the abundance of data supporting its use, CPXT is considered a critical and required element of the evaluation of noninotrope dependent patients who are being considered for heart transplant and/or LVAD support. Mancini and coworkers were the first to definitively demonstrate its utility in this regard when they demonstrated that patients with peak $VO <14$ mL/kg/min could safely have transplantation deferred, whereas those with lower values had a significant mortality risk unless nonpharmacologic intervention such as transplantation was performed. These findings have been corroborated by other investigators and various additional cut-points have been suggested to identify a higher risk cohort of patients needing intervention including peak $VO <10$ mL/kg/min, identifying a group with 1-year mortality rates of at least 60%.

There are numerous other elements of the CPXT that have been shown to provide additional prognostic information such as **VE/VCO$_2$ slope** as well as AT $<40\%$ of the peak VO_2. The combination of peak VO_2 <14 and VE/VCO$_2$ >34 has been shown to be a better indicator of high risk than either component alone. It is important to realize that this information must be taken into consideration along with the other components of CPXT, specifically with an RER >1.0 indicating adequate patient effort. The caveat to this is that there are certain situations in which potentially lethal exercise limitations may occur at or below an RER <1.0, and these would still be expected to represent high-risk situations potentially indicating a need to proceed with transplantation or LVAD support. Examples include significant low-threshold ischemia and severe ventricular arrhythmias.

Evaluation of the Patient With Unexplained Breathlessness and Fatigue

CPXT is an especially underutilized modality in assessing patients who present with ill-defined or unexplained exercise limitations. It can provide an objective and quantitative assessment of the true degree of exercise impairment by comparing achieved peak VO_2 to age- and sex-matched controls. This can additionally be used in a serial fashion to quantify the degree of response to any therapy delivered or simply to plot the course of the limitation over time. Malingering, or inadequate effort, can be documented by assessing whether the patient achieves anaerobic threshold and the final RER at peak exercise (RER <1.0 typically indicates inadequate effort, 1.0 to 1.1 fair effort, 1.1 to 1.2 good effort, and >1.2 excellent effort). Certain conditions that make this latter assessment unreliable were noted in the section dedicated to Respiratory Exchange Ratio.

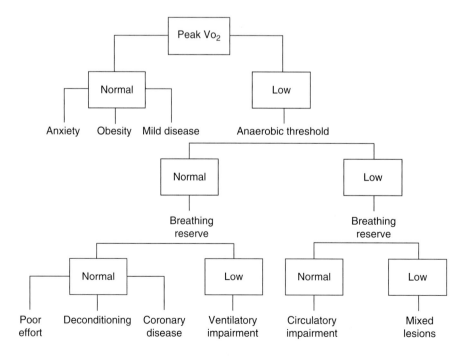

Figure 14.3 *Algorithm for determination of underlying cause of cardiopulmonary impairment.*

The ability of CPXT to discriminate between ventilatory and circulatory limitation can help clarify the underlying cause of the abnormality or at least direct further investigation toward an intrinsic pulmonary or cardiac disorder. There have been several approaches to clarifying the differential diagnosis between a predominantly ventilatory versus circulatory diagnosis. One such algorithm in the literature is displayed in **Figure 14.3**. A peak VO_2 <85% of predicted normal peak VO_2. If AT is <40% of **predicted** peak VO_2 and breathing reserve is preserved (>30%), this points toward a cardiovascular derangement, whereas AT >40% of predicted peak VO_2 and breathing reserve of <30% would indicate primarily ventilatory impairment. Additionally, oxygen desaturation during exercise would typically indicate primary pulmonary disease as this is not an expected finding with severe circulatory dysfunction alone (unless pulmonary edema or significant pulmonary hypertension is present). A patient with low peak VO_2, normal AT, and a normal breathing reserve would typically indicate muscle deconditioning. VE/VCO_2 slope is also useful in discriminating between functional impairment due to cardiopulmonary disease versus that primarily due to muscle deconditioning. Under normal conditions, VE/VCO_2 rises linearly at a slope of 23° to 28° until AT is reached. This slope becomes steeper in the setting of significant heart failure, pulmonary vascular disease, interstitial lung disease, or chronic obstructive disease, whereas it will typically remain normal in the setting of exercise limitation due to muscle deconditioning.

Unfortunately, in practice, not all patients fit perfectly in one of the buckets as there are often comorbid conditions and abnormalities in an individual patient. However, these guidelines can serve to identify the primary limiting factor and document quantitatively and reproducibly the severity of this limitation. Additionally, serial testing can be very useful to objectively quantify the course of the disease process over time.

Other Indications for CPXT

Additional areas where CPXT has utility include the assessment of patients with chronic valvular heart disease, perioperative risk assessment, and disability determination. In patients with moderate-severe chronic valvular disease, decisions regarding surgical intervention may be facilitated by determination of the severity of functional impairment. In this setting, CPXT can be useful in assessing the reportedly "asymptomatic" patient to determine if there is identifiable functional impairment and to confirm that circulatory dysfunction is the underlying cause. Levy et al demonstrated specifically that reduced peak VO_2 and elevated VE/VCO_2 slope were particularly valuable prognostic markers in patients with apparently asymptomatic severe aortic stenosis, while others have demonstrated that elevated VE/VCO_2 slope portends excess mortality in individuals with severe aortic stenosis despite an asymptomatic state and preserved ejection fraction. Such findings therefore should be considered in approaching these patients with earlier surgical intervention. In patients with severe functional impairment evident, peak VO_2 <14 mL/kg/min, and VE/VCO_2 slope >34, consideration of the risk of operative valve repair or replacement (especially in the evaluation of mitral regurgitation) may be tempered by the perceived benefits of transplantation or mechanical ventricular support. CPXT is also useful in the assessment of lung cancer patients being considered for resection. In a review by Beckles et al., those patients with peak VO_2 >20 mL/kg/min were not found to be at risk for postoperative complications as a result of resection, those with peak VO_2 <15 mL/kg/min were at increased risk, and those <10 mL/kg/min were at very high risk. An additional indication for CPXT is the assessment of patients with reported disability. In this setting, CPXT can be useful to objectively measure the degree of functional impairment and to rule out the possibility of malingering utilizing information gleaned from achievement of AT and analysis of RER. Numerous additional potential indications for CPXT exist but are beyond the scope of this brief review.

Conclusion

Cardiopulmonary exercise testing is an underutilized modality in the assessment of a wide range of clinical scenarios. Its benefits rest in the highly objective, reproducible, and quantitative nature of the information derived and in its ability to discriminate between cardiac and ventilatory limitation as well as rule out the contribution of malingering and skeletal muscle deconditioning. The broadest applications for use include the assessment of breathlessness and fatigue of uncertain primary etiology as well as in the assessment of patients with chronic systolic heart failure. In the latter scenario, it should be considered a critical element of the evaluation of severity of disease and is the most powerful tool available in the assessment of prognosis.

Bibliography

1. Beckles MA, Spiro SG, Colice GL, Rudd RM. The physiologic evaluation of patients with lung cancer being considered for resectional surgery. *Chest*. 2003;123(1 suppl):105S-114S.
2. Bolliger CT, Jordan P, Soler M, et al. Exercise capacity as a predictor of postoperative complications in lung resection candidates. *Am J Respir Crit Care Med*. 1995;151:1472-1480.
3. Gauzzi M, Arena R, Halle M, Piepoli M, Myers J, Lavie CJ. 2016 Focused update: clinical recommendations for cardiopulmonary exercise testing data assessment in specific patient populations. *Circulation*. 2016;133:e694-e711.
4. Gauzzi M, Bandera F, Ozemek C, Systrom D, Arena R. *J Am Coll Cardiol*. 2017;70:1618-1636.
5. Levy F, Fayad N, Jeu A, et al. The value of cardiopulmonary exercise testing in individuals with apparently asymptomatic severe aortic stenosis: a pilot study. *Arch Cardiovasc Dis*. 2014;107:519-528.
6. Mancini DM, Eisen H, Kussmaul W, Mull R, Edmunds LH Jr., Wilson JR. Value of peak exercise oxygen consumption for optimal timing of cardiac transplantation in ambulatory patients with heart failure. *Circulation*. 1991;82:778-786.

7. Messika-Zeitoun D, Johnson BD, Nkomo V, et al. Cardiopulmonary exercise testing determination of functional capacity in mitral regurgitation: physiologic and outcome implications. *J Am Coll Cardiol.* 2006;47:2521-2527.

8. Milani RV, Lavie CJ, Mehra MR. Cardiopulmonary exercise testing: how do we differentiate the cause of dyspnea? *Circulation.* 2004;110:e27-e31.

9. Milani RV, Lavie CJ, Mehra MR, Ventura HO. Understanding the basics of cardiopulmonary exercise testing. *Mayo Clin Proc.* 2006;81(12):1603-1611.

10. Neuberg GW, Friedman SH, Weiss MB, Herman MV. Cardiopulmonary exercise testing: the clinical value of gas exchange data. *Arch Intern Med.* 1988;148:2221-2226.

11. Parassuraman S, Schwarz K, Gollop ND, Loudon BL, Frenneaux MP. Healthcare Professional's guide to cardiopulmonary exercise testing. *Br J Cardiol.* 2015;22:156.

12. Shimizu M, Myers J, Buchanan N, et al. The ventilatory threshold: method, protocol, and evaluator agreement. *Am Heart J.* 1991;111:900-916.

13. Wasserman K, Hansen J, Sue DY, et al. *Appendix A: Symbols and Abbreviations, in "Principles of Exercise Testing and Interpretation".* 5th ed. Philadelphia: Lipincott Williams and Wilkins; 2012:542-544.

14. Weber KT, Kinasewitz GT, Janicki JS, Fishman AP. Oxygen utilization and ventilation during exercise in patients with chronic cardiac failure. *Circulation.* 1982;65:1213-1223.

15

Stress Nuclear Imaging in the Evaluation of Suspected Coronary Artery Disease

Dante J. Graves, MD, FACC

Stress Nuclear Cardiac Imaging

Stress nuclear imaging is well established as a testing modality in the evaluation of suspected coronary artery disease (CAD), with over 40 years of data correlation. It compares well in effectiveness with other imaging modalities.[1,2] Its main usefulness is in patients with abnormal electrocardiogram (ECG) and intermediate pretest risk for CAD. Both exercise and pharmacologic stress can be used, with treadmill exercise being the preferred method.

Contraindications for nuclear stress imagining include:
- Unstable angina
- Decompensated heart failure
- Systolic blood pressure >220 mm Hg
- Diastolic blood pressure >110 mm Hg
- Uncontrolled cardiac arrhythmia
- Severe symptomatic aortic stenosis
- Acute pulmonary embolus
- Acute pericarditis
- Severe pulmonary hypertension
- Acute myocardial infarction <4 days

Method

Resting nuclear images are first obtained using a technetium99-based tracer injected intravenously. Then, following exercise or pharmacologic stress with a target of 85% of maximal heart rate, a second injection of technetium99 is given to obtain stress images. During stress, blood pressure, heart rate, and ECG are monitored continually. The ejection fraction calculation is done based on poststress images. Indications for early termination of the test include severe angina, marked dyspnea, near syncope, signs of poor perfusion, ST depression greater than 2 mm, sustained supraventricular or ventricular tachycardia, development of left bundle branch block (LBBB), drop in blood pressure greater than 10 mm Hg, or development of severe hypertension (>230/115 mm Hg).

For patients who are unable to exercise, the choice of pharmacologic stressors includes dipyridamole, regadenoson, and dobutamine. Additionally, pharmacologic stress is useful for patients with LBBB, pacemaker, previous coronary bypass graft, or severe lung disease. Patients must be fasting for pharmacologic stress and must avoid caffeine intake for 24 hours before testing if a vasodilating agent (dipyridamole, regadenoson) will be used.

Results

Hemodynamic and electrocardiographic data are reviewed, providing important prognostic information. Image review uses a 16-segment model to evaluate transient ischemic dilatation, pulmonary uptake, and perfusion mismatch. Patients are classified as low, intermediate, or high risk according to the amount of ischemia found. High-risk patients have multiple or large perfusion deficits in multiple coronary territories, extensive defects with reversibility, increased lung uptake, and/or transient left ventricular dilatation. Those patients whose nuclear stress test is normal have less than 1% rate of major adverse cardiac events over the following 1 year.[2]

Summary

Stress nuclear imaging is a useful modality in the evaluation of suspected CAD, particularly in patients with intermediate pretest probability. It provides valuable prognostic information, especially concerning functional ischemia and myocardial viability.

References

1. Henzlova M, Duvall WC, Einstein AJ, et al. American society of nuclear cardiology imaging guidelines for SPECT nuclear cardiology procedures. Stress protocols, and tracers. *J Nucl Cardiol.* 2016;23(3):606-639.

2. Klocke F, Baird M, Lorell B, et al. ACC/AHA/ASNC guidelines for the clinical use of cardiac radionuclide imaging executive summary: a report of the American College of Cardiology/American Heart Association task force on practice guidelines. *J Am Coll Cardiol.* 2003;42:1318-1333.

16

Stress Echocardiography in the Evaluation of Suspected Coronary Artery Disease

Dante J. Graves, MD, FACC

Cardiovascular disease is the number one killer of Americans. Although the clinician has many options available to evaluate and diagnose coronary artery disease (CAD) before the patient has experienced a major cardiac event, the first process in the evaluation of CAD is a thorough history and physical examination. If disease is suspected at this point, to select further testing the clinician should keep in mind the principles of Bayesian analysis.[1] Pretest probability is paramount in detecting true disease.

As discussed in earlier chapters, a plain exercise treadmill test (ETT) is useful in patients who have a normal electrocardiogram (ECG) and the ability to exercise. Many more patients will not fit this category and will require further testing with imaging modalities. Imaging testing using stress echocardiography and stress nuclear studies is most useful in patients with intermediate cardiac risk. Using imaging we can detect ischemic heart disease, assess the severity of known lesions, evaluate the effects of pharmacologic therapy, and assess overall work capacity, all information vital in establishing diagnosis and prognosis.

Stress Echo: Patient Selection

Several studies have been published concerning the usefulness of stress echocardiography in the diagnosis of CAD.[2] Accuracy ranges from 80% to 90%, with sensitivity of 85% and specificity 77% in properly selected patients.[3] The most appropriate patients for stress echo are those with intermediate cardiac risk AND:

- Abnormal ST-T waves
- Left ventricular hypertrophy with repolarization
- Bundle branch block (left or right)
- Right ventricular pacemaker
- Patient taking digoxin
- Wolff-Parkinson-White syndrome

Contraindications to stress echo are:

- Unstable angina
- Decompensated heart failure
- Systolic blood pressure >220 mm Hg
- Diastolic blood pressure >110 mm Hg
- Uncontrolled cardiac arrhythmia
- Severe symptomatic aortic stenosis
- Acute pulmonary embolus
- Acute pericarditis
- Severe pulmonary hypertension
- Acute myocardial infarction < 4 days

Once stress echocardiography is selected, there are several options for the type of stress used. Exercise treadmill, with a goal of 85% of maximal heart rate, is the first option if the patient is able to exercise. Although less optimal, another option is exercise on a stationary bicycle. If exercise is not possible owing to musculoskeletal or severe lung disease, pharmacologic stress may be contemplated using one of two different pharmacologic agents: dobutamine, the most commonly used, which acts as a positive inotrope, or dipyridamole, a vasodilator.

Method

In performing exercise echo, first, baseline imaging is obtained, looking at ejection fraction and valve structure. Baseline ECG is also evaluated. The patient's blood pressure, heart rate, and ECG are continually monitored during stress. Clinical condition, including angina or anginal equivalent symptoms, are assessed. Indications for terminating a stress echo study early are uncontrolled hypertension

(>220/110 mm Hg), hypotension (drop of >10 mm Hg from baseline), the emergence of malignant arrhythmia or severe angina, or patient request. Peak exercise (or peak pharmacologic stress) echo images are obtained to evaluate wall motion, left ventricular (LV) size, and LV function. A 16-segment model is used to score the various echocardiographic findings.

Results

Exercise capacity can be evaluated by metabolic equivalents of exercise reached; this has prognostic significance. Abnormal blood pressure or heart rate response during the test is an important indicator of CAD, as is malignant arrhythmia.

Duke Treadmill Score (DTS) should be calculated for studies involving treadmill exercise[4]:

DTS = Exercise time − 5x (ST depression) − 4x (angina scale)
Angina scale: none = 0, nonlimiting angina = 1, limiting angina = 2

A DTS greater than or equal to +5 is considered low risk. Those with +4 to −10 scores are considered moderate risk, and a score of −11 or lower indicates high risk of CAD.[3]

Imaging data obtained with stress echo include LV performance, LV size, wall motion thickening, and wall motion abnormality. Along with the hemodynamic data, these parameters provide prognostic as well as diagnostic information in patients with suspected CAD. A 16-segment wall motion score is used to evaluate and report findings. Patients may be categorized into low, intermediate, or high risk based on the extent of wall motion abnormalities found on stress echo and their exercise capacity. A normal stress echo indicates a less than 1% major adverse cardiac event rate over the next year.[5]

Summary

Stress echocardiography is a low-cost, readily available test that is comparable with other image modalities for the diagnosis of CAD. The importance of patient selection cannot be overemphasized. Patients at intermediate risk for CAD are most likely to benefit from stress echocardiography.

Future Use

In the near future, contrast echocardiography, endocardial border definition, and perfusion studies will provide new depth of information for stress echocardiography. In advanced cardiac echo laboratories, stress bicycle echocardiography is already being used to evaluate the functional severity of valvular heart disease.

References

1. Detrano R, Yiannika J, Salcedo E, et al. Bayesian probability analysis: a prospective demonstration of its clinical utility in diagnosing coronary disease. *Circulation*. 1984;69(3):541-547.
2. Crouse LJ, Harbrecht JJ, Vaceyjhet, et al. Exercise echo as a screening test for coronary artery disease and correlation with coronary angiography. *Am J Cardiol*. 1991;67:1213.
3. Fleischmann K, Hunink M, Kuntz K, et al. Exercise echocardiography or exercise SPECT imaging. *JAMA*. 1998;280(10):013-920.
4. Mark DB, Hlatky M, Harell FE, et al. Exercise treadmill score for predicting prognosis in coronary artery disease. *Ann Med*. 1987;106:793-800.
5. Sawada S, Ryan T, Conley M, et al. Prognostic value of normal exercise echocardiogram. *Am Heart J*. 1990;120:49-52.

17

Cardiovascular Computed Tomography

Andrew O. Zurick III, MD, FACC, FASE, FSCMR

Cardiovascular Computed Tomography

For decades, investigators have sought to develop novel technologies that would allow rapid, noninvasive imaging of the heart. One such technology that has evolved rapidly in the past several decades has been cardiovascular computed tomography (CCT). Current-generation, modern CCT now permits highly detailed visualization of the coronary artery walls and lumen and provides assessment of cardiac function, valvular structures and prosthetic materials, pericardium, left atrial anatomy, congenital heart disease, pulmonary arterial and venous anatomy, and diseases of the aorta. Additionally, advancements in artificial intelligence and machine learning now permit noninvasive assessment of coronary artery physiologic function with the advent of computed tomography (CT)-based fractional flow reserve (FFR-CT).

Technology and Data Acquisition Techniques

Imaging the heart and coronary arteries with CT is an extremely technically challenging undertaking and requires sophisticated hardware and software analysis tools. Major difficulties arise because of cardiac and respiratory motion and the relatively small size of the coronary arteries, moving structures, with branches of interest in the range of 2 to 4 mm in diameter. The coronary arteries show rapid cyclic motion throughout the cardiac cycle—essentially moving in three dimensions with each heartbeat.

Over its relatively short history, several different CT scanner technologies have been used for cardiac imaging. Electron beam CT (EBCT), initially introduced in the mid-1970s, utilizes an electron source reflected onto a stationary tungsten target to generate x-rays, allowing for very rapid scan times. EBCT is well suited for cardiac imaging because of its high temporal resolution (50-100 ms) with an estimated slice thickness of 1.5 to 3 mm and the ability to scan the heart in a single breath hold. The primary use of this technique was to evaluate coronary arterial vessel wall calcium volume and density, generating a patient-specific calcium score. EBCT has since been largely supplanted by multidetector CT (MDCT) technology, which consists of a mechanically rotated x-ray source within a cylindrical gantry, with a multirow, collimated, detector located 180° opposite, that permits the simultaneous acquisition of more data ("slices"). 0.625 mm collimator rows provide for markedly increased spatial resolution and for complete acquisition of data during one breath hold. Current-generation MDCT offers improved spatial and temporal resolution, thereby making coronary CT angiography (CCTA) feasible, reproducible, and highly accurate.

CCTA was initially performed using MDCT machines capable of obtaining only four to eight slices per scan. As the technology has advanced, z-axis coverage has continued to improve; now 256-slice (and higher) scanners are available that allow acquisition of higher-resolution images without the requirement for long breath holds or extremely slow heart rates. It is currently recommended that computed tomography angiography (CTA) be performed using a minimum of a 64-slice scanner. Newer technology allows up to 320 to 512 anatomic slices to be simultaneously acquired during a single gantry rotation. With a minimal slice thickness of 0.5 to 0.625 mm, an entire heart can be imaged in a single heartbeat. Despite improved scanner hardware, most current-generation CT scanners can achieve temporal resolution approaching 140 ms but still cannot reach what can be obtained routinely in a cardiac catheterization laboratory, where fluoroscopy provides temporal resolution closer to 33 ms. To overcome the necessity of a slow heart rate, one vendor has placed two x-ray sources in the scanner gantry (so-called dual source imaging) at 90° angles to one another. This technology offers an improved temporal resolution, even with heart rates approaching 100 bpm and greater.

In the past, for coronary CTA using a single x-ray source scanner, it was typically necessary to obtain images with heart rates less than 65 bpm. Most commonly, an oral or intravenous β-blocker is given to slow the heart rate. Newer-generation scanners have somewhat loosened these rigid low heart rate requirements, although the adage still holds when imaging the heart that slower tends to be better. Coronary CTA requires intravenous administration of a contrast agent to opacify the lumen of the coronary arteries. The intravenous contrast agents used for CTA carry the same dose-dependent risks in patients with renal dysfunction as contrast agents used for cardiac catheterization, as well as the risk of an allergic reaction to iodine. Respiratory motion is minimized by patient breath holds up to 10 seconds, depending on scanner generation and patient body size. The most common data acquisition protocol utilizes a spiral mode involving continuous data acquisition during constant rotation of the x-ray tube inside the gantry, while the patient is advanced on the table through the scanner. To minimize radiation exposure, data acquisitions can be performed in sequential mode ("step and shoot"). This involves acquisition of single transaxial slices, sequentially, as a patient is advanced incrementally through the scanner.

Excessive cardiac motion can lead to blurring of the contours of the coronary vessels. For this reason, a regular heart rate is necessary for optimal imaging of the coronary arteries. Relative contraindications to performing CTA include the presence of frequent ectopic beats or atrial fibrillation. Coordinating data acquisition with the cardiac cycle involves either prospective electrocardiogram (ECG)-triggering or retrospective ECG-gating. In prospective triggering, data are acquired in a specific portion of the cardiac cycle, typically late diastole, based on simultaneous ECG recordings. In retrospective gating, data are collected during the entire cardiac cycle. Postprocessing then allows only data from specific periods of the cardiac cycle to be used for image reconstruction, as is needed.

Clinical Indications

Coronary Artery Calcium Score

Coronary artery calcium (CAC) has emerged as a robust marker of subclinical atherosclerosis and a powerful prognostic tool. CAC scoring utilizes no contrast and readily detects calcium because of its high x-ray attenuation coefficient (or CT number) measured in Hounsfield units (HU) (Figure 17.1). The Agatston scoring system assigns a calcium score based on maximal CT number and the area of calcium deposits.[1] More recently, analysis of several large clinical datasets has confirmed that the coronary artery calcium score is a robust predictor of coronary events, particularly in the asymptomatic patient population, independent of traditional risk factors.[2,3] In at least one study, calcium score was more predictive than C-reactive protein and standard risk factors for predicting coronary artery disease (CAD) events.[4]

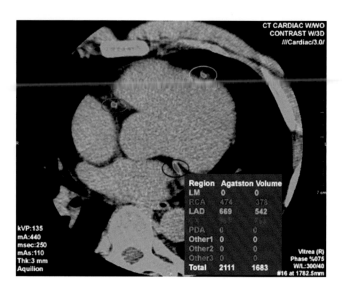

Figure 17.1 *Calcium score computed tomography.*

The coronary calcium score is derived by identifying coronary arterial tree segments that have attenuation characteristics (HU) greater than a certain value (100-130 depending on software and patient size) that correlate with the attenuation due to calcium. These calcified lesions are scored by size and density with a weighting factor for increasing density. Discrete lesions are scored separately, and the density of calcium within each lesion is graded from one to four according to the HU. The sums of all the lesions are totaled to arrive at a single coronary calcium score. In general, the higher the score, the greater the amount of calcified plaque within the arterial tree. There is a positive correlation of cardiac events with this score. It is important to remember, however, that exclusively noncalcified coronary artery plaques have been reported in up to 4% of asymptomatic patients.[2]

The Multiethnic Study of Atherosclerosis (MESA) group published a series of articles suggesting that the calcium score is an independent risk factor for cardiac events.[5] Also, MESA's website (https://www.mesa-nhlbi.org/calcium/input.aspx) has the capacity to allow comparison of an individual patient's calcium score against their large database. This score takes into account age, sex, and race and generates a percentile compared with the database studies. The presence of a high calcium score may prompt clinicians to use more aggressive therapy as if they were reclassified in a higher risk group or to convince patients who are reluctant to take drugs such as statins to take their disease more seriously. Recent studies have shown that a zero coronary artery calcium score demonstrated an annual event rate in asymptomatic subjects of only 0.11% (10-year risk of only 1.1%).[2] Among asymptomatic patients, the incidence of abnormal nuclear stress testing is 1.3%, 11.3%, and 35.2% for calcium scores <100, 101 to 400, and >400, respectively.[6] Studies of serial calcium scanning have noted that calcified plaque progression is significantly and independently associated with a worse overall prognosis.[2]

Coronary Artery Imaging (CCTA)

Chest pain is a common clinical problem and one of the most common complaints of individuals presenting for urgent medical evaluation. One of the most important, life-threatening causes of chest pain is CAD. Although cardiac catheterization is the best method to assess for the presence of hemodynamically significant obstructive CAD, it is impractical as a screening test. It is invasive and costly, can be especially dangerous in some subsets of patients, and when used broadly as a screening tool is performed on a substantial number of patients who have no significant obstructive CAD and/or whose chest pain is unrelated to cardiac causes. Approximately 10% to 25% of the patients who are referred for invasive coronary angiography are found to have normal coronary arteries or nonobstructive CAD.[7] Furthermore, prior meta-analysis has now demonstrated poorer prognosis and increased numbers of hard cardiac end points with non-obstructive CAD compared with normal coronary arteries.[8]

CCTA utilizes intravenous contrast to differentiate vessel lumen from vessel wall (**Figure 17.2**). In 2010, the American College of Cardiology (ACC) and many other societies with interests in cardiac imaging put together recommendations of appropriateness criteria for utilization of cardiac CTA that include appropriate and inappropriate uses of this technology.[9] The most common appropriate utilization is diagnostic study of patients presenting with chest pain who do not have significant ECG changes or elevated cardiac biomarkers but have an intermediate probability of CAD. At experienced centers with careful data acquisition, sensitivities range from 83% to 99% and specificities from 93% to 98% with remarkably high estimated negative predictive value (95%-100%),

indicating that CCTA may be used to reliably rule out the presence of significant flow-limiting coronary atherosclerotic disease.[10] It should be pointed out that CCTA would be inappropriate for patients at high risk for or with other indications of cardiac ischemia such as elevated biomarkers or significant ECG changes. Those patients should be referred immediately for invasive imaging. Currently there is no indication for performing CCTA in asymptomatic patients. Indeed, the appropriateness criteria recommend against the use of CCTA in the asymptomatic population until further evidence suggests that it would positively affect outcomes.

Bypass graft imaging is more easily accomplished than coronary artery imaging because of the larger size of bypass grafts (particularly saphenous vein grafts) and less rapid movement of bypass grafts as compared with native coronary arteries. The patency or occlusion of grafts can be determined by the presence or absence of distal target vessel contrast enhancement.[11] Imaging internal mammary grafts is often more difficult because of artifacts caused by metallic clips near the grafts. Imaging of coronary artery stents is challenging because of artifacts caused by metal that can obscure visualization of the coronary artery lumen. Studies evaluating CCTA to assess in-stent restenosis have been somewhat disappointing, yielding sensitivities of 54% to 83%.[12] Stents less than 3.0 mm in diameter are much more likely to be difficult to evaluate. An additional important application of CCTA is in patients with congenital abnormalities of their coronary arteries, including anomalous coronary artery origins and the presence of intramyocardial bridges (coronary arteries that, for a portion of their course, are not epicardial but rather covered by a layer of myocardial tissue) (**Figure 17.3**).

The past several years have seen many new developments in CCTA technology focusing not just on the coronary artery anatomy but also evaluating simultaneously for functional data on the presence or absence of myocardial ischemia. There have been several publications in the past few years that have focused on the use of CCT for myocardial perfusion imaging, transluminal attenuation gradients and corrected coronary opacification indexes and fractional flow reserve calculated from resting CCTA data (FFR-CT).[13] At the time of this writing, Heartflow is the only US Food and Drug Administration–approved vendor providing FFR-CT analysis utilizing artificial intelligence and machine learning. Several studies have now demonstrated good agreement between FFR-CT and invasive FFR (**Figure 17.4**).

STRUCTURAL HEART EVALUATION

Through appropriate timing of intravenous chamber contrast enhancement, extensive cardiac morphologic and functional information can be obtained by CCT. Myocardial mass and ventricular function can be estimated with a high level of accuracy. CCT can also provide a detailed morphologic picture of left atrium and left atrial appendage anatomy—information that can be useful before planned catheter ablation for atrial fibrillation or device implantation in the left atrial appendage.[14]

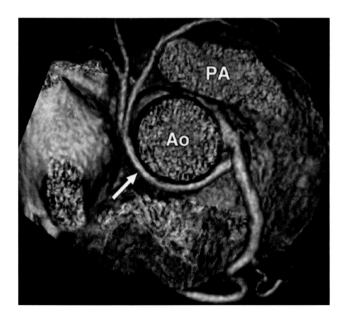

Figure 17.2 *Three-dimensional volume-rendered coronary computed tomography angiography demonstrating anomalous right coronary artery origin arising from the left main, passing posterior to the aorta. Ao, aorta; PA, pulmonary artery.*

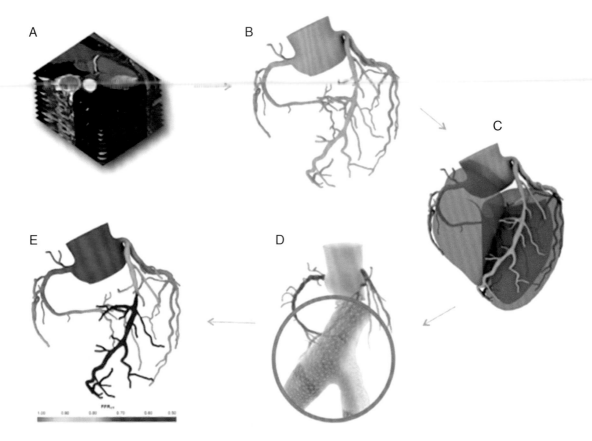

Figure 17.3 *Fractional flow reserve computed tomography (FFR-CT). A, Coronary CT angiography image dataset, acquired using standard imaging protocol. B, Image segmentation produces an anatomic model of the root of aorta and epicardial coronary arteries, including all second- and third-order branchings to approximately 1 mm in diameter. C, Physiologic model of coronary flow with specified inflow and outflow boundary conditions is created. Resting coronary flow is based on left ventricular myocardial volume extracted from CT image data and the microcirculation model is based on epicardial vessel size. D, Computational fluid dynamics methods are used to simulate coronary blood flow under maximal hyperemia with simultaneous computation of coronary pressure and flow at millions of discrete points throughout the coronary tree. E, Three-dimensional display of FFR-CT values in each coronary artery and its branches with color coding of numerical FFR-CT values as shown on the scale.*

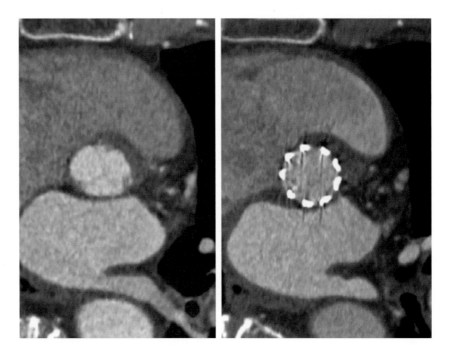

Figure 17.4 *Pre- and post–transcatheter aortic valve replacement computed tomography.*

Three-dimensional anatomic data obtained by CCT can be fused with electrical mapping data acquired in the electrophysiology laboratory and greatly facilitates the procedure.

The past several years have seen an explosive growth in the utilization of transcatheter therapies for the treatment of valvular and structural heart disease. Advancement in transcatheter aortic valve replacement (TAVR) technology has relied heavily on appropriate aortic annular sizing data obtained with CCT (Figure 17.4). Studies have now demonstrated that accurate three-dimensional aortic annular sizing assessment with CCT results in reduced paravalvular regurgitation, which has been associated with increased mortality following these procedures. In 2012, the Society of Cardiovascular Computed Tomography released guidelines for the use of CCT before TAVR.[15] Furthermore, several new therapies on the horizon for mitral and tricuspid valve repair will also rely heavily on preprocedural CCT for accurate sizing and morphologic assessment.

Limitations

CCT involves exposure to radiation and the potential for radiation-related risk (particularly related to the risk of cancer induction).[16] Radiation exposure (effective dose) is quantified in millisieverts (mSv). Patient radiation doses are dependent on tube current (milliamperes) and tube voltage (kiloelectron volts), as well as the duration of radiation exposure and patient body size. Current-generation CT scanners are now able to perform ECG-gated cardiac imaging with 1 to 2 mSv. For comparison purposes with CCT, typical gated cardiac single-photon emission tomography carries a higher radiation dose (effective dose = 10-15 mSv), as does conventional coronary angiography carries a lower radiation dose (effective dose = 6 mSv). ECG-correlated tube current modulation (reduction of tube current in systole) with retrospectively gated studies can reduce radiation exposure by 30% to 50%. Retrospectively gated studies have more recently been supplanted by prospectively triggered studies that limit radiation exposure to a single portion of the cardiac cycle, further decreasing overall patient radiation exposure. Additionally, improvements in iterative reconstruction techniques have also been developed that also further reduce patient radiation exposure. Although the risk from the radiation is low, it does mean that CCT is not well suited for use as a screening test on a regular or repeated basis. The Society of Cardiovascular Computed Tomographyreleased guidelines in 2011 that offered a comprehensive overview of cardiovascular CT radiation.[17]

In addition, allergic contrast reactions are reported in 0.2% to 0.7% of patients receiving nonionic contrast materials. In the absence of preexisting renal disease, the risk of renal dysfunction due to iodinated contrast administration is low.

Future Directions

Our utilization of CT technology has increased significantly over the past 3 decades from nearly 3 million CT scans in 1980 to more than 62 million CT scans in 2007.[16] Current CCT use has not resulted in broad replacement for conventional coronary angiography, but in appropriately selected patients, it may serve as a useful alternative, even more so now with the continued development of FFR-CT technologies, permitting both the assessment of coronary artery anatomy and function, all in a single resting study. Dual-source CCT has improved temporal resolution, and 320-detector row coronary CTA now allows imaging of the entire heart in a single heartbeat. Continued advancements in artificial intelligence technologies and machine learning will also play an increasing role in the use of cardiac CT in the coming decade.

References

1. Agatston AS, Janowitz WR, Hildner FJ, et al. Quantification of coronary artery calcium using ultrafast computed tomography. *J Am Coll Cardiol*. 1990;15(4):827-32.
2. Hecht HS. Coronary artery calcium scanning: past, present, and future. *JACC Cardiovasc Imaging*. 2015;8(5):579-596.
3. Hecht HS, Narula J. Coronary artery calcium scanning in asymptomatic patients with diabetes mellitus: a paradigm shift. *J Diabetes*. 2012;4(4):342-350.
4. Schmermund A, Voigtlander T. Predictive ability of coronary artery calcium and CRP. *Lancet*. 2011;378(9792):641-643.
5. Detrano R, Guerci AD, Carr JJ, et al. Coronary calcium as a predictor of coronary events in four racial or ethnic groups. *N Engl J Med*. 2008;358(13):1336-1345.
6. Engbers EM, Timmer JR, Ottervanger JP, et al. Prognostic value of coronary artery calcium scoring in addition to single-photon emission computed tomographic myocardial perfusion imaging in symptomatic patients. *Circ Cardiovasc Imaging*. 2016;9(5).
7. Patel MR, Dai D, Hernandez AF, et al. Prevalence and predictors of nonobstructive coronary artery disease identified with coronary angiography in contemporary clinical practice. *Am Heart J*. 2014;167(6):846-852.e2.
8. Huang FY, Huang BT, Lv WY, et al. The prognosis of patients with nonobstructive coronary artery disease versus normal arteries determined by invasive coronary angiography or computed tomography coronary angiography: a systematic review. *Medicine (Baltimore)*. 2016;95(11):e3117.
9. Taylor AJ, Cerqueira M, Hodgson JM, et al. ACCF/SCCT/ACR/AHA/ASE/ASNC/NASCI/SCAI/SCMR 2010 appropriate use criteria for cardiac computed tomography. A report of the American College of Cardiology Foundation Appropriate Use Criteria Task Force, the Society of Cardiovascular Computed Tomography, the American College of Radiology, the American Heart Association, the American Society of Echocardiography, the American Society of Nuclear Cardiology, the North American Society for Cardiovascular Imaging, the Society for Cardiovascular Angiography and Interventions, and the Society for Cardiovascular Magnetic Resonance. *J Cardiovasc Comput Tomogr*. 2010;4(6):407.e1-407.e33.
10. Stein PD, Yaekoub AY, Matta F, Sostman HD. 64-slice CT for diagnosis of coronary artery disease: a systematic review. *Am J Med*. 2008;121(8):715-725.
11. Frazier AA, Qureshi F, Read KM, et al. Coronary artery bypass grafts: assessment with multidetector CT in the early and late postoperative settings. *Radiographics*. 2005;25(4):881-896.
12. Oncel D, Oncel G, Tastan A, Tamci B. Evaluation of coronary stent patency and in-stent restenosis with dual-source CT coronary angiography without heart rate control. *AJR Am J Roentgenol*. 2008;191(1):56-63.
13. Goncalves Pde A, Rodríguez-Granillo GA, Spitzer E, et al. Functional evaluation of coronary disease by CT angiography. *JACC Cardiovasc Imaging*. 2015;8(11):1322-35.

14. Wang DD, Eng M, Kupsky D, et al. Application of 3-dimensional computed tomographic image guidance to WATCHMAN implantation and impact on early operator learning curve: single-center experience. *JACC Cardiovasc Interv.* 2016;9(22):2329-2340.

15. Achenbach S, Delgado V, Hausleiter J, et al. SCCT expert consensus document on computed tomography imaging before transcatheter aortic valve implantation (TAVI)/transcatheter aortic valve replacement (TAVR). *J Cardiovasc Comput Tomogr.* 2012;6(6):366-380.

16. Brenner DJ, Hall EJ. Computed tomography–an increasing source of radiation exposure. *N Engl J Med.* 2007;357(22):2277-2284.

17. Halliburton SS, Abbara S, Chen MY, et al. SCCT guidelines on radiation dose and dose-optimization strategies in cardiovascular CT. *J Cardiovasc Comput Tomogr.* 2011;5(4):198-224.

18

Cardiovascular Magnetic Resonance Imaging

Andrew O. Zurick III, MD, FACC, FASE, FSCMR

Cardiac Magnetic Resonance Imaging

Cardiac magnetic resonance imaging (CMR) is a robust noninvasive imaging technique. Through electromagnetic manipulation of biologic hydrogen protons, CMR can provide assessment of cardiac structure, function, perfusion, tissue characterization, blood flow velocity, cardiac masses, valvular heart disease, pericardial disease, and vascular disease. Continued improvements in hardware and pulse sequence design have allowed for improved image quality, speed of data acquisition, and reliability, further increasing the usefulness of CMR for clinical applications. CMR is similar to echocardiography in that neither utilizes ionizing radiation to acquire high-resolution images, avoiding the exposures inherent in invasive coronary angiography, computed tomography, and single photon emission tomography imaging. CMR is capable of assessing cardiac morphology in any number of *x*, *y*, and *z* axis orientations. In addition, the large field of view in CMR imaging allows assessment of both cardiac and noncardiac pathologies.

Technology of CMR

Magnetic resonance imaging (MRI) (including CMR) is based on the electromagnetic manipulation of biologic hydrogen protons. Hydrogen is the most abundant element present within the human body, present within all tissues, whether in water, adipose tissue, or soft tissue. Each water molecule contains two hydrogen nuclei, each with a single proton, and they behave like tiny magnets. Proton spins can be aligned by application of a powerful magnetic field in the $\beta(0)$ direction, given the appropriate frequency via the Larmor equation ($f = \gamma\beta$; where f is the precessional frequency, β is the magnet field strength, and γ is the gyromagnetic ratio). A second radiofrequency electromagnetic field can then be briefly applied and then rapidly discontinued. As protons return to their original alignment after the electromagnetic field is turned off ("relaxation"), they generate a net magnetization that decays to its former position with energy loss in the form of a radio signal that can be detected with a radiofrequency antenna and quantified. Image tissue contrast depends on differences in the decay of net magnetization in the longitudinal plane (T_1) and transverse plane (T_2). Through the application of additional electromagnetic fields (gradient fields), radio waves coming from the body can be spatially encoded, allowing localization within an imaging plane.

Data Acquisition Sequences and Techniques

CMR utilizes two basic imaging sequences: *spin echo* ("dark blood") and *gradient echo* ("bright blood"). Spin echo sequences are commonly used for multislice anatomic imaging, providing clear delineation of the mediastinum, cardiac chambers, and great vessels. Alternatively, gradient echo sequences are used more often for physiologic assessment of function through cine acquisitions. Because of higher possible imaging speeds, gradient echo is more appropriately used for ventricular function and myocardial perfusion assessment and valvular assessment. *Phase contrast imaging* (PCI) allows quantitative flow velocity and volume flow assessment. All cardiac and most vascular CMR sequences require cardiac electrocardiogram (ECG)-gating. Through data acquisition of segments at different phases of the cardiac cycle, a cine image loop can be created tracking cardiac motion. Perfusion imaging, through the use of intravenous contrast agents, permits assessment of tissue vascularity. In the case of vasodilator stress perfusion imaging, assessment of myocardial ischemia is possible (**Figure 18.1**). Inotropic stress imaging, typically with intravenous dobutamine, allows assessment of new regional wall motion abnormalities. Predominantly gadolinium-based contrast agents, chelated to other nontoxic molecules for clinical use, are utilized for imaging the cardiovascular system.

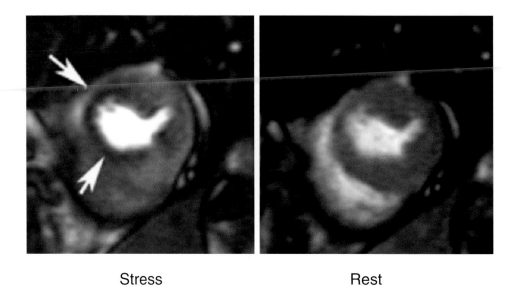

Stress   Rest

Figure 18.1 *Stress perfusion MRI depicting subendocardial hypoperfusion (arrows) of the mid septum on stress image (left) representative of LAD (left anterior descending coronary artery) territory myocardial ischemia. Image at right is corresponding rest perfusion image showing normal perfusion.*

Clinical Indications

VENTRICULAR FUNCTION

CMR is highly accurate and reproducible, providing clinically useful measurements of cardiac wall thickness, chamber volumes, myocardial mass, and systolic contractile function. CMR is recognized as the "gold standard" for assessment of left and right ventricular function. Left ventricular ejection fraction, left ventricular end-diastolic volume, left ventricular end-systolic volume, stroke volume, cardiac output, and left ventricular mass can all be reliably quantified. Left ventricular diastolic function can also be reliably interrogated using PCI.

ISCHEMIC HEART DISEASE

CMR is the most sensitive cardiac imaging modality for the assessment of myocardial viability and the extent of myocardial infarction. It is the imaging modality of choice for patients in whom there is a question about whether the distribution of a planned revascularization is viable or not. For this application, compared with nuclear imaging, CMR is much more sensitive in detecting subendocardial viability (and lack of viability) and, obviously, CMR does not require radiation exposure for patients. Gadolinium is excluded from intact myocardial cell membranes and thus is useful in defining areas of infarction. Correlation with anatomic specimens suggests a sensitivity and specificity above 95%. Delayed hyperenhancement (DHE) protocols, most often using phase sensitive inversion recovery imaging, are based on the high signal intensity ("bright") that results from T_1 time shortening due to gadolinium contrast localization within scar tissue (**Figure 18.2**). Alternatively, first-pass perfusion images that appear hypointense are probably a combination of ischemic and infarcted tissues. The highest

likelihood of recovery of contractility impairment exists when the transmural infarction extent, as assessed by DHE, is less than 50% transmural.[1] Additionally, anomalous coronary arteries can be identified through the use of CMR. In particular, CMR is well suited to demonstrate the relationship of anomalous coronary arteries to other vascular structures (the aorta and main pulmonary artery) and thus to make decisions on the need and timing of surgery.

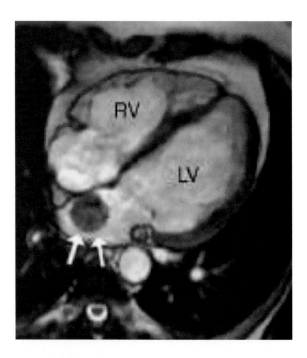

Figure 18.2 *Steady-state free precession (SSFP) image depicting iso-intense (arrows) mass attached to the inter-atrial septum highly suspicious for myxoma. LV, left ventricle; RV, right ventricle.*

AORTIC DISEASE

CMR has rapidly evolved into a clinically reliable, reproducible modality to evaluate the aorta and its primary branch vessels. Gadolinium-enhanced three-dimensional CMR angiography is an extremely rapid technique that can accurately depict aortic pathology. Serial monitoring of chronic aortopathy can be performed safely, without continued radiation exposure, with CMR angiography. Additionally, in patients with concurrent aortic valve regurgitation and aortic pathology, PCI helps to serially monitor aortic regurgitant volumes and fractions to assess for interval changes.[2]

CARDIOMYOPATHIES

CMR is an important tool in the evaluation of dilated cardiomyopathy, hypertrophic cardiomyopathy, and infiltrative disorders. It provides accurate assessment of ventricular function in patients with dilated cardiomyopathies. DHE CMR has a niche role in helping to differentiate heart failure related to dilated cardiomyopathy from CAD. Even so, the distinction is not perfect. More than 10% of patients with dilated nonischemic cardiomyopathy have gadolinium enhancement that is identical in appearance to that seen in patients with CAD. As T1 mapping techniques and pulse sequences continue to improve, characterization of cardiomyopathies will also continue to evolve.

In hypertrophic cardiomyopathy, CMR can accurately localize hypertrophy, particularly when echocardiography data are equivocal. Cine images can also demonstrate systolic anterior motion of the anterior mitral valve leaflet and dynamic outflow tract obstruction, useful measures in selecting an optimal therapeutic approach in this patient population. More recent data indicate that increased DHE scar burden in patients with hypertrophic cardiomyopathy is correlated with an increased risk of arrhythmia or sudden cardiac death.[3] CMR also has a role in the evaluation of patients with suspected infiltrative cardiomyopathies. Sarcoidosis is an infiltrative granulomatous disease pathologically known to nonuniformly involve the myocardium. This patchy distribution tends to result in a moderate to high number of false-negative cardiac biopsy results. When an initial biopsy result is negative in patients with suspected cardiac sarcoidosis, one must consider the benefits of repeated biopsy procedures, given the risks inherent in this procedure. CMR DHE imaging can depict areas of interstitial changes and granulomatous disease. In patients with a high pretest probability for cardiac sarcoidosis, CMR can potentially serve as a reliable screening tool obviating the need for biopsy, particularly if the diagnosis of sarcoidosis has been confirmed by biopsy of noncardiac tissue. Amyloid infiltration in the myocardium may show diffusely increased signal intensity with DHE imaging sequences. Additionally, the combination of ventricular hypertrophy without ECG concordance, atrial wall thickening, valve thickening, pericardial and pleural effusion, and restrictive diastolic filling pattern can collectively raise the clinical suspicion for infiltrative cardiac amyloidosis.[4] CMR is also capable of confirming the diagnosis of arrhythmogenic right ventricular dysplasia, a diagnosis that historically is based on meeting several major and minor criteria. Use of contrast agents and DHE imaging may permit detection of fibrofatty right ventricular free wall infiltration and regional right ventricular wall motion abnormalities and assessment of indexed right ventricular volume, observations that increases specificity for this otherwise difficult diagnosis.

CARDIAC MASSES

CMR is the imaging modality of choice for the evaluation of cardiac masses because of the ability to perform tissue characterization. Spin-echo imaging provides excellent images for the evaluation of the presence, extent, attachment site, and secondary effects of cardiac mass lesions. CMR has a proven role in the identification of intracardiac thrombi, primary and secondary cardiac tumors, and pericardial cysts (**Figure 18.3**).

PERICARDIAL DISEASES

CMR permits assessment of pericardial effusion, constrictive pericarditis, pericardial cysts, and congenital absence of the pericardium. Normal pericardium thickness on CMR is 1 to 4 mm. Functional and structural abnormalities of the pericardium can be reliably assessed through the use of CMR imaging. Pericardial DHE imaging has been demonstrated to correlate with active pericardial inflammation and neovascularization.[5] Additionally, free breathing cine imaging can demonstrate increased ventricular interdependence suggestive of constrictive pericarditis. Failure to see slippage between the visceral and parietal pericardial layers suggests fibrosis, scarring, or connections between these two normally separate tissue layers. CMR has also proven useful in the evaluation of pericardial cysts.

VALVULAR HEART DISEASE

CMR has become a valuable complementary technique for evaluating the severity of valvular heart disease. Through a combination of steady-state free precession (SSFP) and PCI,

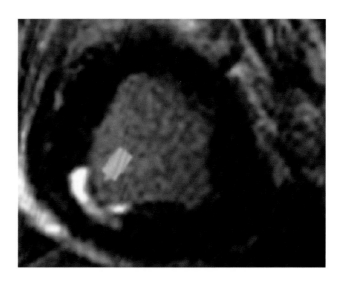

Figure 18.3 *Cardiac magnetic resonance imaging. Left atrial myxoma.*

CMR can provide a comprehensive valvular assessment. Although echocardiography is capable of superior temporal resolution, is more accessible, and is less labor-intensive, CMR is capable of imaging flow in three dimensions (x, y, and z planes), more accurate for measuring absolute flow volumes, and feasible in patients whose body habitus precludes obtaining optimal echocardiographic images. In valvular regurgitant lesions, PCI can provide exact quantifications of regurgitant volume and fraction. In patients with aortic stenosis, planimetry of the aortic valve provides accurate measurements rather than geometric estimations available via echocardiography and catheterization techniques. Additionally, CMR provides accurate measurement of peak transstenotic jet velocities that are orthogonal to the valve, not merely across it.

CONGENITAL HEART DISEASE

CMR is an ideal imaging modality for the assessment of congenital heart disease, providing superior anatomic imaging coupled with functional interrogation and reproducibility. In the evaluation of great vessel abnormalities, CMR is the gold standard, particularly for conditions such as aortic coarctation. Through velocity mapping of the coarctation jet, a pressure gradient across the area of narrowing can be determined. Atrial septal defects can often be visualized on direct SSFP imaging, and through the use of PCI, estimate of Qp/Qs ratio can be calculated, noninvasively. Tetralogy of Fallot, including overriding aorta, membranous ventricular septal defect, right ventricular hypertrophy, and infundibular or pulmonary stenosis, can be completely characterized before and after correction. Additionally, as is often the case with patients who have required surgical Tetralogy repair, CMR is an excellent tool for monitoring patients for progressive pulmonary valvular regurgitation and right ventricular dilation. CMR is also capable of reliably depicting anomalous coronary artery origins and their relation to other cardiac structures and the great vessels.

Safety, Risks, and Contraindications

Because of the physical nature of CMR, magnetic field generation poses a risk to patients of moving metallic, ferromagnetic projectiles while physically inside the scanner. Care must be taken to ensure protocols are in place to minimize this risk. Most prosthetic heart valves, vascular stents including coronary artery stents, and orthopedic implants are safe to be imaged using CMR. Recent data have also demonstrated that, in appropriately selected patients with implantable cardiac electronic devices, MRI can be safely performed as well.[6] In all cases in which there is a question on device MRI safety, the website www.mrisafety.com is a robust source of compiled information on the topic.

Future Directions

CMR has advanced rapidly in the past decade, and the clinical applications for its use continue to evolve. Ultrafast imaging through improved magnet design will continue to improve the logistic constraints associated with CMR. CMR holds promise for further assessment and characterization of atherosclerotic plaque burden and composition, and research is active in this area.

References

1. Kim RJ, Hillenbrand HB, Judd RM. Evaluation of myocardial viability by MRI. *Herz*. 2000;25(4):417-430.
2. Bolen MA, Popovic ZB, Rajiah P, et al. Cardiac MR assessment of aortic regurgitation: holodiastolic flow reversal in the descending aorta helps stratify severity. *Radiology*. 2011;260(1):98-104.
3. Kwon DH, Desai MY. Cardiac magnetic resonance in hypertrophic cardiomyopathy: current state of the art. *Expert Rev Cardiovasc Ther*. 2010;8(1):103-111.
4. Krombach GA, Hahn C, Tomars M, et al. Cardiac amyloidosis: MR imaging findings and T1 quantification, comparison with control subjects. *J Magn Reson Imaging*. 2007;25(6):1283-1287.
5. Zurick AO, Bolen MA, Kwon DH, et al. Pericardial delayed hyperenhancement with CMR imaging in patients with constrictive pericarditis undergoing surgical pericardiectomy: a case series with histopathological correlation. *JACC Cardiovasc Imaging*. 2011;4(11):1180-1191.
6. Nazarian S, Hansford R, Rahsepar AA, et al. Safety of magnetic resonance imaging in patients with cardiac devices. *N Eng J Med*. 2017;377:2555-2564.

19

Carotid Ultrasound

Alfred S. Callahan III, MD

Carotid atherostenosis is a cause of acute ischemic stroke through flow failure from local occlusion or activated plaque resulting in arterial to arterial embolism. Treatment of symptomatic stenotic plaques by surgical or endovascular means has been shown to provide benefit.[1,2] However, atherosclerotic plaque precedes stenosis by many decades. Carotid ultrasonography has been shown to identify carotid stenosis and also provide information about nonstenotic plaque.[3]

Advances in B-mode imaging permit assessment of the carotid arterial wall. Routine studies show the three components of the arterial wall (**Figure 19.1**) in the far wall of the common, internal and external carotid arteries. Such measurements of the intima and media thickness have been used in multiple studies for future vascular risk stratification.[4,5] Although initially the distal 2 cm of the common carotid artery was measured, currently a different approach is utilized.

It made little sense to measure a single segment of the common carotid artery when plaque was visible at the carotid bifurcation where it is more prevalent. From a biologic perspective, the use of B-mode imaging to identify plaque prior to stenosis might provide earlier identification of risk and permit programs of risk reduction.

The utility of carotid plaque identification was shown in the Framingham Off-Spring study. When plaque was defined as an intima-media thickness of 1.5 mm or greater, there was improvement in risk stratification beyond the Framingham Risk Score improving net reclassification.[6] Plus, measuring for plaque was technically easier than measuring the distance (height) of the blood intimal interface to the media-adventitia interface of the distal 2 cm of the common carotid artery.

However, the use of a "cut point" for plaque may not make biologic sense because lipid accumulation is time dependent.

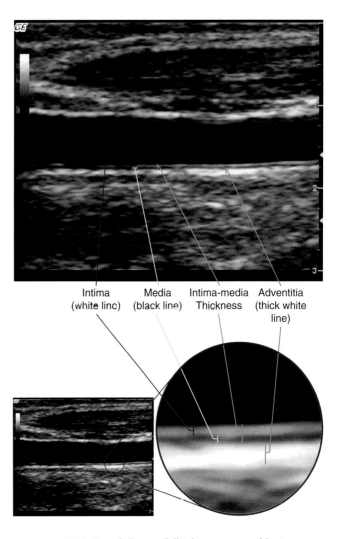

| Intima (white line) | Media (black line) | Intima-media Thickness | Adventitia (thick white line) |

Figure 19.1 *B-mode image of distal common carotid artery.*

A subject with a measure of 1.49 mm must surely be reclassified as having plaque when measured again after a year or so. If so, then subject went from no-plaque to plaque during the period of observation. Biologically, it makes better sense to consider the measure as an individual number, ie, quantitatively rather than categorically.

In more recent studies such as the Bioimage trial,[7] plaque was identified as a localized increase in intima-media thickness that is 50% larger than the surrounding 1 cm, a 0.5 mm encroachment into the lumen, or 1.5 mm or greater in thickness. The underlying presumption was that plaque was a localized collection of lipid in the subendothelial space rather than a specific number.

The Bioimage study compared plaque at any location in the common, internal or external carotid arteries against coronary artery calcium scores (CAC) and had clinical vascular events as the primary endpoint (MACE). Both baseline measures of CAC and plaque showed a relationship to future vascular risk. As either measure increased at baseline, then there was an increased risk of a vascular outcome during study time (Figure 19.2). Ultrasound measures were helpful in the 32% of the population with 0 CAC scores. The utility of identification of carotid plaque and its amount was proven to have benefit in predicting coronary endpoints as well as stroke.

Although the Bioimage trial utilized carotid plaque burden (CPB) for identification of plaque, the technology for this measure is not widely available. A post-hoc study of their dataset utilizing maximum carotid plaque thickness has been shown to produce comparable results.[8] Measurement of the summit of plaques can be accomplished with available ultrasound devices.

When a population without clinical vascular disease and most often not taking lipid-lowering therapy is studied, then unique populations are identified when plaque is plotted against entry LDL levels. As is seen in Figure 19.3, there are large numbers of subjects making plaques with LDL <100 mg/dL and occasional subjects with LDL >200 mg/dL who do not make plaque. The former population has lipid ingress with a small gradient of LDL across the arterial wall, whereas the latter population appears to be "galvanized" against their larger gradient. It is not known how long such galvanization might continue.

Other studies have looked at the morphology of the plaque surface and also the contents of the walls.[9] Alternative technologies including pixel distribution analysis, 3D ultrasonography, contrast enhanced ultrasonography, plaque strain measurement, and IVUS (intravascular ultrasound) are under investigation and have yet to find widespread clinical utility.[10]

Another way to consider carotid wall measures as a predictor of risk is the rate of lipid ingress or growth of plaque volume. Because at birth there is minimal thickness, it might be reasonable to consider plaque growth as a linear function of age in years. The maximum carotid wall thickness in any location is used as the numerator and divided by age in years. One then is able to calculate a rate of growth in mm/y which is called CIMTAR.

If the entire population can be divided into those with and without vascular risk (ie, lifetime vascular risk), then studying a normal population can help determine a rate "cut point" of plaque formers versus nonformers. The literature would suggest that a rate of 0.016 mm/y may have utility[11] (Figure 19.4). One potential advantage of a rate measure is the elimination of age-specific tables of normal wall thickness.

Serial measures of the maximum wall thickness may serve to guide risk reduction programs. The relative benefit shown in most statin trials has been 30% suggesting significant residual risk despite treatment. If annual measures of maximum carotid wall thickness continue to show an increase, then modification of treatment seems reasonable. The expected rate of plaque growth is found from CIMTAR. Optimal treatment should produce stabilization of maximum wall thickness/maximal plaque thickness or its regression. When plaque thickness or summits continue to increase despite best medical therapy, then vascular risk has not been mitigated.

Limitations to carotid wall measures include large neck sizes resulting in an arterial depth beyond the reaches of a 8 to 12 mHz probe, angled or looping arteries resulting in poor angles of insonation, heavily calcified plaques producing distal shadowing (signal absence), lateral wall plaques, patients with severe cervical spondylosis and stiff necks that cannot be rotated for optimal visualization, and extensive vascular calcification producing shadowing. Rarely, the examination has to be conducted in the sitting position, which adds technical difficulty.

Because the examination is operator dependent, high-quality data for risk stratification require a laboratory committed to careful and professional works. It is far easier to use carotid examinations looking for stenosis than to measure wall thickness at its largest identifying plaque. A stenotic plaque can be nearly an order of magnitude larger than wall thickness. To search for stenosis most laboratories rely on color flow analysis and quickly examine the visualized carotid tree for color shift. An identified area of color change can then be interrogated for velocity measures while the B-mode image is included afterward. It takes a patient technician to search the artery for plaque and then measure it at multiple points.

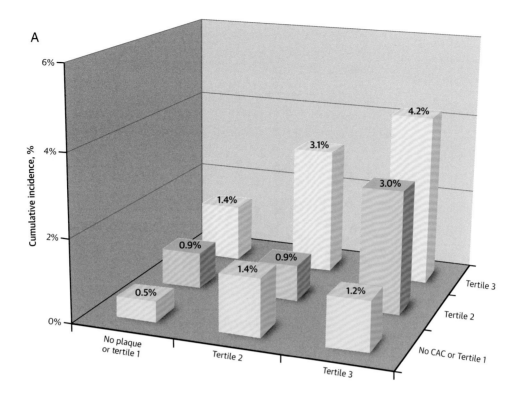

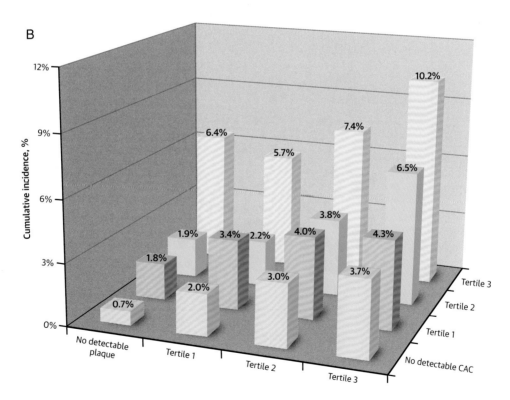

Figure 19.2 *Three-year rates for MACE endpoints by carotid and coronary atherosclerosis A, Primary MACE rates; B, secondary MACE rates. (From Baber U, et al. Prevalence, impact, and predictive value of detecting subclinical coronary and carotid atherosclerosis in asymptomatic adults: the BioImage study.* J Am Coll Cardiol. *2015;65(11):1065-1074.)*

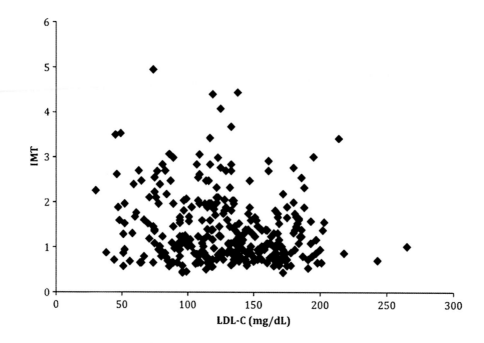

Figure 19.3 *LDL-C versus IMT—all patients (r = 0.17, P = .002). For patients not taking lipid-lowering therapy: r = 0.12, P = .07. LDL-C, low-density lipoprotein cholesterol; IMT, intima-media thickness. (From Callahan AS, Szarek M, Patton JW, et al. Maximum carotid artery wall thickness and risk factors in a young primary prevention population.* Brain and Behavior. *2012:1-5.)*

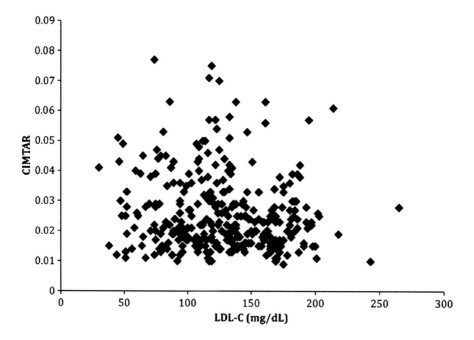

Figure 19.4 *LDL-C versus CIMTAR—all patients (r = 0.12, P = .03). For patients not taking lipid-lowering therapy: r = 0.06, P = .38. LDL-C, low-density lipoprotein cholesterol; CIMTAR, carotid intima-media thickness accretion rate. (From Callahan AS, Szarek M, Patton JW, et al. Maximum carotid artery wall thickness and risk factors in a young primary prevention population.* Brain and Behavior. *2012:1-5.)*

Summary

Identification of plaque formation by carotid wall measures of maximum intima-media thickness regardless of arterial location permits stratification of risk without or with risk factors and may guide treatments to reduce residual risk.

References

1. North American Symptomatic Carotid Endarterectomy Trial Collaborators; Barnett HJM, Taylor DW, Haynes RB, et al. Beneficial effect of carotid endarterectomy in symptomatic patients with high-grade carotid stenosis. *N Engl J Med.* 1991;325(7):445-453.

2. Brott TG, Hobson RW II, Howard G, et al. Stenting versus endarterectomy for treatment of carotid-artery stenosis. *N Engl J Med.* 2010;363(1):11-23. doi:10.1056/NEJMoa0912321. Epub 2010 May 26.

3. Walker MD, Marler JR, Goldstein M, et al. Endarterectomy for asymptomatic carotid artery stenosis. Executive Committee for the Asymptomatic Carotid Atherosclerosis Study. *JAMA.* 1995;273(18):1421-1428.

4. O'Leary DH, Polak JF, Kronmal RA, Manolio TA, Burke GL, Wolfson SK Jr. Carotid-artery intima and media thickness as a risk factor for myocardial infarction and stroke in older adults. Cardiovascular Health Study Collaborative Research Group. *N Engl J Med.* 1999;340(1):14-22.

5. Chambless LE, Heiss G, Folsom AR, et al. Association of coronary heart disease incidence with carotid arterial wall thickness and major risk factors: the Atherosclerosis Risk in Communities (ARIC) Study, 1987-1993. *Am J Epidemiol.* 1997;146(6):483-494.

6. Polak JF, Pencina MJ, Pencina KM, O'Donnell CJ, Wolf PA, D'Agostino RB Sr. Carotid-wall intima-media thickness and cardiovascular events. *N Engl J Med.* 2011;365(3):213-221. doi:10.1056/NEJMoa1012592.

7. Baber U, Mehran R, Sartori S, et al. Prevalence, impact, and predictive value of detecting subclinical coronary and carotid atherosclerosis in asymptomatic adults: the BioImage study. *J Am Coll Cardiol.* 2015;65(11):1065-1074. doi:10.1016/j.jacc.2015.01.017.

8. Sillesen H, Sartori S, Sandholt B, Baber U, Mehran R, Fuster V. Carotid plaque thickness and carotid plaque burden predict future cardiovascular events in asymptomatic adult Americans. *Eur Heart J Cardiovasc Imaging.* 2018;19(9):1042-1050. doi:10.1093/ehjci/jex239.

9. Schmidt C, Fagerberg B, Wikstrand J, Hulthe J; RIS Study Group. Multiple risk factor intervention reduces cardiovascular risk in hypertensive patients with echolucent plaques in the carotid artery. *J Intern Med.* 2003;253(4):430-438.

10. Cires-Drouet RS, Mozafarian M, Ali A, Sikdar S, Lal BK. Imaging of high-risk carotid plaques: ultrasound. *Semin Vasc Surg.* 2017;30(1):44-53. doi:10.1053/j.semvascsurg.2017.04.010. Epub 2017 April 27.

11. Callahan AS III, Szarek M, Patton JW, et al. Maximum carotid artery wall thickness and risk factors in a young primary prevention population. *Brain and Behavior.* 2012:1-5.

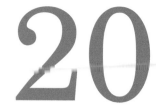

Complete and Advanced Cardiovascular Laboratory Testing

Mark C. Houston, MD, MS, MSc, FACP, FAHA, FASH, FACN, FAARM, ABAARM, DABC

A complete cardiovascular (CV) blood panel with both routine and advanced testing should be done to evaluate all of the top 25 modifiable risk factors and begin to address many of the complete list of 400 coronary heart disease (CHD) risk factors. Cardiovascular genomics and CV gene expression testing that may predict CHD risk should also be included in this evaluation (Tables 20.1-20.3).[1-5] If these tests are done, then the stratification of CHD risk is more accurate and treatment is more personalized and has more precision. This approach will reduce CHD events better by recognizing and treating previously underevaluated CHD risk factors and thus closing the "CHD GAP."

Table 20.1

TOP 25 MODIFIABLE CORONARY HEART DISEASE RISK FACTORS

- Hypertension (24-h ABM)
- Dyslipidemia (advanced lipid analysis)
- Hyperglycemia, metabolic syndrome, insulin resistance, and diabetes mellitus
- Obesity
- Smoking
- Hyperuricemia
- Renal disease
- Elevated fibrinogen
- Elevated serum iron
- Trans fatty acids and refined carbohydrates
- Low dietary omega-3 fatty acids
- Low dietary potassium and magnesium with high sodium intake
- Inflammation: increased hsCRP, MPO, interleukins
- Increased oxidative stress and decreased defense
- Increased immune dysfunction
- Lack of sleep
- Lack of exercise
- Stress, anxiety, and depression
- Homocysteinemia
- Subclinical hypothyroidism
- Hormonal imbalances in both genders
- Chronic clinical or subclinical infections
- Micronutrient deficiencies: numerous ones such as low vitamin D, K, E, and CoQ10
- Heavy metals
- Environmental pollutants

ABM, ambulatory blood pressure monitor; hsCRP, high-sensitivity C-reactive protein; MPO, myeloperoxidase.

Table 20.2

COMPLETE LIST OF ROUTINE AND ADVANCED CARDIOVASCULAR LABORATORY TESTS

- Complete blood count with differential
- Urinalysis
- Complete metabolic profile (CMP 12)
- Advanced lipid profile
- APO B, APO AI and AII
- Complete thyroid panel: Free T4, T3, TSH, RT3, thyroid antibodies
- Magnesium
- Iron, total iron-binding capacity, and ferritin
- Fibrinogen
- hsCRP
- Homocysteine
- Uric acid
- Microalbuminuria
- Gamma-glutamyl transpeptidase and hepatic profile
- Myeloperoxidase
- Cardiovascular genomics
- Toxicology and heavy metal screen: Spot or 24-h urine or blood
- Vitamin D3
- Fasting C peptide, hemoglobin AIC, insulin, proinsulin, 2-h glucose tolerance test
- Plasma renin activity and aldosterone
- Free testosterone, sex hormone-binding globulin, estradiol, estriol, progesterone, dehydroepiandrosterone (DHEA and DHEAS)
- Electrocardiogram
- Cardiopulmonary exercise test
- Chest x-ray
- Computerized arterial pulse wave analysis
- Endothelial Function Testing (ENDOPAT)
- Ankle brachial index at rest and with exercise
- Micronutrient testing
- Omega-3 index
- APO E
- Telomere test
- Body impedance analysis
- ECHO
- Carotid duplex and carotid intimal medial thickness
- Computerized CT angiogram
- Coronary artery calcium
- Retinal scan
- Rest and exercise blood pressure
- 24-h ambulatory blood pressure monitor
- CORUS gene expression testing
- PULS cardiac testing

APO, apolipoprotein; hsCRP, high-sensitivity C-reactive protein.

Table 20.3

GENERAL CLASSES FOR CORONARY HEART DISEASE RISK FACTORS

1. Genomics, SNPs, and epigenetics
2. Gender and age
3. Inflammation
4. Oxidative stress
5. Vascular immune dysfunction
6. Infections
7. Metabolic and nutritional
8. Toxins
9. Psychological and neurological
10. Sleep disturbances
11. Lack of exercise
12. Structural and hemodynamic
13. Hormonal

SNP, single-nucleotide polymorphism.

References

1. Houston Mark C. *What Your Doctor May Not Tell You About Heart Disease. The Revolutionary Book that Reveals the Truth Behind Coronary Illnesses and How You Can Fight Them. Grand Central Life and Style*. New York, NY, Hachette Book Group; 2012.
2. Houston MC. Nutrition and nutraceutical supplements in the treatment of hypertension. *Expert Rev Cardiovasc Ther*. 2010;8:821-833.
3. Houston MC, Basile J, Bestermann WH, et al. Addressing the global cardiovascular risk of hypertension, dyslipidemia, and insulin resistance in the southeastern United States. *Am J Med Sci*. 2005;329(6):276-291.
4. Bestermann W, Houston MC, Basile J, et al. Addressing the global cardiovascular risk of hypertension, dyslipidemia, diabetes mellitus, and the metabolic syndrome in the southeastern United States, part II: treatment recommendations for management of the global cardiovascular risk of hypertension, dyslipidemia, diabetes mellitus, and the metabolic syndrome. *Am J Med Sci*. 2005;329(6):292-305.
5. Houston M. The role of nutraceutical supplements in the treatment of dyslipidemia. *J Clin Hypertens (Greenwich)*. 2012;14(2):121-132.

Section 7

SPECIAL POPULATIONS AND CARDIOVASCULAR DISEASE

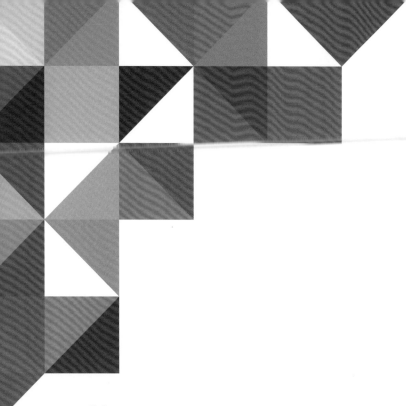

21

Integrative Management of Hypertension: Pathophysiology, Epidemiology, Clinical Aspects, Diagnosis, Prevention, and Treatment With Nutrition, Nutritional Supplements, Lifestyle, and Drugs

Mark C. Houston, MD, MS, MSc, FACP, FAHA, FASH, FACN, FAARM, ABAARM, DABC

Introduction

Cardiovascular disease (CVD) remains the leading cause of death in the United States, is the most common reason for visits to primary care physicians with over 20 billion USD expenditure annually in antihypertensive drug costs, and is one of the top five coronary heart disease (CHD) risk factors.[1-19] There are over 100 million people in the United States with hypertension based on new hypertension guidelines.[19] In numerous clinical trials, pharmacotherapy will control blood pressure (BP) and reduce stroke, CHD, myocardial infarction (MI), congestive heart failure (CHF), and renal disease.[16,17] However, some hypertensive patients either refuse to take drugs or prefer to treat with nutrition or nutritional supplements, if appropriate, as recognized by national and international guidelines.[1-20]

Hypertension is a consequence of micro- and macronutrient insufficiencies, abnormal vascular biology, reduced bioavailability of nitric oxide (NO), and the three finite vascular responses to injury that include inflammation, oxidative stress, and vascular immune dysfunction[2-5,11-14] (Figure 21.1). These abnormalities coexist and interact with genetics, epigenetics, nutrient-gene expression, and other environmental and lifestyle factors.[2-5,11-14] Hypertension is the "correct" but chronic dysregulated response of these infinite insults to the endothelium with gene expression patterns in which the vascular system becomes an innocent bystander.[2-5,11-14]

Hypertension is one of several responses of the blood vessel to endothelial dysfunction (ED), cardiac smooth muscle, vascular dysfunction, and abnormalities of both microvascular function and structure, which may precede the development of hypertension by decades. This consequently leads to vascular and cardiac hypertrophy, remodeling, functional and structural network rarefaction, decreased vasodilatory reserve, altered media to lumen ratio, stiffness, loss of arterial elasticity, fibrosis, increased pulse pressure, elevated pulse wave velocity (PWV), and increased augmentation index (AI) (Figure 21.2).[2-5,11-14] Significant functional, then structural microvascular impairment begins before elevations in BP in normotensive offspring of hypertensive parents.[2-5,11-14]

As the BP increases, a bidirectional feedback occurs that exacerbates and perpetuates the cardiovascular functional and structural abnormalities. Macronutrients and micronutrients are crucial in the regulation of BP and subsequent cardiovascular target organ damage (TOD)[2-5,11-14] and are more common in patients with hypertension than in the general population.[2-5,11-14] The appropriate measurement, interpretation, and treatment of these nutrient deficiencies may effectively lower BP and improve ED, vascular and cardiac functional and structural abnormalities, and CV events.[2-5,11-14]

This chapter will primarily review the role of nutrition and selected nutraceutical supplements, minerals, vitamins, anti-inflammatory agents, natural immune modulators, and antioxidants in the treatment of hypertension.

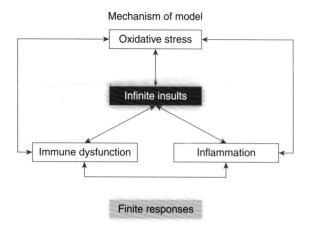

Mechanism of model

Figure 21.1 *Infinite insults to the blood vessel result in only three finite responses of inflammation, oxidative stress, and vascular immune dysfunction.*

Epidemiology and Pathophysiology

The human genome is 99.9% identical to our Paleolithic ancestors, but the changes in modern nutrition and macronutrient and micronutrient intake impair our ability to reduce CVD[21] (Table 21.1). Vascular biology assumes a pivotal role in the initiation

Table 21.1

CONTRASTING THE INTAKE OF NUTRIENTS INVOLVED IN VASCULAR BIOLOGY. EVOLUTIONARY NUTRITIONAL IMPOSITIONS

Nutrient	Paleolithic Intake	Modern Intake
Potassium	>10,000 mEq/d (256 g)	150 mEq/d (6 g)
Sodium	<50 mmol/d (1.2 g)	175 mmol/d (4 g)
Sodium/potassium ratio	<0.13/d	>0.67/d
Fiber	>100 g/d	9 g/d
Protein	37%	20%
Carbohydrate	41%	40%-50%
Fat	22%	30%-40%
Polyunsaturated/saturated fat ratio	1.4	0.4

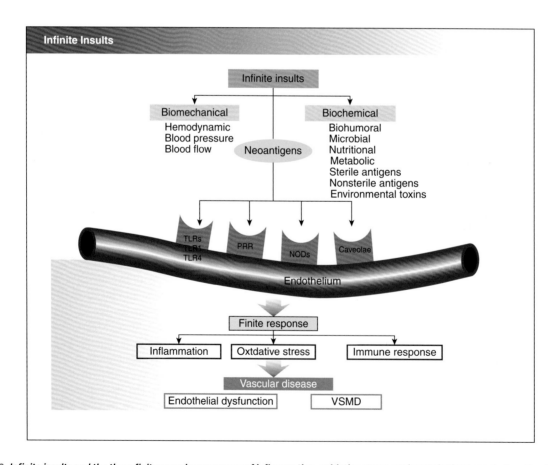

Figure 21.2 *Infinite insults and the three finite vascular responses of inflammation, oxidative stress, and vascular immune dysfunction lead to endothelial dysfunction and cardiac and vascular dysfunction.*

and perpetuation of hypertension.[2-5,11-14] Radical oxygen species (ROS) coupled with impaired oxidative defense, inflammatory mediators, vascular immune dysfunction, and loss of nitric oxide bioavailability contribute to hypertension through complex nutrient-gene interactions.[2-5,11-14,22-32] The high Na$^+$/K$^+$ ratio of modern diets, the reduced intake of magnesium, fiber, protein, and omega-3 fatty acids with increased consumption of omega-6 fatty acids, saturated fat (SFA), and trans fatty acids (TFA) have contributed to hypertension.[2-5,11-14,21]

The Three Finite Vascular Responses and Cardiovascular Disease (Figures 21.1 and 21.2)

Oxidative Stress, Inflammation, and Vascular Immune Dysfunction

Oxidative stress is an imbalance of ROS with a decrease in antioxidant defenses that contributes to hypertension in humans based on genetics and environment.[2-5,11-14,23-37] The predominant ROS produced is superoxide anion, which is generated by numerous cellular sources, will uncouple endothelium-derived NO synthase (U-eNOS) and reduce nitric oxide bioavailability, induces ED, and increases BP.[24,27] Antioxidant deficiency and excess free radical production have been implicated in human hypertension in epidemiologic, observational, and interventional studies.[29-31] These degrade NO, influence eicosanoid metabolism, and increase catecholamine levels in serum and urine.[2-5,11-14,24,26,27] The interrelations of neurohormonal systems, oxidative stress, and CVD are shown in Figure 21.3.

Acute and chronic inflammation with abnormal vascular immune responses and pattern recognition receptors (PRRs) and toll-like receptors (TLRs) are involved in hypertension.[2-5,11-14,33-50] Low levels of IL-10 (interleukin 10) and increased levels of high-sensitivity C-reactive protein (hs-CRP), numerous inflammatory cytokines such as interleukins (IL-6, IL-1b, IL-2, and IL-8), and tumor necrosis factor alpha (TNF-α) are excellent markers for hypertension and hypertensive-related TOD, such as CHD, CHF, and increased carotid intima-media thickness (IMT).[2-5,11-14,33-50] Elevated hs-CRP is both a risk marker and risk factor for hypertension and CVD.[2,38,39] Increases in hs-CRP of over 3 µg/mL may increase BP rapidly that is proportional to the serum hs-CRP level.[38,39] Nitric oxide and endothelial nitric oxide synthase (eNOS) are inhibited by hs-CRP.[38,39] The angiotensin 2 receptor (AT2R), which increases NO when stimulated, normally counterbalances AT1R but it is downregulated or blocked by hs-CRP.[2,38,39] Angiotensin II (A-II) is inflammatory, atherogenic, increases oxidative stress and vascular immune dysfunction, and upregulates many of the cytokines.[2,44,49]

Innate and adaptive immune responses induce hypertension by numerous mechanisms that include angiotensin II, antibodies to the AT1R, cytokine and chemokine production, PRR and TLR activation, central nervous system (CNS) stimulation, and renal damage.[2-4,35,36,40-50] Monocytes cross the endothelial lining, invade the subintimal layer, transform into macrophages and various T-cell subtypes that regulate BP, cause vascular damage, and promote vascular immune dysfunction.[41] Angiotensin II activates immune cells directly and in the CNS via T cells, macrophages, and dendritic cells and promotes cell infiltration into target organs.[41,44,49] Activation of the AT1R and PPAR (peroxisome proliferator-activated

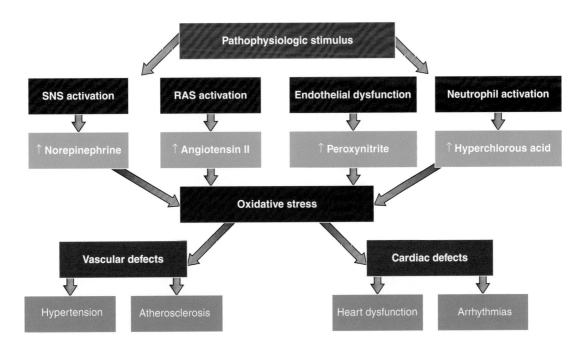

Figure 21.3 *The neurohormonal and oxidative stress systems with interactions on cardiac and vascular muscle.*

receptor) gamma receptors that are expressed on CD4+ T lymphocytes releases TNF-α, interferon, and interleukins within the vascular wall.[41,50] Interleukin 17 (IL-17) produced by T-17 cells may play a pivotal role in the genesis and perpetuation of hypertension caused by angiotensin II.[41]

The Balance of Hypertension

Hypertension is a balance of vascular damage and repair that is mediated through the three finite responses: angiotensin II, endothelin, and aldosterone (**Figures 21.4** and **21.5**).[2-5,11-14] The vascular protection and repair is mediated by nitric oxide and bone marrow–derived endothelial progenitor cells (EPCs).[2-5,11-14] The endothelium maintains communication and homeostasis between the circulating blood cells and the vascular media by modulation of the permeability, contractile state, proliferation, migratory response, and the redox state in the vascular media and modulates platelet function, coagulation, monocyte and leukocyte adhesion, inflammation, oxidative stress and immune responses in the blood[2-5,11-14] (**Figures 21.6** and **21.7**).

Treatment of Hypertension With Nutritional Supplements

A large number of nutraceutical supplements, antioxidants, vitamins, minerals, and natural compounds in food produce physiologic effects that mimic specific classes of

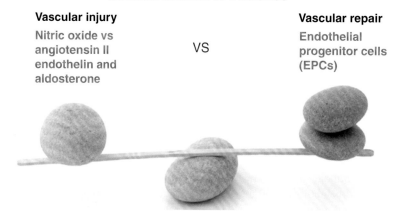

Vascular disease is a balance

Vascular injury

Nitric oxide vs angiotensin II endothelin and aldosterone

VS

Vascular repair

Endothelial progenitor cells (EPCs)

Figure 21.4 *Cardiovascular disease is a balance of vascular injury and vascular repair. (Adapted from Houston MC.* Vascular Biology in Clinical Practice. *Hanley & Belfus: Philadelphia, PA; 2000 and Houston MC.* Handbook of Hypertension. *Wiley- Blackwell: Oxford, UK; 2009.)*

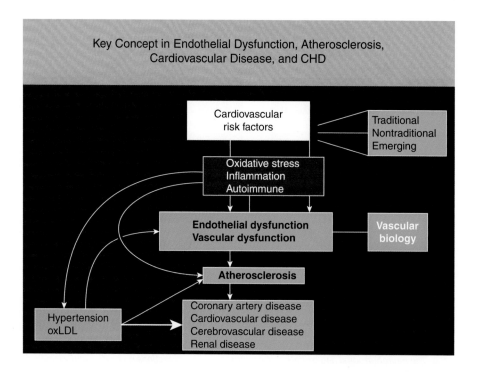

Figure 21.5 *The three finite responses and vascular biology play a key role between CHD risk factors, endothelial and CV dysfunction, and CVD. (From Houston MC.* Handbook of Hypertension. *Wiley- Blackwell: Oxford, UK; 2009. Copyright © 2009 Mark Houston.)*

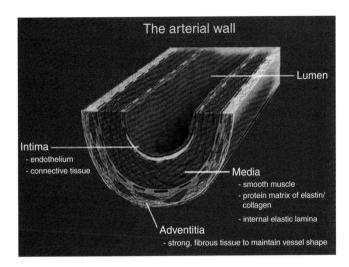

Figure 21.6 *The blood vessel structure: endothelium, smooth muscle, and adventitia. (Modified from Ross R. Atherosclerosis—an inflammatory disease.* N Engl J Med. *1999;340:115-126 and Mulvany MJ, et al. Structure and function of small arteries.* Physiol Rev. *1990;70:921-961.)*

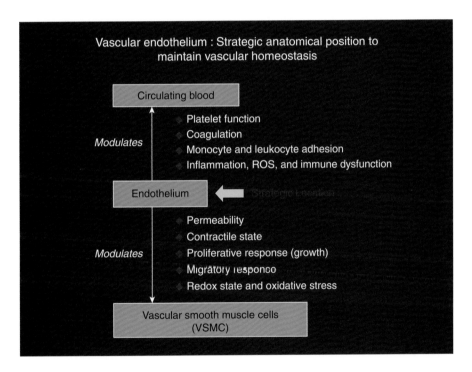

Figure 21.7 *The endothelium has a strategic location and function to maintain communication and homeostasis between the circulating blood elements and the vascular smooth muscle. (Adapted from Houston MC.* Vascular Biology in Clinical Practice. *Hanley & Belfus: Philadelphia, PA; 2000 and Houston MC.* Handbook of Hypertension. *Wiley- Blackwell: Oxford, UK; 2009.)*

antihypertensive medications, improve vascular biology, and decrease BP.[2-14] These natural compounds can be classified into the major antihypertensive drug groups such as diuretics, beta blockers, central alpha agonists (CAAs), calcium channel blockers (CCBs), angiotensin-converting enzyme inhibitors (ACEIs), and angiotensin receptor blockers (ARBs)[2-14] (Table 21.2). Numerous clinical nutrition studies have demonstrated the efficacy of dietary interventions for the prevention and treatment of hypertension. These include Dietary Approaches to Stop Hypertension (DASH 1 and DASH 2), the Mediterranean diet, Trials of Hypertension Prevention

(TOHP 1 and TOHP 2), Trial of Nonpharmacologic Intervention in the Elderly (TONE), Treatment of Mild Hypertension (TOMHS), INTERMAP, INTERSALT, Premier, Vanguard, and others.[2-5,10-14,51,52]

Sodium (Na⁺)

Increased dietary sodium intake is associated with hypertension, CVA, left ventricular hypertrophy (LVH), diastolic dysfunction (DD), CHD, MI, renal insufficiency, proteinuria, arterial stiffness, platelet dysfunction, and increased

Table 21.2

NATURAL ANTIHYPERTENSIVE COMPOUNDS CATEGORIZED BY ANTIHYPERTENSIVE CLASS

Antihypertensive Therapeutic Class (Alphabetical listing)	Foods and Ingredients Listed by Therapeutic Class	Nutrients and Other Supplements Listed by Therapeutic Class
Angiotensin converting enzyme inhibitors	Egg yolk Fish (specific): 　Bonito 　Dried salted fish 　Fish sauce 　Sardine muscle/protein 　Tuna Garlic Gelatin Hawthorne berry Isoflavones/flavonoids Milk products (specific): 　Casein 　Sour milk 　Whey (hydrolyzed) Protein Sake Sea vegetables (kelp) Seaweed (Wakame) Sesame (also ET1) Wheat germ (hydrolyzed) Zein (corn protein)	Melatonin Omega-3 fatty acids Pomegranate Probiotics Pycnogenol Quercetin Zinc
Angiotensin receptor blockers	Celery Fiber Garlic MUFA	Coenzyme Q-10 Gamma-linolenic acid NAC Oleic acid Resveratrol Potassium Taurine Vitamin C Vitamin B6 (pyridoxine)
Beta blockers	Hawthorne berry	
Calcium channel blockers	Celery Garlic Hawthorn berry MUFA	Alpha lipoic acid Calcium Magnesium (PGE,NO) N-acetylcysteine Oleic acid Omega-3 fatty acids: 　Eicosapentaenoic acid 　Docosahexaenoic acid Taurine Vitamin B6 Vitamin C Vitamin E
Central alpha agonists (reduce sympathetic nervous system activity)	Celery Fiber Garlic Protein	Coenzyme Q-10 Gamma-linolenic acid Potassium Probiotics Restriction of sodium Taurine Vitamin C Vitamin B6 Zinc

Table 21.2

NATURAL ANTIHYPERTENSIVE COMPOUNDS CATEGORIZED BY ANTIHYPERTENSIVE CLASS—CONT'D

Antihypertensive Therapeutic Class (Alphabetical listing)	Foods and Ingredients Listed by Therapeutic Class	Nutrients and Other Supplements Listed by Therapeutic Class
Direct renin inhibitors		Vitamin D
Direct vasodilators	Beets (NO, ED) Celery Cocoa (NO, ED) Cooking oils with monounsaturated fats Fiber Garlic Hesperidin and OJ Lycopene food (NO, ED) MUFA Soy Teas: green and black	Alpha-linolenic acid Arginine Calcium Carnitines (eNOS,NO) Flavonoids Grape seed extract Lycopene (NO, ED) Magnesium Melatonin (NO, ED) Omega-3 fatty acids (NO, ED) Potassium (NO, ED) Taurine Vitamin C Vitamin E
Diuretics	Celery Fiber Hawthorn berry Protein	Calcium Coenzyme Q-10 Fiber Gamma-linolenic acid ʟ-carnitine Magnesium Potassium Taurine Vitamin B6 Vitamin C Vitamin E: high gamma/delta tocopherols and tocotrienols

sympathetic nervous system (SNS) activation. A reduction in dietary sodium intake lowers BP and the risk of all of these diseases.[2-5,10-15,18,19,53-61] Decreasing dietary sodium intake in hypertensive patients, especially the salt-sensitive patients, lowers BP by 4 to 6/2 to 3 mm Hg proportional to the amount of sodium restriction[54] and may prevent or delay hypertension in high-risk patients.

Salt sensitivity, defined as a >10% increase in mean arterial pressure (MAP) with salt loading, increases the BP response to dietary salt intake in 51% of hypertensive patients.[57,58] Cardiovascular events may be more common in salt-sensitive patients compared with salt-resistant patients, independent of BP level.[57,58] Decreasing sodium intake to below 1500 to 2300 mg/d was associated with lower BP and a decrease in all-cause mortality, whereas increasing the intake to >2300 mg/d was associated with an increase in all-cause mortality and CVD.[56]

Sodium promotes hypertension by increasing endothelial cell stiffness; reducing the size and pliability of endothelial cells; decreasing eNOS and NO production; elevating asymmetric dimethyl arginine (ADMA), oxidative stress, and TGF-β; and abolishing the AT 2 receptor–mediated

vasodilation.[59,60,62] All of these effects are increased in the presence of aldosterone, which mimics these same pathophysiologic changes.[59,60,63] Endothelial cells act as **vascular salt sensors**.[59,60]

A balance of sodium with potassium and magnesium improves BP control and lowers cardiovascular and cerebrovascular events.[2,63-67] Increasing the sodium to potassium ratio increases BP and the risk of CVD, but increasing the potassium to sodium ratio lowers BP and CVD risk.[64-67] A potassium/sodium ratio of 4:1 is recommended with a daily dietary sodium intake of 1500 mg and a dietary potassium intake of 6000 mg.[2,64-67]

Potassium

Increased dietary potassium intake reduces BP and CVD.[64-71] The minimal recommended intake of K^+ is 4700 mg/d (120 mmol) with a K^+/Na^+ ratio 4-5:1.[64-71] Potassium supplementation at 60 mmol of KCl per day for 12 weeks significantly reduced SBP −5.0 mm Hg in 150 Chinese subjects.[68] Prospective studies in a meta-analysis found that 1.64 g or more per day of potassium intake resulted in a 21% lower risk of stroke ($P = .0007$) and a lower risk of CHD and total CVD. In another meta-analysis, potassium supplementation resulted in modest but significant reductions in both SBP −4.25 mm Hg and DBP 2.53 mm Hg.[70] Studies indicate a dose-related reduction in BP of 4.4/2.5 mm Hg to 8/4.1 mm Hg with potassium supplementation with doses between 60 to 120 mmol per day.[2-14,64-71] Increased dietary potassium reduces CHD, MI, CHF, LVH, diabetes mellitus (DM), and cardiac arrhythmias independent of BP reduction.[68] The incidence of CVA is reduced proportional to BP reduction but also is independent of the BP reduction.[2-14,64-71] Chronic serum levels of potassium below 4.0 meq/dL increase CVD mortality, ventricular tachycardia, ventricular fibrillation, and CHF.[2-14,64-71] Red blood cell potassium is a better indication of total body stores than serum potassium,[2-14] and it lowers NADPH oxidase, which reduces oxidative stress and inflammation.[2-14,64-71]

For each 1000 mg increase of daily dietary potassium, the all-cause mortality is reduced by 20% and for each 1000 mg decrease of daily dietary sodium intake all-cause mortality is decreased by 20%.[64] The recommended daily dietary intake of potassium is 6 g in hypertensive patients with normal renal function, those not taking potassium-retaining medications, or in those with some other contraindication.[2-14,64-71] Potassium sources include dark green leafy vegetables and fruits, nutritional supplements such as "No Salt" (KCL) substitutes, pure potassium powders or capsules or combined potassium/magnesium powders or capsules, and prescription KCL.[2-4]

Magnesium (Mg⁺⁺)

There is an inverse relationship between dietary magnesium intake and BP.[65,72-76] In clinical trials an increased dietary magnesium of 500 to 1000 mg/d lowers BP, but compared with dietary potassium intake the BP results are less.[65,72-76] Significant reductions in BP of 5.6/2.8 mm Hg, as documented by 24-hour ambulatory BP monitoring, home and office blood BP readings, usually take about 2 months.[72] A meta-analysis of trials found that Mg⁺⁺ supplementation of over 370 mg daily reduced BP 3 to 4 ± 2 mmHg/2.5 ± 1 mm Hg.[75] A more recent meta-analysis (34 trials and 2028 participants) showed that Mg⁺⁺ supplementation dosed at 368 mg/d for 3 months reduced BP 2.00/1.78 mm Hg[74]. The combination of high potassium and magnesium combined with a low sodium intake potentiates the antihypertensive effects in both treated and untreated hypertensive subjects .[65,72-76] Magnesium also competes with Na⁺ and calcium on vascular smooth muscle binding sites, simulates the effects of CCBs, and increases nitric oxide levels and endothelial function.[2,72-76]

Intracellular erythrocyte levels of magnesium are a more accurate assessment of total body stores compared to serum levels.[2,65,76] Magnesium formulations chelated to an amino acid, especially magnesium with taurine provides additional BP reduction.[2,65,76] Transdermal preparations of magnesium and magnesium salt baths are also effective.[2,65,76] A

high-magnesium diet or magnesium supplements must be used with caution in patients taking medications that promote magnesium retention, in those with known renal insufficiency or those with other contraindications to high doses of magnesium intake.[2,65,76]

Calcium (Ca⁺⁺)

Calcium supplementation is not recommended as an effective means to reduce BP until more studies are done on specific populations and age groups and the proper formulation and dose is identified.[77-80] The only exception is that calcium may reduce the risk of preeclampsia and its comorbidities for both mother and fetus.[80]

Zinc (Zn⁺⁺)

Low serum zinc levels correlate with hypertension and other CV problems.[2,81,82] There is an inverse correlation between BP, serum Zn⁺⁺, and Zn⁺⁺-dependent enzyme-lysyl oxidase activity in hypertensive subjects.[2,82] Zinc is transported into cardiac and vascular muscle and other tissues by metallothionein.[81] Genetic deficiencies of metallothionein lead to intramuscular zinc deficiencies and hypertension.[81] Zinc reduces the oxidative stress, inflammation, and immune dysfunction and balances the RAAS (renin-angiotensin-aldosterone system) and SNS.[1,2,57,58,81,82] Dietary zinc intake should be approximately 50 mg per day and levels should be monitored.[1]

Protein

Lower blood pressure is associated with an increased intake of animal protein and plant-based protein depending on the type of fat present in animal protein.[2,6,83-113] Lean or wild animal protein with a higher content of essential omega-3 fatty acids and reduced saturated fats improves hypertension.[84-87,113] Dietary protein intake 30% above the mean had a 3.0/2.5 mm Hg lower BP compared to protein intake 30% below the mean (81 vs. 44 g/d).[2,83]

In a meta-analysis of 40 RCTs compared with carbohydrate, dietary animal and vegetable protein intake was associated with significant changes in mean BP 1.2/0.6 mm Hg.[6,86]

In a randomized crossover study of 352 prehypertension and stage I hypertension subjects, soy protein and milk protein significantly reduced SBP 2.0 and 2.3 mm Hg, respectively with no change in DBP compared to a high–glycemic index diet.[87] Soy protein intake of 25 g/d over 3 years was associated with lower BP of 1.9/0.9 mm Hg in 45,694 Chinese women.[99] Randomized clinical trials and meta-analysis of soy protein in hypertensive subjects indicate an average reduction in BP of 5.9/3.3 mm Hg.[9 9-101,103,104,106] The recommended daily intake of fermented soy is 25 g.[2]

Whey protein, milk peptides, fermented milk, and casein significantly lower BP in humans.[2,6,88-93,102,108-113] Administration of 20 g/d of hydrolyzed whey protein lowered BP within 6 weeks by 8.0/5.5 mm Hg.[89] Milk peptides are rich in ACEI peptides which lower BP approximately 4.8/2.2 mm Hg with doses of 5 to 60 mg/d.[2,6,88-93,102] Powdered fermented milk containing *Lactobacillus helveticus and active ACEI peptides* dosed at 12 g daily significantly reduced BP by 11.2/6.5 mm Hg in 1 month.[90]

Administration of 20 g of hydrolyzed whey protein to hypertensive subjects lowered BP 11/7 mm Hg compared to controls within 1 week.[93] The WHEY2Go trial[108] was a double-blinded, randomized, 3-way-crossover, controlled intervention study of 42 participants who were randomly assigned to consume 56 g of whey protein, 56 g of calcium caseinate, or 54 g of maltodextrin (control)/day for 8 weeks separated by a 4-week washout.

The 24-hour ambulatory blood pressure monitoring (ABM) reductions in BP were 3.9/2.5 mm Hg ($P = .05$); the peripheral and central SBP fell 5.7 mm Hg ($P = .007$) and −5.4 mm Hg ($P = .012$), respectively, after whey protein consumption compared with the control group.[108] Whey protein improves endothelial function, stimulates opioid receptors, and improves PWV.

Marine collagen peptides (MCPs) derived from deep sea fish have antihypertensive activity.[94-96] Bonito protein (*Sarda orientalis*) from the tuna and mackerel family has natural ACEI inhibitory peptides and lowers BP 10.2/7 mm Hg with a dose of 1.5 g daily.[95] Administration of MCPs in a double-blind placebo-controlled trial of 100 hypertensive-diabetic subjects for 3 months significantly reduced DBP and MAP (mean arterial pressure).[94]

Sardine muscle protein lowered BP 9.7/5.3 mm Hg ($P < .05$) over 4 weeks in 29 hypertensive subjects at a dose of 3 mg of VAL-TYR (a sardine muscle concentrated extract).[97] A vegetable drink with sardine protein hydrolysates also reduced BP by 8/5 mm Hg over 13 weeks.[98]

The daily recommended intake of protein from all sources is 1.0 to 1.5 g/kg body weight, depending on exercise level, gender, age, hepatic and renal function, medications such as proton pump inhibitors and H_2 blockers, and concomitant medical diseases.[2]

L-Arginine

L-arginine lowers BP in humans with a low side effect profile and to levels similar to the DASH diet.[114-126] L-arginine and endogenous methylarginines are the primary precursors for the eNOS to produce nitric oxide (NO).[114-120]

Intracellular arginine levels far exceed the K(m) of eNOS under normal physiological conditions, but endogenous NO formation depends on extracellular arginine concentration. NO production by endothelial cells is closely coupled to cellular arginine transport mechanisms to regulate NO-dependent functions such as increasing renal vascular flow, renal perfusion, renal tubular NO bioavailability, and BP.[119]

Parenteral and oral L-arginine administration in hypertensive and normotensive subjects lowers BP significantly at doses of 10 to 12 g/d in food or as a supplement lowers BP by about 6.2/6.8 mm Hg in both office and 24-hour ABM readings.[114,115,121,123,124] Arginine administered at 4 g

daily significantly lowered BP in gestational hypertension, reduced concomitant antihypertensive, therapy and improved maternal and neonatal outcomes with normal delivery time.[121,122] The combination of arginine (1200 mg per day) and N-acetylcysteine (600 mg bid) administered over 6 months to hypertensive patients with type 2 diabetes lowered SBP and DBP ($P < .05$).[123] Arginine may have a pro-oxidative effect and increase in mortality in patients with advanced atherosclerosis, CHD, acute coronary syndrome, or MI[125]. Pending more studies, arginine is best avoided in these situations.

Taurine

Taurine is a conditionally essential sulfur-based amino acid that is efficacious for the treatment of hypertension and a variety of CVDs by reducing SNS activity, plasma norepinephrine, plasma and urinary epinephrine.[2-5,14,127-133] In addition, taurine increases urinary sodium and water excretion, atrial natriuretic factor, NO bioavailability, improves ED, and increases EPCs, while it decreases plasma renin activity (PRA), A-II, and aldosterone.[2-5,127-129] Nineteen hypertensive subjects administered 6 g of taurine resulted in lowered BP by 9/4.1 mm Hg ($P < .05$) in 7 days.[128] In a randomized, double-blind, placebo-controlled study over 12 weeks in 120 prehypertensive individuals, taurine supplementation (1.6 g/d) significantly improved endothelial function and decreased the clinic and 24-hour ambulatory BP reading 7.2/2.6 mm Hg and 4.7/1.3 mm Hg, respectively.[132] In another 4-month study of 97 prehypertensive individuals, 1.6 g/d of taurine significantly decreased the clinic and 24-hour ambulatory BPs, improved endothelium-vasodilation, and reduced the carotid IMT.[132]

In a DBRPC study of 42 hypertensive subjects evaluated over 1 month, a combination powder dietary supplement was given once daily.[133] The supplement included 6 g of taurine, vitamin C (as magnesium ascorbate) at 1000 mg, grape seed extract at 150 mg, magnesium ascorbate at 87 mg, vitamin B6 (pyridoxine HCl) at 100 mg, vitamin D 3 at 2000 IU, and biotin at 2 mg. The active group had a reduction in BP of 16/11.35 mm Hg ($P < .001$) at week 4. The recommended dose of taurine is 1.5 to 6 g/d as a single dose or as divided doses.[2,127-133]

Omega-3 Fats and Selected Omega-6 Fats

Omega-3 fatty acids derived from food or nutritional supplements produce a dose-related reduction in BP and CVD in published human studies.[2-14,113,134-149]

A meta-analysis of 70 RCTs found that, compared with placebo, the consumption of omega-3 PUFAs (0.3-15 g/d) for 4 to 26 weeks significantly reduced BP 1.5/1.0 mm Hg.[143] The largest BP reductions were in untreated hypertensive subjects (SBP = −4.5 [95% CI −6.1, −2.8] mmHg; DBP = −3.0 [95% CI −4.3, −1.7] mm Hg).[143] A second meta-analysis of RCTs found that omega-3 fatty acid supplementation for 6 to 105 weeks at 900 to 3000 mg/d improved the PWV ($P < .01$) and arterial compliance ($P < .001$).[144]

DHA is more effective than EPA in reducing the BP by an average of 8/5 mm Hg and also lowering the resting heart rate by 6 beats per minute and improving heart rate variability.[2-14,134-136,139-141]

Administration of EPA and DHA is preferred to ALA because of minimal conversion to these longer chain omega-3 fatty acids.[2-14,135,137] The consumption of coldwater fish three times per week reduces BP because of the combination of protein and omega-3 fatty acids.[2-14,107,135] In patients with chronic kidney disease, 4 g of omega-3 fatty acids significantly lowered 24-hour BP (ABM) by 3.3/2.9 mm Hg compared to placebo ($P < .0001$).[136] The omega-6 fatty acids, gamma-linolenic acid (GLA) and dihomo-gamma-linolenic acid (DGLA), reduce BP and prevent elevations in BP induced by saturated fats.[140] GLA blocks stress-induced hypertension, lowers aldosterone levels, decreases the adrenal AT1R density and affinity, and increases the vasodilating prostaglandins E 1 (PGE1) and PGE 2.[2-14,140]

The omega-3 fatty acids reduce CHD and MI[149]; increase eNOS and NO; improve endothelial function; reduce arterial stiffness; decrease PWV, insulin resistance, and plasma norepinephrine; suppress ACE activity; and increase parasympathetic tone at doses of 900 to 3000 mg daily.[2-14,134,142,145] The recommended daily dose is 3000 to 5000 mg/d of combined DHA and EPA in a ratio of 3 parts EPA to 2 parts DHA with 50% of this dose as GLA combined with gamma/delta tocopherol at 100 mg/g of DHA and EPA to get the RBC membrane and omega-3 index at 8%.[2-5] There are no adverse effects or safety concerns at these recommended doses.[2-14]

Monounsaturated Fatty Acids: Olive Oil, Mediterranean Diet, Omega-9 Fats, Oleic Acid, and Olive Leaf Extract

The Mediterranean diet (MedDiet), which is rich in olive oil and olive leaf extracts (OLEs), reduces BP and CVD in most clinical trials.[2-14,150-172] In an open study over 2 months, 40 borderline hypertensive monozygotic twins given either 500 or 1000 mg/d of OLE had significant reductions in BP of 6/5 mm Hg (500 mg of OLE) and 13/5 mm Hg reduction (1000 of OLE) compared to controls.[170] In another RDBPC trial, the BP decreased 8/6 mm Hg ($P < .01$) in office and 24-hour ABM, and the need for antihypertensive medications was reduced by 48% in the MUFA group ($P < .005$).[150] EVOO (extra virgin olive oil) lowered the SBP by 14 mm Hg in elderly hypertensive patients ($P < .01$).[151,152] Extra virgin olive oil contains lipid-soluble phytonutrients such as nitrates and polyphenols, which lower BP by reducing oxidative stress and oxLDL, blocking the AT1R, altering RAAS and endothelin gene expression, increasing nitric oxide levels and endothelial-induced vasodilation, and blocking calcium channels similar to a CCB.[147,150,154,161-163] EVOO with a total phenol content of at least 161 mg/kg at 20 to 40 g (2-4 tablespoons) per day will significantly lower SBP in about 3 weeks. EVOO with 300 mg/kg of total phenols may also decrease DBP.[2-5,167]

A total of 166 elderly subjects were prescribed a MedDiet or their habitual diet (HabDiet; control) for 6 months.[171] The MedDiet, compared with the HabDiet, lowered SBP by 1.1 mm Hg and improved flow-mediated vasodilation (FMD) at 6 months ($P = .01$). The INTERMAP trial found that dietary monounsaturated fatty acid intake, especially oleic acid from vegetable sources, may contribute to prevention and control of adverse blood pressure levels in general populations.[172]

In the European Prospective Investigation into Cancer and Nutrition (EPIC) study (20,343 subjects), the intake of EVOO and polyphenols documented an inverse relationship with SBP and DBP.[168] In the Prevention with Mediterranean Diet (PREDIMED) trial that included 7447 patients at high risk for CVD, the participants on the Mediterranean diet supplemented with EVOO had a significantly lower DBP than those in the control group (1.5 mm Hg).[169]

OLE has a dose-dependent reduction in BP with a range of 4/3 to 11/5 mm Hg with both office BP measurements and 24-hour ABM.[164-166,170] A total of 60 prehypertensive male subjects in a 6-week study with OLE demonstrated a reduction in BP about 4/3 mm Hg.[164] Olive (*Olea europaea*) leaf extract, at the dosage regimen of 500 mg twice daily was similarly effective in lowering SBP and DBP in subjects with stage-1 hypertension compared to captopril, given at its effective dose of 12.5 to 25 mg twice daily (reduction of about 11/5 mm Hg).[166]

Vitamin C

Dietary intake of vitamin C and plasma ascorbate concentration in humans are inversely correlated to blood pressure.[2-14,173-193] The administration of vitamin C orally and intravenously reduces BP in clinical trials.[2-14,173-193] Thirty-one patients were randomized to 500, 1000, or 2000 mg of oral vitamin C daily with a mean reduction in BP by 4.5/2.8 mm Hg ($P < .05$).[190] There was no difference between the three vitamin C groups indicating that 500 mg daily or 250 mg twice per day is sufficient to reduce BP.[190] In a meta-analysis of 29 trials with a median dose of vitamin C of 500 mg/d and a median duration of 2 months, there was a significant reduction in BP of 3.84/1.48 mm Hg ($P = .04$).[193] Published clinical trials show that vitamin C at a dose of 250 mg twice daily reduces BP by an average of 7/4 mm Hg.[2-14,173-193] Vitamin C is a potent water-soluble antioxidant and electron-donor that recycles vitamin E and other antioxidants and enhances total antioxidant capacity.[173] In elderly patients with refractory hypertension already on maximum pharmacologic therapy, 600 mg of vitamin C daily lowered the BP by an additional 20/16 mm Hg.[182] Plasma ascorbate is inversely correlated with BP in healthy, normotensive individuals, and those with the lowest initial ascorbate serum levels have the best BP reduction.[2-5,183,189] The SBP and 24 ABM show the most significant reductions with chronic oral administration of vitamin C.[2,177-182] Block et al.,[183] in a depletion-repletion study of vitamin C, demonstrated an inverse correlation of plasma ascorbate levels, SBP and DBP. In a meta-analysis of 13 clinical trials with 284 patients, vitamin C at 500 mg per day over 6 weeks reduced BP 3.9/2.1 mm Hg.[184] Hypertensive subjects have significantly lower plasma ascorbate levels compared to normotensive subjects (40 vs. 57 µmol/L, respectively).[186,193] A serum level of 100 µmol/L is recommended for optimal BP lowering.[2-5]

Vitamin E

Very few clinical studies demonstrated improved BP with the various types of tocopherols or tocotrienols.[2,194-198] Patients with type 2 diabetes mellitus on prescription medications with controlled BP (average BP of 136/76 mm Hg) were administered mixed tocopherols containing 60% gamma, 25% delta, and 15% alpha tocopherols.[194] The BP increased by 6.8/3.6 mm Hg in the study patients on the mixed tocopherols ($P < .0001$) and increased even more in those subjects taking alpha tocopherol (BP increased 7/5.3 mm Hg, $P < .0001$).[194] The BP increase was likely due to drug interactions with tocopherols via cytochrome P 450—3A4 and 4F2 that decreased the effective serum levels of the antihypertensive medications.[194] Gamma tocopherol has an antihypertensive and natriuretic effect through the inhibition of the 70pS potassium channel in the thick ascending limb of the loop of Henle.[195] Both alpha and gamma tocopherol improve insulin sensitivity and enhance adiponectin expression via a PPAR gamma–dependent processes, which has the potential to lower BP and serum glucose.[196]

In a retrospective analysis and data from NHNS, the medium and high tertiles of vitamin E intake were associated with a significantly lower odds ratio for hypertension, 0.73 and 0.81, respectively.[197] Fifty-eight individuals with type 2 diabetes given 500 mg/d of RRR-α-tocopherol, 500 mg/d of mixed tocopherols, or placebo for 6 weeks did not significantly alter the rate of daytime or nighttime SBP, DBP, or pulse pressure variation compared with placebo ($P > .05$).[198] If vitamin E has an antihypertensive effect, it is probably small and may be limited to untreated hypertensive patients and those with vitamin E deficiency, known vascular disease, mild volume overload, or other concomitant problems such as diabetes or hyperlipidemia.[2-5,194-198]

Vitamin D

Vitamin D3 has variable BP-lowering effects.[2-5,199-216] Vitamin D may have an independent and direct role in the regulation of BP, insulin metabolism, and dysglycemia,[199-211] but the results have not been consistent in prospective studies or in meta-analysis in which there has been little or no significant BP reduction.[212,213,215] If the vitamin D level is below 30 ng/mL, the circulating PRA levels are higher, which increases angiotensin II and elevates BP.[209] The lowest quartile of serum vitamin D has a 52% incidence of hypertension versus the highest quartile, which has a 20% incidence.[209] Compared with a 25-hydroxyvitamin D > 30 ng/mL, a 25-hydroxyvitamin D < 20 ng/mL was associated with a greater hypertension risk (OR: 1.225 [95% CI: 1.010-1.485],

$P = .04$).[209] In another study during a median follow-up of 2 years, 42.6% of the cohort developed hypertension.[211] This meta-analysis including seven prospective studies of 53,375 participants showed a significant association between vitamin D deficiencies and incident hypertension (HRs = 1.23, $P = .002$).[211] A recent meta-analysis from eight randomized controlled trials (RCTs), who received treatment with vitamin D for more than 3 months, showed that vitamin D supplementation slightly decreased the SBP by 1.964 mmHg ($P = .016$), but the DBP did not change.[213] Compared to placebo, there was also no statistical difference in SBP lowering by vitamin D supplementation.[213] Vitamin D 3 markedly suppresses renin transcription by a VDR-mediated mechanism via the JGA apparatus, which alters electrolyte balance, volume, and BP[2,201] Vitamin D reduces ADMA, suppresses pro-inflammatory cytokines, increases nitric oxide, improves endothelial function and arterial elasticity, and decreases vascular smooth muscle hypertrophy.[202-209]

The hypotensive effect of vitamin D was inversely related to the pretreatment serum levels of 1,25(OH)$_2$ D$_3$ and has additive blood pressure reduction when used concurrently with antihypertensive medications.[210]

Blacks have significantly higher rates of hypertension than whites and lower circulating levels of 25-hydroxyvitamin D.[216] In a 3-month study of placebo, 1000, 2000, or 4000 international units of cholecalciferol per day, the difference in SBP between baseline and 3 months was +1.7 mm Hg for those receiving placebo, −0.66 mm Hg for 1000 U/d, −3.4 mm Hg for 2000 U/d, and −4.0 mm Hg for 4000 U/d of cholecalciferol (−1.4 mm Hg for each additional 1000 U/d of cholecalciferol; $P = .04$). For each 1 ng/mL increase in plasma 25-hydroxyvitamin D, there was a significant 0.2 mm Hg reduction in SBP ($P = .02$).[216] There was no effect of cholecalciferol supplementation on DBP ($P = .37$). Vitamin D levels are lower in patients with nondipping hypertension.[214] A vitamin D level of 60 ng/mL is recommended for optimal BP reduction and CV risk reduction.[2-5]

Vitamin B6 (Pyridoxine)

Low serum vitamin B6 (pyridoxine) levels are associated with hypertension in humans.[2-5,217-221] High-dose vitamin B6 significantly lowered BP 14/10 mm Hg ($P < .005$) and serum catecholamine levels ($P < .05$) in a placebo-controlled study of 20 hypertensive subjects who were administered vitamin B6 at 5 mg/kg/d for 4 weeks.[218]

In a placebo-controlled trial over 12 weeks, 800 mg lipoic acid and 80 mg pyridoxine lipoic acid and pyridoxine, urinary albumin, serum malondialdehyde (MDA), and SBP decreased significantly in the supplement group compared with the placebo group ($P < .05$).[221] Serum NO increased in the supplement group compared with the placebo group ($P < .05$). No statistically significant differences were observed between the two groups in mean changes of serum endothelin-1, glucose, and DBP.[221]

Vitamin B6 thus has similar action to CAAs, diuretics, and CCBs.[2-5] The recommended dose is 200 mg/d orally.[2-5]

Flavonoids: Resveratrol and Pomegranate

Flavonoids (flavonols, flavones, and isoflavones) are potent free radical scavengers that prevent atherosclerosis, promote vascular relaxation, and have antihypertensive properties.[1,2,3]

Resveratrol administration to humans reduces AI, improves arterial compliance, and lowers central arterial pressure when administered as 250 mL of either regular or dealcoholized red wine.[224-228] Aortic AI fell 6.1% with the dealcoholized red wine and 10.5% with regular red wine; central arterial pressure was reduced by dealcoholized red wine by 7.4 and 5.4 mm Hg by regular red wine. Resveratrol increases FMD in a dose-related manner, improves ED, prevents uncoupling of eNOS, and blocks the effects of angiotensin II.[224-228] The recommended dose is 250 mg per day of trans-resveratrol.[2-5,226]

Pomegranate (*Punica granatum* L.) reduces serum ACE activity by 36%, improves endothelial function, lowers BP, and reduces carotid IMT.[2-4,229-232] A meta-analysis from eight RCTs showed significant reductions in both systolic (4.96 mm Hg, $P < .001$) and diastolic BP ($P = .021$) after 6 oz of pomegranate juice consumption.[229]

Lycopene

Lycopene produces a significant reduction in BP, serum lipids, and oxidative stress markers.[2-14,233-239] Dietary sources include grapefruit, watermelon, tomatoes, guava, pink apricots, and papaya.[2-14,233-239] Patients with grade I hypertension given a tomato lycopene extract (10 mg lycopene/day) for 2 months lowered BP by 9/7 mm Hg ($P < .01$).[233,235] Tomato extract administered to 31 hypertensive subjects over 3 months lowered BP 10/4 mm Hg.[234] Patients on antihypertensive agents including ACEI, CCB, and diuretics had an additional significant BP reduction of 5.4/3 mm Hg over 6 weeks when administered a standardized tomato extract.[235] Meta-analysis of the effect of lycopene on SBP showed a significant BP-reducing effect (mean SBP change ± SE: −5.60 ± 5.26 mm Hg, $P = .04$).[238] The doses ranged from 10 to 25 mg/d of lycopene in these trials.[238] Other studies have not shown changes in blood pressure with lycopene.[236] The recommended daily intake of lycopene is 10 to 25 mg in food or in a supplement form, but it is not clear which has the best effect on BP and CVD risk.[239] However, present data suggest that supplemental forms of lycopene are superior for BP reduction.[239]

Coenzyme Q-10 (Ubiquinone)

CoQ-10 (ubiquinone) has consistent and significant antihypertensive effects in hypertensive subjects.[2-14,240-257] CoQ-10 increases eNOS and NO and improves endothelial function and vascular elasticity.[2-14,249,250] CoQ-10 serum levels decrease with age, chronic disease, oxidative stress, dyslipidemia, CHD, hypertension, DM, statin and beta blocker use, exercise, and atherosclerosis.[2-14,249,250,255] Compared with normotensive patients, essential hypertensive patients have a higher incidence of CoQ-10 serum deficiency (39% vs. 6% of

controls).[2-5,243,252,255] In a 12-week RDBPCT of subjects with isolated systolic hypertension (ISH) (165/81-82 mm Hg), CoQ-10 administered orally at 60 mg twice daily reduced SBP 18 mm Hg ($P < .01$) and DBP 2.6 mm Hg (NS).[242] The serum level increased by 2.2 µg/dL ($P < .01$). There was a 55% response rate defined as a reduction in SBP of over 4 mm Hg. The responders had an average reduction in SBP of 26 mm Hg.[242] The therapeutic serum level of CoQ-10 should be 3 µg/mL.[2,208,240,243,251,252] This dose is usually 3 to 5 mg/kg/d of CoQ-10.[1-5,240,245,251,252] Combining a targeted intracellular cardiac CoQ-10 (MitoQ10) and low-dose losartan provides additive therapeutic benefit, significantly attenuating development of hypertension, increasing NO levels, and reducing LVH in the spontaneously hypertensive rat (SHRSP).[256] In addition, MitoQ10 mediates a direct antihypertrophic effect on rat cardiomyocytes in vitro.

Patients with the lowest CoQ-10 serum levels may have the best antihypertensive response to supplementation.[2-5,242] The average reduction in BP is about 15/10 mm Hg with office readings (range of 11-17/8-10 mm Hg)[2-5,240-257] and 18/10 mm Hg with 24-hour ABM ($P < .0001$).[243,257] The antihypertensive effect peaks at 4 weeks, then the BP remains stable during long-term treatment,[2-5,242] but within 2 weeks after discontinuation of CoQ-10 the antihypertensive effect dissipates.[2-5,242] The reduction in BP and systemic vascular resistance (SVR) are correlated with the pretreatment and posttreatment levels of CoQ-10 and the percent increase in serum levels.[2-5,242,243] About 50% of patients respond to oral supplemental CoQ-10.[2-5,242] Patients administered CoQ-10 with enalapril have better 24-hour ABM control compared to enalapril monotherapy and better endothelial function.[248] Approximately 50% of patients on antihypertensive drugs may be able to stop between one and three agents. A recent meta-analysis that suggested that CoQ-10 did not reduce BP is seriously flawed and biased in its data selection.[246] The literature is supportive of significant reductions in BP in human clinical trials.[2-5,240-245,247-255,257] Adverse effects have not been seen in patients in the literature.[2-5,240-245,247-255,257]

Alpha Lipoic Acid

Recent research has evaluated the role alpha lipoic acid (ALA) in the treatment of hypertension, especially as part of the metabolic syndrome.[2-5,178,258-263] Lipoic acid reduces oxidative stress, inflammation, and serum aldehydes, closing calcium channels which leads to vasodilation, improved endothelial function, and lower BP.[2-5,178,258-263] Urinary albumin excretion is stabilized in DM subjects given 600 mg of ALA compared to placebo for 18 months ($P < .05$).[262] In a double-blind crossover study of 36 patients with CHD given 200 mg of lipoic acid with 500 mg of acetyl-L-carnitine twice daily for 8 weeks,[261] there was a 2% increase in brachial artery diameter and a decrease in SBP from 151 ± 20 to 142 ± 18 mm Hg ($P < .03$) with no change in DBP.[261] However, patients with metabolic syndrome had a reduction in SBP from 139 ± 21 to 132 +/- 15 mm Hg ($P < .03$) and DBP from 76 ± 8 to 73 ± 8 mm Hg ($P < .06$).[261] In a 2 month double-blind crossover study of 40 patients with DM and stage I hypertension, quinapril 40 mg daily versus quinapril 40 mg with lipoic acid 600 mg daily reduced urinary albumin excretion by 30% and 53%, respectively ($P < .005$), the BP was reduced significantly by 10 % in both groups, and the FMD increased 58% with quinapril and 116% with the combination ($P < .005$).[260] The HOMA-IR decreased 19% with quinapril and 40% with quinapril with lipoic acid ($P < .005$). The combined administration of lipoic acid and pyridoxine improves albuminuria in patients with diabetic nephropathy.[263] The recommended dose is 100 to 200 mg per day of R-lipoic acid with biotin 2 to 4 mg per day to prevent biotin depletion with long-term use of lipoic acid. R-lipoic acid is recommended instead of the L isomer because of its preferred use by the mitochondria.[2-5]

Pycnogenol

Pycnogenol is a bark extract from the French maritime pine and it significantly reduces BP in human trials.[2-14,221,264-271] Pycnogenol administered at 200 mg/d lowered SBP .27 mmHg ($P < .05$) and DBP fell 1.8 mm Hg (NS).[263] The antihypertensive effect is mediated by an ACEI effect, reduction in ET-1, increases in NO and prostaglandins, reduction in inflammation and oxidative stress, and improvement in endothelial function.[2-14,221,264-271] Other studies have shown reductions in BP and a decreased need for ACEI and CCB.[2-5,221,264,266,268]

Garlic

Meta-analysis and clinical trials of garlic administration have shown consistent reductions in BP in hypertensive patients both on antihypertensive medications and those not antihypertensive medications with an average reduction in BP of 7 to 16/5 to 9 mm Hg.[272-282] Garlic is a vasodilator with ACEI activity and calcium channel blocking activity and increases nitric oxide.[2-14,277] In a DBRPCT over 3 months, subjects given 900 mg of aged garlic extract with 2.4 mg of S-allylcysteine reduced SBP by 10.2 mm Hg ($P = .03$).[274] In another DBRPC trial of 81 prehypertensive and mild hypertensive patients given 300 mg of garlic homogenate for 12 weeks, the BP reduction was 6.6 to 7.5/4.6 to 5.2 mm Hg.[275] Aged garlic extract at 480 mg per day had the best BP reduction of 11.8 ± 5.4 mm Hg ($P = .006$).[276] Garlic improves central blood pressure, central pulse pressure, mean arterial pressure, augmentation pressure, PWV, and arterial stiffness.[280]

Seaweed

Wakame seaweed (*Undaria pinnatifida*) is the most popular, edible seaweed in Japan.[283] A daily dose of 3.3 g of dried Wakame for 4 weeks significantly reduced BP by 14 + 3/5 + 2 mm Hg ($P < .01$).[284] In a study of 62 middle-aged, male subjects with mild hypertension given a potassium-loaded, ion-exchanging sodium-adsorbing, potassium-releasing seaweed preparation, significant BP reductions occurred at 4 weeks on 12 and 24 g/d ($P < .01$).[285] The MAP fell 11.2 mm Hg ($P < .001$) in the sodium-sensitive subjects and 5.7 mm Hg ($P < .05$) in the sodium-insensitive subjects, correlating with PRA.

Seaweed and sea vegetables contain 771 minerals and rare earth elements, fiber, and alginate in a colloidal form.[283-285] Wakame has ACEI activity from at least four parent tetrapeptides and possibly their dipeptide and tripeptide metabolites, especially those containing the amino acid sequence Val-Tyr, Ile-Tyr, Phe-Tyr, and Ile-Try in some combination.[283,286,287] Its long-term use in Japan has demonstrated its safety.

Cocoa: Dark Chocolate

Dark chocolate (100 g) and cocoa with a high content of polyphenols (30 mg or more) significantly reduces blood pressure in various meta-analysis and clinical prospective trials.[2-14,288-299] A meta-analysis of 173 hypertensive subjects given cocoa for 2 weeks lowered BP 4.7/2.8 mm Hg ($P = .002-.006$).[288] Fifteen subjects given 100 g of dark chocolate with 500 mg of polyphenols for 15 days had a 6.4 mm Hg reduction in SBP ($P < .05$).[289] Cocoa at a dose of 30 mg of polyphenols lowered BP in prehypertensive and stage I hypertensive patients by 2.9/1.9 mm Hg at 18 weeks ($P < .001$).[290] Two meta-analysis of 13 trials and 10 trials with a total of 297 patients found a significant reduction in BP of 3.2/2.0 mm Hg and 4.5/3.2 mm Hg respectively.[292,295] The BP reduction is the greatest in those with the highest baseline BP and those with a least 50% to 70 % cocoa at doses of 6-100 g/d.[2-5,288-292,295]

A meta-analysis in 2012 that included 20 DBRPCTs involving 856 mostly healthy participants found a statistically significant BP-reducing effect of flavanol-rich cocoa products, compared with control, in short-term trials of 2 to 18 weeks duration (mean difference in SBP –2.8 mm Hg, $P = .005$; mean difference in DBP – 2.2 mm Hg, $P = .006$].[299] The participants were given 30-1080 mg of flavanols (mean 545.5 mg) in 3.6 to 105.0 g of cocoa products per day in the active intervention group.[299] Cocoa improves insulin resistance, nitric oxide production, and endothelial function in patients with or without hyperglycemia.[289,295-298]

Melatonin

Melatonin demonstrates significant antihypertensive effects in humans in numerous double-blind randomized placebo-controlled clinical trials as single therapy or in conjunction with antihypertensive medications.[266,300-326] Melatonin induces inhibition of plasma A-II levels both centrally and in the peripheral tissues.[6,313-315,318] Melatonin levels are reduced by shortened sleep cycle of less than 6 hours, shift work, age, brief light exposure after darkness, trespass light, beta blockers, and benzodiazepines.[318] Melatonin lowers nocturnal BP in diabetic and nondiabetic hypertensive patients, in those with CHD and improves the dipping pattern in patients with nocturnal nondipping status.[301-307,309,311] In a DBRPCXO study, chronic administration (3 weeks) of melatonin at 2.5 mg before bedtime in hypertensive men, not taking any antihypertensive medications, lowered nocturnal BP by 6/4 mm Hg, reduced day-night amplitudes of SBP by 15% and DBP by 25%, improved sleep, and reduced cortisol levels.[300]

In meta-analysis DBPC RCTs, that included 221 participants treated with controlled-release melatonin 2 to 5 mg/night for 7 to 90 days, there was a significant decrease in night BP of 6.1/3.5 mm Hg ($P = .009$).[323]

Grape Seed Extract

Grape seed extract (GSE) produces a significant reduction in BP in clinical trials and meta-analyses.[2-5,327-331] GSE in variable doses and variable amounts of resveratrol was administered to subjects in nine randomized trials, meta-analysis of 390 subjects and demonstrated a significant reduction in SBP of 1.54 mm Hg ($P < .02$) but no reduction in DBP.[327] Significant reduction in BP of 11/8 mm Hg ($P < .05$) occurs with the 300 mg/d in 1 month.[328] A meta-analysis in 2016 reviewed 16 clinical trials with 810 subjects.[330] There were significant reductions in BP with GSE 6/3 mm Hg ($P = .001$) especially in young patients and those with obesity or metabolic syndrome.[330] A single-center, randomized, two-arm, double-blinded, placebo-controlled, 12-week, parallel study was conducted in 36 middle-aged adults with prehypertension.[331] Subjects consumed a juice containing placebo or 300 mg/d GSE, 150 mg twice daily, for 6 weeks preceded by a 2-week placebo run-in and followed by 4-week no-beverage follow-up.[331] GSE significantly reduced SBP by 56% ($P = .012$) and DBP by 47% ($P = .049$).[331] BP returned to baseline after the 4-week discontinuation period of GSE beverage. The higher the initial BP, the greater was the response.

Dietary Nitrates and Nitrites: Beetroot Juice and Extract

The Mediterranean and DASH diets and the ingestion of fruits and vegetables rich in inorganic nitrate (NO_3^-) are effective methods for elevating vascular nitric oxide (NO) levels through formation of an NO_2^- intermediate that reduces BP, improves arterial compliance and endothelial function.[6,332-342]

The pathway for NO generation involves the activity of facultative oral microflora and the gastric/enterosalivary cycle to facilitate the reduction of inorganic NO_3^-, ingested in the diet, to inorganic NO_2^-. This NO_2^- eventually enters the circulation where, through the activity of numerous and distinct NO_2^- reductases, it is chemically reduced to NO.[6,332,333]

Raw or cooked beets, beet juice or extract, or dark green leafy vegetables (kale and spinach) are concentrated sources of inorganic nitrates. This is the alternate pathway to the arginine NO/eNOS pathway mediated though eNOS. Beet juice at a dose of 250 mL/d reduces BP within 30 to 60 minutes in normotensive, prehypertensive, or mild hypertensive subjects.[334,335] Meta-analysis of DBRPCTs show that daily beetroot juice consumption of 5.1 to 45 mmol (321-2790 mg) over a period of 2 hours to 15 days is associated with dose-dependent changes in SBP (mean reduction − 4.4 mm Hg, $P < .001$).[336] In a blinded placebo-controlled crossover study, the acute effects of an orally disintegrating lozenge that generates nitric oxide (NO) in the oral cavity evaluated the effects on BP response, endothelial function, and vascular compliance in 30 unmedicated hypertensive patients with average baseline BP of 144 ± 3/91 ± 1 mm Hg.[337]

Nitrate supplementation versus placebo resulted in a significant decrease of 4/5 mm Hg ($P < .002$) from baseline after 20 minutes. In addition, there was a further significant reduction of 6 mm Hg in both systolic and diastolic pressure after 60 minutes ($P < .0001$ vs. baseline). After a half hour of a single dose, there was a significant improvement in vascular compliance as measured by AI and, after 4 hours, a statistically significant improvement in endothelial function as measured by the EndoPAT (Itamar Medical, Franklin, MA).[337] In another DBRPC study of 68 drug-naive and treated patients with hypertension a daily dietary supplementation was given for 4 weeks with either dietary nitrate (250 mL daily, as beetroot juice) or a placebo (250 mL daily, as nitrate-free beetroot juice) after a 2-week run-in period and followed by a 2-week washout.[334] Daily supplementation with dietary nitrate was associated with reduction in BP measured by three different methods. Mean reduction in clinic BP was 7.7/2.4 mm Hg (3.6-11.8/0.0-4.9, $P < .001$ and $P = .050$).

Twenty-four-hour ambulatory BP was reduced by 7.7/5.2 mm Hg (4.1-11.2/2.7-7.7, $P < .001$ for both). Home BP was reduced by 8.1/3.8 mm Hg (3.8-12.4/0.7-6.9, $P < .001$ and $P < .01$).[334] There was no evidence of tachyphylaxis, and the study supplement was well tolerated. Endothelial function improved by ≈ 20% ($P < .001$) and arterial stiffness was reduced by 0.59 m/s (0.24-0.93, $P < .01$) after dietary nitrate consumption with no change after placebo.[334]

In a randomized crossover study of 24 hypertensive subjects, raw beet juice was administered for 2 weeks followed by cooked beets.[340] After 2 weeks, both groups had a washout for 2 weeks then switched to the alternative treatment. Each participant consumed 250 mL/d of beet juice or 250 g/d of cooked beets. FMD was significantly ($P < .05$) increased and systolic and diastolic BP were significantly ($P < .05$) decreased with beet juice and cooked beet.[340]

Based on these studies there is a dose-related response to SBP, DBP, endothelial function, and other vascular parameters with beet juice, beet extract, raw and cooked beets.[332-342] The consumption of dietary nitrate at 0.1 mmol/kg of body weight per day (high intake of F and V at 4-6 servings a day) reduces SBP and DBP about 3.5 to 4.0 mm Hg and this effect is potentiated by vitamin C and polyphenols.[332-342]

Vegetables are the primary source of nitrates (80%-85%).[341,342] About 500 mg of beetroot juice with 45 mmol/L or 2.79 g/L of inorganic nitrate lowers BP 10.4/8.1 mm Hg and increases FMD 30%.[341,342] Beetroot tends to be dosed based on the nitrate content, with around 0.1 to 0.2 mmol/kg (6.4-12.8 mg/kg) being the target for nitrate consumption. This is about 436 mg for a 150-lb person, which is comparable to half a kilogram (500 g) of the beetroots themselves (wet weight).[341,342]

Teas

Green tea, black tea, and their respective extracts of active components have demonstrated reduction in BP in human clinical trials and meta-analysis.[343-353] In a DBRPCT of 379 hypertensive subjects given green tea extract 370 mg/d for 3 months, BP was reduced significantly by 4/4 mm Hg. [347]

A meta-analysis of regular consumption of either green or black tea for 4 to 24 weeks (2-6 cups/d) reduced BP significantly. Green tea lowered SBP by 2.1 mm Hg and DBP by 2.0 mm Hg, while black tea reduced SBP by 1.4 and DBP by 1.1 mm Hg.[343] A small 4-week crossover, RDBPCT of 21 women administered 1500 mg of green tea extract (GTE, containing 780 mg of polyphenols) or a matching placebo for 4 weeks, with a washout period of 2 weeks between treatments, had significant reductions in SBP.[351] The 24-hour ABM showed an overall decrease in SBP of 3.6 mm Hg, daytime reduction of 3.61 mm Hg, and nighttime reduction of 3.9 mm Hg.[351] There was no reduction in DBP. A meta-analysis of 10 trials with 834 subjects noted a reduction in BP of 2.36/1.77 mm Hg with green and black tea in 3 months. The best results were with noncaffeinated tea. The required amount is about 500 mg flavonoid content (2 cups of tea/day).[353] Green tea lowers SVR and induces microvascular vasodilation.[347,352]

L-Carnitine and Acetyl-L-Carnitine

Carnitine has mild systemic antihypertensive effects by upregulation of eNOS and inhibition of RAAS.[2-5,354-364] Endothelial function, NO, and oxidative defense are improved, while oxidative stress and BP are reduced.[354-358]

Human studies on the effects of L-carnitine and acetyl-L-carnitine are limited, with minimal to no change in blood pressure.[2-5,359-364] In patients with metabolic syndrome, acetyl-L-carnitine at 1 g bid over 8 weeks improved dysglycemia and reduced SBP by 7 to 9 mm Hg, but DBP was significantly decreased only in those with higher glucose levels.[365] Low carnitine levels are associated with a nondipping BP pattern in type 2 DM.[364] The clinical role of carnitine in hypertension and CVD must be carefully evaluated as carnitine may increase trimethylamine oxidase (TMAO) via the gut microbiome, which is associated with atherosclerosis and CHD.[365] Doses of 2 to 3 g twice per day are recommended if carnitine is used.[2-5]

Fiber

The clinical trials with various types of fiber to reduce BP have been inconsistent.[2-5,366-371] Soluble fiber, guar gum, guava, psyllium, flaxseed, and oat bran may reduce BP and decrease the need for antihypertensive medications in hypertensive subjects, diabetic subjects, and hypertensive-diabetic subjects especially when incorporated into the Mediterranean diet.[2-5,366-371] In a meta-analysis, dietary fiber intake was associated with a significant −1.65 mm Hg reduction in DBP but a nonsignificant −1.15 mm Hg reduction in SBP.[366] However, a significant reduction in both SBP and DBP was observed in trials conducted among patients with hypertension (5.95/4.20 mm Hg) and in trials with a duration of ≥8 weeks (BP 3.12/2.57 mm Hg).[366] In a recent meta-analysis of 14 RCTs, flaxseed, which is a rich dietary source of α-linolenic acid, lignans, and fiber, documented to lower BP by 1.8/1.6 mm Hg (P = .003).[371]

Sesame

Sesame has been shown to reduce BP in several small randomized, placebo-controlled human studies over 30 to 60 days.[372-380] Sesame lowers BP alone[181-185] or in combination with nifedipine,[180,184] diuretics, or beta blockers.[181,185] In a group of 13 mild hypertensive subjects, 60 mg of sesamin for 4 weeks lowered SBP 3.5 mm Hg (P < .044) and DBP 1.9 mm Hg (P < .045).[182] Black sesame meal at 2.52 g/d over 4 weeks in 15 subjects reduced SBP by 8.3 mm Hg (P < .05), but there was a nonsignificant reduction in DBP of 4.2 mm Hg.[183] Sesame oil at 35 g/d significantly lowered central BP within 1 hour and also maintained BP reduction chronically in 30 hypertensive subjects, reduced heart rate, arterial stiffness, AI, PWV, and hs-CRP.[380] Also, sesame oil improved NO and antioxidant capacity while it decreased endothelin-I.[380] In addition, sesame lowers serum glucose, HgbA1C, and LDL-C; increases HDL; reduces oxidative stress markers; and increases glutathione, SOD, GPx, CAT, vitamins C, E, and A.[180,181,183-185] The active ingredients are natural ACEIs such as sesamin, sesamolin, sesaminol glucosides, furofuran lignans, which also suppress NF-kappa B and inflammatory cytokine production.[186,187] All of these effects lower inflammation, decrease oxidative stress, improve oxidative defense, improve endothelial function, vasodilate, and reduce BP.[186,187]

Hesperidin

Hesperidin significantly lowered DBP 3 to 4 mm Hg (P < .02) and improved microvascular endothelial reactivity in 24 obese hypertensive male subjects in a randomized, controlled crossover study over 4 weeks for each of three treatment groups consuming 500 mL of orange juice, hesperidin. or placebo.[381]

N-Acetylcysteine

N-acetylcysteine (NAC) and L-arginine (ARG) in combination reduces endothelial activation and BP in hypertensive patients with and without type 2 DM.[123,382-384] In 24 subjects with type 2 DM and hypertension treated for 6 months with placebo or NAC with ARG, both systolic and diastolic BP were significantly reduced (P = .05).[123] Nitric oxide and endothelial postischemic vasodilation increased.[123] NAC increases NO via IL-1b and increases iNOS mRNA, increases glutathione by increasing cysteine levels, reduces the affinity for the AT1 receptor by disrupting disulfide groups, blocks the L-type calcium channel, lowers homocysteine, and improves carotid IMT.[123,382-384] The recommended dose is 500 to 1000 mg twice a day.

Hawthorne

Hawthorne extract has been used for centuries for the treatment of hypertension, CHF, and other CVDs, but the studies are limited and are not convincing of any significant clinical responses.[485,486] In a recent four-period crossover design, dose-response study of 21 subjects with prehypertension or mild hypertension over 3.5 days did not show changes in FMD or BP on standardized extract with 50 mg of oligomeric procyanidin per 250 mg extract with 1000, 1500, or 2500 mg of the extract.[385] Hawthorne showed noninferiority of ACEI and diuretics in the treatment of 102 patients with NYHC II CHF over 8 weeks.[387] Patients with hypertension and type 2 DM on medications for BP and DM that were randomized to 1200 mg of hawthorne extract for 16 weeks showed significant reductions in DBP of 2.6 mm Hg ($P = .035$).[388] Thirty-six mildly hypertensive patients administered 500 mg of hawthorne extract for 10 weeks and showed a nonsignificant trend in DBP reduction ($P = .081$) compared with placebo.[389] Hawthorne acts like an ACEI, BB (beta blocker), CCB, and diuretic. More studies are needed to determine the efficacy, long-term effects, and dose of hawthorne for the treatment of hypertension.

Quercetin

Quercetin is an antioxidant flavonol found in apples, berries, and onions that reduces BP in hypertensive individuals,[390-392] but the hypotensive effects do not appear to be mediated by changes in HS-CRP, TNF-α, ACE activity, ET-1, NO, vascular reactivity, or FMD.[390] Quercetin is metabolized by CYP 3A4 and should be used with caution in patients on drugs metabolized by this cytochrome system.[390-392] Quercetin was administered to 12 hypertensive men at an oral dose of 1095 mg with reduction in mean BP by 5 mm Hg, SBP by 7 mm Hg, and DBP by 3 mm Hg.[390] Forty-one prehypertensive and stage I hypertensive subjects were enrolled in a randomized, double-blind, placebo-controlled, crossover study with 500 mg of quercetin per day versus placebo.[391] In the stage I hypertensive patients, the BP was reduced by 7/5 mm Hg ($P < .05$).[391] Quercetin administered to 93 overweight or obese subjects at 150 mg/d (plasma levels of 269 nmol/L) over 6 weeks lowered SBP 2.9 mm Hg in the hypertensive group and up to 3.7 mm Hg in SBP in the patients 25 to 50 years of age.[392] The recommended dose of quercetin is 500 mg twice daily.

Probiotics

Gut dysbiosis in hypertension is characterized by a gut microbiome that are less diverse with an increased Firmicutes/Bacteroidetes ratio, a decrease in acetate- and butyrate-producing bacteria, and an increase in lactate-producing bacterial populations. There are several meta-analysis in humans that support the role of probiotic supplementation to reduce blood pressure.[109,393-395]

One meta-analysis of RCTs suggested that consuming probiotics result a modest lowering of BP with a potentially greater effect with an elevated baseline BP, when multiple species of probiotics are consumed, the duration of the intervention is ≥ 8 weeks and the daily dose is ≥ 10^{11} colony-forming units.[393]

Another meta-analysis of 14 RCTs, involving 702 participants, showed that, compared with placebo, probiotic fermented milk produced a slight but significant reduction of 3.1/1.1 mm Hg in BP. Subgroup analyses suggested a slightly greater effect on SBP in hypertensive than in normotensive participants.[109] In a meta-analysis of 11 eligible randomized controlled trial (n = 641), probiotic consumption significantly decreased SBP (WMD [weighted mean difference], −3.28 mm Hg; 95% confidence interval [CI], −5.38 to −1.18) and DBP (WMD, −2.13 mm Hg; 95% CI, −4.5 to 0.24), in type 2 diabetic patients compared with placebo.[394]

Hypertension may be caused by many factors including hypercholesterolemia, chronic inflammation, and inconsistent modulation of the RAAS that are modified by probiotics.[395-397]

Drug Therapy for Hypertension [2-5,11-15,398,399]

The 2017 ACC/AHA Guidelines for the Prevention, Detection, Evaluation, and Management of Hypertension in Adults provides the following summary[398]:

1. **Classification of blood pressure: Four new BP categories based on the average of two or more in-office blood pressure readings**.

   Normal: <120 mm Hg systolic BP (SBP) and <80 mm Hg diastolic BP (DBP)

   Elevated: 120 to 129 mm Hg SBP and <80 mm Hg DBP

   Stage 1 hypertension: 130 to 139 mm Hg SBP or 80 to 89 mm Hg DBP

   Stage 2 hypertension: ≥140 mm Hg SBP or ≥90 mm Hg DBP

2. **Prevalence of high blood pressure**: Substantially higher prevalence of HBP under the new guideline, 46% of US adults versus 32%, based on the JNC 7 definition. However, for most US adults meeting the new definition of hypertension that would not meet the JNC 7 definition, nonpharmacological treatment is recommended. Because most people between 130 to 139 mm Hg SBP or 80 to 89 mm Hg DBP will not require medication to treat their hypertension; there will only be a small increase in the percentage of US adults for whom antihypertensive medication is recommended in conjunction with lifestyle modification. Commit to helping your patients by implementing a BP improvement program.

3. **Treatment of high blood pressure**: All patients with blood pressures above normal should be treated with nonpharmacological interventions. For most

adults these include consuming a heart-healthy diet such as DASH, reducing sodium intake, increasing physical activity, limiting alcohol consumption, and losing weight for those who are overweight. Pharmacological interventions: Use of BP-lowering medications is recommended based on stage of hypertension, an individual's medical history, or estimated 10-year CVD risk ≥10% using the ACC/AHA Risk Estimator.

4. **Blood pressure goal for people with high blood pressure**: For adults with confirmed hypertension and known CVD, or 10-year ASCVD event risk of 10% or higher, a BP goal of less than 130/80 mm Hg is recommended. For adults without additional markers of increased CVD risk, a BP goal of less than 130/80 mm Hg may also be reasonable. The totality of the available information provides evidence that a lower BP target is generally better than a higher BP target. The SBP target recommended in the new guideline (<130 mm Hg) is higher than that which was used in the SPRINT trial (<120 mm Hg). Learn how to improve blood pressure control rates

5. **Use self-measured blood pressure monitoring (SMBP)** to diagnose, reassess, and activate patients with high blood pressure: SMBP refers to the regular measurement of BP by an individual, at their home or elsewhere outside the clinic setting. SMBP can be used for confirmation of hypertension diagnosis based on elevated office readings and for titration of BP-lowering medication, in conjunction with telehealth counseling or clinical interventions. SMBP can help differentiate between sustained, white coat, and masked hypertension. SMBP can also be used for reassessment of patients (at 1-, 3-, 6-, or 12-month intervals) per new guideline recommendations

The selection of antihypertensive drug therapy should be based on all of the following considerations[2-5,11-15]:
- Level of blood pressure
- Presence of other CHD risk factors
- Calculation of CHD risk with COSHEC, ACC/AHA, or Rasmussen risk calculator that indicates high risk
- Presence of clinical CVD TOD
- Presence of other preclinical tests for vascular damage such as EndoPAT, CAPWA, CAC, CORUS, Carotid Duplex, CPET, ECHO, autonomic function testing
- Presence of clinical symptoms related to BP such as headache, chest pain at rest or with exercise and dyspnea, etc.
- PRA, aldosterone and ARR (aldosterone renin ratio). Low renin hypertension (LRH) has an increased intravascular volume (volume dependent) with a PRA < 0.65 ng/mL/h. This represents about 30% of hypertensive patients. High renin hypertension (HRH) has a decreased intravascular volume with a PRA > 0.65 ng/mL/h. This is about 70% of hypertensive patients. The ARR (pg/mL/ng/mL/h) helps to

further establish if the patient has LRH or HRH as follows:
  ARR over 80 is LRH or primary hyperaldosteronism
  ARR over 40 is probably LRH with a sensitivity and specificity of 100% and 92% for primary aldosteronism
  ARR less than 10 is HRH
  ARR between 10 and 40: not sure

The measurement of PRA and aldosterone plasma levels may be done in a random ambulatory setting, is most accurate in drug naïve patients, does not require alterations in patient position, time of day, or sodium intake, etc.

However, the levels of PRA will be altered by concomitant antihypertensive medications, which requires more sophisticated interpretation.
- Nutritional depletion evaluation
- Demographics
- Subsets of hypertension: individualized treatment
- Genetic phenotype (SNP)
  1. Those that predispose an individual to hypertension in some or all conditions
  2. Those that predict response to a drug or nutrient.

Aggressive, early BP reduction results in the best CVD reduction. The recommended new BP goal is 120/80 mm Hg.[2-5,11-15] The 24-hour ABM and with brachial and central BP are recommended over office or home brachial BP to assess dipping status, nocturnal BP, lability, BP load, BP surges, and mean BP.

Noninvasive vascular testing for functional and structural abnormalities of the vasculature should be done such as pulse wave analysis, AI central BP, ED, and arterial compliance. Nocturnal BP drives the risk for CVD. If a patient is a nondipper, then medications should be administered at night. This approach will reduce CV events to a greater extent compared with giving the medications in the morning.

Initial therapy in most hypertensive patients should be amlodipine/ACEI or amlodipine/ARB combinations, as these have the best reductions in BP and CV TOD.[2-5,11-15] However, this selection will depend on the PRA:
- Low renin hypertension is best treated with CCBs, diuretics, serum aldosterone receptor antagonists like spironolactone and eplerenone (SARA).
- High renin hypertension (HRH) is best treated with RAS or renin drugs such as ACEIs, ARBs, direct renin inhibitors (DRIs), certain BBs, or CAAs

Long-acting ACEIs with tissue selectivity are preferred. This would include all of the ACEIs except captopril, enalapril, and lisinopril. An ARB with high affinity for the AT 1 receptor and longer effect on both BP and vascular protection is preferred. These would include most of the ARBs except losartan. The DHP-CCBs such as amlodipine or nifedipine are preferred over verapamil or diltiazem.

Indapamide is diuretic of choice for a third drug, then chlorthalidone. However, HCTZ alone or in combination with other agents should be avoided because of its lack of efficacy in reducing CVD and CHD, increase in glucose and risk of type 2 DM, inducing an abnormal lipid profile, increasing homocysteine, and causing numerous nutritional deficiencies and other metabolic problems such as hypokalemia, hypomagnesemia, and hyponatremia.[2-5,11-15]

Nebivolol (vasodilating and increases nitric oxide) and carvedilol (an alpha/beta blocker with antioxidant activity) are the beta blockers of choice. One should avoid other older beta blockers for hypertension as they do not reduce CVD or CHD compared with the other antihypertensive agents. Renin inhibitors (DRI) are appropriate for add-on treatment except that it should not be given with an ACEI or an ARB. An ACEI should not be administered with an ARB. Spironolactone 12.5 to 25 mg QD is very effective in resistant hypertension or in patients with low renin hypertension or those with the genetic SNP CYP11 B2. Amiloride 5 to 20 mg/d is very effective in patients with hyperactive epithelial sodium channel with a genetic SNP CYP4A11 or low renin hypertension.

If the patient develops edema on a CCB, then the best treatment to reduce the edema is with ACEI or ARB not a diuretic. Also giving the CCB at night may reduce edema during the day. Drugs that may increase serum potassium should be monitored carefully if administered simultaneously (ACEI, ARB, spironolactone, eplerenone, amiloride) and also used carefully in those with renal impairment. Rationale combinations are preferred, which have different mechanisms of action such as ACEI or ARB with CCB, diuretic, and a vasodilating beta blocker. The addition of spironolactone or amiloride will depend on the BP and clinical setting as well as PRA, ARR levels, and genetics.

Clinical Considerations

A comprehensive clinical approach to the categories and clinical use of nutraceutical supplements is detailed in Tables 21.2 and 21.3.

Several of the strategic combinations of nutraceutical supplements with antihypertensive drugs have been shown to lower BP more than the medication alone.[2-5] These are:
- Pycnogenol with ACEI
- Lycopene with various antihypertensive medications
- R-lipoic acid with ACEI
- Vitamin C with CCBs
- N-acetylcysteine with arginine
- Garlic with ACEI, diuretics, and beta blockers
- Coenzyme Q-10 with ACEI and CCB

Many antihypertensive drugs may cause nutrient depletions that can actually interfere with their antihypertensive action or cause other metabolic adverse effects manifest through the laboratory results with clinical symptoms.[400,401] Diuretics decrease potassium, magnesium, phosphorous, sodium, chloride, folate, vitamin B6, zinc, iodine, and coenzyme Q-10; increase homocysteine, calcium, and creatinine; and elevate serum glucose by inducing insulin resistance. Beta blockers reduce coenzyme Q-10, and ACEI and ARBs reduce zinc.[400,401]

Clinical monitoring of blood pressure is required as well as patient awareness that dietary and supplemental interventions need to be taken as consistently as medications. Additional laboratory tests can inform clinical decision-making such as the measurement of intracellular micronutrients in lymphocytes, antioxidant capacity, oxidative stress, inflammation biomarkers such as hs-CRP, PRA, and serum aldosterone followed by repletion of all micronutrient depletions with selected higher doses of nutritional supplements based on the clinical studies that have been reviewed.[402]

Summary

- Vascular biology such as endothelial, vascular, and cardiac smooth muscle dysfunction plays a primary and pivotal role in the initiation and perpetuation of hypertension.
- Nutrient-gene interactions and epigenetics are predominant factors in promoting beneficial or detrimental effects in cardiovascular health and hypertension.
- Oxidative stress, inflammation, and vascular immune dysfunction initiate and propagate hypertension and cardiovascular disease.
- Nutrition, natural whole food, nutraceutical supplements, antioxidants, anti-inflammatory agents, vitamins, and minerals can prevent, control, and treat hypertension through numerous vascular biology mechanisms and may mimic the effects of the various antihypertensive drug classes.
- There is a role for the selected use of single and combined nutraceutical supplements, vitamins, antioxidants, and minerals in the treatment of hypertension based on prospective randomized placebo-controlled studies and meta-analysis as a complement to optimal nutrition and other lifestyle modifications.
- A clinical approach which incorporates optimal nutrition with scientifically proven nutraceutical supplements, exercise, weight reduction, smoking cessation, alcohol and caffeine restriction, and other lifestyle strategies can be systematically and successfully incorporated into clinical practice for the prevention and treatment of hypertension (Tables 21.2 and 21.3).
- BP should be lowered aggressively and early with a combination of nutrition, supplements, lifestyle changes, and drugs.
- Antihypertensive drugs should be directed at both BP and CVD reduction with improvement in vascular function and structure.
- ACEI, ARB, indapamide and DHP-CCB, nebivolol, carvedilol, and spironolactone are preferred drugs than HCTZ and the older beta blockers. Logical combinations are recommended.

Table 21.3

AN INTEGRATIVE APPROACH TO THE TREATMENT OF HYPERTENSION

Intervention Category	Therapeutic Intervention	Daily Intake
Diet characteristics	DASH I, DASH II-Na⁺, or PREMIER diet	Diet type
	Sodium restriction	1500 mg
	Potassium	5000-10,000 mg
	Potassium/sodium ratio	>4:1
	Magnesium	1000 mg
	Zinc	50 mg
Macronutrients	*Protein*: Total intake from nonanimal sources, organic lean or wild animal protein, or coldwater fish	30% of total calories, which is 1.5-1.8 g/kg body weight
	Whey protein	30 g
	Soy protein (fermented sources are preferred)	30 g
	Sardine muscle concentrate extract	3 g
	Milk peptides (VPP and IPP)	30-60 mg
	Fat	30% of total calories
	Omega-3 fatty acids	2-3 g
	Omega-6 fatty acids	1 g
	Omega-9 fatty acids (MUFA)	4 tablespoons (40 g) of EVOO or nuts
	Saturated fatty acids from wild game, bison, or other lean meat	<10% total calories
	Polyunsaturated to saturated fat ratio	>2.0
	Omega 3 to omega 6 ratio	1.1-1.2
	Synthetic trans fatty acids	None (completely remove from diet)
	Nuts in variety	*4 servings*
	Carbohydrates as primarily complex carbohydrates and fiber	40% of total calories
	Oatmeal or	60 g
	Oat bran or	40 g
	Beta-glucan or	3 g
	Psyllium	7 g
Specific foods	Garlic as fresh cloves or aged Kyolic garlic	4 fresh cloves (4 g) or 600 mg aged garlic taken twice daily
	Sea vegetables, specifically dried wakame	3.0-3.5 g
	Lycopene as tomato products, guava, watermelon, apricots, pink grapefruit, papaya or supplements	10-20 mg
	Dark chocolate	100 g
	Pomegranate juice or seeds	8 ounces or one cup
	Sesame	60 mg sesamin or
	Beet juice	2.5 grams sesame meal

(Continued)

Table 21.3

AN INTEGRATIVE APPROACH TO THE TREATMENT OF HYPERTENSION—CONT'D

Intervention Category	Therapeutic Intervention	Daily Intake
	Green tea or EGCG extract	
	Carnitine	500 grams 60 oz of 500 mg bid 2-6 g/d
Exercise	Aerobic	20 min daily at 4200 KJ/wk
	Resistance	40 min/d
Weight reduction	Body mass index <25 Waist circumference: <35 inches for women <40 inches for men Total body fat: <22% for women <16% for men	Lose 1-2 pounds per week and increase the proportion of lean muscle

Other lifestyle recommendations	Alcohol restriction:
	  Among the choice of alcohol, red wine
	    is preferred because of its vasoactive
	    phytonutrients.
		<20 g/d
		Wine <10 ounces
		Beer <24 ounces
		Liquor <2 ounces

	Caffeine restriction or elimination depending on CYP 1A2 450 SNP	<100 mg/d
	Tobacco and smoking	Stop
Medical considerations	Medications which may increase blood pressure	Minimize use when possible, such as by using disease-specific nutritional interventions
Supplemental foods and nutrients	Alpha lipoic acid with biotin	100-200 mg twice daily
	Amino acids: Arginine	2 g twice daily
	Carnitine	1-2 g twice daily
	Taurine	1-3 g twice daily
	Chlorogenic acids	150-200 mg
	Coenzyme Q-10	100 mg once to twice daily
	Grape seed extract Hawthorne extract	300 mg 500 mg twice a day
	Melatonin (long acting) N-acetyl-cysteine (NAC) Olive leaf extract (oleuropein)	3 mg 500 mg twice a day 500 mg twice a day
	Pycnogenol	200 mg
	Quercetin	500 mg twice a day
	Probiotics	11,10 CFU
	Resveratrol (trans)	250 mg
	Vitamin B6	100 mg once to twice daily
	Vitamin C	250-500 mg twice daily
	Vitamin D3	Dose to raise 25-hydroxyvitamin D serum level to 60 ng/mL
	Vitamin E as mixed tocopherols	400 IU

References

1. Wesa KM, Grimm RH Jr. Recommendations and guidelines regarding the preferred research protocol for investigating the impact of an optimal healing environment on patients with hypertension. *J Altern Complement Med.* 2004;10(suppl 1):S245-S250.

2. Houston M. The role of nutrition and nutraceutical supplements in the treatment of hypertension. *World J Cardiol.* 2014;6(2): 38-66.

3. Houston M. Nutrition and nutraceutical supplements for the treatment of hypertension: part 1. *J Clin Hypertens.* 2013;15:752-757.

4. Houston M. Nutrition and nutraceutical supplements for the treatment of hypertension: part II. *J Clin Hypertens.* 2013;15:845-851.

5. Houston M. Nutrition and nutraceutical supplements for the treatment of hypertension: part III. *J Clin Hypertens.* 2013;15:931-937.

6. Borghi C, Cicero AF. Nutraceuticals with a clinically detectable blood pressure-lowering effect: a review of available randomized clinical trials and their meta-analyses. *Br J Clin Pharmacol.* 2017;83(1):163-171.

7. Sirtori CR, Arnoldi A, Cicero AF. Nutraceuticals for blood pressure control. *Rev Ann Med.* 2015;47(6):447-456.

8. Cicero AF, Colletti A. Nutraceuticals and blood pressure control: results from clinical trials and meta-analyses. *High Blood Press Cardiovasc Prev.* 2015;22(3):203-213.

9. Turner JM, Spatz ES. Nutritional supplements for the treatment of hypertension: a practical guide for clinicians. *Curr Cardiol Rep.* 2016;18(12):126.

10. Caligiuri SP, Pierce GN. A review of the relative efficacy of dietary, nutritional supplements, lifestyle and drug therapies in the management of hypertension. *Crit Rev Food Sci Nutr.* 2017;57:3508-3527.

11. Houston MC, Fox B, Taylor N. *What Your Doctor May Not Tell You About Hypertension. The Revolutionary Nutrition and Lifestyle Program to Help Fight High Blood Pressure.* New York, NY: AOL Time Warner, Warner Books; September 2003.

12. Houston MC. *Handbook of Hypertension.* Oxford, UK: Wiley-Blackwell; 2009.

13. Houston MC. *What Your Doctor May Not Tell You About Heart Disease.* New York, NY: Grand Central Press; February 2012.

14. Sinatra S, Houston M, eds. *Nutrition and Integrative Strategies in Cardiovascular Medicine.* Boca Raton, FL: CRC Press; 2015.

15. The seventh report of the Joint National Committee on Prevention, Detection, Evaluation, and Treatment of High Blood Pressure (JNC-7). *JAMA.* 2003;289:2560-2572.

16. Thomopoulos C, Parati G, Zanchetti A. Effects of blood pressure lowering on outcome incidence in hypertension: 7. Effects of more vs. less intensive blood pressure lowering and different achieved blood pressure levels - updated overview and meta-analyses of randomized trials. *J Hypertens.* 2016;34(4):613-622.

17. Ettehad D, Emdin CA, Kiran A, et al. Blood pressure lowering for prevention of cardiovascular disease and death: a systematic review and meta-analysis. *Lancet.* 2016;387(10022):957-967.

18. ESH/ESC Task Force for the Management of Arterial Hypertension. 2013 Practice guidelines for the management of arterial hypertension of the European Society of Hypertension (ESH) and the European Society of Cardiology (ESC): ESH/ESC Task Force for the Management of Arterial Hypertension. *J Hypertens.* 2013;31:1925-1938.

19. Flack JM, Calhoun D, Schiffrin EL. The new ACC/AHA hypertension guidelines for the prevention, detection, evaluation, and management of high blood pressure in adults. *Am J Hypertens.* 2018;31(2):133-135.

20. Appel LJ; American Society of Hypertension Writing Group. ASH position paper: dietary approaches to lower blood pressure. *J Am Soc Hypertens.* 2009;3:321-331.

21. Eaton SB, Eaton SB III, Konner MJ. Paleolithic nutrition revisited: a twelve-year retrospective on its nature and implications. *Eur J Clin Nutr.* 1997;51:207-216.

22. Layne J, Majkova Z, Smart EJ, Toborek M, Hennig B. Caveolae: a regulatory platform for nutritional modulation of inflammatory diseases. *J Nutr Biochem.* 2011;22:807-811.

23. Dandona P, Ghanim H, Chaudhuri A, Dhindsa S, Kim SS. Macronutrient intake induces oxidative and inflammatory stress: potential relevance to atherosclerosis and insulin resistance. *Exp Mol Med.* 2010;42(4):245-253.

24. Kizhakekuttu TJ, Widlansky ME. Natural antioxidants and hypertension: promise and challenges. *Cardiovasc Ther.* 2010;28(4):e20-e32.

25. Houston MC. New insights and approaches to reduce end organ damage in the treatment of hypertension: subsets of hypertension approach. *Am Heart J.* 1992;123:1337-1367.

26. Nayak DU, Karmen C, Frishman WH, Vakili BA. Antioxidant vitamins and enzymatic and synthetic oxygen-derived free radical scavengers in the prevention and treatment of cardiovascular disease. *Heart Dis.* 2001;3:28-45.

27. Ritchie RH, Drummond GR, Sobey CG, De Silva TM, Kemp-Harper BK. The opposing roles of NO and oxidative stress in cardiovascular disease. *Pharmacol Res.* 2017;116:57-69.

28. Russo C, Olivieri O, Girelli D, et al. Antioxidant status and lipid peroxidation in patients with essential hypertension. *J Hypertens.* 1998;16:1267-1271.

29. Tse WY, Maxwell SR, Thomason H, et al. Antioxidant status in controlled and uncontrolled hypertension and its relationship to endothelial damage. *J Hum Hypertens.* 1994;8:843-849.

30. Galley HF, Thornton J, Howdle PD, Walker BE, Webster NR. Combination oral antioxidant supplementation reduces blood pressure. *Clin Sci.* 1997;92:361-365.

31. Dhalla NS, Temsah RM, Netticadam T. The role of oxidative stress in cardiovascular diseases. *J Hypertens.* 2000;18:655-673.

32. Loperena R, Harrison DG. Oxidative stress and hypertensive diseases. *Med Clin North Am.* 2017;101(1):169-193.

33. Pietri P, Vlachopoulos C, Tousoulis D. Inflammation and arterial hypertension: from pathophysiological links to risk prediction. *Curr Med Chem.* 2015;22(23):2754-2761.

34. Amer MS, Elawam AE, Khater MS, Omar OH, Mabrouk RA, Taha HM. Association of high-sensitivity C reactive protein with carotid artery intimamedia thickness in hypertensive older adults. *J Am Soc Hypertens.* 2011;5(5):393-400.

35. Kvakan H, Luft FC, Muller DN. Role of the immune system in hypertensive target organ damage. *Trends Cardiovasc Med.* 2009;19(7):242-246.

36. Rodriquez-Iturbe B, Franco M, Tapia E, Quiroz Y, Johnson RJ. Renal inflammation, autoimmunity and salt-sensitive hypertension. *Clin Exp Pharmacol Physiol.* 2012;39(1):96-103.

37. Mansego ML, Solar Gde M, Alonso MP, et al. Polymorphisms of antioxidant enzymes, blood pressure and risk of hypertension. *J Hypertens.* 2011;29(3):492-500.

38. Vongpatanasin W, Thomas GD, Schwartz R, et al. C-reactive protein causes downregulation of vascular angiotensin subtype 2 receptors and systolic hypertension in mice. *Circulation.* 2007;115(8):1020-1028.

39. Razzouk L, Munter P, Bansilal S, et al. C reactive protein predicts long-term mortality independently of low-density lipoprotein cholesterol in patients undergoing percutaneous coronary intervention. *Am Heart J.* 2009;158(2):277-283.

40. Tian N, Penman AD, Mawson AR, Manning RD Jr, Flessner MF. Association between circulating specific leukocyte types and blood pressure. The atherosclerosis risk in communities(ARIC) study. *J Am Soc Hypertens.* 2010;4(6):272-283.

41. Muller DN, Kvakan H, Luft FC. Immune-related effects in hypertension and target-organ damage. *Curr Opin Nephrol Hypertens.* 2011;20(2):113-117.

42. Leibowitz A, Schiffin EL. Immune mechanisms in hypertension. *Curr Hypertens Rep.* 2011;13(6):465-472.

43. Xiong S, Li Q, Liu D, Zhu Z. Gastrointestinal tract: a promising target for the management of hypertension. *Curr Hypertens Rep.* 2017;19:(4):31.

44. Caillon A, Mian MO, Fraulob-Aquino JC, et al. Cells mediate angiotensin II-induced hypertension and vascular injury. *Circulation.* 2017;135:2155-2162. doi:10.1161/CIRCULATIONAHA.116.016971.

45. Rudemiller NP, Crowley SD. The role of chemokines in hypertension and consequent target organ damage. *Pharmacol Res.* 2017;119:404-411.

46. De Ciuceis C, Agabiti-Rosei C, Rossini C, et al. Relationship between different subpopulations of circulating CD4+ T lymphocytes and microvascular or systemic oxidative stress in humans. *Blood Press.* 2017;26:1-9.

47. Caillon A, Schiffrin EL. Role of inflammation and immunity in hypertension: recent epidemiological, laboratory, and clinical evidence. *Curr Hypertens Rep.* 2016;18(3):21.

48. Abais-Battad JM, Dasinger JH, Fehrenbach DJ, Mattson DL. Novel adaptive and innate immunity targets in hypertension. *Pharmacol Res.* 2017;120:109-115. pii:S1043-6618(16)30860-X. doi:10.1016/j.phrs.2017.03.015.

49. Biancardi VC, Bomfim GF, Reis WL, Al-Gassimi S, Nunes KP. The interplay between Angiotensin II, TLR4 and hypertension. *Pharmacol Res.* 2017;120:88-96. pii:S1043-6618(16)30910-0. doi:10.1016/j.phrs.2017.03.017.

50. Justin Rucker A, Crowley SD. The role of macrophages in hypertension and its complications. *Pflugers Arch.* 2017;469(3-4):419-430.

51. Miller ER III, Erlinger TP, Appel LJ. The effects of macronutrients on blood pressure and lipids: an overview of the DASH and OmniHeart trials. *Curr Atheroscler Rep.* 2006;8:460-465.

52. Pérez-López FR, Chedraui P, Quadro JL. Effects of the Mediterranean diet on longevity and age-related morbid conditions. *Maturitas.* 2009;64:67-79.

53. Cutler JA, Follmann, Allender PS. Randomized trials of sodium reduction: an overview. *Am J Clin Nutr.* 1997;65:643S-651S.

54. Sacks FM, Svetkey LP, Vollmer WM, et al. Effects on blood pressure of reduced dietary sodium and the Dietary Approaches to Stop Hypertension (DASH) diet. DASH-Sodium Collaborative Research Group. *N Engl J Med.* 2001;344(1):3-10.

55. Messerli FH, Schmieder RE, Weir MR. Salt: a perpetrator of hypertensive target organ disease? *Arch Intern Med.* 1997;157:2449-2452.

56. Merino J, Guasch-Ferré M, Martínez-González MA, et al. Is complying with the recommendations of sodium intake beneficial for health in individuals at high cardiovascular risk? Findings from the PREDIMED study. *Am J Clin Nutr.* 2015;101(3):440-448.

57. Weinberger MH. Salt sensitivity of blood pressure in humans. *Hypertension.* 1996;27:481-490.

58. Morimoto A, Usu T, Fujii T, et al. Sodium sensitivity and cardiovascular events in patients with essential hypertension. *Lancet.* 1997;350:1734-1737.

59. Kanbay M, Chen Y, Solak Y, Sanders PW. Mechanisms and consequences of salt sensitivity and dietary salt intake. *Curr Opin Nephrol Hypertens.* 2011;20(1):37-43.

60. Toda N, Arakawa K. Salt-induced hemodynamic regulation mediated by nitric oxide. *J Hypertens.* 2011;29(3):415-424.

61. Rust P, Ekmekcioglu C. Impact of salt intake on the pathogenesis and treatment of hypertension. *Adv Exp Med Biol.* 2017;956:61-84.

62. Foulquier S, Dupuis F, Perrin-Sarrado C, et al. High salt intake abolishes AT(2)-mediated vasodilation of pial arterioles in rats. *J Hypertens.* 2011;29(7):1392-1399.

63. Feis J, Oberleithner H, Kusche-Vihrog K. Menage a trios: aldosterone, sodium and nitric oxide in vascular endothelium. *Biochim Biophys Acta.* 2010;1802(12):1193-1202.

64. Yang Q, Liu T, Kuklina EV, et al. Sodium and potassium intake and mortality among US adults: Prospective data from the third national health and nutrition examination survey. *Arch Int Med.* 2011;171(13):1183-1191.

65. Houston MC, Harper KJ. Potassium, magnesium, and calcium: their role in both the cause and treatment of hypertension. *J Clin Hypertens.* 2008;10(7 suppl 2):3-11.

66. Perez V, Chang ET. Sodium-to-potassium ratio and blood pressure, hypertension, and related factors. *Adv Nutr.* 2014;5:712-741.

67. Filippini T, Violi F, D'Amico R, Vinceti M. The effect of potassium supplementation on blood pressure in hypertensive subjects: A systematic review and metaanalysis. *Int J Cardiol.* 2017;230:127-135.

68. Gu D, He J, Xigui W, Duan X, Whelton PK. Effect of potassium supplementation on blood pressure in Chinese: a randomized, placebo controlled trial. *J Hypertens.* 2001;19:1325-1331.

69. D'Elia L, Barba G, Cappuccio FP, Strazzullo P. Potassium intake, stroke, and cardiovascular disease a meta-analysis of prospective studies. *J Am Coll Cardiol.* 2011;57:1210-1219.

70. Poorolajal J, Zeraati F, Soltanian AR, Sheikh V, Hooshmand E, Maleki. Oral potassium supplementation for management of essential hypertension: a meta-analysis of randomized controlled trials. *PLoS One.* 2017;12(4):e0174967. doi:10.1371/journal.pone.0174967.

71. Houston MC. The importance of potassium in managing hypertension. *Curr Hypertens Rep.* 2011;13(4):309-317.

72. Widman L, Wester PO, Stegmayr BG, Wirell MP. The dose dependent reduction in blood pressure through administration of magnesium: a double- blind placebo controlled cross-over trial. *Am J Hypertens.* 1993;6:41-45.

73. Laurant P, Touyz RM. Physiological and pathophysiological role of magnesium in the cardiovascular system: implications in hypertension. *J Hypertens.* 2000;18:1177-1191.

74. Zhang X, Li Y, Del Gobbo LC, et al. Effects of magnesium supplementation on blood pressure: a meta-analysis of randomized double-blind placebo-controlled trials. *Hypertension.* 2016;68(2):324-333.

75. Kass L, Weekes J, Carpenter L. Effect of magnesium supplementation on blood pressure: a meta-analysis. *Eur J Clin Nutr.* 2012;66:411-418.

76. Houston MC. The role of magnesium in hypertension and cardiovascular disease. *J Clin Hyperten.* 2011;13:843-847.

77. Cormick G, Ciapponi A, Cafferata ML, Belizán JM. Calcium supplementation for prevention of primary hypertension. *Cochrane Database Syst Rev.* 2015;(6):CD010037. doi:10.1002/14651858.CD010037.

78. Resnick LM. Calcium metabolism in hypertension and allied metabolic disorders. *Diabetes Care.* 1991;14:505-520.

79. Garcia Zozaya JL, Padilla Viloria M. Alterations of calcium, magnesium, and zinc in essential hypertension: their relation to the renin-angiotensin-aldosterone system. *Invest Clin.* 1997;38:27-40.

80. Hofmeyr GJ, Lawrie TA, Atallah AN, Duley L. Calcium supplementation during pregnancy for preventing hypertensive disorders and related problems. *Cochrane Database Syst Rev.* 2010;8:CD001059.

81. Shahbaz AU, Sun Y, Bhattacharya SK, et al. Fibrosis in hypertensive heart disease: molecular pathways and cardioprotective strategies. *J Hypetens.* 2010;28:S25-S32.

82. Bergomi M, Rovesti S, Vinceti M, Vivoli R, Caselgrandi E, Vivoli G. Zinc and copper status and blood pressure. *J Trace Elem Med Biol.* 1997;11:166-169.

83. Stamler J, Elliott P, Kesteloot H, et al. Inverse relation of dietary protein markers with blood pressure. Findings for 10,020 men and women in the Intersalt Study. Intersalt Cooperative Research Group. International study of salt and blood pressure. *Circulation.* 1996;94:1629-1634.

84. Altorf-van der Kuil W, Engberink MF, Brink EJ, et al. Dietary protein and blood pressure: a systematic review. *PLoS One.* 2010;5(8);e121 02-e12117.

85. Jenkins DJ, Kendall CW, Faulkner DA, et al. Long-term effects of a plant-based dietary portfolio of cholesterol-lowering foods on blood pressure. *Eur J Clin Nutr.* 2008;62(6):781-788.

86. Rebholz CM, Friedman EE, Powers LJ, Arroyave WD, He J, Kelly TN. Dietary protein intake and blood pressure: a meta-analysis of randomized controlled trials. *Am J Epidemiol.* 2012;176(S7):S27-S43.

87. He J, Wofford MR, Reynolds K, et al. Effect of dietary protein supplementation on blood pressure: a randomized controlled trial. *Circulation.* 2011;124(5):589-595.

88. FitzGerald RJ, Murray BA, Walsh DJ. Hypotensive peptides from milk proteins. *J Nutr.* 2004;134(4):980S-988S.

89. Pins JJ, Keenan JM. Effects of Whey peptides on cardiovascular disease risk factors. *J Clin Hypertens.* 2006;8(11):775-782.

90. Aihara K, Kajimoto O, Takahashi R, Nakamura Y. Effect of powdered fermented milk with *Lactobacillus helveticus* on subjects with high-normal blood pressure or mild hypertension. *J Am Coll Nutr.* 2005;24(4):257-265.

91. Gemino FW, Neutel J, Nonaka M, Hendler SS. The impact of lactotripeptides on blood pressure response in stage 1 and stage 2 hypertensives. *J Clin Hypertens.* 2010;12(3):153-159.

92. Geleijnse JM, Engberink MF. Lactopeptides and human blood pressure. *Curr Opin Lipidol.* 2010;21(1):58-63.

93. Pins J, Keenan J. The antihypertensive effects of a hydrolyzed whey protein supplement. *Cardiovasc Drugs Ther.* 2002;16(suppl):68.

94. Zhu CF, Li GZ, Peng HB, Zhang F, Chen Y, Li Y. Therapeutic effects of marine collagen peptides on Chinese patients with type 2 diabetes mellitus and primary hypertension. *Am J Med Sci.* 2010;340(5):360-366.

95. De Leo F, Panarese S, Gallerani R, Ceci LR. Angiotensin converting enzyme (ACE) inhibitory peptides: production and implementation of functional food. *Curr Pharm Des.* 2009;15(31):3622-3643.

96. Lordan S, Ross P, Stanton C. Marine bioactives as functional food ingredients: potential to reduce the incidence of chronic disease. *Mar Drugs.* 2011;9(6):1056-1100.

97. Kawasaki T, Seki E, Osajima K, et al. Antihypertensive effect of valyl-tyrosine, a short chain peptide derived from sardine muscle hydrolyzate, on mild hypertensive subjects. *J Hum Hypertens.* 2000;14:519-523.

98. Kawasaki T, Jun CJ, Fukushima Y, Seki E. Antihypertensive effect and safety evaluation of vegetable drink with peptides derived from sardine protein hydrolysates on mild hypertensive, high-normal and normal blood pressure subjects. *Fukuoka Igaku Zasshi.* 2002;93(10):208-218.

99. Yang G, Shu XO, Jin F, et al. Longitudinal study of soy food intake and blood pressure among middle-aged and elderly Chinese women. *Am J Clin Nutr.* 2005;81(5):1012-1017.

100. Teede HJ, Giannopoulos D, Dalais FS, Hodgson J, McGrath BP. Randomised, controlled, cross-over trial of soy protein with isoflavones on blood pressure and arterial function in hypertensive patients. *J Am Coll Nutr.* 2006;25(6):533-540.

101. Welty FK, Lee KS, Lew NS, Zhou JR. Effect of soy nuts on blood pressure and lipid levels in hypertensive, prehypertensive and normotensive postmenopausal women. *Arch Inter Med.* 2007;167(10):1060-1067.

102. Mohanty DP, Mohapatra S, Misra S, Sahu P, Saudi S. Milk derived bioactive peptides and their impact on human health – a review. *J Biol Sci.* 2016;23(5):577-583.

103. Nasca MM, Zhou JR, Welty FK. Effect of soy nuts on adhesion molecules and markers of inflammation in hypertensive and normotensive postmenopausal women. *Am J Cardiol.* 2008;102(1):84-86.

104. He J, Gu D, Wu X, et al. Effect of soybean protein on blood pressure: a randomized, controlled trial. *Ann Intern Med.* 2005;143(1):1-9.

105. Hasler CM, Kundrat S, Wool D. Functional foods and cardiovascular disease. *Curr Atheroscler Rep.* 2000;2(6):467-75.

106. Liu XX, Li SH, Chen JZ, et al. Effect of soy isoflavones on blood pressure: a meta-analysis of randomized controlled trials. *Nutr Metab Cardiovasc Dis.* 2012;22:463-470.

107. Begg DP, Sinclari AJ, Stahl LA, Garg ML, Jois M, Weisinger RS. Dietary proteins level interacts with omega-3 polyunsaturated fatty acid deficiency to induce hypertension. *Am J Hyperten.* 2009;23:125-128.

108. Fekete ÁA, Giromini C, Chatzidiakou Y, Givens DI, Lovegrove JA. Whey protein lowers blood pressure and improves endothelial function and lipid biomarkers in adults with prehypertension and mild hypertension: results from the chronic Whey2Go randomized controlled trial. *Am J Clin Nutr.* 2016;104(6):1534-1544.

109. Dong JY, Szeto IM, Makinen K, et al. Effect of probiotic fermented milk on blood pressure: a meta-analysis of randomised controlled trials. *Br J Nutr.* 2013;110:1188-1194.

110. Cicero AF, Gerocarni B, Laghi L, Borghi C. Blood pressure lowering effect of lactotripeptides assumed as functional foods: a meta-analysis of current available clinical trials. *J Hum Hypertens.* 2011;25:425-436.

111. Cicero AF, Aubin F, Azais-Braesco V, Borghi C. Do the lactotripeptides isoleucine-proline-proline and valine-proline-proline reduce systolic blood pressure in European subjects? A meta-analysis of randomized controlled trials. *Am J Hypertens.* 2013;26:442-449.

112. Cicero AF, Rosticci M, Gerocarni B, et al. Lactotripeptides effect on office and 24-h ambulatory blood pressure, blood pressure stress response, pulse wave velocity and cardiac output in patients with high-normal blood pressure or first-degree hypertension: a randomized double-blind clinical trial. *Hypertens Res.* 2011;34:1035-1040.

113. Morris MC. Dietary fats and blood pressure. *J Cardiovasc Risk.* 1994;1:21-30.

114. Siani A, Pagano E, Iacone R, Iacoviell L, Scopacasa F, Strazzullo P. Blood pressure and metabolic changes during dietary L-arginine supplementation in humans. *Am J Hypertens.* 2000;13:547-551.

115. Vallance P, Leone A, Calver A, Collier J, Moncada S. Endogenous dimethyl-arginine as an inhibitor of nitric oxide synthesis. *J Cardiovasc Pharmacol.* 1992;20:S60-S62.

116. Ruiz-Hurtado G, Delgado C. Nitric oxide pathway in hypertrophied heart: new therapeutic uses of nitric oxide donors. *J Hypertens.* 2010;28(suppl 1):56-61.

117. Sonmez A, Celebi G, Erdem G, et al. Plasma apelin and ADMA levels in patients with essential hypertension. *Clin Exp Hypertens.* 2010;32(3):179-183.

118. Michell DL, Andrews KL, Chin-Dusting JP. Endothelial dysfunction in hypertension: the role of arginase. *Front Biosci (Schol Ed).* 2011;3:946-960.

119. Rajapakse NW, Mattson DL. Role of L-arginine in nitric oxide production in health and hypertension. *Clin Exp Pharmacol Physiol.* 2009;36(3):249-255.

120. Tsioufis C, Dimitriadis K, Andrikou E, et al. ADMA, C-reactive protein and albuminuria in untreated essential hypertension: a cross-sectional study. *Am J Kidney Dis.* 2010;55(6):1050-1059.

121. Facchinetti F, Saade GR, Neri I, Pizzi C, Longo M, Volpe A. L-Arginine supplementation in patients with gestational hypertension: a pilot study. *Hypertens Pregnancy.* 2007;26(1):121-130.

122. Neri I, Monari F, Sqarbi L, Berardi A, Masellis G, Facchinetti F. L-Arginine supplementation in women with chronic hypertension: impact on blood pressure and maternal and neonatal complications. *J Matern Fetal Neonatal Med.* 2010;23(12):1456-1460.

123. Martina V, Masha A, Gigliardi VR, et al. Long-term N-acetylcysteine and L-arginine administration reduces endothelial activation and systolic blood pressure in hypertensive patients with type 2 diabetes. *Diabetes Care.* 2008;31(5):940-944.

124. Ast J, Jablecka A, Bogdanski I, Krauss H, Chmara E. Evaluation of the antihypertensive effect of L-arginine supplementation in patients with mild hypertension assessed with ambulatory blood pressure monitoring. *Med Sci Monit.* 2010;16(5):CR266-CR271.

125. Schulman SP, Becker LC, Kass DA, et al. L arginine therapy in acute myocardial infraction: the vascular interaction with age in myocardial infarction (VINTAGE MI) randomized clinical trial. *JAMA.* 2006;295(1):58-64.

126. Dong JY, Qin JQ, Zhang ZL, et al. Effect of oral L-arginine supplementation on blood pressure: a meta-analysis of randomized, double-blind, placebo-controlled trials. *Am Heart J.* 2011;162:959-965.

127. Huxtable RJ. Physiologic actions of taurine. *Physiol Rev.* 1992;72:101-163.

128. Fujita T, Ando K, Noda H, Ito Y, Sato Y. Effects of increased adrenomedullary activity and taurine in young patients with borderline hypertension. *Circulation.* 1987;75:525-532.

129. Huxtable RJ, Sebring LA. Cardiovascular actions of taurine. *Prog Clin Biol Res.* 1983;125:5-37.

130. Tanabe Y, Urata H, Kiyonaga A, et al. Changes in serum concentrations of taurine and other amino acids in clinical antihypertensive exercise therapy. *Clin Exp Hypertens.* 1989;11:149-165.

131. Yamori Y, Taguchi T, Mori H, Mori M. Low cardiovascular risks in the middle age males and females excreting greater 24-hour urinary taurine and magnesium in 41 WHO-CARDIAC study populations in the world. *J Biomed Sci.* 2010;17(suppl 1):s21-s26.

132. Wang B, Li Y, Sun F, et al. Taurine supplementation lowers blood pressure and improves vascular function in prehypertension: randomized, double-blind, placebo-controlled study. *Hypertension.* 2016;67(3):541-549.

133. Houston Mark C. Combination nutraceutical supplement lowers blood pressure in hypertensive individuals. *Integr Med.* 2019;12(3):22-28.

134. Mori TA, Bao DQ, Burke V, Puddey IB, Beilin LJ. Docosahexaenoic acid but not eicosapentaenoic acid lowers ambulatory blood pressure and heart rate in humans. *Hypertension.* 1999;34:253-260.

135. Bønaa KH, Bjerve KS, Straume B, Gram IT, Thelle D. Effect of eicosapentaenoic and docosahexanoic acids on blood pressure in hypertension: a population-based intervention trial from the Tromso study. *N Engl J Med.* 1990;322:795-801.

136. Mori TA, Burke V, Puddey I, Irish A. The effects of omega 3 fatty acids and coenzyme Q 10 on blood pressure and heart rate in chronic kidney disease: a randomized controlled trial. *J Hypertens.* 2009;27(9):1863-1872.

137. Ueshima H, Stamler J, Elliot B, Brown CQ. Food omega 3 fatty acid intake of individuals (total, linolenic acid, long chain) and their blood pressure: INTERMAP study. *Hypertension.* 2007;50(20):313-319.

138. Mon TA. Omega 3 fatty acids and hypertension in humans. *Clin Exp Pharmacol Physio.* 2006;33(9):842-846.

139. Liu JC, Conkin SM, Manuch SB, Yao JK, Muldoon MF. Long-chain omega-3 fatty acids and blood pressure. *Am J Hypertens.* 2011;24(10):1121-1126.

140. Engler MM, Schambelan M, Engler MB, Goodfriend TL. Effects of dietary gamma-linolenic acid on blood pressure and adrenal angiotensin receptors in hypertensive rats. *Proc Soc Exp Biol Med.* 1998;218(3):234-237.

141. Sagara M, Njelekela M, Teramoto T, et al. Effects of docoahexaenoic acid supplementation on blood pressure, heart rate, and serum lipid in Scottish men with hypertension and hypercholesterolemia. *Int J Hypertens.* 2011;8:8091-8098.

142. Colussi G, Catena C, Novello M, Bertin N, Sechi LA Impact of omega-3 polyunsaturated fatty acids on vascular function and blood pressure: Relevance for cardiovascular outcomes. *Nutr Metab Cardiovasc Dis.* 2017;27(3):191-200.

143. Miller PE, Van Elswyk M, Alexander DD. Long-chain omega-3 fatty acids eicosapentaenoic acid and docosahexaenoic acid and blood pressure: a meta-analysis of randomized controlled trials. *Am J Hypertens.* 2014;27:885-896.

144. Pase MP, Grima NA, Sarris J. Do long-chain n-3 fatty acids reduce arterial stiffness? A meta-analysis of randomised controlled trials. *Br J Nutr.* 2011;106:974-980.

145. Cicero AF, Ertek S, Borghi C. Omega-3 polyunsaturated fatty acids: their potential role in blood pressure prevention and management. *Curr Vasc Pharmacol.* 2009;7:330-337.

146. Minihane AM, Armah CK, Miles EA, et al. Consumption of fish oil providing amounts of eicosapentaenoic acid and docosahexaenoic acid that can be obtained from the diet reduces blood pressure in adults with systolic hypertension: a retrospective analysis. *J Nutr.* 2016;146(3):516-523.

147. Rodriguez-Leyva D, Weighell W, Edel AL, et al. Potent antihypertensive action of dietary flaxseed in hypertensive patients. *Hypertension.* 2013 Dec;62(6):1081-1089.

148. Saravanan P, Davidson NC, Schmidt EB, Calder PC. Cardiovascular effects of marine omega-3 fatty acids. *Lancet.* 2010;376(9740):540-550.

149. Alexander DD, Miller PE, Van Elswyk ME, Kuratko CN, Bylsma LC. A meta-analysis of randomized controlled trials and prospective cohort studies of eicosapentaenoic and docosahexaenoic long-chain omega-3 fatty acids and coronary heart disease risk. *Mayo Clin Proc.* 2017;92(1):15-29.

150. Ferrara LA, Raimondi S, d'Episcopa I. Olive oil and reduced need for antihypertensive medications. *Arch Intern Med.* 2000;160:837-842.

151. Perona JS, Canizares J, Montero E, Sanchez-Dominquez JM, Catala A, Ruiz Gutierrez V. Virgin olive oil reduces blood pressure in hypertensive elderly patients. *Clin Nutr.* 2004;23(5):1113-1121.

152. Perona JS, Montero E, Sanchez-Dominquez JM, Canizares J, Garcia M, Ruiz-Gutierrez V. Evaluation of the effect of dietary virgin olive oil on blood pressure and lipid composition of serum and low-density lipoprotein in elderly type 2 subjects. *J Agric Food Chem.* 2009;57(23):11427-11433.

153. Lopez-Miranda J, Perez-Jimenez F, Ros E, et al. Olive oil and health: summary of the II International Conference on Olive oil and health consensus report, Jaen and Cordoba (Spain) 2008. *Nutr Metab Cardiovasc Dis.* 2010;20(4):284-294.

154. Thomsen C, Rasmussen OW, Hansen KW, Vesterlund M, Hermansen K. Comparison of the effects on the diurnal blood pressure, glucose, and lipid levels of a diet rich in monounsaturated fatty acids with a diet rich in polyunsaturated fatty acids in type 2 diabetic subjects. *Diabet Med.* 1995;12:600-606.

155. Sofi F, Abbate R, Gensini GF, Casini A. Accruing evidence on benefits of adherence to the Mediterranean diet on health: an updated systematic review and meta-analysis. *Am J Clin Nutr.* 2010;92(5):1189-1196.

156. Estruch R, Ros E, Salas-Salvadó J, et al. Primary prevention of cardiovascular disease with a Mediterranean diet. *N Engl J Med.* 2013;368(14):1279-1290.

157. Nadtochiy SM, Redman EK. Mediterranean diet and cardioprotection: the role of nitrite, polyunsaturated fatty acids, and polyphenols. *Nutrition.* 2011;27(7-8):733-44.

158. Salas-Salvadó J, Bulló M, Estruch R, et al. Prevention of diabetes with Mediterranean diets: a subgroup analysis of a randomized trial. *Ann Intern Med.* 2014;160(1):1-10.

159. Lopez S, Bermudez B, Montserrat-de la Paz S, Jaramillo S, Abia R, Muriana FJ. Virgin olive oil and hypertension. *Curr Vasc Pharmacol.* 2016;14(4):323-329.

160. Martín-Peláez S, Castañer O, Konstantinidou V, et al. Effect of olive oil phenolic compounds on the expression of blood pressure-related genes in healthy individuals. *Eur J Nutr.* 2017;56(2):663-670.

161. Storniolo CE, Casillas R, Bulló M, et al. A Mediterranean diet supplemented with extra virgin olive oil or nuts improves endothelial markers involved in blood pressure control in hypertensive women. *Eur J Nutr.* 2017;56(1):89-97.

162. Hohmann CD, Cramer H, Michalsen A, et al. Effects of high. phenolic olive oil on cardiovascular risk factors: A systematic review and meta-analysis. *Phytomedicine.* 2015;22(6):631-640.

163. Doménech M, Roman P, Lapetra J, et al. Mediterranean diet reduces 24-hour ambulatory blood pressure, blood glucose, and lipids: one-year randomized, clinical trial. *Hypertension.* 2014;64(1):69-76.

164. Lockyer S, Rowland I, Spencer JP, Yaqoob P, Stonehouse W. Impact of phenolic-rich olive leaf extract on blood pressure, plasma lipids and inflammatory markers: a randomized controlled trial. *Eur J Nutr.* 2017;56(4):1421-1432.

165. Cabrera-Vique C, Navarro-Alarcón M, Rodríguez Martínez C, Fonollá-Joya J. Hypertensive effect of an extract of bioactive compounds olive leaves preliminary clinical study. *Nutr Hosp.* 2015;32(1):242-249. Available from: https://www.ncbi.nlm.nih.gov/pubmed/21036583-comments.

166. Susalit E, Agus N, Effendi I, et al. Olive (Olea europaea) leaf extract effective in patients with stage-1 hypertension: comparison with Captopril. *Phytomedicine.* 2011;18(4):251-258.

167. Flynn M, Wang S. Olive oil as medicine: the effect on blood pressure. *Rep UCD Olive Cent.* December 2015.

168. Psaltopoulou T, Naska A, Orfanos P, Trichopoulos D, Mountokalakis T, Trichopoulou A. Olive oil, the Mediterranean diet, and arterial blood pressure: the Greek European Prospective Investigation into Cancer and Nutrition (EPIC) study. *Am J Clin Nutr.* 2004;80:1012-1018.

169. Toledo E, Hu FB, Estruch R, et al. Effect of the Mediterranean diet on blood pressure in the PREDIMED trial: results from a randomized controlled trial. *BMC Med.* 2013;11:207.

170. Perrinjaquet-Moccetti T, Busjahn A, Schmidlin C, Schmidt A, Bradl B, Aydogan C. Food supplementation with an olive (Olea uropaea L.) leaf extract reduces blood pressure in borderline hypertensive monozygotic twins. *Phytother Res.* 2008;22:1239-1242.

171. Hodgson JM, Woodman R, Bryan J, Wilson C, Murphy KJ. A Mediterranean diet lowers blood pressure and improves endothelial function: results from the MedLey randomized intervention trial. *Am J Clin Nutr.* 2017;105(6):1305-1313. pii:ajcn146803.

172. Miura K, Stamler J, Brown IJ, et al. Relationship of dietary monounsaturated fatty acids to blood pressure: the International Study of Macro/Micronutrients and Blood Pressure. *J Hypertens.* 2013;31(6):1144-1150.

173. Sherman DL, Keaney JF, Biegelsen ES, et al. Pharmacological concentrations of ascorbic acid are required for the beneficial effect on endothelial vasomotor function in hypertension. *Hypertension.* 2000;35:936-941.

174. Ness AR, Khaw K-T, Bingham S, Day NE. Vitamin C status and blood pressure. *J Hypertens.* 1996;14:503-508.

175. Duffy SJ, Bokce N, Holbrook. Treatment of hypertension with ascorbic acid. *Lancet.* 1999;354:2048-2049.

176. Enstrom JE, Kanim LE, Klein M. Vitamin C intake and mortality among a sample of the United States population. *Epidemiology.* 1992;3:194-202.

177. Block G, Jensen CD, Norkus EP, Hudes M, Crawford PB. Vitamin C in plasma is inversely related to blood pressure and change in blood pressure during the previous year in young black and white women. *Nut J.* 2008;17(7):35-46.

178. Hatzitolios A, Iliadis F, Katsiki N, Baltatzi M. Is the antihypertensive effect of dietary supplements via aldehydes reduction evidence based: A systemic review. *Clin Exp Hypertens.* 2008;30(7):628-639.

179. Mahajan AS, Babbar R, Kansai N, Agarwai SK, Ray PC. Antihypertensive and antioxidant action of amlodipine and Vitamin C in patients of essential hypertension. *J Clin Biochem Nutr.* 2007;40(2):141-147.

180. Ledlerc PC, Proulx CD, Arquin G, Belanger S. Ascorbic acid decreases the binding affinity of the AT! Receptor for angiotensin II. *Am J Hypertens.* 2008;21(1):67-71.

181. Plantinga Y, Ghiadone L, Magagna A, Biannarelli C. Supplementation with vitamins C and E improves arterial stiffness and endothelial function in essential hypertensive patients. *Am J Hypertens.* 2007;20(4):392-397.

182. Sato K, Dohi Y, Kojima M, Miyagawa K. Effects of ascorbic acid on ambulatory blood pressure in elderly patients with refractory hypertension. *Arzneimittelforschung.* 2006;56(7):535-540.

183. Block G, Mangels AR, Norkus EP, Patterson BH, Levander OA, Taylor PR. Ascorbic acid status and subsequent diastolic and systolic blood pressure. *Hypertension.* 2001;37:261-267.

184. McRae MP. Is vitamin C an effective antihypertensive supplement? A review and analysis of the literature. *J Chiropr Med.* 2006;5(2):60-64.

185. Simon JA. Vitamin C and cardiovascular disease: a review. *J Am Coll Nutr.* 1992;11(2):107-125.

186. Ness AR, Chee D, Elliott P. Vitamin C and blood pressure—an overview. *J Hum Hypertens.* 1997;11(6):343-350.

187. Trout DL. Vitamin C and cardiovascular risk factors. *Am J Clin Nutr.* 1991;53(1 suppl):322S-325S.

188. Ried K, Travica N, Sali A. The acute effect of high-dose intravenous vitamin C and other nutrients on blood pressure: a cohort study. *Blood Press Monit.* 2016;21(3):160-167.

189. Buijsse B, Jacobs DR Jr, Steffen LM, Kromhout D, Gross MD. Plasma ascorbic acid, a priori diet quality score, and incident hypertension: a prospective cohort study. *PLoS One.* 2015;10(12).

190. Hajjar IM, George V, Sasse EA, Kochar MS. A randomized, double-blind, controlled trial of vitamin C in the management of hypertension and lipids. *Am J Ther.* 2002;9(4):289-293.

191. National Center for Health Statistics, Fulwood R, Johnson CL, Bryner JD. *Hematological and Nutritional Biochemistry Reference Data for Persons 6 Months-74 Years of Age: United States, 1976-80.* Washington, DC; US Public Health Service; 1982. Vital and Health Statistics series 11, No. 232, DHHS publication No. (PHS) 83-1682.

192. McCartney DM, Byrne DG, Turner MJ. Dietary contributors to hypertension in adults reviewed. *Ir J Med Sci.* 2015;184:81-90.

193. Juraschek SP, Guallar E, Appel LJ, Miller ER 3rd. Effects of vitamin C supplementation on blood pressure: a meta-analysis of randomized controlled trials. *Am J Clin Nutr.* 2012;95:1079-1088.

194. Ward NC, Wu JH, Clarke MW, Buddy IB, Vitamin E. Effects on the treatment of hypertension in type 2 diabetics. *J Hypertens.* 2007;227:227-234.

195. Murray ED, Wechter WJ, Kantoci D, et al. Endogenous natriuretic factors 7: Biospecificity of a natriuretic gamma-tocopherol metabolite LLU alpha. *J Pharmacol Exp Ther.* 1997;282(2):657-662.

196. Gray B, Swick J, Ronnenberg AG. Vitamin E and adiponectin: proposed mechanism for vitamin E-induced improvement in insulin sensitivity. *Nutr Rev.* 2011;69(3):155-161.

197. Kuwabara A, Nakade M, Tamai H, Tsuboyama-Kasaoka N, Tanaka K. The association between vitamin E intake and hypertension: results from the re-analysis of the National Health and Nutrition Survey. *J Nutr Sci Vitaminol (Tokyo).* 2014;60(4):239-245.

198. Hodgson JM, Croft KD, Woodman RJ, et al. Effects of vitamin E, vitamin C and polyphenols on the rate of blood pressure variation: results of two randomised controlled trials. *Br J Nutr.* 2014;112(9):1551-1561.

199. Hanni LL, Huarfner LH, Sorensen OH, Ljunghall S. Vitamin D is related to blood pressure and other cardiovascular risk factors in middle-aged men. *Am J Hypertens.* 1995;8:894-901.

200. Bednarski R, Donderski R, Manitius L. Role of Vitamin D in arterial blood pressure control. *Pol Merkur Lekarski.* 2007;136:307-310.

201. Li YC, Kong H, Wei M, Chen ZF. 1,25 Dihydroxyvitamin D 3 is a negative endocrine regulator of the renin angiotensin system. *J Clin Invest.* 2002;110(2):229-238.

202. Ngo DT, Sverdlov AL, McNeil JJ, Horowitz JD. Does vitamin D modulate asymmetric dimethylargine and C-reactive protein concentrations?. *Am J Med.* 2010;123(4):335-341.

203. Rosen CJ. Clinical practice. Vitamin D insufficiency. *N Engl J Med.* 2011;364(3):248-254.

204. Boldo A, Campbell P, Luthra P, White WB. Should the concentration of Vitamin D be measured in all patients with hypertension?. *J Clin Hypertens.* 2010;12(3):149-52.

205. Pittas AG, Chung M, Trikalinos T, et al. Systematic review: Vitamin D and cardiometabolic outcomes. *Ann Intern Med.* 2010;152(5):307-314.

206. Movano Peregrin C, Lopez Rodriguez R, Castilla Castellano MD. Vitamin D and hypertension. *Med Clin (Barc).* 2012;138(9):397-401.

207. Motiwala S, Want TJ. Vitamin D and cardiovascular disease. *Curr Opin Nephrol Hypertens.* 2011;20(4):345-353.

208. Cosenso-Martin LN, Vitela-Martin JF. Is there an association between vitamin D and hypertension. *Recent Pat Cardiovasc Drug Discov.* 2011;6(2):140-147.

209. Bhandari SK, Pashayan S, Liu IL, et al. 25-hydroxyvitamin D levels and hypertension rates. *J Clin Hypertens.* 2011;13(3):170-177.

210. Pfeifer M, Begerow B, Minne HW, Nachtigall D, Hansen C. Effects of a short-term vitamin D (3) and calcium supplementation on blood pressure and parathyroid hormone levels in elderly women. *J Clin Endocrinol Metab.* 2001;86:1633-1637.

211. Qi D, Nie XL, Wu S. Vitamin D and hypertension: prospective study and meta-analysis. *PLoS One.* 2017;12(3):e0174298.

212. McMullan CJ, Borgi L, Curhan GC, Fisher N, Forman JP. The effect of vitamin D on renin-angiotensin system activation and blood pressure: a randomized control trial. *J Hypertens.* 2017;35(4):822-829.

213. Qi D, Nie X, Cai J The effect of vitamin D supplementation on hypertension in non-CKD populations: A systemic review and meta-analysis. *Int J Cardiol.* 2017;227:177-186.

214. Yilmaz S, Sen F, Ozeke O, et al. The relationship between vitamin D levels and nondipper hypertension. *Blood Press Monit.* 2015;20(6):330-334.

215. Beveridge LA, Struthers AD, Khan F, et al. Effect of vitamin D supplementation on blood pressure: a systematic review and meta-analysis incorporating individual patient data. *JAMA Intern Med.* 2015;175(5):745-754.

216. Forman JP, Scott JB, Ng K, et al. Effect of vitamin D supplementation on blood pressure in blacks. *Hypertension.* 2013;61(4):779-785.

217. Keniston R, Enriquez JI Sr. Relationship between blood pressure and plasma vitamin B$_6$ levels in healthy middle-aged adults. *Ann NY Acad Sci.* 1990;585:499-501.

218. Aybak M, Sermet A, Ayyildiz MO, Karakilcik AZ. Effect of oral pyridoxine hydrochloride supplementation on arterial blood pressure in patients with essential hypertension. *Arzneimittelforschung.* 1995;45:1271-1273.

219. Paulose CS, Dakshinamurti K, Packer S, Stephens NL. Sympathetic stimulation and hypertension in the pyridoxine-deficient adult rat. *Hypertension.* 1988;11(4):387-391.

220. Dakshinamurti K, Lal KJ, Ganguly PK. Hypertension, calcium channel and pyridoxine (vitamin B6). *Mol Cel Biochem.* 1998;188(1-2):137-148.

221. Hosseini S, Lee J, Sepulveda RT, et al. A randomized, double blind, placebo-controlled, prospective 16 week crossover study to determine the role of pycnogenol in modifying blood pressure in mildly hypertensive patients. *Nutr Res.* 2001;21:1251-1260.

222. Moline J, Bukharovich IF, Wolff MS, Phillips R. Dietary flavonoids and hypertension: is there a link? *Med Hypotheses.* 2000;55:306-309.

223. Knekt P, Reunanen A, Järvinen R, Seppänen R, Heliövaara M, Aromaa A. Antioxidant vitamin intake and coronary mortality in a longitudinal population study. *Am J Epidemiol.* 1994;139:1180-1189.

224. Karatzi KN, Papamichael CM, Karatizis EN, et al. Red wine acutely induces favorable effects on wave reflections and central pressures in coronary artery disease patients. *Am J Hypertens.* 2005;18(9):1161-1167.

225. Biala A, Tauriainen E, Siltanen A, et al. Resveratrol induces mitochondrial biogenesis and ameliorates Ang II- induced cardiac remodeling in transgenic rats harboring human renin and angiotensinogen genes. *Blood Press.* 2010;19(3):196-205.

226. Wong RH, Howe PR, Buckley JD, Coates AM, Kunz L, Berry NM. Acute resveratrol supplementation improves flow-mediated dilatation in overweight obese individuals with mildly elevated blood pressure. *Nutr Metab Cardiovasc Dis.* 2011;21:851-856.

227. Bhatt SR, Lokhandwala MF, Banday AA. Resveratrol prevents endothelial nitric oxide synthase uncoupling and attenuates development of hypertension in spontaneously hypertensive rats. *Eur J Pharmacol.* 2011;667(1-3):258-264.

228. Rivera L, Moron R, Zarzuelo A, Galisteo M. Long-term resveratrol administration reduces metabolic disturbances and lowers blood pressure in obese Zucker rats. *Biochem Pharmacol.* 2009;77(6):1053-1063.

229. Sahebkar A Ferri C, Giorgini P, Bo S, Nachtigal P, Grassi D. Effects of pomegranate juice on blood pressure: A systematic review and meta-analysis of randomized controlled trials. *Pharmacol Res.* 2017;115:149-161.

230. Tjelle TE, Holtung L, Bøhn SK, et al. Polyphenol-rich juices reduce blood pressure measures in a randomised controlled trial in high normal and hypertensive volunteers. *Br J Nutr.* 2015;114(7):1054-1063.

231. de Jesús Romero-Prado MM, Curiel-Beltrán JA, Miramontes-Espino MV, CardonaMuñoz EG, Rios-Arellano A, Balam-Salazar LB. Dietary flavonoids added to pharmacological antihypertensive therapy are effective in improving blood pressure. *Basic Clin Pharmacol Toxicol.* 2015;117(1):57-64. https://www.ncbi.nlm.nih.gov/pubmed/23519910-comments.

232. Asgary S, Sahebkar A, Afshani MR, Keshvari M, Haghjooyjavanmard S, Rafieian-Kopaei M. Clinical evaluation of blood pressure lowering, endothelial function improving, hypolipidemic and anti-inflammatory effects of pomegranate juice in hypertensive subjects. *Phytother Res.* 2014;28(2):193-199.

233. Paran E, Engelhard YN. Effect of lycopene, an oral natural antioxidant on blood pressure. *J Hypertens* 2001;19:S74.

234. Engelhard YN, Gazer B, Paran E. Natural antioxidants from tomato extract reduce blood pressure in patients with grade-1 hypertension: a double blind placebo controlled pilot study. *Am Heart J.* 2006;151(1):100.

235. Paran E, Novac C, Engelhard YN, Hazan-Halevy I. The effects of natural antioxidants form tomato extract in treated but uncontrolled hypertensive patients. *Cardiovasc Durgs Ther.* 2009;23(2):145-151.

236. Reid K, Frank OR, Stocks NP. Dark chocolate or tomato extract for prehypertension: a randomized controlled trial. *BMC Complement Altern Med.* 2009;9:22.

237. Paran E, Engelhard Y. Effect of tomato's lycopene on blood pressure, serum lipoproteins, plasma homocysteine and oxidative stress markers in grade I hypertensive patients. *Am J Hypertens.* 2001;14:141A.

238. Ried K, Fakler P. Protective effect of lycopene on serum cholesterol and blood pressure: Meta-analyses of intervention trials. *Maturitas.* 2011;68(4):299-310.

239. Burton-Freeman B, Sesso HD. Whole food versus supplement: comparing the clinical evidence of tomato intake and lycopene supplementation on cardiovascular risk factors. *Adv Nutr.* 2014;5(5):457-485.

240. Langsjoen PH, Langsjoen AM. Overview of the use of Co Q 10 in cardiovascular disease. *Biofactors.* 1999;9:273-284.

241. Singh RB, Niaz MA, Rastogi SS, Shukla PK, Thakur AS. Effect of hydrosoluble coenzyme Q10 on blood pressure and insulin resistance in hypertensive patients with coronary heart disease. *J Hum Hypertens.* 1999;12:203-208.

242. Burke BE, Neustenschwander R, Olson RD. Randomized, double-blind, placebo-controlled trial of coenzyme Q10 in isolated systolic hypertension. *South Med J.* 2001;94:1112-1117.

243. Rosenfeldt FL, Haas S, Krum H, Hadu A. Coenzyme Q 10 in the treatment of hypertension: a meta-analysis of the clinical trials. *J Hum Hypertens.* 2007;21(4):297-306.

244. Singh RB, Niaz MA, Rastogi SS, Shukia PK, Thakur AS. Effect of hydrosoluble coenzyme Q 10 on blood pressures and insulin resistance in hypertensive patients with coronary artery disease. *J Hum Hypertens.* 1999;13(3):302-308.

245. Ankola DD, Viswanas B, Bhardqaj V, Ramarao P, Kumar MN. Development of potent oral nanoparticulate formulation of coenzyme Q10 for treatment of hypertension: can the simple nutritional supplement be used as first line therapeutic agents for prophylaxis/therapy? *Eur J Pharm Biopharm* 2007:67(2):361-369.

246. Ho MJ, Li EC, Wright JM. Blood pressure lowering efficacy of coenzyme Q10 for primary hypertension. *Cochrane Database Syst Rev.* 2016;3:CD007435.

247. Ho MJ, Bellusci A, Wright JM. Blood pressure lowering efficacy of coenzyme Q10 for primary hypertension. *Cochrane Database Syst Rev.* 2009;(4):CD007435.

248. Mikhin VP, Kharchenko AV, Rosliakova EA, Cherniatina MA. Application of coenzyme Q(10) in combination therapy of arterial hypertension. *Kardiologiia.* 2011;51(6):26-31.

249. Tsai KL, Huang YH, Kao CL, et al. A novel mechanism of coenzyme Q10 protects against human endothelial cells from oxidative stress-induced injury by modulating NO-related pathways. *J Nutr Biochem.* 2012;23(5):458-468.

250. Sohet FM, Delzenne NM. Is there a place for coenzyme Q in the management of metabolic disorders associated with obesity? *Nutr Rev.* 2012;70(11):631-641.

251. Digiesi V, Cantini F, Oradei A, et al. Coenzyme Q10 in essential hypertension. *Mol Aspects Med.* 1994;15(suppl):s257-s263.

252. Langsjoen P, Langsjoen P, Willis R, Folkers K. Treatment of essential hypertension with coenzyme Q10. *Mol Aspects Med.* 1994;15(suppl):S265-S272.

253. Trimarco V, Cimmino CS, Santoro M, et al. Nutraceuticals for blood pressure control in patients with high-normal or grade 1 hypertension. *High Blood Press Cardiovasc Prev.* 2012;19(3):117-122.

254. Young JM, Florkowski CM, Molyneux SL, et al. A randomized, double-blind, placebo-controlled crossover study of coenzyme Q10 therapy in hypertensive patients with the metabolic syndrome. *Am J Hypertens.* 2012;(2):261-270.

255. Kontush A, Reich A, Baum K, et al. Plasma ubiquinol-10 is decreased in patients with hyperlipidaemia. *Atherosclerosis.* 1997;129(1):119-126.

256. McLachlan J, Beattie E, Murphy MP, et al. Combined therapeutic benefit of mitochondria-targeted antioxidant, MitoQ10, and angiotensin receptor blocker, losartan, on cardiovascular function. *J Hypertens.* 2014;32(3):555-564.

257. Rosenfeldt F, Hilton D, Pepe S, Krum H. Systematic review of effect of coenzyme Q10 in physical exercise, hypertension and heart failure. *Biofactors.* 2003;18(1-4):91-100.

258. McMackin CJ, Widlansky ME, Hambury NM, Haung AL. Effect of combined treatment with alpha lipoic acid and acetyl carnitine on vascular function and blood pressure in patients with coronary artery disease. *J Clin Hypertens.* 2007;9:249-255.

259. Salinthone S, Schillace RV, Tsang C, Regan JW, Burdette DN, Carr DW. Lipoic acid stimulates cAMP production via G protein-coupled receptor-dependent and independent mechanisms. *J Nutr Biochem.* 2011;22(7):681-690.

260. Rahman ST, Merchant N, Hague T, et al. The impact of lipoic acid on endothelial function and proteinuria in Quinapril-treated diabetic patients with stage I hypertension: results from the quality study. *J Cardiovasc Pharmacol Ther.* 2012;17(2):139-145.

261. Huang YD, Li N, Zhang WG, et al. The effect of oral alpha-lipoic acid in overweight/obese individuals on the brachial-ankle pulse wave velocity and supine blood pressure: a randomized, crossover, double-blind,placebo-controlled trial. *Zhonghua Liu Xing Bing Xue Za Zhi.* 2011;32(3):290-296.

262. Morcos M, Borcea V, Isermann B, et al. Effect of alpha-lipoic acid on the progression of endothelial cell damage and albuminuria in patients with diabetes mellitus: an exploratory study. *Diabetes Res Clin Prac.* 2001;52(3):175-183.

263. Noori N, Tabibi H, Hosseinpanah F, Hedayati M, Nafar M. Effects of combined lipoic acid and pyridoxine on albuminuria, advanced glycation end-products, and blood pressure in diabetic nephropathy. *Int J Vitam Nutr Res.* 2013;83(2):77-85.

264. Zibadi S, Rohdewald PJ, Park D, Watson RR. Reduction of cardio-vascular risk factors in subjects with type 2 diabetes by pycnogenol supplementation. *Nutr Res.* 2008;28(5):315-320.

265. Liu X, Wei J, Tan F, Zhou S, Wurthwein G, Rohdewald P. Pycnogenol French maritime pine bark extract improves endothelial function of hypertensive patients. *Life Sci.* 2004;74(7):855-862.

266. Van der Zwan LP, Scheffer PG, Teerlink T. Reduction of myeloper-oxidase activity by melatonin and pycnogenol may contribute to their blood pressure lowering effect. *Hypertension.* 2010;56(3):e35.

267. Cesarone MR, Belcaro G, Stuard S, et al. Kidney flow and function in hypertension: protective effects of pyconogenol in hypertensive participants- a controlled study. *J Cardiovasc Pharmacol Ther.* 2010;15(1):41-46.

268. Gulati OP. Pycnogenol in metabolic syndrome and related disorders. *Phytother Res.* 2015;29(7):949-968. https://www.ncbi.nlm.nih.gov/pubmed/25391252-comments.

269. Hu S, Belcaro G, Cornelli U, et al. Effects of pycnogenol on endo-thelial dysfunction in borderline hypertensive, hyperlipidemic, and hyperglycemic individuals: the borderline study. *Int Angiol.* 2015;34(1):43-52.

270. Enseleit F, Sudano I, Périat D, et al. Effects of pycnogenol on endo-thelial function in patients with stable coronary artery disease: a double-blind, placebo-controlled, cross-over study. *Eur Heart J.* 2012;33(13):1589-1597.

271. Luzzi R, Belcaro G, Hosoi M, et al. Normalization of cardiovascular risk factors in peri-menopausal women with Pycnogenol®. *Minerva Ginecol.* 2017;69(1):29-34.

272. Simons S, Wollersheim H, Thien T. A systematic review on the influ-ence of trial quality on the effects of garlic on blood pressure. *Neth J Med.* 2009;67(6):212-219.

273. Reinhard KM, Coleman CI, Teevan C, Vacchani P. Effects of garlic on blood pressure in patients with and without sys-tolic hypertension: a meta-analysis. *Ann Pharmacother.* 2008;42(12):1766-1771.

274. Reid K, Frank OR, Stocks NP. Aged garlic extract lowers blood pres-sure in patients with treated but uncontrolled hypertension: a random-ized controlled trial. *Maturitas.* 2010;67(2):144-150.

275. Nakasone Y, Nakamura Y, Yamamoto T, Yamaguchi H. Effect of a traditional Japanese garlic preparation on blood pressure in prehypertensive and mildly hypertensive adults. *Exp Ther Med.* 2013;5(2):399-405.

276. Ried K, Frank OR, Stocks NP. Aged garlic extract reduces blood pressure in hypertensives: a dose-response trial. *Eur J Clin Nutr.* 2013;67(1):64-70.

277. Shouk R, Abdou A, Shetty K, Sarkar D, Eid AH. Mechanisms under-lying the antihypertensive effects of garlic bioactives. *Nutr Res.* 2014;34(2):106-115.

278. Stabler SN, Tejani AM, Huynh F, Fowkes C. Garlic for the prevention of cardiovascular morbidity and mortality in hypertensive patients. *Cochrane Database Syst Rev.* 2012;(8):CD007653.

279. Mahdavi-Roshan M, Nasrollahzadeh J, Mohammad Zadeh A, Zahedmehr A. Does garlic supplementation control blood pressure in patients with severe coronary artery disease? A clinical trial study. *Iran Red Crescent Med J.* 2016;18(11):e23871.

280. Ried K, Travica N, Sali A. The effect of aged garlic extract on blood pressure and other cardiovascular risk factors in uncontrolled hypertensives: the AGE at Heart Trial. *Integr Blood Press Control.* 2016;9:9-21.

281. Varshney R, Budoff MJ. Garlic and heart disease. *J Nutr.* 2016;146(2):416S-421S.

282. Xiong XJ, Wang PQ, Li SJ, Li XK, Zhang YQ, Wang J. Garlic for hypertension: a systematic review and meta-analysis of randomized controlled trials. *Phytomedicine.* 2015;22(3):352-361.

283. Suetsuna K, Nakano T. Identification of an antihypertensive peptide from peptic digest of wakame (*Undaria pinnatifida*). *J Nutr Biochem.* 2000;11:450-454.

284. Nakano T, Hidaka H, Uchida J, Nakajima K, Hata Y. Hypotensive effects of wakame. *J Jpn Soc Clin Nutr.* 1998;20:92.

285. Krotkiewski M, Aurell M, Holm G, Grimby G, Szczepanik J. Effects of a sodium-potassium ion-exchanging seaweed preparation in mild hypertension. *Am J Hypertens.* 1991;4:483-488.

286. Sato M, Oba T, Yamaguchi T, et al. Antihypertensive effects of hydro-lysates of wakame (*Undaria pinnatifida*) and their angiotnesin-1-converting inhibitory activity. *Ann Nutr Metab.* 2002;46(6):259-267.

287. Sato M, Hosokawa T, Yamaguchi T, et al. Angiotensin I converting enzyme inhibitory peptide derived from wakame (*Undaria pinnati-fida*) and their antihypertensive effect in spontaneously hypertensive rats. *J Agric Food Chem.* 2002;50(21):6245-6252.

288. Taubert D, Roesen R, Schomig E. Effect of cocoa and tea intake on blood pressure: a meta-analysis. *Arch Intern Med.* 2007;167(7):626-634.

289. Grassi D, Lippi C, Necozione S, Desideri G, Ferri C. Short-term administration of dark chocolate is followed by a significant increase in insulin sensitivity and a decrease in blood pressure in healthy persons. *Am J Clin Nutr.* 2005;81(3):611-614.

290. Taubert D, Roesen R, Lehmann C, Jung N, Schomig E. Effects of low habitual cocoa intake on blood pressure and bioactive nitric oxide: a randomized controlled trial. *JAMA.* 2007;298(1):49-60.

291. Cohen DL, Townsend RR. Cocoa ingestion and hypertension-another cup please? *J Clin Hypertens.* 2007;9(8):647-648.

292. Reid I, Sullivan T, Fakler P, Frank OR, Stocks NP. Does chocolate reduce blood pressure? A meta-analysis. *BMC Med.* 2010;8:39-46.

293. Egan BM, Laken MA, Donovan JL, Woolson RF. Does dark choco-late have a role in the prevention and management of hypertension? Commentary on the evidence. *Hypertension.* 2010;55(6):1289-1295.

294. Desch S, Kobler D, Schmidt J, et al. Low vs higher-dose dark choc-olate and blood pressure in cardiovascular high-risk patients. *Am J Hypertens.* 2010;23(6):694-700.

295. Desch S, Schmidt J, Sonnabend M, et al. Effect of cocoa products on blood pressure: systematic review and meta analysis. *Am J Hypertens.* 2010;23(1):97-103.

296. Grassi D, Desideri G, Necozione S, et al. Blood pressure is reduced and insulin sensitivity increased in glucose intolerant hypertensive subjects after 15 days of consuming high-polyphenol dark chocolate. *J Nutr.* 2008;138(9):1671-1666.

297. Grassi D, Necozione S, Lippi C, et al. Cocoa reduces blood pressure and insulin resistance and improved endothelium-dependent vasodila-tion in hypertensives. *Hypertension.* 2005;46(2):398-405.

298. Grassi D, Desideri G, Necozione S, et al. Protective effects of flavanol-rich dark chocolate on endothelial function and wave reflec-tion during acute hyperglycemia. *Hypertension.* 2012;60:827-832.

299. Ried K, Sullivan TR, Fakler P, Frank OR, Stocks NP. Effect of cocoa on blood pressure. *Cochrane Database Syst Rev.* 2012;8:CD008893.

300. Scheer FA, Van Montfrans GA, van Someren EJ, Mairuhu G, Buijs RM. Daily nighttime melatonin reduces blood pressure in male patients with essential hypertension. *Hypertension.* 2004;43(2):192-197.

301. Cavallo A, Daniels SR, Dolan LM, Khoury JC, Bean JA. Blood pressure response to melatonin in type I diabetes. *Pediatr Diabetes.* 2004;5(1):26-31.

302. Cavallo A, Daniels SR, Dolan LM, Bean JA, Khoury JC. Blood pressure-lowering effect of melatonin in type 1 diabetes. *J Pineal Res.* 2004;36(4):262-266.

303. Cagnacci A, Cannoletta M, Renzi A, Baldassari F, Arangino S, Volpe A. Prolonged melatonin administration decreases nocturnal blood pressure in women. *Am J Hypertens.* 2005;18(12 Pt 1):1614-1618.

304. Grossman E, Laudon M, Yalcin R, et al. Melatonin reduces night blood pressure in patients with nocturnal hypertension. *Am J Med.* 2006;119(10):898-902.

305. Rechcinskl T, Kurpese M, Trzoa E, Krzeminska-Pakula M. The influence of melatonin supplementation on circadian pattern of blood pressure in patients with coronary artery disease-preliminary report. *Pol Arch Med Wewn.* 2006;115(6):520-528.

306. Merkureva GA, Ryzhak GA. Effect of the pineal gland peptide preparation on the diurnal profile of arterial pressure in middle-aged and elderly women with ischemic heart disease and arterial hypertension. *Adv Gerontol.* 2008;21(1):132-142.

307. Zaslavskai RM, Scherban EA, Logvinenki SI. Melatonin in combined therapy of patients with stable angina and arterial hypertension. *Klin Med (Mosk).* 2009;86:64-67.

308. Zamotaev IN, Enikeev AK, Kolomets NM. The use of melaxen in combined therapy of arterial hypertension in subjects occupied in assembly line production. *Klin Med (Mosk).* 2009;87(6):46-49.

309. Rechcinski T, Trzos E, Wierzbowski-Drabik K, Krzeminska-Pakute M, Kurpesea M. Melatonin for nondippers with coronary artery disease: assessment of blood pressure profile and heart rate variability. *Hypertens Res.* 2002;33(1):56-61.

310. Kozirog M, Poliwczak AR, Duchnowicz P, Koter-Michalak M, Sikora J, Broncel M. Melatonin treatment improves blood pressure, lipid profile and parameters of oxidative stress in patients with metabolic syndrome. *J Pineal Res.* 2011;50(3):261-266.

311. Zeman M, Dulkova K, Bada V, Herichova I. Plasma melatonin concentrations in hypertensive patients with the dipping and nondipping blood pressure profile. *Life Sci.* 2005;75(16):1795-1803.

312. Jonas M, Garfinkel D, Zisapel N, Laudon M, Grossman E. Impaired nocturnal melatonin secretion in non-dipper hypertensive patients. *Blood Press.* 2003;12(1):19-24.

313. Simko F, Pechanova O. Potential roles of melatonin and chronotherapy among the new trends in hypertension treatment. *J Pineal Res.* 2009;47(2):127-133.

314. Cui HW, Zhang ZX, Gao MT, Liu Y, Su AH, Wang MY. Circadian rhythm of melatonin and blood pressure changes in patients with essential hypertension. *Zhonghua Xin Xue Guan Bing Za Zhi.* 2008;36(1):20-23.

315. Ostrowska Z, Kos-Kudla B, Marek B, et al. Circadian rhythm of melatonin in patients with hypertension. *Pol Merkur Lekarski.* 2004;17(97):50-54.

316. Shatilo VB, Bondarenke EV, Amtoniuk-Shcheglova IA. Pineal gland melatonin-producing function in elderly patients with hypertensive disease: age peculiarities. *Adv Gerontol.* 2010;23(4):530-542.

317. Forman JP, Curhan GC, Schemhammer ES. Urinary melatonin and risk of incident hypertension among young women. *J Hypetens.* 2010;28(3):336-351.

318. Li HL, Kang YM, Yu L, Xu HY, Zhao H. Melatonin reduces blood pressure in rats with stress-induced hypertension via GABAA receptors. *Clin Exp Pharmacol.* 2009;36(4):436-440.

319. Simko F, Paulis L. Melatonin as a potential antihypertensive treatment. *J Pineal Res.* 2007;42(4):319-322.

320. Irmak MK, Sizlan A. Essential hypertension seems to result from melatonin-induced epigenetic modifications in area postrema. *Med Hypthesis.* 2006;66(5):1000-1007.

321. De-Leersnyder H, de Biois MC, Vekemans M, et al. Beta(1) adrenergic antagonists improve sleep and behavioural disturbances in a circadian disorder, Smith-Magenis syndrome. *J Med Genet.* 2010;38(9):586-90.

322. Rodella LF, Favero G, Foglio E, et al. Vascular endothelial cells and dysfunctions: role of melatonin. *Front Biosci.* 2013;5:119-129.

323. Grossman E, Laudon M, Zisapel N. Effect of melatonin on nocturnal blood pressure: meta-analysis of randomized controlled trials. *Vasc Health Risk Manag.* 2011;7:577-584.

324. Scheer FA, Morris CJ, Garcia JI, et al. Repeated melatonin supplementation improves sleep in hypertensive patients treated with beta-blockers: a randomized controlled trial. *Sleep.* 2012;35:1395-1402.

325. Zaslavskaya RM, Lilitsa GV, Dilmagambetova GS, et al. Melatonin, refractory hypertension, myocardial ischemia and other challenges in nightly blood pressure lowering. *Biomed Pharmacother.* 2004;58(S1):S129-S134.

326. Sun H, Gusdon AM, Qu S. Effects of melatonin on cardiovascular diseases: progress in the past year. *Curr Opin Lipidol.* 2016;27(4):408-413.

327. Feringa HH, Laskey DA, Dickson JE, Coleman CI. The effect of grape seed extract on cardiovascular risk markers: a meta-analysis of randomized controlled trials. *J Am Diet Associ.* 2011;111(8):1173-1181.

328. Sivaprakasapillai B, Edirisinghe K, Randolph J, Steinberg F, Kappagoda T. Effect of grape seed extract on blood pressure in subjects with the metabolic syndrome. *Metabolism.* 2009;58(12):1743-1746.

329. Edirisinghe I, Burton-Freeman B, Tissa Kappagoda C. Mechanism of the endothelium-dependent relaxation evoked by grape seed extract. *Clin Sci (Lond).* 2008;114(4):331-337.

330. Zhang H, Liu S, Li L, et al. The impact of grape seed extract treatment on blood pressure changes: a meta-analysis of 16 randomized controlled trials. *Medicine (Baltimore).* 2016;95(33):e4247.

331. Park E, Edirisinghe I, Choy YY, Waterhouse A, Burton-Freeman B. Effects of grape seed extract beverage on blood pressure and metabolic indices in individuals with pre-hypertension: a randomised, double-blinded, two-arm, parallel, placebo-controlled trial. *Br J Nutr.* 2016;115(2):226-238.

332. Clements WT, Lee SR, Bloomer RJ. Nitrate ingestion: a review of the health and physical performance effects. *Nutrients.* 2014;6:5224-5264.

333. Kapil V, Milsom AB, Okorie M, et al. Inorganic nitrate supplementation lowers blood pressure in humans: role for nitrite-derived NO. *Hypertension.* 2010;56:274-281.

334. Kapil V, Khambata RS, Robertson A, Caulfield MJ, Ahluwalia A. Dietary nitrate provides sustained blood pressure lowering in hypertensive patients: a randomized, phase 2, double-blind, placebo-controlled study. *Hypertension.* 2015;65:320-327.

335. Coles LT, Clifton PM. Effect of beetroot juice on lowering blood pressure in free-living, disease-free adults: a randomized, placebo-controlled trial. *Nutr J.* 2012;11:106.

336. Siervo M, Lara J, Ogbonmwan I, Mathers JC. Inorganic nitrate and beetroot juice supplementation reduces blood pressure in adults: a systematic review and meta-analysis. *J Nutr.* 2013;143:818-826.

337. Houston M. Acute effects of an oral nitric oxide supplement on blood pressure, endothelial function, and vascular compliance in hypertensive patients. *J Clin Hypertens (Greenwich).* 2014;16(7):524-529.

338. Hobbs DA, Kaffa N, George TW, Methven L, Lovegrove JA. Blood pressure-lowering effects of beetroot juice and novel beetroot-enriched bread products in normotensive male subjects. *Br J Nutr.* 2012;108(11):2066-2074.

339. Kapil V, Pearl V, Ghosh S, Ahluwalia A. Inorganic nitrate ingestion improves vascular compliance but does not alter flow-mediated dilatation in healthy volunteers. *Nitric Oxide.* 2012;26(4):197-202.

340. Asgary S, Afshani MR, Sahebkar A, et al. Improvement of hypertension, endothelial function and systemic inflammation following short-term supplementation with red beet (Beta vulgaris L.) juice: a randomized crossover pilot study. *J Hum Hypertens.* 2016;30(10):627-632.

341. Bryan NS. Application of nitric oxide in drug discovery and development. *Expert Opin Drug Discov.* 2011;6(11):1139-1154.

342. Machha A, Schechter AN. Inorganic nitrate: a major player in the cardiovascular health benefits of vegetables? *Nutr Rev.* 2012;70(6):367-372.

343. Liu G, Mi XN, Zheng XX, Xu YL, Lu J, Huang XH. Effects of tea intake on blood pressure: a meta-analysis of randomised controlled trials. *Br J Nutr.* 2014;112:1043-1054.

344. Hodgson JM, Puddey IB, Burke V, Beilin LJ, Jordan N. Effects on blood pressure of drinking green and black tea. *J Hypertens.* 1999;17:457-463.

345. Kurita I, Maeda-Yamamoto M, Tachibana H, Kamei M. Antihypertensive effect of Benifuuki tea containing O-methylated EGCG. *J Agric Food Chem.* 2010;58(3):1903-1908.

346. McKay DL, Chen CY, Saltzman E, Blumberg JB. *Hibiscus sabdariffa* L. tea (tisane) lowers blood pressure in pre-hypertensive and mildly hypertensive adults. *J Nutr*. 2010;140(2):298-303.

347. Bogdanski P, Suliburska J, Szulinska M, Stepien M, Pupek-Musialik D, Jablecka A. Green tea extract reduces blood pressure, inflammatory biomarkers, and oxidative stress and improves parameters associated with insulin resistance in obese, hypertensive patients. *Nutr Res* 2012;32(6):421-427.

348. Hodgson JM, Woodman RJ, Puddey IB, Mulder T, Fuchs D, Croft KD. Short-term effects of polyphenol-rich black tea on blood pressure in men and women. *Food Funct*. 2013;4(1):111-115.

349. Medina-Remón A, Estruch R, Tresserra-Rimbau A, Vallverdú-Queralt A, Lamuela-Raventos RM. The effect of polyphenol consumption on blood pressure. *Mini Rev Med Chem*. 2013;13(8):1137-1139.

350. Jiménez R, Duarte J, Perez-Vizcaino F. Epicatechin: endothelial function and blood pressure. *J Agric Food Chem*. 2012;60(36):8823-8830.

351. Nogueira LP, Nogueira Neto JF, Klein MR, Sanjuliani AF. Short-term effects of green tea on blood pressure, endothelial function, and metabolic profile in obese prehypertensive women: a crossover randomized clinical trial. *J Am Coll Nutr*. 2017;36(2):108-115.

352. Wasilewski R, Ubara EO, Klonizakis M. Assessing the effects of a short-term green tea intervention in skin microvascular function and oxygen tension in older and younger adults. *Microvasc Res*. 2016;107:65-71.

353. Yarmolinsky J, Gon G, Edwards P. Effect of tea on blood pressure for secondary prevention of cardiovascular disease: a systematic review and meta-analysis of randomized controlled trials. *Nutr Rev*. 2015;73(4):236-246.

354. Houston MC. Treatment of hypertension with nutraceuticals, vitamins, antioxidants and minerals. *Expert Rev Cardiovasc Ther*. 2007;5:681-691.

355. Miguel-Carrasco JL, Monserrat MT, Mate A, Vázquez CM. Comparative effects of captopril and l-carnitine on blood pressure and antioxidant enzyme gene expression in the heart of spontaneously hypertensive rats. *Eur J Pharmacol*. 2010;632(1-3):65-72.

356. Zambrano S, Blanca AJ, Ruiz-Armenta MV, et al. ʟ-Carnitine protects against arterial hypertension-related cardiac fibrosis through modulation of PPAR-γ expression. *Biochem Pharmacol*. 2013;85(7):937-944.

357. Vilskersts R, Kuka J, Svalbe B, et al. Administration of L-carnitine and mildronate improves endothelial function and decreases mortality in hypertensive Dahl rats. *Pharmacol Rep*. 2011;63(3):752-762.

358. Mate A, Miguel-Carrasco JL, Monserrat MT, Vázquez CM. Systemic antioxidant properties of L-carnitine in two different models of arterial hypertension. *J Physiol Biochem*. 2010;66(2):127-136.

359. Digiesi V, Cantini F, Bisi G, Guarino G, Brodbeck B. L-carnitine adjuvant therapy in essential hypertension. *Clin Ter*. 1994;144:391-395.

360. Ghidini O, Azzurro M, Vita G, Sartori G. Evaluation of the therapeutic efficacy of L-carnitine in congestive heart failure. *Int J Clin Pharmacol Ther Toxicol*. 1988;26(4):217-220.

361. Digiesi V, Palchetti R, Cantini F. The benefits of L-carnitine therapy in essential arterial hypertension with diabetes mellitus type II. *Minerva Med*. 1989;80(3):227-231.

362. Ruggenenti P, Cattaneo D, Loriga G, et al. Ameliorating hypertension and insulin resistance in subjects at increased cardiovascular risk: effects of acetyl-L-carnitine therapy. *Hypertension*. 2009;54(3):567-574.

363. Martina V, Masha A, Gigliardi VR, et al. The therapeutic prospects of using L-carnitine to manage hypertension-related organ damage. *Drug Discov Today*. 2010;15(11-12):484-492.

364. Korkmaz S, Yıldız G, Kılıçlı F, et al. Low L-carnitine levels: can it be a cause of nocturnal blood pressure changes in patients with type 2 diabetes mellitus? *Anadolu Kardiyol Derg*. 2011;11(1):57-63.

365. Velasquez MT, Ramezani A, Manal A, Raj DS. Trimethylamine N-Oxide: The Good, the Bad and the Unknown. *Toxins (Basel)*. 2016;8(11):1-12.

366. He J, Whelton PK. Effect of dietary fiber and protein intake on blood pressure: a review of epidemiologic evidence. *Clin Exp Hypertens*. 1999;21:785-796.

367. Pruijm M, Wuerzer G, Forni V, Bochud M, Pechere-Bertschi A, Burnier M. Nutrition and hypertension: more than table salt. *Rev Med Suisse*. 2010;6(282):1715-1720.

368. Cicero AF, Derosa G, Manca M, Bove M, Borghi C, Gaddi AV. Different effect of psyllium and guar dietary supplementation on blood pressure control in hypertensive overweight patients: a six-month, randomized clinical trial. *Clin Exp Hypertens*. 2007;29:383-394.

369. Pal S, Khoussousi A, Binns C, Dhaliwal S, Radavelli-Bagatini S. The effects of 12-week psyllium fibre supplementation or healthy diet on blood pressure and arterial stiffness in overweight and obese individuals. *Br J Nutr*. 2012;107:725-734.

370. Houston MC. Nutrition and nutraceuticals supplements in the treatment of hypertension. *Prog Cardiovasc Dis*. 2005;47:396-449.

371. Caligiuri SP, Edel AL, Aliani M, Pierce GN. Flaxseed for hypertension: implications for blood pressure regulation. *Curr Hypertens Rep*. 2014;16:499.

372. Sankar D, Sambandam G, Ramskrishna Rao M, Pugalendi KV. Modulation of blood pressure, lipid profiles and redox status in hypertensive patients taking different edible oils. *Clin Chim Acta*. 2005;355(1-2):97-104.

373. Sankar D, Rao MR, Sambandam G, Pugalendi KV. Effect of sesame oil on diuretics or beta-blockers in the modulation of blood pressure, athropometry, lipid profile and redox status. *Yale J Biol Med*. 2006;79(1):19-26.

374. Miyawaki T, Aono H, Toyoda-Ono Y, Maeda H, Kiso Y, Moriyama K. Anti-hypertensive effects of sesamin in humans. *J Nutr Sci Vitaminol (Toyko)*. 2009;55(1):87-91.

375. Wichitsranoi J, Weerapreeyakui N, Boonsiri P, et al. Antihypertensive and antioxidant effects of dietary black sesame meal in pre-hypertensive humans. *Nutr J*. 2011;10(1):82-88.

376. Sudhakar B, Kalaiarasi P, Al-Numair KS, Chandramohan G, Rao RK, Pugalendi KV. Effect of combination of edible oils on blood pressure, lipid profile, lipid peroxidative markers, antioxidant status, and electrolytes in patients with hypertension on nifedipine treatment. *Saudi Med J*. 2011;32(4):379-385.

377. Sankar D, Rao MR, Sambandam G, Pugalendi KV. A pilot study of open label sesame oil in hypertensive diabetics. *J Med Food*. 2006;9(3):408-412.

378. Harikumar KB, Sung B, Tharakan ST, et al. Sesamin manifests chemopreventive effects through the suppression of NF-kappa-B-regulated cell survival, proliferation, invasion and angiogenic gene products. *Mol Cancer Res*. 2010;8(5):751-761.

379. Nakano D, Ogura K, Miyakoshi M, et al. Antihyptensive effect of angiotensin I- converting enzyme inhibitory peptides from a sesame protein hydrolysate in spontaneously hypertensive rats. *Biosci Biotechnol Biochem*. 2006;70(5):1118-1126.

380. Karatzi K, Stamatelopoulos K, Lykka M, et al. Acute and long-term hemodynamic effects of sesame oil consumption in hypertensive men. *J Clin Hypertens (Greenwich)*. 2012;14(9):630-636.

381. Morand C, Dubray C, Milenkovic D, et al. Hesperidin contributes to the vascular protective effects of orange juice: a randomized crossover study in healthy volunteers. *Am J Clin Nutr*. 2011;93(1):73-80.

382. Jiang B, Haverty M, Brecher P. N-acetyl-L-cysteine enhances interleukin-1beta-induced nitric oxide synthase expression. *Hypertension*. 1999;34(4 Pt 1):574-579.

383. Vasdev S, Singal P, Gill V. The antihypertensive effect of cysteine. *Int J Angiol*. 2009;18(1):7-21.

384. Meister A, Anderson ME, Hwang O. Intracellular cysteine and glutathione delivery systems. *J Am Coll Nutr*. 1986;5(2):137-151.

385. Asher GN, Viera AJ, Weaver MA, Dominik R, Caughey M, Hinderliter AL. Effect of hawthorn standardized extract on flow mediated dilation in prehypertensive and mildly hypertensive adults: a randomized, controlled cross-over trial. *BMC Complement Altern Med*. 2012;12:26-30.

386. Koçyildiz ZC, Birman H, Olgaç V, Akgün-Dar K, Melikoğlu G, Meriçli AH. Crataegus tanacetifolia leaf extract prevents L-NAME-induced hypertension in rats: a morphological study. *Phytother Res*. 2006;20(1):66-70.

387. Schröder D, Weiser M, Klein P. Efficacy of a homeopathic Crataegus preparation compared with usual therapy for mild (NYHA II) cardiac insufficiency: results of an observational cohort study. *Eur J Heart Fail.* 2003;5(3):319-326.

388. Walker AF, Marakis G, Simpson E, et al. Hypotensive effects of hawthorn for patients with diabetes taking prescription drugs: a randomised controlled trial. *Br J Gen Pract.* 2006;56(527):437-443.

389. Walker AF, Marakis G, Morris AP, Robinson PA. Promising hypotensive effect of hawthorn extract: a randomized double-blind pilot study of mild, essential hypertension. *Phytother Res.* 2002;16(1):48-54.

390. Larson A, Witman MA, Guo Y, et al. Acute, quercetin-induced reductions in blood pressure in hypertensive individuals are not secondary to lower plasma angiotensin-converting enzyme activity or endothelin-1: nitric oxide. *Nutr Res.* 2012;32(8):557-564.

391. Edwards RL, Lyon T, Litwin SE, Rabovsky A, Symons JD, Jalili T. Quercetin reduces blood pressure in hypertensive subjects. *J Nutr.* 2007;137(11):2405-2411.

392. Egert S, Bosy-Westphal A, Seiberl J, et al. Quercetin reduces systolic blood pressure and plasma oxidised low-density lipoprotein concentrations in overweight subjects with a high-cardiovascular disease risk phenotype: a double-blinded, placebo-controlled cross-over study. *Br J Nutr.* 2009;102(7):1065-1074.

393. Khalesi S, Sun J, Buys N, Jayasinghe R. Effect of probiotics on blood pressure: a systematic review and meta-analysis of randomized, controlled trials. *Hypertension.* 2014;64:897-903.

394. Hendijani F, Akbari V. Probiotic supplementation for management of cardiovascular risk factors in adults with type II diabetes: A systematic review and meta-analysis. *Clin Nutr.* 2018;37(2):532-541. pii:S0261-5614(17)30065-1. doi:10.1016/j.clnu.2017.02.015.

395. Robles-Vera I, Toral M, Romero M, et al. Antihypertensive effects of probiotics. *Curr Hypertens Rep.* 2017;19(4):26.

396. de Sousa VP, Cavalcanti Neto MP, Magnani M, et al. New insights on the use of dietary polyphenols or probiotics for the management of arterial hypertension. *Front Physiol.* 2016;7:448-460.

397. Dalili ED, Lee RM, Cho HH. Current perspectives on antihypertensive probiotics. *Probiotics Antimicrob Proteins.* 2017;9(2):91-101.

398. Whelton PK, Carey RM, Aronow WS, et al. ACC/AHA/AAPA/ABC/ACPM/AGS/APhA/ASH/ASPC/NMA/PCNA guideline for the prevention, detection, evaluation, and management of high blood pressure in adults: a report of the American College of Cardiology/American Heart Association Task Force on Clinical Practice Guidelines. *Hypertension.* 2018;71(6):e13-e115. doi:10.1161/HYP.0000000000000065.

399. Wright JM, Musini VM, Gill R. First-line drugs for hypertension. *Cochrane Database Syst Rev.* 2018;4:CD001841. doi:10.1002/14651858.CD001841.pub3.

400. Trovato A, Nuhlicek DN, Midtling JE. Drug-nutrient interactions. *Am Fam Physician.* 1991;44(5):1651-1658.

401. McCabe BJ, Frankel EH, Wolfe JJ, eds. *Handbook of Food-Drug Interactions.* Boca Raton, FL: CRC Press; 2003.

402. Houston MC. The role of cellular micronutrient analysis and minerals in the prevention and treatment of hypertension and cardiovascular disease. *Ther Adv Cardiovasc Dis.* 2010;4:165-183.

22

Nutrition, Nutritional Supplements, and Drugs in the Management of Dyslipidemia

Mark C. Houston, MD, MS, MSc, FACP, FAHA, FASH, FACN, FAARM, ABAARM, DABC and Sergio Fazio, MD, PhD

Brief Summary

The combination of a lipid-lowering diet and scientifically proven nutritional supplements and drugs has the ability to significantly reduce total cholesterol (TC) and low-density lipoprotein (LDL) cholesterol (LDL-C) levels; decrease LDL particle concentration (LDL-P); increase LDL particle size; lower triglycerides (TG), remnant particles, very-low-density lipoprotein (VLDL), and lipoprotein (a) levels; increase total high-density lipoprotein (HDL) cholesterol (HDL-C) and HDL particle concentration (HDL-P); provide beneficial effects on HDL subfractions; and improve HDL functionality. In addition, inflammation, oxidative stress, and abnormal vascular immune responses are decreased as a result of these interventions. In several prospective clinical trials, coronary heart disease (CHD) rates have been reduced with optimal nutrition and/or administration of several nutritional supplements, including omega-3 fatty acids (FAs), red yeast rice (RYR), alpha-linolenic acid (ALA), berberine, and niacin. Other studies have shown additional reduction in CHD events using a statin with an omega-2 FA and with drugs such as ezetimibe and monoclonal antibodies against PCSK9. An integrative program of nutrition, nutritional supplements, and lipid-lowering drugs represents the most scientifically valid and most efficacious approach for the treatment of dyslipidemia. This new approach to decrease dyslipidemia-induced vascular disease goes beyond the present traditional evaluation and management of an altered standard lipid panel or even advanced lipid testing with particle number and particle size, to the recognition and treatment of the multiple mechanisms that are secondary to or synergistic with dyslipidemia in the development of atherosclerosis and CHD.

Introduction

The combination of a lipid-lowering diet with the judicious use of scientifically proven nutritional supplements and lipid-lowering drugs has the ability to significantly reduce TC and LDL-C; decrease LDL particle number (LDL-P); increase LDL particle (LDL-P) size; lower TG, remnant particles, VLDL, and lipoprotein (a) levels; and increase HDL-C and HDL particle number (HDL-P), while providing a beneficial effect on HDL subfractions and HDL functionality. In addition, vascular inflammation, oxidative stress, and vascular immune responses are also decreased with aggressive lipid management. In several prospective clinical trials, CHD, myocardial infarction (MI), and cardiovascular disease (CVD) events have been reduced by nutraceutical supplements utilized. Other trials show additional improvement in CHD events when lipid-lowering drugs such as statins are supplemented with nutraceuticals such as omega-3 FAs or niacin. This chapter will review the role of nutrition, nutritional supplements, and lipid-lowering drugs that favorably improve dyslipidemia and address the myriad steps and mechanisms involved in lipid-mediated atherosclerosis and clinical cardiovascular events such as MI and stroke.

Pathophysiology

Dyslipidemia is a major risk factor for CHD, along with hypertension, diabetes mellitus (DM), smoking, and obesity.[1] The mechanisms by which certain plasma lipids induce vascular damage are complex, but from a pathophysiologic viewpoint these include vascular inflammation, oxidative stress with reduced oxidative defense, and vascular immune dysfunction.[2-4] These pathophysiologic mechanisms lead to endothelial dysfunction (ED) and vascular smooth muscle dysfunction (VSMD) with loss of arterial elasticity and compliance. In addition, coronary artery obstruction, coronary artery ED, and coronary artery spasm cause cardiac myocyte dysfunction. The consequences are CHD, MI, and cerebrovascular accidents (CVAs).[4]

The causes of dyslipidemia include genetic inheritance and a number of acquired conditions such as poor nutrition, visceral obesity, numerous comorbidities, and the use of pharmacological agents such as nonselective and nonvasodilating beta blockers and diuretics (including hydrochlorothiazide and chlorthalidone), anti-retrovirals, retinoids and rexinoids, steroids, and sex hormones.[5] In addition, tobacco use, DM, hypothyroidism and other metabolic dysfunctions, an abnormal gut microbiome, acute and chronic infections, heavy metals, toxins, and lack of exercise also may induce dyslipidemia.[5] Often there are both genetic and acquired factors at play. For example, several genetic phenotypes, such as the common apolipoprotein E (apoE) polymorphism, regulate intestinal absorption of dietary fat and result in variable serum lipid responses to diet, thus controlling the risk for CHD and MI.[6,7] In addition, variations in the HDL proteome, involving players such as paroxonase-1 (PON-1), scavenger receptor B-1 (SR –BI), SCARB-1, and apolipoprotein C3 (APO C3), influence the risk for CHD and MI.[8] The Sortilin I allele variants on Chromosome 1p13 increase LDL-C and CHD risk by 29%.[9] More recently, a polygenic risk score has been developed to identify common variants in a number of genes modulating lipid metabolism in a single individual. An elevated risk score explains many cases of familial hypercholesterolemia not due to mutations in the LDL receptor.[10]

Recent studies suggest that dietary cholesterol intake has a minimal effect on serum cholesterol levels and on rates of CHD and MI, and that only saturated fats (SFAs) with a carbon length of C12 or greater have adverse effects on serum lipids and CHD risk.[5,11-17] However, consumption of monounsaturated (MUFAs) and polyunsaturated fats (PUFAs) has a favorable influence on serum lipids and CHD risk. Increased refined carbohydrate intake adversely affects serum lipoproteins and their subfractions more than do short-chain SFAs with carbon length of C-10 and less. Refined carbohydrates and sugars have significant effects on insulin resistance and adverse effects on LDL-C, LDL-P, LDL-P size, VLDL, TG, total HDL-C, HDL-P, HDL subfractions, HDL functionality, vascular inflammation, oxidative stress, and vascular immune function. All of these lipid changes from sugar intake contribute more to CHD risk than do short-chain SFAs.[5,11-17]

The validity of the long-standing "**Diet Heart Hypothesis**," which suggests that dietary SFAs and dietary cholesterol increase the risk of CHD and MI has been questioned.[12-14] However, dietary trans fatty acids (TFAs) do have definite adverse lipid effects and increase the risk of sudden death, MI, CVD, and CHD. The TFAs suppress transforming growth factor beta responsiveness, and this facilitates the deposition of cholesterol in vascular tissue.[12,14-16] In contrast, PUFAs and omega-3 FAs, such as docosahexaenoic acid (DHA) and eicosapentaenoic acid (EPA), and MUFAs improve serum lipids and reduce CHD and MI risk.[5,11-17]

Expanded lipid profiles (advanced lipid testing) that measure lipids, lipid subfractions, particle size, particle number, and apolipoprotein B and A are preferred over the standard lipid panel that measures only the TC, LDL-C, TG, and HDL-C (**Figure 22.1**). Expanded lipid profiles are offered by numerous commercial laboratories, including Boston Labs, Berkeley Labs, LabCorps, and Quest Diagnostics. These expanded lipid profiles have been shown to improve CHD risk profiling, better predict CHD and MI events, and allow a more accurate assessment of the lipid changes that occur with exercise, weight loss or weight gain, lifestyle changes, and use of nutritional supplements or pharmacotherapy.[18,19] CHD risk assessment, identification of the mechanisms of dyslipidemia-induced vascular disease, and evaluation of efficacy of natural or drug treatment are vastly improved

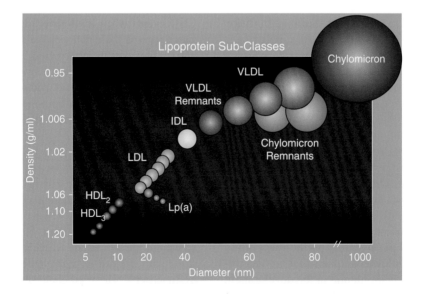

Figure 22.1 *The various lipoprotein particles are shown with nuclear magnetic resonance (NMR). High-density lipoprotein (HDL), low-density lipoprotein (LDL), intermediate-density lipoprotein (IDL), very-low-density lipoprotein (VLDL), and chylomicrons.*

by using the new expanded lipid profiles.[18,19] In addition, new concepts in assessing dysfunctional or inflammatory HDL-C[20] directly or indirectly by measuring reverse cholesterol transport,[21] lipoprotein-associated phospholipase A2, platelet-activating factor acetylhydrolase, high-sensitivity C-reactive protein (hsCRP), and myeloperoxidase levels[22] will add to the intervention toolkit and allow improved assessment of CHD and MI risk.

An understanding of the pathophysiological steps and mechanisms in dyslipidemia-induced vascular damage and atheroma plaque formation that goes beyond measurement of lipid levels or even expanded lipid profiles allows for the treatment of dyslipidemia and prevention of CHD and MI to be conducted in a more logical and efficacious manner (**Figure 22.2**). The ability to interfere with most steps and mechanisms in this pathway will allow more specific approaches and treatments to reduce vascular injury, improve vascular repair systems, and maintain and restore vascular health. Native LDL, especially large type A LDL, is not usually atherogenic unless it accumulates in very high concentrations or is oxidized or otherwise modified. However, effective pinocytosis mechanisms allow macrophage ingestion of native LDL-C in the setting of chronic infection or inflammation, which could account for up to 30% of the foam cell formation in the subendothelium.[23,24] Identifying maneuvers to decrease modified LDL forms such as oxidized (oxLDL) and glycated (glyLDL) or glyco-oxidized LDL (gly-oxLDL) would represent a gigantic next step toward a revolution in the management of this common condition. In addition, it would be important to have instruments to decrease the uptake of modified LDL-C into macrophages by the SR-A and CD 36 scavenger receptors (SR) and to decrease inflammatory and oxidative stress and abnormal vascular immune responses. All of these approaches would reduce vascular damage beyond just treating LDL-C levels.[25-31] There are at least 45 potential mechanisms that can be treated in the pathways involving dyslipidemia-induced vascular damage. We now know that lowering of serum hsCRP, an inflammatory marker and mediator, leads to fewer cardiovascular events independent of reductions in LDL-C cholesterol.[30]

Treatment

Overview

Many patients cannot tolerate or will not in principle use pharmacologic treatments such as statins, fibrates, bile-acid binders, ezetimibe, or PCSK9 inhibitors to treat dyslipidemia.[5] Other patients with definitive indications for use of statins and other antilipid therapies prefer their use for many reasons such as cost, convenience, and proven efficacy. The most informed patients prefer to use an integrative approach to lipid management as clinical trials indicate an improved risk reduction in CHD and MI with combinations of nutraceuticals and drugs.

Drug-induced side effects (myopathy, myositis, rhabdomyolysis, abnormal liver function tests, neuropathy, memory loss, mental status changes, decreased focus and concentration, gastrointestinal disturbances, glucose intolerance or type 2 DM) are the largest reason why patients find lipid management notoriously disagreeable.[32-35] With prolonged or high-dose usage of statin medications, patients may experience other clinical symptoms such as chronic fatigue, exercise-induced fatigue with myalgias and muscle weakness, reduced exercise tolerance, and loss of lean muscle mass. In addition, there may be reductions in both serum and tissue levels of coenzyme Q 10, carnitine, copper, zinc, creatine, vitamin E (tocopherols and tocotrienols), vitamin D, vitamin A, vitamin K2, selenium, selenoproteins, heme A, steroid, and sex hormone. Statins also may reduce the conversion of thyroxine (T4) to free tri-idothyronine (T3) by inhibiting the deiodinase enzyme, resulting in hypothyroidism.[5,32,36-43] The newer PCSK9 inhibitors are free of most of these adverse effects because they are monoclonal antibodies and therefore they do not penetrate cells, are not metabolized by the liver, and are not perceived as xenobiotics by the body.[44]

New treatment approaches that combine weight loss, reductions in visceral and total body fat with increases in lean muscle mass, optimal aerobic and resistance exercise, and scientifically proven nutrition, use of nutritional supplements, and lipid-lowering drugs will improve serum lipids and reduce vascular inflammation, oxidative stress, abnormal vascular immune dysfunction, ED, and VSMD. In addition, both surrogate markers for vascular disease and rates of clinical end points such as CHD and MI are reduced in clinical trials.[5] This chapter will review nutrition, nutritional supplements, and lipid-lowering drugs in the treatment of dyslipidemia and dyslipidemia-induced vascular disease. The reader is referred to an extensive body of literature on the role of exercise, weight loss, and other lifestyle treatments for dyslipidemia.

Nutrition

FRAMINGHAM HEART STUDY AND SEVEN COUNTRIES STUDY

Nutrition has long been recognized as an important modality for managing and preventing dyslipidemia and other risk factors for CVD, MI, and CHD.[45] The Framingham Heart Study (FHS) and Seven Countries studies (SCS) found associations between increased LDL-C and TC levels with increased risk of CVD, and between elevated levels of HDL-C and decreased risk of CVD. An association between CVD and dietary fat consumption was also identified at that time, and a general link was established between Western diet, lipid levels, CHD, and CVD.[46-48] The FHS initially included a cohort of 5209 healthy, mostly Caucasian residents of Framingham, Massachusetts, aged 30 to 60 years, and then added a second cohort of 5124 offspring in 1971. The last FHS cohort included 500 minorities.[49] It should be noted that this is an epidemiologic, hypothesis-generating study with a small number of subjects of a single race. The ability to apply these conclusions to a broader population was to be verified later.

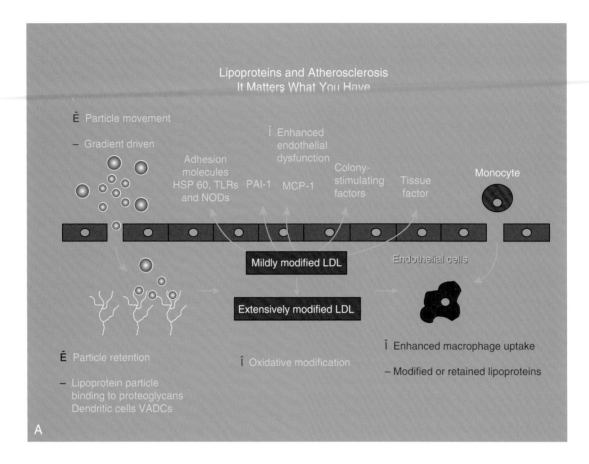

Atherosclerotic Plaque Formation

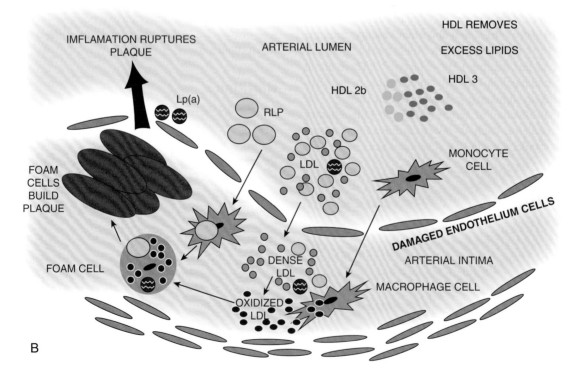

Figure 22.2 *A and B lipoproteins and atherosclerosis and atherosclerotic plaque formation. Proposed mechanisms of actions of nutraceuticals and statins in the dyslipidemia-induced atherosclerotic vascular disease pathway to the development of an atherosclerotic plaque. Diagrammed here are the various steps in the uptake of LDL-C, modification, macrophage ingestion with scavenger receptors, foam cell formation, oxidative stress, inflammation, autoimmune cytokines, and chemokine production.*

The SCS was a large prospective study that evaluated nutrition and lifestyle habits in 12,000 middle-aged men in Asia, Northern Europe, Southern Europe, and the United States. This study found a link between a high-fat diet and increased risk of CVD. The SCS has been criticized as to its validity because of selection bias and forced premises. It should also be noted that the high-fat diet consumed at that time was rich in TFA and long-chain SFA. Intake of omega-3 FA and MUFA was associated with a reduced risk of CHD. The SCS thus should not have bundled all dietary fats together in the link to increased risk of CVD.

PRITIKIN DIET

The Pritikin diet is a low-fat diet based primarily on vegetables, grains, and fruits with total fat supplying 10% of energy needs.[50,51] Studies of this diet suggested that the dietary fat content reduced CVD and reduced LDL-C and TG and increased HDLC when coupled with a regular exercise program.[52] It cannot be concluded that any one modality in this program was the primary reason for the CVD and lipid outcomes. A plant-based diet with exercise could have been the primary reason for the positive outcomes, more than the dietary fat reduction per se.

ORNISH DIET

The Ornish diet[53] started from a randomized controlled trial (RCT) that had as its 1-year and 5-year end points LDL-C level, number of anginal episodes, and angiography-based regression of coronary stenosis.[54-56] It was based on a combined intensive therapeutic approach of diet, exercise, and other lifestyle changes. The diet consisted of a low-fat, whole foods vegetarian diet with 10% of total energy as fat, drastic reduction (10 mg/d) in dietary cholesterol, increased intake of complex carbohydrates (fiber and plant-based nutrition), and minimal intake of simple sugars. Lifestyle modifications included moderate aerobic exercise, stress reduction, smoking cessation, and group psychosocial support. Compared with the control group, the experimental group had statistically significant reduction in LDL-C, a lower frequency of angina episodes, and regression of coronary artery stenosis at years 1 and 5. In contrast, the control group had minimal reduction in LDL-C, a significant increase in the frequency of angina episodes, and an increase in coronary artery stenosis. The dietary fat reduction here was primarily in long-chain SFA and TFA, which are now known to increase CHD risk. There was a concomitant increase in the intake of omega-3 FAs and MUFAs. The effects due to reduced consumption of these types of fats in combination with a plant-based diet, more fiber, and lower simple sugars are consistent with those of other studies using the same nutritional components, also showing a reduction in CHD rates. The comprehensive approach of nutrition, exercise, stress reduction, and smoking cessation, although certainly efficacious, does not allow one to pinpoint any single treatment as the primary reason for the clinical findings.

THERAPEUTIC LIFESTYLE CHANGES DIET

The National Heart, Lung, and Blood Institute (NHLBI) and the Adult Treatment Panel III of the National Cholesterol Education Program (ATP III) recommends the Therapeutic Lifestyle Changes (TLC) nutritional program with dietary SFA of <7% of total energy, dietary cholesterol of <200 mg/d, 10 to 25 g/d of viscous fiber, and 2 g/d of plant sterols/stanols.[57,58] A randomized crossover study of 36 moderately hypercholesterolemic subjects treated over a period of 1 month compared the TLC diet (28% total fat, <7% SFA, 66 mg cholesterol/1000 kcal) with a Western diet (38% total fat, 15% SFA, 164 mg cholesterol/1000 kcal. Compared with the Western diet, the TLC diet significantly reduced plasma levels of both LDL-C (by 11%) and HDL-C (by 7%), with no significant effect on TG or the TC/HDL-C ratio.[59] These net lipid changes are not impressive as the decrease in LDL was negated by the decrease in HDL. The lack of change in the TC/HDL ratio would predict no change in CHD risk over time. Moreover, in the 15-year Women's Health Initiative, a multicenter randomized clinical trial of 48,835 postmenopausal women, a diet low in fat (20% of total calories), high in fruits and vegetables (five or more servings/d), and high in grains (six or more servings/d) did not show an effect on CVD rates or improvement in lipid profile. The type of fat reduction and the relatively low intake of fruits and vegetables could account for the negative CV outcomes.[60] The addition of plant sterols in the TLC could also have biased the results in that study.

OMNIHEART TRIAL

The Optimal Macronutrient Intake for Heart Health trial (OmniHeart trial) investigated the effect of a Mediterranean-style diet on plasma lipids and blood pressure.[49] In this randomized controlled intervention crossover study of generally healthy adults, three diets were compared for 6 weeks in each of the three groups (total 18 weeks): a carbohydrate-rich diet, a protein-rich diet, and a diet rich in MUFAs. The MUFA diet did not change LDL-C levels but increased HDL-C levels, the protein-rich diet decreased LDL-C and HDL-C levels, and all three diets reduced serum TG. After adjustment for potential confounders, an OMNIHEART score higher by 1 point was associated with systolic/diastolic BP differences of $-1.0/-0.5$ mm Hg (both $P < .001$). Findings were comparable for men and women, for nonhypertensive participants, and with adjustment for antihypertensive treatment. The trial could not assess the effects on CHD as it was too short and underpowered with only 164 subjects.

PORTFOLIO DIET

The Portfolio diet[61-66] is a vegetarian version of the low-fat TLC diet, with the addition of soluble fiber, nuts, soy protein, and plant sterols. In a 1-month randomized control feeding trial, the Portfolio diet was compared with the TLC control diet.[61] The LDL-C fell an average of 35.0% compared with 12.1% on the control diet. A follow-up study found that the Portfolio diet reduced LDL-C equal to a statin medication.[64]

In a subsequent study of hyperlipidemic adults who were followed for 1 year on the Portfolio diet, about 50% had reductions in LDL-C of >20%.[62] Increasing the MUFA content increased the HDL-C levels without changing LDL-C.[65] In the largest RCT of the Portfolio diet to date, LDL-C levels in those following this diet were significantly lower than in those following a low-saturated-fat diet.[66] Once again, the addition of plant sterols with fiber and more plant-based nutrition likely resulted in improved lipid profiles over the basic nutritional suggestions of just low-fat dieting in the TLC diet.

MEDITERRANEAN DIETS

The Mediterranean-style diet is characterized by a high intake of vegetables, fruits, bread and other cereal grains, potatoes, legumes, nuts, and seeds. MUFA with extra-virgin olive oil (EVOO) and nuts are the primary fats consumed, which is typically 15% to 20% of total calories. Animal product intake, such as meat, poultry, fish, dairy, and eggs, is low to moderate, and wine consumption is regular but in moderation.[67] Several clinical trials on the Mediterranean-style diet and CVD are discussed subsequently.

LYON DIET HEART STUDY

The Lyon Diet Heart Study was the first intervention trial to investigate the effect of a Mediterranean-style diet on CVD risk. This randomized single-blind secondary prevention trial was conducted in a single center in the Lyon region of France and included over 600 participants with prior MI.[68-70] The primary outcome measurement (fatal or nonfatal MI) was significantly reduced by the intervention over the 4-year study period. CV outcomes including recurrent stable angina and restenosis of grafts were decreased by 47%, whereas the composite of MI, cardiovascular death, and major secondary events was decreased by 67%. These changes were independent of serum lipid changes, which were not significantly different between the groups. The design introduced changes to the usual Mediterranean diet consumed in southern Europe that the study is not generally considered an appropriate test of the efficacy of that diet on CVD risk. For example, the diet was 30.5% fat, with 12.5% as MUFA, much lower than the 15% to 20% MUFA content in the diet of southern Europe. Furthermore, the diet was enriched in ALA, an omega-3 polyunsaturated fat, rather than the usual MUFA oleic acid.

INDIAN HEART STUDY

The Indian Heart Study was a case-control study of 350 Indian subjects with ischemic heart disease on the effect of a Mediterranean-style diet enriched in ALA.[71] The control group was advised on smoking cessation, stress management regular exercise, and reduction of dietary fat and alcohol. Compared with the control group at the 1-year follow-up, the treatment group had a 38% reduction in nonfatal MI and a 32% reduction in fatal MI. There was a significant and dose-dependent inverse association between vegetable intake and CHD risk. The inverse association was stronger for green leafy vegetables; in multivariate analysis, persons consuming a median of 3.5 servings/wk had a 67% lower relative risk (RR, 0.33; 95% confidence interval [CI], 0.17, 0.64; P for trend = 0.0001) than did those consuming 0.5 servings/wk. Controlling for other dietary covariates did not alter the association. Cereal intake was also associated with a lower risk. Use of mustard oil, which is rich in alpha-linolenic acid, was associated with a lower risk than was the use of sunflower oil (for use in cooking: RR, 0.49 [95% CI, 0.24-0.99]; for use in frying, RR, 0.29 [95% CI, 0.13-0.64]). Diets that are rich in vegetables and use of mustard oil could contribute to the lower risk of CHD among Indians.

There are numerous other diets that have been recommended for weight management and blood sugar or lipid control. These include the Atkins diet; South Beach diet; ketogenic diet; Paleo diet; vegetarian, vegan, or plant-based diet; the Esselstyn diet; and the fasting mimicking diet. All of these will be discussed in other chapters. Of all these diets, the fasting mimicking diet shows the best results for control of weight, glucose, lipids, stem cell production, and possibly slowing the aging process.

Nutrigenomics

The importance of nutrigenomic effects on serum lipids, DM, CHD, MI, CVD, ASCVD, hypertension, inflammation, oxidative stress, immune function, and cancer have all been demonstrated in numerous clinical trials such as the FUNGENUT study, the GEMINAL study, and the PREDIMED study.[72-79] These are discussed in the following sections.

FUNGENUT Study

Diet changes can influence both phenotypic outcomes and gene expression.[72] The Functional Genomics and Nutrition (FUNGENUT) Study of Finnish subjects with metabolic syndrome was conducted over 3 months, and participants were randomly assigned to either a low-glycemic-load rye-pasta diet to curtail postprandial insulin response or a high-glycemic-load oat-wheat-potato diet promoting a high postprandial insulin response. Gene expression was determined on samples of subcutaneous adipose tissue.[72]

In the low-glycemic-load rye-pasta group, the insulinogenic index improved and 71 genes were downregulated, including genes involved in insulin signaling and apoptosis. In the high-glycemic-load oat-wheat-potato diet group, 62 genes were upregulated, such as those promoting oxidative stress and inflammation.[72]

The GEMINAL Study

The Gene Expression Modulation by Intervention with Nutrition and Lifestyle (GEMINAL)[73] study reported changes in gene expression in 30 men with low-risk prostate cancer after a 3-month intensive diet-and-lifestyle intervention. The intervention consisted of a low-fat, plant-based diet; moderate exercise; stress management; and psychosocial group support. Microarray analysis of gene expression in prostate biopsies taken before and after the intervention detected 453 downregulated genes, many associated with tumorigenesis, as a result of the intensive diet-lifestyle intervention.

PREDIMED Study

In the PREDIMED study,[74] three diets were evaluated for their effects on gene expression. The control diet was a low-fat TLC diet; the experimental diets were a Mediterranean-style diet enhanced with either EVOO or mixed nuts. The Mediterranean-style diets, particularly the EVOO, decreased expression of genes related to inflammation, foam cell formation, and thrombosis.

Another cohort of the PREDIMED study[75] investigated these same three diets over a 3-year period to determine the effects on body weight parameters of a variant of the IL6 gene (IL6 −174G>C, rs1800795) that overproduces this proinflammatory cytokine and is associated with increased body weight, waist circumference, and serum lipid levels. The change in weight was numerically greatest in the EVOO group but was not statistically significant between groups. When the population was stratified by genotype (GG+GC versus CC), the CC group experienced greater weight loss irrespective of diet type. Interestingly, these individuals had greater adiposity at baseline but lost significantly more weight than those with one or two copies of the G allele ($P = .002$). In the CC group the nut diet actually led to weight gain.

Analyses of intermediate markers of cardiovascular risk demonstrated beneficial effects of the Mediterranean diet on blood pressure, lipid profiles, lipoprotein particles, DM, inflammation, oxidative stress, and carotid atherosclerosis, as well as on the expression of proatherogenic genes.[76-79] Nutrigenomics studies also demonstrated favorable interactions of a Mediterranean diet with cyclooxygenase-2 (COX-2), interleukin-6 (IL-6), apolipoprotein A2 (APOA2), cholesteryl ester transfer protein plasma (CETP), transcription factor 7-like 2 (TCF7L2), beta adrenergic receptor gene (ADR B2), interleukin (IL7R), interferon (IFN gamma), monocyte chemotactic protein (MCP), and tumor necrosis factor (TNF) alpha gene polymorphisms.[76-79]

Nutritional Conclusions and Recommendations

Despite some apparent conflicts in these studies, owing to variations in amount and types of fats, simple sugars, complex carbohydrates, fiber, and the use of plant sterols, one can draw fairly solid conclusions from these nutritional interventions:

1. TFAs increase LDL-C and TG, reduce HDL-C, and increase CHD risk.
2. FAs that are C-12 and longer increase LDL-C and TG and may increase or not change HDL-C. They are associated with an increased risk of CHD. Shorter-chain FAs of C-10 and below instead lower LDL-C and TG, increase HDL-C, and are not associated with an increased risk for CHD.
3. Increased dietary intake of simple sugars increases LDL-C and TG and lowers HDL-C and is associated with an increased risk of CHD.
4. Omega-3 FAs and MUFAs lower LDL-C and TG, increase HDL-C, and reduce CHD risk. They also have effects that are independent of serum lipids that decrease CHD risk.

Specific Foods, Nutrients, and Dietary Supplements

Omega-3 Fatty Acids

Observational, epidemiologic, and controlled clinical trials of dietary omega-3 FAs have shown significant reductions in serum TG, VLDL, and LDL-P and variable changes in LDL-C, along with an increase in HDL-C, HDL particle size, and HDL-P, all of which are associated with major reductions in all CVD events.[5,80-87] The Diet and Reinfarction Trial (DART) demonstrated a decrease in mortality of 29% in men post MI. In DART, 2033 men who had recovered from MI were allocated to receive advice on each of three dietary factors: a reduction in fat intake with an increased ratio of polyunsaturated to saturated fat, an increase in fatty fish intake, and an increase in cereal fiber intake. The advice on fat was not associated with any difference in mortality. The subjects advised to eat fatty fish had a 29% reduction in 2-year all-cause mortality. This effect, which was significant, was not altered by adjusting for potential confounding factors. Subjects given fiber advice had a slightly higher mortality (not significant). The 2-year incidence of reinfarction plus death from ischemic heart disease was not significantly affected by any of the dietary regimens. A modest intake of fatty fish (two or three portions per week) may reduce mortality in men who have recovered from MI.

The Gruppo Italiano per lo Studio della Sopravvivenza nell'Infarto Miocardico (GISSI) enrolled 11,324 patients surviving an MI (less than 3 months). The patients were randomly assigned supplements of n-3 PUFA (1 g daily, n = 2836), vitamin E (300 mg daily, n = 2830), both (n = 2830), or none (control, n = 2828) for 3.5 years. The primary combined efficacy end point was death, nonfatal MI, and stroke. Treatment with n-3 PUFA, but not vitamin E, significantly lowered the risk of the primary end point (relative risk decrease 10%). There was a decrease in total mortality of 20%. CV deaths decreased by 30%, and sudden death was reduced by 45%. The Kuopio Ischemic Heart Disease Risk Factor Study[5,80,81] was a prospective population study of 871 men aged 42 to 60 years who had no clinical CHD at baseline examination. A total of 194 men had a fatal or nonfatal acute coronary event during follow-up. In a Cox proportional hazards' model adjusting for other risk factors, men in the highest quintile of serum DHA in all FAs had a 44% reduced risk ($P = .014$) of acute coronary events compared with men in the lowest quintile. Men in the highest quintile who had a low hair content of mercury had a 67% reduced risk ($P = .016$) of acute coronary events compared with men in the lowest quintile and with a high hair content of mercury. There was no association between EPA levels and the risk of acute coronary events. Fish oil–derived FAs reduce the risk of acute coronary events. However, a high mercury content in fish could attenuate this protective effect.[5,80,81] The range of omega-3 FA was from 500 to 1000 mg/d in these studies and included both food and supplemental sources.

Omega-3 FAs reduce CHD progression, stabilize plaque, reduce coronary artery stent restenosis, and reduce graft restenosis.[5,82] In the Japan EPA Lipid Intervention Study (JELIS), the addition of 1.8 g of EPA to a statin resulted in an additional 19% relative risk reduction (RRR) in major coronary events and nonfatal MI and a 20% decrease in CVA.[5,83] A recent very large meta-analysis of 825,000 subjects[80] included 18 RCTs and 16 prospective cohort studies examining the combination of EPA + DHA from foods or supplements and CHD, including MI, sudden cardiac death, coronary death, and angina.

In the RCTs, there was a nonstatistically significant reduction in CHD risk of 6% with EPA + DHA (summary relative risk elements = 0.94; 95% CI, 0.85-1.05).

However, subgroup analyses of data from these RCTs indicate a statistically significant CHD risk reduction with the combination of EPA + DHA (dose range of 340 mg/d to 5000 mg/d) among higher-risk populations with TG levels over 150 mg/dL (16% reduction in CHD) and/or LDL-C over 130 mg/dL (14% reduction in CHD). A meta-analysis of data from these 16 prospective cohort studies resulted in a statistically significant decrease in CHD of 18% for higher intakes of EPA + DHA from diet and supplement and risk of any CHD event.

Although the value is not statistically significant, a 6% reduced risk of any CHD event was observed among RCTs, a finding supported by a statistically significant 18% reduced risk of CHD among the prospective cohort studies. From a clinical perspective, these results indicate that EPA + DHA are associated with reducing CHD risk to a greater extent in populations with elevated TG levels or LDL-C, which affect a significant portion of the general adult population in the United States.[80] In addition, a significant reduction in CHD rates in patients with known CHD was reported for a dietary intake over 1000 mg daily of combined DHA and EPA with a longer duration of treatment.

EPA and DHA in combination demonstrate a dose-related reduction in VLDL and TG of up to 50%, with a decrease in total TC, and ApoB, and a slight increase in LDL size and increase in HDL-C, HDL-P, and HDL size at the very high dose of 5 g/d. Lower doses, used by most, have less favorable effects on lipids.[5,84-87] Despite a small increase in LDL-C in some subjects, the other lipid changes were beneficial and reduced the risk of CHD and MI. Patients with LDL-C over 100 mg/dL usually have reductions in total LDL-C, and those that are below 80 mg/dL have mild increases.[86] The rate of entry of VLDL particles into the circulation is decreased by omega-3, and the lowering of APOCIII allows lipoprotein lipase to be more active. There was also a decrease in remnant chylomicrons and remnant lipoproteins.[5,85] Omega-3 fats are

also anti-inflammatory and antithrombotic and lower blood pressure, heart rate, and improve heart rate variability.[5,80]

Insulin resistance is improved and there are slight decreases or no significant changes in fasting glucose or hemoglobin A1c with long-term supplementation with omega-3 FA at doses up to 5000 mg/d.[5,88] The combination of plant sterols and omega-3 FAs appears to be synergistic in improving lipids and inflammation.[87]

A recent meta-analysis of omega-3 FA and CVD has suggested no beneficial effect on CHD.[89] This is at variance with the Mayo Clinic meta-analysis as well as the large body of published literature showing improved CHD risk with omega-3 FA. The more recent meta-analysis included only 10 trials involving 77,917 individuals compared with 34 trials and 825,000 subjects in the Mayo Clinic meta-analysis. Its limitations include:

- Exclusion of data with arbitrary selection of studies: 500 individuals for at least 1 year (1-6.2 years) and no minimum dose of omega-3 required. Included both RCTs[8] and open-label studies.[2] Only 10 studies included with a total of 77,917 individuals.
- Many studies used nontherapeutic, low doses of DHA and EPA. The EPA dose ranged from 226 to 800 mg/d and the DHA dose 0 to 1700 mg/d. Most studies used <1800 mg EPA/DHA in the high-risk CV population. Only three studies used >1800 mg EPA/DHA per day.
- There was no monitoring of blood or tissue levels of omega-3 FAs, no compliance evaluations, and no omega-3 index data showing achievement of the minimal therapeutic level of 8%.
- The studies with best results used the higher doses of DHA and EPA.
- The larger studies with over 10,000 subjects and those consuming 1000 mg or more of omega-3 FA all had reductions in CV events (JELIS R and P, GISSI-P).
- There were insufficient numbers of subjects in many studies to show any CV effect.
- The quality of DHA/EPA may not have been good or it was not mentioned. Omega-3 FA was from the ester form in 9/10 trials.
- CV morbidity and mortality was nominally lower in most of the studies, which suggests that benefits favor treatment.

In another recent Cochrane analysis of 79 RCTs with 112,059 subjects, the authors concluded that increasing consumption of EPA and DHA has little to no effect on mortality or CV health.[90]

RCTs that lasted at least 12 months were evaluated and compared supplementation and/or advice to increase LCn3 or ALA intake versus usual or lower intake. It included 79 RCTs with trials of 12 to 72 months' duration and included adults at varying cardiovascular risk, mainly in high-income countries. Most studies assessed LCn3 supplementation with capsules, but some used LCn3- or ALA-rich or enriched foods or dietary advice compared with placebo or usual diet.

Meta-analysis and sensitivity analyses suggested little or no effect of increasing LCn3 on all-cause mortality

(RR, 0.98; 95% CI, 0.90 to 1.03; 92,653 participants; 8189 deaths in 39 trials), cardiovascular mortality (RR, 0.95; 95% CI, 0.87 to 1.03; 67,772 participants; 4544 CVD deaths in 25 RCTs), cardiovascular events (RR, 0.99; 95% CI, 0.94 to 1.04; 90,378 participants; 14,737 events in 38 trials), CHD mortality (RR, 0.93; 95% CI, 0.79 to 1.09; 73,491 participants; 1596 CHD deaths in 21 RCTs), stroke (RR, 1.06; 95% CI, 0.96 to 1.16; 89,358 participants; 1822 strokes in 28 trials), or arrhythmia (RR, 0.97; 95% CI, 0.90 to 1.05; 53,796 participants; 3788 events in 28 RCTs). There was a suggestion that LCn3 reduced CHD events (RR, 0.93; 95% CI, 0.88 to 0.97; 84,301 participants; 5469 events in 28 RCTs); however, this was not maintained in sensitivity analyses.

Increasing ALA intake does not impact all-cause mortality (RR, 1.01; 95% CI, 0.84 to 1.20; 19,327 participants; 459 deaths, five RCTs) and cardiovascular mortality (RR, 0.96; 95% CI, 0.74 to 1.25; 18,619 participants; 219 cardiovascular deaths, four RCTs), although it may slightly benefit CHD events (RR, 1.00; 95% CI, 0.80 to 1.22; 19,061 participants; 397 CHD events, four RCTs).

There was no evidence that increasing LCn3 or ALA altered serious adverse events, adiposity, or lipids, although LCn3 slightly reduced TG and increased HDL. The authors actually show a 5% to 7% reduction in CHD mortality with omega-3 FAs despite their negative conclusion. There are potential limitations and sources of variability that should be noted in all meta-analyses. The individual RCTs differed in terms of CHD prevalence at baseline, the EPA + DHA dosage provided, follow-up duration, and the methods of patient selection and randomization. The benefit of n-3 LCPUFA intake is likely to accrue over time, but RCTs of longer duration may suffer from poorer compliance with dietary supplementation. The variable use of terminology specific to CHD outcomes, or a lack of specificity required to discern CHD from broader CVD outcomes, is problematic. Many of the RCTs lacked statistical power to detect an effect because of relatively small sample sizes and/or few observed events due to the increased survival rate associated with current standards of care. Finally, most RCTs did not measure the baseline intake of EPA + DHA from the diet nor did they track EPA + DHA intake from sources other than that supplemented during the course of study, thus making it impossible to determine whether background dietary EPA + DHA intake affected the relationship between supplemental EPA + DHA and CHD.

Neither *JAMA* nor the Cochrane analysis has the validity of the Mayo Clinic meta-analysis, which included more appropriate types of studies, more than 825,000 subjects, better analysis, and less bias. Based on all published clinical trials, RCTs, cohort studies, and meta-analysis, these are the most valid conclusions regarding omega-3 FA dietary intake and CHD.

1. CHD is reduced by 16% in patients with TG over 150 mg/dL.
2. CHD is reduced by 14% in patients with LDL-C over 130 mg/dL.
3. DHA and EPA over 1000 mg/d significantly reduce CHD in both primary and secondary prevention settings.
4. A longer duration of treatment results in a greater reduction in CHD.
5. Secondary prevention trials with known CHD have shown more robust reductions of CHD event rates.

Flax

Flax seeds and flax lignan complexed with SDG (secoisolariciresinol diglucoside) have been shown in several meta-analyses to reduce TC and LDL-C by 5% to 15%, Lp(a) by 14%, and TG by up to 36%, with either no change or a slight reduction in HDL.[5,91-93] These properties do not apply to flax seed oil. Flax seeds contain fiber and lignans that reduce the levels of 7 alpha hydroxylase and acyl CoA cholesterol transferase to decrease LDL-C, TG, and Lp(a).[5,91-93] Flax seeds and ALA are anti-inflammatory, increase endothelial nitric oxide synthase (eNOS), improve ED, decrease vascular smooth muscle hypertrophy, reduce oxidative stress, and reduce the risk of CHD.[5,91-93] The dose required for these effects is from 14 to 40 g of flax seed per day.[5,91-93]

Monounsaturated Fats

MUFAs such as those in olive oil, especially EVOO, and nuts reduce LDL-C by 5% to 10%, lower TG 10% to 15%, increase HDL 5%, improve HDL function, increase cholesterol efflux capacity (CEC), and decrease oxLDL. In addition, MUFAs reduce vascular inflammation and oxidation; decrease IL-23, IL-8, intracellular adhesion molecule, vascular cell adhesion molecule, and TNF alpha; improve ED; lower blood pressure; and decrease thrombosis. The net effect is to reduce the incidence of CHD by 30% (PREDIMED diet).[5,74,75,94-96] In a study of 195 subjects,[95] replacing SFAs with MUFAs or n-6 PUFAs did not affect the percentage change in flow-mediated dilatation (primary end point) or other measures of vascular reactivity, but the substitution of SFAs with MUFAs attenuated the increase in night systolic blood pressure (−4.9 mm Hg, P = .019) and reduced E-selectin (−7.8%, P = .012). Replacement of SFAs with MUFAs or n-6 PUFAs lowered fasting serum TC (−8.4% and −9.2%, respectively), LDL-C (−11.3% and −13.6%, respectively), and the TC/HDL ratio (−5.6% and −8.5%, respectively) (P ≤ .001). These changes in LDL-C equate to an estimated 17% to 20% reduction in CVD mortality. MUFAs are one of the most potent agents to reduce oxLDL.[5] The equivalent of three to four tablespoons (30-40 g) per day of EVOO in MUFA content is recommended for the maximum effect in conjunction with omega-3 FAs. The best ratio of EVOO to combined DHA and EPA is about 5:1.[5] The polyphenol content of EVOO is important for its overall lipid and CV effects. However, the caloric intake of this amount of MUFA must be balanced with the other beneficial effects.

Garlic

Numerous placebo-controlled clinical trials in humans indicate reductions in TC and LDL-C of about 9% to 12% with a standardized extract of allicin and ajoene[5,97] at doses of 600 to 900 mg/d. However, many studies have been poorly controlled and used different types and doses of garlic, which have given inconsistent results.[5,97] The best form of garlic is the CV formulation of aged garlic. Garlic reduces intestinal cholesterol absorption and inhibits enzymes involved in cholesterol synthesis.[5,97] In addition, garlic lowers blood pressure, has fibrinolytic and antiplatelet activity, reduces oxLDL, and may decrease coronary artery calcification.[5,97,98]

Green Tea

Catechins, especially epigallocatechin gallate (EGCG), as green tea or in supplement form, may improve the lipid profile by interfering with micellar solubilization of cholesterol in the gastrointestinal tract and reducing its absorption.[5] In addition, EGCG reduces FA gene expression, inhibits HMG-CoA reductase, increases mitochondrial energy expenditure, reduces oxLDL, increases paroxonase (PON-1), upregulates the LDL receptor, decreases ApoB secretion, mimics the action of insulin, improves ED, and decreases body fat.[5,99-102] A meta-analysis of 14 clinical trials shows that EGCG at 224 to 674 mg/d or 60 oz of green tea per day minimally reduced TC (7 mg/dL) and LDL-C (2 mg/dL) ($P < .001$ for both).[102] Recent studies have confirmed similar reductions in TC and LDL-C in postmenopausal women.[99] There is no significant change in HDL or TG levels.[102] The recommended dose is a standardized EGCG extract 500 to 700 mg/d or green tea 12 to 60 oz/d.

Orange Juice

In one human study, 750 mL of concentrated orange juice per day over 2 months decreased LDL-C by 11% and had positive effects on ApoB, TG, and HDL (up by 21%).[103] The effects are due to polymethoxylated flavones, hesperidin naringin, pectin, and essential oils.[103] Additional studies are needed to verify these data.

Pomegranate Juice and Seeds

Pomegranate seeds and juice increase PON-1 binding to HDL-C, increase PON-2 and HDL-C, lower the TG/HDL ratio, and decrease TG.[104-109] As a potent antioxidant, it increases total antioxidant status, lowers oxLDL, decreases antibodies to oxLDL, inhibits platelet function, reduces glycosylated LDL, decreases macrophage LDL uptake, and reduces lipid deposition in the arterial wall.[104-109] Pomegranate juice at 6 oz/d and seeds at ¼ cup twice a day, decrease progression of carotid artery intimal medial thickness (IMT) and stabilize or reduce carotid artery plaque, especially in those with the higher levels of serum TG and HDL-C.[104-109] In addition, it may reduce blood pressure at the above-mentioned doses within 2 months, especially in subjects with the highest levels of oxidative stress. Consuming about 6 to 8 oz of pomegranate juice or ¼ to ½ cup of seeds per day is recommended.

Sesame

Sesame seeds and oil at 40 g/d reduces LDL-C by 9% through inhibition of intestinal absorption and increased biliary secretion of cholesterol.[110,111] Sesame also decreases HMG-CoA reductase activity, upregulates the LDL receptor gene and the 7-alpha hydroxylase gene expression and **sterol regulatory element-binding proteins (SREBP)** 2 genes.[110,111] A randomized placebo-controlled crossover study of 26 postmenopausal women who consumed 50 g of sesame powder daily for 5 weeks had a 5% decrease in TC and a 10% decrease in LDL-C.[110]

Soy

Numerous studies have shown mild improvements in serum lipids with consumption of soy-containing foods at doses of about 30 to 50 g/d.[5,112,113] In most studies the average reduction in TC is 9.3%, LDL-C decreased 4% to 12.9%, TG fell 10.5%, and HDL increased 2.4%.[5,112,113] However, the studies are conflicting because of differences in the type and dose of soy used (fermented, powders, foods, etc.) in many of the clinical trials, as well as nonstandardized methodologies.[5,112,113] Soy decreases the micellar content and absorption of lipids through a combination of fiber, isoflavones (genistein, glycitein, daidzein), and phytoestrogens.[5,112,113] The greatest reduction is seen with soy-enriched isoflavones with soy protein.

Nutrients and Dietary Supplements

New important scientific information and clinical studies are required to understand the present role of these natural agents in the management of dyslipidemia.[5,79] Several clinical trials show excellent reductions in serum lipids and risk of CHD with niacin, omega-3 FAs, RYR, fiber, and alpha linolenic acid-ALA.[5,79,98,114] Smaller studies show reductions in surrogate vascular markers such as carotid intima-media thickness and obstruction, plaque progression, stabilization and regression, coronary artery calcium (CAC) score, generalized atherosclerosis, and endothelial function with numerous other nutritional supplements.[5,79,98,114] The mechanisms by which nutritional supplements exert their effects are variable and will be discussed in detail with each of the supplements in the following text (**Table 22.1**).

Citrus Bergamot

Citrus bergamot has been evaluated in several clinical prospective trials in humans. In doses of 1000 mg/d, citrus bergamot lowers LDL-C up to 36% and TG by 39%, whereas it increases HDL-C by 40%.[115,116] Citrus bergamot inhibits HMG-CoA reductase, increases cholesterol and bile acid excretion, and reduces radical oxygen species and oxLDL.[115,116] The active ingredients include naringin, neroeriocitrin, neohesperidin, poncerin, rutin, neodesmin, rhoifolin, melitidine, and brutelidine.[115,116]

Curcumin

Curcumin is one of the phenolic compounds in turmeric and curry.[5,117] It induces changes in the expression of genes involved in cholesterol synthesis such as LDL receptor

Table 22.1

NUTRIENTS FOR THE TREATMENT OF DYSLIPIDEMIA-INDUCED VASCULAR DISEASE[5]

Mechanism	Food or Nutrient Therapy (Alphabetically by Mechanism)
Inhibit LDL oxidation	Citrus bergamot Coenzyme Q 10 Curcumin Epigallocatechin gallate Flavonoids Garlic Glutathione Grape seed extract Lycopene Monounsaturated fatty acids Niacin Oleic acid Pantethine Polyphenols Pomegranate Pycnogenol Quercetin Red wine Resveratrol Sesame Tangerine extract Tocotrienols and tocopherols (γ and δ)
Inhibit LDL glycation	Carnosine Histidine Kaempferol Morin Myricetin Organosulfur compounds Pomegranate Rutin
Reduce LDL	Astaxanthin Berberine Citrus bergamot Curcumin Epigallocatechin gallate Flax seed Garlic Gamma linolenic acid Lycopene Monounsaturated fatty acids Niacin Omega-3 fatty acids Orange juice Pantethine Plant sterols Quercetin Red yeast rice Resveratrol Sesame Soluble fiber Tocotrienols (gamma/delta)

Table 22.1

NUTRIENTS FOR THE TREATMENT OF DYSLIPIDEMIA-INDUCED VASCULAR DISEASE—CONT'D

Mechanism	Food or Nutrient Therapy (Alphabetically by Mechanism)
Convert dense LDL B to large LDL A	Niacin Omega-3 fatty acids Plant sterols
Reduce intestinal cholesterol absorption	Berberine Epigallocatechin gallate Fiber Flax seeds Garlic Plant sterols Sesame Soy
Inhibit HMG CoA reductase	Berberine Citrus bergamot Curcumin Epigallocatechin gallate Gamma-linolenic acid Garlic Lycopene Omega-3 fatty acids Pantethine Plant sterols Red yeast rice Sesame Tocotrienols (gamma/delta)
Reduce lipoprotein (a)	Berberine Coenzyme Q10 Curcumin Flax seed l-Arginine L-Carnitine L-Lysine N-acetylcysteine Niacin Omega-3 fatty acids Proline Quercetin Tocotrienols (γ and δ) Vitamin C
Reduce triglycerides	Astaxanthin Berberine Citrus bergamot Coenzyme Q 10 Fiber Flax seed Krill oil Monounsaturated fatty acids Niacin Omega-3 fatty acids Orange juice Pantethine Red yeast rice Resveratrol

(Continued)

Table 22.1

NUTRIENTS FOR THE TREATMENT OF DYSLIPIDEMIA-INDUCED VASCULAR DISEASE—CONT'D

Mechanism	Food or Nutrient Therapy (Alphabetically by Mechanism)
Increase total HDL and HDL 2 b levels and convert HDL 3 to HDL 2 and 2 b	Astaxanthin Citrus bergamot Coenzyme Q 10 Curcumin Krill oil Lycopene Monounsaturated fatty acids Niacin Omega-3 fatty acids Orange juice Pantethine Pomegranate Red yeast rice Resveratrol
Alter scavenger receptor NADPH oxidase and oxLDL uptake into macrophages	*N*-acetylcysteine Resveratrol
Increase reverse cholesterol transport	Anthocyanadins Coenzyme Q 10 Curcumin Flavonoids Glutathione Lycopene Monounsaturated fatty acids Niacin Plant sterols Phosphatidyl serine Quercetin Resveratrol
Decrease LDL particle number	Berberine Niacin Omega-3 fatty acids Red yeast rice
Reduce inflammation	Curcumin Flax seed Glutathione Monounsaturated fatty acids Niacin Omega-3 fatty acids Plant sterols Quercetin Resveratrol
Lower apolipoprotein B	Astaxanthin Berberine Epigallocatechin gallate Niacin Omega-3 fatty acids Plant sterols Red yeast rice

Table 22.1

NUTRIENTS FOR THE TREATMENT OF DYSLIPIDEMIA-INDUCED VASCULAR DISEASE—CONT'D

Mechanism	Food or Nutrient Therapy (Alphabetically by Mechanism)
Increase apolipoprotein A-1	Niacin Coenzyme Q 10
Upregulate the LDL receptor	Berberine (PCSK9 inhibition) Curcumin (PCSK9 inhibition) Epigallocatechin gallate Fiber Niacin (PCSK9 inhibition) Plant sterols Quercetin (PCSK9 inhibition) Sesame Soy Tocotrienols (γ and δ)
Increase PON-1 and PON-2	Epigallocatechin gallate Lycopene Quercetin Pomegranate Resveratrol Glutathione
Increase bile acid excretion	Berberine Citrus bergamot Fiber Resveratrol Probiotics Plant sterols Sesame
Reduce fibrinogen	Red yeast rice Plant sterols *L reuteri*
Reduce TNF alpha	Monounsaturated fatty acids Omega-3 fatty acids Plant sterols Red yeast rice
Reduce CAMs	Curcumin Luteolin Lycopene Monounsaturated fatty acids Niacin Resveratrol
Reduce NADPH oxidase	Berberine *N*-acetylcysteine Niacin Resveratrol Red yeast rice
Reduce myeloperoxidase	Curcumin Niacin Pomegranate

Table 22.1

NUTRIENTS FOR THE TREATMENT OF DYSLIPIDEMIA-INDUCED VASCULAR DISEASE—CONT'D

Mechanism	Food or Nutrient Therapy (Alphabetically by Mechanism)
Increase adiponectin and lower leptin	Curcumin Niacin Omega-3 fatty acid (PPAR) Red yeast rice
Improve insulin sensitivity	Berberine Curcumin Epigallocatechin gallate Lycopene (PPAR) Omega-3 fatty acid (PPAR) Quercetin (PPAR) Red yeast rice
Reduce MMP	Red yeast rice Luteolin

CAM, cell adhesion molecule; HDL, high-density lipoprotein; LDL, low-density lipoprotein; MMP, metalloproteinases; NADPH, nicotinamide adenine dinucleotide phosphate; PON, paroxonase; PPAR, peroxisome proliferator-activated receptors; TNF, tumor necrosis factor.

mRNA, HMG-CoA reductase, SREBP, cholesterol 7 alpha hydroxylase, peroxisome proliferator-activated receptors (PPARs), liver X receptor (LXR), activated protein kinase (AMPK), the ATP-binding cassette transporters (ABCA1 and ABCG1), the receptors for reverse cholesterol transport, and CEC.[5,117] In one human study of 10 patients consuming 500 mg/d of curcumin, the HDL increased 29% and TC fell 12%.[5,117] This needs confirmation in larger randomized clinical trials.

Guggulipids

Guggulipids are resins from the mukul myrrh tree (*Commiphora mukul*) that contain active lipid-lowering compounds called guggulsterones.[5,118,119] These increase hepatic LDL receptors and bile acid secretion and decrease cholesterol synthesis in animal experiments.[5,118] However, controlled human clinical trials have not shown these agents to be effective in improving serum lipids.[118,119] One study of 103 subjects given 50 to 75 mg of guggulsterones per day for 8 weeks actually had a 5% increase in LDL-C; no change in TC, TG, or HDL-C; and insignificant reductions in Lp(a) and hsCRP.[118] Guggulipids are not recommended at this time pending more studies in humans.

Lycopene

Lycopene has been shown in tissue culture to inhibit HMG-CoA reductase, increase PON-1 and HDL-C, improve HDL functionality, decrease oxLDL, induce Rho inactivation, increase PPAR gamma and LXR receptor activities, and increase reverse cholesterol transport and CEC with ATP binding cassette (ABCA1) and caveolin 1 expression.[120,121] There are no prospective clinical trials with lycopene, tomatoes, or tomato extract on CHD risk reduction to date.

Niacin (Vitamin B3)

Niacin has a dose-related effect (1-4 g/d) on serum lipids and CVD.[5,122-128] Niacin reduces TC, LDL-C, ApoB, LDL-P, TG, and VLDL. Niacin increases LDL size from small type B to large type A; increases HDL by 15% to 35%; increases HDL-P, especially the protective and larger HDL 2b particle; and increases APO A1 by 15% to 35%.[5,122-128] The average changes in lipids in the dose range of 1 to 4 g/d are TC, 20% to 25% decrease; LDL-C and ApoB, 10% to 25% decrease; and LDL-P, 10% to 25% reduction, with an increase in LDL size. Niacin reduces Lp(a) 25% to 35%, lowers TG 20% to 25% with a decrease in VLDL size, improves HDL functionality, inhibits proprotein convertase subtilisin/kexin type 9 (PCSK9), and lowers oxLDL. The inhibition of PCSK9 and increases in RCT and CEC all may contribute to its antiatherogenic effects.[125,126]

These dose-related changes range from approximately 10% to 30% for each lipid level as noted earlier.[5,122,123] Many of the antiatherosclerotic effects of niacin may be independent of the favorable effects on serum lipids.[5,123,127] Niacin increases TG lipolysis in adipose tissue, increases Apo-B degradation, reduces the fractional catabolic rate of HDL-ApoA-1, inhibits platelet function, induces fibrinolysis, decreases cytokines, inhibits inflammation, decreases cell adhesion molecules, increases adiponectin, and has potent antioxidant activities.[5,122,123]

Randomized controlled clinical trials such as the Coronary Drug Project (CDP), HDL-Atherosclerosis Treatment Study (HATS), Arterial Biology for the Investigation of the Treatment Effects of Reducing Cholesterol (ARBITER 2 and 6), Oxford Niaspan Study, Familial Atherosclerosis Treatment Study (FATS), Cholesterol Lowering Atherosclerosis Studies (CLAS I and CLAS II), and Air Force Regression Study (AFRS) have shown reduction in coronary events, decreases in coronary atheroma, carotid necrotic core and atheroma, and carotid IMT as monotherapy or in combination with other antilipid therapies and superiority to some antilipid agents.[5,122-127] Eleven trials of 9959 subjects found that niacin use was associated with significant reductions in the composite end points of any CVD event (odds ratio [OR], 0.66; 95% CI, 0.49 to 0.89; $P = .007$) and even major CHD (OR, 0.75; 95% CI, 0.59 to 0.96; $P = .02$). No significant association was observed between niacin therapy and stroke incidence (OR, 0.88; 95% CI, 0.5 to 1.54; $P = .65$).[125] The magnitude of on-treatment HDL-C difference between treatment arms was not significantly associated with the magnitude of the effect of niacin on outcomes.[125]

In a meta-analysis of 13 trials (N = 35,206), niacin led to significant increases in serum HDL-C levels by 21.4% (95%

CI, 5.11-13.51) from baseline trial enrollment.[124] Niacin treatment was associated with a trend toward lower risk of cardiovascular mortality (RR, 0.91; 95% CI, 0.81-1.02), coronary death (RR, 0.93; 95% CI, 0.78-1.10), nonfatal MI (RR, 0.85; 95% CI, 0.73 1.0), revascularization (coronary and noncoronary) (RR, 0.83; 95% CI, 0.65-1.06), and stroke (RR, 0.89; 95% CI, 0.72-1.10), compared with control. The recent negative findings in the AIM-HIGH and HPS 2 THRIVE studies[127,128] do not detract from positive results in previous trials.

The AIM-HIGH study was designed to test whether extended-release niacin added to intensive statin therapy, as compared with statin therapy alone, would reduce the risk of CV events in patients with established atherosclerotic CV disease (defined as stable coronary, cerebrovascular, or peripheral arterial disease) and atherogenic dyslipidemia (low baseline levels of HDL-C < 40 mg/dL for men; <50 mg/dL for women, and elevated triglyceride levels 150 to 400 mg/dL). A total of 3414 patients, 45 years or older, were randomly assigned to receive high-dose (1500-2000 mg) extended-release niacin or placebo. Both groups received simvastatin adjusted to maintain LDL-C level below 80 mg/dL. The primary end point was the composite of death from CHD, nonfatal MI, ischemic stroke, hospitalization (>23 hours) for an acute coronary syndrome (ACS), or symptom-driven coronary or cerebral revascularization. Secondary end points included the composite of death from CHD, nonfatal MI, ischemic stroke, or hospitalization for a "high-risk" ACS (characterized by accelerating ischemic symptoms or prolonged chest pain with electrocardiographic evidence of ischemia or biomarker values greater than two times the upper limit of the normal range); death from CHD; and nonfatal MI, ischemic stroke, or death from CV causes. The study was terminated after a mean follow-up period of 3 years owing to lack of clinically meaningful efficacy. Over 3 years, HDL-C levels increased by 9.6 mg/dL (35%) in the niacin group compared with 4.2 mg/dL (9.8%) in the placebo group ($P < .001$), whereas TG levels decreased by 28.6% in the niacin group compared with 8.1% in the placebo group. The use of aspirin, beta-blockers, and inhibitors of renin angiotensin system was similar in both groups. Niacin was discontinued after randomization in 25.4% compared with 20.1% in the placebo. The primary end point occurred in 16.4% in the niacin group and in 16.2% in the placebo group (hazard ratio with niacin, 1.02; 95% CI, 0.87-1.21, $P = .8$). There was no statistically significant difference in the composite secondary end point between patients assigned to niacin and those assigned to placebo (hazard ratio, 1.08; 95% CI, 0.87 to 1.34, $P = .49$). Among the components of the primary end point, an unexpected increase in the rate of ischemic stroke was noticed in the niacin group (1.6%) compared with the placebo group (0.9%). The primary problem with the AIM-HIGH study was the patient selection bias. All patients were taking statins with very low LDL levels of about 60 mg/dL or less. At this level of LDL-C the ability of any additional antilipid agent is not likely to show any additional significant reduction in CHD.

HPS2-THRIVE was a study of an investigational drug (Tredaptive, Merck) containing **both** extended-release niacin (ERN) (Niaspan) and the drug laropiprant, a selective antagonist of the prostaglandin D2 receptor subtype 1 (DP1R), which partially blocks the dermal flushing response to niacin. HPS2-THRIVE randomized 25,673 high-risk patients who could tolerate niacin to either placebo or ERN plus laropiprant (ERNL). The study subjects were all taking simvastatin 40 mg/d. The primary end point was the time to first major vascular event (MVE), defined as the composite of nonfatal MI or coronary death, any stroke, or any arterial revascularization.

The primary composite end point of MVEs was not significantly reduced (risk ratio, 0.96; 95% CI, 0.90-1.03, $P = .3$) in the active arm. "Serious adverse events" were found in 3% more subjects in the active arm, although most were "minor hyperglycemic problems." Myopathy generally was uncommon (0.34%/y) but was 4-fold higher overall in the active arm and 10-fold higher among Chinese subjects.

The study subjects had excellent baseline control of serum lipids on statin therapy (simvastatin 40 mg/d) with an average LDL-C of 63 mg/dL, HDL of 44 mg/dL, and TG of 125 mg/dL. The National Lipid Association (NLA) in the March 2013 position paper stated that in HPS2-THRIVE: "niacin was clinically irrelevant in the average study subject, and there was substantial subgroup heterogeneity." However, the investigators "tested a drug in patients who, on average, had no indication to take it." MVE reduction with ERNL was strongly predicted by baseline LDL-C (heterogeneity $P = .02$), with apparent net benefit if LDL-C was above 58 mg/dL at study entry. Thus, this study population was not likely to have any significant CVD reduction. In addition to the early data from the Coronary Drug Project (CDP),[5,6] which showed significant reductions in cardiovascular events when niacin was used **alone** in individuals with documented heart disease as well as in many other niacin trials, there are documented benefits of additive therapy on top of statins when LDL-C or triglyceride remain elevated and HDL remains low.

Nevertheless, there were several positive effects of treated patients on ERNL, including reductions in weight, blood pressure, lipoprotein(a); a significant reduction in arterial vascularization procedures ($P = .03$); and significant reduction in CV risk in the subgroup with the higher baseline LDL-C level. ($P = .02$) The adherence rate was poor at 1 year and at completion of the study, which may have altered hard CV outcomes. The average age was 64.9 years, and the patients studied were mostly men. The data cannot be totally extrapolated to a younger population or perhaps to women.

The claim that in HPS2 THRIVE niacin induced more harm than statin alone is baseless. However, the study did show increases in serious adverse events (3.7% absolute excess adverse events), including myalgia (0.7% $P < .001$), new-onset diabetes (1.3%, $P < .001$), gastrointestinal problems (1.0% $P < .001$), skin problems (0.3%, $P < .003$), infections (1.4%, $P < .001$), and bleeding (0.7%, $P < .001$). The dose of niacin was high and fixed, resulting in dose-related adverse effects. About 43% of the study subjects were Chinese. This influenced many of the adverse effects, especially myopathy and skin eruptions. As noted in the paper, "the absolute risk of myopathy in the placebo group was higher in China than in Europe and the relative risk with ERNL versus placebo was 5.2 in China, as compared to 1.5 in Europe. This is 10x greater in China participants, with 50 cases per 10,000, compared to 3 cases per 10,000 in Europe."

The investigational drug laropiprant has documented mechanisms of harm similar to that of the Cox-2 inhibitors and nonsteroidal anti-inflammatory drugs to which it is related, as well as many other potential adverse effects. Laropiprant with aspirin or clopidogrel induces a prolongation of bleeding time and an inhibitory effect on platelet aggregation ex vivo in healthy subjects and in patients with dyslipidemia.

These studies are too far from reality. It is unlikely that niacin (or any other HDL-C-raising medications) would be prescribed in practice to patients with a lipoprotein profile similar to that in these studies before randomization. In the HPS2-THRIVE study, average baseline LDL-C was 63 mg/dL, HDL-C was 44 mg/dL, and TG was 125 mg/dL before study drug treatment. Of further concern, MVE reduction in the niacin-laropiprant group was strongly predicted by baseline LDL-C ($P = .02$), with apparent clinical benefit if baseline LDL-C level was above 58 mg/dL. Indeed, it might not be expected to get clinical benefit if patients were on the flat part of the event curve. Patients in the placebo group in AIM-HIGH study had received 50 mg immediate-release niacin in each placebo tablet to mask the identity of treatment to patients or study personnel. Per protocol, the placebo group in all studies received also high dose of statin with or without ezetimibe. The early termination of the AIM-HIGH might not allow detection of positive results.

The effective dosing range of niacin is from 500 to 4000 mg/d. The niacin dose should be gradually increased, starting at 100 mg/d, and administered at meal time. Niacin-induced flushing can be reduced by giving a daily dose of 81 mg aspirin taken with a quercetin supplement at 500 to 1000 mg/d. Niacin should not be taken within 6 hours of alcohol.[5] Only vitamin B3 niacin is effective for dyslipidemia. The no-flush (inositol hexanicotinate) does not improve lipid profiles and is not recommended.[5] The potential side effects of niacin include hyperglycemia, hyperuricemia, gout, hepatitis, flushing, rash, pruritus, hyperpigmentation, hyperhomocysteinemia, gastritis, ulcers, bruising, tachycardia, and palpitations.[5,122,123] At lower doses of niacin, these side effects are not common.

Pantethine

Pantethine is the disulfide derivative of pantothenic acid and is metabolized to cystamine-SH, which is the active form for treating dyslipidemia.[5] Over 28 clinical trials have shown consistent and significant improvement in serum lipids. TC is decreased 15%, LDL-C falls by 20%, ApoB is decreased 27.6%, and TGs are reduced by 36.5% over 4 to 9 months. HDL-C and APO A1 are increased 8%.[5,129-133] The effects on lipids are slow to occur and have a peak effect at 4 months but may take up to 6 to 9 months. Pantethine reduces lipid peroxidation of LDL-C and decreases lipid deposition, intimal thickening, and fatty streak formation in the aorta and coronary arteries.[5,129-133] Pantethine inhibits cholesterol synthesis and accelerates FA metabolism in the mitochondria by inhibiting hepatic acetyl-CoA carboxylase; increases CoA in the cytoplasm, which stimulates the oxidation of acetate at the expense of FA and cholesterol synthesis; and increases Krebs cycle activity.[5,129-133] In addition, cholesterol esterase activity increases and HMG-CoA reductase activity is decreased. There is 50% inhibition of FA synthesis and 80% inhibition of cholesterol synthesis.[5] It has an additive effect when used with RYR, statins, niacin, and fibrates.[5,129-133] The recommended effective dose is 450 mg twice a day with or without food.[5,129-133]

Plant Sterols (Phytosterols)

The plant sterols are naturally occurring cholesterol-like compounds with different side chain substitutions that give them unique properties. These include B-sitosterol (the most abundant), campesterol, and stigmasterol (4-desmethyl sterols of the cholestane series) and the stanols, which are saturated sterols.[5,134-136] The plant sterols are much better absorbed than the plant stanols. The daily intake of plant sterols in the United States is about 150 to 400 mg/d, mostly from soybean oil and from various nuts.[5,134-136] Consumption of these compounds results in a dose-dependent reduction in serum lipids.[135] TC is decreased 8% and LDL-C is decreased 10% (range 6%-15%) with no change in TG and HDL-C, from doses of 2 to 3 g/d in divided doses with meals.[5,134,135] A recent meta-analysis of 84 trials showed that an average intake of 2.15 g/d reduced LDL-C by 8.8% with no improvement with higher doses.[135] They are additive with other antilipid therapies such as statins, niacin, fibrates, and curcumin. The mechanism of action is primarily to a decrease the incorporation of dietary and biliary cholesterol into micelles due to lowered micellar solubility of cholesterol, which reduces cholesterol absorption and increases bile acid secretion. In addition, there is an interaction with enterocyte ATP-binding cassette transport proteins (ABCG8 and ABCG 5) that directs cholesterol back into the intestinal lumen.[5,134] The only difference between cholesterol and sitosterol is that an additional ethyl group is present at position C-24 in sitosterol, which is responsible for its poor absorption. The plant sterols have a higher affinity than cholesterol for micelles.

The plant sterols are also anti-inflammatory and decrease the levels of proinflammatory cytokines such as interleukins (IL-6, IL1b) and TNF alpha, as well as hsCRP, LpPLA 2, and fibrinogen; however, these effects vary among the various phytosterols.[136] Other potential mechanisms include modulation of signaling pathways, activation of cellular stress responses, cellular growth arrest, reduction of Apo B 48 secretion from intestinal and hepatic cells, reduction of cholesterol synthesis with suppression of HMG-CoA reductase and cytochrome P 450 (CYP7A1), interference with sterol receptor element binding protein (SREBP), and promotion of reverse cholesterol transport via ABCA1 and ABCG1.[136] The biological activity of phytosterols is both cell-type and sterol specific.[134]

The plant sterols can interfere with absorption of lipid-soluble compounds such as the fat-soluble vitamins and carotenoids (vitamins A D, E, K, and alpha carotene).[5] Some studies have shown reduction in atherosclerosis progression, reduced carotid IMT, and decreased plaque progression, but the results have been conflicting.[5] There are no studies on CHD or other CVD outcomes. The recommended dose is about 2 to 2.5 g/d (average 2.15 g/d). Patients who have the rare homozygote mutations of sitosterolemia and abnormal ATP-binding cassette are hyperabsorbers of sitosterol (absorbing 15%-60% instead of the normal 5%) and will develop premature atherosclerosis. The patients can be identified with genetic testing and should avoid plant sterols.

Policosanol

Policosanol is a sugarcane extract of eight aliphatic alcohols that has undergone extensive clinical studies with variable results.[5,137-140] Most of the earlier studies that showed positive results were performed in Cuba, and these have been questioned as to their validity.[5,138] More recent double-blind placebo-controlled clinical trials have not shown any significant improvement in any measured lipids, including TC, LDL-C, TG, or HDL-C. A recent small study (14 subjects, underpowered) suggested that policosanol may improve HDL-C functionality, increase paraoxonase (PON), lower glucose, reduce uric acid, decrease blood pressure and the oxidative stress marker malondialdehyde, and improve the lipid profile.[137] Other studies have found that policosanol may enhance the effects of statins and improve hepatic function.[140] Policosanol is not recommended at this time for the treatment of any form of dyslipidemia pending more definitive studies with a larger study population.[5,138,139]

Tocotrienols

Tocotrienols are a family of unsaturated forms of vitamin E termed alpha, beta, gamma, and delta tocotrienols.[5,141,142] The gamma and delta tocotrienols lower TC up to 17%, LDL-C by 24%, ApoB by 15%, and Lp(a) by 17% with minimal changes or a slight increase in HDL-C and Apo-A1 in 50% of subjects at doses of 200 mg/d given at night with food.[5,141,142] In addition, the LDL-C receptor is augmented and the tocotrienols exhibit antioxidant activity.[5,141,142] The gamma/delta from of tocotrienols inhibits cholesterol synthesis by suppression of HMG-CoA reductase activity by two posttranscriptional actions.[5,141,142] These include increased controlled degradation of the reductase protein and decreased efficiency of translation of HMG-CoA reductase mRNA. These effects are mediated by sterol binding of the reductase enzyme to the endoplasmic reticulum membrane proteins call INSIGS. The tocotrienols have natural farnesylated analogues of tocopherols that give them their effects on HMG-CoA reductase.[141]

The tocotrienol dose is important because increased dosing will induce its own metabolism and reduce effectiveness, whereas lower doses are not as effective.[5] Also, concomitant intake within 12 hours of alpha tocopherol reduces tocotrienol absorption. Increased intake of alpha tocopherol over 20% of the total tocopherol intake may interfere with the lipid lowering effect.[5,141] Tocotrienols are metabolized by successive beta oxidation, then catalyzed by the CYP 450 enzymes 3A4 and CYP 4F2.[5] The combination of a statin with gamma/delta tocotrienols further reduces LDL-C cholesterol by 10%.[141] The tocotrienols block the adaptive response of upregulation of HMG-CoA reductase secondary to competitive inhibition by the statins.[5,141] Tocotrienols lower hsCRP, advanced glycation end products, cell adhesion molecules, and thrombotic risk and suppress matrix metalloproteinases.[142] In addition, they suppress, regress, and slow the progression of atherosclerosis, stabilize atherosclerotic plaques, and reduce the risk of cardiac events in established CHD.[142] Carotid artery stenosis regression has been reported in about 30% of subjects given tocotrienols over 18 months. They also slow the progression of generalized atherosclerosis.[5,142] The recommended dose is 200 mg of gamma delta tocotrienol at night with food.

Red Yeast Rice

RYR (*Monascus purpureus*) is a fermented product of rice that contains monocolins, which inhibit cholesterol synthesis via HMG-CoA reductase and thus has "statinlike" properties.[5,143,144] RYR also contains sterols, isoflavones, and MUFAs. At 2400 mg/d LDL-C is reduced 22% ($P < .001$) and TG falls 12% with little change in HDL-C.[5,143,144] A meta-analysis by Xiong showed that RYR reduced LDL 17.6% ($P < 0,01$) and increased HDL 4.2% ($P < .001$) at doses of up to 1600-mg/d dose.[144] In addition, the CV mortality was decreased by 30% ($P < .005$) and total mortality by 33% ($P < .0003$) in the treated subjects. The overall primary end points for MI and death are decreased by 45% ($P < .001$).[5,144] Numerous previous controlled clinical trials of RYR showed similar effects.[5] RYR lowers metalloproteinases 2 and 3, leptin, insulin resistance, hsCRP, tissue factor, NADPH oxidase, thrombosis, caveolin-1, TNF-alpha, pulse wave velocity, and angiotensin II and decreases the risk of abdominal aortic aneurysms.[5,143,144] RYR increases nitric oxide and eNOS.[5,143,144] A highly purified and certified RYR must be used to avoid potential renal damage induced by a mycotoxin, citrinin.[5,144] The recommended dose is 2400 to 4800 mg of a standardized RYR at night with food. No adverse clinical effects have been reported with long-term use. Reductions in coenzyme Q 10 may occur in predisposed patients and those given prolonged high-dose RYR because of its weaker statinlike effect. RYR provides an alternative to patients with statin-induced myopathy or other statin-induced adverse effects.[5,143,144]

Resveratrol

Resveratrol reduces oxLDL-C; inhibits ACAT activity and cholesterol ester formation; increases bile acid excretion; reduces TC, TG, and LDL-C; and increases PON-1 activity and HDL-C. In vitro studies showed that resveratrol inhibits NADPH oxidase in macrophages and blocks the uptake of modified LDL-C by CD36 SR (scavenger receptors).[5] N-acetylcysteine (NAC) has this same effect on CD 36 SR and should be used in conjunction with resveratrol.[5] The dose of trans-resveratrol is 250 mg/d and that of NAC is 1000 mg once or twice a day.[5]

Vitamin C

Vitamin C supplementation lowers serum LDL-C and TG.[145] A meta-analysis of 13 RCTs in subjects given at least 500 mg of vitamin C daily for 3 to 24 weeks found a reduction in LDL-C cholesterol of 7.9 mg/dL ($P < .0001$) and a decrease of TG by 20.1 mg/dL ($P < .003$). HDL-C did not change. The reductions in LDL-C and TG were greatest in those with the highest initial lipid levels and the lowest serum vitamin C levels.[146] High-dose vitamin C is part of a therapeutic regimen to neutralize the negative effects of elevated Lp(a) levels.

Berberine

Berberine, an alkaloid present in plant roots, rhizomes, and stem barks, is effective as either monotherapy or in combination with other nutritional supplements to improve serum lipids.[147-150] In one study, at 3 months, with berberine at 500 mg twice a day TC decreased by 29%, LDL-C fell 25%, and TG were reduced by 35%.[148] A meta-analysis of 11 trials in 874 subjects demonstrated significant reductions in TC (23 mg/dL), LDL-C (25 mg/dL), and TG (44 mg/dL) and an increase in HDL-C (2 mg/dL).[149] Berberine suppresses PCSK9 expression and increases hepatic LDL R (mRNA/protein) 2.6- to 3.5-fold, reduces cholesterol absorption, increases biliary excretion of LDL, inhibits HMG-CoA reductase, decreases FA synthesis, and increases FA oxidation.[147-149] Berberine is additive for the reduction of LDL-C, TC, and TG with ezetimibe, RYR, and phytosterols.[147-150] Berberine may inhibit CYP enzymes and increase serum levels of statins. The recommended dose of berberine HCL is 500 to 1000 mg/d.

Combination Therapies[151-156]

A prospective open-label human clinical trial of 30 patients for 2 months showed significant improvement in serum lipids using a proprietary product (LS) with a combination of pantethine, plant sterols, EGCG, and gamma/delta tocotrienols.[157] The TC fell 14%, LDL-C decreased 14%, VLDL dropped 20%, and small dense LDL-C particles fell 25% (type III and IV).[147] In another study using the same proprietary product with RYR 2400 to 4800 mg/d and niacin 500 mg/d, the TC fell 34%, LDL-C decreased by 34%, LDL-C particle number fell 35%, VLDL dropped 27%, and HDL-C increased 10%.[151]

The most recent study of a proprietary lipid-lowering product (LC) found significant improvement in the expanded lipid profile particle numbers, size, and total lipid levels, and inflammatory markers.[152] Forty participants were recruited for a single-center, double-blind randomized, placebo-controlled

trial. The 40 participants were randomly assigned to receive either the proprietary multi-ingredient lipid-lowering supplement (LC) n = 20 or placebo n = 20. The trial consisted of a screening visit, a 2-week run-in, and a 4-month treatment period. Results from the trial showed that the LC significantly reduced TC, LDL-C, VLDL-C, oxLDL.

Apo B, TG, LDL-P heart rate, and diastolic blood pressure were compared with placebo at 1 month and 4 months. The LC significantly increased HDL-P and LDL particle size from dense type III and IV to larger type I and II LDL particle compared with placebo at 1 month and 4 months. In addition, LC significantly lowered hsCRP, TNF-α, and IL-6 within the treatment group from baseline. There were no adverse effects noted in the treatment group after 4 months of supplementation.

Clinical studies indicate a RRR of CVD mortality with omega-3 FAs of 0.68, with resins of 0.70, and with statins of 0.78.[153] Combining statins with omega-3 FAs further decreases CHD by 19%.[83] The combination of gamma/delta tocotrienols with a statin reduces LDL-C an additional 10%.[140] Plant sterols with omega-3 FAs have synergistic lipid-lowering and anti-inflammatory effects.[87] Future studies are needed to evaluate various other combinations on serum lipids, surrogate vascular end points, and CHD and CVD morbidity and mortality.[154-156]

Pharmacologic Therapies

Although the drug arsenal for lipid management has traditionally been scant, unlike that for hypertension and diabetes, the use of natural molecules has always been an integral part of drug discovery and clinical management in this area of medicine. It should suffice to remind the reader that: (1) niacin (vitamin B3) was the very first "drug" approved to treat lipids in the late 1950s; (2) statins are derivatives of a molecule found in nature in fungi and bacteria, and also available as supplement in RYR; (3) prescription omega-3 fats are extracted from fish just like their supplemental counterparts; (4) fibrates are derivatives of FAs; and (5) monoclonal antibodies against PCSK9 fall in the category of natural products, because they are fully human IgG molecules. The next few paragraphs will quickly cover the main mechanisms of action, indications for use, expected effects and adverse events, and vascular benefits of the drugs approved for the management of dyslipidemia. One has to keep in mind that use of drugs is neither an alternative nor a primary element of management, as drugs and supplements work well together, many patients reject the use of artificial molecules, and vascular benefits are believed to be secondary to adjustment of lipid levels, irrespective of the modality used. The best outcome for the patient is when the naturopathic or integrative physician and the classically trained provider collaborate to design a regimen that contains as many elements of lifestyle changes and natural supplements as needed and as few medications as possible at the lowest effective doses, the most cost-effective program that is compatible with reaching standard-of-care goals. Although the natural lipid-lowering agents have been covered extensively earlier, here we will summarize the essential practical knowledge for all the drugs approved by the FDA separated by main lipid effect: (1) cholesterol-lowering agents (resins, statins, ezetimibe, PCSK9 inhibitors) and (2) triglyceride-lowering agents (niacin, fibrates, omega-3 fats). A recent review we published on the lipid-lowering landscape provides additional information.[158]

Resins

These agents are not absorbed by the intestine and act by binding bile acids and impeding their reabsorption, thus triggering hepatic neosynthesis of bile acids from cholesterol derived from plasma LDL.[159] They have been in the market for decades and sold as generic drugs for many years, although they continue to be expensive and usually not well covered by insurance. Cholestyramine and colestipol are known to interfere with the absorption of other drugs, and for this reason they must be taken alone and not with other agents. In addition, because their action depends on the presence of bile in the intestine, these medications must be timed in connection with a meal. Colesevelam is the newest member of the class and the only one to also have an indication for diabetes management.[160] Unlike the others, it does not interfere with other drugs and does not need to be timed with meal. Resins reduce LDL-C by about 20% at full dose (several grams per day), have no effect on HDL, and may increase TG levels in those susceptible, such as insulin-resistant patients. This effect is due to the upregulation of the nuclear receptor FXR in the liver. Although resins are safe, they are generally poorly tolerated because of constipation, difficulty of swallowing many large pills or a gritty solution, and cost considerations. Some of the resins have been used in early clinical trials (before statins) and have shown evidence of moderate cardiovascular benefits.[161] They can be combined with statins or ezetimibe, although most patients would be better off instead following dietary and supplemental regimens that also can ensure a 20% LDL reduction.[162] Additional reasons to prefer resins is when there is need to combat pruritus due to liver failure[163] or to help manage diarrhea from different causes.[164]

Statins

This is the "drug" that everybody has in mind when discussing cholesterol drugs. Statins inhibit HMG-CoA reductase in the liver, the rate-limiting enzyme for cholesterol synthesis. Because cholesterol is essential for the survival of liver cells, this inhibition triggers a response from hepatocytes to increase the expression of their LDL receptor to capture more LDL from plasma, hence inducing LDL lowering.[165] Statins also affect TG and HDL levels, although modestly, and do not influence Lp(a) or LDL size, although LDL-P falls concomitantly with LDL-C. Concomitant use of statins with omega-3 FAs and/or niacin may increase LDL size, lower Lp(a), and augment LDL-C and LDL-P lowering. Statins are the reason why the cholesterol hypothesis of atherosclerosis-based

CVD has become universally accepted, as a plethora of clinical trials have shown benefits in primary and secondary prevention populations.[166] This knowledge was congealed by the American Heart Association (AHA)/American College of Cardiology (ACC) cholesterol guidelines of 2013, when the standard for clinical management became the use of the right statin at the right dose for the right patient.[167] The highest-risk patients should be treated either with atorvastatin 40 or 80 mg or rosuvastatin 20 or 40 mg. Most anything else in terms of statin type and dose will suffice to address lower-risk individuals. These guidelines have been recently revised to accommodate for the use of nonstatin agents and to reinstate LDL-C goal achievement.[168] Statins are blessed by low cost and ease of use but damned by an unusually high rate of intolerance, fear of side effects, and other forms of aversion. All statins except for pitavastatin are now generic and covered by insurance for little to no copay. However, it is estimated that over 20% of patients in need of statin will either not accept it at all or not continue it for long.[169] The partial failure of statins to become a universally acceptable staple for CVD risk management has opened the way for other agents that contribute to bring LDL to goal. As we discussed earlier, a patient not willing or able to take a statin may respond well to a combination strategy that includes other drugs, dietary factors, and supplements. It must be emphasized that the trend created by the ACC/AHA 2013 guidelines, which supported the necessity of statin coverage to manage risk, has been short lived and has more recently reverted to a consensus view that achieving the LDL goal is what ultimately protects the patient. Natural ways to achieve a protective LDL-C level are expected to be superior to any pharmacologic intervention.

Ezetimibe

This oral agent works by blocking the intestinal cholesterol receptor and therefore reduces intestinal absorption of both dietary and biliary cholesterol.[170] Ezetimibe is a generic medication taken orally once a day and at the fixed dose of 10 mg/d. It has a nearly exclusive effect on LDL-C, which is reduced on average by 15% to 20%. Very little to no changes are produced by this drug on TG, HDL, and Lp(a) levels. Ezetimibe had a troubled history because it was approved by the FDA in the absence of evidence of clinical benefits, and thus for many years it was seen as an expensive and ineffective add-on or alternative to statins. Then it became subject of intense scrutiny and criticism when the ENHANCE trial published results showing no effect of adding ezetimibe to simvastatin on carotid intima-media thickness in low-risk individuals.[171] More recently, the IMPROVE-IT trial rescued its image but not enough to turn it into a blockbuster, as the effect of adding ezetimibe to simvastatin on CVD events was a relative risk reduction of less than 10% over 7 years, statistically significant but clinically unimpressive.[172] Today, there has been a resurgence of ezetimibe because insurances favor its addition to the lipid-lowering regimen before approving a PCSK9 inhibitor.[173,174] It remains a reasonable choice for subjects needing less than 20% LDL reduction, although this can also be easily accomplished with natural interventions. There is no evidence that ezetimibe alone (for example, in patients who refuse to take a statin) has any effects on CVD event rates.

PCSK9 Inhibitors

These are injectable monoclonal antibodies (fully human IgG) self-administered with subcutaneous injection via automated prefilled pen either once or twice a month. There are two drugs in this class, evolocumab and alirocumab, but they are similar and accomplish the same effect, ie, they bind to PCSK9 in the circulation and block it from performing its physiologic action as destroyer of the LDL receptor.[175] Most subjects prefer the twice-a-month dosing, because this is done with a single pen action, whereas the monthly dosing requires more complex procedures (either three consecutive injections for one or the use of a device that slowly delivers a larger amount for the other). The antibody is injected in vast excess to the ligand, and thus a few hours after injection there is no free PCSK9 available in the blood. Because PCSK9 is the physiologic inducer of LDL receptor degradation, its blockade allows for the LDL receptors in the liver to recycle without challenge, thus greatly enhancing their ability to internalize plasma LDL, and leading to plasma LDL-C drops between 55% and 70% on top of any prior reductions obtained with a statin. This has changed the panorama of lipid management, as now it is possible to completely wipe away the LDL-C component of risk, and having instead to face the paradoxical scenario of the patient complaining or concerned because LDL-C levels are too low (often below 25 mg/dL). PCSK9i are approved for subjects with familial hypercholesterolemia and those with preexisting CVD and LDL-C not at goal on maximally tolerated therapy. These categories cover as many as 9 million Americans, but these two drugs combined have been prescribed to less than 100,000 people in the 4 years since initial approval. Reasons for this low uptake include: (1) lack of familiarity by both doctors and patients with injectable drugs for cholesterol management; (2) perception that the drug is needed only if one has to achieve tremendous reductions in LDL-C (say >50%); (3) concerns about cost to patients and the health care system; (4) insurance denials and Medicare coinsurance (the so-called donut hole) requirements.

Both PCSK9i available in the market have proven clinical benefits[176,177] when added to a statin and have shown the following: (1) Driving LDL to an average of 35 mg/dL produces additional benefits in the range of 15% risk reduction of MI, stroke, and CVD death. (2) No side effects are emerging to limit acceptance, and these drugs are well tolerated by patients who cannot take a statin because of myalgia. (3) The residual risk after maximal LDL control remains unexpectedly high, and thus there is no hope to use the LDL-lowering strategy to stop the epidemic of MIs. This final point is as important as it is sobering, and it highlights the value of a healthy lifestyle and of maintenance

of cardiovascular health. Once you start growing coronary plaques, you can do little to prevent an MI even if you drive LDL-C to near nothing.

Niacin

This agent has been covered plenty already in this chapter as vitamin B3. Here we want to simply highlight the practical takes on the most recent evidence from clinical trials. First of all, the available choices include regular (immediate release), slow-release, extended-release (the only prescription formulation, now generic), and no-flush (inositol hexanicotinate) niacin.[178] The last one should never be used because it does not release niacin to the circulation (remember, no-flush means no-niacin). The others are equally effective on affecting lipid levels (TG −30%, HDL +20%, LDL-C −20%, Lp(a) −25%) but different on the extent and duration of flushing. Although historically doses of regular niacin would go up to 6000 mg/d, more recently providers have adjusted to small doses of 250 to 1000 mg/d. For slow- and extended-release formulations the maximal dose is 2000 mg, but again most patients will take doses lower than 1000 mg/d. Even though the AIM-HIGH and HPS2-THRIVE studies have shown no value from adding benefit to statin therapy in high-risk subjects with LDL at goal and low HDL, there is still potential for different niacin formulations to be of value in reducing risk in patients needing additional LDL-C or Lp(a) reduction.

Fibrates

These agents have been in the market for a long time and have been exclusively used for control of TG, particularly in patients at risk of acute pancreatitis (TG > 500 mg/dL). The two available molecules in the United States are gemfibrozil (600 mg twice a day) and fenofibrate or fenofibric acid (120-200 mg/d fixed dose depending on formulation).[179] Fibrates reduce TG levels by up to 40% and can have moderate effects on HDL (+10%) and LDL (−10%). After the primary prevention trial called Helsinki Heart Study (HHS) and the secondary prevention trial called VA-HIT, each showing cardiovascular benefits from gemfibrozil alone in the pre-statin era (HHS) or in subjects with LDL not needing statin control (VA-HIT), fibrates have had an unimpressive run in trials where the background therapy was a statin.[180,181] In the two most prominent studies, FIELD and ACCORD, high-CVD-risk diabetic patients did not receive benefits from adding fenofibrate to simvastatin.[182,183] Even though subgroup analyses showed a significant CVD risk reduction among those with the highest TG levels, the lack of effect in the treated population as a whole has prohibited the inclusion of either fibrate therapy or aggressive TG control as part of the mandate for CVD risk management in modern clinical guidelines. Today fibrates are reserved for extreme hypertriglyceridemia, and preference is given to fenofibrate because of its ability to be combined with a statin with minimal risk for pharmacokinetic interaction and side effects. Gemfibrozil is not recommended in subjects taking a statin.[184]

Prescription Omega-3 Fats

Two formulations in the market compete with the vast offering of supplements, a generic purified mixture of EPA and DHA and a branded formulation of pure EPA, both used at the fixed dose of 4 g/d. These medications are approved, just like the fibrates, for the treatment of extreme hypertriglyceridemia (TG > 500 mg/dL) to reduce the risk of pancreatitis.[185] Omega-3 fats reduce TG levels by up to 45% and have minimal effects on HDL. The EPA/DHA drug tends to raise LDL-C levels significantly in the absence of a statin, whereas the EPA-only drug does not affect or even reduces LDL-C levels.[186,187] Clinical trials of omega-3 formulations containing both EPA and DHA have not been able to convincingly show CVD benefits, whereas the EPA-only drug has had two successful clinical studies reporting significant benefits on top of statin therapy, the JELIS and the REDUCE-IT trials. In JELIS, 1.8 g/d of EPA in subjects taking a low-dose statin was sufficient to reduce TG levels minimally (10%) and CVD risk substantially (20%). In addition, CVD benefits were magnified in subjects whose starting lipids included high TG and low HDL.[188,189] More recently, the REDUCE-IT trial has shown a tremendous 25% CVD risk reduction in statin-treated subjects with a history of diabetes and/or prior MI with the use of 4 g of purified EPA.[190] Again, the effect occurred with minimal TG reduction and with no relation between degree of TG control and CVD benefits. It is thus possible that the value of omega-3 fats in general, and EPA in particular, is not linked to TG control, but to one or more of the many additional vascular effects exerted by these natural agents.

Future Perspectives

Advances in the understanding of the pathophysiology and causes of dyslipidemia and dyslipidemia-induced CVD[191-197] coupled with new diagnostic CV biomarkers, genetics, microbiome analysis,[198] and noninvasive testing will allow for more personalized treatment in the future. The most common secondary causes for dyslipidemia are:

1. Chronic inflammatory macronutrient and micronutrient intake (metabolic endotoxemia)
2. Chronic infections (all types, including bacteria, virus, fungi, tuberculosis, and parasites)
3. Heavy metals (mercury, cadmium, lead, arsenic) and other toxins

It is estimated that approximately 70% of secondary dyslipidemia is due to one of these three etiologies. All patients with dyslipidemia should be evaluated and treated for these causes as well as the traditional metabolic causes such as hypothyroidism, renal and liver disease, and autoimmunity and secondary causes such as dietary factors and drugs affecting lipids. Proper therapy for the underlying cause can often correct the dyslipidemia over time. Such therapies would include optimal diets, probiotics, prebiotics, anti-infectives, improvement in the natural immune function, and chelation therapy in addition to the drugs discussed previously, if ever needed.

Summary and Conclusions

The combination of a lipid-lowering diet, select foods, nutraceutical supplements, and lipid-lowering drugs have the ability to reduce TC and LDL-C by 65% or more, decrease LDL-C particle number, increase LDL-C particle size, lower TG and VLDL, and increase total HDL-C and HDL-P, and improve HDL functionality. In addition, vascular inflammation, oxidative stress, and immune responses are decreased and vascular target organ damage, atherosclerosis, CHD, and CVD are reduced by many of the dietary interventions, RYR, omega-3 FAs, niacin, statins, or a combination of these (Table 22.2). The LDL-P is the primary lipid component that drives the risk for CHD and MI. RYR, omega-3 FAs, niacin, and berberine are effective in reducing LDL-P and increasing small dense LDL size. Statins will decrease LDL-P approximately 30% to 50% of the time, and the new PCSK9 inhibitors are effective on

---

Table 22.2

SUMMARY OF NUTRACEUTICAL SUPPLEMENTS AT RECOMMENDED DOSES FOR THE TREATMENT OF DYSLIPIDEMIA

- Red yeast rice: 2400-4800 mg at night with food
- Plant sterols: 2.5 g/d
- Berberine: 500 mg/d to twice d
- Niacin (nicotinic acid B3: 500 to 3000 mg/d as tolerated pretreated with quercetin, apples, ASA. Take with food and avoid alcohol. Never interrupt therapy
- Omega-3 fatty acids with EPA/DHA at 3/2 ratio: 4 g/d with GLA at 50% of total EPA and GLA and gamma/delta tocopherol
- Gamma delta tocotrienols: 200 mg hs
- Aged garlic—Kyolic standardized 600 mg twice a day
- Sesame 40 g/d
- Phosphatidyl serine: 300 mg twice a day
- Pantethine: 450 mg twice a day
- MUFA: 20 to 40 g/d (EVOO 4 tablespoons per day)
- Lycopene: 20 mg/d
- Luteolin: 10 per day
- Astaxanthin: 15 mg/d
- Trans-resveratrol: 250 mg/d
- NAC: 500 mg twice a day
- Carnosine: 500 mg twice a day
- Citrus bergamot: 1000 mg/d
- Quercetin: 500 mg twice a day
- Probiotics standardized: 15-50 billion organisms twice a day
- Curcumin: 500-1000 mg twice a day
- EGCG: 500-1000 mg twice a day or 60-100 ounces of green tea per day
- Pomegranate: 1/4-1/2 cup of seeds/d or 6 ounces of juice per day

DHA, docosahexaenoic acid; EGCG, epigallocatechin gallate; EPA, eicosapentaenoic acid; EVOO, extra-virgin olive oil; MUFA, monounsaturated fatty acid; NAC, N-acetylcysteine.

both LDL-C and LDL-P but limited in scope to the patients at the highest risk of CVD. Recent new proprietary nutritional supplements have combined many of these supplements to favorably affect all the components of the advanced lipid profile as well as interrupt many of the 45 mechanisms involved in

dyslipidemia and dyslipidemia-induced vascular disease. This approach broadens treatment options by leveraging the effects of diet, food, nutritional supplements, and lipid-lowering drugs to the underlying, complex pathophysiology of lipid-induced vascular damage.

References

1. Kannel WB, Castelli WD, Gordon T, et al. Serum cholesterol, lipoproteins and risk of coronary artery disease. The Framingham Study. *Ann Intern Med.* 1971;74:1-12.
2. Houston MC. Nutrition and nutraceutical supplements in the treatment of hypertension. *Expert Rev Cardiovasc Ther.* 2010;8:821-833.
3. Tian N, Penman AD, Mawson AR, Manning RD Jr, Flessner MF. Association between circulating specific leukocyte types and blood pressure: the atherosclerosis risk in communities (ARIC) study. *J Am Soc Hypertens.* 2010;4(6):272-283.
4. Ungvari Z, Kaley G, de Cabo R, Sonntag WE, Csiszar A. Mechanisms of vascular aging: new perspectives. *J Gerontol A Biol Sci Med Sci.* 2010;65(10):1028-1041.
5. Houston M. The role of nutrition and nutritional supplements in the treatment of dyslipidemia. *Clin Lipidol.* 2014;9(3):333-335.
6. Plourde M, Vohl MC, Vandal M, Couture P, Lemieux S, Cunnane SC. Plasma n-3 fatty acid supplement is modulated by apoE epsilon 4 but not by the common PPAR-alpha L162 polymorphism in men. *Br J Nutr.* 2009;102:1121-1124.
7. Neiminen T, Kahonen M, Viiri LE, Gronroos P, Lehtimaki T. Pharmacogenetics of apoliproprotein E gene during lipid-lowering therapy: lipid levels and prevention of coronary heart disease. *Pharmacogenomics.* 2008;9(10):1475-1486.
8. Shih DM, Lusis AJ. The roles of PON 1 and PON 2 in cardiovascular disease and innate immunity. *Curr Opin Lipidol.* 2009;20(4):288-292.
9. Calkin AC, Tontonoz P. Genome-wide association studies identify new targets in cardiovascular disease. *Sci Transl Med.* 2010;2(48):48.
10. Talmud PJ, Shah S, Whittall R, et al. Use of low-density lipoprotein cholesterol gene score to distinguish patients with polygenic and monogenic familial hypercholesterolaemia: a case-control study. *Lancet.* 2013 Apr 13;381(9874):1293–1301.doi: 10.1016/S0140-6736(12)62127-8.
11. Djousse L, Caziano JM. Dietary cholesterol and coronary artery disease: a systematic review. *Curr Atheroscler Rep.* 2009;11(6):418-422.
12. Houston M. The role of noninvasive cardiovascular testing, applied clinical nutrition and nutritional supplements in the prevention and treatment of coronary heart disease. *Ther Adv Cardiovasc Dis.* 2018;12(3):85-108.
13. Erkkila A, de Mello VD, Riserus U, Laaksonen DE. Dietary fatty acids and cardiovascular disease: an epidemiological approach. *Prog Lipid Res.* 2008;47(3):172-187.
14. Houston M, Minich D, Sinatra ST, Kahn JK, Guarneri M. Recent science and clinical application of nutrition to coronary heart disease. *J Am Coll Nutr.* 2018;37(3):169-187.
15. Mozaffarian D, Willet WC. Trans fatty acids and cardiovascular risk: a unique cardiometabolic imprint. *Curr Atheroscler Rep.* 2007;9(6):486-493.
16. Chen CL, Tetri LH, Neuschwander-Tetri BA, Huang SS, Huang JS. A mechanism by which dietary trans fats cause atherosclerosis. *J Nutr Biochem.* 2011;22:649-655.
17. Siri-Tarino PW, Sun Q, Hu FB, Krauss RM. Saturated fat, carbohydrate and cardiovascular disease. *Am J Clin Nutr.* 2010;91(3):502-509.
18. Otvos JD, Mora S, Shalaurova I, Greenland P, Mackey RH, Goff DC Jr. Clinical implications of discordance between low-density lipoprotein cholesterol and particle number. *J Clin Lipidol.* 2011;5(2):105-113.
19. Hodge AM, Jenkins AJ, English DR, O'Dea K, Giles GG. NMR Determined lipoprotein subclass profile is associated with dietary composition and body size. *Nutr Metab Cardiovasc Dis.* 2011;21(8):603-609.
20. Asztalos BF, Tani M, Schaefer E. Metabolic and functional of HDL subspecies. *Curr Opin Lipidol.* 2011;22:176-185.
21. Khera AV, Cuchel M, de la Llera-Moya M, et al. Cholesterol efflux capacity, high-density lipoprotein function, and atherosclerosis. *N Engl J Med.* 2011;64:127-135.
22. Karakas M, Koenig W, Zierer A, et al. Myeloperoxidase is associated with incident coronary heart disease independently of traditional risk factors: results form the MONICA/KORA Augsburg study. *J Intern Med.* 2012;271(1):43-50.
23. Lamarche B, Tchernof A, Mooriani S, et al. Small, dense low-density lipoprotein particles as a predictor of the risk of ischemic heart disease in men. Prospective results from the Quebec Cardiovascular Study. *Circulation* 1997;95(1);69-75.
24. Kruth HS. Receptor-independent fluid-phase pinocytosis mechanisms for induction of foam cell formation with native low density lipoprotein particles. *Curr Opin Lipidol.* 2011;22(5):386-393.
25. Zhao ZW, Zhu XL, Luo YK, Lin CG, Chen LL. Circulating Soluble lectin-like oxidized low-density lipoprotein receptor-1 levels are associated with angiographic coronary lesion complexity in patients with coronary artery disease. *Clin Cardiol.* 2011;34(3):172-177.
26. Ehara S, Ueda M, Naruko T, et al. Elevated levels of oxidized low density lipoprotein show a positive relationship with the severity of acute coronary syndromes. *Circulation.* 2001;103(15): 1955-1960.
27. Hansson GK. Inflammation, atherosclerosis, and coronary artery disease. *N Engl J Med.* 2005;352(16):1685-1695.
28. Harper CR, Jacobson TA. Using apolipoprotein B to manage Dyslipidemic patients: time for a change? *Mayo Clin Proc.* 2010; 85(5):440-445.
29. Curtiss LK. Reversing atherosclerosis? *N Engl J Med.* 2009;360(11): 1144-1146.
30. Ridker PM, Danielson E, Fonseca FA, et al. Rosuvastatin to prevent vascular events in men and women with elevated C-reactive protein. *N Engl J Med.* 2008;359(21):2195-2207.
31. Shen GX. Impact and mechanism for oxidized and glycated Lipoproteins on generation of fibrinolytic regulators from vascular endothelial cells. *Mol Cell Biochem.* 2003;246(1-2):69-74.
32. Krishnan GM, Thompson PD. The effects of statins on skeletal muscle strength and exercise performance. *Curr Opin Lipidol.* 2010;21(4):324-328.
33. Mills EJ, Wu P, Chong G, et al. Efficacy and safety of statin treatment for cardiovascular disease: a network meta-analysis of 170,255 patients from 76 randomized trials. *QJM.* 2011;104(2): 109-124.
34. Mammen AL, Amato AA. Statin myopathy: a review of recent progress. *Curr Opin Rheumatol.* 2010;22(6):544-550.
35. Russo MW, Scobev M, Bonkovsky HL. Drug-induced liver injury associated with statins. *Semin Liver Dis.* 2009;29(4):412-422.
36. Moosmann B, Behl C. Selenoproteins, cholesterol-lowering drugs, and the consequences: revisiting of the mevalonate pathway. *Trends Cardiovasc Med.* 2004;14(7):273-281.
37. Liu CS, Lii CK, Chang LL, et al. Atorvastatin increases blood ratios of vitamin E/low-density lipoprotein cholesterol and coenzyme Q10/low-density lipoprotein cholesterol in hypercholesterolemic patients. *Nutr Res.* 2010;30(2):118-124.
38. Wyman M, Leonard M, Morledge T. Coenzyme Q 10: a therapy for hypertension and statin-induced myalgia?. *Clev Clin J Med.* 2010;77(7):435-442.
39. Mortensen SA. Low coenzyme Q levels and the outcome of statin treatment in heart failure. *J Am Coll Cardiol.* 2011;57(14):1569.

40. Shojaei M, Djalali M, Khatami M, Siassi F, Eshraghian M. Effects of carnitine and coenzyme Q 10 on lipid profile and serum levels of lipoprotein (a) in maintenance hemodialysis patients on statin therapy. *Iran J Kidney Dis*. 2011;5(20):114-118.

41. Gupta A, Thompson PD. The relationship of Vitamin D deficiency to statin myopathy. *Atherosclerosis*. 2011;215(1):23-29.

42. Avis HJ, Hargreaves IP, Ruiter JP, Land JM, Wanders RJ, Wijburg FA. Rosuvastatin lowers coenzyme Q 10 levels, but not mitochondrial adenosine triphosphate synthesis, in children with familial hypercholesterolemia. *J Pediatr*. 2011;158(3):458-462.

43. Kiernan TJ, Rochford M, McDermott JH. Simvastatin induced Rhapdomyloysis and an important clinical link with hypothyroidism. *Int J Cardiol*. 2007;119(3):374-376.

44. Shapiro MD, Tavori H, Fazio S. PCSK9: from basic science discoveries to clinical trials. *Circ Res*. 2018;122(10):1420-1438. doi:10.1161/CIRCRESAHA.118.311227. Review. PubMed PMID:29748367; PubMed Central. PMCID: PMC5976255.

45. Van Horn L, McCoin M, Kris-Etherton PM, et al. The evidence for dietary prevention and treatment of cardiovascular disease. *J Am Diet Assoc*. 2008;108:287-331.

46. Dawber TR, Meadors GF, Moore FE. Epidemiological approaches to heart disease: the Framingham Study. *Am J Public Health*. 1951;41:279-286.

47. Keys A. Coronary heart disease in seven countries. *Circulation*. 1970;41(suppl 1):1-21.

48. Keys A, Menotti A, Karvonen MJ, et al. The diet and 15-year death rate in the Seven Countries Study. *Am J Epidemiol*. 1986;124:903-915.

49. Appel LJ, Sacks FM, Carey VJ, et al. Effects of protein, monounsaturated fat, and carbohydrate intake on blood pressure and serum lipids: results of the OmniHeart randomized trial. *JAMA*. 2005;294:2455-2464.

50. Pritikin N. Dietary factors and hyperlipidemia. *Diabetes Care*. 1982;5:647-648.

51. Pritikin N. The Pritikin diet. *JAMA*. 1984;251:1160-1161.

52. Barnard RJ, Lattimore L, Holly RG, et al. Response of non-insulin-dependent diabetic patients to an intensive program of diet and exercise. *Diabetes Care*. 1982;5:370-374.

53. Ornish D, Scherwitz LW, Doody RS, et al. Effects of stress management training and dietary changes in treating ischemic heart disease. *JAMA*. 1983;249:54-59.

54. Ornish D, Brown SE, Scherwitz LW, et al. Can lifestyle changes reverse coronary heart disease? The Lifestyle Heart Trial. *Lancet*. 1990;336:129-133.

55. Ornish D, Scherwitz LW, Billings JH, et al. 1998. Intensive lifestyle changes for reversal of coronary heart disease. *JAMA* 280: 2001-2007. Erratum in: *JAMA*, 1999;281:1380.

56. Chainani-Wu N, Weidner G, Purnell DM, et al. Changes in emerging cardiac biomarkers after an intensive lifestyle intervention. *Am J Cardiol*. 2011;108:498-507.

57. Expert Panel on Detection, Evaluation, and Treatment of High Blood Cholesterol in Adults. Executive summary of the third report of the National Cholesterol Education Program (NCEP) expert panel on detection, evaluation, and treatment of high blood cholesterol in adults (adult treatment panel III). *JAMA*. 2001;285:2486-2497. Available at http://www.nhlbi.nih.gov/guidelines/cholesterol/atp3upd04.htm. Accessed November 27, 2011.

58. Lichtenstein AH, Appel LJ, Brands M, et al. Summary of American Heart Association diet and lifestyle recommendations revision 2006. *Arterioscler Thromb Vasc Biol*. 2006;26:2186-2191.

59. Lichtenstein AH, Ausman LM, Jalbert SM, et al. Efficacy of a Therapeutic Lifestyle Change/Step 2 diet in moderately hypercholesterolemic middle-aged and elderly female and male subjects. *J Lipid Res*. 2002;43:264-273.

60. Howard BV, Van Horn L, Hsia J. Low-fat dietary pattern and risk of cardiovascular disease: the Women's Health Initiative Randomized Controlled Dietary Modification Trial. *JAMA*. 2006;295:655-666.

61. Jenkins DJ, Kendall CW, Marchie A, et al. The effect of combining plant sterols, soy protein, viscous fibers, and almonds in treating hypercholesterolemia. *Metabolism*. 2003;52:1478-1483.

62. Jenkins DJ, Kendall CW, Faulkner DA, et al. Assessment of the longer-term effects of a dietary portfolio of cholesterol-lowering foods in hypercholesterolemia. *Am J Clin Nutr*. 2006;83:582-591.

63. Jenkins DJ, Kendall CW, Faulkner D, et al. A dietary portfolio approach to cholesterol reduction: combined effects of plant sterols, vegetable proteins, and viscous fibers in hypercholesterolemia. *Metabolism*. 2002;51:1596-1604.

64. Jenkins DJ, Kendall CW, Marchie A, et al. Effects of a dietary portfolio of cholesterol-lowering foods vs lovastatin on serum lipids and C-reactive protein. *JAMA*. 2003;290:502-510.

65. Jenkins DJ, Chiavaroli L, Wong JM, et al. Adding monounsaturated fatty acids to a dietary portfolio of cholesterol-lowering foods in hypercholesterolemia. *CMAJ*. 2010;182:1961-1967.

66. Jenkins DJ, Jones PJ, Lamarche B, et al. Effect of a dietary portfolio of cholesterol-lowering foods given at 2 levels of intensity of dietary advice on serum lipids in hyperlipidemia: a randomized controlled trial. *JAMA*. 2011;306:831-839.

67. Kris-Etherton P, Eckel RH, Howard BV, et al. AHA Science Advisory: Lyon Diet Heart Study. Benefits of a Mediterranean-style, National Cholesterol Education Program/American Heart Association step I dietary pattern on cardiovascular disease. *Circulation*. 2001;103:1823-1825.

68. de Lorgeril M, Renaud S, Mamelle N, et al. Mediterranean alpha-linolenic acid-rich diet in secondary prevention of coronary heart disease. *Lancet*. 1994;343:1454-1459. Erratum in: *Lancet*. 1994;345:738.

69. de Lorgeril M, Salen P, Martin JL, et al. Mediterranean diet, traditional risk factors, and the rate of cardiovascular complications after myocardial infarction: final report of the Lyon Diet Heart Study. *Circulation*. 1999;99:779-785.

70. de Lorgeril M, Salen P. The Mediterranean diet: rationale and evidence for its benefit. *Curr Atheroscler Rep*. 2008;10:518-522.

71. Rastogi T, Reddy KS, Vaz M, et al. Diet and risk of ischemic heart disease in India. *Am J Clin Nutr*. 2004;79:582-592.

72. Kallio P, Kolehmainen M, Laaksonen DE, et al. Dietary carbohydrate modification induces alterations in gene expression in abdominal subcutaneous adipose tissue in persons with the metabolic syndrome: the FUNGENUT Study. *Am J Clin Nutr*. 2007;85:1417-1427.

73. Ornish D, Magbanua MJ, Weidner G, et al. Changes in prostate gene expression in men undergoing an intensive nutrition and lifestyle intervention. *Proc Natl Acad Sci USA*. 2008;105:8369-8374.

74. Llorente-Cortés V, Estruch R, Mena MP, et al. Effect of Mediterranean diet on the expression of pro-atherogenic genes in a population at high cardiovascular risk. *Atherosclerosis*. 2010;208:442-450.

75. Razquin C, Martinez JA, Martinez-Gonzalez MA, et al. A Mediterranean diet rich in virgin olive oil may reverse the effects of the -174G/C IL6 gene variant on 3-year body weight change. *Mol Nutr Food Res*. 2010;54(suppl 1):S75-S82.

76. Ros E, Martínez-González MA, Estruch R, Salas-Salvadó J, Fitó M, Martínez JA. Mediterranean diet and cardiovascular health: teachings of the PREDIMED study. *Adv Nutr*. 2014;5(3):330S-336S.

77. Castañer O, Corella D, Covas MI, et al. In vivo transcriptomic profile after a Mediterranean diet in high-cardiovascular risk patients: a randomized controlled trial. *Am J Clin Nutr*. 2013;98(3):845-853.

78. Konstantinidou V Covas MI, Sola R, Fitó M. Up-to date knowledge on the in vivo transcriptomic effect of the Mediterranean diet in humans. *Mol Nutr Food Res*. 2013;57(5):772-783.

79. Estruch R, Ros E, Salas-Salvadó J, et al. Primary prevention of cardiovascular disease with a Mediterranean diet. *N Engl J Med*. 2013;368(14):1279-1290.

80. Alexander DD, Miller PE, Van Elswyk ME, Kuratko CN, Bylsma LC. A meta-analysis of randomized controlled trials and prospective cohort studies of eicosapentaenoic and docosahexaenoic long-chain omega-3 fatty acids and coronary heart disease risk. *Mayo Clin Proc*. 2017;92(1):15-29.

81. Rissanen T, Voutilainen S, Nyyssonen K, Lakka TA, Salonen JT. Fish oil-derived fatty acids, docosahexaenoic acid and docosapentaenoic acid and the risk of acute coronary events: the Kuopio ischaemic heart disease risk factor study. *Circulation*. 2000;102(22):2677-2679.

82. Davis W, Rockway S, Kwasny M. Effect of a combined therapeutic approach of intensive lipid management, omega 3 fatty acid supplementation, and increased serum 25(OH) D on coronary calcium scores in asymptomatic adults. *Am J Ther.* 2009;16(4):326-332.

83. Yokoyama M, Origasa H, Matsuzaki M, et al. Effects of eicosapentaenoic acid on major coronary events in hypercholesterolaemic patients (JELIS): a randomised open-label, blinded endpoint analysis. *Lancet.* 2007;369(9567):1090-1098.

84. Ryan AS, Keske MA, Hoffman JP, Nelson EB. Clinical Overview of algal-docosahexaenoic acid: effects on triglyceride levels and other cardiovascular risk factors. *Am J Ther.* 2009;16(2):183-192.

85. Kelley DS, Siegal D, Vemuri M, Chung GH, Mackey BE. Docosahexaenoic acid supplementation decreases remnant-like particle cholesterol and increases the (n-3) index in hypertriglyceridemic men. *J Nutr.* 2008;138(1):30-35.

86. Maki KC, Dicklin MR, Davidson MH, Doyle RT, Ballantyne CM, Combination of prescription Omega -3 with Simvastatin (COMBOS) Investigators. Baseline lipoprotein lipids and low-density lipoprotein cholesterol response to prescription omega-3 acid ethyl ester added to Simvastatin therapy. *Am J Cardiol.* 2010;105(10):1409-1412.

87. Micallef MA, Garg ML. The lipid-lowering effects of phytosterols and (n-3) polyunsaturated fatty acids are synergistic and complementary in hyperlipidemic men and women. *J Nutr.* 2008;138(6):1085-1090.

88. Mori TA, Burke V, Puddey IB, et al. Purified eicosapentaenoic and docosahexaenoic acids have differential effects on serum lipids and lipoproteins, LDL particle size, glucose and insulin in mildly hyperlipidemic men. *Am J Clin Nutr.* 2000;71(5):1085-1094.

89. Aung T, Halsey J, Kromhout D. Associations of omega-3 fatty acid supplement use with cardiovascular disease risks: meta-analysis of 10 trials involving 77 917 individuals. *JAMA Cardiol.* 2018;3(3):225-234.doi:10.1001/jamacardio.2017.5205.

90. http://cochranelibrary-wiley.com/wol1/doi/10.1002/14651858.CD012345.pub2/full.

91. Prasad K. Flaxseed and cardiovascular health. *J Cardiovasc Pharmacol.* 2009;54(5):369-377.

92. Bioedon LT, Balkai S, Chittams J, et al. Flaxseed and cardiovascular risk factors: results from a double-blind, randomized controlled clinical trial. *J Am Coll Nutr.* 2008;27(1):65-74.

93. Mandasescu S, Mocanu V, Dascalita AM, et al. Flaxseed supplementation in hyperlipidemic patients. *Rev Med Chir Soc Med Nat Lasi.* 2005;109(3):502-506.

94. Bester D, Esterhuyse AJ, Truter EJ, van Rooven J. Cardiovascular effects of edible oils: a comparison between four popular edible oils. *Nutr Res Rev.* 2010;23(2):334-348.

95. Vateradou K, Weech M, Altowaijri H, et al. Replacement of saturated with unsaturated fats had no impact on vascular function but beneficial effects on lipid biomarkers, E-selectin, and blood pressure: results from the randomized, controlled Dietary Intervention and VAScular function (DIVAS) study. *Am J Clin Nutr.* 2015;102(1):40-48.

96. Bogani P, Gali C, Villa M, Visioli F. Postprandial anti-inflammatory and antioxidant effects of extra virgin olive oil. *Atherosclerosis.* 2007;190(1):181-186.

97. Reid K. Garlic lowers blood pressure in hypertensive individuals, regulates serum cholesterol, and stimulates immunity: an updated meta-analysis and review. *J Nutr.* 2016;146(2):389S-396S.

98. Ried K Toben C, Fakler P. Effect of garlic on serum lipids: an updated meta-analysis. *Nutr Rev.* 2013;71(5):282-99.

99. Samavat H, Newman AR Wang R, Yuan JM, Wu AH, Kurzer MS. Effects of green tea catechin extract on serum lipids in postmenopausal women: a randomized, placebo-controlled clinical trial. *Am J Clin Nutr.* 2016;104(6):1671-1682.

100. Tinahones FJ, Rubio MA, Garrido-Sanchez L, et al. Green tea reduces LDL oxidizability and improves vascular function. *J Am Coll Nutr.* 2008;27(2):209-213.

101. Brown AL, Lane J, Holyoak C, Nicol B, Mayes AE, Dadd T. Health effects of green tea catechins in overweight and obese men: a randomized controlled cross-over trial. *Br J Nut.* 2011;7:1-10.

102. Zheng XX, Xu YL, Li SH, Liu XX, Hui R, Huang XH. Green Tea intake lowers fasting serum total and LDL cholesterol in adults: a

103. Cesar TB, Aptekman NP, Araujo MP, Vinagre CC, Maranhao RC. Orange juice decreases low-density lipoprotein cholesterol in hypercholesterolemic subjects and improves lipid transfer to high-density lipoprotein in normal and hypercholesterolemic subjects. *Nutr Res.* 2010;30(10):689-694.

104. Mirmiran P, Fazeli MR, Asghari G, Shafiee A, Azizi F. Effect of pomegranate seed oil on hyperlipidaemic subjects: a double-blind placebo-controlled clinical trial. *Br J Nutr.* 2010;104(3):402-406.

105. Fuhrman B, Volkova N, Aviram M. Pomegranate juice polyphenols increase recombinant paroxonase-1 binding to high density lipoprotein: studies in vitro and in diabetic patients. *Nutrition.* 2010;26(4):359-366.

106. Avairam M, Rosenblat M, Gaitine D, et al. Pomegranate juice consumption for 3 years by patients with carotid artery stenosis reduces common carotid intima-media thickness, blood pressure and LDL oxidation. *Clin Nutr.* 2004;23(3):423-433.

107. Mattiello T, Trifiro E, Jotti GS, Pulcinelli FM. Effects of pomegranate juice and extract polyphenols on platelet function. *J Med Food.* 2009;12(2):334-339.

108. Aviram M, Dornfeld L, Rosenblat M, et al. Pomegranate juice consumption reduces oxidative stress, atherogenic modifications to LDL, and platelet aggregation: studies in humans and in atherosclerotic apolipoprotein E-deficient mice. *Am J Clin Nutr.* 2000;71(5):1062-1076.

109. Davidson MH, Maki KC, Dicklin MR, et al. Effects of consumption of pomegranate juice on carotid intima-media thickness in men and women at moderate risk for coronary heart disease. *Am J Cardiol.* 2009;104(7):936-942.

110. Devarajan S, Singh R, Chatterjee B, Zhang B, Ali A. A blend of sesame oil and rice bran oil lowers blood pressure and improves the lipid profile in mild-to-moderate hypertensive patients. *J Clin Lipidol.* 2016;10(2):339-349.

111. Namiki M. Nutraceutical functions of sesame: a review. *Crit Rev Food Sci Nutr.* 2007;47(7):651-673.

112. Sacks FM, Lichtenstein A, Van Horn L, et al. Soy protein, isoflavones, and cardiovascular health: an American Heart Association Science Advisory for professionals from the Nutrition Committee. *Circulation.* 2006;113(7):1034-1044.

113. Harland JI, Haffner TA. Systemic review, meta-analysis and Regression of randomized controlled trials reporting an association between an intake of circa 25 g soya protein per day and blood cholesterol. *Atherosclerosis.* 2008;200(1):13-27.

114. Houston MC. Juice powder concentrate and systemic blood pressure, progression of coronary artery calcium and antioxidant status in hypertensive subjects: a pilot study. *Evid Based Complement Alternat Med.* 2007;4(4):455-462.

115. Toth PP, Patti AM, Nikolic D, et al. Bergamot reduces plasma lipids, atherogenic small dense LDL, and subclinical atherosclerosis in subjects with moderate hypercholesterolemia: a 6 months prospective study. *Front Pharmacol.* 2016;6:299.

116. Mollace V, Sacco I, Janda E, et al. Hypolipidemic and hypoglycaemic activity of bergamot polyphenols: from animal models to human studies. *Fitotherapia.* 2011;82(3):309-316.

117. Soni KB, Kuttan R. Effect of oral curcumin administration on serum peroxides and cholesterol levels in human volunteers. *Indian J Physiol Pharmacol.* 1992;36(4):273-275.

118. Ulbricht C, Basch E, Szapary P, et al. Guggul for hyperlipidemia: a review by the Natural Standard Research Collaboration. *Complement Ther Med.* 2005;13(4):279-290.

119. Nohr LA, Rasmussen LB, Straand J. Resin from the Mukul Myrrh tree, guggul, can it be used for treating hypercholesterolemia: a randomized, controlled study. *Complement Ther Med.* 2009;17(1):16-22.

120. McEneny J, Wade L, Young IS, et al. Lycopene intervention reduces inflammation and improves HDL functionality in moderately overweight middle-aged individuals. *J Nutr Biochem.* 2013 Jan;24(1):163-168.

121. Palozza P, Simone R, Gatalano A, Parrone N, Monego G, Ranelletti F. Lycopene regulation of cholesterol synthesis and efflux in human macrophages. *J Nutr Biochem.* 2011;22:971-978.

122. Ruparelia N, Digby JE, Choudhury RP. Effects of niacin on atherosclerosis and vascular function. *Curr Opin Cardiol.* 2011;26(1):66-70.

123. Al-Mohissen MA, Pun SC, Frohlich JJ. Niacin: from mechanisms of action to therapeutic uses. *Mini Rev Med Chem.* 2010;10(3):204-217.

124. Garg A, Sharma A, Krishnamoorthy P, et al. Role of niacin in current clinical practice: a systematic review. *Am J Med.* 2017;130(2):173-187.

125. Lavigne PM, Karas RH. The current state of niacin in cardiovascular disease prevention: a systematic review and meta-regression. *J Am Coll Cardiol.* 2013;61(4):440-446.

126. Khera AV, Qamar A, Reilly MP, Dunbar RL, Rader DJ. Effects of niacin, statin, and fenofibrate on circulating proprotein convertase subtilisin/kexin type 9 levels in patients with dyslipidemia. *Am J Cardiol.* 2015;115(2):178-182.

127. Houston M, Pizzorno J. "Niacin doesn't work and is harmful/" proclaim the headlines. Yet another highly publicized questionable study to discredit integrative medicine. *Integr Med.* 2014;13(5): 8-11.

128. AIM HIGH Investigators. The role of niacin in raising high density lipoprotein cholesterols to reduce cardiovascular events in patients with atherosclerotic cardiovascular disease and optimally treated low density lipoprotein cholesterol: baseline characteristics of study participants. The Atherothrombosis Intervention in Metabolic syndrome with low HDL/high triglycerides: impact on Global Health outcomes (AIM-HIGH) trial. *Am Heart J.* 2011;161(3):538-543.

129. McRae MP. Treatment of hyperlipoproteinemia with pantethine: a review and analysis of efficacy and tolerability. *Nutr Res.* 2005;25:319-333.

130. Kelly G. Pantethine: a review of its biochemistry and therapeutic applications. *Altern Med Rev.* 1997;2:365-377.

131. Rumberger JA, Napolitano J, Azumano I, Kamiya T, Evans M. Pantethine, a derivative of vitamin B(5) used as a nutritional supplement, favorably alters low-density lipoprotein cholesterol metabolism in low- to moderate-cardiovascular risk North American subjects: a triple-blinded placebo and diet-controlled investigation. *Nutr Res.* 2011;31(8):608-615.

132. Evans M, Rumberger JA, Azumano I, Napolitano JJ, Citrolo D, Kamiya T. Pantethine, a derivative of vitamin B5, favorably alters total, LDL and non-HDL cholesterol in low to moderate cardiovascular risk subjects eligible for statin therapy: a triple-blinded placebo and diet-controlled investigation. *Vasc Health Risk Manag.* 2014;10:89-100.

133. Pantethine. Monograph. *Altern Med Rev.* 2010;15(3):279-282.

134. Plat J, Baumgartner S, Mensink RP. Mechanisms underlying the health benefits of plant sterol and stanol ester consumption. *J AOAC Int.* 2015;98(3):697-700.

135. Demonty I, Ras RT, van der Knaap HC, et al. Continuous dose response relationship of the LDL cholesterol lowering effect of phytosterol intake. *J Nutr.* 2009;139(2):271-284.

136. Sabeva NS, McPhaul CM, Li X, Cory TJ, Feola DJ, Graf GA. Phytosterols differently influence ABC transporter expression, cholesterol efflux and inflammatory cytokine Secretion in macrophage foam cells. *J Nutr Biochem.* 2011;22:777-783.

137. Kim JY Kim SM, Kim SJ, Lee EY Kim JR Cho KH. Consumption of policosanol enhances HDL functionality via CETP inhibition and reduces blood pressure and visceral fat in young and middle-aged subjects. *Int J Mol Med.* 2017;39(4):889-899.

138. Berthold HK, Unverdorben S, Degenhardt R, Bulitta M, Gourni, Berthold I. Effect of policosanol on lipid levels among patients with hypercholesterolemia or combined hyperlipidemia: a randomized controlled trial. *JAMA.* 2006;295(19):2262-2269.

139. Greyling A, De Witt C, Oosthuizen W, Jerling JC. Effects of a policosanol supplement on serum lipid concentrations in hypercholesterolemic and heterozygous familial hypercholesterolaemic subjects. *Br J Nutr.* 2006;95(5):968-975.

140. Solomenchuk TM, Vosukh V, Bedzay A, Koval VG, Chepka IM, Trotsko VV. Efficiency of concomitant use of policosanol and rosuvastatin in patients with stable coronary artery disease and moderate hepatic dysfunction. *Lik Sprava.* 2015;(7-8):29-37.

141. Qureshi AA, Sami SA, Salser WA, Khan FA. Synergistic effect of tocotrienol-rich fraction (TRF 25) of rice bran and lovastatin on lipid parameters in hypercholesterolemic humans. *J Nutr Biochem.* 2001;12(6):318-329.

142. Prasad K. Tocotrienols and cardiovascular health. *Curr Pharm Des.* 2011;17(21):2147-2154.

143. Cicero AFG. Red yeast rice, monacolin K, and pleiotropic effects. *Recenti Prog Med.* 2018;109(2):154e-157e.

144. Xiong X, Wang P, Li X, Zhang Y, Li S. The effects of red yeast rice dietary supplement on blood pressure, lipid profile, and C-reactive protein in hypertension: a systematic review. *Crit Rev Food Sci Nutr.* 2017;57(9):1831-1851.

145. McRae MP. Vitamin C supplementation lowers serum low-density cholesterol and triglycerides: a meta-analysis of 13 randomized controlled trials. *J Chiropr Med.* 2008;7(2):48-58.

146. McRae MP. The efficacy of Vitamin C supplementation on reducing total serum cholesterol in human subjects: a review of 51 experimental trials. *J Chiropr Med.* 2006;5(1):2-12.

147. Sahebkar A, Watts GF. Mode of action of berberine on lipid metabolism: a new-old phytochemical with clinical applications? *Curr Opin Lipidol.* 2017;28(3):282-283.

148. Kong W, Wei J, Abidi P, et al. Berberine is a novel cholesterol-lowering drug working through a unique mechanism distinct from statins. *Nat Med.* 2004;10(12):1344-1351.

149. Dong H, Zhao Y, Zhao L, Lu F. The effects of berberine on blood lipids: a systemic review and meta-analysis of randomized controlled trials. *Planta Med.* 2013;79(6):437-446.

150. McCarty MF, O'Keefe JH, DiNicolantonio JJ. Red yeast rice plus berberine: practical strategy for promoting vascular and metabolic health. *Altern Ther Health Med.* 2015;21(suppl 2):40-45.

151. Personal communication from Mark Houston MD, Hypertension Institute, Nashville, TN. Unpublished data on combination nutritional supplements for the treatment of dyslipidemia. 2017.

152. Houston M, Rountree R, Lamb J, Phipps S, Meng S, Zhang R. A placebo-controlled trial of a proprietary lipid-lowering nutraceutical supplement in the management of dyslipidemia. *J Biol Regul Homeost Agents.* 2016;30(4):1115-1123.

153. Studer M, Briel M, Leimenstoll B, Glass TR, Bucher HC. Effect of different anti-lipidemic agents and diets on mortality: a systemic review. *Arch Int Med.* 2005;165(7):725-730.

154. Nijjar PS, Burke FM, Bioesch A, Rader DJ. Role of dietary supplements in lowering low-density lipoprotein cholesterol: a review. *J Clin Lipidol.* 2010;4:248-258.

155. Cicero AFG, Colletti A, Bajraktari G, et al. Lipid lowering nutraceuticals in clinical practice: position paper from an International Lipid Expert Panel. *Arch Med Sci.* 2017;13(5):965-1005.

156. Mannarino MR, Ministrini S, Pirro M. Nutraceuticals for the treatment of hypercholesterolemia. *Eur J Intern Med.* 2014;25(7):592-599.

157. Houston M, Sparks W. Effect of combination pantethine, plant sterols, green tea extract, delta-tocotrienol and phytolens on lipid profiles in patients with hyperlipidemia. *JANA.* 2010;13(1): 15-20.

158. Shapiro MD, Fazio S. From lipids to inflammation: new approaches to reducing atherosclerotic risk. *Circ Res.* 2016;118(4):732-749. doi:10.1161/CIRCRESAHA.115.306471. Review. PubMed PMID:26892970.

159. Out C, Groen AK, Brufau G. Bile acid sequestrants: more than simple resins. *Curr Opin Lipidol.* 2012;23(1):43-55. doi:10.1097/MOL.0b013e32834f0ef3. Review. PubMed PMID:22186660.

160. Elkeles RS. Colesevelam for Type 2 diabetes mellitus: an abridged Cochrane review. *Diabet Med.* 2014;31(7):880. doi:10.1111/dme.12424. Review. PubMed PMID:24588426.

161. Ross S, D'Mello M, Anand SS, et al. Effect of bile acid sequestrants on the risk of cardiovascular events: a mendelian randomization analysis. 2015;8(4):618-627. 1161/CIRCGENETICS.114.000952. Epub 2015 June 4.

162. Vasudevan AR, Jones PH. Effective use of combination lipid therapy. *Curr Cardiol Rep.* 2005;7(6):471-479. Review. PubMed PMID:16256018.

163. Düll MM, Kremer AE. Management of chronic hepatic itch. *Dermatol Clin*. 2018;36(3):293-300. doi:10.1016/j.det.2018.02.008. Epub 2018 May 1. Review. PubMed PMID:29929600.

164. Kumpf VJ. Pharmacologic management of diarrhea in patients with short bowel syndrome. *JPEN J Parenter Enteral Nutr*. 2014;38(1 suppl):38S-44S. doi:10.1177/0148607113520618. Epub 2014 January 24. Review. PubMed PMID:24463352.

165. Taylor F, Huffman MD, Macedo AF, et al. Statins for the primary prevention of cardiovascular disease. *Cochrane Database Syst Rev*. 2013;(1):CD004816. doi:10.1002/14651858.CD004816.pub5. Review. PubMed PMID:23440795.

166. Hadjiphilippou S, Ray KK. Cholesterol-lowering agents. *Circ Res*. 2019;124(3):354-363. doi:10.1161/CIRCRESAHA.118.313245. PubMed PMID:30702991.

167. Stone NJ, Robinson JG, Lichtenstein AH, et al. 2013 ACC/AHA guideline on the treatment of blood cholesterol to reduce atherosclerotic cardiovascular risk in adults: a report of the American College of Cardiology/American Heart Association Task Force on Practice Guidelines. *J Am Coll Cardiol*. 2014;63(25 pt B):2889-2934. doi:10.1016/j.jacc.2013.11.002. Epub 2013 November 12. Erratum in: *J Am Coll Cardiol*. 2015;66(24):2812. *J Am Coll Cardiol*. 2014;63(25 pt B):3024-3025. PubMed PMID:24239923.

168. Grundy SM, Stone NJ, Bailey AL, et al. 2018 AHA/ACC/AACVPR/AAPA/ABC/ACPM/ADA/AGS/APhA/ASPC/NLA/PCNA guideline on the management of blood cholesterol: executive summary. *Circulation*. 2018;139(25):CIR0000000000000624. doi:10.1161/CIR.0000000000000624. [Epub ahead of print]. PubMed PMID:30565953.

169. Banach M, Stulc T, Dent R, Toth PP. Statin non-adherence and residual cardiovascular risk: there is need for substantial improvement. *Int J Cardiol*. 2016;225:184-196. doi:10.1016/j.ijcard.2016.09.075. Epub 2016 September 26. Review. PubMed PMID:27728862.

170. Bays HE, Moore PB, Drehobl MA, et al. Effectiveness and tolerability of ezetimibe in patients with primary hypercholesterolemia: pooled analysis of two phase II studies. *Clin Ther*. 2001;23(8):1209-1230. Erratum in: *Clin Ther*. 2001;23(9):1601. PubMed PMID:11558859.

171. Kastelein JJ, Akdim F, Stroes ES, et al. Simvastatin with or without ezetimibe in familial hypercholesterolemia. *N Engl J Med*. 2008;358(14):1431-1443. doi: 10.1056/NEJMoa0800742. Epub 2008 March 30. Erratum in: *N Engl J Med*. 2008;358(18):1977. PubMed PMID:18376000.

172. Cannon CP, Blazing MA, Giugliano RP, et al. Ezetimibe added to statin therapy after acute coronary syndromes. *N Engl J Med*. 2015;372(25):2387-2397. doi:10.1056/NEJMoa1410489. Epub 2015 June 3.

173. Kaufman TM, Duell PB, Purnell JQ, Wójcik C, Fazio S, Shapiro MD. Application of PCSK9 inhibitors in practice: challenges and opportunities. *Circ Res*. 2017;121(5):499-501. doi:10.1161/CIRCRESAHA.117.311532. PubMed PMID:28819040.

174. Kaufman TM, Warden BA, Minnier J, et al. Application of PCSK9 inhibitors in practice. *Circ Res*. 2019;124(1):32-37. doi:10.1161/CIRCRESAHA.118.314191. PubMed PMID:30605414; PubMed Central PMCID:PMC6319384.

175. Rosenson RS, Hegele RA, Fazio S, Cannon CP. The evolving future of PCSK9 inhibitors. *J Am Coll Cardiol*. 2018;72(3):314-329. doi:10.1016/j.jacc.2018.04.054. Epub 2018 July 9. Review. PubMed PMID:30012326.

176. Sabatine MS, Giugliano RP, Keech AC, et al. Evolocumab and clinical outcomes in patients with cardiovascular disease. *N Engl J Med*. 2017;376(18):1713-1722. doi:10.1056/NEJMoa1615664. Epub 2017 March 17.

177. Schwartz GG, Steg PG, Szarek M, et al. Alirocumab and cardiovascular outcomes after acute coronary syndrome. *N Engl J Med*. 2018;379(22):2097-2107. doi:10.1056/NEJMoa1801174. Epub 2018 November 7. PubMed PMID:30403574.

178. Superko HR, Zhao XQ, Hodis HN, Guyton JR. Niacin and heart disease prevention: engraving its tombstone is a mistake. *J Clin Lipidol*. 2017;11(6):1309-1317. doi:10.1016/j.jacl.2017.08.005. Epub 2017 August 24. Review. PubMed PMID:28927896.

179. Jakob T, Nordmann AJ, Schandelmaier S, Ferreira-González I, Briel M. Fibrates for primary prevention of cardiovascular disease events. *Cochrane Database Syst Rev*. 2016;11:CD009753. Review. PubMed PMID:27849333.

180. Frick MH, Elo O, Haapa K, et al. Helsinki Heart Study: primary-prevention trial with gemfibrozil in middle-aged men with dyslipidemia. Safety of treatment, changes in risk factors, and incidence of coronary heart disease. *N Engl J Med*. 1987;317(20):1237-1245.

181. Rubins HB, Robins SJ, Collins D, et al. Gemfibrozil for the secondary prevention of coronary heart disease in men with low levels of high-density lipoprotein cholesterol. Veterans Affairs High-Density Lipoprotein Cholesterol Intervention Trial Study Group. *N Engl J Med*. 1999;341(6):410-418. PubMed PMID:10438259.

182. Keech A, Simes RJ, Barter P, et al. Effects of long-term fenofibrate therapy on cardiovascular events in 9795 people with type 2 diabetes mellitus (the FIELD study): randomised controlled trial. *Lancet*. 2005;366(9500):1849-1861. Erratum in: *Lancet*. 2006;368(9545):1415. Erratum in: Lancet. 2006;368(9545):1420. PubMed PMID:16310551.

183. ACCORD Study Group; Ginsberg HN, Elam MB, Lovato LC, et al. Effects of combination lipid therapy in type 2 diabetes mellitus. *N Engl J Med*. 2010;362(17):1563-1574. doi:10.1056/NEJMoa1001282. Epub 2010 March 14. Erratum in: *N Engl J Med*. 2010;362(18):1748. PubMed PMID:20228404; PubMed Central PMCID:PMC2879499.

184. Schneck DW, Birmingham BK, Zalikowski JA, et al. The effect of gemfibrozil on the pharmacokinetics of rosuvastatin. *Clin Pharmacol Ther*. 2004;75(5):455-463. PubMed PMID:15116058.

185. Roth EM, Bays HE, Forker AD, et al. Prescription omega-3 fatty acid as an adjunct to fenofibrate therapy in hypertriglyceridemic subjects. *J Cardiovasc Pharmacol*. 2009;54(3):196-203. doi:10.1097/FJC.0b013e3181b0cf71. PubMed PMID:19597368.

186. Mosca L, Ballantyne CM, Bays HE, et al. Usefulness of icosapent ethyl (eicosapentaenoic acid ethyl ester) in women to lower triglyceride levels (results from the MARINE and ANCHOR trials). *Am J Cardiol*. 2017;119(3):397-403. doi: 10.1016/j.amjcard.2016.10.027. Epub 2016 November 1. PubMed PMID:27939227.

187. Ballantyne CM, Bays HE, Philip S, et al. Icosapent ethyl (eicosapentaenoic acid ethyl ester): effects on remnant-like particle cholesterol from the MARINE and ANCHOR studies. *Atherosclerosis*. 2016;253:81-87. doi:10.1016/j.atherosclerosis.2016.08.005. Epub 2016 August 20. PubMed PMID:27596132.

188. Yokoyama M, Origasa H, Matsuzaki M, et al. Effects of eicosapentaenoic acid on major coronary events in hypercholesterolaemic patients (JELIS): a randomised open-label, blinded endpoint analysis. *Lancet*. 2007;369(9567):1090-1098. Erratum in: Lancet. 2007;370(9583):220. PubMed PMID:17398308.

189. Saito Y, Yokoyama M, Origasa H, et al. Effects of EPA on coronary artery disease in hypercholesterolemic patients with multiple risk factors: sub-analysis of primary prevention cases from the Japan EPA Lipid Intervention Study (JELIS). *Atherosclerosis*. 2008;200(1):135-140. doi: 10.1016/j.atherosclerosis.2008.06.003. Epub 2008 June 19. Erratum in: Atherosclerosis. 2009 May;204(1):233. PubMed PMID:18667204.

190. Bhatt DL, Steg PG, Miller M, et al. Cardiovascular risk reduction with icosapent ethyl for hypertriglyceridemia. *N Engl J Med*. 2019;380(1):11-22. doi:10.1056/NEJMoa1812792. Epub 2018 November 10.

191. Feng X, Zhang Y, Xu R, et al. Lipopolysaccharide up-regulates the expression of Fcalpha/mu receptor and promotes the binding of oxidized low-density lipoprotein and its IgM antibody complex to activated human macrophages. *Atherosclerosis*. 2010;208(2):396-405.

192. Wiesner P Choi SH, Almazan F, et al. Low doses of lipopolysaccharide and minimally oxidized low-density lipoprotein cooperatively activate macrophages via nuclear factor kappa B and activator protein-1: possible mechanism for acceleration of atherosclerosis by subclinical endotoxemia. *Circ Res*. 2010;107(1):56-65.

193. Han R. Plasma lipoproteins are important components of the immune system. *Microbiol Immunol*. 2010;54(4):246-253.

194. Park K, Seo E. Toenail mercury and dyslipidemia: interaction with selenium. *J Trace Elem Med Biol.* 2017;39:43-49.

195. Zhou Z, Lu YH, Pi HF, et al. Cadmium exposure is associated with the prevalence of dyslipidemia. *Cell Physiol Biochem.* 2016;40(3-4):633-643.

196. Oladipo OO, Ayo JO, Ambali SF, Mohammed B, Aluwong T. Dyslipdemia induced by chronic low dose co-exposure to lead, cadmium and manganese in rats: the role of oxidative stress. *Environ Toxicol Pharmacol.* 2017;53:199-205.

197. Kim K. Blood cadmium concentration and lipid profile in Korean adults. *Environ Res.* 2012;112:225-229.

198. Jones ML, Martoni CJ, Prakash S. Cholesterol lowering and inhibition of sterol absorption by Lactobacillus reuteri NCIMB 30242: a randomized controlled trial. *Eur J Clin Nutr.* 2012;66(11), 1234-1241.

23

Coronary Heart Disease Risk Factors, Coronary Heart Disease, Congestive Heart Failure, and Metabolic Cardiology

Stephen T. Sinatra, MD, FACC, FACN, CNS and Mark C. Houston MD, MS, MSc, FACP, FAHA, FASH, FACN, FAARM, ABAARM, DABC

Abstract

Approximately 80% of coronary heart disease (CHD) can be prevented by optimal nutrition coupled with exercise, weight management, mild alcohol intake, and avoidance of all tobacco products. A limit has been reached in our ability to decrease the incidence of CHD utilizing the traditional diagnostic evaluation and prevention and treatment strategies for the top five cardiovascular (CV) risk factors that include hypertension, diabetes mellitus, dyslipidemia, obesity, and smoking. Approximately 50% of patients continue to have CHD or myocardial infarction (MI) despite the presently defined "normal" levels of the top five CHD risk factors. This is often referred to as the "**CHD gap**." There are numerous external insults that damage the cardiovascular system that result in three finite cardiovascular responses: vascular inflammation, vascular oxidative stress, and vascular immune vascular dysfunction. These three finite vascular responses cause functional or structural damage to the vascular system and preclinical and eventually clinical CHD. This article will review the emerging science of infinite vascular insults that cause the three vascular finite responses and the implications for diagnostic testing, prevention, and treatment of CHD and cardiovascular disease (CVD). The discussion will include the use of advanced and updated CV risk scoring systems, new and redefined CHD risk factors and biomarkers, micronutrient testing, cardiovascular genetics, nutrigenomics, genetic expression testing, and noninvasive cardiovascular testing.

Introduction

CVD remains the number one cause of morbidity and mortality in the United States.[1,2] The annual cost, direct and indirect, of treating CVD is approximately $320 billion USD.[2]

Every one in three deaths in the United States is due to CVD with over 2200 citizens dying from MI or stroke daily.[2-5]

Clinical studies suggest that a limit has been reached in the ability to reduce CHD and CVD.[1] About 80% of CHD can be prevented by optimal nutrition, optimal exercise, optimal weight and body fat, mild alcohol intake, and avoiding smoking.[1] More than 400 CHD risk factors have been defined.[2] The three finite responses of the cardiovascular system to the infinite insults include vascular inflammation, vascular oxidative stress, and vascular immune dysfunction. Laboratory measurement of the finite responses allows the physician "to backtrack" and determine the "why" or the genesis of CHD and CVD, remove the insult(s), and initiate optimal prevention and treatment methodologies to meet defined clinical, noninvasive testing, and laboratory goals.

Prevention and treatment strategies must be directed at these three finite vascular responses while reducing the allostatic load of the 400 or more CHD risk factors and biomarkers.[2]

The traditional diagnostic testing, evaluation, prevention, and treatment strategies for the top five cardiovascular risk factors (hypertension, diabetes, dyslipidemia, obesity, and smoking) have resulted in a **CHD gap**.[4] Approximately 50% of patients admitted to a hospital with acute coronary syndrome (ACS) or MI have "normal" levels of the top five CHD risk factors.[2,5] The "cholesterol-centric" approach to prevent CHD is clearly important, but the other risk factors must be redefined and treated early and aggressively. Simultaneously, the clinician should measure and treat the three finite cardiovascular responses. Advances in the direct assessment of the top five risk factors and the refinement of their definitions are often not utilized by physicians so that optimal prevention and treatment strategies for CHD are not clinically applied.[2] Physicians should also evaluate new CHD risk scoring systems, novel and redefined CHD risk biomarkers and risk factors, micronutrient testing, cardiovascular genetics, nutrigenomics, genetic expression testing, and noninvasive cardiovascular testing, which will allow cardiovascular medicine to become more personalized and precise.

Revolutionizing the Treatment of Coronary Heart Disease

Addressing cell membrane physiology and identification of dysfunction represents the first step in the prevention and treatment of CHD. Cell membranes are the primary barrier between the external milieu (attacked by various hemodynamic or biochemical insults) and the internal cell organelles. The interaction of the various insults with the endothelial vascular receptors such as pattern recognition receptors (PRR), nod-like receptors (NLR), toll-like receptors (TLR), and caveolae determine the signaling transduction into the cell.[2] The external insults stimulate these inflammatory vascular receptors directly or through epitopes.[2]

Any cell membrane insult, such as hypertension, alterations in hemodynamics, modified low-density lipoprotein cholesterol (LDL-C), glucose, advanced glycosylation end products, microbes, internal tissue breakdown, toxins, heavy metals, homocysteine, or the other CHD risk factors, results in a reaction diffusion wave (tsunami effect) throughout the cell membrane that may disrupt cell receptors and the signaling mechanisms with subsequent membrane damage and dysfunction.[6,7] Depending on the biological fatty acid makeup of the cell membrane with trans fats (TFAs), saturated fats (SFAs), monounsaturated fats (MUFAs), or omega-3 fats (PUFAs), the responses will vary. Fluidity within the cell membrane (MUFA, PUFA) dampens injury at the site of the insult as well as throughout the rest of the cell membrane. However, stiff cell membranes (SFA, TFA) will exacerbate local and distant cell membrane dysfunction and damage. In addition, a heightened response (*metabolic memory*) from the inflammatory/oxidative stress/immune cascade can create additional cell dysfunction and damage.[6,7] The acute response to cell injury is defensive, short lived, regulated, and appropriate, but with chronic insults of any type, the vascular inflammatory, oxidative stress, and immune responses become dysregulated and dysfunctional to the point that there is damage to the cardiovascular system. In this regard, the blood vessel becomes an "innocent bystander" to its own defense mechanisms that lead to functional and structural cardiovascular injury then to preclinical CHD and clinical CHD.[2] The maladaptation of the renin-angiotensin-aldosterone system (RAAS), sympathetic nervous system, and the inflammatory/oxidative stress/immune pathways contribute to the cardiovascular dysfunction and disease.[2]

The CHD risk factors have well-defined clinical goals that indicate the "normal" level at which the risk for CHD is minimal. There exists a continuum of risk of CHD with all risk factors such that a "true" normal level can be somewhat misleading.[2,8-13] Normal blood pressure (BP) is now defined

as 120/80 mm Hg.[8,12] The new ACC/AHA Hypertension Guidelines are as follows[12]:

Systolic, Diastolic Blood Pressure (mm Hg)	2017 ACC/AHA
120-129 and <80	Elevated BP
130-139 or 80-89	Stage 1 hypertension
140-159 or 90-99	Stage 2 hypertension
>160 or >100	Stage 3 hypertension

Dyslipidemia is defined as an LDL-C greater than 100 mg/dL depending on the clinical setting, and glucose intolerance is defined as a fasting glucose over 99 mg/dL.[2] However, the continuum of risk starts at even lower levels for BP, LDL-C, and glucose, as well as for most of the other CHD risk factors.[2] The risk for CHD actually starts with a fasting glucose of 75 mg/dL. For each 1 mg/dL increase in fasting blood sugar (FBS), the risk for CHD and MI increase by 1%.[2,9-12] The risk for CHD starts at a BP level of 110/70 mm Hg. For every 20/10 mm Hg increase in BP the risk for CHD is doubled.[2,12,13] As the LDL-C increases over 60 mg/dL there is a gradual reduction in endothelial nitric oxide (NO) as well as risk for CHD.[2,13]

The concept of **"translational vascular medicine"** correlates CHD risk factors with the actual presence of CVD. The question is whether or not measured CHD risk factors accurately translate into cardiovascular pathology that can be evaluated by noninvasive or invasive vascular testing. Conversely, does the absence of measured CHD risk factors accurately define the absence of cardiovascular pathology or cardiovascular health? Evaluation of this correlation requires more sophisticated technology and advanced CHD risk factor analysis combined with comprehensive CHD risk factor scoring systems such as those of **COSEHC**[13,14] and **Rasmussen**[15] (Tables 23.1 and 23.2).

THE ENDOTHELIUM, ENDOTHELIAL FUNCTION AND DYSFUNCTION

The endothelium is a very thin lining of vascular cells forming an interface between the arterial lumen and the vascular smooth muscle (VSM).[2,4,16] Endothelial dysfunction occurs when nitric oxide bioavailability is reduced, which leads to vascular inflammation, oxidative stress, immune dysfunction, abnormal vascular growth, vasoconstriction, increased permeability, thrombosis, and CHD.[2,4,16,17]

LDL-C has a primary role in the development of atherosclerotic plaque formation starting at birth (Figure 23.1).[18] LDL-C migrates from the blood into the subendothelial layer and attaches to proteoglycans and becomes modified, antigenic, and toxic primarily via oxidation of LDL (oxLDL) and glycation of LDL (glyLDL).[18] The modified LDLs produce numerous cytokines and chemokines that attract monocytes into the subendothelial layer, which transform into macrophages. The modified LDL is taken up by scavenger receptors (SRA) on the macrophage cell membranes, which transform into foam cells, then fatty streaks, and eventually form a coronary artery

Table 23.1

COSHEC CV SCORING SYSTEM

- **Absolute Risk:** probability of an adverse event occurring in an individual within a defined period of time
- **Relative Risk:** probability of an adverse event happening in an individual compared with average or normal individuals sharing similar demographics other than the risk factor

High Cardiovascular Risk

- **Relative Risk** $\geq$ **60th percentile**
- **Absolute Risk: Risk score** $\geq$ **40** $\geq$ **2.3% risk of CV death/5 y**

Approximate 60th Percentile Relative Risk Scores

Men	Age Range (years)	Women
29	35-39	18
32	40-44	21
<u>36</u>	45-49	27
40	50-54	31
44	55-59	<u>36</u>
48	60-64	41
53	65-69	45
57	70-74	49

- Men at age 50 y = relative risk of $\geq$ 60th percentile
- Women at age 60 y = relative risk of $\geq$ 60th percentile

Women (12 CHD risk factors)
- Age (years)
- Cigarette smoking
- Systolic blood pressure (mm Hg)
- Total cholesterol concentration (mg/dL)
- Height (inches)
- Creatinine concentration (mg/dL)
- Homocysteine (µmol/L)
- Prior MI
- Prior stroke
- LVH
- Diabetes
- Nondiabetic, FBS (mg/dL)

Men (17 CHD risk factors)
- Being male
- Age (years)
- Cigarette smoking
- Systolic blood pressure (mm Hg)
- Total cholesterol concentration (mg/dL)
- LDL cholesterol (mg/dL)
- HDL cholesterol (mg/dL)
- Triglyceride (mg/dL)
- Height (inches)
- Creatinine concentration (mg/dL)
- Homocysteine (µmol/L)
- Prior MI
- Family history of MI pre-60
- Prior stroke
- LVH
- Diabetes
- Nondiabetic, FBS (mg/dL)

Table 23.1

COSHEC CV SCORING SYSTEM—CONT'D

Calculated Risk Score	% dying from cardiovascular disease in 5 y
0	0.04
5	0.07
10	0.11
15	0.19
20	0.31
25	0.51
30	0.84
35	1.4
40	2.3
45	3.7
50	6.1
55	9.8
60	15.6

CHD, coronary heart disease; CV, cardiovascular; FBS, fasting blood sugar; HDL, high-density lipoprotein; LDL, low-density lipoprotein; LVH, left ventricular hypertrophy; MI, myocardial infarction.

plaque (stable plaque or a soft rupture-prone plaque) that can result in an MI. Approximately 45 different steps exist in this process of dyslipidemia-induced vascular disease that can be interrupted with nutrition, nutritional supplements, and drugs.[18] Endothelial dysfunction, arterial pathology, cardiac dysfunction, and CHD represent a delicate balance of vascular injury (angiotensin II and endothelin), vascular protection with nitric oxide, and vascular repair from endothelial progenitor cells, produced by the bone marrow.[2,4,6]

THE PATHOPHYSIOLOGY OF CARDIOVASCULAR DISEASE

The primary causes of CHD are the three finite responses that are generated from the large number of allostatic environmental insults coupled with cardiovascular genetics, nutrigenomics, metabolomics, proteomics, and gene expression patterns. The three finite vascular responses are vascular oxidative stress, vascular inflammation, and vascular immune dysfunction.

Apart from targeting the derangements in lipid metabolism, blood pressure, glucose, and obesity, therapeutic modulation to regulate chronic inflammation, oxidative stress, and the immune system response may prove to be a promising strategy in the management of atherosclerosis and CHD.

Oxidative Stress

Oxidative stress is an imbalance of radical oxygen species (ROS) and radical nitrogen species (RNS) with a decrease in antioxidant defenses that contribute to CHD.[2-4,19] In CHD, ROS and RNS are increased in the vasculature and

Table 23.2

RASMUSSEN CV SCORING SYSTEM

- Disease score 0-2: no CV events in 6 y
- Disease score 3-5: 5% CV events in 6 y
- Disease score over 6: 15% CV events in 6 y
- Superior to Framingham risk score
- Variables measured: CAPWA, blood pressure at rest and exercise, LV mass by ECHO, microalbuminuria, BNP, retinal score, carotid IMT, and ultrasound and EKG

Test	Normal	Borderline	Abnormal
Score for each test	0	1	2
Large artery elasticity		(age and genderdependent)	
Small artery elasticity		(age and genderdependent)	
Resting BP (mm Hg)	SBP <130 and DBP <85	SBP 130-139 or DBP 85-89	SBP ≥140 or DBP ≥90
Treadmill exercise BP (mm Hg)	SBP increase <30 and SBP ≤169	SBP increase 30-39 or SBP 170-179	SBP increase ≥40 or SBP ≥180
Optic fundus photography retinal vasculature	A/V ratio >3:5	A/V ratio ≤3:5 or mild A/V crossing changes	A/V ratio ≤1.2 or A/V nicking
Carotid IMT		(age and genderdependent)	
Microalbuminuria (mg/mmol)	≤0.6	0.61-0.99	≥1.00
Electrocardiogram	No abnormalities	Nonspecific abnormality	Diagnostic abnormality
LV ultrasound LVMI (g/m²)	<120	120-129	≥130
NT-proBNP (pg/dL)	<150	150-250	>250

BNP, brain natriuretic peptide; CAPWA, computerized arterial pulse wave analysis; CV, cardiovascular; DBP, diastolic blood pressure; ECHO, echocardiogram; EKG, electrocardiogram; IMT, intimal medial thickness; LV, left ventricular; SBP, systolic blood pressure.

kidneys.[2-4,19] The predominate ROS produced is superoxide anion, which is generated by numerous cellular sources, especially increases in angiotensin-II levels with an increased stimulation of the angiotensin I receptor (AT1 R).[2-4,19] The interaction of superoxide anion with nitric oxide (NO) will partially or completely eliminate NO. In addition, there may be uncoupling of endothelium-derived NO synthase (eNOS) and production of downstream ROS, such as peroxynitrite, hydroxyl ion, and hydrogen peroxide, which induce more vascular damage.[2-4,19] All of these events lead to a reduction in NO bioavailability, endothelial dysfunction, loss of vascular compliance, vascular and cardiac smooth muscle hypertrophy, hypertension, vascular oxidative stress, vascular inflammation, vascular immune dysfunction, CHD, and MI.[2,19]

Inflammation

Increased inflammation in the vasculature and kidney can be assessed by measuring inflammatory markers such as high-sensitivity C-reactive protein (hsCRP), leukocytosis with increased neutrophils and decreased lymphocytes, increased levels of cytokines and chemokines such as interleukins (IL-6 and IL-1B), interferon gamma, and tumor necrosis factor

(TNF) alpha.[2-4,20-23] In addition, there is an increased activity of the RAAS, especially angiotensin II and aldosterone, in the arteries and kidneys with stimulation of the PRR, NLR, and TLR.[2-4,20-23] Elevation of hsCRP is both a risk factor and risk marker for CHD.[20] Nitric oxide and eNOS are inhibited by hsCRP, which increases the risk of hypertension, CHD, and MI.[20] The hsCRP is produced in the liver from the precursor cytokines of IL-6, IL-1b, and TNF alpha from various systemic sources such as adipose tissue, macrophages, the heart, and the vasculature.

Vascular Immune Dysfunction

The immune system is involved in the pathogenesis of hypertension, atherosclerosis, and CHD in the general population.[2-4,22-31] The immune system contributes to the pathogenesis of hypertension, CVD, and CHD via action in the kidney, the vasculature, and the brain, such that immunomodulation may represent a novel approach to reduce these CV complications.[2-4,22-31] Emerging evidence points to a role of adaptive cellular immunity in the development of CHD, CVD, and hypertension, especially expansion of proinflammatory and antiapoptotic and cytotoxic CD4+ and CD28null T cells, which are closely associated with incident CVD in

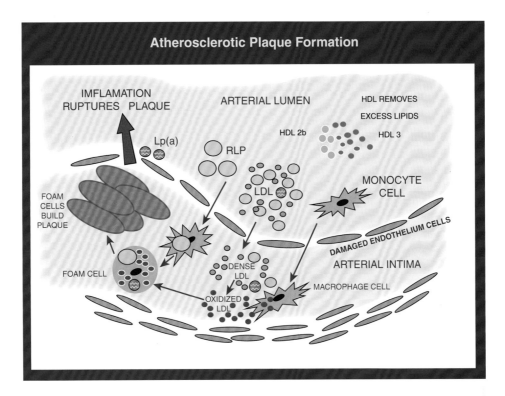

Figure 23.1 *The pathogenesis of atherosclerotic plaque formation. The movement of low-density lipoprotein cholesterol (LDL-C) into the subintimal layer is followed by modification of the LDL-C, uptake by macrophages and then inflammation, oxidative stress and vascular immune dysfunction that leads to fatty streaks, foam cells and complex plaque formation, and finally thrombosis with acute myocardial infarction. HDL, high-density lipoprotein; Lp(a), lipoprotein a; RLP, remnant lipoprotein.*

various study populations.[2-4,22-31] Autoimmune dysfunction of both the arteries and kidneys occurs with leukocytosis and involvement of CD4+ (T-helper cells) and CD 8+ (cytotoxic T-cells) to induce hypertension and CHD.[2-4,22-31] Innate and adaptive immune responses induce both hypertension and CHD by numerous mechanisms that include angiotensin II, cytokines, chemokines, interferon gamma, TGF-beta, interleukins, monocytes, macrophages, T cells, dendritic cells, ROS, PPR, TLR, and NLR activation and increase in sympathetic tone.[2-4,22-31] Monocytes cross the endothelial lining, invade the subintimal layer, and transform into macrophages and various T-cell subtypes that promote vascular damage and vascular immune dysfunction.[22-31] Activation of the AT1R expressed on CD4+T lymphocytes release TNF alpha, interferon, and interleukins within the vascular wall; increases blood pressure; and allows for progression of vascular immune dysfunction.[2-4,22-31] T-lymphocytes impair natriuresis by suppression of renal NOS 3 and COX-2, which increases intravascular volume and blood pressure.[23]

Figure 23.2 illustrates the interconnection of the external insults and the vascular receptors (PRR, NLR, TLR, caveolae) on the endothelium.[30,31] These insults are divided into two major categories; biomechanical (blood pressure, pulse pressure, shear stress, and oscillatory pressure) within the arterial system and external biochemical factors that include dietary factors, various biohumoral and metabolic factors, microbes, sterile and nonsterile antigens, and environmental toxins.[30,31]

INTERRUPTING THE FINITE PATHWAYS

Reducing the allostatic load; interrupting the insult-vascular receptor interaction to the PPR, NLR, TLR, and caveolae; and disruption of the downstream mediators are paramount to a successful prevention and treatment regimen for CHD. Numerous scientifically validated nutritional or dietary components and nutraceutical supplements have great promise in this regard.[31] These will be discussed in detail in the treatment section.

Preventing and treating CHD and establishing cardiovascular ecology and balance involve utilizing a more complex and logical approach such as dynamic systems biology, functional and metabolic medicine, CV genetics, nutrigenomics, and gene expression testing. As one might expect with a complex network of physiological interactions underlying vascular responsiveness and development of CHD, a single genetic cause has not been identified. Instead, as many as 30 separate loci are associated with MI and CHD. The majority of these involve inflammatory pathways, but only a minority of those 30 loci relate to the top five cardiovascular risk factors.[3]

Atherosclerosis and Endothelial Dysfunction

Atherosclerosis and endothelial dysfunction are postprandial diseases.[32] The consumption of sodium chloride (NaCl), refined carbohydrates (CHO), sugars, starches, and some but not all SFA and TFA will promote glucotoxicity,

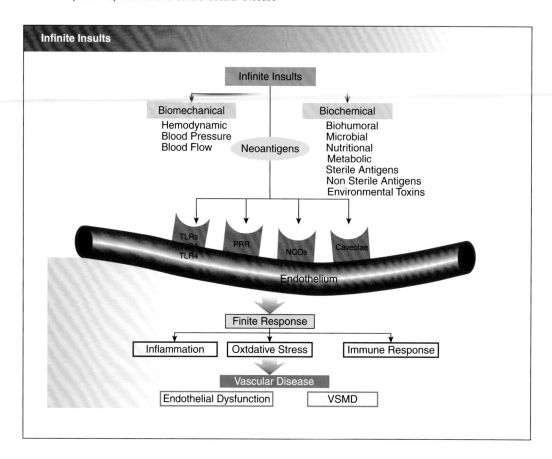

Figure 23.2 *Biochemical and biomechanical insults that interact with vascular receptors (pattern recognition receptors [PRR], nod-like receptors [NLR], toll-like receptors [TLR], caveolae) to induce the three finite responses of vascular inflammation, oxidative stress, and vascular immune dysfunction, which lead to endothelial dysfunction and vascular smooth muscle (VSM) and cardiac dysfunction.*

triglyceride toxicity, vascular metabolic endotoxemia, inflammation, oxidative stress, and vascular immune dysfunction that may persist long after the initial insult. This may also result in an exaggerated response (*metabolic memory*) with repeated or chronic dietary insults.[6,32] Fortunately, studies have shown that eating a diet rich in low-glycemic foods; low in refined CHO, sugars, and starches; low in NaCl; high in potassium and magnesium; and enriched with MUFA, PUFA, polyphenols, and antioxidants can help to prevent the postprandial endothelial dysfunction and endotoxemia.[18] Early evidence of CHD in the form of fatty streaks in the aorta and coronary arteries has been documented in children in the first and second decades of life and in postmortem examinations of teenagers and war victims (**Figure 23.3**).[2] The CVD is subclinical for decades before any cardiovascular events.[2,4,16] Endothelial dysfunction is the earliest functional abnormality, followed later by changes in arterial compliance of small resistance arteries and then larger conduit arteries with loss of elasticity leading to hypertension, VSM hypertrophy, diastolic dysfunction (DD), left ventricular hypertrophy (LVH), congestive heart failure (CHF) and CHD.[17]

Figure 23.4 shows the progression from subintimal coronary atherosclerosis to obstructive CHD. The coronary artery on the left is normal; the one in the center demonstrates mild

subintimal disease with increased intimal medial thickening (IMT) but a normal and unchanged arterial lumen. This extraluminal disease and inflammation would be captured using computed tomography angiogram (CTA) or intravascular ultrasound but missed by conventional coronary arteriogram (**Figure 23.5**). The image on the right in **Figure 23.4** illustrates extensive extraluminal and intraluminal obstructive CHD. Most MIs occur with mild stenosis of the coronary arteries.[2,4,16]

Some of the Top CHD Risk Factors and the CHD Gap Hypertension, Dyslipidemia, and Diabetes Mellitus

The "CHD gap" is related to incorrect definitions, assessment, and treatment of the top five CHD risk factors; the lack of assessment and treatment of the other 395 risk factors; not performing various noninvasive cardiovascular tests; genomic CV individuality; and possibly other unknown factors.[2]

Hypertension

A 24-hour ambulatory blood pressure monitor accurately measures blood pressure and CV risk and predicts CHD

Sequences in Progression of Artherosclerosis

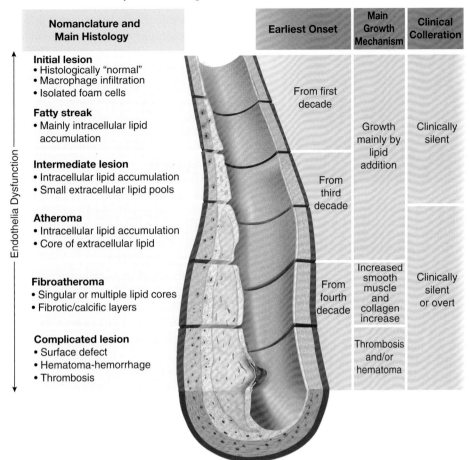

Figure 23.3 *Atherosclerosis progression. This illustrates the beginning of atherosclerosis from the initial lesion to the intermediate lesion to the final complicated lesion and plaque formation.*

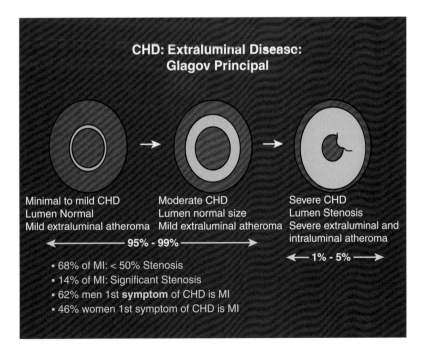

Figure 23.4 *Progression of subintimal coronary atherosclerosis to obstructive coronary heart disease. The initial extraluminal disease cannot be seen by coronary angiogram but only with computed tomography scans (CTA) or cardiac magnetic resonance imaging and angiography. CHD, coronary heart disease; MI, myocardial infarction.*

Angiographically Inapparent Atheroma

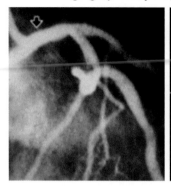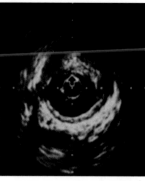

Figure 23.5 *Coronary heart disease that is not detectable by angiogram (left) because it is initially extraluminal but is evident using intravascular ultrasound (right). (Adapted from Topol E, Nissen S. Our preoccupation with coronary luminology.* Circulation. *1995;92(8):2333-2342.)*

and other CV target organ damage and is superior to office BP and home BP monitors.[2,16] Measurements of nocturnal BP and dipping status (normal is a 10% reduction from the mean daytime BP during the night), BP surges, BP load (normal is below 140/90 mm Hg in 15% of the total BP measurements), and BP variability are superior to office BP readings as a predictor of CHD risk.[2,16] Excessive dipping is associated with an increased risk of ischemic stroke, and reverse dipping is associated with an increased risk of intracerebral hemorrhage.[2,16] Nocturnal blood pressure is clinically more important than daytime blood pressure and drives CV target organ damage (a 27/15-mm Hg difference is optimal).[2,16] Morning blood pressure surges (both the level and rate of BP rise) increase the risk of ischemic stroke, MI, and LVH.[2,16] Hypertension is marker for vascular endothelial dysfunction with reduced nitric oxide bioavailability, but the vascular damage and disease is increased in a bidirectional manner.[17] This means that as NO decreases the vascular damage increases and as vascular damage increases there is more reduction in NO bioavailability. The items that should always be considered when evaluating blood pressure include[16]:

- A normal blood pressure is 120/80 mm Hg, but there is a continuum of risk for CHD starting at 110/70 mm Hg.
- Each increase of 20/10 mm Hg doubles CHD.
- Before age 50 years, the diastolic blood pressure is a better predictor of CHD risk.
- After age 50 years, the systolic blood pressure is a better predictor of CHD risk.
- A 24-hour ABM is more accurate than office blood pressure measurements and should be the standard of care for defining blood pressure, CHD risk, and treatment options, as well as time of administration of antihypertensive drugs.
- Mercury sphygmomanometers are preferred. Electronic arm units are accurate if done correctly and validated. The wrist or finger monitors are not as accurate and should not be used as the basis for a hypertension diagnosis or management.

Dyslipidemia

Dyslipidemia should be evaluated using advanced lipid profiles to determine treatment and predict individual CHD risk more accurately.[18,22,23] An advanced lipid profile will measure:

- Total cholesterol
- LDL-C
- LDL-P (LDL particle number), which drives CHD risk
- LDL size. The dense type B LDL is more atherogenic compared with the large type A LDL
- Modified LDL (oxidized, glycated, glyco-oxidized, and acetylated)
- Apolipoprotein (APO) B and apolipoprotein A
- Lipoprotein a: Lp(a)
- Total high-density lipoprotein (HDL-C)
- HDL particle number (HDL-P)
- HDL size and HDL mapping with the five types of HDL
- Dysfunctional HDL
- Reverse cholesterol transport and cholesterol efflux capacity
- Myeloperoxidase (MPO)
- Apolipoprotein C-III (APO-CIII)
- Very low-density lipoprotein (VLDL-C) and triglyceride (TG)
- Large VLDL
- VLDL-P particle number
- Remnant particles

The primary CHD risk related to LDL-C is LDL-P and apolipoprotein B.[13,18,33,34] Dense LDL is also predictive but only if LDL-P is elevated above the normal level.[13,18,33,34] Oxidized LDL is also associated with increased CHD. HDL-P is more protective for CHD and more predictive than total HDL for reducing CHD risk. The larger HDL type 2b is also an important protective mechanism.[13,18,33,34] Although the smaller pre-beta HDLs are more efficient at reverse cholesterol transport, the larger HDL may be more protective for CHD as it will decrease inflammation, oxidative stress, and immune dysfunction. It is also important to analyze dysfunctional HDL with MPO.[13,18,33,34] Patients who have a HDL of 85 mg/dL or more often have dysfunctional HDL that may not be protective.[33,34] The VLDL, especially large VLDL, triglycerides, and remnant particles are very atherogenic and thrombogenic.[18]

Dysglycemia, Insulin Resistance, and Diabetes Mellitus

An FBS of over 75 mg/dL increases CHD by 1% for each 1 mg/dL increase in FBS and induces endothelial dysfunction.[2,9-11] A 2-hour glucose tolerance test (GTT) over 110 mg/dL increases CHD by 2% for each 1 mg/dL over 110 mg/dL.[2,9-11] The current definition of an abnormal 2-hour GTT is >140 mg/dL. Hyperinsulinemia is also an independent risk factor for CHD.[2,9-11] Calculating a **Homeostatic Model Assessment of Insulin Resistance** (HOMA-IR) score will provide additional insight into the clinical presence of insulin resistance. Multiplying the FBS and fasting insulin level and dividing by 405 will give an excellent estimate of HOMA-IR.

A normal HOMA-IR is less than 1.0, mild insulin resistance is between 1.0 and 2.0, and over 2.0 is severe insulin resistance. Insulin resistance creates inflammation, reduces NO levels, and causes endothelial dysfunction and vascular disease through the mitogen-activated protein kinase pathway, which induces hypertension, inflammation, atherogenesis, and CHD.[2] On the other hand, the phosphatidylinositol 3-kinase pathway is anti-inflammatory, antihypertensive, and antiatherogenic, which reduces CHD.[2]

Noninvasive Testing

Fortunately, many noninvasive tests exist that will determine cardiovascular pathology before clinical CHD[2] (Table 23.3). One of the best validated early detection tests for functional abnormalities of the endothelium is the EndoPAT, which determines endothelial function and dysfunction.[35-37] The EndoPAT measures postocclusion brachial artery hyperemia, which is an excellent indirect measure of nitric oxide (NO) bioavailability and endothelial dysfunction in the coronary arteries. The EndoPAT predicts accurately the future risk for hypertension, CHD, unstable angina, CVD, CHF,

MI, cardiac death, hospitalization, coronary artery bypass graft, stent restenosis, the presence of plaque in the coronary arteries that are rupture prone, peripheral arterial disease (PAD), and cerebrovascular accidents (CVAs) beyond the Framingham risk scoring (FRS).[36-38] In a study 528 of patients with high risk for CV events over 5 years, the EndoPAT reactive hyperemia index (RHI) was measured before and after coronary angiogram.[39] The RHI, brain natriuretic peptide (BNP), and CV score by SYNTAX were independent risk predictors for all future CV events, such as MI, CV death, unstable angina, ischemic CVA, coronary artery bypass graft (CABG), CHF, and PAD. When RHI was added to FRS, BNP, and SYNTAX, the net reclassification index was significantly improved by 27.5% with a significant increase in the C-statistic from 0.728 to 0.766. A normal RHI is over 1.67.[39]

The computerized arterial pulse wave analysis (**CAPWA**) (**CV profiler**) also predicts future CHD by measuring large and small arterial compliance.[40-43] The C2 compliance identifies the presence of endothelial dysfunction and small resistance artery stiffness in the microvascular circulation, the very small arterioles, and medium sized arteries (range 4-9 µm). The C1 compliance is a measure of the elastic behavior of the aorta and larger arteries (range 8-17 µm). Lower numbers of C1 and C 2 compliance indicate diseased arteries, arterial stiffness, and decreased arterial compliance of the vascular wall and endothelial dysfunction. These are all age and gender adjusted. The CAPWA improves risk stratification beyond usual risk factors, including microalbuminuria, echocardiogram (ECHO), and carotid IMT. A low C2 and increased pulse wave velocity (PWV) predict CHD.

The **carotid IMT** predicts future risk of CHD and CVA.[44-46] Normal values without any plaque present must be adjusted for age and gender. A carotid IMT of less than 0.6 mm is normal to low risk, 0.6 to 0.7 mm is moderate risk, and 0.7 to 0.95 mm is high risk for future CVD. The normal IMT accretion rate (CIMTAR) is less than 0.016 mm/yr. Carotid IMT reflects not only early atherosclerosis but also nonatherosclerotic compensatory enlargement with largely medial hypertrophy as a result of smooth muscle cell hyperplasia and fibrocellular hypertrophy. Carotid IMT correlates well with CHD risk factors and future CV events such as CHD, MI (transient ischemic attack, and stroke. The risk for MI is 1.26 (95% confidence interval [CI], 1.21-1.30) per one standard deviation (SD) of common carotid artery IMT difference and 1.15 (95% CI, 1.12-1.17) per 0.10 mm of common carotid artery IMT difference over 5 years.[46] The risk for stroke is 1.32 (95% CI, 1.27-1.38) per one SD common of carotid artery IMT difference and 1.18 (95% CI, 1.16-1.21) per 0.10 mm common of carotid artery IMT difference over 5 years.[46]

Fundus examination of retinal arterioles with SLDF (scanning laser doppler flowmetry) correlates highly with micromyographic biopsies of the medial lumen ratio in subcutaneous small arteries. Retinal pathology indicates microvascular disease even after adjustment of renal dysfunction and traditional CVD risk factors. Retinal microvascular

Table 23.3

NONINVASIVE CARDIOVASCULAR TESTING

Functional Tests
EndoPAT (endothelial dysfunction [ED], augmentation index [AI], and heart rate variability [HRV])
CAPWA (computerized arterial pulse wave analysis)
HRV: Heart rate variability (HRV) and HRRT (heart rate recovery time)
EKG and treadmill test (TMT)
CPET (cardiopulmonary exercise test)
MCG (magnetocardiography)
Autonomic dysfunction testing
Structural tests
Carotid IMT/duplex (intimal medial thickness) and plaque
CT angiogram (CTA)
CAC (coronary artery calcium scoring)
Cardiac MRI (CMRI)
ECHO: rest and exercise
ABI (ankle brachial index): rest and exercise
Retinal scan and OPA (ocular pulse amplitude)
Other tests
Cardiac PET, SPECT
FDG-PET/CT: vascular inflammation/plaque/biologic activity
PET/CT/F-NaF for coronary plaque/inflammation/morphology
PET/MRI for coronary plaque morphology and inflammation
IVUS: intravascular ultrasound
Coronary angiogram

CT, computed tomography; FDG, F18 fluoro deoxy glucose; MRI, magnetic resonance imaging; PET, positron emission tomography; SPECT, single-photon emission computed tomography.

endothelial dysfunction assessed with flicker light of retinal veins and arteries is a nitric oxide–dependent phenomenon and predicts hypertension and CVD and CHD.[47-50]

Coronary artery calcification (CAC) is associated more strongly than carotid IMT with the risk of incident CHD in 6698 subjects over 5.3 years. The CAC predicted a CHD risk increase of 2.1-fold per one SD, whereas the carotid IMT predicted a CHD risk increase of 1.3-fold per one SD.[51] CAC progression over 15% annually predicts an increase in CHD risk with a 17-fold increase in CHD.[52-55] A baseline CAC score predicts CHD risk beyond traditional risk factors, and a CAC score of over 300 has a hazard ratio of CHD of 10. A positive CAC increases the risk of major cardiac events by 6- to 35-fold. CAC correlates not only with traditional risk factors but also with increased oxidative stress, autoantibodies to oxLDL, APO-B-immune complexes, glycemic load, and glycemic index.[52-55]

The risk of major CV events or death increases in a graded manner with the degree of coronary atherosclerosis as defined by **computerized tomographic angiogram (CTA)** even in the absence of high-grade coronary artery stenosis. Coronary CTA detects approximately twice as many coronary segments with plaque compared with coronary angiograms. This results in 52% of patients being assigned to a greater risk category.[56-58]

The **multifunction cardiogram (MCG)** is a computational electrophysiologic system to detect abnormal stress and strain between the myocardium (viscoelastic solid) and intracardiac blood flow (non-Newtonian fluid at low and intermediate shearing states) from a two-lead (II and V5) resting ECG. The MCG detects myocardial ischemia in an 82-second analysis.[59-62] This maps the heart's electrical activity to predict early CHD, ACS, MI, and arrhythmias. The sensitivity is 88% and specificity is 88% (range 80%-100%) for the early diagnosis of CHD depending on the degree of stenosis in some studies[62-81] but less specific and sensitive in other trials.[60]

Other noninvasive CV tests include the cardiac exercise ECHO, CEPT (cardiopulmonary exercise testing), exercise treadmill, various cardiac nuclear medicine scans, and magnetic resonance imaging and angiography for coronary plaque and obstruction. The fluorine-18-2-flouro-2-deoxy D-glucose positron emission tomography and computed tomography (FDG-PET/CT) is used to define cardiac arterial inflammation and biologic activity as FDG accumulates in activated immune cells such as macrophages and T cells due to increase glycolysis. It predicts CAC/CHD events. The PET and cardiac CT with sodium fluoride (PET/CT/F-Na-F) predicts coronary plaque and inflammation and the PET/MR predicts coronary artery plaque and inflammation.[63-65]

The **micronutrient testing** for functional deficiencies of nutrients (Spectracell, Houston, TX, USA) is valuable to assess nutritional status and provide a more scientific rationale for nutrition and nutritional supplement treatment of CHD and hypertension.[66] This is a lymphocyte assay that measures the status of 28 micronutrients for the previous 6 months. A recent study found that approximately 62% of hypertensive subjects could taper or discontinue pharmacologic therapy utilizing an aggressive micronutrient replacement program in conjunction with other lifestyle changes.[66]

Complete and Advanced Cardiovascular Laboratory Testing

A complete CV blood panel with advanced testing should be done to evaluate all of the top 25 modifiable risk factors and begin to address many of the complete list of 400 CHD risk factors. Cardiovascular genomics and CV gene expression testing that may predict CHD risk should also be included in this evaluation (Tables 23.4 and 23.5).[2,4,13,14,18]

Treatment

Interrupting the Finite Pathways at the PRR Level With Nutraceuticals

One of the many keys to the successful prevention and treatment of CVD is not only the recognition of all the new and emerging CHD risk factors but also the identification

Table 23.4

TWENTY-FIVE TOP MODIFIABLE CORONARY HEART DISEASE RISK FACTORS

- Hypertension (24 h ABM)
- Dyslipidemia (advanced lipid analysis)
- Hyperglycemia, metabolic syndrome, insulin resistance, and diabetes mellitus
- Obesity
- Smoking
- Hyperuricemia
- Renal disease
- Elevated fibrinogen
- Elevated serum iron
- Trans fatty acids and refined carbohydrates
- Low dietary omega-3 fatty acids
- Low dietary potassium and magnesium with high sodium intake
- Inflammation: increased hs-CRP, MPO, interleukins
- Increased oxidative stress and decreased defense
- Increased immune dysfunction
- Lack of sleep
- Lack of exercise
- Stress, anxiety, and depression
- Homocysteinemia
- Subclinical hypothyroidism
- Hormonal imbalances in both genders
- Chronic clinical or subclinical infections
- Micronutrient deficiencies: numerous ones such as low vitamin D, K, E, CoQ10
- Heavy metals

ABM, ambulatory blood pressure monitor; hs-CRP, high-sensitivity C-reactive protein; MPO, myeloperoxidase.

Table 23.5

COMPLETE LIST OF ADVANCED CARDIOVASCULAR LABORATORY TESTS

- Complete blood count (CBC) with differential
- Urinalysis
- Complete metabolic profile (CMP 12)
- Advanced lipid profile
- APO B, APO AI and AII
- Complete thyroid panel: Free T4, T3, TSH, RT3, thyroid antibodies
- Magnesium
- Iron, total iron binding capacity (TIBC) and ferritin
- Fibrinogen
- hs-CRP
- Homocysteine
- Uric acid
- Microalbuminuria
- Gammaglutamyl transpeptidase (GGTP) and hepatic profile
- Myeloperoxidase (MPO)
- Cardiovascular genomics
- Toxicology and heavy metal screen: Spot or 24-h urine or blood
- Vitamin D3
- Fasting C peptide, hemoglobin AIC, insulin, proinsulin, 2-h glucose tolerance test (GTT)
- Plasma renin activity (PRA) and aldosterone
- Free testosterone, sex hormone binding globulin (SHBG), estradiol, estriol, progesterone, dehydroepiandrosterone (DHEA and DHEAS)
- Electrocardiogram (EKG)
- CPET: cardiopulmonary exercise test
- Chest x-ray
- Computerized arterial pulse wave analysis (CAPWA)
- Endothelial Function Testing (EndoPAT)
- Ankle brachial index (ABI) at rest and with exercise
- Micronutrient testing (MNT)
- Omega-3 index
- APO E
- Telomere test
- Body impedance analysis
- ECHO
- Carotid duplex and carotid intimal medial thickness (IMT)
- Computerized CT angiogram (CTA)
- Coronary artery calcium (CAC)
- Retinal scan
- Rest and exercise blood pressure
- 24-h ambulatory blood pressure monitor (ABM)
- CORUS gene expression testing
- PULS cardiac testing

of treatments that will interrupt the pathways that connect the risk factors to the PRR. There are many scientifically proven nutraceuticals and dietary nutrients that block the PRRs[32]:

- Curcumin (turmeric): blocks TLR 4, NOD 1, and NOD 2
- Cinnamaldehyde (cinnamon): blocks TLR 4
- Sulforaphane (broccoli): blocks TLR 4

- Resveratrol (nutritional supplement, red wine, grapes): blocks TLR 1
- Epigallocatechin gallate (green tea): blocks TLR 1
- Luteolin (celery, green pepper, rosemary, carrots, oregano, oranges, olives): blocks TLR 1
- Quercetin (tea, apples, onion, tomatoes, capers): blocks TLR 1
- Chrysin: blocks TLR 1

Nutritional Interventions

MEDITERRANEAN DIET: TRADITIONAL MEDITERRANEAN DIET

In the 4.8-year primary prevention (**PREDIMED**), the rate of major cardiovascular events from MI, CVA, or total CV deaths was reduced by 30% with nuts and 30% with extra-virgin olive oil (EVOO). The reduction in CVA was 39% ($P <$ .003) with a 33% reduction from EVOO and a 46% reduction from nuts. The reduction in MI was 23% ($P = $ .25) with a 20% reduction from EVOO and a 26% reduction from nuts. Total CV deaths were reduced by 17% ($P = $ .8).[68-87] New-onset type 2 diabetes mellitus was decreased by 40% with EVOO and 18% with mixed nuts.[67,68] This reduction was associated with decreases in hsCRP and IL-6. The high content of nitrate (NO_3), at an average of 400 mg/d, is converted to nitrite (NO_2), which eventually forms nitric oxide.[69] Also the increased amount of omega-3 FA, good omega-6 FA, and polyphenols (such as quercetin, resveratrol, and catechins in grapes and wine) provides many of the beneficial outcomes in CHD.[69]

Secondary prevention post MI in the **Lyon Heart Study**[70] demonstrated significant reductions in all events including cardiac death, nonfatal MI, unstable angina, CVA, CHF, and hospitalization at 4 years using the Mediterranean-style diet supplemented with alpha-linolenic acid compared with a prudent Western diet. Compared with the control diet, the Mediterranean-style diet demonstrated a 76% lower risk of cardiac death and nonfatal MI during the study period.

Olive oil was associated with a decreased risk of overall mortality and an important reduction in CVD mortality in a large Mediterranean cohort of 40,622 subjects.[71] For each increase in olive oil by 10 g there was a 13% decrease in CV mortality. In the highest quartile of olive oil intake, there was a 44% decrease in CV mortality. One of the mechanisms by which the traditional Mediterranean diet, particularly if supplemented with EVOO at 50 g/d, can exert CV health benefits is through changes in the transcriptomic response of genes related to cardiovascular risk that include genes for atherosclerosis, inflammation, oxidative stress, vascular immune dysfunction, type 2 diabetes mellitus, and hypertension.[72-75] This includes genes for adrenergic beta 2 receptor (ADR-B2), interleukin 7 receptor, gamma interferon, monocyte chemotactic protein, TNF alpha, IL-6, and hsCRP.[62-65] In summary, the TMD has been shown to have the following effects:

- Lowers blood pressure.
- Improves serum lipids: lowers TC, LDL-C, and TG; increases HDL-C; lowers oxLDL and Lp(a); improves LDL-C size; and lowers LDL-P to a less atherogenic profile.

- Improves type 2 diabetes mellitus and dysglycemia.
- Improves oxidative defense and reduces oxidative stress: F-2 isoprostanes and 8 hydroxy D-guanosine.
- Reduces inflammation: lowers hsCRP, IL-6, soluble cell adhesion molecules and vascular cell adhesion molecules.
- Reduces thrombosis and factor VII after meals.
- Improves BNP.
- Increases nitrates and nitrites.
- Improves membrane fluidity.
- Reduces MI, CHD, and CVA.
- Reduces homocysteine.

DASH DIETS (DASH 1 AND 2)

The DASH diets reduce BP and CHD. Both DASH 1 and DASH 2 emphasize fruits, vegetables, whole grains, beans, fiber, low-fat dairy products, poultry, fish, seeds, and nuts but limit red meat, sweets, and sugar-containing beverages while increasing the intake of potassium, magnesium, and calcium but with variable restriction in dietary sodium.[76-78] Both DASH diets reduce blood pressure within 4 weeks by about 10/5 mm Hg or more, which is at least as effective as one antihypertensive medication. In the Nurses' Health Study (NHS), adherence to the DASH dietary pattern was associated with a lower risk of CHD by 14% in those with the highest adherence to the diet.[78]

PORTFOLIO DIET

The first Portfolio Diet was given to 34 patients with dyslipidemia treated with three diets for 1 month each in random order.[79]
- Control diet: very low saturated fat
- Diet 2: control diet plus lovastatin 20 mg
- Diet 3 (Portfolio): plant sterols, soy foods, almonds, viscous fibers, okra, eggplant
  The results showed the following:
- Control diet: reduced LDL-C by 8.5%
- Diet 2: reduced LDL-C by 33.3% and TG by 11%
- Portfolio Diet: reduced LDL-C by 29.6% and TG by 9.3%

The second Portfolio Diet[80] performed over a 6-month period with 351 subjects included a low saturated fat diet as the control arm, which reduced LDL-C by 3%. The dietary portfolio with variable counseling showed an LDL-C reduction of 13.1%. The dietary portfolio with two clinic visits resulted in an LDL-C decrease of 13.1%.

The dietary portfolio with seven clinic visits had an LDL-C reduction of 13.8%.

Dietary Summary

A combination of the Mediterranean and/or DASH diet, in our opinion, is the most supportive dietary consideration. We prefer a higher-fat, generous-protein, and moderate-carbohydrate diet, such as approximately 30% protein, 30% MUFA and omega-3 FA, limited SFA and no TFA, minimal refined carbohydrates (CHO) (less than 50 g), and more complex CHO (40%). In addition, consume 0.1 mmol/kg of body weight/d of dietary nitrates and nitrites. Ingest at least 10 multicolored servings of fruits and vegetables fruits (four servings) (berries) and vegetables (six servings) with dark green leafy vegetables. Do caloric restriction at 12.5% and

a 12.5 % energy expenditure with a 12-hour overnight fast. Also consume smaller meals more frequently with antioxidants at each meal. Minimal caffeine depending on CYP 1A2 status. The DASH 2 and Mediterranean diets achieve many of these recommendations.

Nutritional Supplements

The following list of nutritional supplements and specific food groups should be considered for the prevention and treatment of CHD.[2,4,16,18]

1. Basic multi/multimineral formula with 5-methyl folate 400 µg/d with B complex vitamins with broad-spectrum vitamin E.
2. Vitamin C sustained release: 250 to 500 mg twice a day (bid).
3. Vitamin K 2 MK 7: 200 to 300 µg/d.
4. Polyphenols: 20 g dark chocolate (>70%) and EGCG 500 mg bid or green tea 32 oz/d (decaffeinated).
5. Quercetin: 500 to 1000 mg/d.
6. Curcumin: 500 to 1000 mg bid.
7. Magnesium—Krebs cycle components—400 to 600 once a day.
8. 500 mg beetroot juice: 45 mmol/L or 2.79 g/L inorganic nitrate per day (see in number 1).
9. Pomegranate seeds: 1/4 cup once or twice per day or pomegranate juice 6 oz/d.
10. R-lipoic acid (RLA) 100 mg/d with biotin 5000 µg/d for GSH (glutathione) and mitochondrial function and acetyl L-carnitine 1000 mg/d for mitochondrial function.
11. NAC (N-acetyl cysteine) 500 mg bid for GSH (glutathione).
12. Whey protein 30 to 40 g/d for GSH (glutathione).
13. Branched-chain amino acids (leucine, valine, isoleucine at 4:1:1 ratio) 5000 mg/d.
14. Trans-resveratrol: up to 250 mg/d.
15. Balanced omega-3 FA (DHA, EPA) 1 to 4 g/d
16. Vitamin D3 to a serum level of 60 to 80 ng/mL.
17. Aged garlic (Kyolic) CV formulation: 600 mg bid.
18. Coenzyme Q 10: Ubiquinone 100 mg or more per day.
19. Lycopene: 10 to 20 mg/d (supplement, tomato, pink grapefruit, watermelon etc).
20. Carnosine: 500 mg bid.
21. Grape seed extract: 200 to 250 mg/d.
22. EGCG: 200 to 250 mg daily.
23. Berberine HCL: 500 mg/d.
24. Probiotics: 50 billion colony-forming units (CFU) per day.

Pharmacologic Treatments

The most important drugs for the prevention and treatment of CHD are shown below.[13,14,16]

1. Angiotensin converting enzyme (ACE) inhibitors (such as perindopril 16 mg/d).
2. Angiotensin receptor blockers (ARB) (such as telmisartan 80 mg/d). The recent data on possible carcinoma appear to have been resolved at this time, but we will await more research.

3. Amlodipine 5 mg/d.
4. Rosuvastatin 5 mg/d or intermittent therapy 2 to 3 times per week.
5. Metformin 500 mg/d.
6. Baby aspirin (ASA) 81 mg in high-risk patients. However, one must weigh the risk of bleeding and efficacy based on age and known CVD risk, such as previous MI, CABG, PCTA, ischemic CVA, and carotid artery obstruction.

Other Interventions[2,4]

1. Exercise 60 min/d for 6 d/wk. Include balanced aerobic and resistance training using the Aerobic, Build, Contour and Tone (ABCT) exercise program.[2]
2. Eight hours of uninterrupted sleep each night.
3. Stress reduction and meditation programs.
4. Ideal body weight and body composition monitored with body impedance analysis: total body fat at or below 16% for men and 22% for women.

Conclusions

There are an infinite number of insults that attack the blood vessel, but there are only three finite responses: vascular inflammation, vascular oxidative stress, and vascular immune dysfunction that lead to CHD. The top five cardiovascular risk factors, as they are currently defined, do not provide an adequate explanation for CHD. To reduce the CHD gap, the top five risk factors require improved definitions, the top 25 modifiable risk factors must be measured and treated, and the other 395 risk factors and mediators must also be incorporated into clinical decision making. Early detection, aggressive prevention, and treatment of CVD are needed to decrease the burden of CVD. This requires immediate, early, and aggressive evaluation of functional CV disease (endothelial dysfunction, arterial compliance) and CVD risk factors and biomarkers before any cardiovascular structural changes occur or clinical CV disease becomes manifest. Improved utilization of new laboratory techniques are required, such as the advanced lipid profiles; 24-hour BP monitoring; and specific tests to identify vascular inflammation with hsCRP, interleukins, TNF alpha, oxidative stress with oxLDL, MPO, and isoprostanes and immune vascular dysfunction with thyroid antibodies and other T cell and B cell immune markers. In addition, vascular translational medicine must be evaluated with new imaging technologies, such as EndoPAT, CAPWA, carotid IMT, MCG, CAC, and CT angiogram.

To truly revolutionize the treatment of CHD, new therapies must address the underlying pathophysiology, CHD risk factors, mediators and their downstream effects, as well as the three finite vascular responses. This will be achievable by using a combination of targeted personalized and precision treatments with genomics, proteomics, metabolomics, nutrition, nutraceutical supplements, vitamins, minerals, antioxidants, anti-inflammatory agents, anti-immunological agents, and drugs. Future studies must measure all of the pertinent CHD risk factors that have been reviewed in this article. Only by addressing all of these factors will CHD be reduced.

Congestive Heart Failure and Metabolic Cardiology

CHF, a common pathological situation for the internist and cardiologist, remains the leading cause of hospitalization in the United States. Since its prevalence continues to increase as the population ages, the amount of human suffering associated with heart failure is enormous and the financial burden placed on society is remarkable. Although there has been some considerable progress in the treatment of heart failure over the past 20 years with diuretics, ACE therapies,[81,82] ARB therapy,[83] beta-receptor blockade,[84,85] and resynchronization therapy,[86-88] heart failure is still associated with an annual mortality of 10%, and 30% to 40%[89,90] of patients die within 1 year of diagnosis. The search for novel and effective treatments such as mitochondrial support and stem cell therapy are becoming some of the most interesting areas of modern investigative cardiology. Adipose-derived stem cell therapy has recently offered new therapeutic strategies and perhaps may be the most attractive missing link in the future treatment of CHF.[91]

The preservation of mitochondrial function and the optimization of energy substrates in the heart have been gaining such momentum as a contemporary therapy.[92,93] Because the failing myocardium is "viable but dysfunctional,"[92] and not irreversibly damaged, treatment options that target the cardiomyocyte itself should be instituted as vulnerable and dysfunctional heart cells can still be rescued.[94] And if we consider the evidence for cardiomyocyte renewal in humans,[95] it makes even more sense to treat the myocardium at cellular and metabolic levels to help bolster progress in supporting the body's intrinsic stem cell wisdom in the direction of regenerative therapy.[95-97]

Although the genesis of heart failure includes multiple factors and many mechanisms, the essence of heart failure as an energy-starved heart running out of fuel identifies the myocardial energetics of the failing heart.[97-99] There is a definite energy disequilibrium between the available energy the heart has and the required energy it has available to fulfill its needs.

Thus, supporting energy substrates in heart cells will be a new cardiological approach that focuses on the biochemistry of cellular energy as "metabolic cardiology."[99] Many physicians are not trained to look at heart disease in terms of cellular biochemistry; therefore, the challenge in any metabolic cardiology discussion is in taking the conversation from the "bench to bedside."[99,100]

Bioenergetics is the study of energy transformation in living organisms used in biochemistry to reference cellular energy. The concentration of adenosine triphosphate (ATP) in the cell and the efficiency of ATP turnover and recycling is central to our appreciation of cellular bioenergetics as a new form of nonpharmaceutical therapy. Once an understanding of how ATP repairs and restores heart cells is realized, targeted biochemical interventions to support ATP production and turnover will be strongly considered by the medical establishment.

We shall learn that the bottom line in the treatment of any form of CVD and especially in CHF is the restoration of the heart's supply of ATP. Cardiac conditions such as angina, CHF, silent ischemia, and DD all cause an ATP deficit. These conditions are both the cause and the result of chronic energy demand in the compromised heart. Over the years, it has been clear to many of our colleagues that the concept of metabolic cardiology is the missing link that has been eluding health professionals for years. It is also the solution in improving quality of life for anyone struggling with symptoms of CHF.

Energy preservation is a key to optimum health and is integral to both a preventive and recovery strategy. Cellular energy levels can actually be measured. Healthy cells pulsate at higher frequencies and have more ATP than diseased cells. Using a cutting-edge imaging technique, MIT researchers actually demonstrated this by studying red blood cells.[101] When researchers compared the vibration of healthy cells with the vibration of unhealthy cells (which were depleted of ATP), they found that the frequencies of the unhealthy cells were 20% lower than that of the healthy cells. The researchers also noted that, when ATP was reintroduced into the unhealthy cells, the vibrations increased back to normal.[101,102]

Dr Sinatra was excited to read about these experiments at MIT, but, admittedly, not surprised. He has treated hundreds of patients using a metabolic approach that is specifically designed to replenish ATP supplies in the body, especially in the heart. Countless times, he witnessed the profound healing that can happen when you give the body the key nutrients it needs to make ATP molecules. Many of his patients who were on heart transplant lists no longer needed donor hearts after a few months or even weeks of treatment, and several were successfully weaned from life support. Hundreds of others improved their cardiovascular health and quality of life, and many even extended their lifespans, all by supporting natural energy production in their own compromised cardiomyocytes.

In cardiology, solving the heart's energy crisis is essential to optimizing cardiovascular function. For decades, heart disease prevention has inadvertently been focused on risk factor modification in an effort to prevent or slow down the onset of cardiac decompensation. Rather, it behooves us to concentrate on the mitochondria and employ nutritional strategies targeting improved ATP synthesis and, therefore, heart function. It is now widely accepted that one characteristic of the failing heart is the persistent and progressive loss of energy. The requirement for energy to support the systolic and diastolic work of the heart is absolute. Therefore, a disruption in cardiac energy metabolism, and the energy supply/demand mismatch that results, can be identified as the pivotal factor contributing to the inability of failing hearts to meet the hemodynamic requirements of the body.[103] In her landmark book, *ATP and the Heart*, Joanne Ingwall, PhD,[104] describes the metabolic process associated with the progression of CHF

and identifies the mechanisms that lead to a persistent loss of cardiac energy reserves as the disease process unfolds.

The heart consumes a tremendous amount of energy approximately 700 mg of ATP (about 10 heartbeats) or more energy per gram than any other organ, and the chemical energy that fuels the heart comes primarily from adenosine triphosphate, or ATP (Figure 23.6). The chemical energy held in ATP is resident in the phosphoryl bonds, with the greatest amount of energy residing in the outermost bond holding the ultimate phosphoryl group to the penultimate group. When energy is required to provide the chemical driving force to fuel a myocyte cell, this ultimate phosphoryl bond is broken and chemical energy is released. The cell then converts this chemical energy to mechanical energy to sustain stretching and contracting, drive ion pump function, synthesize large and small molecules, and perform other necessary activities of the cell.

The consumption of ATP in the enzymatic reactions that release cellular energy yields the metabolic by-products adenosine diphosphate (ADP) and inorganic phosphate (Pi) (Figure 23.7). A variety of metabolic mechanisms has evolved within the cell to provide rapid rephosphorylation of ADP to restore ATP levels and maintain the cellular energy pool. But these metabolic mechanisms are disrupted in CHF, tipping the balance in a manner that creates a chronic energy supply/demand mismatch that results in an energy deficit.

The normal nonischemic heart is capable of maintaining a stable ATP concentration despite large fluctuations in work load and energy demand. In a normal heart, the rate of cellular ATP synthesis via rephosphorylation of ADP closely matches ATP utilization. The primary site of cellular ATP rephosphorylation is the mitochondria, where fatty acid and carbohydrate metabolic products flush down the oxidative phosphorylation pathways. The heart is richly endowed with

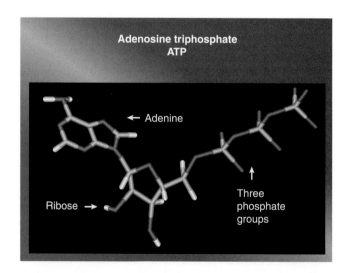

Figure 23.6 *Adenosine triphosphate (ATP) is composed of an adenine ring, d-ribose, and three phosphate groups. The severance of the last chemical bond attached the last phosphate group to ATP releases the chemical energy that is converted to mechanical energy to perform work of the cell.*

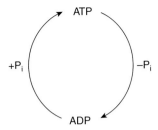

Figure 23.7 *When ATP is used, the remaining by-products are adenosine diphosphate (ADP) and inorganic phosphate (P). ADP and P$_i$ can then recombine to form ATP in the cellular processes of energy recycling. When oxygen and food (fuel) are available, energy recycling occurs and the lack of oxygen or mitochondrial dysfunction severely limits the cell's ability to recycle its energy supply.*

mitochondria where approximately 30% of cardiomyocyte volume is occupied by these powerhouses of energy. The content of ATP in heart cell mitochondria progressively falls in CHF, frequently reaching and then stabilizing at levels that are 25% to 30% lower than normal.[105,106] The fact that ATP diminishes in the failing heart means that the metabolic network responsible for maintaining the balance between energy supply and demand is no longer functioning normally in these hearts.

The mechanism explaining energy depletion in heart failure is the loss of energy substrates and the delay in their resynthesis. In conditions in which energy demand outstrips supply, ATP is consumed at a rate that is faster than it can be restored via oxidative phosphorylation or the alternative pathways of ADP rephosphorylation. The cardiac muscle cell has a continuing need for energy, so it will use all its ATP stores and then break down the by-product, adenosine diphosphate (ADP), to pull the remaining energy out of this compound as well. What is left is adenosine monophosphate (AMP).

An increase in the concentration of AMP is incompatible with sustained cellular function. It is quickly broken apart, and the by-products are washed out of the cell. When the by-products of AMP catabolism are driven out of the cell, they are lost forever (**Figure 23.8**). It takes a considerable amount of time to replace these lost energy substrates even when the cell is fully perfused with oxygen again.

Energy Starvation in the Failing Heart

The long-term mechanism explaining the loss of ATP in CHF is the decreased capacity for ATP synthesis relative to ATP demand. In part, the disparity between energy supply and demand in hypertrophied and failing hearts is associated with a shift in the relative contribution of fatty acid versus glucose oxidation to ATP synthesis. The major consequence of the complex readjustment toward carbohydrate metabolism is that the total capacity for ATP synthesis decreases. At the same time, the demand for ATP continually increases as hearts work harder to circulate blood in the face of the increased filling pressures that are associated with CHF and hypertrophy.

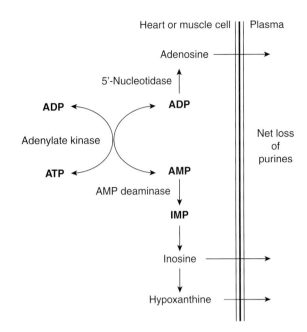

Figure 23.8 *When the cellular concentration of ATP falls and ADP levels increase, two molecules of ADP can combine. This reaction provides one ATP, giving the cell additional energy, and one AMP. The enzyme adenylate kinase (also called myokinase) catalyzes this reaction. The AMP formed in this reaction is then degraded, and the by-products are washed out of the cell resulting in the loss of these vital purines, which decreases the cellular energy pool even further.*

The net result of this energy supply/demand mismatch is a decrease in the absolute concentration of ATP in the failing heart, and this decrease in absolute ATP level is reflected in a lower energy reserve in the failing and hypertrophied heart. A declining energy reserve is directly related to heart function, with diastolic function being the first to be affected, followed by systolic function, and finally global performance (**Figure 23.9**). In ischemic or hypoxic hearts, the cell's ability to match ATP supply and demand is disrupted leading to both depletion of the cardiac energy pool and dysfunction in mitochondrial ATP turnover mechanisms. When ATP levels drop, diastolic heart function deteriorates.

DD is an early sign of myocardial failure despite the presence of normal systolic function and preserved ejection fraction. Higher concentrations of ATP are required to activate calcium pumps necessary to facilitate cardiac relaxation and promote diastolic filling. This observation leads to the conclusion that, in absolute terms, more ATP is needed to fill the heart with blood than to empty it, consistent with Starling's law that requires more energy in diastole than in systole. The absolute requirement for ATP in the context of cardiac conditions in which energy is depleted makes a metabolic therapeutic approach such a reasonable intervention. Since DD occurs in clinical situations of high blood pressure, mitral valve prolapse, and infiltrative cardiomyopathy, several segments of the population, and particularly woman, are afflicted by it.

In our experience, pharmaceutical drugs do not remedy the heart in diastole, so it makes sense to use a nutraceutical support in any patient you may suspect to have DD. The

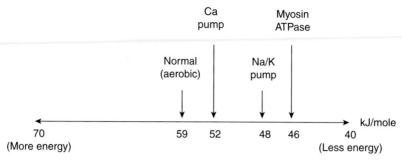

Figure 23.9 *Cellular energy levels can be measured as the free energy of hydrolysis of ATP, or the amount of chemical energy available to fuel cellular function. Healthy, normal hearts contain enough energy to fuel all the cellular functions with a contractile reserve for use in emergency. Cellular mechanisms used in calcium management and cardiac relaxation require the highest level of available energy. Sodium/potassium pumps needed to maintain ion balance are also significant energy consumers. The cellular mechanisms associated with contraction require the least amount of cellular energy; thus, more energy is required to fill the heart than to empty the heart.*

earlier signs of DD include fatigue and shortness of breath, and it takes a knowledgeable physician to suspect it in any patient with high blood pressure or in any patient with shortness of breath as a predominant symptom. Easily observable, echocardiographic abnormalities are diagnostic of DD. The treatment of DD involves a metabolic cardiology approach that help cardiomyocytes meet their absolute need for ATP to preserve diastolic and pulsatile cardiac function while maintaining mitochondrial, cellular, and tissue viability. After treating hundreds of patients in our clinics, the mystery and therapeutic challenge of DD has been unraveled in metabolic cardiology. We shall now investigate the individual components of such a metabolic cardiology program as an alternative strategy in the management of diastolic and congestive heart failure.

Energy Nutrients for Congestive Heart Failure

D-RIBOSE (RIBOSE)

The effect of the pentose monosaccharide, D-ribose, in cardiac energy metabolism has been evaluated since the 1970s, with clinical studies describing its value as an adjunctive therapy in ischemic heart disease first appearing in 1991. Ribose is a naturally occurring simple carbohydrate that is found in every living tissue, and natural synthesis is via the oxidative pentose phosphate pathway of glucose metabolism. Ribose, like coenzyme Q10 (CoQ10) and carnitine, is synthesized in the body.

As a pentose, ribose is not used by cells as a primary energy fuel. Unlike glucose, ribose is preserved for the important metabolic task of stimulating purine nucleotide synthesis and salvage for the production of ATP. Approximately 98% of consumed ribose is quickly absorbed into the bloodstream and is circulated to remote tissue with no first pass effect by the liver. As ribose passes through the cell membrane it is phosphorylated by membrane-bound ribokinase before entering the pentose phosphate pathway downstream of the gatekeeper enzymes. In this way, the administered ribose is able to increase intracellular 5-phosphorribosy1-1-pyrophosphate (PRPP) concentration and initiate purine nucleotide synthesis and salvage.

The study of ribose in CHF was first reported in the *European Journal of Heart Failure* in 2003.[107] Until that time, the clinical benefit for ribose in CVD was largely confined to its increasing role in treating coronary artery disease and other ischemic heart diseases, where its benefit has been well established. The reported double-blind, placebo-controlled, crossover study included patients with chronic coronary artery disease and New York Heart Association (NYHA) class II/III CHF. Patients underwent two treatment periods of 3 weeks each, during which either oral ribose (5 g three times a day [t.i.d.]) or placebo (glucose; 5 g t.i.d.) was administered. Following a 1-week washout period, the alternate test supplement was administered for a subsequent 3-week test period. Before and after each 3-week trial period, assessment of myocardial function was made by echocardiography and the patient's exercise capacity was determined using a stationary exercise cycle. Participants also completed a quality-of-life questionnaire. Ribose administration significantly enhanced all indices of diastolic heart function and exercise tolerance and was also associated with an improved quality of life score. By comparison, none of these parameters were changed with glucose (placebo) treatment.[107]

Indeed, in our experience, the magic of D-ribose is its efficacy in DD. In a recent review article, the clinical benefits of D-ribose in ischemic CVD was revealed. Because myocardial ischemia lowers ATP levels and is reflected in increasing DD, D-ribose as a pentose support has been shown in pilot clinical studies to enhance the recovery of ATP levels while improving DD at the same time.[108]

In another small cohort study using D-ribose, an improvement in tissue Doppler velocity (E') demonstrated a beneficial trend in 64% of the patients, suggesting that D-ribose supports patients with DD.[109]

Many patients experience typical and atypical chest symptoms as well as generalized weakness following stent and angioplasty procedures. When temporary ischemia occurs in the myocardium following balloon inflation, ATP levels drop. It may take the body several days to make up the deficit with de novo ATP synthesis. In our experience, ribose has been a significant factor in supporting energy substrate levels that enhance ATP production thus alleviating symptoms in these patients. Temporary or prolonged ischemia results in lower myocardial energy levels. Increasing the cardiac energy level not only improves symptoms and function but also may delay vulnerable changes in a variety of CHF conditions. This therapeutic advantage ribose provides in improving cardiac index and left ventricular function suggests its value as an adjunct to traditional therapy for ischemia and CHF.

Because D-ribose administration creates favorable physiological parameters on cardiac function and has been shown to enhance the recovery of high-energy phosphates following myocardial ischemia, it was hypothesized that D-ribose could improve cardiological indices for off-pump coronary artery bypass procedures.[110] In a retrospective analysis of 366 patients undergoing off-pump coronary artery bypass surgery (CABS), 308 received D-ribose as a perioperative metabolic protocol. Patients given D-ribose had a greater improvement in cardiac index post revascularization compared with non-D-ribose patients (37% versus 17% $P < .0001$).[48] The research has suggested that a larger randomized placebo-controlled prospective trial be considered to further test the hypothesis that ribose can be considered standard management in myocardial ischemia.[110]

Researchers and practitioners using ribose in cardiology and internal medicine practices recommend a dose range of 10 to 15 g/d as metabolic support for CHF or other cardiac ailments. In our experience, patients are placed on a regimen of 5 g/dose three times a day for any form of CHF and/or myocardial ischemia. Individual doses of greater than 10 g are not recommended because high single doses of a hygroscopic carbohydrate may cause mild gastrointestinal discomfort or transient lightheadedness. Because ribose has a lower glycemic index, it should be administered with meals or mixed in beverages containing a secondary carbohydrate source when administered to diabetic patients prone to hypoglycemia.

In conclusion, D-ribose has been instrumental in alleviating symptoms of shortness of breath and easy fatigability in our patients experiencing CHF and hypertensive CVD with and without left ventricular hypertrophy. D-Ribose along with CoQ10, L-carnitine, and magnesium (awesome foursome) has reduced considerable suffering in our patients. Because the clinical efficacy of these nutraceuticals has been appreciated by many health care practitioners, the University of Kansas Medical Center is participating in a 250 randomized patient study that will evaluate the clinical benefits of D-ribose and CoQ10 (to be completed March 2020). We shall now discuss CoQ10 as the second arm of metabolic cardiology.

COENZYME Q10 AND THE HEART

CoQ10 or ubiquinone, so named for its ubiquitous nature in cells, is a fat-soluble compound that functions as an antioxidant and coenzyme in the energy-producing pathways. As an antioxidant, the reduced form of CoQ10 inhibits lipid peroxidation in both cell membranes and serum LDL and also protects proteins and DNA from oxidative damage. CoQ10 also has membrane-stabilizing activity. However, its bioenergetic activity and electron transport function for its role in ATP oxidative phosphorylation is probably its most important function.

The electron transport chain is a series of oxidation-reduction (REDOX) chemical reactions that allow the mitochondria to transform the food you eat into energy (ATP). The electrons need CoQ10 to make their way down the electron transport chain or ATP production slows, causing a decrease in energy production, an increase in free radicals, and potentially disease or even death.

Although CoQ10 is found in high concentrations in the liver, kidney, and lung, the heart requires the highest levels of ATP activity because it is continually aerobic and contains more mitochondria per gram than any other tissue in the body. Because mitochondrial dysfunction, diminished REDOX capacity, and lower CoQ10 levels have been a feature of heart failure, it makes sense to offer CoQ10 to enhance contractile dynamics in the failing heart.[111] Tissue deficiencies and low serum blood levels of CoQ10 have also been reported across a wide range of CVDs, including DD, hypertension, aortic valvular disease, and coronary artery disease, and research suggests that CoQ10 support may be indicated in these disease conditions.[112]

In patients with CHF or dilated cardiomyopathy, we generally use higher doses of CoQ10 in ranges of at least 300 mg or more to get a biosensitive result requiring a blood level at least greater than 2.5 µg/mL and preferably 3.5 µg/mL.[113] In a previous analysis in three patients with refractory CHF, higher doses of CoQ10 were required to get such a biosensitive or therapeutic result.[114]

In an investigation at the Lancisi Heart Institute in Italy, researchers studied 23 patients with a mean age of 59 years, using a double-blind, placebo-controlled, crossover design. Patients were assigned to receive 100 mg of oral CoQ10 three times a day plus supervised exercise training. The study concluded that CoQ10 supplementation improved functional capacity, endothelial function, and left ventricular contractility in CHF without any side effects.[115]

In a previous long-term study of 424 patients with systolic and/or DD in the presence of CHF, dilated cardiomyopathy, or hypertensive heart disease, a dose of 240 mg/d maintained blood levels of CoQ10 above 2.0 µg/mL and allowed 43% of the participants to discontinue one to three conventional drugs over the course of the study.[116] Patients were followed for an average of 17.8 months, and during that time, a mild case of nausea was the only reported side effect. This long-term study clearly shows CoQ10 to be a safe and effective adjunctive treatment of patients with systolic and/or diastolic left ventricular dysfunction with or without CHF, dilated cardiomyopathy, or hypertensive heart disease.

These results are further confirmed by an investigation involving 109 patients with hypertensive heart disease and isolated DD showing that CoQ10 supplementation resulted in clinical improvement, lowered elevated blood pressure, enhanced diastolic cardiac function, and decreased myocardial thickness in 53% of study patients.[117]

In 2008, New Zealand researchers studied the relationship of plasma CoQ10 levels and survival in patients with chronic heart failure. In their cohort of 236 patients[118] (mean age 77 years), they concluded that plasma CoQ10 concentrations were an independent predictor of mortality. The higher blood levels were the best predictors for survival, and lower concentrations of plasma CoQ10 might be detrimental in the long-term prognosis of CHF. Because CoQ10 depletion is associated with worse outcomes in CHF, the authors suggested further controlled intervention studies on CoQ10 supplementation.

Several years later, the most impressive analysis of CoQ10 and survival in patients with severe heart failure was reproduced in the Q-SYMBIO study.[119] In this double-blind, placebo-controlled trial involving 420 patients with moderate to severe heart failure, subjects treated with 300 mg of CoQ10 supplementation (ubiquinone) or placebo were evaluated. Although there were no changes in short-term end points, the long-term benefits were considerable. There was a significant reduction in the incidence of major adverse cardiovascular events in the CoQ10 group: 15% in the CoQ10 group versus 26% in the placebo group. There was also a significant reduction in overall mortality: 9% in the CoQ10 group versus 16% in the placebo group and in cardiovascular mortality and heart failure hospitalizations. The study strongly suggests that CoQ10 is a major nutraceutical to improve survival in chronic heart failure. Although ACE inhibitors and beta blockers have shown to have efficacy in heart failure, CoQ10 is the nonpharmaceutical nutrient of choice in chronic CHF or the energy-starved heart.[119]

This effect of CoQ10 administration on 32 heart transplant candidates with end-stage CHF and cardiomyopathy was designed to determine if CoQ10 could improve the pharmacological bridge to transplantation and the results showed three significant findings.[120] First, following 6 weeks of CoQ10 therapy the study group showed elevated blood levels from an average of 0.22 to 0.83 mg/L*, an increase of 277% (*please note that different laboratories in other countries have different standardizations of CoQ10). By contrast, the placebo group measured 0.18 mg/L at the onset of the study and 0.178 mg/L at 6 weeks. Second, the study group showed significant improvement in 6-minute walk test distance, shortness of breath, NYHA functional classification, fatigue, and episodes of waking for nocturnal urination. No such changes were found in the placebo group. These results strongly show that CoQ10 therapy may augment pharmaceutical treatment of patients with end-stage CHF and cardiomyopathy.[120]

Two other CoQ10 studies deserve merit in the consideration of left ventricular dysfunction. In one small study of 28 patients with ischemic left ventricular systolic dysfunction, taking 300 mg of CoQ10 supplement per day versus 28 placebo controls, 8 weeks of supplementation improved mitochondrial functioning and brachial flow-mediated dilatation.[121] The researchers concluded that CoQ10 improved endothelial function via reversal of mitochondrial dysfunction in patients with diminished ejection fraction. Serum levels of TNF alpha were also reduced.[121]

In another double-blind, placebo-controlled trial[122] among elderly Swedish citizens, 443 patients were administered selenium and CoQ10 versus placebo. There was a significant reduction in mortality in the active group 5.9% versus 12.6% in controls. In addition, N-terminal pro-B-type natriuretic peptide (NT-Pro-Bnp) and echocardiographic measurements were significantly improved.

CoQ10 has also demonstrated a considerable impact on the lipid marker Lp(a), which is perhaps one of the major risk factors in the development of inflammatory coronary artery disease. In a meta-analysis of six small trials, including subjects with type 2 diabetes, coronary artery disease, obesity, hypertriglyceridemia, and systolic dysfunction, as well as hemodialysis patients, CoQ10 supplementation 100 to 300 mg/d was associated with Lp(a) reduction 3.54 mg/dL, $P < .001$.[123]

The effect of CoQ10 supplementation on another inflammatory marker, high-sensitivity C-reactive protein (hs-CRP), was most recently studied in a meta-analysis of randomized trials.[124] In patients with CVD who took CoQ10 for more than 12 weeks with baseline serum levels of hs-CRP of greater than 3 mg/L, a beneficial effect was realized. Thus, it makes sense to utilize CoQ10 to assuage any biomarkers of inflammation, including IL-6[125] in patients with any form of CVD, including CHF.[121,124,125] In another study, ubiquinone supplementation at a dose of 300 mg/d significantly decreased the serum level of TNF alpha.[125]

COENZYME Q10 VARIETALS—UBIQUINONE, UBIQUINOL, AND MITOQ

Ever since CoQ10 was first isolated by Dr Frederick Crane and colleagues in 1957,[126] scientists have been conducting hundreds of clinical studies on this intriguing nutrient. Over the last few years, there has been some considerable debate about which form of CoQ10 should be utilized in clinical practice as the ubiquinol/ubiquinone controversy continues. Quite frankly, we feel that the use of ubiquinone versus ubiquinol does not really matter, and a high-quality bioavailable form of ubiquinone in some cases may be preferred to a high-quality ubiquinol.

For example, a case study in the *Alternative Medicine Journal*[127] is illustrative in a long-distance runner who meticulously recorded better times on ubiquinone over ubiquinol. Dr Sinatra also conducted an unpublished study in 12 patients with a crossover design involving ubiquinone versus ubiquinol in which blood levels were slightly higher on ubiquinol. However, a Connecticut woman weight lifter had such profound fatigue and diminished ability in competition on ubiquinol that she literally wanted to drop out of the study. When he convinced her that it was only a few more weeks for the washout to be completed, she agreed to go on ubiquinone in which she reported profound energy and stamina. We really cannot explain why there is such a discrepancy in energy and endurance in these competitive endeavors. However, because most clinical trials have been conducted with ubiquinone over ubiquinol, it makes sense to utilize ubiquinone as ubiquinol is considerably more costly both to the manufacturer as well as the patient. Because ubiquinone and ubiquinol shift from one form to another inside the body, the most important aspect is clinical response. This was obviously demonstrated in the last two statistically significant major trials on CoQ10 (Q-SYMBIO and KiSEL).[119,122] We believe that if a clinical benefit is not realized with the reduced or the oxidative varietal of CoQ10, despite an optimal blood level analysis, switching the compound should strongly be considered.

To complicate the ubiquinone/ubiquinol controversy, another form of CoQ10 referred to as MitoQ surfaced within the last several years. MitoQ is a mitochondria-Quinol reactive oxygen species moiety linked to triphenylphosphonium, a lipophilic compound that easily crosses the membranes and accumulates in the mitochondrial matrix as a function of membrane potential.[93]

Because CoQ10 has been utilized in clinical practice for almost 50 years, it is reasonable that multiple varietals of CoQ10 preparations have been studied. Massive marketing campaigns for ubiquinone, ubiquinol, and MitoQ may have caused confusion for both clinicians and their patients about what form of the compound to consider. Again, we feel that a high-quality ubiquinone that has demonstrated superior bioavailability in blood analysis studies is the most logical and ethical situation to consider. In the final analysis, because different forms of CoQ10 can be converted to one form or another, it makes sense to consider the most affordable and bioavailable compound. Certainly, more research regarding MitoQ and other forms of CoQ10 is reasonable, and it may take a considerable amount of research to see if one compound is indeed clinically better than another.

To complicate the confusion regarding different forms of CoQ10, a recent investigation suggested that the gamma cyclodextrin complex form of CoQ10 is a powerful nutraceutical for additional antiaging and health improvements.[128] Certainly, the most important aspect of CoQ10 is its bioavailability, and the CoQ10 gamma cyclodextrin complex has major improvements in plasma concentrations of CoQ10. Thus, we feel that any CoQ10 formulation with a gamma cyclodextrin complex may perhaps be the most bioavailable form of CoQ10 to consider.

To summarize, CoQ10 is one of the body's most important endogenous compounds as a powerful antioxidant and membrane stabilizer as well as a critical electron donor for mitochondrial cellular production. Multiple controlled studies have confirmed our observations in decades of utilizing CoQ10 applications in thousands of patients. It is the most efficacious, bioenergetic, and therapeutic compound we have ever discovered in the treatment and management of CHF with and without hypertensive CVD.

L-CARNITINE

Carnitine is derived naturally in the body from the amino acids lysine and methionine. Biosynthesis occurs in a series of metabolic reactions involving these amino acids, complemented with niacin, vitamin B_6, vitamin C, and iron.

The principal role of carnitine is to facilitate the transport of fatty acids across the inner mitochondrial membrane to initiate beta-oxidation. The inner mitochondrial membrane is normally impermeable to activated coenzyme A (CoA) esters. To affect transfer of the extracellular metabolic by-product acyl-CoA across the cellular membrane, the mitochondria delivers its acyl unit to the carnitine residing in the inner mitochondrial membrane. Carnitine (as acetyl-carnitine) then transports the metabolic fragment across the membrane and delivers it to coenzyme A residing inside the mitochondria. This process of acetyl transfer is known as the carnitine shuttle, and the shuttle also works in reverse to remove excess acetyl units from the inner mitochondria for disposal. Excess acetyl units that accumulate inside the mitochondria disturb the metabolic burning of fatty acids.

Thus, nature created carnitine to serve as a freight train or ferry boat to carry fatty acids into the mitochondria. More importantly, it is not only the burning of fat in the mitochondria that fuels the energy for ATP but also the fact that as a high-energy organism, we humans produce a lot of toxic waste. This is where the carnitines are so absolutely phenomenal and instrumental, especially in cardiac health. Not only do these carnitines shuttle in the fatty acids to be burned in the mitochondria as fuel but they also shuttle out the toxic metabolites.

Other crucial functions of intracellular carnitine include the metabolism of branched-chain amino acids, ammonia detoxification, and lactic acid clearance from tissue. Carnitine also exhibits antioxidant and free radical scavenger properties.

The relationship between carnitine availability and heart tissue, carnitine metabolism, and the heart and carnitine's impact on left ventricular function has been extensively studied. In the first study of carnitine tissue levels and CHF, the myocardial tissue from 25 cardiac transplant recipients with end-stage CHF and 21 control donor hearts was analyzed for concentrations of total carnitine, free carnitine, and carnitine derivatives. Compared with controls, the concentration of carnitines in the heart muscle of heart transplant recipients was significantly lower in patients, and the level of carnitine in the tissue was directly related to ejection fraction. This study concluded that carnitine deficiency in the heart tissue might be directly related to heart function.[129]

The second study measured plasma and urinary levels of L-carnitine in 30 patients with CHF and cardiomyopathy and compared them with 10 control subjects with no heart disease.[130] Results showed that patients with CHF had higher plasma and urinary levels of carnitine, suggesting that carnitine was being released from the challenged heart muscle cells. Similarly, the results showed that the level of plasma and urinary carnitine was related to the degree of left ventricular systolic dysfunction and ejection fraction, showing that elevated plasma and urinary carnitine levels, indices of carnitines being leeched out of compromised cardiomyocytes, might represent measurable physiological markers for myocardial damage and impaired left ventricular function.

More recently, free L-carnitine levels and its derivative palmitoyl-carnitine were increased in patients with CHF and correlated with NT-Pro-BNP and NYHA functional class status. In this study of 183 patients with heart failure and 111 healthy controls, higher levels of palmitoyl-carnitine were also associated with more adverse outcomes. The authors believed these findings suggested prognostic value and recommended additional investigational analysis of L-carnitine administration in candidates with heart failure.[131]

A meta-analysis in the Mayo Clinic's proceedings 2013 reviewed the benefits of L-carnitine and cardiovascular function.[132] Thirteen clinical trials involving 3629 patients post-MI were evaluated. L-Carnitine benefits were attributed to the ability of L-carnitine to limit infarct size, stabilize membranes, and improve compromised cellular energy production. The major improvements in these vulnerable post-MI patients showed not only a reduction of angina symptoms by 40% and reduced arrhythmia by 60% but also a striking reduction in all-cause death by 27%.[132]

This Mayo Clinic's analysis is contrary to the trimethamine-N-oxide (TMAO) investigations that have emerged in the medical literature in the past few years. In a recent rodent model, low-dose TMAO Rx reduced DD and heart fibrosis in hypertensive rats.[133] Indeed, the TMAO hypothesis may be in a cross fire, and the research needs further investigation.[134] When one considers the longevity merits of the Mediterranean and Okinawan diets abundant in proteins, sea foods, and other TMAO-raising properties, it just does not make sense to restrict and modify the diet over such inconclusive evidence. Hopefully, newer research will bring clarity into the controversial concept.

To summarize, without carnitine, fats that are a high-energy fuel for the heart cannot be converted to ATP. The heart uses free fatty acids as its main energy source, and the only way for long-chain fatty acids to get to the inner mitochondrial membrane where energy is produced is via the carnitine shuttle. Thus, the addition of L-carnitine is an important contribution in the synergy of metabolic cardiology.

MAGNESIUM—SWITCHING ON THE ENERGY ENZYMES

Magnesium is an essential mineral that is critical for energy-requiring processes, in protein synthesis, membrane integrity, nervous tissue conduction, neuromuscular excitation, muscle contraction, hormone secretion, maintenance of vascular tone, and intermediary metabolism. Deficiency may lead to changes in neuromuscular, cardiovascular, immune, and hormonal function; impaired energy metabolism; and reduced capacity for physical work. Magnesium deficiency is now considered to contribute to many diseases, and the role for magnesium as a therapeutic agent is expanding. A published German study[135] brings this point into focus.

Researchers in this study evaluated a random population of about 16,000 people, who were assigned to subgroups based on gender, age, and state of health. Low blood levels of magnesium, or hypomagnesemia, was identified in 14.5% of all persons examined, and suboptimal levels were found in yet another 33.7%, a total of 58.2%, more than half of those evaluated.[135] Thus, low-magnesium situations are more common than we think.

Magnesium deficiency, which is better detected by mononuclear blood cell magnesium than by the standard serum level performed at most hospitals, predisposes patients with acute MI to excessive mortality and morbidity.

Unless we have adequate levels of magnesium in our cells, the cellular processes of energy metabolism cannot function. Small changes in magnesium levels can have a large effect on heart and blood vessel function. Although magnesium is found in most foods, particularly beans, figs, and vegetables, deficiencies are increasing. Softened water, depleted soils, and a trend toward lower vegetable consumption are the culprits contributing to these rising deficiencies.

Taurine

The use of taurine in CHF may help to reduce human suffering especially if a traditional metabolic cardiology approach is not ideal. Taurine is a nonessential amino acid that stabilizes cellular membranes in the heart. Several citations on taurine came out in the 1980s by Japanese researchers suggesting that 2 g three times a day may have benefit in CHF.[136] In our experience, we agree with this concept especially because we have had patients with diverse cardiovascular disorders who have improved on taurine when usual metabolic approaches were not successful.[137]

Summary

The energy-starved heart is often not considered by physicians who treat cardiac disease on a day-to-day basis. ACE inhibitors and angiotensin receptor II blockers improve survival in ischemic and nonischemic heart failure and should be considered as a conventional approach in any patient with heart failure. However, therapies that target the cardiomyocyte itself must also be employed[95] as it has been shown that, although cardiomyocytes in the failing heart are metabolically compromised, their function can be potentially improved and restored.[95]

Physicians must consider the biochemistry of "pulsation." It is critically important to treat both the molecular and cellular components of the heart when managing CHF. Remember, one characteristic of the failing heart is the persistent and progressive loss of cellular energy substrates and abnormalities in cardiac bioenergetics that directly compromise diastolic performance, with the capacity to impact global cardiac function. We think that the heart is all about ATP and the restoration of the heart's energy reserve. "Metabolic Cardiology" addresses the biochemical interventions that directly improve energy substrates and therefore energy metabolism in heart cells. In simple terms, sick hearts leak out and lose vital ATP, and the endogenous restoration of ATP cannot keep pace with the relentless depletion of energy substrates especially in situations of ischemia. When ATP levels drop, diastolic function, the most important precursor of CHF, deteriorates. Because epidemiological studies suggest that DD is present in

more than half of patients admitted to hospitals with CHF,[138] it makes sense to target myocardial energetics with effective modalities that truly work. Energizing diastole and myocyte metabolism is the most effective therapy for diastolic heart failure and some day may be the standard of care for CHF.[99,100]

D-Ribose, CoQ10, L-carnitine, and magnesium all act to promote cardiac energy metabolism and help normalize myocardial adenine nucleotide concentrations. These naturally occurring compounds exert a physiological benefit that positively impacts DD, hypertensive heart failure, CHF, and congestive cardiomyopathy. Acknowledging metabolic support for the heart provides the missing link that has been eluding physicians for decades and offers great potential for the future treatment of CVD.

References

1. Yusuf S, Hawken S, Ounpuu S, et al. Effect of potentially modifiable risk factors associated with myocardial infarction in 52 countries (the INTERHEART study): case-control study. *Lancet*. 2004;364(9438):937-952.
2. Houston Mark C. *What Your Doctor May Not Tell You About Heart Disease. The Revolutionary Book that Reveals the Truth Behind Coronary Illnesses and How You Can Fight Them. Grand Central Life and Style*. New York, NY: Hachette Book Group; 2012.
3. O'Donnell CJ, Nabel EG. Genomics of cardiovascular disease. *N Engl J Med*. 2011;365(22):2098-2109.
4. Houston MC. Nutrition and nutraceutical supplements in the treatment of hypertension. *Expert Rev Cardiovasc Ther*. 2010;8:821-833.
5. ACCORD Study Group; Gerstein HC, Miller ME, Genuth S, et al. Long-term effects of intensive glucose lowering on cardiovascular outcomes. *N Engl J Med*. 2011;364(9):818-828.
6. Youssef-Elabd EM, McGee KC, Tripathi G. Acute and chronic saturated fatty acid treatment as a key instigator of the TLR-mediated inflammatory response in human adipose tissue, in vitro. *J Nutr Biochem*. 2012;23:39-50.
7. El Khatib N, Génieys S, Kazmierczak B, Volpert V. Mathematical modelling of atherosclerosis as an inflammatory disease. *Philos Transact A Math Phys Eng Sci*. 2009;367(1908):4877-4886.
8. Ko MJ, Jo AJ, Park CM, Kim HJ, Kim YJ, Park DW. Level of blood pressure control and cardiovascular events: SPRINT criteria versus the 2014 hypertension recommendations. *J Am Coll Cardiol*. 2016;67(24):2821-2831.
9. Coutinho M, Gerstein HC, Wang Y, Yusuf S. The relationship between glucose and incident cardiovascular events. A meta-regression analysis of published data from 20 studies of 95,783 individuals followed for 12.4 years. *Diabetes Care*. 1999;22(2):233-240.
10. Balkau B, Shipley M, Jarrett RJ, et al. High blood glucose concentration is a risk factor for mortality in middle-aged nondiabetic men. 20-year follow-up in the Whitehall Study, the Paris Prospective Study, and the Helsinki Policemen Study. *Diabetes Care*. 1998;21(3):360-367.
11. Pereg D, Elis A, Neuman Y, Mosseri M, Lishner M, Hermoni D. Cardiovascular risk in patients with fasting blood glucose levels within normal range. *Am J Cardiol*. 2010;106(11):1602-1605.
12. Carey RM, Whelton PK, 2017 ACC/AHA Hypertension Guideline Writing Committee. Prevention, detection, evaluation, and management of high blood pressure in adults: synopsis of the 2017 American College of Cardiology/American Heart Association Hypertension Guideline. *Ann Intern Med*. 2018;168(5):351-358.
13. Houston MC, Basile J, Bestermann WH, et al. Addressing the global cardiovascular risk of hypertension, dyslipidemia, and insulin resistance in the southeastern United States. *Am J Med Sci*. 2005;329(5):276-291.
14. Bestermann W, Houston MC, Basile J, et al. Addressing the global cardiovascular risk of hypertension, dyslipidemia, diabetes mellitus, and the metabolic syndrome in the southeastern United States, part II: treatment recommendations for management of the global cardiovascular risk of hypertension, dyslipidemia, diabetes mellitus, and the metabolic syndrome. *Am J Med Sci*. 2005;329(6):292-305.
15. Duprez DA, Florea N, Zhong W, et al. Vascular and cardiac functional and structural screening to identify risk of future morbid events: preliminary observations. *J Am Soc Hypertens* 2011;5(5):401-409.
16. Houston Mark C. *Handbook of Hypertension*. Oxford, UK: Wiley-Blackwell; 2009.
17. Della Rocca DG, Pepine CJ. Endothelium as a predictor of adverse outcomes. *Clin Cardiol*. 2010;33(12):730-732.
18. Houston M. The role of nutraceutical supplements in the treatment of dyslipidemia. *J Clin Hypertens (Greenwich)*. 2012;14(2):121-132.
19. Siti HN, Kamisah Y, Kamsiah J. The role of oxidative stress, antioxidants and vascular inflammation in cardiovascular disease (a review). *Vascul Pharmacol*. 2015;71:40-56.
20. Razzouk, Munter P, Bansilal S, et al. C reactive protein predicts long-term mortality independently of low-density lipoprotein cholesterol in patients undergoing percutaneous coronary intervention. *Am Heart J*. 2009;158(2):277-283.
21. Martinez BK, White CM. The emerging role of inflammation in cardiovascular disease. *Ann Pharmacother*. 2018;52(8):801-809.
22. Epelman S, Liu PP, Mann DL. Role of innate and adaptive immune mechanisms in cardiac injury and repair. *Nat Rev Immunol*. 2015;15(2):117-129.
23. Wen Y, Crowley SD. Renal effects of cytokines in hypertension. *Curr Opin Nephrol Hypertens*. 2018;27(2):70-76.
24. Van Laecke S, Malfait T, Schepers E, Van Biesen W. Cardiovascular disease after transplantation: an emerging role of the immune system. *Transpl Int*. 2018;31(7):689-699.
25. Petrie JR, Guzik TJ, Touyz RM. Diabetes, hypertension, and cardiovascular disease: clinical insights and vascular mechanisms. *Can J Cardiol*. 2018;34(5):575-584.
26. Caillon A, Mian MO, Fraulob-Aquino JC, et al. Gamma delta T cells mediate angiotensin II-induced hypertension and vascular injury. *Circulation*. 2017;135(22):2155-2162.
27. Solanki A, Bhatt LK, Johnston TP. Evolving targets for the treatment of atherosclerosis. *Pharmacol Ther*. 2018;187:1-12.
28. De Ciuceis C, Agabiti-Rosei C, Rossini C, et al. Relationship between different subpopulations of circulating CD4+ T lymphocytes and microvascular or systemic oxidative stress in humans. *Blood Press*. 2017;26(4):237-245.
29. Justin Rucker A, Crowley SD. The role of macrophages in hypertension and its complications. *Pflugers Arch*. 2017;469(3-4):419-430.

30. Ritchie RH, Drummond GR, Sobey CG, De Silva TM, Kemp-Harper BK. The opposing roles of NO and oxidative stress in cardiovascular disease. *Pharmacol Res.* 2017;116:57-69.

31. Lundberg AM, Yan ZQ. Innate immune recognition receptors and damage-associated molecular patterns in plaque inflammation. *Curr Opin Lipidol.* 2011;22(5):343-349.

32. Zhao L, Lee JY, Hwang DH. Inhibition of pattern recognition receptor-mediated inflammation by bioactive phytochemicals. *Nutr Rev.* 2011;69(6):310-320.

33. Mah E, Bruno RS. Postprandial hyperglycemia on vascular endothelial function: mechanisms and consequences. *Nutr Res.* 2012;32(10):727-740.

34. Fazio S, Linton MF. High-density lipoprotein therapeutics and cardiovascular prevention. *J Clin Lipidol.* 2010;4(5):411-419.

35. van der Steeg WA, Holme I, Boekholdt SM, et al. High-density lipoprotein cholesterol, high-density lipoprotein particle size, and apolipoprotein A-I: significance for cardiovascular risk: the IDEAL and EPIC-Norfolk studies. *J Am Coll Cardiol.* 2008;51(6):634-642.

36. Matsuzawa Y, Sugiyama S, Sugamura K, et al. Digital assessment of endothelial function and ischemic heart disease in women. *J Am Coll Cardiol.* 2010;55(16):1688-1696.

37. Bonetti PO, Pumper GM, Higano ST, Holmes DR Jr, Kuvin JT, Lerman A. Noninvasive identification of patients with early coronary atherosclerosis by assessment of digital reactive hyperemia. *J Am Coll Cardiol.* 2004;44(11):2137-2141.

38. Hamburg NM, Keyes MJ, Larson MG, et al. Cross-sectional relations of digital vascular function to cardiovascular risk factors in the Framingham Heart Study. *Circulation.* 2008;117(19):2467-2474.

39. Schoenenberger AW, Urbanek N, Bergner M, Toggweiler S, Resink TJ, Erne P. Associations of reactive hyperemia index and intravascular ultrasound-assessed coronary plaque morphology in patients with coronary artery disease. *Am J Cardiol.* 2012;109(12):1711-1716.

40. Matsuzawa Y, Sugiyama S, Sumida H, et al. Peripheral endothelial function and cardiovascular events in high-risk patients. *J Am Heart Assoc.* 2013;2(6):e000426.

41. Prisant LM, Pasi M, Jupin D, Prisant ME. Assessment of repeatability and correlates of arterial compliance. *Blood Press Monit.* 2002;7(4):231-235.

42. Cohn JN, Hoke L, Whitwam W, et al. Screening for early detection of cardiovascular disease in asymptomatic individuals. *Am Heart J.* 2003;146(4):679-685.

43. Nelson MR, Stepanek J, Cevette M, Covalciuc M, Hurst RT, Tajik AJ. Noninvasive measurement of central vascular pressures with arterial tonometry: clinical revival of the pulse pressure waveform? *Mayo Clin Proc.* 2010;85(5):460-472.

44. Hashimoto J, Ito S. Some mechanical aspects of arterial aging: physiological overview based on pulse wave analysis. *Ther Adv Cardiovasc Dis.* 2009;3(5):367-378.

45. Johnsen SH, Mathiesen EB. Carotid plaque compared with intima-media thickness as a predictor of coronary and cerebrovascular disease. *Curr Cardiol Rep.* 2009;11(1):21-27.

46. Bots ML, Taylor AJ, Kastelein JJ, et al. Rate of change in carotid intima-media thickness and vascular events: meta-analyses cannot solve all the issues. A point of view. *J Hypertens.* 2012;30(9):1690-1696.

47. Lorenz MW, Markus HS, Bots ML, Rosvall M, Sitzer M. Prediction of clinical cardiovascular events with carotid intima-media thickness: a systematic review and meta-analysis. *Circulation.* 2007;115(4):459-467.

48. Rizzoni D, Porteri E, Duse S, et al. Relationship between media-to-lumen ratio of subcutaneous small arteries and wall-to-lumen ratio of retinal arterioles evaluated noninvasively by scanning laser Doppler flowmetry. *J Hypertens.* 2012;30(6):1169-1175.

49. Ying GS, Maguire M, Pistilli M, et al. Association between retinopathy and cardiovascular disease in patients with chronic kidney disease (from the Chronic Renal Insufficiency Cohort [CRIC] Study). *Am J Cardiol.* 2012;110(2):246-253.

50. Virdis A, Savoia C, Grassi G, et al. Evaluation of microvascular structure in humans: a "state-of-the-art" document of the Working Group on Macrovascular and Microvascular Alterations of the Italian Society of Arterial Hypertension. *J Hypertens.* 2014;32(11):2120-2129.

51. Al-Fiadh AH, Wong TY, Kawasaki R, et al. Usefulness of retinal microvascular endothelial dysfunction as a predictor of coronary artery disease. *Am J Cardiol.* 2015;115(5):609-613.

52. Folsom AR, Kronmal RA, Detrano RC, et al. Coronary artery calcification compared with carotid intima-media thickness in the prediction of cardiovascular disease incidence: the Multi-Ethnic Study of Atherosclerosis (MESA). *Arch Intern Med.* 2008;168(12):1333-1339.

53. Choi Y, Chang Y, Ryu S, et al. Relation of dietary glycemic index and glycemic load to coronary artery calcium in asymptomatic korean adults. *Am J Cardiol.* 2015;116(4):520-526.

54. Ahmadi N, Tsimikas S, Hajsadeghi F, et al. Relation of oxidative biomarkers, vascular dysfunction, and progression of coronary artery calcium. *Am J Cardiol.* 2010;105(4):459-466.

55. Raggi P, Callister TQ, Shaw LJ. Progression of coronary artery calcium and risk of first myocardial infarction in patients receiving cholesterol-lowering therapy. *Arterioscler Thromb Vasc Biol.* 2004;24(7):1272-1277.

56. Criqui MH, Denenberg JO, Ix JH, et al. Calcium density of coronary artery plaque and risk of incident cardiovascular events. *JAMA.* 2014;311(3):271-278.

57. Schmermund A, Elsässer A, Behl M, et al. Comparison of prognostic usefulness (three years) of computed tomographic angiography versus 64-slice computed tomographic calcium scanner in subjects without significant coronary artery disease. *Am J Cardiol.* 2010;106(11):1574-1579.

58. Ochs MM, Siepen FA, Fritz T, et al. Limits of the possible: diagnostic image quality in coronary angiography with third-generation dual-source CT. *Clin Res Cardiol.* 2017;106(7):485-492.

59. Rong J, Bai SR, Chen YL, He C. Increased detection of coronary atherosclerosis on 320-slice computed tomographic angiography with burden of cardiovascular risk factors and complications in patients with type 2 diabetes. *J Diabetes Complications.* 2016;30(3):494-500.

60. Kawaji T, Kimura T. The diagnostic performance of Multifunction Cardiogram (MCG) in functional myocardial ischemia. *Ann Noninvasive Electrocardiol.* 2015;20(5):508-510.

61. Kawaji T, Shiomi H, Morimoto T, et al. Noninvasive detection of functional myocardial ischemia: Multifunction Cardiogram Evaluation in Diagnosis of Functional Coronary Ischemia Study (MED-FIT). *Ann Noninvasive Electrocardiol.* 2015;20(5):446-453.

62. Kandori A, Ogata K, Miyashita T, et al. Subtraction magnetocardiogram for detecting coronary heart disease. *Ann Noninvasive Electrocardiol.* 2010;15(4):360-368.

63. Kwon H, Kim K, Lee YH, et al. Non-invasive magnetocardiography for the early diagnosis of coronary artery disease in patients presenting with acute chest pain. *Circ J.* 2010;74(7):1424-1430.

64. Greenwood JP, Herzog BA, Brown JM, et al. Prognostic value of cardiovascular magnetic resonance and single-photon emission computed tomography in suspected coronary heart disease: long-term follow-up of a prospective, diagnostic accuracy cohort study. *Ann Intern Med.* 2016;165(1):1-9.

65. Emami H, Tawakol A. Noninvasive imaging of arterial inflammation using FDG-PET/CT. *Curr Opin Lipidol.* 2014;25(6):431-437.

66. Houston MC. The role of cellular micronutrient analysis, nutraceuticals, vitamins, antioxidants and minerals in the prevention and treatment of hypertension and cardiovascular disease. *Ther Adv Cardiovasc Dis.* 2010;4(3):165-183.

67. Sofi F, Abbate R, Gensini GF, Casini A. Accruing evidence on benefits of adherence to the Mediterranean diet on health: an updated systematic review and meta-analysis. *Am J Clin Nutr.* 2010;92(5):1189-1196.

68. Estruch R, Ros E, Salas-Salvadó J, et al. Primary prevention of cardiovascular disease with a Mediterranean diet. *N Engl J Med.* 2013;368(14):1279-1290.

69. Nadtochiy SM, Redman EK. Mediterranean diet and cardioprotection: the role of nitrite, polyunsaturated fatty acids, and polyphenols. *Nutrition.* 2011;27(7-8):733-744.

70. de Lorgeril M, Salen P, Martin JL, Monjaud I, Delaye J, Mamelle N. Mediterranean diet, traditional risk factors, and the rate of cardiovascular complications after myocardial infarction: final report of the Lyon Diet Heart Study. *Circulation.* 1999;99(6):779-785.

71. Buckland G, Mayén AL, Agudo A, et al. Olive oil intake and mortality within the Spanish population (EPIC-Spain). *Am J Clin Nutr.* 2012;96(1):142-149.

72. Castañer O, Corella D, Covas MI, et al. In vivo transcriptomic profile after a Mediterranean diet in high-cardiovascular risk patients: a randomized controlled trial. *Am J Clin Nutr.* 2013;98(3):845-853.

73. Konstantinidou V, Covas MI, Sola R, Fitó M. Up-to date knowledge on the in vivo transcriptomic effect of the Mediterranean diet in humans. *Mol Nutr Food Res.* 2013;57(5):772-783.

74. Corella D, Ordovás JM. How does the Mediterranean diet promote cardiovascular health? Current progress toward molecular mechanisms: gene-diet interactions at the genomic, transcriptomic, and epigenomic levels provide novel insights into new mechanisms. *Bioessays.* 2014;36(5):526-537.

75. Salas-Salvadó J, Bulló M, Estruch R, et al. Prevention of diabetes with Mediterranean diets: a subgroup analysis of a randomized trial. *Ann Intern Med* 2014;160(1):1-10.

76. Appel LJ, Moore TJ, Obarzanek E, et al. A clinical trial of the effects of dietary patterns on blood pressure. DASH Collaborative Research Group. *N Engl J Med.* 1997;336(16):1117-1124.

77. Sacks FM, Svetkey LP, Vollmer WM, et al. Effects on blood pressure of reduced dietary sodium and the Dietary Approaches to Stop Hypertension (DASH) diet. DASH-Sodium Collaborative Research Group. *N Engl J Med.* 2001;344(1):3-10.

78. Fung TT Chiuve SE, McCullough ML, Rexrode KM, Logroscino G, Hu FB. Adherence to a DASH-style diet and risk of coronary heart disease and stroke in women. *Arch Intern Med.* 2008;168(7):713-720.

79. Jenkins DJ, Kendall CW, Marchie A, et al. Direct comparison of a dietary portfolio of cholesterol-lowering foods with a statin in hypercholesterolemic participants. *Am J Clin Nutr.* 2005;81(2):380-387.

80. Jenkins DJ, Jones PJ, Lamarche B, et al. Effect of a dietary portfolio of cholesterol-lowering foods given at 2 levels of intensity of dietary advice on serum lipids in hyperlipidemia: a randomized controlled trial. *JAMA.* 2011;306(8):831-839.

81. The CONSENSUS Trial Study Group. Effects of enalapril on mortality on mortality in severe congestive heart failure: results of the Cooperative North Scandinavian Enalapril Survival Study (CONSENSUS). *N Engl J Med.* 1987;316:1429-1435.

82. Pfeffer MA, Braunwalk E, Moye LA, et al. Effect of captopril on mortality and morbidity in patients with left ventricular dysfunction after myocardial infarction: results of the Survival and Ventricular Enlargement Trial. *N Engl J Med.* 1992;327:669-677.

83. Hunt SA, American College of Cardiology; American Heart Association Task Force on Practice Guidelines (Writing Committee to Update the 2001 Guidelines for the Evaluation and Management of Heart Failure). ACC/AHA 2005 guideline update for the diagnosis and management of chronic heart failure in the adult: a report of the American College of Cardiology/American Heart Association Task Force on Practice Guidelines (Writing Committee to Update the 2001 Guidelines for the Evaluation and Management of Heart Failure). *J Am Coll Cardiol.* 2005;46(6):e1-e82.

84. CIBIS Investigators and Committees. A randomized trial of B-blockade in heart failure: the Cardiac Bisoprolol Insufficiency Study (CIBIS). *Circulation.* 1994;90:1765-1773.

85. Packer M, Bristow MR, Cohn JN, et al. The effect of carvedilol on morbidity and mortality in patients with chronic heart failure. *N Engl J Med.* 1996;334:1349-1355.

86. Agnetti N, Kaludercic LA, Kane ST, et al. Modulation of mitochondrial proteome and improved mitochondrial function by biventricular pacing of dyssynchronous failing hearts. *Circ Cardiovasc Genet.* 2010;3:78-87.

87. Kitaizumi K, Yukiiri K, Masugata H, et al. Positron emission tomographic demonstration of myocardial oxidative metabolism in a case of left ventricular restoration after cardiac resynchronization therapy. *Circ J.* 2008;72:1900-1903.

88. Christenson SD, Chareonthaitawee P, Burnes JE, et al. Effects of simultaneous and optimized sequential cardiac resynchronization therapy on myocardial oxidative metabolism and efficiency. *J Cardiovasc Electrophysiol.* 2008;19:125-132.

89. McMurray JJ, Pfeffer MA. Heart failure. *Lancet.* 2005;365:1877-1889.

90. Gheorghiade M, Peterson ED. Improving postdischarge outcomes in patients hospitalized for acute heart failure syndromes. *JAMA.* 2011;305:2456-2457.

91. Ma T, Sun J, Zhao Z, et al. A brief review: adipose-derived stem cells and their therapeutic potential in cardiovascular disease. *Stem Cell Res Ther.* 2017;8(1):124.

92. Stanley WC, Hoppel CL. Mitochondrial dysfunction in heart failure: potential for therapeutic interventions? *Cardiovasc Res.* 2000;45:805-806.

93. Bayeva M, Gheorghiade M, Ardehali H. Mitochondria as a therapeutic target in heart failure. *J Am Coll Cardiol.* 2013;61(6):599-610.

94. Ardehali H, Sabbah HN, Burke MA, et al. Targeting myocardial substrate metabolism in heart failure: potential for new therapies. *Eur J Heart Fail.* 2012;14:120-129.

95. Bergmann O, Bhardwaj RD, Bernard S, et al. Evidence for cardiomyocyte renewal in humans. *Science.* 2009;324:98-102.

96. Parmacek MS, Epstein JA. Cardiomyocyte renewal. *N Engl J Med.* 2009;361(1):86-88.

97. Ingwall JS, Weiss RG. Is the failing heart energy starved? On using chemical energy to support cardiac function. *Circ Res.* 2004;95:135-145.

98. Neubauer S. The failing heart – An engine out of fuel. *N Engl J Med.* 2007;356(11):1140-1151.

99. Sinatra ST. Metabolic Cardiology: the missing link in cardiovascular disease. *Altern Ther Health Med.* 2009;15(2):48-50.

100. Sinatra ST. *The Sinatra Solution/Metabolic Cardiology.* Laguna Beach: Basic Health Publications; 2011.

101. Fitzgerald M. Vibrating cells disclose their ailments. MIT Technology Review; September 9, 2008. Available at https://www.technologyreview.com/s/410793/vibrating-cells-disclose-their-ailments/. Accessed December 26, 2017.

102. Trafton A. Chemical energy influences tiny vibrations of red blood cell membranes. Phys Org; December 21, 2009. Available at https://phys.org/news/2009-12-chemical-energy-tiny-vibrations-red.html. Accessed December 26, 2017.

103. Ingwall JS. On the hypothesis that the failing heart is energy starved: lessons learned from the metabolism of ATP and creatine. *Curr Hypertens Rep.* 2006;8:457-464.

104. Ingwall JS. *ATP and the Heart.* Boston: Kluwer Academic Publishers; 2002.

105. Barth E, Stammler G, Speiser B, et al. Ultrastructural quantitation of mitochondria and myofilaments in cardiac muscle from 10 different animal species including man. *Mol Cell Cardiol.* 1992;24(7):669-681.

106. Bashore TM, Magorien DJ, Letterio J, et al. Histologic and biochemical correlates of left ventricular chamber dynamics in man. *J Am Coll Cardiol.* 1987;9:734-742.

107. Omran H, Illien S, MacCarter D, et al. D-ribose improves diastolic function and quality of life in congestive heart failure patients: a prospective feasibility study. *Eur J Heart Fail.* 2003;5:615-619.

108. Shecterle LM, Terry KR, St Cyr JA. Potential clinical benefits of D-ribose in ischemic cardiovascular disease. *Cureus.* 2018;10(3):e2291.

109. Bayram M, St Cyr JA, Abraham WT. D-ribose aids heart failure patients with preserved ejection fraction and diastolic dysfunction – a pilot study. *Ther Adv Cardiovasc Dis.* 2015;9(3):56-65.

110. Perkowski DJ, Wagner S, Schneider JR. A targeted metabolic protocol with D-ribose for off-pump coronary artery bypass procedures: a retrospective analysis. *Ther Adv Cardiovasc Dis.* 2011;5(4):185-192.

111. Sheeran FL, Pepe S. Mitochondrial bioenergetics and dysfunction in failing heart. *Adv Exp Med Biol.* 2017;982:65-80.

112. Langsjoen PH, Langsjoen AM. Overview of the use of CoQ10 in cardiovascular disease. *Biofactors.* 1999;9(2-4):273-284.

113. Sinatra ST. Letter to the editor: coenzyme Q10 and congestive heart failure. *Ann Intern Med.* 2000;133(9):745-746.

114. Sinatra ST. Coenzyme Q10: a vital therapeutic nutrient for the heart with special application in congestive heart failure. *Conn Med.* 1997;61(11):707-711.

115. Belardinelli R, Mucaj A, Lacalaprice F, et al. Coenzyme Q10 and exercise training in chronic heart failure. *Eur Heart J.* 2006;27(22):2675-2681.

116. Langsjoen PH, Langsjoen P, Willis R, et al. Usefulness of coenzyme Q10 in clinical cardiology: a long-term study. *Mol Aspects Med.* 1994;15:S165-S175.

117. Langsjoen P, Willis R, Folkers K. Treatment of essential hypertension with coenzyme Q10. *Mol Aspects Med.* 1994;15 suppl:265-272.

118. Molyneux S, Florkowski C, George P, et al. Coenzyme Q10: an independent predictor of mortality in chronic heart failure. *JACC.* 2008;52(18):1435-1441.

119. Mortensen SA. The effect of coenzyme Q10 on morbidity and mortality in chronic heart failure: results from Q-SYMBIO: a randomized double-blind trial. *JACC-Heart Fail.* 2014;2(6):641-649.

120. Berman M, Erman A, Ben-Gal T, et al. Coenzyme Q10 in patients with end-stage heart failure awaiting cardiac transplantation: a randomized, placebo-controlled study. *Clin Cardiol.* 2004;27:295-299.

121. Dai YL, Luk TH, Yiu KH, et al. Reversal of mitochondrial dysfunction by coenzyme Q10 supplement improves endothelial function in patients with ischaemic left ventricular systolic dysfunction: a randomized controlled trial. *Atherosclerosis.* 2011;216(2):395-401.

122. Alehagen U, Johansson P, Bjornstedt M, et al. Cardiovascular mortality and N-terminal-proBNP reduced after combined selenium and coenzyme Q10 supplementation: a 5-year prospective randomized double-blind placebo-controlled trial among elderly Swedish citizens. *Int J Cardiol.* 2013;167(5):18680-18686.

123. Sahebkar A, Simental-Mendia LE, Stefanutti C, et al. Supplementation with coenzyme Q10 reduces plasma lipoprotein(a) concentrations but not other lipid indices: a systematic review and meta-analysis. *Pharmacol Res.* 2016;105:198-209.

124. Aslani Z, Shab-Bidar S, Fatahi S, et al. Effect of coenzyme Q10 supplementation on serum of high sensitivity c-reactive protein level in patients with cardiovascular diseases: a systematic review and meta-analysis of randomized controlled trials. *Int J Prev Med.* 2018;9:82.

125. Lee B, Huang Y, Chen S, et al. Effects of coenzyme Q10 supplementation on inflammatory markers (high-sensitivity C-reactive protein, interleukin-6, and homocysteine) in patients with coronary artery disease. *Nutrition.* 2012;28(7-8):767-772.

126. Crane FL, Hatefi Y, Lester RL, et al. Isolation of a quinone from beef heart mitochondria. *Biochim Biophys Acta.* 1957;25(1):220-221.

127. Misner B. Coenzyme Q10 effects the endurance of the runner performance: a case report. *Alt Med.* 2011;2(12).

128. Uekaji Y, Terao K. Coenzyme Q10 – gamma cyclodextrin complex is a powerful nutraceutical for anti-aging and health improvements. *Biomed Res Clin Prac.* 2017;2(1):1-5

129. El-Aroussy W, Rizk A, Mayhoub G, et al. Plasma carnitine levels as a marker of impaired left ventricular functions. *Mol Cell Biochem.* 2000;213(1-2):37-41.

130. Narin F, Narin N, Andac H, et al. Carnitine levels in patients with chronic rheumatic heart disease. *Clin Biochem.* 1997;30(8):643-645.

131. Ueland T, Svardal A, Oie E, et al. Disturbed carnitine regulation in chronic heart failure: increased plasma levels of palmitoyl-carnitine are associated with poor prognosis. *Int J Cardiol.* 2013;167(5):1892-1899.

132. DiNicolantonio JD. L-carnitine in the secondary prevention of cardiovascular disease: systemic review and meta-analysis. *Mayo Clinic Proceed.* 2013;88(6):544-551.

133. Huc T, Drapala A, Gawrys M, et al. Chronic, low-dose TMAO treatment reduces diastolic dysfunction in heart fibrosis in hypertensive rats. *Am J Physiol Heart Circ Physiol.* September 28, 2018. In press.

134. Cho CE, Caudill MA. Trimethylamine-N-Oxide: friend, foe, or simply caught in the cross-fire? *Trends Endocrinol Metab.* 2017;28(2):121-130.

135. Schimatschek HF, Rempis R. Prevalence of hypomagnesemia in an unselected German population of 16,000 individuals. *Magnes Res.* 2001;14(4):283-290.

136. Azuma J, Sawamura A, Awata N, et al. Therapeutic effect of taurine in congestive heart failure: a double-blind crossover trial. *Clin Cardiol.* 1985;8(5):276-282.

137. Xu Y, Arneja A, Tappia P, et al. The potential health benefits of taurine in cardiovascular disease. *Exp Clin Cardiol.* 2008;13(2):57-65.

138. Schwartz K, Siddiqi N, Singh S, et al. The breathing heart: mitochondrial respiratory chain dysfunction in cardiac disease. *Int J Cardiol.* 2014;171(2):134-143.

24

Sex Hormones in Women

Pamela W. Smith, MD, MPH, MS

This chapter will begin by examining the major sex hormone in a woman's body, which is estrogen, produced mainly by the ovaries. Women have estrogen receptor sites throughout their system, including the brain, muscles, bone, bladder, gut, uterus, ovaries, vagina, breasts, eyes, heart, lungs, and blood vessels, to name a few. Estrogen has 400 critical functions, some of which are the following[1-13]:

- Stimulates the production of choline acetyltransferase, an enzyme that prevents Alzheimer disease
- Increases metabolic rate
- Improves insulin sensitivity
- Regulates body temperature
- Helps prevent muscle damage
- Helps maintain muscle
- Improves sleep
- Reduces risk of cataracts
- Helps maintain the elasticity of arteries
- Dilates small arteries
- Increases blood flow
- Inhibits platelet stickiness
- Decreases the accumulation of plaque on arteries
- Enhances magnesium uptake and utilization
- Maintains the amount of collagen in the skin
- Decreases blood pressure
- Decreases low-density lipoprotein and prevents its oxidation
- Helps maintain memory
- Increases reasoning and new ideas
- Helps with fine motor skills
- Increases the water content of skin and is responsible for its thickness and softness
- Enhances the production of nerve growth factor
- Increases high-density lipoprotein by 10% to 15%
- Reduces the overall risk of heart disease by 40% to 50%
- Decreases lipoprotein(a)
- Acts as a natural calcium channel blocker to keep arteries open

- Enhances energy
- Improves mood
- Increases concentration
- Maintains bone density
- Helps prevent glaucoma
- Increases sexual interest
- Reduces homocysteine
- Decreases wrinkles
- Protects against macular degeneration
- Decreases the risk of colon cancer
- Helps prevent tooth loss
- Aids in the formation of neurotransmitters in the brain such as serotonin, which decreases depression, irritability, anxiety, and pain sensitivity
- Increases glucose and oxygen transport to the neurons
- Maintains the blood-brain barrier
- Protects neurons
- Increases the production of choline acetyltransferase, which is needed for the production of acetylcholine, the main neurotransmitter of memory

Progesterone is another sex hormone synthesized by the ovaries that has many functions in a woman's body[1,14-19]:

- Balances estrogen
- Has a positive effect on her sleeping pattern
- Helps build bone
- Helps prevent anxiety, irritability, and mood swings
- Helps bladder function
- Regulates the smooth muscle in the gut so that the body can break down food into nutrients that are absorbed to be used elsewhere in the body

Testosterone falls into a class of hormones called androgens, which are commonly referred to as "male" hormones, but they are present in women as well. Testosterone is made in the ovaries, and a small amount is also made in the adrenal glands. It has numerous functions[20-25]:

- Decreases bone deterioration
- Decreases excess body fat

- Aids with pain control
- Elevates norepinephrine in the brain consequently having an antidepressant effect
- Helps maintain memory
- Increases muscle mass and strength
- Increases muscle tone
- Increases sense of emotional well-being, self-confidence, and motivation
- Increases sexual interest

It is paramount that women maintain hormonal balance, of all of their steroid hormones, throughout their lifetime to help maintain optimal function as well as to aid in pain control.

Sex Hormones in Males

Testosterone is the main sex hormone produced by the male. It is produced by the Leydig cells in the testes, and a small amount is also produced in the adrenal glands. Men have hormone receptors in several locations in their body. Testosterone has many functions including the following[26-40]:

- Important for sexual interest
- Involved in the making of protein and muscle formation
- Helps manufacture bone
- Improves oxygen uptake throughout the body
- Helps control blood sugar
- Needed for normal sperm development
- Regulates acute hypothalamic pituitary adrenal responses under dominance challenge
- Helps regulate cholesterol
- Helps maintain a powerful immune system
- Aids in mental concentration
- Improves mood
- Helps protect the brain against Alzheimer disease
- Regulates the population of thromboxane A2 receptors on megakaryocytes and platelets and consequently platelet aggregation
- Aids in pain control

Progesterone also has functions in a male's body[41]:
- Influences spermiogenesis
- Sperm capacitation/acrosome reaction
- Testosterone biosynthesis in the Leydig cells
- Blocking of gonadotropin secretion
- Sleep improvement
- Regulates immune system
- Positive cardiovascular effects
- Regulates kidney function
- Affects adipose tissue
- Regulates behavior
- Affects the respiratory system

Androgens aromatize into estrogens via the enzyme aromatase. Estrogens, at low levels, are important for a male to help maintain memory and bone structure.[42]

Pregnenolone in Women and Men

Pregnenolone makes estrogen, progesterone, testosterone, dehydroepiandrosterone (DHEA), and cortisol in both men and women. It also has the following functions[43-47]:

- Regulates the balance between excitation and inhibition in the nervous system
- Increases resistance to stress
- Improves energy both physically and mentally
- Enhances nerve transmission
- Reduces pain and inflammation
- Blocks the production of acid-forming compounds
- Modulates the neurotransmitter gamma aminobutyric acid
- Helps to repair nerve damage
- Promotes mood elevation
- Modules *N*-methyl-D-aspartate receptors
- Regulates pain control, learning, memory, and alertness

Adrenal Hormones in Women and Men

DHEA (dehydroepiandrosterone), which is made in adrenal glands and a small amount in the brain and the skin has many wonderful functions in both women and men, including the following[48-53]:

- Breaks down into estrogen and testosterone
- Decreases cholesterol
- Decreases formation of fatty deposits
- Prevents blood clots
- Increases bone growth
- Promotes weight loss
- Increases brain function
- Increases lean body mass
- Increases sense of well-being
- Helps one deal with stress
- Supports the immune system
- Helps the body repair and maintain tissues
- Decreases allergic reactions
- Lowers triglycerides

Cortisol, which is likewise made in the adrenal glands, is one of the most valuable hormones in the body. It is essential for life. If the body stops manufacturing it, the individual will shortly expire. Therefore, it is preferentially made from pregnenolone over the remainder of the steroidogenic pathway owing to its overwhelming importance in the body. Cortisol has the following functions[54-70]:
- Balances blood sugar
- Controls weight
- Regulates immune system response
- Modulates the stress reaction
- Regulates sleep
- Involved in protein synthesis
- Controls mood and thoughts
- Influences testosterone/estrogen ratio
- Influences DHEA/insulin ratio

- Affects pituitary/thyroid/adrenal system
- Regulates bone turnover rate
- Participates with aldosterone in sodium reabsorption

- Is an anti-inflammatory
- Regulates pain control

References

1. Smith P. *What You Must Know About Women's Hormones.* Garden City Park, NY: Square One Publishers; 2010.
2. Fink G, Sumner BE, Rosie R, Grace O, Quinn JP. Estrogen control of central neurotransmission: effect on mood, mental state, and memory, *Cell Mol Neurobiol.* 1996;16(3):325-344.
3. Felson D, Cummings SR. Aromatase inhibitors and the syndrome of arthralgias with estrogen deprivation. *Arthritis Rheum.* 2005;52:2594-2598.
4. Di Paolo T. Modulation of brain dopamine transmission by sex steroids. *Rev Neurosci.* 2005;3:27-41.
5. Miller V, et al. Vascular effects of estrogen and progesterone. In: Fraser J, ed. *Estrogens and Progestogens in Clinical Practice.* New York: Harcourt Publishers; 2000.
6. Miller V, Duckles SP. Vascular actions of estrogens: functional implications. *Pharmacol Rev.* 2008;60(2):210-241.
7. Stirone C, Duckles SP, Krause DN, Procaccio V. Estrogen increases mitochondrial efficiency and reduces oxidative stress in cerebral blood vessels. *Mol Pharmacol.* 2005;68:959-965.
8. Duckles S, Krause DN, Stirone C, Procaccio V. Estrogen and mitochondria: a new paradigm for vascular protection? *Mol Interv.* 2006;6:26-35.
9. Nike E, Nakano M. Estrogens as antioxidants. *Methods Enzymol.* 1990;186:330.
10. Puder J, Freda PU, Goland RS, Wardlaw SL. Estrogen modulates the hypothalamic-pituitary-adrenal and inflammatory cytokine responses to endotoxin in women. *J Clin Endocrinol Metab.* 2001;86(6):2403-2408.
11. Xu H, Gouras GK, Greenfield JP, et al. Estrogen reduces neuronal generation of Alzheimer's B-amyloid peptides. *Nat Med.* 1998;4(4):447-451.
12. Weiland N. Estradiol selectively regulates against binding sites on the N-methyl-d-aspartate receptor complex in the CA1 region of the hippocampus. *Endocrinology.* 1992;131:662-668.
13. Wise P, Dubal DB, Wilson ME, Rau SW, Böttner M. Minireview: neuroprotective effects of estrogen—new insights in mechanisms of action. *Endocrinol.* 2001;142(3):969-973.
14. Carmody B, Arora S, Wakefield MC, Weber M, Fox CJ, Sidawy AN. Progesterone inhibits human infragenicular arterial smooth muscle cell proliferation induced by high glucose and insulin concentrations. *J Vasc Surg.* 2002;36(4):833-838.
15. Rosano G, Webb CM, Chierchia S , et al. Natural progesterone, but not medroxyprogesterone acetate, enhances the beneficial effect of estrogen on exercise-induced myocardial ischemia in postmenopausal women. *J Am Coll Cardiol.* 2000;36(7):2154-2159.
16. Prior J. Progesterone as a bone-tropic hormone. *Endocr Rev.* 1990;11:386-398.
17. Taylor D. Perimenstrual symptoms and syndromes: Guidelines for symptom management and self-care. *Obstetrics Gynecol.* 2005;595):228-241.
18. Solomon C, Hu FB, Dunaif A, et al. Long or irregular menstrual cycle as a marker for the risk of type 2 diabetes mellitus. *JAMA.* 2001;286(19):2421-2426.
19. Stein D. The case for progesterone. *Ann NY Acad Sci.* 2005;1052:152-159.
20. Almeida O. Sex playing with the mind. Effects of oestrogen and testosterone on mood and cognition. *Arch Neuropsych.* 1999;57(3A):701-706.
21. Ehrenreish H, Halaris A, Ruether E, Hüfner M, Funke M, Kunert H. Psychoendocrine sequelae of chronic testosterone deficiency. *J Psychiatr Res.* 1999;33(5):379-397.
22. Davis S, et al. Testosterone influences libido and well-being in women. *Curr Opin Obstet Gynecol.* 1997;9(3):177-180.
23. Brincat M, Moniz CF, Studd JW, Darby AJ, Magos A, Cooper D. Sex hormones and skin collagen content in postmenopausal women. *Br Med Jour.* 1983;287(6402):1337-1338.
24. Rohr U. The impact of testosterone imbalance on depression and women's health. *Maturitas.* 2002;41(suppl 1):S25-S46.
25. Monjo M, Rodríguez AM, Palou A, Roca P. Direct effects of testosterone, 17 beta-estradiol, and progesterone on adrenergic regulation in cultured brown adipocytes: potential mechanism for gender-dependent thermogenesis. *Endocrinol.* 2003;144(11):4923-4930.
26. Annewieke W, de Jong FH, Grobbee DE, Pols HA, Lamberts SW. Measures of bioavailable serum testosterone and estradiol and their relationships with muscle strength, bone density, and body composition in elderly men. *J Clin Endo Met.* 2000;85(9):3276-3282.
27. Swerdloff R, Wang C. Androgen deficiency and aging in men. *West J Med.* 1993;159(5):579-585.
28. Vermuelen A. Androgens in the aging male. *J Clin Endocrin Met.* 1991;73(2):221-224.
29. Menta P, Jones AC, Josephs RA. The social endocrinology of dominance: basal testosterone predicts cortisol changes and behavior following victory and defeat. *J Pers Soc Psychol.* 2008;94(6):1078-1093.
30. Ajayi A, Mathur R, Halushka PV. Testosterone increases human platelet thromboxane A-2 receptor density and aggregation responses. *Circulation.* 1995;91(11):2742-2747.
31. Webb C, McNeill JG, Hayward CS, de Zeigler D, Collins P. Effects of testosterone on coronary vasomotor regulation in men with coronary heart disease. *Circulation.* 1999;100(16):1690-1696.
32. Channer K, Jones TH. Cardiovascular effects of testosterone: implications of the "male menopause?" *Heart.* 2003;89(2):121-122.
33. Yaffe K, Lui LY, Zmuda J, Cauley J. Sex hormones and cognitive function in older men. *J Am Geriatr Soc.* 2002;50:707-712.
34. Thilers P, Macdonald SW, Herlitz A. The association between endogenous free testosterone and cognitive performance: a population based study in 35 to 90 year-old men and women. *Psychoneuroendocrinology.* 2006;31:565-576.
35. Guder G, Frantz S, Bauersachs J, Allolio B, Ertl G, Angermann CE, Störk S. Low circulating androgens and mortality risk in heart failure. *Heart.* 2010;96:504-509.
36. Torkler S, Wallaschofski H, Baumeister SE, et al. Inverse association between total testosterone concentrations, incident hypertension and blood pressure. *Aging Male.* 2011;14(3):176-182.
37. Hyde Z, Norman PE, Flicker L, et al. Low free testosterone predicts mortality from CVD but not other causes: the health in men study. *J Clin Endocriol Met.* 2012;97(1):179.
38. Rizza R. Androgen effect on insulin action and glucose metabolism. *Mayo Clin Proc.* 2000;75 Suppl:S61-S64.
39. Stellato R, Feldman HA, Hamdy O, Horton ES, McKinlay JB. Testosterone, sex hormone-binding globulin, and the development of type 2 diabetes in middle-aged men: prospective results from the Massachusetts male aging study. *Diabetes Care.* 2000;23(4):490-494.
40. Ma R, So WY, Yang X, et al. Erectile dysfunction predicts coronary heart disease in type 2 diabetes. *J Am Coll Cardiol.* 2008;51:2045-2050.
41. Oettel M, Mukhopadhyay AK. Progesterone: the forgotten hormone in men? *Aging Male.* 2004;7(3):236-257.
42. Gibbs R, Gabor R. Estrogen and cognition: applying preclinical findings to clinical perspectives. *J Neurosci Res.* 2003;74(5):637-643.
43. Akwa Y, Young J, Kabbadj K, et al. Neurosteroids: biosynthesis, metabolism, and function of pregnenolone and dehydroepiandrosterone in the brain. *J Steroid Biochem Mol Biol.* 1991;40(1-3):71-81.

44. Havlikova H, Hill M, Hampl R, Stárka L. Sex and age-related changes in epitestosterone in relation to pregnenolone sulfate and testosterone in normal subjects. *Jour Clin Endocrinol Met.* 2002;87(5):2225-2237.

45. Labrie F, Bélanger A, Cusan L, Gomez JL, Candas B. Marked decline in serum concentrations of adrenal C19 sex steroid precursors and conjugated androgen metabolites during aging. *J Clin Endocrinol Metab.* 1997;82(8):2396-2402.

46. Mayo W, Le Moal M, Abrous DN. Pregnenolone sulfate and aging of cognitive functions: behavioral, neurochemical, and morphological investigations. *Horm Behav.* 2001;40(2):215-217.

47. Vallee M, Mayo W, Le Moal M. Role of pregnenolone, dehydroepiandrosterone and their sulfate esters on learning and memory in cognitive aging. *Brain Res Rev.* 2001;37(1-2):301-312.

48. De Bruin V, Vieira MC, Rocha MN, Viana GS. Cortisol and dehydroepiandrosterone sulfate plasma levels and their relationship to gaining, cognitive function, and dementia. *Brain Cogn.* 2002;50(2):316-323.

49. Buffington C, Pourmotabbed G, Kitabchi AE. Case report: amelioration of insulin resistance in diabetes with dehydroepiandrosterone. *Am J Med Sci.* 1993;306(5):320-324.

50. Villareal D, Holloszy JO. Effect of DHEA on abdominal fat and insulin action in elderly women and men. *JAMA.* 2004;292:2243-2248.

51. Watson R, Huls A, Araghinikuam M, Chung S. Dehydroepiandrosterone and diseases of aging. *Drugs Aging.* 1996;9(4):274-291.

52. Yamaguchi Y, Tanaka S, Yamakawa T, et al. Reduced serum dehydroepiandrosterone levels in diabetic patients with hyperinsulinaemia. *Endocrinol (Oxf).* 1998;49(3):377-383.

53. Barrett-Conner E, et al. A prospective study of dehydroepiandrosterone sulfate, mortality, and cardiovascular disease. *NEJM.* 1986;37(9):1035.

54. Carlson L, Sherwin BB. Relationships among cortisol (CRT), dehydroepiandrosterone-sulfate (DHEAS), and memory in longitudinal study of healthy elderly men and women. *Neurobiol Aging.* 1999;20(3):315-324.

55. Whitworth J, Williamson PM, Mangos G, Kelly JK. Cardiovascular consequences of cortisol excess. *Vasc Health Risk Manage.* 2005;1(4):291-299.

56. Kelly J, Mangos G, Williamson PM, Whitworth JA. Cortisol and hypertension. *Clin Exp Pharmacol Physiol.* 1998;25:S51-S56.

57. Hamer M, Steptoe A. Cortisol responses to mental stress and incident hypertension in healthy men and women. *J Clin Endocrinol Metab.* 2012;97(1):E29-E34.

58. Hamer M, Endrighi R, Venuraju SM, Lahiri A, Steptoe A. Cortisol responses to mental stress and the progression of coronary artery calcification in healthy men and women. *PLoS One.* 2012;7(2):e31356.

59. Hewagalamulage S, Lee TK, Clarke IJ, Henry BA. Stress, cortisol, and obesity: a role for cortisol responsiveness in identifying individuals prone to obesity. *Domest Anim Endocrinol.* 2016;56 Suppl:S112-S120.

60. Rosmond R, Björntorp P. The hypothalamic-pituitary-adrenal axis activity as a predictor of cardiovascular disease, type 2 diabetes and stroke. *J Inter Med.* 2000;247(2):188-197.

61. Krajnak K. Potential contribution of work-related psychosocial stress to the development of cardiovascular disease and Type II diabetes: a brief review. *Environ Health Insights.* 2014;8(suppl 1):41-45.

62. Nijm J, Jonasson L. Inflammation and cortisol response in coronary artery disease. *Ann Med.* 2009;41(3):224-233.

63. Jonasson L, Grauen Larsen H, Lundberg AK, et al. Stress-induced release of the S100A8/A9 alarmin is elevated in coronary artery disease patients with impaired cortisol response. *Sci Rep.* 2017;791:17545.

64. Fantidis P, Perez De Prada T, Fernandez-Ortiz A, et al. Morning cortisol production in coronary heart disease patients. *Eur J Clin Invest.* 2002;32(5):304-308.

65. Ronaldson A, Kidd T, Poole L, et al. Diurnal cortisol rhythm is associated with adverse cardiac events and mortality in coronary artery bypass patients. *J Clin Endocrinol Metab.* 2015;100(10):3676-3682.

66. Elenkov I. Systemic stress-induced Th2 shift and its clinical implications. *Intern Rev Neurobiol.* 2002;52:163-186.

67. Cohen S. Psychological stress and susceptibility to upper respiratory infections. *Am J Respir Crit Care Med.* 1995;152(4 pt 2):53-58.

68. Kunz-Ebrecht S, Mohamed-Ali V, Feldman PJ, Kirschbaum C, Steptoe A. Cortisol responses to mild psychological stress are inversely associated with proinflammatory cytokines. *Brain Behav Immun.* 2003;17(5):373-383.

69. Ohlin B, Nilsson PM, Nilsson JA, Berglund G. Chronic psychological stress predicts long-term cardiovascular morbidity and mortality in middle-aged men. *Eur Heart J.* 2004;25(10):867-873.

70. Yehuda R, Golier JA, Kaufman S. Circadian rhythm of salivary cortisol in holocaust survivors with and without PTSD. *Am J Psychiatr.* 2005;162:998-1000.

25

Thyroid and Adrenal Influences on the Cardiovascular System

Erik Lundquist, MD, ABFM, AboIM, IFMCP and Annalouise O'Connor, BS, PhD

The endocrine system is a complex and sophisticated dance of hormones and their influence on end organ targets within the human body. This dance begins often in the brain and is influenced by a sophisticated biofeedback mechanism. The endocrine system is made up of multiple different glands that produce these hormones throughout the body. Outside and environmental influences have a significant impact on the release of stimulating hormones, the receptors they bind to, and the effectiveness of the stimulation on their target. The key to the dance of the endocrine system is to try to bring balance to the system.

For purposes of this chapter we will be focusing on the hypothalamus-pituitary-adrenal-thyroid (HPAT) axis and the influence this system has on the cardiovascular system. The purpose of the cardiovascular system is to supply oxygen and nutrients throughout the body. The cardiovascular system is affected by the endocrine system. The endocrine system in turn is dependent on the cardiovascular system for the delivery of its hormones to appropriate target tissues. This symbiotic and synergistic relationship ties these two systems together intimately. One cannot survive without the other.

This chapter will be divided into two sections, one on the thyroid and one on the adrenals.

The following are the objectives of this chapter:

- Understand the function and metabolism of hormones and neurotransmitters as they relate to the thyroid and adrenal systems.
- Explain how thyroid and adrenal hormones impact the cardiovascular system.
- Identify the laboratory tests available and how to use these to understand the production, transport, receptor sensitivity, and metabolism of the hormones and neurotransmitters involved with the adrenal and thyroid systems.
- Examine the impact that stress has on the cardiovascular system as mediated through different adrenal and thyroid hormonal influences.

- Review the evidence behind targeted nutritional and lifestyle treatments to optimize thyroid and adrenal function, particularly in how they relate to the cardiovascular system.

Signs and Symptoms of Thyroid Dysfunction

The thyroid system has a multifaceted impact on the heart and vascular system, and changes in thyroid hormone status has knock-on effects to many aspects of this system including lipid metabolism, heart rate and contractility, endothelial function, vascular resistance, and blood pressure control.[1] Additionally, a change in thyroid status, specifically hypothyroidism, is linked to an increased risk of metabolic syndrome and type 2 diabetes, which pose additional cardiovascular risk.[2] Indeed, thyroid dysfunction, both overt and subclinical, and hyper- and hypothyroidism increase the risk of heart failure, cardiovascular events, and death.[1]

The prevalence of thyroid disorders is fairly substantial in the United States. The spectrum of thyroid disorders include hypothyroidism, hyperthyroidism, and autoimmune thyroiditis, which can be manifested as hypothyroidism, as with Hashimoto disease, or hyperthyroidism, as with Graves disease. Because so many individuals with thyroid dysfunction are undertreated or undiagnosed it is important for their cardiac minded clinician to understand the prevalence, symptoms, and disorders associated with thyroid dysfunction.

According to the Colorado thyroid disease prevention study that measured individuals with a thyroid stimulating hormone (TSH) above 4.5, there are approximately 30 to 35 million individuals in the United States with thyroid disorders. Of those, approximately half are undiagnosed. Of those who are diagnosed, approximately 10 to 14 million have Hashimoto disease (a form of autoimmune thyroiditis resulting in hypothyroidism) and a much smaller portion have Graves disease, which is another form of autoimmune thyroiditis resulting in hyperthyroidism. A large portion of these individuals are women, with some studies estimating as high as 80%.[3]

Thyroid hormones also help to regulate core body temperature, maintain proper brain metabolism, manage body energy expenditure and heat generation, and influence body composition and weight and digestive tract function.

Symptoms associated with hypothyroidism include the following:

- Cold intolerance and cold hands and feet
- Menstrual irregularities and infertility
- Fatigue
- Weight gain
- Constipation
- Hair loss
- Dry skin
- Frequency of urination
- Mental fog, dizziness, and depression
- Bradycardia
- Arthralgias and myalgias (seen mostly with patients with Hashimoto disease)

Hypothyroid symptoms can include the following:
- Heat intolerance
- Diarrhea/loose stools
- Rapid weight loss
- Goiter and thyromegaly
- Anxiety and insomnia
- Tachycardia, palpitations, and arrhythmias
- Tremors and muscle fasciculations
- Hair changes, such as hair loss

Thyroid Physiology and Metabolism

Thyrotropin releasing hormone (TRH) is released by the hypothalamus in response to external cues and biofeedback by thyroxine levels in the blood.[4] TRH then binds to receptors on the anterior pituitary, which stimulates the release of thyrotropin, or TSH.[4] TSH then binds to receptors on the thyroid gland, stimulating production of enzymes needed in thyroid hormone synthesis (such as protease, peptidase, and peroxidase), as well as the production and release of thyroglobulin into the colloid of the thyroid gland. At this point, binding of iodine to tyrosine residues on thyroglobulin is required for the production of thyroxine (T4) and triiodothyronine (T3). TSH binding stimulates iodide transport into the cell via sodium iodide (I-) symporters that sit on the surface of the thyroid follicular cells. Iodide is then oxidized to form iodine (I2) by thyroid peroxidase. Iodine is then taken up into the colloid of the thyroid gland where it binds to tyrosine residues on thyroglobulin for the production of T4 or T3.[5]

T4 and T3 are then released into the blood where 99% is quickly bound by thyroid binding globulin. Approximately 80% to 90% of all thyroid hormone production is in the form of T4. T4 is considered a "storage" thyroid hormone and must be reduced to the more active T3 before it can be utilized by the cells and tissues of the body. Enzymes that reduce thyroid hormones by removing an iodine molecule are known as the deiodinases. There are three primary types of selenium-dependent iodothyronine deiodinases (known as D1, D2, D3) that are responsible for thyroid hormone metabolism.[5] To properly treat thyroid disorders as well as to order and interpret thyroid function testing, it is critical to understand how thyroid hormones are metabolized and what physiologic and external factors can have influences on their metabolism. For this reason, an in-depth discussion has been included in this chapter.

Both D1 and D3 are intercellular enzymes, located on the plasma membrane of cells that affect the conversion of circulating T4 and T3. D1 influences an increase in cellular metabolism because it reduces T4 to the potently active form of thyroid hormone, T3. D3 influences a decrease in cellular metabolism by reducing T4 to the mostly inhibitory form of reverse triiodothyronine (rT3). Both fT3 and rT3 can bind to the same receptors within the nucleus of the cell to either promote gene expression and therefore increase cellular metabolism, in the case of fT3, or inhibit gene expression and decrease cellular metabolism, as in the case of rT3. I find it helpful to think of fT3 as the gas and rT3 as the brakes.

D1 also reduces rT3 to diiodothyronine (T2), reducing the potential for a decrease in metabolism from circulation. In humans, it appears that D1 has a much greater affinity for rT3 than for T4; thus its primary purpose is to reduce circulating levels of rT3. D1 is found mostly in the liver, kidneys, and thyroid. D1 is induced by T3, vitamin A (in the form of retinoic acid), cyclic AMP, and TSH. D1 is downregulated by selenium deficiency, fasting, some cancers, and chronic inflammation, particularly interleukin-6 and interleukin-1 beta. **It can be inhibited by some pharmaceutical drugs, notably amiodarone, propranolol, propylthiouracil, dexamethasone, and ipodate.**

D3 converts circulating fT3 to the significantly less potent metabolite T2; it also converts T4 to reverse T3 decreasing a potential for an increase in metabolism stimulated by circulating fT3. The body's production of D3 diminishes after birth and is found mostly in the brain and pituitary. During gestation it is produced by the placenta where its primary role is believed to be associated with protecting the fetus from hyperthyroid states. However, certain disease processes can upregulate D3, causing altered cellular metabolism and release of growth factors such as TGF-beta. Other factors that may influence D3 production include starvation, some cancers, and hyperthyroidism.[6,7]

Deiodinase type 2, D2, is found intracellularly within the endoplasmic reticulum primarily in the central nervous system, pituitary, thyroid, bone, brown adipose tissue, and skeletal muscle. Owing to its location inside the cytosolic compartment, the activity of D2 is a primary determinant of intracellular T3 availability and thyroid receptor occupancy within the nucleus. Although T3 generated from the activity of D1 is known to equilibrate rapidly with the plasma, D2-generated T3 remains within the cell and takes several hours to equilibrate with plasma. It is upregulated by the sympathetic nervous system, high-fat diet, as well as cyclic AMP. Its primary physiological role is hypothalamic-pituitary feedback as well as thermogenesis in brown adipose tissue. It also helps to increase plasma levels of T3.

Lastly, certain types of bacteria help in the recirculation of T3 from the inactive conjugated forms, T3 sulfate and T3 glucuronide. This can account for up to 20% of circulating T3 in healthy individuals. Gut dysbiosis, small intestinal bacterial overgrowth, and leaky gut can significantly reduce this contribution leading to an increase in excreted T3 in the conjugated form.[8]

Thyroid Function Testing

To evaluate thyroid hormone status, plasma testing is available for total T4, free T4, total T3, free T3, reverse T3, and T3 uptake. To evaluate antibodies that can influence thyroid function, the following tests are available through most commercial laboratory tests: thyroid peroxidase antibody (TPO Ab), thyroglobulin (TG Ab) antibody, TSH receptor antibody (TR Ab), thyroid stimulating immunoglobulin (TSI), and thyroid-binding globulin inhibitory immunoglobulin (TBII).

The following are considered to be positive indicators of Hashimoto disease: TPO Ab, TG Ab.

The following are considered to be positive indicators of Graves disease: TR Ab, TBII.

Also, owing to the critical nature of the following minerals and vitamins in thyroid function it is recommended to test their serum and/or urine levels. These include red blood cell (RBC) selenium, RBC zinc, RBC magnesium, iodine, ferritin, vitamin D, and vitamin A. A discussion of the value of each of these will be detailed later in the chapter.

Other laboratory tests to consider would include adrenal function testing (to be discussed later in the chapter) and sex hormone function testing, because of their influence on the thyroid system as well as the cardiovascular system.

Specialty laboratory testing would include nutritional evaluation (examples include NutrEval by Genova Diagnostics, Micronutrient Test by Spectracell), iodine loading tests (Hakala Labs), heavy-metal testing (Genova, Doctor's Data, Thorne, Great Plains Labs, ZRT Labs), and gastrointestinal function testing (Genova, Salveo, Vibrant, GI Map). Infections that may be contributing to autoimmune disorders may include *Yersinia enterocolitica*, *Helicobacter pylori*, *Borrelia burgdorferi* (Lyme disease), and Epstein-Barr virus.

Laboratory Interpretation

One of the big challenges and controversies with thyroid function testing has been the interpretation of TSH as the primary measurement of thyroid function. Historically we have been taught that, if the TSH was elevated, greater than the upper limits of normal, then this was a problem likely associated with hypothyroidism. The next test was to check a total T4 to see if it was low, normal, or elevated. If it was elevated, typically >4.5 mIU/L, then it was assumed that the individual had primary hyperthyroidism with the pituitary gland releasing too much

TSH, overstimulating the thyroid gland to produce too much T4. This was most likely secondary to a pituitary adenoma. But if the T4 level was normal, this was described as subclinical hypothyroidism. If the T4 level was below normal, typically < 0.9 ng/dL, then the individual had hypothyroidism and should be treated with synthetic bioidentical T4 medication.

Dr Dennis St. John O'Reilly analyzed the evidence and the history surrounding the concept of using TSH concentration as a measurement of T4 replacement. It became clear through his analysis that early in the 1970s TSH was being used on theoretical grounds but without proper assessment, as an indicator of clinical thyroid status. He stated, "the overlap between the statistically derived normal and abnormal ranges is accepted in diagnostic test, giving rise to faults positive and false negative results. These concepts have not been applied to measurements of thyroid stimulating hormone. Rather than accepting that the test can be fallible, we transfer the problem to the patient." Meaning, that if a patient is experiencing hypothyroid symptoms yet has a normal TSH level, then the problem must be something else (ie, in the patient's head) and not that his thyroid function is abnormal.[9]

There is currently little to no scientific data on the relative importance of biochemical thyroid function testing and its association with clinical symptoms and signs when addressing and assessing thyroid dysfunction. The secretion of TSH is influenced by multiple factors other than direct negative feedback inhibition by either T4 or T3. Although we have some understanding of euthyroid sick syndrome or nonthyroid illness with critical care patients and its effects on intracellular thyroid metabolism, changes in TSH, T4, T3, and reverse T3 concentrations during other systemic illnesses are poorly understood.

The National Health and Nutrition Examination Survey III (NHANES) evaluated levels of TSH, T4, and thyroid antibodies in the US population from 1988 to 1994. The results of the study identified that 80% of the 17,000 people evaluated had a serum TSH below 2.5 mIU/L. Hashimoto disease, evidenced by positive TPO antibodies, had a prevalence that was lowest (<3%) when the TSH was between 0.1 and 1.5 mIU/L in women and 0.1 to 2.0 mIU/L in men. In individuals who had a TSH >20 mIU/L, positive TPO antibodies were seen in over 50% of the individuals. The reference limits of TSH may be skewed by individuals with occult autoimmune thyroid dysfunction but who test negative for TPO antibodies. Thyroglobulin antibodies were not checked in the study.[10,11]

The utility of evaluating serum T3 levels has also been grossly under recommended. In fact, practice guidelines from the American Association of Clinical Endocrinologists in collaboration with the American Thyroid Association published the following in their most recent guidelines. "Serum T3 measurement, whether total or free, has limited utility in hypothyroidism because levels are often normal due to hyper stimulation of the remaining functioning thyroid tissue by elevated TSH and to up-regulation of type 2 iodothyronine deiodinase. Moreover, levels of T3 are low in the absence of thyroid disease in patients with severe illness because of reduced peripheral conversion of T4 to T3 and increase in activation of thyroid hormone."[12]

The T3/rT3 Ratio

Looking at the T3/rT3 ratio helps to identify cellular hormone bioavailability and status and how this may impact overall physical function. A study of elderly men highlighted how rT3 is related to overall physical function. The results demonstrated that serum rT3 levels increased significantly with age and with the presence of comorbidities. A low T3/rT3 ratio was associated with a lower physical performance score, independent of their chronic disease. Low levels of free T4 were related to a better 4-year survival, suggesting possible adaptive mechanisms to prevent excessive catabolism of skeletal muscle and other tissue. The authors concluded "the T3/rT3 ratio is the most useful marker for tissue hypothyroidism and as a marker of diminished cellular functioning." This shows the value of these tests and does not support the most recent position of the American Association of Clinical Endocrinologists of no recommendations for routine testing of reverse T3.[13]

Another study of T3/rT3 was conducted in subjects with and without type 2 diabetes (n = 140) to see if there was an increase in cardiovascular events associated with nonthyroid illness. Type 2 diabetes is commonly associated with nonthyroid illness, a condition with normal TSH and T4 levels but often with intracellularly low T3 levels and elevated reverse T3 levels. When the two groups were compared, those with type 2 diabetes with a history of cardiovascular events were noted to have low levels of total T3, free T3, and T3/rT3 ratios despite having higher free T4 and similar TSH levels when compared with the control group. The inflammatory biomarker serum amyloid A levels correlated positively with reverse T3 levels and inversely with T3/rT3 levels. This study demonstrates that T3/rT3 levels can be used as an independent marker for cardiovascular event risk.[14]

WHY CHECK FOR THYROID ANTIBODIES?

Autoimmune thyroiditis is one of the most common autoimmune diseases in the United States with some estimates as high as 7% to 8% of the population, roughly 24 million individuals, and is the most common cause of hypothyroidism.[15] A retrospective cohort analysis of 1100 patients with newly diagnosed Hashimoto disease and 4609 non-Hashimoto controls in the Taiwan National Health Insurance Research Database reported that the risk of developing coronary heart disease (CHD) was significantly greater in women under 49 years with Hashimoto disease compared with controls. This increased risk was not observed in men. After adjusting for comorbidities, Hashimoto disease was an independent risk factor for CHD; however, the risk was enhanced when diagnosis was combined with hypertension or hyperlipidemia. Untreated Hashimoto disease or T4 treatment for less than 1 year carried the highest CHD risk[16] (Table 25.1).

CAVEATS OF LABORATORY TESTING

Serum levels of mineral are kept relatively constant. RBC mineral status can shed more light on the functional requirements of certain minerals.

When testing for iodine, urine is a best functional test and then serum; however, if serum levels are low, you can assume that total body levels are low. Also, serum is much more convenient than collecting a first morning void or a 24-hour urine sample for your patients.

Table 25.1

SUMMARY OF LABORATORY TESTS AVAILABLE FOR ASSESSMENT OF THYROID STATUS AND RELEVANT REFERENCE RANGES

Laboratory Test (These are Based on Laboratory Values From Quest Diagnostics)	Optimal Level	Normal Range
TSH	<2.5 mIU/L (consider <1.5 for AIT)	0.4-4.5 mIU/L
FT4	>1.2 ng/dL	0.8-1.8 ng/dL
TT4	>8 µg/dL	5.1-11.9 µg/dL
fT3	>3.0 pg/mL	2.3-4.2 pg/mL
TT3	>120 ng/dL	76-181 ng/dL
rT3	<20 ng/dL	8-25 ng/dL
TT3/rT3	>6	

- Iodine: serum >80 for Quest, >65 Labcorp
- Ferritin: serum >50-70
- Vitamin D: serum >50-70
- RBC selenium: >200 (>240 if supplementing with iodine)

AIT, amiodarone-induced thyrotoxicosis; FT3, free triiodothyonine; FT4, free thyroxine; RBC, red blood cell; rT3, reverse triiodothyronine TT3, total triiodothyonine; TT4, total thyroxine.

When performing urine iodine testing it is important to keep in mind that the kidneys excrete approximately 90% of ingested iodine. If a 24-hour urine collection is not practical, a random urinary iodine to creatinine ratio can be used instead. A medium of 50 to 100 μg of iodine per liter is considered mild iodine deficiency, 20 to 49 μg of iodine per liter is moderate deficiency, and less than 20 μg of iodine per liter signifies severe deficiency.[17]

Thyroid Influences on the Cardiovascular System

Thyroid hormones have pleiotropic effects on the cardiovascular system. Both hypothyroidism and hyperthyroidism are associated with increased cardiovascular risk markers as summarized in the following. Key aspects of risk will be examined in more detail later in this chapter.

- Hypothyroid[18]:
  - Impaired cardiac contractility and diastolic function
  - Systolic and diastolic congestive heart failure
  - Increased systemic vascular resistance
  - Diastolic hypertension
  - Decreased endothelial-derived relaxation factor
  - Dyslipidemia
  - Coronary heart disease and myocardial infarction
  - Increased C-reactive protein
  - Increased homocysteine
- Hyperthyroid[18]:
  - Palpitations
  - Coronary heart disease and angina
  - Exercise intolerance
  - Atrial fibrillation, atrial flutter, and premature atrial contractions (PACs)
  - Ventricular arrhythmias, premature ventricular contractions (PVCs), ventricular tachycardia, and fibrillation
  - Exertional dyspnea
  - Cardiac hypertrophy
  - Systolic hypertension
  - Peripheral edema
  - Hyperdynamic precordium
  - Congestive heart failure

Impact of Hypothyroidism on Lipid and Lipoprotein Metabolism

Thyroid hormones regulate lipid and lipoprotein metabolism and act as part of a system to regulate the balance between lipid synthesis and lipid clearance and degradation, helping to fine-tune the availability of lipids to meet the body's needs. Hypothyroidism has been linked with plasma cholesterol since the 1930s and was considered a marker for levothyroxine treatment response before assays for TSH and FT4 were readily available.[19] Hypothyroidism shifts the system to one favoring lipid synthesis over degradation and clearance, and this is reflected in a more atherogenic lipid profile.[20] Cross talk between these atherogenic lipid changes and other adverse

consequences of hypothyroidism, including obesity[21] and reduced antioxidant capacity,[22] contribute to an environment of increased cardiovascular risk.[1] The adverse changes in lipoprotein and lipid metabolism are summarized in **Table 25.2**. The general pattern observed is that lipid status worsens in parallel to rising TSH concentrations. Although lipid abnormalities are present with subclinical hypothyroidism, these become increasingly evident with progression to overt hypothyroidism.[20]

THYROID FUNCTION AND LOW-DENSITY LIPOPROTEIN METABOLISM

The lipid profile of hypothyroid patients is characterized by an increase in plasma total- and low-density lipoprotein (LDL)-cholesterol (LDL-C).[20] Some studies also report an increase in small dense LDL (sdLDL)[23] and higher levels of lipid peroxidation[24] and higher circulating oxidized LDL (oxLDL).[23,25] Published data on LDL particle number (LDL-P) in hypothyroidism are lacking. Thyroid hormone is known to stimulate the expression of the LDL receptor (LDL-R) in the liver via increasing SREBP-2 and/or by direct effects on LDL-R promoter sites.[26,27] Studies in model systems show that reduced signaling in hypothyroid states decreases the number of LDL-R in the liver[28] resulting in reduced clearance of LDL from circulation.[19] Additionally, levels of proprotein convertase subtilisin/kexin type 9 serine protease (PCSK9) are increased with hypothyroidism, but normalization of levels is observed by correction of thyroid status in humans.[29] In addition to regulating the LDL-R and clearance

Table 25.2

ADVERSE LIPID CHANGES REPORTED IN PATIENTS WITH HYPOTHYROIDISM

	Change With Hypothyroidism
Total cholesterol	Increased
LDL-C	Increased
sdLDL	Increased
oxLDL	Increased
apoB	Increased
Hepatic LDL receptor expression	Reduced
Lp(a)	Increased
Triglycerides	Normal to increased
Postprandial triglycerides	Increased
HDL-C	Normal to slight increase
HDL-2	Increased
Enzymes linked to HDL functionality	Reduced

apoB, apolipoprotein B; HDL-C, high-density lipoprotein cholesterol; LDL-C, low-density lipoprotein cholesterol; Lp(a), lipoprotein (a).

of LDL-C, thyroid hormone also reduces the production of apolipoprotein B (apoB), and loss of thyroid hormone signaling in hypothyroid states is associated with an increase in apoB production, which is reversed in humans with normalization of thyroid status.[29,30] The potential for impaired LDL clearance as a result of reduced expression of the LDL-R and upregulation of PCSK9, as well as the increased synthesis of apoB, is considered to underpin the increased LDL-C in circulation associated with hypothyroidism.

THYROID FUNCTION AND HIGH-DENSITY LIPOPROTEIN AND REVERSE CHOLESTEROL TRANSPORT

Hypothyroidism is not generally associated with a change in high-density lipoprotein cholesterol (HDL-C),[19] although differences in HDL composition are reported, notably an increase in HDL2 subparticles (the more protective form of HDL particles) and apo-A1.[31,32] This increase in HDL2 count can be reduced with treatment leading to euthyroidism. These changes in HDL particle number are thought to be related to induction of hepatic lipase (HL) enzyme by thyroid hormone. High HL activity is associated with small, dense LDL particles and with reduced HDL2 cholesterol levels seen in hyperthyroidsm.[33] The reduction in HDL2 during treatment correlates with an increase in the activity of HL during normalization of thyroid status in humans.[32] This relationship between reduced HL and increased HDL2 particles has been demonstrated in studies in other populations also.[33] Despite this apparent increase in protective HDL, other studies in animal models have shown that hypothyroidism can lead to an increase in oxidized LDL with a reduction in reverse cholesterol transport (RCT). Thyroid hormone is involved in the regulation of SR-B1, and treatment of hypothyroidism with thyroid hormone analogues in these models leads to upregulation of SR-B1 expression.[34] SR-B1 is an enzyme involved in the efflux of cholesterol from macrophages to HDL, a critical step in RCT.[34] The activity of paraoxonase-1 (PON-1), an enzyme associated with HDL in plasma involved in protecting against LDL oxidation and supporting HDL functionality, was shown to be reduced in both subclinical and overt hypothyroid patients compared with controls.[35,36] A study in patients who underwent thyroidectomy due to thyroid carcinoma demonstrated that cholesterol efflux capacity was reduced in the overt hypothyroid state and remained low with radioactive iodine therapy.[37] Further studies to understand the impact of hypothyroidism and reverse cholesterol transport and HDL function are needed; however, the evidence suggests that HDL functionality may be impaired in these patients.

THYROID HORMONE AND CHOLESTEROL ELIMINATION

A final step in reverse cholesterol transport can be considered the removal of cholesterol from the body through bile. Overall, thyroid hormone stimulates the conversion of cholesterol to bile acids in the liver, and therefore, the excretion of cholesterol from the liver, by increasing the expression of cholesterol 7 alpha hydroxylase (CYP7A1), the rate limiting enzyme in cholesterol breakdown and bile acid synthesis, and other transporters (ABCG5 and ABCG8) that promote the movement of cholesterol into bile.[19] Lack of thyroid hormone may reduce the breakdown and turnover of cholesterol in the liver and increase the cholesterol content of the liver.[20] Additionally, TSH itself has been reported to regulate hepatic lipid metabolism in model systems and may suppress bile acid synthesis,[38,39] although more in vivo evidence is needed. Although studies have cast doubt over the role of bile acid synthesis[19] changes driving the lipid abnormalities seen in human hypothyroidism,[40,41] reduced bile flow as evidenced by bile duct stone procedures and blockages in this patient cohort have been reported.[42,43]

THYROID FUNCTION AND TRIGLYCERIDES

Hypothyroidism is associated with an increase in plasma triglycerides in some studies, and postprandial hypertriglyceridemia, which is considered more atherogenic than fasting levels,[44,45] has been demonstrated to be increased, with one study showing that patients with TSH >5 mIU/L had a sevenfold increased risk of postprandial hypertriglyceridemia.[46] Apolipoprotein B48, a marker of intestinally derived triglycerides, was also increased in overt hypothyroidism compared with controls during the postprandial period.[47] These changes in triglyceride metabolism can compound issues with HDL and LDL metabolism discussed earlier. For example, hypertriglyceridemia can lead to reduced anti-inflammatory capacity of HDL[48] and reduced capacity for HDL to deliver cholesterol esters to hepatic cells.[49]

Some but not all studies have suggested that thyroid hormone stimulates lipoprotein lipase (LPL).[19] Reduced LPL could reduce the clearance of triglyceride-rich lipoproteins from circulation,[50] which may explain the increased postprandial triglyceridemia identified in hypothyroid states. Thyroid hormone also controls the release of VLDL-TG from the liver, and reduced thyroid hormone signaling in hypothyroidism increases hepatic VLDL-TG secretion, which can negatively impact plasma triglyceride concentration.[19] HL is sensitive to thyroid hormone status, and hypothyroidism is associated with a reduction in HL activity, which can be recovered by thyroid hormone replacement therapy.[34] A decline in HL activity can impair the chemical composition of isolated LDL particles owing to triglyceride enrichment.[20] In hypothyroidism, hypertriglyceridemia appears to develop as a result of impaired removal of endogenous triglyceride and increased hepatic production of triglyceride.[20]

Hypothyroidism is associated with, in addition to changes in synthesis and clearance, an accumulation of triglyceride within the liver, leading to an increased risk of nonalcoholic fatty liver disease and nonalcoholic steatohepatitis in this population.[51] Mechanistically, thyroid hormone enhances the activity of HLs, lipophagy, and mitochondrial biogenesis and oxidation of fatty acids, the primary processes utilized by the liver to reduce steatosis.[34] Therefore, a reduction in thyroid hormone signaling can impair the process by which triglyceride and fatty acids are metabolized and cleared from within the liver. Additionally, TSH itself may stimulate lipogenesis,[38] and in addition to T3 and T4, 3,5-diiodothyronine (T2) influences hepatic lipid metabolism through non-THR-mediated signaling.[34]

THYROID FUNCTION AND LP(a)

Lp(a) levels are seen to be increased in hypothyroid patients,[52,53] although the mechanisms are not fully understood. Lp(a) is higher in overt compared with subclinical hypothyroidism and controls and responds to T4 therapy.[52]

SUMMARY

Overall, the available data show that dyslipidemia is prevalent in hypothyroidism and that restoration of thyroid hormone levels improves lipid abnormalities.[19]

Physicians should check for hypothyroidism in patients with raised LDL. Hypothyroidism has been reported in 4.2% to 5.2% of patients with hyperlipidemia,[54-56] suggesting that thyroid failure may go undetected, and testing patients with hyperlipidemia for hypothyroidism is warranted to guide clinical intervention.[12,57-59] This may be in contrast to current clinical practices, as recent evidence suggests that, in newly diagnosed hyperlipidemia, only 50% of patients are typically screened for hypothyroidism.[55]

Studies have demonstrated that subclinical hypothyroidism is linked to a small increased risk of cardiovascular disease (CVD)[60,61] and coronary heart disease events and mortality,[62,63] particularly in younger patients (<50 years old),[63] those with TSH >10 mIU/L,[62] and those with increased cardiovascular risk.[60]

Although there are currently no randomized controlled trials to suggest that treatment with thyroid hormones will lead to reduced CV risk or dyslipidemia in individuals with subclinical hypothyroidism, given the data suggesting that correcting the thyroid hormone abnormality can lower biomarkers that carry an elevated CV risk, treatment may be warranted to prevent potential long-term risks.

Hypothyroidism and Heart Failure

Thyroid hormone plays a key role in the regulation of cardiac function and peripheral circulation, with thyroid hormone signaling impacting cardiovascular hemodynamics, cardiac filling, myocardial contractility, and systemic vascular resistance. Loss of thyroid hormone signaling and hypothyroidism is a risk factor for the development of heart failure. Prospective cohort studies in the United States and Europe demonstrate that the risk of heart failure events is increased in individuals with subclinical hypothyroidism, even after adjustment for other cardiovascular risk factors.[64] In patients with heart failure, the presence of hypothyroidism (including subclinical hypothyroidism) is associated with an increased risk of all-cause mortality and cardiac mortality and/or hospitalization compared with euthyroid patients with heart failure.[65] TSH has been associated with progression of heart failure in patients with condition, and patients with modestly increased TSH above 5.5mIU/L were at greater risk of heart failure progression (defined as mortality after hospitalization or transplant).[66]

As stated earlier, thyroid hormone has a wide-ranging impact on the heart and vasculature. In the heart, thyroid hormone drives a gene expression program that regulates aspects

of contraction and relaxation. Thyroid hormone increases the expression of the gene encoding cardiac myosin heavy chain-alpha (MHCα) and reduces the expression of the gene encoding the beta isoform MHCβ, leading to an enhanced velocity of contraction.[67] The upregulation of β-1 adrenergic receptor gene expression is also involved in enhancing contraction velocity, as well as in increasing the heart rate.[67] Thyroid hormone signaling leads to upregulation of SERCA2, a calcium pump involved in muscle relaxation, and leads to downregulation of the SERCA2 inhibitor phospholamban (PLN), leading to an overall increase in the velocity of the diastolic relaxation.[67] Additionally, thyroid hormone suppresses cardiac fibrosis through a combination of downregulating collagen gene expression and upregulating metalloproteinases and upregulates the expression of Na/K-transporting ATPases.[67]

Thyroid hormone signaling contributes to reduced systemic vascular resistance and upregulating the expression of a number of molecules and pathways involved in vasodilation in the endothelial and vascular smooth muscle cells of the vasculature. Thyroid hormone actives nitric oxide synthase in vascular smooth muscle cells,[68] and endothelial nitric oxide is also thought to play a role in thyroid hormone–induced vasodilation.[69] In animal models, T3 increased adrenomedullin, a vasodilatory peptide,[70,71] and has also been shown to increase other vasodilatory molecules.[72,73]

The cardiac changes observed in hypothyroid states are summarized in **Table 25.3**. In subclinical hypothyroidism, the abnormalities in cardiac function observed are the same but less severe than those showed in the overt form.

A decrease in signaling of many of the known thyroid hormone direct and indirect targets have been demonstrated in animal models of hypothyroidism. Several studies have demonstrated these mechanisms in humans also. For example, the expression of the gene encoding MHCα was shown to be reduced and expression of the gene encoding MHCβ

Table 25.3

SUMMARY OF CARDIAC CHANGES IN HYPOTHYROID STATES[67]

Cardiac output	Reduced
Heart rate	Reduced
Contractility	Reduced
Diastolic function	Impaired
Systolic function	Impaired particularly with exercise
Systemic vascular resistance	Increased
Nitric oxide	Reduced
Carotid intima-media thickness	Increased
Diastolic blood pressure	Increased
Cardiac fibrosis	Present

was increased in human cardiac tissue from a patient with hypothyroidism and heart failure, and these gene expression changes as well as cardiac function were reversed with restoration of euthyroid.[74] Endothelium-derived NO has also been shown to be impaired in patients with hypothyroidism[75] and improves with thyroid hormone replacement.[76,77]

HYPOTHYROIDISM, CARDIAC REMODELING AND REACTIVATION OF A FETAL GENE EXPRESSION PROGRAM

One interesting finding related to hypothyroidism-related heart failure is the reactivation of a fetal gene expression pattern and how this contributes to reduced cardiac function.[78]

Cardiac remodeling can occur in response to stressors such as ischemia, mechanical loading, and metabolic alterations. Initially this response helps to maintain cardiac function and creates a low-energy state, which is thought to protect the damaged myocardium. However, over time a sustained remodeling response is viewed as maladaptive, leading to a decline in cardiac function.[78] One of the characteristics of this stress-induced remodeling is a dedifferentiation of cardiac cells driven by a reactivation of a "fetal gene expression program." Indeed, this initially adaptive and protective dedifferentiation in response to stress is thought to be a prerequisite for regeneration after stress.[79] However, a redifferentiation "deficit" may result in heart failure, and particularly thyroid deficit-related heart failure.[78] Pathways controlling dedifferentiation and redifferentiation in response to stress appear to be at least in part driven by thyroid hormone. The thyroid hormone system is an ancestral hormone system and plays a role in tissue remodeling after injury in many tissues and species, including in cardiac dedifferentiation/redifferentiation following stress.[78] This was shown clearly in experiments that inhibited thyroid hormone signaling in cardiomyocytes, leading to dedifferentiation and a switch to a fetal pattern of gene expression, including myosin isoform expression (increase in MHC-β).[80-82] However, importantly these cells retain the ability to redifferentiate with T3 treatment.[81]

LOW-T3 SYNDROME AND HEART FAILURE

Altered thyroid hormone bioavailability has been documented in cardiac patients with thyroid disorders. This is most commonly seen as reduced T3 and an increase in rT3 (inactive metabolite) with normal or low TSH. This low-T3 syndrome (also known as euthyroid sick syndrome or nonthyroid illness syndrome) is considered a coordinated systemic reactions to illness and has been reported in 20% to 30% of patients with heart failure.[83-85] Low-T3 syndrome negatively impacts prognosis for patients following myocardial infarction and coronary bypass surgery and during the progression of heart failure.[86,87] Altered peripheral thyroid hormone bioavailability is associated with a high incidence of cardiac events and a greater risk of heart transplantation.[83,84,88,89] The precise mechanisms of low-T3 syndrome are not known; however, alterations in enzyme activity involved in T4 to T3 conversion and T3 to rT3 conversion,[78] in addition to change in TSH or TRH section, or in thyroid hormone binding or transport into tissues have all been implicated.[67]

LOCAL CARDIAC HYPOTHYROIDISM IN HEART FAILURE

Hypothyroidism can also occur locally in the heart during heart failure, independent of serum levels of thyroid hormones, and LV function appears to be more closely related to thyroid cardiac levels than serum thyroid hormone levels in heart failure.[67] Several mechanisms have been suggested to explain the change in local thyroid hormone concentrations, and upregulation of D3 in heart failure, reduction in uptake of thyroid hormone into tissue, change in TH receptor expression within cardiomyocytes have all been implicated in local reduction in thyroid hormone and signaling in heart failure.[67]

SUMMARY

AHA/ACC Guidelines for the Diagnosis and Management of Heart Failure in Adults recommend that thyroid function tests be evaluated in all newly presenting patients with heart failure, and whether determining the cause of heart failure, that current and history of thyroid disorder be evaluated. Thyroid disorders should be treated. Reevaluation of thyroid function should be triggered by any new atrial fibrillation or exacerbation of ventricular arrhythmias.[90]

Clinical studies suggest TH supplementation may improve cardiac function in heart failure.[67]

Hyperthyroid and Hypertension

The impact of thyroid hormone on vascular resistance discussed earlier in addition to the positive inotropic effect and increased heart rate can lead to enhanced cardiac output commonly seen in patients with hyperthyroidism.[1] Additionally, the impact of thyroid hormones on the renin-angiotensin-aldosterone system is also related to cardiac output. Thyroid hormones reduce vascular resistance, which stimulates renin release and sodium reabsorption, leading to increased venous return to the heart and an increase in blood volume of 5.5%,[1,91] and ultimately an increase in cardiac output, which can be up to 300% higher in patients with overt hyperthyroidism.[92]

These hemodynamic changes can increase systolic blood pressure,[92] and studies indicate that patients with hyperthyroidism have significantly higher systolic blood pressure compared with euthyroid controls.[93-95] Systolic blood pressure, as well as cardiac output, is reduced with antithyroid treatment.[95] Blunted nocturnal decline in blood pressure has also been reported in some small studies to occur in hyperthyroid states.[96-98] In contrast to the blood pressure changes that occur in overt hyperthyroidism, studies have generally indicated that subclinical hyperthyroidism does not increase the risk of hypertension.[99]

Pulmonary hypertension has been reported in 35% to 65% of hyperthyroid individuals[100-103] and can be corrected following total thyroidectomy.[104] Pulmonary hypertension that occurs in thyroid disorders is considered to have unclear and/or multifactorial mechanisms.[105] Despite the pathogenic mechanisms being unknown, several hypotheses have been outlined. First, the increase in cardiac output and elevated circulatory volume lead to an increased and rapid venous return to the right ventricle causing pressure overload and consequent increase in pulmonary arterial pressure. This hemodynamic stress can cause endothelium shear stress within the pulmonary system, creating endothelial dysfunction and downstream vasoconstriction in pulmonary beds.[106] Direct action of thyroid hormones on pulmonary vascular system has been demonstrated,[107,108] and pulmonary vascular remodeling in hyperthyroid states promoting pulmonary hypertension has been suggested.[106] Second, an autoimmunity-induced pulmonary hypertension has been proposed. Levels of TSH receptor antibodies in Graves disease (which accounts for up to 80% of hyperthyroid cases[109]) have been shown to be positively associated with pulmonary arterial pressure,[102] and vascular endothelial changes secondary to the autoimmune inflammatory environment have been proposed to play a role in the development of pulmonary hypertension.[110] More clinical studies are needed in individuals diagnosed with hypertension or pulmonary hypertension to further understand the specific causes.

The hemodynamic changes that occur with thyroid hormone excess if left untreated can negatively influence cardiac morphology and function. Long-term hyperthyroidism can lead to left ventricle hypertrophy, arterial stiffness, and reduced diastolic function and left ventricle performance.[111] Exercise intolerance, a sign that the heart cannot further accommodate the increased cardiac demand required in physical activity, can be considered one of the primary signs of heart failure in hyperthyroidism.[111] These changes in cardiac performance can couple with the loss of sinus rhythm (discussed later) to increase the risk and progression of heart failure in these patients. Hyperthyroidism (overt and subclinical) is associated with an increased risk of heart failure, but the degree of heart failure is influenced by other factors including age, duration and cause of hyperthyroidism, and the presence of other cardiovascular risk markers.[111]

Hyperthyroid and Sinus Tachycardia and Atrial Fibrillation

The inotropic and chronotropic effects of thyroid hormones on the heart, in addition to the negative impact of thyroid hormone excess on vascular function overtime, can lead to rhythm disturbances.

Sinus tachycardia is the most common rhythm disturbance seen in hyperthyroid patients[112,113] but can be overshadowed clinically by an increased risk of atrial fibrillation.

Hyperthyroidism increases the risk of atrial fibrillation,[114] and the overall prevalence of atrial fibrillation in hyperthyroidism has been reported at 13.8% (compared with 2.3% of a control euthyroid population).[113] The risk of developing atrial fibrillation in hyperthyroidism is increased in men, older people, and those with coexistent CVD diagnosis.[115] Several studies show a positive correlation between plasma T4 and atrial fibrillation risk,[1] and patients treated with levothyroxine causing exogenous subclinical hyperthyroidism have an increased risk of dysrhythmic events.[1] Treatment to normalize thyroid hormone levels reverses atrial fibrillation.[1] Atrial fibrillation in hyperthyroid patients increases the risk of developing cerebrovascular and pulmonary embolism.[111]

Treatment for Thyroid Disorders

Thyroid Replacement Therapy

Almost all negative impacts on the cardiovascular system can be improved by correcting low thyroid hormone levels. The addition of T4 for hypothyroidism, and TPO or deiodinase inhibitors (such as methimazole or propylthiouracil) for treatment of hyperthyroidism, is a common treatment. However, treating the system of thyroid dysfunction, such as with T3, nutritional support (with diet and nutritional supplements), as well as avoiding and eliminating environmental toxins and heavy metals can more holistically support thyroid status and function and the cardiovascular system as well.

For the past 80 years, levothyroxine (L-T4) has been the primary source for thyroid replacement therapy. With the inception of commercial TSH testing, levothyroxine has been dosed to get TSH levels in the normal range versus treating clinic symptoms of hypothyroidism. T4 stimulates myocardial metabolism increasing oxygen demand, which can in some susceptible older individuals carry a small risk of inducing cardiac arrhythmias, angina pectoris, or myocardial infarction. A study from 1961 of the effects of initiating thyroid hormone on hypothyroid patients with angina found improvements in chest pain in up to 40% of patients.[116,117] Other studies suggest an increased risk of hospitalization with ischemic heart disease due to poorly treated hypothyroidism as evidenced by suboptimal TSH levels in those admitted. Therefore, appropriate use of T4 therapy may decrease angina as well as the risk for ischemic cardiac events requiring hospitalization.

As discussed earlier, circulating T4 has a negative feedback on the hypothalamus decreasing TSH production; however, it does not impact the conversion of T4 to T3 intracellularly. Therefore, it is a poor choice for treating nonthyroid illness caused by chronic diseases or low T3 syndrome as manifested by a poor T3/rT3 ratio. Utilizing liothyronine or a combination treatment of T4/T3 with a synthetic or natural desiccated thyroid glandular may be a better treatment of poor conversion of T4 to T3.

Liothyronine (L-T3) comes in 5 and 25 μg doses and is easily absorbed and, unlike its predecessor, does not require to be taken on an empty stomach. Although its drug label suggests that its half-life is 18 hours, clinically it seems to reach a peak within 6 to 8 hours after intake. Therefore, this author and others in the integrative world have found twice and thrice a day dosing to be more effective than once daily dosing. Strictly using L-T3 therapy has been helpful at lowering rT3 levels by inducing D1 activity to convert more rT3 to T2. L-T4 can also be used in combination with L-T3 to more readily mimic physiological levels, which are believed to be at a 13:1 to 20:1 ratio according to the European Thyroid association.[118]

Natural desiccated thyroid (NDT) is standardized to 38 μg T4 and 9 μg of T3 per gram (60 or 65 mg depending on brand). Owing to reports of fluctuating dosages of T4 and T3 from refill to refill, NDT is not recommended by most Endocrinology or Thyroid societies. However, most prescription brands (Armour, Nature-throid, NP Thyroid) have been meeting US Pharmacopeia guidelines for over 100 years. When converting from L-T4 to NDT the standard of 100 µg = 1 g is typically used. There are not any good head-to-head studies showing superiority of NDT to LT4 therapy in the literature currently. However, in a small study published in the *Journal of Clinical Metabolism* in 2013 and posted on the American Thyroid Association website, NDT appeared to be at least as effective as L-T4 for symptoms and neurocognitive outcomes, as there was no significant different between the treatments for these variables. About 49% of the 70 patients who tried both L-T4 and NDT preferred NDT over L-T4 therapy, with 23% stating no preference. The authors concluded that the small amount of weight loss (3 lbs on average) seen while taking NDT versus L-T4 may have led to the preference. Subjects reported great improvements in their subjective assessment of symptoms of hypothyroidism while taking the NDT.[119]

TARGETED NUTRITIONAL SUPPLEMENTS

The following nutrients have been identified as essential or play a role in the production of thyroid hormones, enhancing cellular sensitivity, as well as in the production and upregulation of the D1 and D2 enzymes that enhance the conversion of T4 to T3. These include but are not limited to iodine, tyrosine, selenium, zinc, iron, and the fat-soluble vitamins (retinoic acid, calcifediol, and alpha-tocopherol), as well as ascorbate, riboflavin, niacin, and pyridoxine. When it comes to reviewing the literature to identify the effectiveness of supplementation with these nutrients to influence thyroid metabolism and hormone balance, the literature is sparse at best. It must be kept in mind that, although the studies that will be reviewed are suggestive and trend toward a positive influence, they are small and not definitive.

SELENIUM

The thyroid gland contains the highest concentration of selenium in the body. It plays an essential role in thyroid hormone metabolism because three enzymes produced in large quantity by the thyroid gland are selenoproteins: the deiodinases, thioredoxin reductase, and glutathione peroxidase. Glutathione peroxidase helps in dealing with oxidative stress within the thyroid gland as well as metabolizing pesticides and helping to clear mercury, chlorine, and bromine, two halogens that compete for iodine-binding sites, disrupting thyroid synthesis. Thioredoxin reductase is a potent antioxidant enzyme that also helps with reducing oxidative influences on the thyroid and regulating the gene expression of certain inflammatory proteins, such as NF-κb. Selenium and iodine together help to regulate certain immune cells involved in the development of thyroid autoimmune disease.[120-122]

Studies done on populations with iodine and selenium deficiency seem to suggest that indiscriminate supplementation of iodine-deficient individuals with iodine can only trigger autoimmune thyroiditis and goiter formation. However, when selenium supplementation is added to iodine in hypothyroid

subjects there is a reduction in inflammation of the thyroid gland, which may lead to a diminution of an iodine-deficient goiter. A review published in 2013 demonstrated that selenium supplementation reduced both thyroglobulin antibodies and TPO antibodies in treated patients (supplementation ranged from 40 to 200 µg/d).[123] There seemed to be an inverse relationship to serum selenium levels and TPO antibodies.[123-125]

ZINC

Zinc also plays a role in optimizing thyroid function. There is evidence to suggest that impaired zinc and/or selenium levels may contribute to a low T3/T4 ratio. Supplementation with both zinc and selenium was associated with modest changes in thyroid hormones, with an earlier normalization of T4 and rT3 plasma levels.[126,127]

The D2 enzyme is a zinc-rich protein. Therefore, zinc deficiency may lead to elevated levels of serum rT3. In a small study of 134 individuals, those with mild to moderate zinc deficiency were treated with oral zinc sulfate at 4 to 10 mg per kilogram of body weight for 12 months. It appears that zinc plays a role in T4 to T3 conversion as both serum fT3 and T3 levels normalized as well as serum rT3 levels reduced. In a more recent study in overweight or obese hypothyroid patients, zinc ± selenium supplementation led to an increase in fT3 levels and the fT3:fT4 ratio compared with placebo. rT3 was not checked in this study. Therefore, zinc supplementation should be considered in low T3 syndrome or nonthyroid illnesses.[128,129]

IODINE

When comparing the National Health and Nutrition Examination Survey (NHANES) data from 1971 with the NHANES III from 1994, an American's median urinary iodine concentration decreased by 50%. The number of Americans that met the threshold of iodine deficiency as defined by the World Health Organization (WHO) based on urinary excretion levels (<100 µg/L) increased by 4.5-fold during this same period. Monitoring of high-risk groups showed that 6.7% of pregnant women and 14.9% of women of childbearing age had a urine excretory level of less than the WHO threshold of severe iodine deficiency (<50 µg/L). Since NHANES III the number of deficient Americans has stabilized but has not improved, with severe iodine deficiency occurring in approximately 9% of the population and mild or greater levels of iodine deficiency occurring in close to 50% of the population.[130,131]

This is similar to what the author has seen in his practice when a review was done on 255 patients with serum testing of iodine from July to December 2014. Of the 255 tests ordered, 133 or 57% were abnormally low (<52, Quest Diagnostic laboratories normal range 52-109). There were 214 or 90% that were considered suboptimal (<80). In 2016, another review was repeated, this time on 442 patients with tests ordered over 12 months with similar results, 277 were abnormally low for 63%, with 427 considered suboptimal accounting for approximately 97% of all tests ordered. It is clear that despite living in a first world country with all of the nutritional benefits available we are still not obtaining adequate iodine intake. This becomes problematic because a majority of cases of overt hypothyroidism are now associated with AIT possibly triggered by an excess of iodine intake in iodine-deficient populations. In fact, hypothyroidism has been shown to be associated with both diets high and low in iodine. Studies have demonstrated that both low and high urinary iodine excretion is associated with hypothyroidism. So the question does iodine cause hypothyroidism and/or AIT is a tough one to answer. The jury is still out.[132,133]

Multiple population studies have demonstrated that, when iodine is introduced to iodine-deficient populations, there is a sudden surge in autoimmune thyroid cases. However, in those studies, selenium was neither tested for nor provided as a supplement. Because selenium has such an important role in combating oxidative stress and modulating immune balance, it is likely that any iodine supplementation given without controlling for adequate selenium levels is problematic and can trigger an autoimmune response on the thyroid gland. Based on the results of the aforementioned selenium studies, plus or minus iodine supplementation, there were improvements in thyroid antibody levels. There are no current studies that have analyzed a randomized controlled experiment with iodine in conjunction with selenium treatment in iodine-deficient populations and its prevalence of autoimmune thyroiditis. The literature is also lacking in any published data analyzing randomized control studies of treating patients with autoimmune thyroiditis with iodine ± selenium and placebo to determine its impact on anti-TG and TPO antibody levels. It is the expert opinion of this author that iodine supplementation should only be given in conjunction with adequate selenium supplementation to protect the thyroid gland from immune dysregulation.[134-137]

HYPERTHYROID AND IODINE

Although propylthiouracil or methimazole continue to be the mainstay of treatment of hyperthyroidism, according to secondary sources, iodine can serve as an adjunct to these prescription drug inhibitors of thyroid function. A saturated solution of potassium iodide, 1 to 5 drops by mouth every 8 hours, or Lugol solution (8 mg of potassium iodide per drop) 2 to 6 drops (1 mL) every 8 hours, has been used with some efficacy to suppress thyroid storm. Lower doses may be used in pregnancy as well.[138]

IRON

Thyroid peroxidase (TPO) is a heme-dependent enzyme; iron deficiency can negatively impact thyroid hormone synthesis owing to a reduction in its activity. Iron deficiency anemia also blunts the efficacy of iodine supplementation. Thyroid function appears to be affected by lower erythrocyte indices caused by low serum iron concentrations leading to small fluctuations in T4/T3 levels. Iron levels were below normal in individuals with subclinical hypothyroidism compared with euthyroid subjects.[122,139]

TYROSINE

Tyrosine seems like an obvious choice for a nutritional supplement to augment thyroid function, but the literature is almost nonexistent in evidence supporting its use for thyroid function. Tyrosine is an amino acid made from phenylalanine and is not only a building block for epinephrine, norepinephrine, and dopamine but also part of the thyroglobulin structure in the thyroid colloid where it binds with iodine to make mono- and diiodothyronine. It is rare to be deficient in tyrosine. However, depletion of tyrosine and phenylalanine led to reduction in plasma T4 and T3, and re-supplementation with tyrosine, in combination with phenylalanine, led to a rapid increase in serum T3, rT3, T4, and freeT4.[140]

FAT-SOLUBLE VITAMINS

Like T3, vitamin A in its active form of retinoic acid and vitamin D in its active form, 1, 25-dihydroxycholecalciferol, exert their effect on gene expression by binding to nuclear receptors. Research suggests that vitamin A may provide a functional support role that may contribute to the regulation of the responsiveness of the genetic binding sites for thyroid hormone. Factors that either lead to vitamin A insufficiency or prevent the conversion of vitamin A to retinoic acid may result in reduced thyroid nuclear signaling.[141,142] The prevalence of vitamin D deficiency was significantly higher in patients with autoimmune thyroiditis compared with healthy individuals. Significantly low levels of vitamin D were documented in patients with autoimmune thyroiditis that were related to the presence of antithyroid antibodies and abnormal thyroid function tests, suggesting the possibility of involvement of vitamin D in the pathogenesis of autoimmune thyroiditis and the advisability of supplementation. In one study, poor vitamin D status was found to play a role in thyroid follicular oncogenesis.[143,144]

VITAMIN SUPPLEMENTATION SUMMARY

Although there seems to be some evidence suggesting the role and evidence for nutritional supplementation for improving overall thyroid function, the evidence is sparse at best for making recommendations on dosing as there are not any placebo-controlled studies of the best dosing schedule for nutrients involved in thyroid metabolism. **Table 25.4** lists the possible nutritional supplement dosing based on expert opinion. Because the all dosing suggestions appear to be safe the potential for benefit drives the recommendation; however, the efficacy is still in question owing to lack of evidence.

Dietary and Lifestyle Influences

CALORIC INTAKE AND DIETARY COMPOSITION

Diet can influence the functionality of thyroid hormone. In very-low-calorie restricted diets (0-500 kcal per day), serum T3 concentrations decrease as a consequence of its reduced production rate from peripheral deiodination of T4. Serum rT3 concentrations markedly increased as a result of its

Table 25.4

EXPERT OPINION RECOMMENDATIONS FOR MICRONUTRIENT SUPPLEMENTATION IN THYROID DISORDERS

Nutrient	Dosing
Iodine (mix of iodine/iodide)	150-6000 µg
Selenium (selenomethionine)	150-300 µg
Zinc	15 -60 mg
Iron bisglycinate	30 -65 mg
Vitamin A (retinyl palmitate)	25,000 IU
Vitamin D$_3$	2000-5000 IU

decreased metabolic clearance rate. During caloric restriction and overeating, serum T4 concentrations and its production and degradation do not appear to be modified. Thus the metabolic changes associated with profound caloric restriction appear to be associated with intracellular changes in deiodinase activity leading to increases in the T4/T3 ratio and elevations in rT3 levels. These effects appear to be related to carbohydrate content as T3 levels are not as affected during an isocaloric diet with adequate carbohydrate compared with a no-carbohydrate diet. This correlation of low T3 with a no-carbohydrate diet seems to be influenced more by blood glucose levels and ketones than by insulin or glucagon changes.[145-147]

Diets rich in minerals, antioxidants, and fat cyber vitamins appear to have the greatest influence on healthy thyroid metabolism. Although there are concerns about consumption of goitrogenic foods (foods that have the potential for increasing thyroid size), most of the studies have been done in animals and with large quantities of brassica vegetables or soy protein. A well-balanced plant-based diet will provide the most benefit at reducing and preventing thyroid disorders.

STRESS

There is a link between the endocrinology of stress response and thyroid function and availability. Circulating cortisol levels are positively correlated with TSH even in healthy young men and women.[148] Recently, hair cortisol levels were shown to be higher in hypothyroid patients compared with euthyroid control.[149] The influence of cortisol on thyroid hormone metabolism was seen more clearly in patients with hypocorticism. In this patient group, T4 was lower and T3 was higher. Furthermore, rT3 was significantly decreased, indicating that cortisol may play a role in the peripheral T4 to T3 conversion and in T4 to rT3 conversion.[150] Similarly, a study administering adrenocorticotropic hormone (ACTH) to induce endogenous glucocorticoid hypersecretion showed an increase in serum rT3.[151]

PHYSICAL ACTIVITY

Thyroid hormone influences skeletal muscle metabolism, for example, by increasing basal and insulin-stimulated glucose transport, oxidative phosphorylation, and Na$^+$/K$^+$-ATPase expression. Some studies show that serum levels of thyroid hormone are increased during physical activity,[152,153] and recent more mechanistic work showed that physical activity increased the expression of thyroid receptor beta 1 expression in skeletal muscle and enhanced the sensitivity of TH target genes to T3 treatment.[154]

Exercise promotes improved thyroid gland secretion mostly from positive influences on the pituitary, can enhance tissue sensitivity to thyroid hormone. and is well known for its stress relieving effects on the HPTA axis. Because of the many benefits of both weight training (which builds muscle mass) and aerobic exercise (which improves the body's use of oxygen) on the system as a whole, exercise is always recommend as part of lifestyle modifications for enhancing thyroid function.

Future Challenges

- Better optimization of low T3 syndrome or nonthyroid disease with use of T3 and NDT to drive increased intracellular levels of T3 and reduced rT3 levels.
- Identification of genetic influences such as polymorphisms for deiodinases that can influence intracellular levels of T3.
- Development of biomarkers that capture intracellular T3 stats, independent of circulating thyroid hormone status.
- Better understanding of influences of environmental hormone disruptors and their impact on thyroid function, specifically as it relates to the cardiovascular system.
- Testing for impact of iodine in combination with selenium for autoimmune thyroiditis.

Signs and Symptoms of Adrenal Gland Dysfunction

Preface

Before starting on the adrenal function and its impact on the cardiovascular system, I just wanted to share that this chapter is based on the bias and opinions of its authors. There is a lot that we still do not understand about how the adrenal hormones affect the cardiovascular system. And there is a lot of room for interpretation, and you will come across conflicting opinions. Do not get discouraged. It is imperative, therefore, that the information that is learned from this chapter be taken into consideration and then placed into context of your evaluation with your patient who sits in front of you. And please do not attempt to implement a specific protocol or an algorithm or a laboratory test to your specific patient's situation. Every patient is unique, and has his or her own genetic expression. Therefore, it is important that you understand the concepts discussed in this chapter (and the other ones for that matter) so that you can apply them while looking at the interaction of all the systems within your patient to best try and create a balance to that particular individual. Although we will discuss different nutritional supplements as well as specific hormones, it should not be assumed that this will be a complete fix for the individual patient. If you have or can gain an appreciation for the intricate hormonal web that is within the endocrine system and how each hormone relates and interacts with the other hormones, glands, and systems with the body, and relate that to the goal of influencing a balance within the system, then we will have done our job.

The other part of the HPAT access is the adrenal gland. Like the thyroid and sex hormones, adrenal hormones are influenced by the negative and positive feedback mechanisms that inhibit or stimulate the hypothalamus. The adrenal gland, pituitary, and hypothalamus constitute a major neuroendocrine system[155] that controls reactions to stress. It helps in regulating many systems within the body, to include digestion, the immune system, mood and emotions, sexuality, and energy storage and expenditure. Most important for this chapter is its influence on the cardiovascular system. It is the common mechanism for interactions among glands, hormones, and parts of the midbrain that mediate the general adaptation syndrome (GAS) introduced by Hans Selye.[156] As there is another chapter in this textbook that will focus on the influence of stress and its impact on the cardiovascular system, this chapter will focus mostly on the hormones released from the adrenal glands and their influence on the cardiovascular system either directly or indirectly.

When in balance, the adrenal gland provides an amazing adaptability to stressful demands placed on the body. This adaptation allows the body to be in a very relaxed, rebuilding state (most often at night during sleep) or in a hyper alert state known as the "flight or fight" response. This prepares the individual to react in an immediate way to increase survivability. However, a prolonged stimulus can lead to an imbalance or dysfunction of the HPAT axis, placing the adrenal gland and thyroid gland in an overactive state. Initially, elevations in glucocorticoids such as cortisol, catecholamines such as epinephrine and norepinephrine, as well as androgens such as dehydroepiandrosterone (DHEA) are observed. This early or arousal stage may last for a few days or months depending on the individual's epigenetic makeup and is similar in what is seen in Cushing syndrome symptomatically. However, unlike in Cushing syndrome, which is often caused by a secretory neoplasm in the pituitary or adrenal gland and is characterized by hypersecretion of glucocorticoids and catecholamines, the adrenal glands continue to adapt to this overactive state from the persistent stressful stimulus. A drop in DHEA production is followed by fluctuations in catecholamines with a persistently elevated cortisol level.[157] This often starts a significant change in mood stability with fluctuations between anxiety and depression. With no recovery available, the persistent demands on adrenal gland production of hormones leads to a flat-line in the production of ACTH and development of secondary adrenal insufficiency.[158] This differs from primary adrenal insufficiency or Addison disease whereby secretion of both cortisol

and aldosterone is lost owing to destruction of the adrenal cortex due to cancer, autoimmunity, infections, or hemorrhage. In secondary adrenal failure or adrenal insufficiency aldosterone secretion is largely intact.[159]

Signs and Symptoms of Adrenal Dysfunction

Symptoms associated with an overactive or hyperstimulated adrenal gland (which leads to increased circulatory levels of adrenaline and cortisol ± DHEA) include:
- Irritability (particularly when hungry) and anxiety
- Night sweats
- Muscle tremors
- Insomnia with or without sleep disturbances
- Hot flashes
- Shakiness between meals with or without sugar cravings
- Headaches
- Muscle aches and pains
- Weight loss
- Frequent bowel movements
- Heart palpitations

Symptoms associated with underactivity or insufficient adrenal gland function (leading to lower levels of circulating cortisol, DHEA, and adrenaline) include:
- Fatigue (typically in the mornings or late afternoons but not all day)
- Low energy
- Increased susceptibility to viral and fungal infections
- Centripetal weight gain
- Depression
- Insomnia with early morning awakenings and nonrestorative sleep
- Slow repair of injuries and wounds
- Dizziness/lightheadedness

Adrenal Physiology and Metabolism

The hypothalamus influence on the adrenal gland, however, can be divided into two parts, the endocrine and the neuroendocrine or autonomic pathways. The endocrine part of the hypothalamus influences the adrenal cortex by producing and releasing corticotropin releasing hormone (CRH) and vasopressin, also known as antidiuretic hormone (ADH).

Although ADH has most of its influence on circulatory volume homeostasis through water reabsorption, its activation by stress and the neuromodulatory influences of the amygdala, hippocampus, and prefrontal cortex on its release from the hypothalamus may play an important role in social behavior, sexual motivation, and pair bonding,[160] as well as possibly leading to induction and differentiation of stem cells into cardiomyocytes promoting heart muscle homeostasis.[161] This influences the release of ACTH from the anterior pituitary. ACTH stimulates all three zones of the adrenal cortex, each releasing a different hormone. The three zones are known as the zona glomerulosa, which releases the mineralocorticoid aldosterone; the zona fasciculata, which releases the glucocorticoids cortisone, deoxycorticosterone, and corticosterone; and lastly the zona reticularis, which produces androgens, including DHEA and DHEA sulfate (DHEAS).

The neuroendocrine pathway works through the sympathetic nervous system (SNS) where it activates the adrenal medulla to release adrenaline or epinephrine. The adrenal glands are responsible for a large majority of the adrenaline that circulates in the body but only for a small percentage of the circulating noradrenaline. Adrenaline and noradrenaline act at adrenoreceptors throughout the body, with effects that include an increase in blood pressure and heart rate.[162] Levels of adrenaline and noradrenaline influence the body's fight or flight response, characterized by a rapid increase in breathing and heart rate, as well as an elevation in blood pressure secondary to constriction of blood vessels in multiple parts of the body. Therefore, this response, which acts primarily on the cardiovascular system, is mediated directly via signals transmitted through the sympathetic nervous system and indirectly via catecholamines secreted from the adrenal medulla.[163]

The following are triggers of the HPA system that lead to an elevation in circulatory cortisol: physical and/or psychological stressors, such as prenatal and/or early childhood trauma; biological toxins that include infections from microbes such as bacteria, yeast, parasites, and mold; environmental and synthetic toxins such as persistent organic pollutants, pesticides, heavy metals; genetic or other factors leading to impaired detoxification pathways (eg, alcohol); persistent exposure to allergens from food, mold, dust, animal products, pollens, and chemicals; as well as a nutritional-insufficient and caloric-excessive diet (**Figure 25.1**).

There are multiple factors that can stimulate the SNS to cause release of adrenaline, but all are a result of stress on the physiological, emotional, or physical state of the body. These include but are not limited to lack of sleep, rapid changes in blood sugar such as hypoglycemia, heat and cold changes, pain, physical trauma such as life-threatening accidents, war, and attacks by others. Emotional responses to fear particularly, and to a lesser extent to anger and frustration as the evidence is not as strong, are direct triggers of adrenaline release via the SNS.[164] Environmental triggers include sympathomimetic drugs or chemicals, such as cocaine and amphetamines, as well as the natural occurring ephedrine found in the Ephedra plant. Another natural stimulant, caffeine, exerts its influence mostly through blocking the breakdown of cyclic adenosine monophosphate (cAMP) by inhibiting phosphodiesterase and can enhance the adrenergic effects of adrenaline.[165] The half-life of epinephrine is approximately 2 minutes. The effect of epinephrine and norepinephrine on the cardiovascular system is mediated through alpha- and beta-adrenergic receptors (ARs). Even dopamine at higher levels activates ARs. Catecholamines increase the heart rate and contractility via β-1Ars; increase in venous return and increase in peripheral resistance are a result of α-AR activation, especially those in the subcutaneous, mucosal, and splenic and renal vascular beds.

Modulation of fluid and electrolytes via reabsorption in the gut (mostly the colon), kidneys, and gallbladder is also an α-AR-mediated response. Metabolically, βAR-mediated glycogenolysis and lipolysis increases fuel sources for the body. Increases in diet-induced and nonshivering thermogenesis occurs via βARs.

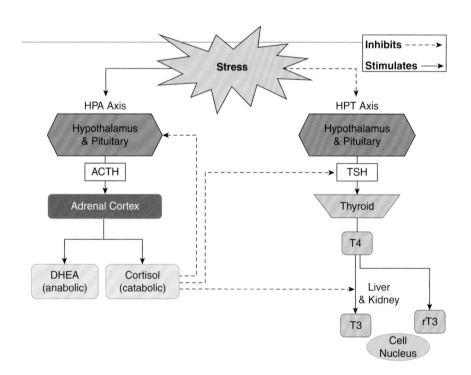

Figure 25.1 *Overview of the impact of stress of the hypothalamic-pituitary-adrenal (HPA) and hypothalamus-pituitary-thyroid (HPT) axes. ACTH, adrenocorticotropic hormone; DHEA, dehydroepiandrosterone; TSH, thyroid stimulating hormone.*

Water and electrolyte metabolism are decreased via sodium excretion, and glomerular filtration is due to direct effects on the kidney by beta receptors. Renin secretion also leads to an increased aldosterone production within the adrenal cortex. Serum potassium may be increased as a result of alpha-mediated effects on the liver but decreased as a result of β-2Ars-mediated effects on smooth muscle. Lastly, hormone secretion is influenced by the same path or adrenal part of the autonomic nervous system or sympathetic nervous system modulating the responses of endocrine systems, including the renin-angiotensin-aldosterone system.

Evaluation of individuals who have adrenal gland dysfunction includes an appropriate history, physical, questionnaires, and laboratory testing. The history would be looking for symptoms as well as potential triggers that have already been mentioned. Examination findings may include striae, buffalo hump, moon faces, orthostatic hypotension, postural tachycardia, and delayed reflexes. Questionnaires such as the Identi-T stress assessment tool[166] can help identify if individuals are exhibiting symptoms of an overactive or underactive response of the HPA axis. It should not be used to diagnose but can be helpful to guide the practitioner in streamlining a complex assessment (**Figure 25.2**).

Scoring the Identi-T Stress Assessment is done as follows:

To determine an **overactive HPA response** add up A, B, and C scores together. A score greater than 35 signifies mild to moderate symptoms consistent with an overactive HPA axis. A score greater than 70 exhibits symptoms consistent with a persistent or chronic stimulatory response. Symptoms, physical manifestations, and metabolic dysfunction found within an HPA Over-Responsiveness Profile include: nervous energy, unable to calm down despite feeling tired, and complaints of being warm. Tissues (tongue, face, mucous membranes) appear normal to red or inflamed. Workaholic type with cardiometabolic health issues.

To determine an **underactive HPA response** add up C, D, and E scores together. A score greater than 35 signifies mild to moderate symptoms consistent with an underactive HPA axis. A score greater than 70 are individuals manifesting symptoms consistent with a persistent suppressive response. Symptoms, physical manifestations, and metabolic dysfunction found within an HPA Under-Responsiveness Profile include: tiredness, weakness, and complaints of persistent cold intolerance (feeling cold regardless of the temperature). Tissues (tongue, face, mucous membranes) appear pale and puffy, although dark circles may appear under the eyes. Dizziness upon standing, hypoglycemia, darkening of the skin, muscle weakness, and weight loss are indications of stress-related adrenal gland insufficiency.

Adrenal Function Testing

There are different tests to determine different aspects of adrenal gland function and hormone homeostasis. Serum testing identifies circulating levels of adrenal hormones. Serum testing is a reflection of adrenal gland production of hormones. Circulating catecholamine levels fluctuate rapidly, and therefore serum testing is not recommended. Salivary testing is

a measurement of the level of adrenal glucocorticoids and androgen hormones found within the tissue. This test helps to measure the tissue sensitivity to the hormones and their ability to cross the cell membrane to get into the salivary glands. Salivary testing is not typically used to measure catecholamines or mineralocorticoids. Urine testing is a representation of the metabolism of adrenal gland hormones. Assessing urine metabolites allows the practitioner an opportunity to evaluate for unhealthy levels of catecholamines, anabolic/catabolic ratios, and levels of steroid precursors.

Serum testing recommendations (production):

- AM Cortisol, DHEA, DHEA-S, pregnenolone, progesterone, aldosterone, androstenedione.
- Additional serum laboratory tests to evaluate indirect and direct mediators of the adrenal gland include high-sensitivity C-reactive protein, gamma glutamyltransferase, vitamin D 25-OH, hemoglobin A1C, insulin-like growth factor-1

Saliva (sensitivity)

- Cortisol: with four measurements to reflect cortisol circadian rhythm (6-8 AM, 10:30-12:30 PM, 2:30-4:30 PM, 8:30-10:30 PM)
- DHEA, pregnenolone, progesterone
- Other hormones: melatonin, testosterone, estradiol, estrone, estriol

Urine (how the body metabolizes adrenal hormones)

- 11-Hydroxy-androsterone, 11-hydroxy-etiocholanolone, 11-keto-androsterone, 11-keto-etiocholanolone, androstanediol, androsterone, DHEA, etiocholanolone, pregnanediol, pregnanetriol, tetrahydrocortisol, tetrahydrocortisone, tetrahydrodeoxycortisol, allo-tetrahydrocortisol, creatinine
- 24-hour urine: Catecholamine tests to consider to rule out pheochromocytoma include adrenaline, noradrenaline, dopamine, metanephrine, normetanephrine, vanillylmandelic acid, homovanillic acid
- Other urine hormone metabolites: 16 alpha-hydroxyestrone, 2-hydroxyestrone, 2-methoxyestrone, 4-hydroxyestrone, 4-methoxyestrone, estradiol, estrone, estriol, testosterone

Other laboratory tests that can influence adrenal gland function:

- 21-Hydroxylase antibodies, 17 hydroxyprogesterone, ACTH

Functional ranges of laboratory tests (target is in upper half or third of normal range):

Serum testing:

- AM Cortisol: >12 normal, >15 optimal
- DHEA > 250 women, >350 men (range 60-1600)
- DHEAS >150 (range 23-266)
- Progesterone: menstruating female >10, postmenopausal >1
- Pregnenolone > 30

Salivary and urine hormone testing will have different ranges based upon different laboratory tests. Recommendation is to look at laboratory test levels for optimal hormone function.

Identi-**T**™ Stress Assessment

Name _____ **Age** _____ **Sex** _____ **Date** _____

Stress is a normal part of life. Every day, we're faced with stimuli, called stressors, which can elicit the body's "fight or flight" response, setting off a cascade of physiological reactions and resulting in emotions ranging from mild to intense. But while occasional stress is natural and even healthy, chronic or acute stress can be harmful.

Please take a few moments to discover your body's response to situations you perceive as stressful. By honestly assessing how you feel, your healthcare provider can create a natural stress relief program for your individual needs.

Directions:

Please read each statement and circle the number 0, 1, 2, or 3 that best describes your feelings or reactions throughout the course of the day. Determine the subtotal score for each section, then determine the total scores for sections A-C and C-E. Some questions may appear redundant between sections. There's a reason for each question. Don't spend much time on any one question.

0 = Never true   1= Seldom true   2= Sometimes true   3= Often true

When under stress for two weeks or longer, I...

Section A:

1.	Get wound up when I get tired and have trouble calming down	0	1	2	3
2.	Feel driven, appear energetic but feel "burned out" and exhausted	0	1	2	3
3.	Feel restless, agitated, anxious, and uneasy	0	1	2	3
4.	Feel easily overwhelmed by emotion	0	1	2	3
5.	Feel emotional — cry easily or laugh inappropriately	0	1	2	3
6.	Experience heart palpitations or a pounding in my chest	0	1	2	3
7.	Am short of breath	0	1	2	3
8.	Am constipated	0	1	2	3
9.	Feel warm, over-heated, and dry all over	0	1	2	3
10.	Get mouth sores or sore tongue	0	1	2	3
11.	Get hot flashes	0	1	2	3
12.	Sleep less than seven hours a night	0	1	2	3
13.	Have trouble falling asleep and staying asleep	0	1	2	3
14.	Worry about high blood pressure, cholesterol, and triglycerides	0	1	2	3
15.	Forget to eat and feel little hunger	0	1	2	3

Total points: _____

Section B:

1.	Find myself worrying about things big and small	0	1	2	3
2.	Feel like I can't stop worrying, even though I want to	0	1	2	3
3.	Feel impulsive, pent up, and ready to explode	0	1	2	3
4.	Get muscle spasms	0	1	2	3
5.	Feel aggressive, unyielding, or inflexible when pressed for time	0	1	2	3
6.	See, hear, and smell things that others do not	0	1	2	3
7.	Stay awake replaying the events of the day or planning for tomorrow	0	1	2	3
8.	Have upsetting thoughts or images enter my mind again and again	0	1	2	3
9.	Have a hard time stopping myself from doing things again and again, like checking on things or rearranging objects over and over	0	1	2	3
10.	Worry a lot about terrible things that could happen if I'm not careful	0	1	2	3

Total points: _____

Section C:

1.	Have muscle and joint pains	0	1	2	3
2.	Have muscle weakness	0	1	2	3
3.	Crave salt or salty things	0	1	2	3
4.	Have multiple points on my body that when touched are tender or painful	0	1	2	3
5.	Have dark circles under my eyes	0	1	2	3
6.	Feel a sudden sense of anxiety when I get hungry	0	1	2	3
7.	Use medications to manage pain	0	1	2	3
8.	Get dizzy when rising or standing up from a kneeling or sitting position	0	1	2	3
9.	Have diarrhea or bouts of nausea with or without vomiting for no apparent reason	0	1	2	3
10.	Have headaches	0	1	2	3

Total points: _____

Figure 25.2 *Identi-T Stress assessment. (© 2011 Metagenics, Inc. All Rights Reserved.)*

Section D:

1. Have trouble organizing my thoughts..0   1   2   3
2. Get easily distracted and lose focus..0   1   2   3
3. Have difficulty making decisions and mistrust my judgment..0   1   2   3
4. Feel depressed and apathetic..0   1   2   3
5. Lack the motivation and energy to stay on task and pay attention 0   1   2   3
6. Am forgetful..0   1   2   3
7. Feel unsettled, restless, and anxious..0   1   2   3
8. Wake up tired and unrefreshed 0   1   2   3
9. Experience heartburn and indigestion 0   1   2   3
10. Catch colds or infections easily 0   1   2   3

Total points: _____

Section E:

1. Feel tired for no apparent reason...0   1   2   3
2. Experience lingering mild fatigue after exertion or physical activity 0   1   2   3
3. Find it difficult to concentrate and complete tasks 0   1   2   3
4. Feel depressed and apathetic..0   1   2   3
5. Feel cold or chilled – hands, feet, or all over – for no apparent reason..0   1   2   3
6. Have little or no interest in sex..0   1   2   3
7. Sweat spontaneously during the day..0   1   2   3
8. Feel puffy and retain fluids...0   1   2   3
9. Sleep more than nine hours a night...0   1   2   3
10. Have poor muscle tone...0   1   2   3
11. Have trouble losing weight 0   1   2   3
12. Wake up tired even though I seem to get plenty of sleep...0   1   2   3
13. Have no energy and feel physically weak...0   1   2   3
14. Am susceptible to colds and the flu 0   1   2   3
15. Feel dragged down by multiple symptoms, such as poor digestion and body aches.........................0   1   2   3

Total points: _____

Add points from sections A, B & C	**Total for A, B & C:** _____
Add points from sections C, D & E	**Total for C, D & E:** _____

LIfestyle and Health Status:

1. Circle the level of stress you experience on the scale of 1-10, 10 being the worst:

    1   2   3   4   5   6   7   8   9   10

2. What do you consider to be the major causes of your stress (for example — spouse, family, friends, work, finances, wedding, pregnancy, legal, commute):

    _____

3. I eat breakfast _____ times a week.   My typical breakfast is: _____

4. I take a multiple vitamin/mineral _____ days per week.   I take a fish oil supplement _____ days per week.

5. I participate in 30 minutes of physical activity such as walking, aerobics (e.g., running), resistance training (e.g., weights, pilates), sports (e.g. biking), or yoga:

    ❑ Daily   ❑ 5-6 times per week   ❑ 3-4 times per week   ❑ 1-2 times per week   ❑ Less than once a week

6. I smoke _____ cigarettes daily.

7. I drink two or more 8 ounce cups of caffeinated coffee or other caffeinated beverages like energy/diet drinks, colas, or black or green teas:

    ❑ Daily   ❑ 5-6 times per week   ❑ 3-4 times per week   ❑ 1-2 times per week   ❑ Less than once a week

8. I drink two or more ounces of alcoholic beverages:

    ❑ Daily   ❑ 5-6 times per week   ❑ 3-4 times per week   ❑ 1-2 times per week   ❑ Less than once a week

9. List your current health problems and any over-the-counter or prescription medications that you are now taking:

    Current health problem(s)   Date of onset   List all current medication(s)

    _____   _____   _____

    _____   _____   _____

    _____   _____   _____

Figure 25.2 *Identi-T Stress assessment (continued). (© 2011 Metagenics, Inc. All Rights Reserved.)*

Adrenal Influences on the Cardiovascular System

Adrenal Excess and Cardiovascular Risk

PRIMARY ALDOSTERONISM

Primary aldosteronism is characterized by aldosterone secretion that is independent of renin and angiotensin II and sodium status.[167] Primary aldosteronism can occur in cases of aldosterone-producing adenomas (~40% of cases) and idiopathic aldosteronism for around 60% of cases. Less than 1% of cases accounted for from unilateral adrenal hyperplasia or familial primary aldosteronism.[168]

The publication in 1955 by Jerome W Conn of the first case of hypertension and hypokalemia associated with elevated aldosteronism, which was subsequently cured by adrenalectomy,[169] kicked off decades of research on the link between aldosterone production and blood pressure regulation.

Mineralocorticoids such as aldosterone play a critical role in regulating extracellular volume homeostasis.[170] Their release is upregulated by blood volume depletion, and they act to increase sodium status through upregulating salt appetite with resultant enhanced salt intake, reducing renal sodium loss by stimulating Na^+ reabsorption and K^+ secretion in the kidney, and curtailing salt loss by stimulating salt reabsorption/absorption in the colon, sweat glands, and salivary glands.[170] A least in part through blood volume expansion, they impact cardiac output and blood pressure.[170] Aldosterone also leads to reduced calcium and magnesium (Ca^{2+} and Mg^{2+}) reabsorption, calciuria and magnesuria.

Primary aldosteronism is **the most common** form of secondary hypertension, and prevalence of primary aldosteronism increases with the severity of hypertension. Primary aldosteronism has an estimated prevalence of 4% among hypertensive patients in primary care and ~10% of hypertensive patients referred to specialized centers.[171,172] Primary aldosteronism reaches its highest prevalence in resistant hypertension, affecting 17% to 23% of patients in this group.[173-176] The severity of aldosteronism also increases with increasing blood pressure. The presence of "unrecognized yet biochemically overt primary aldosteronism" can be detected in 13% to 14% of normotensive individuals,[177,178] and although these individuals may be able to handle the additional blood volume short-term, longitudinal studies over 5 years have shown that 85% of normotensive patients with primary aldosteronism develop frank hypertension in contrast to 23% of normotensive individuals without primary aldosteronism.[177]

However, hypertension is not the only cardiovascular consequence of primary aldosteronism, and aldosterone has vascular actions beyond its impact on sodium reabsorption and subsequent effect on blood pressure control. Observational studies have demonstrated that individuals with primary aldosteronism have a greater risk for developing coronary artery disease, atrial fibrillation, stroke, and left ventricular hypertrophy compared with matched controls with a comparable degree of blood pressure elevation, and patients with primary aldosteronism have a greater cardiac mortality risk.[167,168] In addition to the well-established role in blood volume regulation, raised mineralocorticoids have other consequences within the vascular system. Mineralocorticoids have been shown to increase endothelial and vascular stiffness,[179] upregulate vascular inflammation,[170] influence tissue calcification,[180] and stimulate cardiac and renal fibrosis.[181] Additionally, mineralocorticoids may contribute to insulin resistance and obesity,[170] which further impact cardiovascular health. Many of these actions are mediated through the mineralocorticoid receptor and can be blunted or prevented by mineralocorticoid receptor antagonists such as spironolactone.

GLUCOCORTICOID EXCESS

Glucocorticoid secretion is a foundational endocrine response to stress, ranging from trauma, sepsis, and ischemia to psychological stress.[182] Under these circumstances, glucocorticoids are involved in a host of adaptive processes that impact metabolism, neurobiology, immunity and inflammation, fluid volume and hemorrhage risk, as well as cardiovascular function.[182]

Acting through both the glucocorticoid receptors and the mineralocorticoid receptors, both of which are widely distributed throughout the cardiovascular system as well as in inflammatory cells that can accumulate in vascular tissue, glucocorticoids can substantially impact cardiovascular risk.[183] Acting via the glucocorticoid receptor, glucocorticoids have been reported to increase contractility, reduce proliferation and migration in vascular smooth muscle, reduce vasodilation and angiogenesis in endothelial cells, and reduce phagocytosis of apoptotic neutrophils in macrophages, as well as contribute to the progression of obesity, hypertension, lipid abnormalities, insulin resistance, and glucose intolerance.[183] Acting via the mineralocorticoid receptors, glucocorticoids have been reported to increase perivascular inflammation in vascular smooth muscle, increase fibrosis within the myocardium, and increase hypertension and a prothrombotic environment.[183]

Although many of the actions of glucocorticoids can be protective in certain times of stress,[182] under conditions of chronic activation the effects of glucocorticoids become maladaptive.

Cortisol regulates blood pressure. In normotensive subjects, administration of ACTH was shown to significantly increase systolic blood pressure and mean arterial pressure, with a modest rise in diastolic blood pressure over a period of 5 days.[184] Chronically raised cortisol levels are associated with hypertension, and approximately 20% of patients treated with long-term exogenous corticosteroids develop hypertension.[185] Deficient inactivation of cortisol due to reduced 11b-HSD2 activity has been identified in patients with essential hypertension.[186]

Glucocorticoids increase the risk of hypertension; in addition, observation studies have highlighted a link between chronic raised glucocorticoids and overall cardiovascular risk. Urinary cortisol levels at the upper end of the normal physiological range were associated with increased cardiovascular risk (Framingham risk score) in a group of nondiabetic individuals.[187] Epidemiological studies describe a link between exogenous glucocorticoid usage and cardiovascular risk. In a study of >50,000 individuals with CVD, and an equal number of matched controls, exposure to oral glucocorticoid therapy (as opposed to inhaled therapies) significantly increased the risk of developing CVD.[188] In a second study in >150,000 individuals, exposure to exogenous glucocorticoids also increased cardiovascular risk, although individuals who had been exposed to supraphysiological doses (>7.5 mg prednisolone or equivalent per day) were seen to be driving this increased risk.[189] Further analysis revealed that exposure to chronic glucocorticoid treatment was most strongly associated with risk of heart failure,[188,189] although additional studies also suggest an increase in atheromatous vascular disease.[183]

Given the awareness of adverse cardiovascular effects, some clinical task forces have begun recommending that the lowest effective dose of corticosteroids for the shortest possible duration should be prescribed in the treatment of active inflammatory joint disorders such as rheumatoid arthritis.[190]

CATECHOLAMINES

Catecholamines are another critical component of the body's physiological and behavioral response to stress.[191] Epinephrine and norepinephrine are cardiac stimulants, increasing myocardial contractile force. Heart rate is also increased through the actions of catecholamines on pacemaker cells.[191] A major impact of catecholamines in the periphery is vasoconstriction of blood vessels, mediated predominantly in small arterioles, but veins and larger arteries also respond.[191] Catecholamines increase fuel availability, and circulating epinephrine increases blood glucose and free fatty acid through multilevel impact on insulin secretion, lipolysis, and gluconeogenesis.[191] This altered metabolic state over a prolonged period of time can create a proatherogenic metabolic environment.[192]

Epinephrine and norepinephrine act through alpha- and beta-adrenergic receptors (ARs) located throughout the body. α1-ARs mediate much of the cardiovascular response to stress, particularly vasoconstriction, and in sustained activation, cardiac remodeling.[191] α1-ARs are located in vascular smooth muscle cells and respond to both epinephrine and norepinephrine and mediate vasoconstriction. α 2-ARs are present in presynaptic nerve terminals of sympathetic nerves, as well as in vascular smooth muscle cells, and again respond to both epinephrine and norepinephrine and mediate vasoconstriction. β-ARs are important in the regulation of heart, smooth muscle contraction and relaxation. β-1ARs are located in the heart and mediate positive inotropic and chronotropic responses and respond to both epinephrine and norepinephrine. β-2ARs are present in vascular smooth muscle cells and mediate vasodilation.[191]

In the heart, normal catecholamine/AR signaling is involved in regulating myocardial contractility and relaxation, as well as heart rate and rhythm. However, persistent AR activation by raised catecholamines leads to maladaptive response and a reversal of these normal effects.[193] Aging, for example, is associated with an increase in circulating catecholamines linked to the effort to maintain cardiac output.[192] As a result of chronic catecholamine stimulation, β-AR responsiveness is altered.[193] Similarly, heart failure is associated with sympathetic nervous system hyperactivation and an increase in catecholamine signaling, which is thought to represent a compensatory mechanism to maintain cardiac output. Over time, however, this persistent stimulation can lead to β-AR dysfunction and decreased cardiac contractility and diminished inotropic reserve.[193] Persistent catecholamine stimulation can also negatively impact left ventricular remodeling and promote fibrosis and angiogenesis.[193]

CUSHING SYNDROME

Cushing syndrome, characterized by excessive glucocorticoids, is an illustration of the maladaptive effects of chronic HPA axis activation. Cushing syndrome is associated with significant metabolic and vascular risk. Cushing syndrome is associated with endothelial dysfunction[194] and an increased risk of stroke.[195] Carotid and aortic artery intima-media thickness (IMT) is significantly increased in patients with Cushing syndrome and associated with premature development of carotid atherosclerotic plaques,[196] and compared with controls, patients with Cushing syndrome have an increased risk for myocardial infarction.[195] Left ventricular dysfunction is more prevalent,[197] and abnormal left ventricular mass has been described.[198] Cushing syndrome's influences on glucose metabolism include increased hepatic glucose production, reduction of glycogen synthesis, decreased insulin-dependent glucose uptake into the periphery, and breakdown of proteins and lipids for glucose production substrates. Owing to the widespread actions of glucocorticoid excess on liver, muscle, adipose tissue, and pancreas, impaired insulin sensitivity and carbohydrate abnormalities as well as dyslipidemia are common findings in patients with Cushing syndrome.[199] Almost two-thirds of patients with Cushing syndrome meet the criteria for metabolic syndrome.[200] These metabolic derangements likely factor into the long-term cardiovascular outcome by accelerating atherosclerosis and vascular remodeling.[185]

It has been estimated that 70% to 85% of adult patients and 50% to 78% of children with Cushing syndrome develop hypertension.[185] The mechanism of hypertension in Cushing syndrome is complex and only partially understood and is not solely related to excess cortisol.[185] Disruption in the renin-angiotensin system in Cushing syndrome has been most robustly studied, and an increase in angiotensin secretion and response has been described.[185] ACE inhibitors have been shown to be effective for blood pressure lowering in patients with Cushing syndrome.[201] Mineralocorticoid receptor hyperactivation in the kidney leading to sodium retention has also been proposed to play a role in hypertension development in patients with very high cortisol levels.[185] Ongoing work on vasodilator regulation in the setting of glucocorticoid excess has shown that eNOS inhibition and reduced arginine availability for nitric oxide synthesis may be related to hypertension in Cushing syndrome[185] (**Table 25.5**).

Table 25.5

SUMMARY OF IMPACT OF ADRENAL EXCESS ON THE CARDIOVASCULAR SYSTEM

Condition	Impact
Primary aldosteronism	• Increased blood volume and cardiac output • Hypertension • Increased risk of coronary artery disease • Increased risk of atrial fibrillation • Increased risk of stroke • Increased risk of left ventricle hypertrophy
Elevated glucocorticoids	• Hypertension • Increased overall cardiovascular risk • Increased risk of heart failure • Cardiometabolic dysfunction (glucose and lipid abnormalities and central obesity)

Elevated catecholamines	• Increased heart rate
	• Vasoconstriction
	• Increased glucose and free fatty acids
	• Persistent elevation lead to maladaptive response
	  • Reduced cardiac contractility
	  • Reduced inotropic reserve
	  • Associated with heart failure

Cushing syndrome	• Endothelial dysfunction • Hypertension • Increased risk of stroke • Increased carotid and aortic intima-media thickness • Premature development of carotid atherosclerotic plaques • Increased risk of myocardial infarction • Left ventricular dysfunction • Insulin and carbohydrate abnormalities • Hypertension • Metabolic syndrome

Adrenal Insufficiency

LOW DHEAS AND CARDIOVASCULAR RISK

DHEAS deficiency has been speculated to contribute to the development of age-related diseases including CVD. Several clinical observational studies have identified a link between plasma DHEAS and vascular dysfunction or pathogenesis.

Participants in the Massachusetts Male Aging Study with lower serum DHEAS at baseline were significantly more likely to develop ischemic heart disease in subsequent years.[202] The Nurses' Health Study reported an independent association between lower circulating DHEAS and increased stroke risk.[203] A study in postmenopausal women identified a link between lower plasma DHEAS and endothelial dysfunction.[204] In Japanese men, lower DHEAS levels were associated with higher carotid IMT scores, an association that was not observed in women.[205] In men undergoing coronary angiography, lower DHEAS was associated with stenosis and the extent of atherosclerosis and was also associated with a greater number of affected coronary vessels.[206]

In patients with existing CVD, lower DHEAS has been linked to poorer prognosis. This relationship between low serum concentration of DHEA and higher morbidity and mortality in patients with CVD has been shown since the 1980s, and a recent systematic review and meta-analysis on the prognostic value of DHEAS levels in patients with existing CVD showed that lower DHEAS concentrations significantly increased the risk of all-cause mortality, as well as both fatal and nonfatal CV events.[207]

The mechanisms through which reduced plasma DHEAS exert cardiovascular risk remain poorly understood. Preclinical models suggest that DHEAS is involved in several antiatherogenic activities, including helping to maintain the oxidative balance within cardiovascular tissue, moderating the proinflammatory response within endothelial cells, inhibiting monocyte adhesion to arterial endothelial cells, reducing platelet aggregation, and inducing a vasodilatory effects on smooth muscle cells,[208] indicating that loss of these effects of DHEAS may be related to the increased cardiovascular risk observed. Supplementation studies with DHEAS in humans are also supportive of the potential vascular benefit, with clinical studies showing improvement in endothelial function.[208]

ADDISON DISEASE

Primary adrenal insufficiency, now termed Addison disease, is estimated to occur in 1 in 10,000 people and is characterized by a reduction in circulating corticosteroids, with a concomitant reduction in mineralocorticoids sometimes observed.[209] Considering the influence of corticosteroids and mineralocorticoids on electrolyte balance and blood volume regulation, it is unsurprising that patients with Addison disease typically present with hyponatremia, hyperkalemia, and depleted intravascular volume.[209] Although cardiovascular complications are most commonly related to hypovolemic hypotension, in untreated adrenal insufficiency, cases of acute addisonian crisis-related reversible cardiomyopathies have been described in both children and adults.[210-215]

Addison disease can also coexist with hypertension, and it has been estimated that hypertension can occur in ~20% of patients with Addison disease.[216] This finding is thought to be secondary to glucocorticoid replacement therapy,[217] as glucocorticoids in supraphysiological doses have been shown to produce hypertension in humans and animals independent of an effect of blood volume or mineralocorticoid receptor expression.[218] The assessment of patients with Addison disease who present with new-onset hypertension should address the possibility of overreplacement with glucocorticoid, with appropriate correction as needed.[217]

Reports of heart failure in Addison disease has been reported, although reports of this connection in the literature are infrequent. An observational study that followed

22 patients with Addison disease for an average of 30 years reported that 7 of 22 (~32%) developed heart failure. However, similar to the connection with hypertension, the authors identified an influence of treatment. Six of the 7 patients who developed heart failure were treated with fludrocortisone, and dose reduction or cessation was effective in managing the heart failure.[219] This connection to fludrocortisone therapy and heart failure has been corroborated in isolated case reports, where withdrawal of fludrocortisone was seen to resolve heart failure[220,221] (**Table 25.6**).

Treatment Options for Adrenal Health

Lifestyle Modifications—Focus on Mind, Body, and Spirit

A multipronged approach to lifestyle modification including a focus on movement, sleep, stress reduction, and prayer/meditation has been shown to benefit adrenal health.

YOGA

Salivary cortisol was seen to significantly reduce in young women following a 1-hour session of both power and stretch yoga.[222] In a systematic review and meta-analysis of 42 studies, interventions that included yoga asanas were associated with reduced evening cortisol, reduced waking cortisol, as well as reduced ambulatory systolic blood pressure, resting rate, higher-frequency heart rate variability, fasting glucose, cholesterol, and LDL cholesterol compared with active control.[223] In a study in healthy volunteers, once weekly 90-minute yoga session was seen to significantly reduce plasma adrenaline compared with control.[224]

PRAYER/MEDITATION

In a study of unemployed adults experiencing high levels of stress (n = 35) participating in a 3-day mindfulness meditation retreat, there was increased functional connectivity in the brain, meaning that brain cells in regions involved in attention and executive control were working together better than they were before the retreat. These changes were not seen in the control group who had participated in a 3-day program where they were told to simply relax, without any focus on mindfulness meditation.[225] A systematic review and meta-analysis including 45 studies of various forms of meditation showed that, when analyzed together, all forms of meditation reduced cortisol as well as blood pressure and heart rate.[226] Integrated Amrita Meditation has been shown to significantly reduce circulating adrenaline concentrations.[227]

MINDFULNESS

In a group of female nurses (age 45-66 years) showing subclinical features of posttraumatic stress disorder (PTSD), 60 minutes of mindfulness-based stretching and deep breathing exercises semiweekly for 8 weeks led to normalization of cortisol levels and reduced symptoms of PTSD.[228]

SLEEP

Sleep dysfunction and dysfunction of the HPA and renin–angiotensin–aldosterone system (RAAS) axes are connected.

Reduced sleep quality has been reported in patients with primary aldosteronism,[229] and within this group, sleep quality in women appears to be more adversely affected than in men.[230] Sleep apnea has been associated with higher aldosterone levels, particularly in patients with hypertension, and stimulation of RAAS activity as a result of obstructive sleep apnea (OSA) has been suggested as one of the mechanisms of how it induces hypertension.[231] Higher daytime cortisol has been linked with sleep disturbance in older adults.[232]

Supporting adequate sleep in those with HPA and RAAS axes dysfunction is an important part of care, as is assessing HPA and RAAS function in those with sleep disturbance including sleep apnea.

Dietary Modifications

Dietary composition can influence cortisol release. A fatty acid profile more in line with a Mediterranean diet (low saturated fat and higher monounsaturated fat) was associated with normal diurnal cortisol pattern.[233] Higher adherence to a diet rich in fruits and vegetables, whole grains, and fish, with moderate to low saturated fat, *trans* fat cholesterol, and refined sugar, was shown to reduce urinary cortisol concentration in women. DHEAS concentrations were also seen to reduce in women, whereas men experienced a reduction in norepinephrine concentrations.[234] Diets richer in flax lignans

Table 25.6

SUMMARY OF IMPACT OF ADRENAL INSUFFICIENCY ON THE CARDIOVASCULAR SYSTEM

Condition	Cardiovascular Impact
Low DHEAS	• Increased risk of ischemic heart disease • Increased risk of stroke • Endothelial dysfunction • Increased carotid intima-media thickness • Increased mortality in existing cardiovascular disease
Addison disease	• Volemic hypotension • Electrolyte disturbances: hyponatremia and hypokalemia • Acute addisonian crisis-related reversible cardiomyopathies • Hypertension (thought to be related to effects of glucocorticoid treatment) • Increased risk of heart failure (infrequently reported; thought to be related to effects of glucocorticoid treatment)

were shown in postmenopausal women with vascular disease to enhance peripheral resistance to stress and reduce circulating cortisol concentrations during a stress challenge.[235]

In addition to focus on background dietary composition, recommendation of a cardioprotective diet rich in phytonutrients without excessive salt intake is prudent. Dietary patterns supporting adequate glucose control are also prudent given the propensity to dysregulated plasma glucose and insulin response with many conditions or adrenal dysfunction.

Vitamin and Mineral Supplementation

Several nutrients as described in the following text have been shown to impact adrenal hormones and the stress response. Considering the impact of adrenal dysfunction on the cardiovascular system, other nutrients associated with cardioprotection, including vitamin D and omega-3 fatty acids, are also warranted in this population.

VITAMIN C

In a study of psychological stress (Trier Social Stress Test consisting of public speaking and mental arithmetic), subjects supplemented with ascorbic acid (3 × 1000 mg/d of sustained-release ascorbic acid) (n = 60) showed a reduced increase in blood pressure and lower subjective stress response as well as a faster salivary cortisol recovery.[236] In animal models, marginal ascorbic acid deficiency has been shown to increase salivary and blood levels of glucocorticoids, specifically plasma cortisol concentrations.[237] The effects have also been shown in the cortisol-response to physical stress. In a study of ultramarathon runners, vitamin C supplementation (1500 mg/d for 7 days before the race, on the day of the race, and 2 days post race) was shown to reduce postrace plasma cortisol compared with the placebo and 500 mg vitamin C groups.[238]

MAGNESIUM

Magnesium deficiency is associated with an intensified adverse reaction to stress.[239] Low magnesium is associated with an increased release of stress hormones under conditions of stress.[240] Magnesium deficiency is also associated with other aspects of cardiometabolic dysfunction and cardiovascular risk.[241,242]

B VITAMINS

Pantothenic acid supplementation was shown to stimulate the ability of adrenal cells to secrete corticosterone and progesterone. Vitamin B5 supplementation of male rats induced adrenal hyperresponsiveness to ACTH stimulation.[243]

Low levels of vitamin B6, B12, and folate are associated with increased homocysteine and risk for coronary heart disease.[244] Thiamine has also shown antistress activity in animals by protecting cardiac tissue from stress-induced ischemia.[245]

PHOSPHATIDYLSERINE

Phosphatidylserine is a phospholipid located within cell membranes. Phosphatidylserine supplementation has been shown to blunt serum cortisol, ACTH, and salivary cortisol levels.[246] In another study, supplementation with phosphatidylserine was shown to normalize ACTH and serum and salivary cortisol in chronically stressed subjects.[247]

Botanical Supplementation

Use of adaptogenic herbs can be beneficial in patients with adrenal dysfunction. Adaptogens are medicinal plants that augment resistance to stress and increase concentration, performance, and endurance during fatigue.[248] Adaptogenic herbs can help to normalize stress response, although certain adaptogenic herbs may be more appropriate in specific hyper- or hypoadrenergic situations.

LIQUORICE AND GLYCYRRHETINIC ACID

Glycyrrhizin is a compound found in the licorice plant. In a crossover clinical study in men and women consuming nonliquorice confectionery (control) or liquorice (3% liquorice extract)-containing confectionary for 1 week, plasma aldosterone was seen to be reduced in the liquorice group.[249] Glycyrrhizin has also been shown to lower levels of cortisol and cortisone, thus decreasing the stress reaction.[250] Licorice ingestion has been shown to inhibit 11bHSD enzyme activity, causing apparent mineralocorticoid excess, and can produce overt hypertension in individuals with genetic background driving low 11bHSD activity.[251]

RHODIOLA ROSEA (ARCTIC ROOT)

In a study of men and women aged 20 to 55 years with a diagnosis of fatigue syndrome (n = 60), *Rhodiola* (standardized to 3% rosavins and 1% salidroside, 200-600 mg one to two times a day) has been shown to improve scores on the Pines burnout scale and the tests of attention showing an overall antifatigue effect with increased mental performance. Particular benefits were seen in the ability to concentrate. A significant reduction in cortisol response to awakening stress was seen compared with control.[252] Additional studies have demonstrated that Rhodiola significantly improves depression, insomnia, and emotional instability[253] and reduced general fatigue under stressful conditions.[254]

The authors' clinical recommendation is to start dosing with *Rhodiola* at 100 mg and increase to a maximum of 400 mg (200 mg 30 minutes before breakfast plus 200 mg 30 minutes before lunch) gradually over a period of 1 to 2 weeks. A possible stimulating effect of *Rhodiola* can be seen in sensitive individuals. If this occurs, a starting dose between 50 to 100 mg is appropriate, and restricting the dose to 1 × 50 mg or 2 × 200 mg per day may be warranted.

SIBERIAN GINSENG (*ELEUTHEROCOCCUS SENTICOSUS*)

Eleutherococcus has been shown to reduce stress-induced cortisol increase and inhibit stress-induced immune suppression in a preclinical stress model.[255]

ASHWAGANDHA (*WITHANIA SOMNIFERA*)

Ashwagandha is a revered "vitalizer" in Ayurvedic medicine and is used as a rejuvenating tonic. Adaptogens are used traditionally for improving stress tolerance, vigor and stamina, convalescence, nervous exhaustion, fatigue, geriatric, debility, physical and mental stress, and insomnia. Contemporary research has confirmed adaptogenic properties of Ashwagandha and shown that it supports HPA axis function.

Ashwagandha moderates the stress response when exposed to chronic environmental stressors, including lessening of symptoms such as depression, increased blood sugar and glucose intolerance, increased cortisol, cognitive deficits, and stomach ulcers.[256,257]

CORDYCEPS SINENSIS (CATERPILLAR MUSHROOM)

A valued medicinal fungus in Chinese medicine, *Cordyceps* is used traditionally to strengthen and rebuild the body after exhaustion or long-term illness and has specific uses for excessive tiredness, persistent cough, impotence, debility, and anemia.[258] Study in rodents showed that administration of an extract of *Cordyceps sinensis* elicited an increase in corticosterone production by adrenal cells.[259] Possible mechanisms of action may increase cortisone production and have additional benefits for glucose and lipid reduction.[260]

PANAX (ASIAN GINSENG)

This is used in traditional medicine to stimulate mental and physical activity, enhance stamina, prevent fatigue, and increase resistance to stress and indicated for individuals who have exhausted reserves.[261] Several studies have demonstrated antianxiety effects of *Panax*.[262] Research has also shown that *Panax* ginseng improves cortisol:DHEAS ratios.[263] In animal models of stress, *Panax* ginseng administration has been shown to increase corticosterone levels and physical endurance in these models.[264] In the cardiovascular system, *Panax* exhibits antiatherosclerotic and antihypertensive activity as well as enhances insulin sensitivity.[265] *Panax* appears to help the adrenal glands recover from chronic stress by improving corticoid response and the corticotropin feedback loops within the HPA axis.[266]

Hormone Support

MELATONIN

Melatonin can be used to indirectly lower cortisol levels. Cortisol and melatonin are considered "mirrored" hormones in that they are closely linked to the circadian rhythm, and cortisol elevates in the morning and melatonin elevates in the evening. Melatonin can help with disturbed circadian cycling and enhance sleep in many individuals with insomnia. Melatonin supplementation has been found to lead to improvements in sleep quality, morning alertness, and reported quality of life.[267]

HYDROCORTISONE

Hydrocortisone supplementation for adrenal insufficiency and Addison disease has been used for a long time. However, recent trends to replace cortisol in a more physiological replication has been a growing trend in recent years. A study in 2010 demonstrated the benefits of following and supporting the cortisol circadian rhythm. However, one of the challenges of using hydrocortisone is that it has a short plasma half-life and therefore patients using this drug can wake with undetectable cortisol levels if they have true Addison disease. Peak cortisol levels are reached after an hour of taking a dose of hydrocortisone.[268] Doses less than 20 mg/d can be used without further adrenal suppression.[269] A 24-hour urine cortisol should be used to measure adequate hydrocortisone support. A typical dosing regimen could be 7.5 to 10 mg between the hours of 6 and 8 AM, followed by 5 to 7.5 mg between 10 AM and 12 PM, and 2.5 mg between 2 and 4 PM. For true Addison disease, doses greater than 20 mg should be considered.[270]

DEHYDROEPIANDROSTERONE

Low circulating levels of DHEA clearly have a negative impact on the cardiovascular system. Although there are no current studies on DHEA supplementation and CVD outcomes, there are several studies in animals that have shown benefit. One particular study showed improvements in pulmonary hypertension and right ventricular function in rats with left-sided heart failure when given DHEA supplementation.[271] This is clearly an area of future research but holds promise. Because of the low risks of using DHEA supplementation, it is the opinion of the author to recommend 25 mg of DHEA in patients who have low circulating levels of DHEA and have heart failure.

Future Challenges

- More research is needed to evaluate the effect of DHEA supplementation on improving cardiovascular risk. Although interesting relationships between diminished DHEAS status and increased cardiovascular risk have been uncovered, long-term supplementation with a focus on hard cardiovascular end points are lacking.
- A greater understanding of where adaptogenic herbs should be combined clinically is needed. Investigation of whether these herbs work together additively or synergistically or indeed should be used in isolation is needed.
- More clinically focused studies are needed to shed light on the impact of a multidisciplinary approach for HPA axis management.

References

1. Jabbar A, Pingitore A, Pearce SH, Zaman A, Iervasi G, Razvi S. Thyroid hormones and cardiovascular disease. *Nat Rev Cardiol.* 2017;14(1):39-55.

2. Biondi B, Kahaly GJ, Robertson RP. Thyroid dysfunction and diabetes mellitus: two closely associated disorders. *Endocr Rev.* 2019;40(3):789-824.

3. Canaris GJ, Manowitz NR, Mayor G, Ridgway EC. The Colorado thyroid disease prevalence study. *Arch Intern Med*. 2000;160(4):526-534.

4. Nillni EA. Regulation of the hypothalamic Thyrotropin Releasing Hormone (TRH) neuron by neuronal and peripheral inputs. *Front Neuroendocrinol*. 2010;31(2):134-156.

5. Peeters RP, Visser TJ. Metabolism of thyroid hormone. In: Feingold KR, Anawalt B, Boyce A, et al, eds. *Endotext*. South Dartmouth, MA: MDText.com, Inc.; 2000.

6. Orozco A, Navarrete-Ramirez P, Olvera A, Garcia GC. 3,5-Diiodothyronine (T2) is on a role. A new hormone in search of recognition. *Gen Comp Endocrinol*. 2014;203:174-180.

7. Leonard JL. Nongenomic actions of thyroid hormone in brain development. *Steroids*. 2008;73(9-10):1008-1012.

8. de Herder WW, Hazenberg MP, Pennock-Schroder AM, Oosterlaken AC, Rutgers M, Visser TJ. On the enterohepatic cycle of triiodothyronine in rats; importance of the intestinal microflora. *Life Sci*. 1989;45(9):849-856.

9. O'Reilly DS. Thyroid function tests—time for a reassessment. *BMJ*. 2000;320(7245):1332-1334.

10. Hollowell JG, Staehling NW, Flanders WD, et al. Serum TSH, T4, and thyroid antibodies in the United States population (1988 to 1994): National Health and Nutrition Examination Survey (NHANES III). *J Clin Endocrinol Metab*. 2002;87(2):489-499.

11. Spencer CA, Hollowell JG, Kazarosyan M, Braverman LE. National Health and Nutrition Examination Survey III Thyroid-Stimulating Hormone (TSH)-thyroperoxidase antibody relationships demonstrate that TSH upper reference limits may be skewed by occult thyroid dysfunction. *J Clin Endocrinol Metab*. 2007;92(11):4236-4240.

12. Garber JR, Cobin R, Gharib H, et al. Clinical practice guidelines for hypothyroidism in adults: cosponsored by the American Association of Clinical Endocrinologists and the American Thyroid Association. *Endocr Pract*. 2012;18(6):988-1028.

13. van den Beld AW, Visser TJ, Feelders RA, Grobbee DE, Lamberts SW. Thyroid hormone concentrations, disease, physical function, and mortality in elderly men. *J Clin Endocrinol Metab*. 2005;90(12):6403-6409.

14. Moura Neto A, Parisi MC, Tambascia MA, Pavin EJ, Alegre SM, Zantut-Wittmann DE. Relationship of thyroid hormone levels and cardiovascular events in patients with type 2 diabetes. *Endocrine*. 2014;45(1):84-91.

15. Betterle C, Zanchetta R. Update on autoimmune polyendocrine syndromes (APS). *Acta Biomed*. 2003;74(1):9-33.

16. Chen WH, Chen YK, Lin CL, Yeh JH, Kao CH. Hashimoto's thyroiditis, risk of coronary heart disease, and L-thyroxine treatment: a nationwide cohort study. *J Clin Endocrinol Metab*. 2015;100(1):109-114.

17. Soldin OP. Controversies in urinary iodine determinations. *Clin Biochem*. 2002;35(8):575-579.

18. Klein I, Danzi S. Thyroid disease and the heart. *Circulation*. 2007;116(15):1725-1735.

19. Feingold K, Brinton EA, Grunfeld C. The effect of endocrine disorders on lipids and lipoproteins. In: Feingold KR, Anawalt B, Boyce A, et al, eds. *Endotext*. South Dartmouth, MA: MDText.com, Inc.; 2000.

20. Duntas LH, Brenta G. A renewed focus on the association between thyroid hormones and lipid metabolism. *Front Endocrinol (Lausanne)*. 2018;9:511.

21. Pearce EN. Thyroid hormone and obesity. *Curr Opin Endocrinol Diabetes Obes*. 2012;19(5):408-413.

22. Resch U, Helsel G, Tatzber F, Sinzinger H. Antioxidant status in thyroid dysfunction. *Clin Chem Lab Med*. 2002;40(11):1132-1134.

23. Bansal SK, Yadav R. A study of the extended lipid profile including oxidized LDL, small dense LDL, lipoprotein (a) and apolipoproteins in the assessment of cardiovascular risk in hypothyroid patients. *J Clin Diagn Res*. 2016;10(6):BC04-BC08.

24. Zha K, Zuo C, Wang A, et al. LDL in patients with subclinical hypothyroidism shows increased lipid peroxidation. *Lipids Health Dis*. 2015;14:95.

25. Geng H, Zhang X, Wang C, et al. Even mildly elevated TSH is associated with an atherogenic lipid profile in postmenopausal women with subclinical hypothyroidism. *Endocr Res*. 2015;40(1):1-7.

26. Lopez D, Abisambra Socarras JF, Bedi M, Ness GC. Activation of the hepatic LDL receptor promoter by thyroid hormone. *Biochim Biophys Acta*. 2007;1771(9):1216-1225.

27. Shin DJ, Osborne TF. Thyroid hormone regulation and cholesterol metabolism are connected through Sterol Regulatory Element-Binding Protein-2 (SREBP-2). *J Biol Chem*. 2003;278(36):34114-34118.

28. Staels B, Van Tol A, Chan L, Will H, Verhoeven G, Auwerx J. Alterations in thyroid status modulate apolipoprotein, hepatic triglyceride lipase, and low density lipoprotein receptor in rats*. *Endocrinology*. 1990;127(3):1144-1152.

29. Bonde Y, Breuer O, Lutjohann D, Sjoberg S, Angelin B, Rudling M. Thyroid hormone reduces PCSK9 and stimulates bile acid synthesis in humans. *J Lipid Res*. 2014;55(11):2408-2415.

30. Goldberg IJ, Huang LS, Huggins LA, et al. Thyroid hormone reduces cholesterol via a non-LDL receptor-mediated pathway. *Endocrinology*. 2012;153(11):5143-5149.

31. Skoczynska A, Wojakowska A, Turczyn B, et al. Serum lipid transfer proteins in hypothyreotic patients are inversely correlated with Thyroid-Stimulating Hormone (TSH) levels. *Med Sci Monit*. 2016;22:4661-4669.

32. Tan KC, Shiu SW, Kung AW. Effect of thyroid dysfunction on high-density lipoprotein subfraction metabolism: roles of hepatic lipase and cholesteryl ester transfer protein. *J Clin Endocrinol Metab*. 1998;83(8):2921-2924.

33. Deeb SS, Zambon A, Carr MC, Ayyobi AF, Brunzell JD. Hepatic lipase and dyslipidemia. *J Lipid Res*. 2003;44(7):1279-1286.

34. Sinha RA, Singh BK, Yen PM. Direct effects of thyroid hormones on hepatic lipid metabolism. *Nat Rev Endocrinol*. 2018;14(5):259-269.

35. Singh S, Dey Sarkar P. Serum lipids, tHcy, hs-CRP, MDA and PON-1 levels in SCH and overt hypothyroidism: effect of treatment. *Acta Biomed*. 2014;85(2):127-134.

36. Azizi F, Raiszadeh F, Solati M, Etemadi A, Rahmani M, Arabi M. Serum paraoxonase 1 activity is decreased in thyroid dysfunction. *J Endocrinol Invest*. 2003;26(8):703-709.

37. Jung KY, Ahn HY, Han SK, Park YJ, Cho BY, Moon MK. Association between thyroid function and lipid profiles, apolipoproteins, and high-density lipoprotein function. *J Clin Lipidol*. 2017;11(6):1347-1353.

38. Yan F, Wang Q, Lu M, et al. Thyrotropin increases hepatic triglyceride content through upregulation of SREBP-1c activity. *J Hepatol*. 2014;61(6):1358-1364.

39. Liu J, Hernandez-Ono A, Graham MJ, Galton VA, Ginsberg HN. Type 1 deiodinase regulates ApoA-I gene expression and ApoA-I synthesis independent of thyroid hormone signaling. *Arterioscler Thromb Vasc Biol*. 2016;36(7):1356-1366.

40. Sauter G, Weiss M, Hoermann R. Cholesterol 7αHydroxylase activity in hypothyroidism and hyperthyroidism in humans. *Horm Metab Res*. 1997;29(4):176-179.

41. Angelin B, Einarsson K, Leijd B. Bile acid metabolism in hypothyroid subjects: response to substitution therapy. *Eur J Clin Invest*. 1983;13(1):99-106.

42. Laukkarinen J, Sand J, Autio V, Nordback I. Bile duct stone procedures are more frequent in patients with hypothyroidism. A large, registry-based, cohort study in Finland. *Scand J Gastroenterol*. 2010;45(1):70-74.

43. Laukkarinen J, Sand J, Saaristo R, et al. Is bile flow reduced in patients with hypothyroidism? *Surgery*. 2003;133(3):288-293.

44. Bansal S, Buring JE, Rifai N, Mora S, Sacks FM, Ridker PM. Fasting compared with nonfasting triglycerides and risk of cardiovascular events in women. *JAMA*. 2007;298(3):309-316.

45. Nordestgaard BG, Benn M, Schnohr P, Tybjaerg-Hansen A. Nonfasting triglycerides and risk of myocardial infarction, ischemic heart disease, and death in men and women. *JAMA*. 2007;298(3):299-308.

46. Tanaci N, Ertugrul DT, Sahin M, et al. Postprandial lipemia as a risk factor for cardiovascular disease in patients with hypothyroidism. *Endocrine*. 2006;29(3):451-456.

47. McGowan A, Widdowson WM, O'Regan A, et al. Postprandial studies uncover differing effects on HDL particles of overt and subclinical hypothyroidism. *Thyroid*. 2016;26(3):356-364.

48. Patel S, Puranik R, Nakhla S, et al. Acute hypertriglyceridaemia in humans increases the triglyceride content and decreases the anti-inflammatory capacity of high density lipoproteins. *Atherosclerosis.* 2009;204(2):424-428.

49. Julia Z, Duchene E, Fournier N, et al. Postprandial lipemia enhances the capacity of large HDL2 particles to mediate free cholesterol efflux via SR-BI and ABCG1 pathways in type IIB hyperlipidemia. *J Lipid Res.* 2010;51(11):3350-3358.

50. Liu G, Xu JN, Liu D, et al. Regulation of plasma lipid homeostasis by hepatic lipoprotein lipase in adult mice. *J Lipid Res.* 2016;57(7):1155-1161.

51. Guo Z, Li M, Han B, Qi X. Association of non-alcoholic fatty liver disease with thyroid function: a systematic review and meta-analysis. *Dig Liver Dis.* 2018;50(11):1153-1162.

52. Tzotzas T, Krassas GE, Konstantinidis T, Bougoulia M. Changes in lipoprotein(a) levels in overt and subclinical hypothyroidism before and during treatment. *Thyroid.* 2000;10(9):803-808.

53. de Bruin TW, van Barlingen H, van Linde-Sibenius Trip M, van Vuurst de Vries AR, Akveld MJ, Erkelens DW. Lipoprotein(a) and apolipoprotein B plasma concentrations in hypothyroid, euthyroid, and hyperthyroid subjects. *J Clin Endocrinol Metab.* 1993;76(1):121-126.

54. Tagami T, Kimura H, Ohtani S, et al. Multi-center study on the prevalence of hypothyroidism in patients with hypercholesterolemia. *Endocr J.* 2011;58(6):449-457.

55. Willard DL, Leung AM, Pearce EN. Thyroid function testing in patients with newly diagnosed hyperlipidemia. *JAMA Intern Med.* 2014;174(2):287-289.

56. Diekman T, Lansberg PJ, Kastelein JJ, Wiersinga WM. Prevalence and correction of hypothyroidism in a large cohort of patients referred for dyslipidemia. *Arch Intern Med.* 1995;155(14):1490-1495.

57. National Cholesterol Education Program Expert Panel on Detection ETreatment of High Blood Cholesterol in Adults. Third Report of the National Cholesterol Education Program (NCEP) Expert Panel on Detection, Evaluation, and Treatment of High Blood Cholesterol in Adults (Adult Treatment Panel III) final report. *Circulation.* 2002;106(25):3143-3421.

58. Jellinger PS, Smith DA, Mehta AE, et al. American association of clinical endocrinologists' guidelines for management of dyslipidemia and prevention of atherosclerosis. *Endocr Pract.* 2012;18(suppl 1):1-78.

59. Ladenson PW, Singer PA, Ain KB, et al. American thyroid association guidelines for detection of thyroid dysfunction. *Arch Intern Med.* 2000;160(11):1573-1575.

60. Moon S, Kim MJ, Yu JM, Yoo HJ, Park YJ. Subclinical hypothyroidism and the risk of cardiovascular disease and all-cause mortality: a meta-analysis of prospective cohort studies. *Thyroid.* 2018;28(9):1101-1110.

61. Floriani C, Gencer B, Collet TH, Rodondi N. Subclinical thyroid dysfunction and cardiovascular diseases: 2016 update. *Eur Heart J.* 2018;39(7):503-507.

62. Rodondi N, den Elzen WP, Bauer DC, et al. Subclinical hypothyroidism and the risk of coronary heart disease and mortality. *JAMA.* 2010;304(12):1365-1374.

63. Razvi S, Shakoor A, Vanderpump M, Weaver JU, Pearce SH. The influence of age on the relationship between subclinical hypothyroidism and ischemic heart disease: a metaanalysis*J Clin Endocrinol Metab.* 2008;93(8):2998-3007.

64. Gencer B, Collet TH, Virgini V, et al. Subclinical thyroid dysfunction and the risk of heart failure events. *Circulation.* 2012;126(9):1040-1049.

65. Ning N, Gao D, Triggiani V, et al. Prognostic role of hypothyroidism in heart failure. *Medicine (Baltimore).* 2015;94(30):e1159.

66. Iacoviello M, Guida P, Guastamacchia E, et al. Prognostic role of sub-clinical hypothyroidism in chronic heart failure outpatients. *Curr Pharm Des.* 2008;14(26):2686-2692.

67. Vale C, Neves JS, von Hafe M, Borges-Canha M, Leite-Moreira A. The role of thyroid hormones in heart failure. *Cardiovasc Drugs Ther.* 2019;33(2):179-188.

68. Carrillo-Sepulveda MA, Ceravolo GS, Fortes ZB, et al. Thyroid hormone stimulates NO production via activation of the PI3K/Akt pathway in vascular myocytes. *Cardiovasc Res.* 2010;85(3):560-570.

69. Hiroi Y, Kim HH, Ying H, et al. Rapid nongenomic actions of thyroid hormone. *Proc Natl Acad Sci USA.* 2006;103(38):14104-14109.

70. Imai T, Hirata Y, Iwashina M, Marumo F. Hormonal regulation of rat adrenomedullin gene in vasculature. *Endocrinology.* 1995;136(4):1544-1548.

71. Isumi Y, Shoji H, Sugo S, et al. Regulation of adrenomedullin production in rat endothelial Cells1. *Endocrinology.* 1998;139(3): 838-846.

72. Tamajusuku AS, Carrillo-Sepúlveda MA, Braganhol E, et al. Activity and expression of ecto-5′-nucleotidase/CD73 are increased by thyroid hormones in vascular smooth muscle cells. *Mol Cell Biochem.* 2006;289(1-2):65-72.

73. Fukuyama K, Ichiki T, Takeda K, et al. Downregulation of vascular angiotensin II type 1 receptor by thyroid hormone. *Hypertension.* 2003;41(3):598-603.

74. Ladenson PW, Sherman SI, Baughman KL, Ray PE, Feldman AM. Reversible alterations in myocardial gene expression in a young man with dilated cardiomyopathy and hypothyroidism. *Proc Natl Acad Sci USA.* 1992;89(12):5251-5255.

75. Lekakis J, Papamichael C, Alevizaki M, et al. Flow-mediated, endothelium-dependent vasodilatation is impaired in subjects with hypothyroidism, borderline hypothyroidism, and high-normal serum thyrotropin (TSH) values. *Thyroid.* 1997;7(3):411-414.

76. Taddei S, Caraccio N, Virdis A, et al. Impaired endothelium-dependent vasodilatation in subclinical hypothyroidism: beneficial effect of levothyroxine therapy. *J Clin Endocrinol Metab.* 2003;88(8):3731-3737.

77. Papaioannou GI, Lagasse M, Mather JF, Thompson PD. Treating hypothyroidism improves endothelial function. *Metabolism.* 2004;53(3):278-279.

78. Mourouzis I, Forini F, Pantos C, Iervasi G. Thyroid hormone and cardiac disease: from basic concepts to clinical application. *J Thyroid Res.* 2011;2011:958626.

79. Odelberg SJ. Inducing cellular dedifferentiation: a potential method for enhancing endogenous regeneration in mammals. *Semin Cell Dev Biol.* 2002;13(5):335-343.

80. Rolfe M, McLeod LE, Pratt PF, Proud CG. Activation of protein synthesis in cardiomyocytes by the hypertrophic agent phenylephrine requires the activation of ERK and involves phosphorylation of tuberous sclerosis complex 2 (TSC2). *Biochem J.* 2005;388(pt 3):973-984.

81. Pantos C, Xinaris C, Mourouzis I, et al. Thyroid hormone receptor alpha 1: a switch to cardiac cell "metamorphosis"? *J Physiol Pharmacol.* 2008;59(2):253-269.

82. Kinugawa K, Jeong MY, Bristow MR, Long CS. Thyroid hormone induces cardiac myocyte hypertrophy in a thyroid hormone receptor α1-specific manner that requires TAK1 and p38 mitogen-activated protein kinase. *Mol Endocrinol.* 2005;19(6):1618-1628.

83. Hamilton MA, Stevenson LW, Luu M, Walden JA. Altered thyroid hormone metabolism in advanced heart failure. *J Am Coll Cardiol.* 1990;16(1):91-95.

84. Opasich C, Pacini F, Ambrosino N, et al. Sick euthyroid syndrome in patients with moderate-to-severe chronic heart failure. *Eur Heart J.* 1996;17(12):1860-1866.

85. Pingitore A, Landi P, Taddei MC, Ripoli A, L'Abbate A, Iervasi G. Triiodothyronine levels for risk stratification of patients with chronic heart failure. *Am J Med.* 2005;118(2):132-136.

86. Friberg L, Werner S, Eggertsen G, Ahnve S. Rapid down-regulation of thyroid hormones in acute myocardial infarction. *Arch Intern Med.* 2002;162(12):1388-1394.

87. Galli E, Pingitore A, Iervasi G. The role of thyroid hormone in the pathophysiology of heart failure: clinical evidence. *Heart Fail Rev.* 2010;15(2):155-169.

88. Ascheim DD, Hryniewicz K. Thyroid hormone metabolism in patients with congestive heart failure: the low triiodothyronine state. *Thyroid.* 2002;12(6):511-515.

89. Iervasi G, Pingitore A, Landi P, et al. Low-T3 syndrome. *Circulation.* 2003;107(5):708-713.

90. Hunt SA, Abraham WT, Chin MH, et al. 2009 Focused update incorporated into the ACC/AHA 2005 Guidelines for the Diagnosis and Management of Heart Failure in Adults A Report of the American College of Cardiology Foundation/American Heart Association task force on practice guidelines developed. *J Am Coll Cardiol.* 2009;53(15):e1-e90.

91. Resnick LM, Laragh JH. Plasma renin activity in syndromes of thyroid hormone excess and deficiency. *Life Sci.* 1982;30(7-8):585-586.

92. Prisant LM, Gujral JS, Mulloy AL. Hyperthyroidism: a secondary cause of isolated systolic hypertension. *J Clin Hypertens (Greenwich).* 2006;8(8):596-599.

93. Saito I, Ito K, Saruta T. The effect of age on blood pressure in hyperthyroidism. *J Am Geriatr Soc.* 1985;33(1):19-22.

94. Saito I, Saruta T. Hypertension in thyroid disorders. *Endocrinol Metab Clin North Am.* 1994;23(2):379-386.

95. Marcisz C, Jonderko G, Kucharz E. Changes of arterial pressure in patients with hyperthyroidism during therapy. *Med Sci Monit.* 2002;8(7):CR502-CR507.

96. Middeke M, Schrader J. Nocturnal blood pressure in normotensive subjects and those with white coat, primary, and secondary hypertension. *BMJ.* 1994;308(6929):630-632.

97. Iglesias P, Acosta M, Sanchez R, Fernandez-Reyes MJ, Mon C, Diez JJ. Ambulatory blood pressure monitoring in patients with hyperthyroidism before and after control of thyroid function. *Clin Endocrinol (Oxf).* 2005;63(1):66-72.

98. Botella-Carretero JI, Gómez-Bueno M, Barrios V, et al. Chronic thyrotropin-suppressive therapy with levothyroxine and short-term overt hypothyroidism after thyroxine withdrawal are associated with undesirable cardiovascular effects in patients with differentiated thyroid carcinoma. *Endocr Relat Cancer.* 2004;11(2):345-356.

99. Cai Y, Ren Y, Shi J. Blood pressure levels in patients with subclinical thyroid dysfunction: a meta-analysis of cross-sectional data. *Hypertens Res.* 2011;34(10):1098-1105.

100. Li JH, Safford RE, Aduen JF, Heckman MG, Crook JE, Burger CD. Pulmonary hypertension and thyroid disease. *Chest.* 2007;132(3):793-797.

101. Armigliato M, Paolini R, Aggio S, et al. Hyperthyroidism as a cause of pulmonary arterial hypertension: a prospective study. *Angiology.* 2006;57(5):600-606.

102. Sugiura T, Yamanaka S, Takeuchi H, Morimoto N, Kamioka M, Matsumura Y. Autoimmunity and pulmonary hypertension in patients with Graves' disease. *Heart Vessels.* 2015;30(5):642-646.

103. Tudoran C, Tudoran M, Vlad M, Balas M, Pop GN, Parv F. *Anatol J Cardiol.* 2018;20(3):174-181.

104. Muthukumar S, Sadacharan D, Ravikumar K, Mohanapriya G, Hussain Z, Suresh RV. A prospective study on cardiovascular dysfunction in patients with hyperthyroidism and its reversal after surgical cure. *World J Surg.* 2016;40(3):622-628.

105. Simonneau G, Gatzoulis MA, Adatia I, et al. Updated clinical classification of pulmonary hypertension. *J Am Coll Cardiol.* 2013;62(25 suppl):D34-D41.

106. Scicchitano P, Dentamaro I, Tunzi F, et al. Pulmonary hypertension in thyroid diseases. *Endocrine.* 2016;54(3):578-587.

107. Al Husseini A, Bagnato G, Farkas L, et al. Thyroid hormone is highly permissive in angioproliferative pulmonary hypertension in rats. *Eur Respir J.* 2013;41(1):104-114.

108. Davis FB, Mousa SA, O'Connor L, et al. Proangiogenic action of thyroid hormone is fibroblast growth factor-dependent and is initiated at the cell surface. *Circ Res.* 2004;94(11):1500-1506.

109. Pokhrel B, Bhusal K. *Graves Disease.* In: *StatPearls.* Treasure Island, FL. StatPearls Publishing, 2019.

110. Nicolls MR, Taraseviciene-Stewart L, Rai PR, Badesch DB, Voelkel NF. Autoimmunity and pulmonary hypertension: a perspective. *Eur Respir J.* 2005;26(6):1110-1118.

111. Biondi B. Mechanisms in endocrinology: heart failure and thyroid dysfunction. *Eur J Endocrinol.* 2012;167(5):609-618.

112. Cacciatori V, Bellavere F, Pezzarossa A, et al. Power spectral analysis of heart rate in hyperthyroidism. *J Clin Endocrinol Metab.* 1996;81(8):2828-2835.

113. Ertek S, Cicero AF. State of the art paper Hyperthyroidism and cardiovascular complications: a narrative review on the basis of pathophysiology. *Arch Med Sci.* 2013;9(5):944-952.

114. Ellervik C, Roselli C, Christophersen IE, et al. Assessment of the relationship between genetic determinants of thyroid function and atrial fibrillation. *JAMA Cardiol.* 2019;4(2):144-152.

115. Frost L, Vestergaard P, Mosekilde L. Hyperthyroidism and risk of atrial fibrillation or flutter. *Arch Intern Med.* 2004;164(15):1675-1678.

116. Keating FR Jr, Parkin TW, Selby JB, Dickinson LS. Treatment of heart disease associated with myxedema. *Prog Cardiovasc Dis.* 1961;3:364-381.

117. Catz B, Russell S. Myxedema, shock and coma. *Arch Intern Med.* 1961;108:407-417.

118. Wiersinga WM, Duntas L, Fadeyev V, Nygaard B, Vanderpump MP. 2012 ETA guidelines: the use of L-T4 + L-T3 in the treatment of hypothyroidism. *Eur Thyroid J.* 2012;1(2):55-71.

119. Hoang TD, Olsen CH, Mai VQ, Clyde PW, Shakir MK. Desiccated thyroid extract compared with levothyroxine in the treatment of hypothyroidism: a randomized, double-blind, crossover study. *J Clin Endocrinol Metab.* 2013;98(5):1982-1990.

120. Dickson RC, Tomlinson RH. Selenium in blood and human tissues. *Clin Chim Acta.* 1967;16(2):311-321.

121. Kohrle J. The trace element selenium and the thyroid gland. *Biochimie.* 1999;81(5):527-533.

122. Zimmermann MB, Kohrle J. The impact of iron and selenium deficiencies on iodine and thyroid metabolism: biochemistry and relevance to public health. *Thyroid.* 2002;12(10):867-878.

123. Drutel A, Archambeaud F, Caron P. Selenium and the thyroid gland: more good news for clinicians. *Clin Endocrinol (Oxf).* 2013;78(2):155-164.

124. Contempre B, Dumont JE, Ngo B, Thilly CH, Diplock AT, Vanderpas J. Effect of selenium supplementation in hypothyroid subjects of an iodine and selenium deficient area: the possible danger of indiscriminate supplementation of iodine-deficient subjects with selenium. *J Clin Endocrinol Metab.* 1991;73(1):213-215.

125. Duntas LH. Environmental factors and thyroid autoimmunity. *Ann Endocrinol (Paris).* 2011;72(2):108-113.

126. Berger MM, Reymond M, Shenkin A, et al. Influence of selenium supplements on the post-traumatic alterations of the thyroid axis: a placebo-controlled trial. *Intensive Care Med.* 2001;27(1):91-100.

127. Olivieri O, Girelli D, Stanzial AM, Rossi L, Bassi A, Corrocher R. Selenium, zinc, and thyroid hormones in healthy subjects. *Biol Trace Elem Res.* 1996;51(1):31-41.

128. Nishiyama S, Futagoishi-Suginohara Y, Matsukura M, et al. Zinc supplementation alters thyroid hormone metabolism in disabled patients with zinc deficiency. *J Am Coll Nutr.* 1994;13(1):62-67.

129. Mahmoodianfard S, Vafa M, Golgiri F, et al. Effects of zinc and selenium supplementation on thyroid function in overweight and obese hypothyroid female patients: a randomized double-blind controlled trial. *J Am Coll Nutr.* 2015;34(5):391-399.

130. Caldwell KL, Makhmudov A, Ely E, Jones RL, Wang RY. Iodine status of the U.S. Population, National Health and Nutrition Examination Survey, 2005-2006 and 2007-2008. *Thyroid.* 2011;21(4):419-427.

131. Hollowell JG, Staehling NW, Hannon WH, et al. Iodine nutrition in the United States. Trends and Public health implications: iodine excretion data from National Health and Nutrition Examination Surveys I and III (1971-1974 and 1988-1994). *J Clin Endocrinol Metab.* 1998;83(10):3401-3408.

132. Duarte GC, Tomimori EK, de Camargo RY, et al. Excessive iodine intake and ultrasonographic thyroid abnormalities in schoolchildren. *J Pediatr Endocrinol Metab.* 2009;22(4):327-334.

133. Laurberg P, Bulow Pedersen I, Knudsen N, Ovesen L, Andersen S. Environmental iodine intake affects the type of nonmalignant thyroid disease. *Thyroid.* 2001;11(5):457-469.

134. Markou KB, Georgopoulos NA, Makri M, et al. Improvement of iodine deficiency after iodine supplementation in schoolchildren of Azerbaijan was accompanied by hypo and hyperthyrotropinemia and increased titre of thyroid autoantibodies. *J Endocrinol Invest.* 2003;26(2 suppl):43-48.

135. Teng W, Shan Z, Teng X, et al. Effect of iodine intake on thyroid diseases in China. *N Engl J Med.* 2006;354(26):2783-2793.

136. van Zuuren EJ, Albusta AY, Fedorowicz Z, Carter B, Pijl H. Selenium supplementation for hashimoto's thyroiditis: summary of a cochrane systematic review. *Eur Thyroid J.* 2014;3(1):25-31.

137. Winther KH, Bonnema SJ, Cold F, et al. Does selenium supplementation affect thyroid function? Results from a randomized, controlled, double-blinded trial in a Danish population. *Eur J Endocrinol*. 2015;172(6):657-667.

138. Benua RS, Becker DV, Hurley JR. Thyroid storm. *Curr Ther Endocrinol Metab*. 1994;5:75-77.

139. Bremner AP, Feddema P, Joske DJ, et al. Significant association between thyroid hormones and erythrocyte indices in euthyroid subjects. *Clin Endocrinol (Oxf)*. 2012;76(2):304-311.

140. Tahara Y, Hirota M, Shima K, et al. Primary hypothyroidism in an adult patient with protein-calorie malnutrition: a study of its mechanism and the effect of amino acid deficiency. *Metabolism*. 1988;37(1):9-14.

141. Higueret P, Pailler I, Garcin H. Vitamin A deficiency and tri-iodothyronine action at the cellular level in the rat. *J Endocrinol*. 1989;121(1):75-79.

142. Feart C, Pallet V, Boucheron C, et al. Aging affects the retinoic acid and the triiodothyronine nuclear receptor mRNA expression in human peripheral blood mononuclear cells. *Eur J Endocrinol*. 2005;152(3):449-458.

143. Kivity S, Agmon-Levin N, Zisappl M, et al. Vitamin D and autoimmune thyroid diseases. *Cell Mol Immunol*. 2011;8(3):243-247.

144. Stepien T, Krupinski R, Sopinski J, et al. Decreased 1-25 dihydroxyvitamin D3 concentration in peripheral blood serum of patients with thyroid cancer. *Arch Med Res*. 2010;41(3):190-194.

145. Roti E, Minelli R, Salvi M. Thyroid hormone metabolism in obesity. *Int J Obes Relat Metab Disord*. 2000;24(suppl 2):S113-S115.

146. Carter JP, Allain J. TRH, reverse T3, and leuenkephalin levels and other physiological changes in a male adult during prolonged fasting. *J Natl Med Assoc*. 1983;75(12):1161-1166.

147. Koppeschaar HP, Meinders AE, Schwarz F. Metabolic responses in grossly obese subjects treated with a very-low-calorie diet with and without triiodothyronine treatment. *Int J Obes*. 1983;7(2):123-131.

148. Walter KN, Corwin EJ, Ulbrecht J, et al. Elevated thyroid stimulating hormone is associated with elevated cortisol in healthy young men and women. *Thyroid Res*. 2012;5(1):13.

149. Abdulateef DS, Mahwi TO. Assessment of hair cortisol in euthyroid, hypothyroid, and subclinical hypothyroid subjects. *Endocrine*. 2019;63(1):131-139.

150. Comtois R, Hebert J, Soucy JP. Increase in T3 levels during hypocorticism in patients with chronic secondary adrenocortical insufficiency. *Acta Endocrinol (Copenh)*. 1992;126(4):319-324.

151. Banos C, Tako J, Salamon F, Gyorgyi S, Czikkely R. Effect of ACTH-stimulated glucocorticoid hypersecretion on the serum concentrations of thyroxine-binding globulin, thyroxine, triiodothyronine, reverse triiodothyronine and on the TSH-response to TRH. *Acta Med Acad Sci Hung*. 1979;36(4):381-394.

152. Mastorakos G, Pavlatou M. Exercise as a stress model and the interplay between the hypothalamus-pituitary-adrenal and the hypothalamus-pituitary-thyroid axes. *Horm Metab Res*. 2005;37(9):577-584.

153. Fortunato RS, Ignácio DL, Padron ÁS, et al. The effect of acute exercise session on thyroid hormone economy in rats. *J Endocrinol*. 2008;198(2):347-353.

154. Lesmana R, Iwasaki T, Iizuka Y, Amano I, Shimokawa N, Koibuchi N. The change in thyroid hormone signaling by altered training intensity in male rat skeletal muscle. *Endocr J*. 2016;63(8):727-738.

155. Nestler EJ, Hyman SE, Malenka RC. *Molecular Neuropharmacology: A Foundation for Clinical Neuroscience*. 2nd ed. New York: McGraw-Hill Medical; 2009.

156. Selye H. *Stress Without Distress*. London: Hodder and Stoughton; 1974.

157. Castinetti F, Morange I, Conte-Devolx B, Brue T. Cushing's disease. *Orphanet J Rare Dis*. 2012;7:41.

158. Yiallouris A, Tsioutis C, Agapidaki E, et al. Adrenal aging and its implications on stress responsiveness in humans. *Front Endocrinol (Lausanne)*. 2019;10:54.

159. Pazderska A, Pearce SH. Adrenal insufficiency – recognition and management. *Clin Med (Lond)*. 2017;17(3):258-262.

160. Insel TR. The challenge of translation in social neuroscience: a review of oxytocin, vasopressin, and affiliative behavior. *Neuron*. 2010;65(6):768-779.

161. Costa A, Rossi E, Scicchitano BM, Coletti D, Moresi V, Adamo S. Neurohypophyseal hormones: novel actors of striated muscle development and homeostasis. *Eur J Transl Myol*. 2014;24(3):3790.

162. Walker BR, Colledge NR, Ralston S, Penman ID, Britton R. *Davidson's Principles and Practice of Medicine*. 22nd ed. Edinburgh; New York: Churchill Livingstone/Elsevier; 2014.

163. Gleitman H, Fridlund AJ, Reisberg D. *Psychology*. 6th ed. New York: W.W. Norton; 2004.

164. Mezzacappa EK, Palmer ES, Palmer SN. Epinephrine, arousal, and emotion: a new look at two-factor theory. *Cogn Emot*. 1999;13(2):181-199.

165. Echeverri D, Montes FR, Cabrera M, Galan A, Prieto A. Caffeine's vascular mechanisms of action. *Int J Vasc Med*. 2010;2010:834060.

166. Metagenics Inc. Identi-T Stress Assessment. 2019:MET1673.

167. Vaidya A, Mulatero P, Baudrand R, Adler GK. The expanding spectrum of primary aldosteronism: implications for diagnosis, pathogenesis, and treatment. *Endocr Rev*. 2018;39(6):1057-1088.

168. Vilela LAP, Almeida MQ. Diagnosis and management of primary aldosteronism. *Arch Endocrinol Metab*. 2017;61(3):305-312.

169. Conn JW. Primary aldosteronism. *J Lab Clin Med*. 1955;45(4):661-664.

170. Lang F. On the pleotropic actions of mineralocorticoids. *Nephron Physiol*. 2014;128(1-2):1-7.

171. Hannemann A, Wallaschofski H. Prevalence of primary aldosteronism in patient's cohorts and in population-based studies – a review of the current literature. *Horm Metab Res*. 2012;44(3):157-162.

172. Plouin PF, Amar L, Chatellier G. Trends in the prevalence of primary aldosteronism, aldosterone-producing adenomas, and surgically correctable aldosterone-dependent hypertension. *Nephrol Dial Transpl*. 2004;19(4):774-777.

173. Calhoun DA, Nishizaka MK, Zaman MA, Thakkar RB, Weissmann P. Hyperaldosteronism among black and white subjects with resistant hypertension. *Hypertension*. 2002;40(6):892-896.

174. Gallay BJ, Ahmad S, Xu L, Toivola B, Davidson RC. Screening for primary aldosteronism without discontinuing hypertensive medications: plasma aldosterone-renin ratio. *Am J Kidney Dis*. 2001;37(4):699-705.

175. Strauch B, Zelinka T, Hampf M, Bernhardt R, Widimsky J Jr. Prevalence of primary hyperaldosteronism in moderate to severe hypertension in the Central Europe region. *J Hum Hypertens*. 2003;17(5):349-352.

176. Eide IK, Torjesen PA, Drolsum A, Babovic A, Lilledahl NP. Low-renin status in therapy-resistant hypertension. *J Hypertens*. 2004;22(11):2217-2226.

177. Markou A, Pappa T, Kaltsas G, et al. Evidence of primary aldosteronism in a predominantly female cohort of normotensive individuals: a very high odds ratio for progression into arterial hypertension. *J Clin Endocrinol Metab*. 2013;98(4):1409-1416.

178. Baudrand R, Guarda FJ, Fardella C, et al. Continuum of renin-independent aldosteronism in normotension. *Hypertension*. 2017;69(5):950-956.

179. Briet M, Schiffrin EL. Vascular actions of aldosterone. *J Vasc Res*. 2013;50(2):89-99.

180. Gao J, Zhang K, Chen J, et al. Roles of aldosterone in vascular calcification: an update. *Eur J Pharmacol*. 2016;786:186-193.

181. Brown NJ. Contribution of aldosterone to cardiovascular and renal inflammation and fibrosis. *Nat Rev Nephrol*. 2013;9(8):459-469.

182. Sapolsky RM, Romero LM, Munck AU. How do glucocorticoids influence stress responses? integrating permissive, suppressive, stimulatory, and preparative actions. *Endocr Rev*. 2000;21(1):55-89.

183. Walker BR. Glucocorticoids and cardiovascular disease. *Eur J Endocrinol*. 2007;157(5):545-559.

184. Whitworth JA, Saines D, Thatcher R, Butkus A, Scoggins BA, Coghlan JP. Blood pressure, renal and metabolic effects of ACTH in normotensive man. *Clin Sci (Lond)*. 1981;61(suppl 7):269s-272s.

185. Isidori AM, Graziadio C, Paragliola RM, et al. The hypertension of Cushing's syndrome. *J Hypertens*. 2015;33(1):44-60.

186. Soro A, Ingram MC, Tonolo G, Glorioso N, Fraser R. Evidence of coexisting changes in 11β-hydroxysteroid dehydrogenase and 5β-reductase activity in subjects with untreated essential hypertension. *Hypertension*. 1995;25(1):67-70.

187. Haas AV, Hopkins PN, Brown NJ, et al. Higher urinary cortisol levels associate with increased cardiovascular risk. *Endocr Connect.* 2019;8(6):634-640.

188. Souverein PC, Berard A, Van Staa TP, et al. Use of oral glucocorticoids and risk of cardiovascular and cerebrovascular disease in a population based case-control study. *Heart.* 2004;90(8):859-865.

189. Wei L, MacDonald TM, Walker BR. Taking glucocorticoids by prescription is associated with subsequent cardiovascular disease. *Ann Intern Med.* 2004;141(10):764-770.

190. Agca R, Heslinga SC, Rollefstad S, et al. EULAR recommendations for cardiovascular disease risk management in patients with rheumatoid arthritis and other forms of inflammatory joint disorders: 2015/2016 update. *Ann Rheum Dis.* 2017;76(1):17-28.

191. Tank AW, Lee Wong D. Peripheral and central effects of circulating catecholamines. *Compr Physiol.* 2015;5(1):1-15.

192. Santulli G, Iaccarino G. Adrenergic signaling in heart failure and cardiovascular aging. *Maturitas.* 2016;93:65-72.

193. de Lucia C, Eguchi A, Koch WJ. New insights in cardiac β-adrenergic signaling during heart failure and aging. *Front Pharmacol.* 2018;9:904.

194. Akaza I, Yoshimoto T, Tsuchiya K, Hirata Y. Endothelial dysfunction A associated with hypercortisolism is reversible in Cushing's syndrome. *Endocr J.* 2010;57(3):245-252.

195. Dekkers OM, Horváth-Puhó E, Jørgensen JOL, et al. Multisystem morbidity and mortality in Cushing's syndrome: a cohort study. *J Clin Endocrinol Metab.* 2013;98(6):2277-2284.

196. Albiger N, Testa R, Almoto B, et al. Patients with Cushing's syndrome have increased intimal media thickness at different vascular levels: comparison with a population matched for similar cardiovascular risk factors. *Horm Metab Res.* 2006;38(6):405-410.

197. Muiesan ML, Lupia M, Salvetti M, et al. Left ventricular structural and functional characteristics in Cushing's syndrome. *J Am Coll Cardiol.* 2003;41(12):2275-2279.

198. Toja PM, Branzi G, Ciambellotti F, et al. Clinical relevance of cardiac structure and function abnormalities in patients with Cushing's syndrome before and after cure. *Clin Endocrinol (Oxf).* 2012;76(3):332-338.

199. Ferrau F, Korbonits M. Metabolic syndrome in Cushing's syndrome patients. *Front Horm Res.* 2018;49:85-103.

200. Chanson P, Salenave S. Metabolic syndrome in Cushing's syndrome. *Neuroendocrinology.* 2010;92(suppl 1):96-101.

201. Cicala MV, Mantero F. Hypertension in Cushing's syndrome: from pathogenesis to treatment. *Neuroendocrinology.* 2010;92(suppl 1):44-49.

202. Feldman HA, Johannes CB, Araujo AB, Mohr BA, Longcope C, McKinlay JB. Low dehydroepiandrosterone and ischemic heart disease in middle-aged men: prospective results from the Massachusetts male aging study. *Am J Epidemiol.* 2001;153(1):79-89.

203. Jimenez MC, Sun Q, Schürks M, et al. Low dehydroepiandrosterone sulfate is associated with increased risk of ischemic stroke among women. *Stroke.* 2013;44(7):1784-1789.

204. Akishita M, Hashimoto M, Ohike Y, et al. Association of plasma dehydroepiandrosterone-sulfate levels with endothelial function in postmenopausal women with coronary risk factors. *Hypertens Res.* 2008;31(1):69-74.

205. Yoshida S, Aihara KI, Azuma H, et al. Dehydroepiandrosterone sulfate is inversely associated with sex-dependent diverse carotid atherosclerosis regardless of endothelial function. *Atherosclerosis.* 2010;212(1):310-315.

206. Herrington DM, Gordon GB, Achuff SC, et al. Plasma dehydroepiandrosterone and dehydroepiandrosterone sulfate in patients undergoing diagnostic coronary angiography. *J Am Coll Cardiol.* 1990;16(6):862-870.

207. Wu TT, Chen Y, Zhou Y, et al. Prognostic value of dehydroepiandrosterone sulfate for patients with cardiovascular disease: a systematic review and meta-analysis. *J Am Heart Assoc.* 2017;6(5).

208. Mannic T, Viguie J, Rossier MF. In vivo and in vitro evidences of dehydroepiandrosterone protective role on the cardiovascular system. *Int J Endocrinol Metab.* 2015;13(2):e24660.

209. Schumaecker MM, Larsen TR, Sane DC. Cardiac manifestations of adrenal insufficiency. *Rev Cardiovasc Med.* 2016;17(3-4):131-136.

210. Krishnamoorthy A, Mentz RJ, Hyland KA, et al. A crisis of the heart. *ASAIO J.* 2013;59(6):668-670.

211. Dimarakis I, Shaw S, Venkateswaran R. Durable left ventricular assist device as a bridge to recovery for addisonian crisis related cardiomyopathy. *J Card Surg.* 2017;32(10):665-666.

212. Wolff B, Machill K, Schulzki I, Schumacher D, Werner D. Acute reversible cardiomyopathy with cardiogenic shock in a patient with addisonian crisis: a case report. *Int J Cardiol.* 2007;116(2):e71-e73.

213. Wiltshire EJ, Wilson R, Pringle KC. Addison's disease presenting with an acute abdomen and complicated by cardiomyopathy. *J Paediatr Child Health.* 2004;40(11):644-645.

214. Conwell LS, Gray LM, Delbridge RG, Thomsett MJ, Batch JA. Reversible cardiomyopathy in paediatric Addison's disease–a cautionary tale. *J Pediatr Endocrinol Metab.* 2003;16(8):1191-1195.

215. Afzal A, Khaja F. Reversible cardiomyopathy associated with Addison's disease. *Can J Cardiol.* 2000;16(3):377-379.

216. Ross IL, Bergthorsdottir R, Levitt N, et al. Cardiovascular risk factors in patients with Addison's disease: a comparative study of South African and Swedish patients. *PLoS One.* 2014;9(6):e90768.

217. Inder WJ, Meyer C, Hunt PJ. Management of hypertension and heart failure in patients with Addison's disease. *Clin Endocrinol (Oxf).* 2015;82(6):789-792.

218. Whitworth JA, Gordon D, Andrews J, Scoggins BA. The hypertensive effect of synthetic glucocorticoids in man: role of sodium and volume. *J Hypertens.* 1989;7(7):537-549.

219. Knowlton AI, Baer L. Cardiac failure in Addison's disease. *Am J Med.* 1983;74(5):829-836.

220. Bhattacharyya A, Tymms DJ. Heart failure with fludrocortisone in Addison's disease. *J R Soc Med.* 1998;91(8):433-434.

221. Willis FR, Byrne GC, Jones TW. Fludrocortisone induced heart failure in Addison's disease. *J Paediatr Child Health.* 1994;30(3):280-281.

222. Sullivan M, Carberry A, Evans ES, Hall EE, Nepocatych S. The effects of power and stretch yoga on affect and salivary cortisol in women. *J Health Psychol.* 2017:1359105317694487.

223. Pascoe MC, Thompson DR, Ski CF. Yoga, mindfulness-based stress reduction and stress-related physiological measures: a meta-analysis. *Psychoneuroendocrinology.* 2017;86:152-168.

224. Lim SA, Cheong KJ. Regular yoga practice improves antioxidant status, immune function, and stress hormone releases in young healthy people: a randomized, double-blind, controlled pilot study. *J Altern Complement Med.* 2015;21(9):530-538.

225. Creswell JD, Taren AA, Lindsay EK, et al. Alterations in resting-state functional connectivity link mindfulness meditation with reduced interleukin-6: a randomized controlled trial. *Biol Psychiatry.* 2016;80(1):53-61.

226. Pascoe MC, Thompson DR, Jenkins ZM, Ski CF. Mindfulness mediates the physiological markers of stress: systematic review and meta-analysis. *J Psychiatr Res.* 2017;95:156-178.

227. Vandana B, Vaidyanathan K, Saraswathy LA, Sundaram KR, Kumar H. Impact of integrated amrita meditation technique on adrenaline and cortisol levels in healthy volunteers. *Evid Based Complement Alternat Med.* 2011;2011:379645.

228. Kim SH, Schneider SM, Bevans M, et al. PTSD symptom reduction with mindfulness-based stretching and deep breathing exercise: randomized controlled clinical trial of efficacy. *J Clin Endocrinol Metab.* 2013;98(7):2984-2992.

229. Velema MS, de Nooijer A, Burgers V, et al. Health-related quality of life and mental health in primary aldosteronism: a systematic review. *Horm Metab Res.* 2017;49(12):943-950.

230. Hanusch FM, Fischer E, Lang K, et al. Sleep quality in patients with primary aldosteronism. *Hormones (Athens).* 2014;13(1):57-64.

231. Jin ZN, Wei YX. *J Geriatr Cardiol.* 2016;13(4):333-343.

232. Morgan E, Schumm LP, McClintock M, Waite L, Lauderdale DS. Sleep characteristics and daytime cortisol levels in older adults. *Sleep.* 2017;40(5):1-11.

233. Garcia-Prieto MD, Tebar FJ, Nicolas F, Larque E, Zamora S, Garaulet M. Cortisol secretary pattern and glucocorticoid feedback sensitivity in women from a Mediterranean area: relationship with anthropometric characteristics, dietary intake and plasma fatty acid profile. *Clin Endocrinol (Oxf).* 2007;66(2):185-191.

234. Mattei J, Bhupathiraju S, Tucker KL. Higher adherence to a diet score based on American Heart Association recommendations is associated with lower odds of allostatic load and metabolic syndrome in Puerto Rican Adults. *J Nutr.* 2013;143(11):1753-1759.

235. Spence JD, Thornton T, Muir AD, Westcott ND. The effect of flax seed cultivars with differing content of α-linolenic acid and lignans on responses to mental stress. *J Am Coll Nutr.* 2003;22(6):494-501.

236. Brody S, Preut R, Schommer K, Schurmeyer TH. A randomized controlled trial of high dose ascorbic acid for reduction of blood pressure, cortisol, and subjective responses to psychological stress. *Psychopharmacology (Berl).* 2002;159(3):319-324.

237. Enwonwu CO, Sawiris P, Chanaud N. Effect of marginal ascorbic acid deficiency on saliva level of cortisol in the Guinea pig. *Arch Oral Biol.* 1995;40(8):737-742.

238. Peters EM, Anderson R, Nieman DC, Fickl H, Jogessar V. Vitamin C supplementation attenuates the increases in circulating cortisol, adrenaline and anti-inflammatory polypeptides following ultramarathon running. *Int J Sports Med.* 2001;22(7):537-543.

239. Cuciureanu MD, Vink R. Magnesium and stress. In: Vink R, Nechifor M, eds. *Magnesium in the Central Nervous System.* Adelaide,AU: University of Adelaide Press; 2011.

240. Seelig MS. Consequences of magnesium deficiency on the enhancement of stress reactions; preventive and therapeutic implications (a review). *J Am Coll Nutr.* 1994;13(5):429-446.

241. Bertinato J, Wang KC, Hayward S. Serum magnesium concentrations in the canadian population and associations with diabetes, glycemic regulation, and insulin resistance. *Nutrients.* 2017;9(3):296.

242. Razzaque MS. Magnesium: are we consuming enough? *Nutrients.* 2018;10(12):1863.

243. Jaroenporn S, Yamamoto T, Itabashi A, et al. Effects of pantothenic acid supplementation on adrenal steroid secretion from male rats. *Biol Pharm Bull.* 2008;31(6):1205-1208.

244. Folsom AR, Nieto FJ, McGovern PG, et al. Prospective study of coronary heart disease incidence in relation to fasting total homocysteine, related genetic polymorphisms, and B vitamins. *Circulation.* 1998;98(3):204-210.

245. Vinogradov VV, Shneider AB, Senkevich SB. Thiamine cardiotropism. *Cor Vasa.* 1991;33(3):254-262.

246. Benton D, Donohoe RT, Sillance B, Nabb S. The influence of phosphatidylserine supplementation on mood and heart rate when faced with an acute stressor. *Nutr Neurosci.* 2001;4(3):169-178.

247. Hellhammer J, Vogt D, Franz N, Freitas U, Rutenberg D. A soy-based phosphatidylserine/ phosphatidic acid complex (PAS) normalizes the stress reactivity of hypothalamus-pituitary-adrenal-axis in chronically stressed male subjects: a randomized, placebo-controlled study. *Lipids Health Dis.* 2014;13:121.

248. Panossian A, Wikman G, Kaur P, Asea A. Adaptogens exert a stress-protective effect by modulation of expression of molecular chaperones. *Phytomedicine.* 2009;16(6-7):617-622.

249. Al-Dujaili EA, Kenyon CJ, Nicol MR, Mason JI. Liquorice and glycyrrhetinic acid increase DHEA and deoxycorticosterone levels in vivo and in vitro by inhibiting adrenal SULT2A1 activity. *Mol Cell Endocrinol.* 2011;336(1-2):102-109.

250. Baker ME, Fanestil DD. Licorice, computer-based analyses of dehydrogenase sequences, and the regulation of steroid and prostaglandin action. *Mol Cell Endocrinol.* 1991;78(1-2):C99-C102.

251. Walker BR, Edwards CR. Licorice-induced hypertension and syndromes of apparent mineralocorticoid excess. *Endocrinol Metab Clin North Am.* 1994;23(2):359-377.

252. Olsson EM, von Scheele B, Panossian AG. A randomised, double-blind, placebo-controlled, parallel-group study of the standardised extract shr-5 of the roots of Rhodiola roseain the treatment of subjects with stress-related fatigue. *Planta Med.* 2009;75(2):105-112.

253. Darbinyan V, Kteyan A, Panossian A, Gabrielian E, Wikman G, Wagner H. Rhodiola rosea in stress induced fatigue - a double blind cross-over study of a standardized extract SHR-5 with a repeated low-dose regimen on the mental performance of healthy physicians during night duty. *Phytomedicine.* 2000;7(5):365-371.

254. Spasov AA, Wikman GK, Mandrikov VB, Mironova IA, Neumoin VV. A double-blind, placebo-controlled pilot study of the stimulating and adaptogenic effect of Rhodiola rosea SHR-5 extract on the fatigue of students caused by stress during an examination period with a repeated low-dose regimen. *Phytomedicine.* 2000;7(2):85-89.

255. Kimura Y, Sumiyoshi M. Effects of various Eleutherococcus senticosus cortex on swimming time, natural killer activity and corticosterone level in forced swimming stressed mice. *J Ethnopharmacol.* 2004;95(2-3):447-453.

256. Bhattacharya SK, Muruganandam AV. Adaptogenic activity of Withania somnifera: an experimental study using a rat model of chronic stress. *Pharmacol Biochem Behav.* 2003;75(3):547-555.

257. Visavadiya NP, Narasimhacharya AV. Hypocholesteremic and antioxidant effects of Withania somnifera (Dunal) in hypercholesteremic rats. *Phytomedicine.* 2007;14(2-3):136-142.

258. Panda AK, Swain KC. Traditional uses and medicinal potential of Cordyceps sinensis of Sikkim. *J Ayurveda Integr Med.* 2011;2(1):9-13.

259. Wang SM, Lee LJ, Lin WW, Chang CM. Effects of a water-soluble extract ofCordyceps sinensis on steroidogenesis and capsular morphology of lipid droplets in cultured rat adrenocortical cells. *J Cell Biochem.* 1998;69(4):483-489.

260. Zhu JS, Halpern GM, Jones K. The Scientific Rediscovery of an Ancient Chinese Herbal Medicine: Cordyceps sinensis Part I. *J Altern Complement Med.* 1998;4(3):289-303.

261. Oliynyk S, Oh S. Actoprotective effect of ginseng: improving mental and physical performance. *J Ginseng Res.* 2013;37(2):144-166.

262. Li X, Xie H, Zhan R, Chen D. Effect of double bond position on 2-phenyl-benzofuran antioxidants: a comparative study of moracin C and iso-moracin C. *Molecules.* 2018;23(4):754.

263. Hiai S, Yokoyama H, Oura H, Yano S. Stimulation of pituitary-adrenocortical system by ginseng saponin. *Endocrinol Jpn.* 1979;26(6):661-665.

264. Singh A, Saxena E, Bhutani KK. Adrenocorticosterone alterations in male, albino mice treated withTrichopus zeylanicus, withania somnifera and Panax ginseng preparations. *Phytother Res.* 2000;14(2):122-125.

265. Radad K, Gille G, Liu L, Rausch WD. Use of ginseng in medicine with emphasis on neurodegenerative disorders. *J Pharmacol Sci.* 2006;100(3):175-186.

266. Avakian EV, Sugimoto RB, Taguchi S, Horvath SM. Effect of Panax ginseng extract on energy metabolism during exercise in rats. *Planta Med.* 1984;50(2):151-154.

267. Wade A, Gembert K, Florea I. A comparative study of the efficacy of acute and continuation treatment with escitalopram versus duloxetine in patients with major depressive disorder. *Curr Med Res Opin.* 2007;23(7):1605-1614.

268. Mah PM, Jenkins RC, Rostami-Hodjegan A, et al. Weight-related dosing, timing and monitoring hydrocortisone replacement therapy in patients with adrenal insufficiency. *Clin Endocrinol (Oxf).* 2004;61(3):367-375.

269. Jefferies WM. Low-dosage glucocorticoid therapy. *Arch Intern Med.* 1967;119(3):265-278.

270. Chan S, Debono M. Review: replication of cortisol circadian rhythm: new advances in hydrocortisone replacement therapy. *Ther Adv Endocrinol Metab.* 2010;1(3):129-138.

271. Zhang YT, Xue JJ, Wang Q, et al. Dehydroepiandrosterone attenuates pulmonary artery and right ventricular remodeling in a rat model of pulmonary hypertension due to left heart failure. *Life Sci.* 2019;219:82-89.

26

Insulin Resistance, Metabolic Syndrome, and Diabetes Mellitus Type 1 and Type 2: Physiology, Pathophysiology, Metabolic Considerations, and Clinical Presentation

Filomena Trindade, MD, MPH, ABOIM, IFMCP, FAARM, ABFM

Introduction

Diabetes mellitus (both type 1 and type 2) is rapidly emerging as one of the biggest health concerns in the United States as well as worldwide. Diabetes mellitus affects more than 180 million people around the world, and this number is anticipated to increase to 300 million by 2025.[1] Recent statistics indicate that the prevalence of diabetes in adults has increased since 1980 in virtually every country of the world with close to a quadrupling of the number of adults worldwide with diabetes.[2] This is particularly significant because the prevalence is especially increasing in countries where the prevalence of common risk factors such as obesity is low. Diabetes is associated with profound implications for disability, mortality, and health care costs. The rates of diabetes have been increasing at alarming rates and correlate with the changes in the nutrient density and quality of our food, our increasing sedentary lifestyle, and changes in our gut microbiome. In addition, global industrialization with the production of plastics, pesticides, synthetic fertilizers, heavy metals, electronic waste, food additives, and endocrine-disrupting chemicals in the environment has drastically altered our food chain.[3] At the root of type 2 diabetes is insulin resistance, which presents as a continuum that should be evaluated in every patient.

Forty percent of children are overweight (meaning a body mass index or BMI of 25 or more and less than 30) and 2 million are morbidly obese (BMI of 30 or greater), exceeding the 99th percentile for weight.[4] The numbers of "adult onset" or type 2 diabetes in children have also climbed astronomically. Over the last two decades there has been over 1000% increase in type 2 diabetes in children.[5] Fifteen years ago 3% of new cases of diabetes in children were type 2 diabetes; now it is 50%.[6] The first study to estimate trends in newly diagnosed cases of type 1 and type 2 diabetes in youth under the age of 20, from the five major racial/ethnic groups in the United States (non-Hispanic whites, non-Hispanic blacks, Hispanics, Asian Americans/Pacific Islanders), and Native Americans found that the combined triggers for the development of type 2 DM were genetic predisposition and environmental factors that result in an immune reaction that destroys pancreatic beta cells.[7] In this study, they noted a significant annual increase in the incidence of type 1 and type 2 diabetes in all racial and ethnic groups except non-Hispanic whites in the period studied from 2002 to 2012.[7]

The causes of type 2 diabetes and insulin resistance are mostly due to environmental and lifestyle factors; meaning it is completely curable and preventable. Even when considering changes in the gut microbiota as the root cause of insulin resistance or diabetes type 1, it is environmental and lifestyle factors that can affect the gut microbiota. Dr Barbara Corkey proposed a model that environmentally induced elevated background levels of insulin, superimposed on a susceptible genetic background, or basal hyperinsulinemia is the root cause of insulin resistance, obesity, and diabetes.[8] Dr David Ludwig has discussed how ubiquitous junk food marketing, lack of opportunities for physically active recreation, and other aspects of modern society promote unhealthful lifestyles in children. Furthermore, he points to how inadequate or unskilled parental supervision can leave children vulnerable to the obesogenic environmental influences in our food. He also discussed the emotional distress and depression, or other psychological problems arising from abuse and neglect that may exacerbate this situation by leading to disordered eating and withdrawal from sports and other social activities which compounds the problem even further.[9]

Dr David Kessler, the former Food and Drug Administration (FDA) director, has described the science of how food is made into drugs leading to neurochemical addiction in his book, *The End of Overeating*. Our children are most susceptible to advertising schemes accounting for one of the reasons for obese children being nutritionally deficient.[10] Another cause of the childhood obesity epidemic is the consumption of energy-rich sugar and high-fructose sweetened drinks.[11]

The focus of this chapter is on early detection and diagnosis of diabetes type 1 and insulin resistance (before insulin resistance progresses to prediabetes or diabetes type 2). We will also review the causes and the physiology of insulin resistance and diabetes type 1 as well as discuss and review treatment options. I hope to provide tools to help clinicians to better diagnose, treat, and hopefully reverse the progression to type 2 diabetes.

Medical Consequences of Metabolic Dysfunction

Cardiovascular disease and diabetes be it type 1 or type 2 are linked to each other through obesity, insulin resistance, inflammation, oxidative stress, and immune dysfunction. People with diabetes suffer vascular disease at much higher rates. It is estimated that diabetics are four times more likely to die of heart disease including coronary heart disease (CHD), myocardial infarction (MI), and congestive heart failure. The rate of cerebrovascular accidents (CVAs) is three to four times higher in diabetics. Patients with prediabetes are also four times more likely to die of heart disease. So "pre" is not really "pre" at all. Consequently, it is the insulin resistance that is the real problem and where our focus should be as clinicians.

The close association of insulin resistance, obesity, inflammation, oxidative stress, and immune dysfunction allows the clinician to diagnose vascular dysfunction early. Appropriate laboratory testing and noninvasive cardiovascular testing gives us the opportunity to diagnose vascular dysfunction in this "pre" stage so we can initiate aggressive prevention and treatment.[9,12]

It has been said over and over again by many researchers that one of the main reasons for the increase in diabetes and insulin resistance is obesity. In my opinion based on clinical review I believe that the opposite is true; that the reason we see such a big increase in obesity is due to insulin resistance. I am not disputing the fact that obesity can lead to insulin resistance; I am saying that a major cause of obesity is due to insulin resistance. I believe the major cause of weight gain is undiagnosed insulin resistance. As clinicians we need to ascertain why and how a patient became insulin resistant, or if they have diabetes type 1 what was the trigger? How and where do we start? How do we identify insulin resistance, and how do we treat it? What is the root cause? Why is a person insulin resistant? Applying medical principles and cutting edge scientific research, it is important to get to the "genesis" of these diseases and answer these questions. This is one of the major objectives in this chapter.

According to Dr Barbara Corkey, insulin resistance actually starts with damage to the pancreatic beta cells leading to hyperinsulinemia and causing insulin resistance.[8] In a publication in 2014, Dr Corkey discusses the role of beta cell toxicity inducing insulin resistance.[13] In this article, she identifies many toxins including food additives, contaminants such as persistent organic pollutants, noncaloric sweeteners, and high-dose nutrients, to name a few, as potential causes of beta cell damage.[13] Hyperinsulinemia and hyperlipidemia are early indicators of metabolic dysfunction, and treating and reversing these abnormalities may prevent the development of more serious metabolic diseases.[14] In my opinion, based on her work and that of other researchers, I firmly believe that undiagnosed insulin resistance in many cases can be the cause of obesity and not the reverse. Obesity can lead to insulin resistance, but one of the main reasons for such high rates of diabetes type 2 may be undiagnosed insulin resistance. The continuum of insulin resistance must be understood, diagnosed, and properly treated and addressed.

The Continuum of Insulin Resistance and Diabetes Type 2

Diabetes Type 2 Exists on a Continuum of Insulin Resistance

Insulin resistance is a condition where insulin becomes less effective at lowering blood sugar. It is the inability of insulin to facilitate glucose uptake into the cell due to poor insulin binding at the insulin receptors. Insulin is unable to be transported to the interior of the cell, which results in increased pancreatic insulin production and hyperinsulinemia well above the normal range. Initially the excess insulin is able to keep serum glucose in the normal range.

Impaired Glucose Tolerance

Impaired glucose tolerance occurs when glucose rises above the normal range as the pancreas continues to overproduce insulin. The rise can be seen after meals or in the fasting state. In many patients, the fasting glucose may be normal, but there is an elevated glucose level after a meal or after a high glycemic load challenge. Serum glucose is elevated but not enough to qualify the patient as prediabetic. These are the patients who have an elevated HgbA1c but may have a normal fasting glucose. This implies that the pancreas is no longer able to keep blood glucose normal after a glucose challenge.

Prediabetes

As the pancreas continues to overproduce insulin, it is no longer able to keep fasting blood glucose in the normal range. This new range needs to be redefined based on new data. However, according to most laboratories and the ADA this is presently defined as fasting blood glucose over 100 mg/dL but less than 126 mg/dL. However, data from NHS about the relationship of fasting blood sugar (FBS) to CHD and MI suggest that risk starts at about 80 mg/dL. If we analyze the data further, several studies have shown that fasting blood sugar (FBG) over 75 is where cardiovascular risk starts, and for each 1 mg% increase in FBG starting at 75 mg%, there is a 1% increase in CV events. Also, for 2-hour oral glucose tolerance test (OGTT), there is a 2% increase in CV events per 1 mg% increase in glucose starting at 110 mg%.[15-17]

Diabetes Mellitus Type 2

Diabetes type 2 is still being defined by most laboratory reference ranges as an FBS of 126 mg/dL or higher, or a random blood sugar of over 200 mg/dL on more than one occasion. However, these values need to be redefined. According to multiple studies, postprandial risk starts at 110 mg/dL and should not be more than 140 mg/dL. Postprandial hyperglycemia predicts CHD better than FBS in both diabetic and normal individuals. Mean amplitude of glucose excursions (MAGE) predicts glucose instability between peaks and nadirs and is the best predictor of CVD.[18] Post challenge hyperglycemia predicts early vascular damage better than fasting glucose and HgbA1C. The 2-hour OGTT is superior to FBG and HgbA1C in predicting vascular disease early in obese and high-risk patients without DM. Also 2-hour OGTT correlates better with carotid IMT and arterial stiffness.[19]

What are the Causes of Diabetes Type 1 and Insulin Resistance

The following is a list I copyrighted and have used to look for the underlying root cause(s) of insulin resistance and diabetes type 1. I also ask the question: How did this person develop insulin resistance, impaired glucose tolerance, prediabetes, diabetes type 2, or diabetes type 1?

Consider the following causes of Insulin Resistance:
- Food allergies and/or sensitivities
- Dysbiosis, leaky gut and gut microbiota
- Food additives or excesses
- Digestive insufficiencies
- Oxidative stress and/or mitochondrial dysfunction
- EMF, dirty electricity
- Toxins (heavy metals, endocrine disruptors, volatile solvents, etc)
- Obesity
- Stress or adrenal fatigue/dysfunction
- Lack of sleep
- Hormone imbalances
- Infections (especially occult-dental, fungal, parasitic, bacterial, viral)
- Nutrient deficiencies/excesses
- Rx drugs (statins and DM, PPIs)
- Genetic predispositions/SNPs
- More than one cause?

We apply this to each patient and personalize our approach. You first ask the question: How did this particular person develop insulin resistance or type 1 diabetes? Remembering that there may be more than one cause. Also, some of the potential causes on the list may contribute in more than one way. For example, obesity can cause insulin resistance because

of increased inflammation and oxidative stress, but it may also cause insulin resistance by changing the gut microbiome.

In diabetes type 1 we know patients have a genetic predisposition, but in order for them to develop the disease they need an environmental trigger and increased permeability in the gut. Basically, the trigger interacts with the genetic predisposition, and in the presence of increased gut permeability they develop the autoimmune disease. There may exist a trio of causes where the genetic predisposition, an environmental trigger, and leaky small intestine act together to develop the autoimmune condition according to Dr Alessio Fasano.[20] Dr Fasano was initially talking about celiac disease but has published articles describing that this is basically what you see in most autoimmune conditions. Consequently, whether we are talking about insulin resistance, type 1 or type 2 diabetes, we need to identify the trigger to get to the root cause. In order to find the root cause or causes we must take a thorough history, perform a complete physical exam as well as obtain the appropriate laboratory evaluations.

Complete History and Physical Examination

Glean as much as you can from the history and physical examination. Chronic conditions from a patient's past medical history can also give you clues. Conditions such as hypertension, polycystic ovarian syndrome, nonalcoholic fatty liver disease (NAFLD), obstructive sleep apnea, elevated uric acid levels, infertility, elevated liver function tests, and breast cancer, to name a few, can be associated with insulin resistance. The higher breast cancer risk associated with greater abdominal visceral obesity may be related to aberrant insulin signaling leading to insulin resistance, hyperinsulinemia, and increased concentrations of endogenous estrogen and androgen. Overall adiposity in women may adversely affect breast cancer risk mainly by greater exposure of mammary epithelial tissue to endogenous estrogen.[21] Consequently, overall adiposity in women does affect their breast cancer risk, but visceral obesity as measured with body composition analysis is preferred as physical habitus and BMI may not accurately reflect body fat.

Gout and high uric acid levels can be a common sign of insulin resistance secondary to high sugar intake and high-fructose corn syrup.[22] NAFLD, the commonest liver problem in the Western world, can be seen in patients with insulin resistance, metabolic syndrome, and prediabetes. NAFLD is the most common cause of elevated liver function without clinical symptoms. Insulin resistance is the cause of NAFLD. One-third of NAFLD cases progress to nonalcoholic steatohepatitis (NASH) and 20% to 25% of NASH cases go on to cirrhosis.[23,24]

The history and physical exam are the first interactions with the patient. Consider how they interact with you and the office staff, but also look for signs of insulin resistance on physical exam such as acanthosis nigricans, which are dark skin folds in the neck, inguinal and axillary areas, and the elbows. Also look for skin pallor, skin coloration, hydration, and lesions. Skin tags or hirsutism even without obesity are also important observations consistent with insulin resistance. Examine the nails because they can give you clues to vitamin and mineral status as well as gastrointestinal and digestion issues. White spots on the nail bed can be a sign of possible zinc deficiency. People with insulin resistance or impaired glucose tolerance or prediabetes can present with peripheral neuropathy. Look in the mouth and pay particular attention to the mucosa. What does the tongue look like? If there is papillary atrophy, it can be associated with riboflavin (B2) and other B vitamin deficiencies. Is there periodontal disease? Are there amalgams? Hidden chronic infections as well as amalgams and general oral health can give us clues to underlying processes and causes. Enhanced tongue fissures (longitudinal and lambda) can be a sign of upregulated gut-associated lymphoid tissue (GALT), which can be seen in both type 1 as well as type 2 diabetes and insulin resistance.[25] The body shape (pear vs apple) in women can also give you an idea as to the underlying processes and root causes. An android body shape is more consistent with increased inflammation through adipocytokine communication and hyperinsulinemia and reduced adiponectin levels. Increased weight around the midsection can be a sign of autonomic dysfunction, anxiety, and elevated cortisol levels. Women who are gynoid can have more risks for hypothalamic-pituitary-thyroid-gonadal dysfunction and more detoxification abnormalities as well as gastrointestinal concerns and food sensitivities. In addition, the extreme gynoid can be associated with estrogen dominance and higher risk for estrogen-related conditions. You also want to look at muscle bulk, hair, and skin. Someone who is exercising regularly and has poor muscle bulk points to the probable existence of a catabolic state.

Laboratory Evaluation

Hemoglobin A1c

Hemoglobin A1C (HgbA1C) measures the 3-month average of fasting and postprandial glucose with about one-third of the HgbA1C from fasting glucose and two-thirds from the postprandial glucose. The risk of CVD is a continuum with increasing levels of HgbA1C starting at a level of 5.4.

If a hemoglobin A1C is 5.4 or higher, the patient has impaired glucose tolerance. At this point it is imperative to preserve beta cell function and aggressively address the underlying cause. Hemoglobin A1C is an independent risk factor for cardiovascular morbidity and mortality: "The predictive value of HbA1c for total mortality was stronger than that documented for cholesterol concentration, body mass index and blood pressure."[26]

HOMA-IR

HOMA-IR is a homeostatic model assessment for insulin resistance. It is a calculation based on plasma levels of fasting glucose and insulin and is used to assess insulin sensitivity. The HOMA-IR is calculated according to the formula:

Fasting insulin (microU/L) × fasting glucose (nmol/L)/22.5.

The HOMA-IR has shown enhanced diagnostic value in the differentiation of patients with NAFLD and healthy individuals.[27] However, there are patients who could have normal fasting insulin levels and normal fasting glucose levels and therefore a normal HOMA-IR and still be insulin resistant. Usually the first value to increase as someone becomes insulin resistant is the postprandial insulin level.

Adiponectin, Insulin, and Pro-insulin and the Three Stages

Adiponectin is an adipose-derived protein. It is protective against atherosclerosis, moderates fat tissue, promotes insulin insensitivity, and decreases hepatic glucose and lipid production. Adiponectin decreases before insulin increases and is the earliest marker of insulin sensitivity. One should also measure insulin, pro-insulin, hemoglobin A1C, fasting glucose, and 2-hour postprandial glucose and 30-minute insulin levels after a 75 g glucose load. In optimal control, adiponectin will be normal, fasting insulin will be 5, hemoglobin A1C would be less than 5.4, and fasting sugar should be less than 81 mg/dL. I have discussed earlier[15-17] regarding the risk of cardiovascular disease and mortality begins at 75 mg/dL. Other studies have shown there is a lower risk of developing diabetes if a fasting blood glucose is less than 81 mg/dL and the risk of diabetes significantly increases when the fasting blood glucose is greater than 87 mg/dL.[28] Furthermore, these higher fasting plasma glucose levels within the normoglycemic range constitute an independent risk factor for type 2 diabetes.[28]

Dr Andreas Pfutzner has developed stages of prediabetes and these have been decreased to three stages, which makes it easier to see the progression.[29] Stage 1 is when adiponectin starts to decrease; in stage 2, insulin is already starting to increase; and in stage 3 the pro-insulin increases.

Not everyone presents in precisely these stages and there are variations. There are some patients who fall between type 1 and type 2, and this is usually due to an underlying autoimmune disease.[30] Remember that manifestations of insulin resistance and metabolic syndrome are all along the continuum of insulin resistance from hyperinsulinemia to prediabetes and diabetes. If someone starts out with insulin resistance and hyperlipidemia, it may be the insulin resistance that is causing the hyperlipidemia, especially elevated triglycerides, and it is the insulin resistance that is increasing the progression to glucose intolerance and prediabetes.

In stage 1, adiponectin is declining and fasting insulin is still normal. Postprandial insulin might be elevated, but the primary determining factor of stage 1 is a normal fasting insulin as the pro-insulin and glucose are normal. Adiponectin is a key link that needs to be restored as much as possible because low adiponectin is a marker for insulin resistance, and the patient is more at risk for dyslipidemia. There is increased risk for vascular injury and increased risk of progression along the continuum toward type II diabetes. Decreasing adiponectin tends to be associated with increasing inflammatory markers.

Stage 1 shows low adiponectin, normal HOMA-IR (remember fasting insulin is normal), normal glucose, normal hemoglobin A1C, normal insulin, and normal pro-insulin.

Stage I treatment includes healthy nutrition and lifestyle changes, with a focus on body composition. Many experts recommend a Mediterranean type diet with a low glycemic index or load.

Stage 2 progresses from stage 1. Adiponectin is decreasing, insulin is starting to increase, and pro-insulin is still normal. There could be early beta cell impairment. There will be a higher HOMA-IR, higher than normal insulin, a high postprandial glucose, but the fasting glucose can be borderline and average glucose may be normal. Usually stage 2 treatment consists of lifestyle changes and supplementation. Pharmacotherapy is not generally started until stage 3 and even then, only if diet, nutrition, lifestyle modification, and nutraceutical support are not effective.

In stage 3 pro-insulin is increasing which indicates that the pancreas is struggling to maintain a normal glucose. The pancreas is releasing large amounts insulin rapidly before the final cleavage to insulin occurs. In stage 3 there is low adiponectin, high HOMA-IR, high insulin, elevated pro-insulin, possibly high glucose, and high hemoglobin A1C.[29,31] There are some patients who can maintain normal or close to normal fasting glucose, even with these numbers. However, a glucose challenge will increase the postprandial glucose level. These patients may not meet the criteria for prediabetes or diabetes. The ADA definition for prediabetes is a fasting glucose level of 100 to 125 mg/dL. The number one treatment aim in a patient in stage 3 is to preserve beta cell function as much as possible. There may be a totally normal fasting glucose, but in most cases the postprandial glucose will increase with a high glycemic load meal. Having patients check postprandial glucose levels also helps the patient learn what particular foods increase their glucose level.

Glucose Challenge

According to researcher David Ludwig, insulin concentration at 30 minutes after glucose consumption has been shown to be a good measure of insulin secretion in humans.[32] By challenging patients with 75 g of glucose and checking them at 1 hour, 2 hours, or even 3 hours, Ludwig discovered that early insulin secretors could slip through the cracks. He set new parameters. At 30 minutes, insulin should be less than 57.5 µIU/mL. Over that, they are insulin resistant. At 2 hours, the insulin level should be 25 and the fasting glucose should be less than 10, but ideally 5 to 7. These criteria are different from the ADA guidelines.

Comprehensive Digestive Stool Analysis and Gut Microbiome

Although genetic factors may play an important role in the susceptibility to DM type 1, the dramatic worldwide increase in prevalence is likely due to changes in the environmental factors. One environmental factor which has gained prominence in recent years is the alterations in gut microbiota, which leads to increased gut permeability and metabolic endotoxemia. Bacterial lipopolysaccharide (LPS), an endotoxin with a unique glycolipid located at the outer membrane of gram negative bacteria can induce inflammation.[33] Comprehensive digestive stool analysis that also evaluates the commensals in

the gut microbiota is an essential part of a laboratory evaluation for both type 1 and type 2 diabetes. This test looks at products of digestion, short chain fatty acids such as butyrate, propionate, and acetate as well as diversity of the commensal organisms, microbiology (including pathogenic bacteria, fungi, parasites as well as the good bacteria such as lactobacillus and *Bifidobacterium*) as well as pancreatic function.

AVP, Cortisol, Copeptin, and Diabetes

Arginine vasopressin (AVP) and corticotrophin releasing hormone (CRH) act on pituitary to release ACTH, and ACTH acts on adrenal to increase release of cortisol. AVP can also directly stimulate the adrenal cortex to release cortisol, through V1a receptors. Psychological stress amplifies the action of AVP on pituitary to release ACTH via action on V1b receptors. The ACTH released through AVP, however, does not respond to negative feedback by serum cortisol unlike the CRH-induced ACTH release, which does respond to cortisol levels.[34,35] In human and animal trials AVP has been shown to affect glucose metabolism and play a role in metabolic disorders. In the liver, AVP can cause elevation of blood glucose via glycolysis, and infusion of AVP causes significant elevation of plasma glucose in subjects with normal serum glucose. AVP stimulates glycogenolysis in the liver by stimulation of glucagon and epinephrine, which in turn cause an increase in glucose levels. In obese male subjects when CRH and AVP are infused, there is an exaggerated pituitary response to the AVP with an increased release of ACTH and a higher cortisol level resulting in hyperglycemia. This AVP role in causing hyperglycemia is not only by acting on islet cells but also through its actin on V1b receptors in the pituitary. This is important in both type 1 and type 2 diabetes. In patients with type 1 DM there is increased secretion of glucagon as there is no inhibition by insulin and thereby increasing glucose levels. Thus, in type 1 DM, even physiological levels of AVP can cause profound increase in blood glucose by stimulating glucagon and resulting in increased production of glucose by the liver.[36,37] AVP is a peptide with a short half-life and difficult to measure. Copeptin is a surrogate marker for AVP. It is easy to measure, is stable, has a long half-life, and levels correlate with plasma AVP levels. Baseline levels of copeptin can predict the incidence of DM without impaired fasting glucose, and the association between copeptin and DM is independent of development of obesity.[38]

Review of Laboratory Testing

Laboratory testing can be divided into initial laboratory evaluations which one should order on the first/initial (Table 26.1) visit and as well as additional ones that are helpful but you may not need to them on the first visit (Table 26.1).

Treatment

Treatment will emphasize the nonpharmacologic aspects. Table.26.2 presents my approach for the treatment of insulin resistance and diabetes type 1. Remember that these

Table 26.1

LABORATORY TESTING FOR INSULIN RESISTANCE

Initial Lab Workup

- Adiponectin
- Pro-insulin
- HgbA1C
- Fasting insulin
- 30-min insulin, 1 h insulin, and a 2 h insulin level, after a 75 g glucose load
- Fasting glucose
- 30-min glucose, 1 h glucose, and 2 h glucose after a 75 g glucose load
- CBC

- C-reactive protein high sensitivity (CRP-HS)
- Uric acid
- Comprehensive metabolic panel
- Comprehensive digestive stool analysis with commensal microbiome evaluation
- GGTP
- Expanded lipoprotein profile including lipid particle numbers
- Comprehensive metabolic panel

Additional Helpful Lab Tests

- 25-OH vitamin D
- Homocysteine
- Lipoprotein(a)
- Copeptin
- CRP-HS
- Apolipoprotein B and apolipoprotein A1

- Gliadin antibody
- Celiac panel
- Celiac genetic panel (HLA-DQ2 and DQ8)
- Salivary cortisol profile
- Lp-PLA2

Table 26.2

INSULIN RESISTANCE TREATMENT PROTOCOL

- Nutritional Support with:
- Wholesome food (fresh, whole, unprocessed, organic, colorful, fermented that includes nuts and seeds with 10 servings of vegetables and 2 servings of Low glycemic-load fruit and an additional 35 g of fiber)
- Personalize the elimination diet according to individual patient needs and clinical exam
- Identify the underlying functional imbalances, prioritize, and address
- Lifestyle modification: individualized stress reduction, alcohol consumption, smoking cessation
- Exercise: tailor to individual patient needs
- Address the gut microbiota: food, probiotics and prebiotics
- Nutritional supplementation: personalized based on clinical exam and laboratory testing
- Mind-body-spirit connection: Find and foster purpose and meaning in life
- Assess need for pharmacological treatment based on functional testing, patient needs, and response to above approach

Decreasing Insulin Stimulation

Dietary modifications that decrease insulin release include high mixed fiber, monounsaturated fatty acids, omega-3 fatty acids, and complex carbohydrates with a low glycemic index and load and high quality protein at every meal and with every snack. All inflammatory foods, including wheat, dairy, soy, corn, and nightshades, should be eliminated.

This would include organic, fresh, whole, unprocessed, and colorful foods, eliminating all trans fats, some saturated fats, and food allergens. The elimination diet, lifestyle modification, exercise, nutritional supplements, stress, and the mind/body/spirit connection are all extremely important and should be addressed on the first visit. Recent data suggest that, in a compromised metabolic state such as type 2 diabetes, a continual snacking routine will cumulatively worsen their glucose control more rapidly than in other individuals because of the greater exposure to endotoxin.[41]

Addressing the Gut Microbiota

The gut microbiota has been considered an environmental factor that can modulate metabolic diseases such as diabetes and obesity.[42] Studies have shown that the gut microbiota differs in composition between lean and obese individuals and that diet, especially high-fat and low-fiber Western diet, dramatically impacts the gut microbiota in a negative way.

factors need to be addressed both at baseline and throughout the course of treatment. The first step is to remove the triggers and mediators looking back to what may have been the underlying root causes. For both, my approach is to decrease insulin stimulation as much as possible, to modify the gut microbiota, and to increase the cellular responsiveness to insulin. When it comes to DM type 1, we know that food sensitivities particularly gluten and dairy have been shown to be triggers. Pancreatic β-cell autoimmunity appears frequently in the first 6 years of life, and its progression toward type 1 diabetes usually occurs in preschoolers or during puberty; the factors investigated as possible triggers are related to early life and the immune system maturation process. In addition to genetics, other factors such as birth delivery mode, diet, infections, dysbiosis, and the use of antibiotics have been associated with DM type I development.[39,40] Management for the patient with insulin resistance includes decreasing insulin stimulation, addressing the gut microbiota, and increasing the cellular responsiveness to insulin.

The gut microbiome profile can be changed within 24 hours via dietary modifications.[43] The gut microbiota can be manipulated by prebiotics, probiotics, and antibiotics. Probiotics affect the microbiota directly by modulating its bacterial content and indirectly through bacteriocins produced by the probiotic bacteria.[44]

Furthermore, studies have found that probiotics have direct effects on glycemic controls in human studies where significant reductions in levels of fasting plasma glucose, postprandial blood glucose, glycated hemoglobin, insulin, insulin resistance, and onset of diabetes.[45]

Increasing Cellular Responsiveness to Insulin

Many phytochemicals can do this. Many phytochemicals work as tissue-specific serum kinase response modulators (SKRMs). These are going to affect cellular communication and cellular signaling. Some dietary phytochemicals that modulate these pathways include berberine, cinnamon, ginseng, quercetin, resveratrol, green tea extract, and hops extract.

Nutrients known to modify insulin responsiveness at the cellular level include chromium, alpha lipoic acid, CoQ10, vitamin D, magnesium, vitamin C, vitamin E, omega-3 fatty acids, vanadium, and SKRMs. A recent study on chromium and insulin resistance on children showed good results using 400 μg chromium chloride.[46]

Micronutrient Recommendations

Chromium: Give 200 μg/daily to 400 μg/daily if insulin resistant. It is likely most effective if deficient, but difficult to test. There are some earlier recommendations to supplement to 1000 μg/d, but this is too high and can potentially be toxic.[47]

Vitamin D: Test 25(OH)D and supplement as appropriate (or supplement 2000-5000 IU/daily). Vitamin D levels should be 50 to 80 ng/mL, depending on whether other medical conditions are present. Increasing vitamin D levels from 10 to 30 ng/mL can improve insulin sensitivity by an amazing 60%. A study showed a positive correlation of 25(OH)D concentration with insulin sensitivity and a negative effect of hypovitaminosis D on beta cell function.

Subjects with hypovitaminosis D are at higher risk of insulin resistance and the metabolic syndrome. Increasing 25(OH)D from 10 to 30 ng/mL can improve insulin sensitivity by 60%.[48]

CoQ10: Supplement in patients with metabolic syndrome, insulin resistance, hypertension, or mitochondrial dysfunction. CoQ10 dose depends on functional levels: optimize to >3 μg/mL in the plasma. In a patient with high oxidative stress or mitochondrial dysfunction, you may need to supplement at a much higher dose. We know that 120 mg/d of coenzyme Q10 improves glycemic control and blood pressure in NIDDM. Also, 200 mg of CoQ10 daily improved HgbA1C and blood pressure in NIDDM patients.[49-52]

Alpha lipoic acid: Doses of 600 to 1800 mg/d of alpha lipoic acid (ALA) can improve insulin sensitivity in patients with type 2 diabetes. And 600 to 1200 mg/d of ALA may improve microcirculation and diabetic polyneuropathy.[53,54]

ALA and CoQ10 are some of the rate-limiting steps in phosphorylation.

Magnesium: Give 200 to 400 mg of chelated magnesium. Likely most effective if deficient, accurate testing is cumbersome. Supplementation if signs and symptoms of deficiency/insufficiency. Epidemiological studies show that high daily Mg intake is predictive of a lower incidence of NIDDM. Poor intracellular Mg concentration is found in NIDDM and in hypertensive patients. Daily Mg administration in NIDDM patients and in insulin-resistant patients restores intracellular Mg concentration and contributes to improve insulin sensitivity and glucose uptake.[55] Magnesium supplementation has been shown to improve insulin sensitivity.[56] Many patients have a hard time absorbing magnesium intracellularly. A buccal swab is the best way to assess intracellular magnesium. Patients with low magnesium are at a slightly higher risk for atrial fibrillation and arrhythmias. Many of these patients may also need potassium. Magnesium glycinate may be preferred in some as it has less effects on the gut in terms of causing loose bowels and is better absorbed plus it also helps with detoxification. A transdermal magnesium gel may be used and have the patient apply it on the bottoms of their feet at bedtime. Epsom salt foot soaks or baths may also be helpful (see Table 26.3).

Table 26.3

MICRONUTRIENT RECOMMENDATIONS

- *Chromium:* If using generally give 200 μg/daily if insulin resistant. Likely most effective if deficient, but difficult to test

- *Vitamin D:* Test 25(OH)D and supplement as appropriate (or supplement 1000-2000) IU/daily

- *Magnesium:* Generally give 200-400 mg. Most effective if deficient, accurate testing is cumbersome. Supplementation if signs and symptoms of deficiency/insufficiency

- *CoQ10 100-200 mg/d:* Generally supplement in patients with metabolic syndrome or diabetes or hypertensive

- *Alpha lipoic acid:* 600 mg bid if diabetic or specifically if peripheral neuropathy. Likely useful at lower dosages in insulin resistant

Conclusion

Diabetes mellitus type 1 and type 2 are rapidly emerging as one of the biggest health concerns in the United States and worldwide. Endocrine disruptors, poor quality food, changes in the gut microbiota, and lifestyle factors are among some of the factors accounting for this rapid rise. As clinicians, we need to glean as much as we can from the patient's history and physical examination in order to ascertain the underlying root causes. When it comes to insulin resistance, being aware of potential causes of pancreatic beta cell damage as well as the continuum of insulin resistance can help in the diagnoses. Early diagnoses aggressive treatment, particularly focusing on diet and lifestyle factors can help us reverse this global health epidemic.

References

1. Mozaffarian D, Benjamin EJ, Go AS, et al. Heart disease and stroke statistics–2015 update: a report from the American Heart Association. *Circulation*. 2015;131:e29-e322.
2. Collaboration NCDRF. Worldwide trends in diabetes since 1980: a pooled analysis of 751 population-based studies with 4.4 million participants. *Lancet*. 2016;387(10027):1513-1530.
3. Velmurugan G, Ramprasath T, Gilles M, et al. Gut microbiota, EDC's and the diabetes epidemic. *Trends Endocrinol Metab*. 2019;28(8):612-625.
4. Lakka HM, Laaksonen DE, Lakka TA, et al. The metabolic syndrome and total and cardiovascular disease mortality in middle-aged men. *JAMA*. 2002;288(21):2709-2716.
5. Ludwig DS, Ebbeling CB. Type 2 diabetes mellitus in children: primary care and public health considerations. *JAMA*. 2001;286(12):1427-1430.
6. Pinhas-Hamiel O, Zeitler P. The global spread of type 2 diabetes mellitus in children and adolescents. *J Pediatr*. 2005;146:693-700.
7. Mayer-Davis EJ, Lawrence JM, Dabelea D, et al. Incidence trends of type 1 and type 2 diabetes among youths, 2002-2012. *NEJM*. 2017;376(15):1419-1429.
8. Corkey BE. Banting Lecture 2011. Hyperinsulinemia: cause or consequence? *Diabetes*. 2012;61(1):4-13.doi:10.2337/db11-1483.
9. Murtagh L, Ludwig DS. State intervention in life-threatening childhood obesity. *JAMA*. 2011;306(2):206-207.
10. Gillis L, Gillis A. Nutrient inadequacy in obese and non-obese youth. *Can Diet Pract Res*. 2005;66(4):237-242.
11. Ludwig DS, Peterson KE, Gortmaker SL. Relation between consumption of sugar-sweetened drinks and childhood obesity: a prospective, observational analysis. *Lancet*. 2001;357:505-508.
12. Blaedel M, Raun K, Boonen HC, Sheykhzade M, Sams A. Early onset inflammation in pre-insulin-resistant diet-induced obese rats does not affect the vasoreactivity of isolated small mesenteric arteries. *Pharmacology*. 2012;90(3-4):125-132. PMID:22832498.
13. Simmons AL, Schlezinger JJ, Corkey BE. What are we putting in our food that is making us fat? Food additives, contaminants, and other putative contributors to obesity. *Curr Obes Rep*. 2014;3(2):273-285.
14. Corkey BE, Erion KA. Hyperinsulinemia: a cause of obesity? *Curr Obes Rep*. 2017;6(2):178-186.
15. Coutinho M, Gerstein HC, Wang Y, Yusuf S. The relationship between glucose and incident cardiovascular events. A metaregression analysis of published data from 20 studies of 95,783 individuals followed for 12.4 years. *Diabetes Care*. 1999;22(2):233-240.
16. Balkau B, Shipley M, Jarrett RJ, et al. High blood glucose concentration is a risk factor for mortality in middle-aged nondiabetic men. 20-year follow-up in the Whitehall Study, the Paris Prospective Study, and the Helsinki Policemen Study. *Diabetes Care*. 1998;21(3):360-367.
17. Pereg D, Elis A, Neuman Y, Mosseri M, Lishner M, Hermoni D. Cardiovascular risk in patients with fasting blood glucose levels within normal range. *Am J Cardiol*. 2010;106(11):1602-1605.
18. Akasaka T, Sueta D, Tabata N, et al. Effects of the mean amplitude of glycemic excursions and vascular endothelial dysfunction on cardiovascular events in nondiabetic patients with coronary artery disease. *J Am Heart Assoc*. 2017;6(5).
19. Schneider MP, Ott C, Ritt M, et al. Postchallenge hyperglycemia is closely related with early vascular damage in overweight and obese patients. *J Hypertens*. 2012;30:147.
20. Fasano A. Surprises from celiac disease. *Scientific Am*. 2009;301(2):54-61.
21. Stoll BA. Upper abdominal obesity, insulin resistance and breast cancer risk. *Int J Obes Relat Metab Disord*. 2002;26(6):747-753.
22. Choi HK, Willet W, Curhan G. Fructose-rich beverages and risk of gout in women. *JAMA*. 2010;304(20):2270-2278.
23. Yun JW, Cho YK, Park JH, et al. Abnormal glucose tolerance in young male patients with nonalcoholic fatty liver disease. *Liver Int*. 2009;29(4):525-529.
24. Guturu P, Duchini A. Etiopathogenesis of nonalcoholic steatohepatitis: role of obesity, insulin resistance and mechanisms of hepatotoxicity. *Int J Hepatol*. 2012;2012:212865.
25. N Sight: Nutrition-Focused Clinical Exams: https://www.ifm.org/learning-center/nsight.
26. Khaw KT, Wareham N, Luben R, et al. Glycated hemoglobin, diabetes, and mortality in men in Norfolk cohort of European prospective investigation of cancer and nutrition (EPIC-Norfolk). *BMJ*. 2001;322(7277):15-18.
27. Salgado AL, Carvalho Ld, Oliveira AC, et al. Insulin resistance index (HOMA-IR) in the differentiation of patients with non-alcoholic fatty liver disease and healthy individuals. *Arq Gastroenterol*. 2010;47(2):165-169.
28. Tirosh A, Shai I, Tekes-Manova D, et al. Normal fasting glucose levels and diabetes type 2 in young men. *NEJM*. 2005;353:1454-1462.
29. Pfutzner A, Weber MM, Forst T. A novel concept for assessment of insulin resistance, beta cell function and chronic inflammation in type 2 diabetes mellitus. *Clin Lab*. 2008;54(11-12):485-490.
30. Gabriel CL, Smith PB, Mendez-Fernandez YV, Wilhelm AJ, Ye AM, Major AS. Autoimmune-mediated glucose intolerance in a mouse model of systemic lupus erythematosus. *Am J Physiol Endocrinol Metab*. 2012;303(11):E1313-E1324.
31. Forst T, Pfützner A. Current laboratory parameters in the differential diagnosis of type 2 diabetes mellitus. Proinsuin, adiponectin and others. *Dtsch Med Wochenschr*. 2006;131(suppl 8):S268-S273. Review.
32. Chaput JP, Tremblay A, Rimm EB, Bouchard C, Ludwig DS. A novel interaction between dietary composition and insulin secretion: effects on weight gain in the Quebec Family Study. *AJCN*. 2008;87:303-309.
33. Aravindhan V, Mohan V, Arunkumar N, Sandhya S, Babu S. Chronic Endotoxemia in subjects with type 1 diabetes mellitus is seen much before the onset of microvascular complications. *PLoS One*. 2015;10(9):e0137618.
34. Mavani G, DeVita MV, Michelis MF. A review of the nonpressor and nonantidiuretic actions of the hormone vasopressin. *Rev Med*. 2015;2(19):1-10.
35. Hiroyama M, Aoyagi T, Fujiwara Y, et al. Hypermetabolism of fat in V1a vasopressin receptor knockout mice. *Mol Endocrinol*. 2007;21(1):247-258.
36. Pasquali R, Gagliardi L, Vicennati V. ACTH and cortisol response to combined corticotropin releasing hormone-arginine vasopressin stimulation in obese males and its relationship to body weight, fat distribution and parameters of the metabolic syndrome. *Int J Obes Relat Metab Disord*. 1999;23(4):419-424.
37. Yibchok-anun S, Abu-Basha EA, Yao CY, Panichkriangkrai W, Hsu WH. The role of arginine vasopressin in diabetes-associated increase in glucagon secretion. *Regul Pept*. 2004;122(3):157-162.
38. Enhorning S, Wang TJ, Nilsson PM, et al. Plasma copeptin and the risk of diabetes mellitus. *Circulation*. 2010;121(19):2102-2108.

39. Larsson EH, Vehik K, Gesualdo P, et al. Children followed in the teddy study are diagnosed with type 1 diabetes at an early stage of disease. *Pediatr Diabetes*. 2014;15:118-126.

40. Atkinson MA, Eisenbarth GS. Type 1 diabetes: new perspectives on disease pathogenesis and treatment. *Lancet*. 2001;358:221-229.

41. Harte AL, Varma MC, Tripathi G, et al. High fat intake leads to acute postprandial exposure to circulating endotoxin in type 2 diabetic subjects. *Diabetes Care*. 2012;35(2):375-382.

42. Greiner T, Backhed F. Effects of the gut microbiota on obesity and glucose homeostasis. *Trends Endocrinol Metab*. 2011;22(4):117-123.

43. Del Chierico F, Vernocchi P, Dallapiccola B, Putignani L. Mediterranean diet and heatlh: food effects on gut microbiota and disease control. *Int J Mol Sci*. 2014;15(7):11678-11699.

44. Million M, Lagier JC, Yahav D, Paul M. Gut bacterial microbiota and obesity. *Clin Microbiol Infect*. 2013;19(4):305-313.

45. Razmpoosh E, Javadi M, Ejtahed HS, et al. Probiotics as beneficial agents in the management of diabetes mellitus: a systemic review. *Diabetes Metab Res Rev*. 2016;32(2):143-168.

46. Kim CW, Kim BT, Park KH, et al. Effects of short-term chromium supplementation on insulin sensitivity and body composition in overweight children: randomized, double-blind, placebo-controlled study. *J Nutr Biochem*. 2011;22(11):1030-1034.

47. Amooee S. Metformin versus chromium picolinate in clomiphene citrate-resistant patients with PCOs: a double-blind randomized clinical trial. *Iran J Reprod Med*. 2013;11(8):611-618.

48. Chiu KC, Chu A, Go VL, Saad MF. Hypovitaminosis D is associated with insulin resistance and beta cell dysfunction. *Am J Clin Nutr*. 2004;79(5):820-825.

49. Yoo JY, Yum KS. Effect of coenzyme Q10 on insulin resistance in korean patients with prediabetes: a pilot single-center, randomized, double-blind, placebo-controlled study. *Biomed Res Int*. 2018;2018:1613247.

50. Singh RB, Niaz MA, Rastogi SS, et al. Effect of hydrosoluble coenzyme Q10 on blood pressures and insulin resistance in hypertensive patients with coronary artery disease. *J Hum Hypertens*. 1999;13(3):203-208.

51. Huang H, Chi H, Liao D, Zou Y. Effects of coenzyme Q10 on cardiovascular and metabolic biomarkers in overweight and obese patients with type 2 diabetes mellitus: a pooled analysis. *Diabetes Metab Syndr Obes*. 2018;11:875-886.

52. Hodgson JM, Watts GF, Playford DA, Burke V, Croft KD. Coenzyme Q10 improves blood pressure and glycaemic control: a controlled trial in subjects with type 2 diabetes. *Eur J Clin Nutr*. 2002;56(11):1137-1142.

53. Jacob S, Ruus P, Hermann R, et al. Oral administration of RAC-alpha-lipoic acid modulates insulin sensitivity in patients with type-2 diabetes mellitus: a placebo- controlled pilot trial. *Free Radic Biol Med*. 1999;27(3-4):309-314.

54. Haak E, Usadel KH, Kusterer K, et al. Effects of alpha-lipoic acid on microcirculation in patients with peripheral diabetic neuropathy. *Exp Clin Endocrinol Diabetes*. 2000;108(3):168-174.

55. Barbagallo M, Dominguez LJ, Galioto A, et al. Role of magnesium in insulin action, diabetes and cardio-metabolic syndrome X. *Mol Aspects Med*. 2003;24(1-3):39-52.

56. Guerrero-Romero F, Tamez-Perez HE, González-González G, et al. Oral magnesium supplementation improves insulin sensitivity in non-diabetic subjects with insulin resistance. A double-blind placebo-controlled randomized trial. *Diabetes Metab*. 2004;30:253-258.

27

The Role of the Gut Microbiome in Cardiovascular Disease

Jill C. Carnahan, MD, ABIHM, ABoIM, IFMCP

Purpose of This Chapter

Defining what is "normal" in healthy microbiota communities is an ongoing process. Currently, there are key players that have already come to light with regards to many diseases. This chapter serves to identify which microorganisms and related mechanisms play a role in cardiovascular disease.

The Role of the Gut Microbiome in Cardiovascular Disease

The gut microbiome regulates and influences many metabolic processes in the body. Research clearly indicates that it has a profound impact on the pathogenesis of cardiovascular disease. The gut microbiota is the collection of 40 trillion microorganisms living in the gastrointestinal tract, whereas the gut microbiome is the collection of total genes of these microorganisms. The cells of the human body are outnumbered by microbial cells 10 to 1 and the genes 150 to 1.[1] These genes are so influential in many biological processes that there has been a major shift in the realm of research to examine these microorganisms as they relate to every function and dysfunction of the body. So far, there is not one chronic disease wherein an imbalance of this ecosystem has not been observed.

The term "gut microbiome" was coined only in 2001,[2] but it was not until 2007 that the science and understanding of the gut microbiome really progressed. Using technology developed for the Human Genome Project, scientists began to realize that the gut microbiome is essential to human health. This resulted in the National Institute of Health's Human Microbiome Project, which set out to catalog the microorganisms living across the various human body's "ecosystems." The differences in diversity of the strains found in the human body are so vast[3] that they dwarf the differences in biodiversity found between a tropical rainforest and a savanna when you combine all their respective flora and fauna.

A unique characteristic of the gut microbiome is that it appears to shift and adapt rapidly depending on what resources are present to meet the metabolic needs of the host. This means it is more important that we map the metabolic pathways (the means of obtaining a by-product) and functions (the by-products themselves) of these organisms, rather than focus on specific strains, because their behavior is dependent on their resources and the presence of other organisms.

It is worth mentioning that some of the language used to describe microorganisms needs to change. Because strains once labeled "pathogenic" are proving to play vital roles in human health when they are in the appropriate numbers and location within the body, the more appropriate term is now considered "opportunistic." Some bacteria are able to be either symbiotic or parasitic depending on the context, which is also called amphibiosis. An example of this is *Helicobacter pylori*[4], which is generally associated with acute gastritis but has been found to also be protective against acid reflux. Another concern is the translocation of particular strains, which can sometimes cause issues. An example of this would be a condition called small intestinal bacterial overgrowth (SIBO), where colonic-type bacteria proliferate in large numbers in the small intestine.

The intricate role of these microorganisms in human biology is so profound, it is appropriate to consider this complex ecosystem as an organ of multiple systems, including:

The endocrine system—The gut microbiota is arguably the largest endocrine organ[5] and capable of producing a wide range of biologically active compounds that may be carried via circulation to distant sites within the host.

The nervous system—The gut microbiota directly influences the development, function, and activity of the enteric nervous system[6] through neurotransmitter synthesis and the physical and chemical stimuli on intrinsic primary afferent neurons[7] throughout the gut lining.

The immune system—The gut microbiota is also integral to maintaining homeostasis in the immune system[8] of the host. It plays an important metabolic role through maintaining cross-talk with the immune system.

Important metabolic functions of the gut microbiome include:

- Breakdown of dietary fiber
- Breakdown of oligosaccharides
- Gas production
- Fermentation
- Production of phenols
- Detoxification
- Mucus production
- Short-chain fatty acid (SCFA) metabolism
- Primary bile acid deconjugation
- Vitamin absorption
- Fats, triglycerides, and cholesterol regulation

Similar to an ecological ecosystem, the best indicators of the overall health of the gut microbiome are richness and diversity. Richness is the number of species within the community, and diversity refers to the richness combined with how evenly distributed the species are. The gut microbiota includes bacteria, viruses, fungi, archaea, and phages. Bacteria are by far the most prominent microorganisms, comprising almost 90% of this ecosystem.[9]

Greater microbial diversity is associated with the body's ability to deal with stressors, such as opportunistic pathogens, dietary, and environmental perturbations. Individuals with disease are more likely[10] to have alterations in their gut microbiome compared with healthy controls. There are strong associations between reduced microbial diversity and illness.

Bacterial colonization during birth plays a major role in the formation and resilience of the gut microbiota. Babies born vaginally colonize with a gut microbiome similar to their mothers' vaginal microbiota, whereas cesarean section-born infants are colonized by bacteria found on the mothers' skin surface. It is well established that cesarean sections are associated with a higher risk of numerous diseases including asthma, food allergy, type 1 diabetes, and obesity[11], and it appears that an altered microbiota is a likely mechanism. Factors that affect diversity throughout life include:

- Genetics
- Stress
- Physiologic processes
- Anatomical structure of the digestive tract
- Diet
- Prebiotic intake
- Probiotic intake
- Antibiotic usage
- Lifestyle
- Living environment

The importance of the gut microbiome and its various roles across human biology makes having an understanding of this "organ" essential for anyone in the medical field. Furthermore, it is critical that medical professionals remain vigilant in continuously educating themselves on the most current research.

Pathophysiology of Cardiovascular Disease As It Relates to the Gut Microbiome

Dysbiosis is the imbalance or maladaptation of the gut microbiome. Low diversity and richness can present as dysbiosis and are associated with higher levels of inflammation[12], higher adiposity, insulin resistance, and dyslipidemia. A 2013 study[13] published in the journal *Nature* studied participants (n = 292) in two characterized groups, delineated by the number of gut microbial genes (gut bacterial richness) with an average 40% difference between low gene count individuals and high gene count individuals. Individuals with low bacterial gene richness (23% of the study population) were characterized by an increase in adiposity, insulin resistance, and dyslipidemia. Additionally, low bacterial richness individuals showed a more pronounced inflammatory phenotype when compared with high bacterial richness individuals. Various metabolic diseases, including type 2 diabetes and obesity, are associated with dysbiosis that is distinguishable by a unique microbiota profile.

Some causes of dysbiosis include:

- Standard American Diet (SAD)—low in fiber, high in fat and simple carbs
- Broad-spectrum antibiotics
- Chronic maldigestion
- Long-term use of proton pump inhibitors
- Chronic constipation
- Suppression of *Lactobacillus, Bifidobacteria,* and secretory immunoglobulin A (sIgA) due to stress, for example, growth of gram-negative organisms (*Yersinia, Pseudomonas*) is stimulated by catecholamines.
- Consumption of genetically modified foods with exposure to glyphosate.

The gut microbiota is an important player in atherogenesis.[14] Specifically, higher levels of Lactobacillales and decreased levels in *Bacteroides* have been associated with coronary artery disease.[15] Metabolism by certain intestinal flora has been linked to the deleterious association between the development of atherosclerotic plaque and egg yolk consumption, due to its choline content. Certain gut microbiota can metabolize choline, phosphatidylcholine[16], and L-carnitine[17] to produce trimethylamine (TMA), which can be oxidized in the liver into trimethylamine N-oxide (TMAO), a proatherogenic metabolite. Inhibiting TMAO production through the gut microbiota has been found to be a promising treatment of atherosclerosis.[18] Owing to the inherent complexity of the gut microbiome and its differences among individuals, this pathway is not the same for everyone. The complex ecology of the gut microbiota and its role in metabolic behavior must be considered. For example, many types of fish are still considered beneficial for cardiovascular patients[19] despite their trimethylamine content. Additionally, L-carnitine may ameliorate metabolic diseases[20] by increasing insulin sensitivity of the skeletal muscle and may reduce ischemic heart disease in some people.

Metabolic Endotoxemia and Cardiovascular Disease

Another major mechanism that causes systemic inflammation in the body and is largely modulated by the gut microbiota and gastrointestinal lining is the development of metabolic endotoxemia[21] brought on by intestinal permeability and lipopolysaccharides (LPS). There is a strong correlation between metabolic endotoxemia and an increased risk of cardiovascular disease, diabetes, and obesity. Metabolic endotoxemia is characterized by insulin resistance and low-grade inflammation.

Intestinal permeability can cause systemic inflammation through translocation of LPS. Intestinal permeability is also known as "leaky gut" and is a reinforcing process that can result in intestinal inflammation, damage to the gut lining, dysregulation of the immune system response, nutrient malabsorption (especially vitamins B12, magnesium, and iron), gastrointestinal issues, multiple food intolerances, and, eventually, autoimmune disease.

LPS are a major component of the outer membrane of gram-negative bacteria and considered endotoxins. If they are absorbed through the gastrointestinal lining, they can elicit systemic inflammation and a strong immune system response. The detection of antibodies against LPS can reveal macromolecule endotoxin infiltration through the intestinal barrier into the systemic circulation. Other indicators of a compromised gastrointestinal lining include occludin, the main component of the proteins that hold together the tight junctions, and zonulin, which is a protein that regulates permeability of the intestine. Detection of antibodies for occludin and zonulin can indicate that tight junctions are breaking down or that normal regulation of tight junctions is compromised, respectively. An assessment of gut barrier damage can be done by measuring these barrier protein antibodies. This detects damage long before there is a dysregulation of the immune system response. This process can be a major driver of inflammation in the body.

Clinical indications that would warrant testing for LPS endotoxemia include:
- Cardiovascular disease
- Obesity
- Metabolic syndrome or diabetes
- Increase in food allergies or sensitivities
- History of celiac disease or other cause of villous atrophy
- Inflammatory bowel disease

- Autoimmune diseases or family history of autoimmune disease
- Neurological conditions such as Parkinson disease or multiple sclerosis
- Mood disorders, such as bipolar disorder, anxiety, or depression
- Cognitive dysfunction, including Alzheimer disease

Causes of increased intestinal permeability include:
- Inflammatory bowel disease
- Nonsteroidal anti-inflammatory drug (NSAID) therapy
- Small intestinal bacterial overgrowth
- Small intestinal fungal overgrowth
- Celiac disease
- Protozoal infections
- Toxic chemical exposure
- Mold or mycotoxin exposure
- Glyphosate consumption
- Severe food allergies or lectin sensitivity
- Chronic alcoholism
- Hypochlorhydria
- Other infections
- Psychological stressors
- Surgery
- Strenuous exercise
- Advanced age
- Nutritional depletions (zinc, vitamin D, vitamin A, butyrate)
- Tobacco use
  Biomarkers of intestinal permeability:
- **Permeability/dysbiosis:** Bacterial endotoxin—LPS, IgG, IgM, IgA
- **Epithelial cell damage:** Actomyosin network—IgA
- **Tight junction damage:** Occludin and zonulin—IgG, IgM, IgA

Metabolic endotoxemia is characterized by:
- Insulin resistance and low-grade inflammation
- An LPS concentration of two to three times the threshold
- An increase in endotoxins during fed states and decrease during fasting states
- An increase in the proportion of LPS-containing microbiota in the gut with a high-fat diet
- Dysregulation of inflammatory processes, triggering weight gain and diabetes, and cytokine production

This mechanism suggests that lowering plasma LPS concentration is a potential strategy for controlling metabolic diseases.

Hypertension and the Gut Microbiome

The gut microbiota and its metabolites have been implicated in the regulation of host physiological functions that can contribute to hypertension, a precursor to cardiovascular disease. As in cardiovascular disease, Firmicutes, *Bacteroides*, Actinobacteria, and Proteobacteria are the microorganisms that play a major role in the pathogenesis of hypertension. Toxic products produced by the gut microbiome, such as TMAO, p-cresol sulfate, and indoxyl sulfate, can contribute to salt sensitivity and affect blood pressure regulation and related epigenetic changes. SCFA receptors are expressed in the kidney and blood vessels and have been reported to function as a regulator of blood pressure (BP).

Specific and observed gut microbiome contributors to hypertension[22]:
- Increased Firmicutes: *Bacteroides* ratio lowers BP
- Increased gut inflammation increases BP
- Increased TMAO and phosphatidyl choline increase BP
- Increased Firmicutes: *Bacteroides* ratio may trigger angiotensin II (A II)-induced hypertension
- Norepinephrine increases virulence factors in gram-negative bacteria

These interactions provide novel therapeutic pathways for BP regulation. The regulation of BP via SCFA receptors has provided new insights into the interactions between the gut microbiota and BP control systems. Other hypertension intervention methods via the gut microbiome worth considering include[23]:
- Angiotensin-converting enzyme inhibitory (ACEI) peptides made by the microbiome via fermentation lower BP.
- *Lactobacilli* are natural ACEI and produce biologically active peptides that inhibit ACE.
- Phenylacetylglutamine, a gut metabolite, is negatively associated with pulse-wave velocity and systolic blood pressure (SBP).
- Probiotics with over 10^{11} CFU of multiple strains administered over 8 weeks decreased SBP and diastolic blood pressure.
- Gut-derived hormones, such as gastrin and glucagon-like peptide-1 (GLP-1), regulate gut sodium reabsorption and renal sodium homeostasis and BP.
- Blockade of the gut Na^+/H^+ exchanger-3 (NHE3) will lower BP.
- Probiotics have been shown to lower BP.

When the brain-gut microbiome axis and the gastrorenal reflex are affected, psychological symptoms may be observed. The absence of some gut microbiota may increase anxiety and decrease dopamine in the frontal cortex, hippocampus, and striatum. There can also be alterations in renal dopamine with salt intake. Finally, changes to the gut microbiome can induce changes in microRNAs, DNA methylation, and acetylation, which can contribute to inflammatory diseases including hypertension and cardiovascular disease.

Periodontal Disease and Cardiovascular Disease

The connection between periodontal microbes and cardiovascular disease has long been observed with no definitive mechanisms identified. LPS-mediated mitochondrial dysfunction[24] is a potential origin of oxidative stress in periodontal patients, as is intestinal permeability. Research indicates that inflammatory responses evoked by the LPS of *Porphyromonas gingivalis* is one key factor in this process. The influence of LPS on fibroblast and peripheral blood mononuclear cells appears to increase reactive oxygen species production while reducing CoQ10 levels and citrate synthase activity. Mitochondrial dysfunction promoted by *Porphyromonas gingivalis* LPS on these cells may also promote oxidative stress and alter cytokine homeostasis.

Specific Microbial Species and Microbiota Composition Associated With Cardiovascular Health Risks

Certain organisms and gut microbiota composition patterns have been associated with cardiovascular disease and metabolic syndrome. Low bacterial richness is associated with a reduction in beneficial butyrate-producing bacteria. Butyrate is an SCFA with potent anti-inflammatory potential. Low bacterial richness is also associated with mucus degradation, potential gut barrier impairment, and an increase in oxidative stress (Table 27.1).

Species and patterns associated with atherosclerosis:
- Low microbial diversity is associated with atherosclerosis.[25]
- *Chryseomonas, Veillonella,* and *Streptococcus* have been found in artery plaques but are believed to originate from the oral cavity and gut.
- Patients with symptomatic atherosclerosis[26] have higher levels of *Collinsella* and lower levels of *Eubacterium* and *Roseburia* in their gut.

Species associated with cardiovascular disease (Table 27.2):
- Increases in the abundance of the family Pseudomonadaceae
- Lower levels of Firmicutes species
- A higher ratio of Pseudomonadaceae to Firmicutes bacteria in coronary heart disease plaque

Table 27.1

SPECIES DIFFERENTIATING BACTERIAL RICHNESS

High Bacterial Richness Species	Low Bacterial Richness Species
Species level:	**Species level:**
• *Faecalibacterium prausnitzii*	• *Bacteroides* sp.
• *Bifidobacterium*	• *Ruminococcus* sp.
• *Lactobacillus*	
• *Alistipes*	
• *Akkermansia*	
Phylum level:	**Phylum level:**
• Verrucomicrobia (eg, *Akkermansia muciniphila*)	• Bacteroidetes
• Actinobacteria	• Proteobacteria

Table 27.2

GENUS/SPECIES OF PROBIOTIC AND ASSOCIATED CARDIOVASCULAR RISK

Genus/Species	Potential Associated Risk
Collinsella	Atherosclerosis
Eubacterium	
Lactobacillus reuteri	High LDL-Cholesterol
Lactobacillus acidophilus	
Lactobacillus plantarum	Atherosclerosis and Triglyceride levels
Prevotella	Potentially increased TMAO levels leading to atherosclerosis
Sporobacter	
Peptostreptococcaceae (family)	
Peptostreptococcaceae incertae sedis	
Clostridiaceae	
Fusibacter	
Lachnospira	
Clostridium	
Clostridiales incertae sedis XII (family)	
Anaerococcus hydrogenalis	
Clostridium asparagiforme	
Clostridium hathewayi	
Clostridium sporogenes	
Escherichia fergusonii	
Proteus penneri	
Providencia rettgeri	
Edwardsiella tarda	

LDL, low-density lipoprotein; TAMO, trimethylamine N-oxide.
Data from Vibrant Wellness Gut Zoomer. www.vibrant-wellness.com. Accessed September 15, 2019

Species associated with diabetes:
- Higher levels of
  - *Lactobacillus gasseri* and *Streptococcus mutans*
  - Certain *Clostridium* species
  - Proteobacteria
- Lower prevalence of butyrate producers:
  - *Roseburia intestinalis* (butyrate producer)
  - *Faecalibacterium prausnitzii*
- Increased expression of microbial genes involved in oxidative stress leading to a proinflammatory signature.
- Reduced expression of genes involved in vitamin synthesis like riboflavin.
- Gut microbiota may increase hepatic production of triglycerides and development of insulin resistance.

- Sulfate-reducing species *Desulfovibrio* was more frequently observed in diabetic patients.
- Dietary fiber improved microbiota-related metabolic functions such as glucose tolerance, insulin sensitivity, and weight gain and reduced low-grade inflammation.

Clinically, low bacterial richness and dysbiosis are associated with:
- Inflammatory bowel disease[27]
- Obesity
- Diabetes
- Nonalcoholic fatty liver disease
- Low-grade inflammation (elevated C-reactive protein)
- Insulin resistance
  - Elevated leptin
  - Decreased adiponectin
- Dyslipidemia
- Hypertension[28]
- High blood pressure

The Effects of Certain Dietary Components on the Gut Microbiota and Cardiovascular Disease

Diet significantly affects the composition and function of the gut microbiome. Specifically, the consumption of high-fiber foods, such as fruits and vegetables high in prebiotic fibers, have been shown[29] to increase bacterial richness and improve clinical symptoms associated with obesity. Even short-term diets alter the microbial community in a predictable manner.[30] A 2010 study[31] found that switching from a low-fat, polysaccharide-rich diet to a high-fat, high-sugar Western diet changed the composition of the microbial community mice with humanized microbiota within 1 day. Through fecal microbial transplantation, the effects of the Western diet were transferred to donor mice where increased adiposity was observed, leading researchers to conclude that the effects came from the microbiota and not merely the diet. It is important to note that we need a better understanding of the extent to which the gut microbiota changes based on diet. It appears that, even though changes can be seen in as little as a day, individuals have a core population that is more resilient to change. This core population has been compared with a microbial "fingerprint" because its signature can allow scientists to identify individuals based on their microbial patterns alone. This microbial pattern bears a resemblance most closely to the mother's gut or skin microbiota depending on the delivery method.

Beyond diet, other factors have been associated with metabolic abnormalities through altering the gut microbiota, including (Table 27.3):
- **Artificial sweeteners**[32]—Noncaloric artificial sweeteners drive the development of glucose intolerance through changing the composition and function of the gut microbiota.
- **Metformin**[33]—Metformin disrupts the bacterial folate cycle resulting in decreased levels of *S*-adenosylmethionine synthase.

Table 27.3

SUMMARY OF DIET-INDUCED DYSBIOSIS

Diet	Bacteria Altered	Effect on Bacteria	References
High fat	*Bifidobacteria* spp.	Decreased (absent)	[45]
High fat and high sugar	*Clostridium innocuum, Catenibacterium mitsuokai* and *Enterococcus* spp.	Increased	[18]
	Bacteroides spp.	Decreased	[18]
Carbohydrate reduced	Bacteroidetes	Increased	[49]
Caloric restricted	*Clostridium coccoides, Lactobacillus* spp. and *Bifidobacteria* spp.	Decreased (growth prevented)	[48]
Complex carbohydrates	*Mycobacterium avium*, subspecies *para tuberculosis* and Enterobacteriaceae	Decreased	[49]
	B. longum subspecies *longum, B. breve* and *B. thetaiotaomicron*	Increased	[53]
Refined sugars	*C. difficile* and *C. perfringens*	Increased	[54,55]
Vegetarian	*E. coli*	Decreased	[56]
High *n-6* PUFA from safflower oil	Bacteroidetes	Decreased	[59,60]
	Firmicutes, Actinobacteria, and Proteobacteria	Increased	[59,60]
	δ-Proteobacteria	Increased	[61]
Animal milk fat	*δ-Proteobacteria*	Increased	[62]

Summary of the Effects of Gut Dysbiosis on Cardiovascular Disease

Balance	Dysbiosis
High beneficial/commensal microbes versus low opportunistic	Low beneficial/commensal microbes versus high opportunistic
Associated lifestyle factors: high-fiber diet, prebiotics, probiotics, immune-potentiating therapeutics, nutraceuticals	**Associated lifestyle factors:** high-fat, high-caloric, high-sugar diets, sedentary lifestyle, excessive antibiotic use
Decreased gut permeability Decreased toxemia and sepsis Decreased proinflammation Increased insulin sensitivity Better gut, metabolic, cardiovascular health	Increased gut permeability Increased toxemia and sepsis Increased proinflammation Decreased insulin sensitivity Poorer gut, metabolic, cardiovascular health

Clinical Presentation of Cardiovascular Disease Driven by Gut Microbiology

A well-functioning gut microbiome is essential to modulating inflammation, suggesting that initial symptoms of dysregulation or dysbiosis could potentially be preclinical symptoms of cardiovascular disease. Gastrointestinal issues could be an early indicator of mechanisms that can contribute to and drive cardiovascular disease, creating a unique opportunity for intervention. Should gastroenterologists check for cardiovascular disease markers? Research suggests so.

Clinical presentation of cardiovascular disease driven by gut microbiology:

- **Exocrine pancreatic insufficiency** (EPI)[34]—EPI should be ruled out in all patients with cardiovascular disease in the presence of overt malnutrition or in the case of persistent gastrointestinal symptoms despite a gluten-free diet.
- Inflammatory bowel disease
- **SIBO**—Symptoms of SIBO include excessive gas, abdominal bloating, distention, diarrhea, and abdominal pain. Few patients with SIBO have chronic constipation over diarrhea. If overgrowth is severe and prolonged, it

Table 27.4

PANCREATIC ELASTASE VALUES

> 350 μg/g	Normal pancreatic function
200-350 μg/g	Declining pancreatic function Consider supplementation
100-200 μg/g	Moderate pancreatic insufficiency Supplement with broad array of pancreatic enzymes
<100 μg/g	Severe pancreatic insufficiency Supplement with broad array of pancreatic enzymes

can interfere with digestion and absorption of food and may result in nutrient deficiencies.

- **Celiac disease**
- **Protozoal infections**
- **Food allergy**
- **Low stomach acid**
- **Diarrhea**
- **Nutritional depletion**

In addition to finding these indicators of dysbiosis and/or a compromised intestinal lining, additional testing can be done to measure the influence of the gut on systemic inflammation, which is potentially contributing to or driving cardiovascular disease.

Current testing to assess gut microbiome-modulated inflammation in cardiovascular patients breaks down into three categories:

1. Digestion and absorption
2. Inflammation and immunology
3. Gastrointestinal microbiota and metabolic markers

Digestion and Absorption (Table 27.4)

- **Pancreatic Elastase 1 (PE1)**—PE1 is a proteolytic enzyme exclusively secreted by the human pancreas and serves as a noninvasive fecal biomarker of pancreatic exocrine function (producing amylase, lipase, and protease). This test is used for initial determination of pancreatic exocrine insufficiency and monitoring of pancreatic exocrine function in patients.[35,36] Replacement of pancreatic enzymes is warranted until PE1 levels rebound (ie, when underlying etiology can be corrected). Prescription and nonprescription formulations are available.
- **Products of Protein Breakdown into Putrefactive SCFAs**—These SCFAs (isovalerate, valerate, and isobutyrate) are produced by bacterial fermentation of proteinaceous material (polypeptides and amino acids) in the distal colon. Elevated levels suggest increased protein material in the distal colon, which

may be due to underlying gastrointestinal conditions such as hypochlorhydria and exocrine pancreatic insufficiency (maldigestion), bacterial overgrowth of the small intestine (SIBO), or gastrointestinal irritation. Levels may also be elevated with increased protein intakes.

Potential causes of inadequate protein digestion and bacterial fermentation and their corresponding tests:

- **Low Hydrochloric (HCl) Acid**—Symptoms include bloating/belching after meals; intolerance for protein; rectal itching; weak, peeling, or cracked fingernails/vertical ridges; adult acne; and undigested food in stool. Potential causes include advanced age (30% of elderly), use of proton pump inhibitors, autoimmunity, fasting, and chronic medical conditions. Consequences include SIBO, dysbiosis, chronic candidal infections, unexplained low ferritin or anemia, and mineral deficiencies: Ca, Mg, Zn, Fe, Cr, Mo, Mn, Cu, B_{12}.
- **Protease insufficiency**—Majority of protein digestion is due to the pancreatic proteases. Trypsin and chymotrypsin are two primary pancreatic proteases, which are synthesized and packaged into secretory vesicles as the inactive proenzymes trypsinogen and chymotrypsinogen.
  - **SIBO**—Breath test for SIBO.
  - **Intolerance to fructose**—Can be counterbalanced with a low FODMAP diet.
- **Fecal Fat**—Fecal fat measurement is an extraction method that provides a quantitative result for the amount of fat in the stool. Excess fecal fat may be due to a lack of bile acids (caused by liver damage, hyperlipidemia drugs, or impaired gallbladder function), disorders that impact pancreatic exocrine function (such as chronic pancreatitis or cystic fibrosis), celiac disease, small bowel bacterial overgrowth, or other conditions and medications.

Inflammation and Immunology (Table 27.5)

- Calprotectin[37] and EPX primary markers of inflammation elevated in:
  - Inflammatory bowel disease
  - Postinfectious irritable bowel syndrome
  - Irritable bowel syndrome
  - Gastrointestinal cancers
  - Certain gastrointestinal infections
  - NSAID enteropathy
  - Food allergy
  - Chronic pancreatitis
- **Eosinophilic Protein X (EPX)**—Benefits of EPX as an inflammation biomarker and test include its release in eosinophil degranulation, sensitivity as a marker of gastrointestinal inflammation and low-level inflammation, possible predictor of relapse in inflammatory bowel disease, and stability of transport up

Table 27.5

CALPROTECTIN VALUES

<50 µg/g	No significant inflammation
50-120 µg/g	Indicates some GI inflammation: IBD, infection, polyps, neoplasia, NSAIDs
> 120 µg/g	Significant inflammation; referral may be needed to determine pathology
>250 µg/g	Active disease present; predicts imminent relapse in treated patients

GI, gastrointestinal; IBD, inflammatory bowel disease; NSAID, nonsteroidal anti-inflammatory drug.

to 7 days.[38-41] EPX can be elevated in inflammatory bowel disease, celiac disease, parasitic infection, allergic reaction. Less common: gastroesophageal reflux disease, chronic diarrhea, chronic alcoholism, protein-losing enteropathy.[42-46]

Gastrointestinal Metabolic Markers

- **Beneficial SCFAs**—Includes acetate, n-butyrate, and propionate, which are produced by anaerobic bacterial fermentation of indigestible carbohydrate (fiber). The role of SCFAs includes providing nutrients for the colonic epithelium; modulating colonic and intracellular pH, cell volume, and other functions associated with ion transport; and regulating proliferation, differentiation, and gene expression.[47] SCFAs may enter the systemic circulation and directly affect metabolism or the function of peripheral tissues. SCFAs can beneficially modulate adipose tissue, skeletal muscle, and liver tissue function. SCFAs may contribute to improved glucose homeostasis and insulin sensitivity.[48]

Prevention and Treatment Strategies

A diet consisting of whole foods high in vegetables and sufficient exercise are common recommendations for those with cardiovascular disease. However, gut microbiome science provides new insights into the various mechanisms behind why these recommendations are beneficial. A diet high in fermentable fibers and plant polyphenols[49] appears to regulate microbial activities within the gut and increase beneficial SCFA[50] production. New insights into microbiota activity support the increased consumption of whole plant foods and provide a scientific rationale for the use of efficacious prebiotics.

Furthermore, the gut microbiota plays a major role in inflammation mediation throughout the body and offers novel treatment strategies through nutrition, nutritional supplements, and lifestyle changes. Targeting the gut microbiota

or related metabolic pathways may offer potential therapeutic benefits to patients with cardiovascular disease.

I. Select interventions for reducing LPS levels:
  - **Quercetin**[51]—Quercetin, a naturally occurring flavonoid, has been shown to downregulate inflammatory responses and provide cardioprotection by inhibiting LPS-induced phosphorylation of stress-activated protein kinases (JNK/SAPK) and p38 MAP kinases.
  - **Curcumin**[52]—Studies indicate that curcumin attenuates LPS-induced cardiac hypertrophy in vivo.
  - **Sulforaphane**[53]—Sulforaphane is a biologically active compound often found in cruciferous vegetables, such as broccoli. Sulforaphane is both anti-inflammatory and has anticancer properties. It has been shown to significantly suppress LPS-induced COX-2 protein and mRNA expression in a dose-dependent manner. In animal studies, sulforaphane activated the nuclear factor-E2-related factor 2 (Nrf2)/antioxidant response element (ARE) pathway in mice with LPS-induced injury.
  - **Resveratrol**[54]—Resveratrol is a naturally occurring stilbenoid phenol with free radical scavenging activity.
  - **EPA/DHA**[55]—EPA and DHA have been shown to downregulate LPS-induced activation of NF-kappaB.
  - **Bifidobacteria**[56]—*Bifidobacterium* is effective in inhibiting LPS-induced intestinal inflammation and could be an intervention for chronic intestinal inflammation. By-products associated with fermentation of prebiotics by *Bifidobacterium*, such as SCFAs (butyrate, propionate, and lactate), positively affect leaky gut and improve tight junctions.

II. Dietary interventions to decrease endotoxemia include:
  - Increase whole plant food.
  - Increase low-mercury fish consumption.
  - Avoid sugar and processed foods.
  - Incorporate intermittent fasting.
  - Increase dietary fiber and prebiotic consumption (especially foods high in oligofructose, inulin, and galactooligosaccharide).
    - Soluble fibers are digested by enzymes into SCFAs.
    - SCFAs constitute approximately 5% to 10% of the energy source in healthy people.
    - Fiber-enriched diets improve insulin sensitivity[57] in lean and obese diabetic subjects.

III. Pancreatic elastase treatment:
  - Smoking cessation
  - Reduced alcohol consumption
  - Small frequent meals
  - Replacement of fat-soluble vitamins
  - Supplemental lipase or pancreatic enzymes (plant-based are not strong enough for severe EPI)
  - Prescription strength enzymes: CREON, ZENPEP, and others

IV. Recommendations for adequate protein digestion and fermentation by anaerobic bacteria include:

- A low FODMAP diet if intolerance to fructose is suspected

V. To increase beneficial SCFAs:
- Increase dietary fiber.
- Use prebiotics and probiotics.
- Take *Saccharomyces boulardii*.

VI. To reduce high levels of beta-glucuronidase:
- Decrease meat intake and increase insoluble fiber.
- Take probiotics.
- Consider *Silybum marianum* for liver support.
- Take calcium-D-glucarate.

VII. **Prebiotics and probiotics are essential**.

VIII. **Probiotics**—An animal study[58] that examined the effects of probiotics on circulating cytokine levels and severity of ischemia/reperfusion injury in the heart found that the leptin-suppressing bacteria *Lactobacillus plantarum 299v* resulted in decreased circulating leptin levels by 41%, smaller myocardial infarcts by 29%, and greater recovery of postischemic mechanical function by 35%, when compared with untreated controls. Finally, a pretreatment with leptin abolished the protective properties of the probiotic. This demonstrated the mechanistic link between microbiota composition and myocardial infarction and demonstrated that probiotic supplementation can have a beneficial effect on those with cardiovascular disease.

IX. **Polyphenol-rich foods** are extensively metabolized[59] by gut bacteria into anti-inflammatory end products. One study found that foods such as coffee and cocoa support a significant effect on the functional ecology of symbiotic partners that can affect the host physiology.

Cacao is a prebiotic for beneficial microbes, including *Bifidobacterium* and lactic acid bacteria. These bacteria ferment the cacao and produce anti-inflammatory compounds.[60]

Coffee consumption[61] attenuated an increase in Firmicutes to Bacteroidetes ratios normally associated with high-fat eating. Coffee also increases levels of SCFAs while lowering branched-chain amino acid.

X. **Mediterranean-style diet recommended**—Lean protein (fish, poultry), nuts, vegetables, and fruit, together with regular physical activity, are recommended to maintain cardiovascular health.

Summary

- The products of the microbiome can have a dramatic effect on risk of developing cardiovascular disease.
- The microbiome may contribute to obesity, insulin resistance, diabetes, hypertension, dyslipidemia, congestive heart failure, myocardial infarction, and coronary artery disease.
- Always check the microbiome and intestinal integrity in a patient who presents with cardiovascular disease.
- It is critical to rule out LPS endotoxemia as a contributing factor in diabetes and cardiovascular disease.
- Assume that intestinal permeability is likely present in patients presenting with cardiovascular or metabolic disorders.
- TMAO can come from choline, phosphatidylcholine, and carnitine and increases heart disease risk. The microbiome metabolism of these compounds is what determines the actual risk.
- Beneficial SCFAs include butyrate, propionate, and acetate and are critical to cardiovascular health.
- Check bile acid metabolism in patients with cardiovascular disease with gut-related symptoms.
- Test for metabolic switches for FXR, PRP, TGR5, glucose metabolism, lipid metabolism, thermogenesis in brown adipose tissue.
- KEY TREATMENT OPTIONS: Mediterranean diet, added soluble and insoluble fiber, fasting-mimicking diet or intermittent fasting, prebiotics, probiotics, butyrate, extra-virgin olive oil, and DMB (dimethylbutanol).

Future Challenges

As the cost of metatranscriptomic or RNA sequencing continues to come down, research of the gut microbiome will continue to improve. Currently, metatranscriptomic technology is the best means we have of analyzing the gut microbiome because of its ability to see the function and pathways of the gut microbiome. Defining what a healthy gut microbiome looks like and its variations among diseases is a meticulous and arduous process that requires a high input of data for accurate statistical analysis.

References

1. Qin J, Li R, Raes J, et al. A human gut microbial gene catalogue established by metagenomic sequencing. *Nature*. 2010;464(7285):59-65. doi:10.1038/nature08821.
2. Ursell L, Metcalf J, Parfrey LW, et al. Defining the human microbiome. *Nutr Rev*. 2013;70(suppl 1):S38-S44. doi:10.1111/j.1753-4887.2012.00493.x.
3. Lozupone CA, Stombaugh JI, Gordon JI, et al. Diversity, stability and resilience of the human gut microbiota. *Nature*. 2012;489(7415):220-230. doi:10.1038/nature11550.
4. Blaser MJ. *Missing Microbes: How the Overuse of Antibiotics is Fueling Our Modern Plagues*. New York: Henry Holt & Company; 2014.
5. Ahlman H, Nilsson O. The gut as the largest endocrine organ in the body. *Ann Oncol*. 2001;12 suppl 2:S63-S68. doi:10.1093/annonc/12.suppl_2.S63.
6. Hyland NP, Cryan JF. Microbe-host interactions: influence of the gut microbiota on the enteric nervous system. *Dev Biol*. 2016;417(2):182-187. doi:10.1016/j.ydbio.2016.06.027.
7. Furness JB, Jones C, Nurgali K, et al. Intrinsic primary afferent neurons and nerve circuits within the intestine. *Prog Neurobiol*. 2004;72(2):143-164. doi:10.1016/j.pneurobio.2003.12.004.
8. Wu H, Wu E. The role of gut microbiota in immune homeostasis and autoimmunity. *Gut Microbes*. 2012;3(1):4-14. doi:10.4161/gmic.19320.

9. Clemente J, Ursell L, Parfrey L, et al. The impact of the gut microbiota on human health: an integrative view. *Cell*. 2012;148(6):1258-1270. doi:10.1016/j.cell.2012.01.035.

10. Shreiner AB, Kao JY, Young VB. The gut microbiome in health and disease. *Cur Opin Gastroenterol*. 2015;31(1):69-75. doi:10.1097/MOG.0000000000000139.

11. Magne F, Silva AP, Carvajal B, et al. The elevated rate of cesarean section and its contribution to non-communicable chronic diseases in Latin America: the growing involvement of the microbiota. *Front Pediatr*. 2017;5:192. doi:10.3389/fped.2017.00192.

12. Fang S, Evans R. Wealth management in the gut. *Nature*. 2013;500:538-539. doi:10.1038/500538a.

13. Le Chatelier E, Neilsen T, Qin J, et al. Richness of human gut microbiome correlates with metabolic markers. *Nature*. 2013;500(7464):541-546. doi:10.1038/nature12506.

14. Jie Z, Xia H, Zhong SL, et al. The gut microbiome in atherosclerotic cardiovascular disease. *Nat Commun*. 2017;8(1):845. doi:10.1038/s41467-017-00900-1.

15. Yamashita T. Intestinal immunity and gut microbiota in atherogenesis. *J Atheroscler Thromb*. 2017;24(2):110-119. doi:10.5551/jat.38265.

16. Wang Z, Klipfell E, Bennett B, et al. Gut flora metabolism of phosphatidylcholine promotes cardiovascular disease. *Nature*. 2011; 472(7341):57-63. doi:10.1038/nature09922.

17. Koeth RA, Wang Z, Levinson BS, et al. Intestinal microbiota metabolism of *L*-carnitine, a nutrient in red meat, promotes atherosclerosis. *Nat Med*. 2013;19(5):576-585. doi:10.1038/nm.3145.

18. Wang Z, Roberts AB, Buffa JA, et al. Non-lethal inhibition of gut microbial trimethylamine production for the treatment of atherosclerosis. *Cell*. 2015;163(7):1585-1595. doi:10.1016/j.cell.2015.11.055.

19. Morris MC, Manson JE, Rosner B, et al. Fish consumption and cardiovascular disease in the physicians' health study: a prospective study. *Am J Epidemiol*. 1995;142(2):166-175. doi:10.1093/oxfordjournals. aje.a117615.

20. Ruggenenti P, Cattaneo D, Loriga G, et al. Ameliorating hypertension and insulin resistance in subjects at increased cardiovascular risk: effects of acetyl-L-carnitine therapy. *Hypertension*. 2009;54(3):567-574. doi:10.1161/HYPERTENSIONAHA.109.132522.

21. Cani PD, Amar J, Iglesias MA, et al. Metabolic endotoxemia initiates obesity and insulin resistance. *Diabetes*. 2007;(7)1761-1772. doi:10.2337/db06-1491.

22. Jose PA, Raj D. Gut microbiota in hypertension. *Curr Opin Nephrol Hypertens*. 2015;24(5):403-409. doi:10.1097/MNH.0000000000000149.

23. Afsar B, Vaziri ND, Aslan G, et al. Gut hormones and gut microbiota: implications for kidney function and hypertension. *J Am Soc Hypertens*. 2016;10(12):954-961. doi:10.1016/j.jash.2016.10.007.

24. Bullon P, Cordero MD, Quiles JL, et al. Mitochondrial dysfunction promoted by Porphyromonas gingivalis lipopolysaccharide as a possible link between cardiovascular disease and periodontitis. *Free Radic Biol Med*. 2011;50(10):1336-1343. doi:10.1016/j.freeradbiomed.2011.02.018.

25. Menni C, Lin C, Cecelja M, et al. Gut microbial diversity is associated with lower arterial stiffness in women. *Eur Heart J*. 2018;39(25):2390-2397. doi:10.1093/eurheartj/ehy226.

26. Karlsson F, Fak F, Nookaew I, et al. Symptomatic atherosclerosis is associated with an altered gut metagenome. *Nat Commun*. 2012;3: 1245. doi:10.1038/ncomms2266.

27. Machiels K, Joossens M, Sabino J, et al. A decrease of the butyrate-producing species Roseburia hominis and Faecalibacterium prausnitzii defines dysbiosis in patients with ulcerative colitis. *Gut*. 2014;63(8):1275-1283. https://www.ncbi.nlm.nih.gov/pubmed/24021287. Accessed October 21, 2018.

28. Yang T, Santisteban MM, Rodriguez V. Gut dysbiosis is linked to hypertension. *Hypertension*. 2015;65(6):1331-1340. doi:10.1161/HYPERTENSIONAHA.115.05315.

29. Cotillard A, Kennedy SP, Kong LC, et al. Dietary intervention impact on gut microbial gene richness. *Nature*. 2013;500(7464):585-588. doi:10.1038/nature12480.

30. David LA, Maurice CF, Carmody RN, et al. Diet rapidly and reproducibly alters the human gut microbiome. *Nature*. 2014;505(7484):559-653. doi:10.1038/nature12820.

31. Turnbaugh PJ, Ridaura VK, Faith JJ, et al. The effect of diet on the human gut microbiome: a metagenomic analysis in humanized gnotobiotic mice. *Sci Transl Med*. 2009;1(6):6ra14. doi:10.1126/scitranslmed.3000322.

32. Suez J, Korem T, Zeevi D, et al. Artificial sweeteners induce glucose intolerance by altering the gut microbiota. *Nature*. 2014;514(7521):181-186. doi:10.1038/nature13793.

33. Cabreiro F, Au C, Leung K. Metformin retards aging in *C. elegans* by altering microbial folate and methionine metabolism. *Cell*. 2013;153(1):228-239. doi:10.1016/j.cell.2013.02.035.

34. Vujasinovic M, Tepes B, Volfrand J, et al. Exocrine pancreatic insufficiency, MRI of the pancreas and serum nutritional markers in patients with coeliac disease. *Postgrad Med J*. 2015;91(1079):497-500. doi:10.1136/postgradmedj-2015-133262.

35. Stein J, Jung M, Sziegoleit A, et al. Immunoreactive elastase I: clinical evaluation of a new noninvasive test of pancreatic function. *Clin Chem*. 1996;42(2):222-226. https://www.ncbi.nlm.nih.gov/pubmed/8595714. Accessed October, xx, 2018.

36. Loser C, Mollgaard A, Folsch UR. Faecal elastase 1: a novel, highly sensitive, and specific tubeless pancreatic function test. *Gut*. 1996;39(4):580-586. doi:10.1136/gut.39.4.580.

37. Pouillis A, Foster R, Mendall MA, et al. Emerging role of calprotectin in gastroenterology. *J Gastroenterol Hepatol*. 2003;18(7):756-762. doi:10.1046/j.1440-1746.2003.03014.x.

38. Carlson M, Raab Y, Peterson C, et al. Increased intraluminal release of eosinophil granule proteins EPO, ECP, EPX, and cytokines in ulcerative colitis and proctitis in segmental perfusion. *Am J Gastroenterol*. 1999;94(7):1876-1883. doi:10.1111/j.1572-0241.1999.01223.x.

39. Bischoff SC, Mayer J, Nguyen QT, et al. Immunohistological assessment of intestinal eosinophil activation in patients with eosinophilic gastroenteritis and inflammatory bowel disease. *Am J Gastroenterol*. 1999;94(12):3521-3529. doi:10.1111/j.1572-0241.1999.01641.x.

40. Hau J, Andersson E, Carlsson HE. Development and validation of a sensitive ELISA for quantification of secretory IgA in rat saliva and faeces. *Lab Anim*. 2001;35(4):301-306. doi:10.1258/0023677011911822.

41. Choi SW, Park CH, Silva TM, et al. To culture or not to culture: fecal lactoferrin screening for inflammatory bacterial diarrhea. *J Clin Microbiol*. 1996;34(4):928-932. https://www.ncbi.nlm.nih.gov/pubmed/8815110. Accessed October 21, 2018.

42. Saitoh O, Kojima K, Sugi K, et al. Fecal eosinophil granule-derived proteins reflect disease activity in inflammatory bowel disease. *Am J Gastroenterol*. 1999;94(12):3513-3520. doi:10.1111/j.1572-0241.1999.01640.x.

43. Liu LX, Chi J, Upton MP, et al. Eosinophilic colitis associated with larvae of the pinworm Enterobius vermicularis. *Lancet*. 1995;346(8972):410-412. doi:10.1016/S0140-6736(95)92782-4.

44. Bischoff SC, Grabowsky J, Manns MP. Quantification of inflammatory mediators in stool samples of patients with inflammatory bowel disorders and controls. *Dig Dis Sci*. 1997;42(2):394-403. https://www.ncbi.nlm.nih.gov/pubmed/9052525. Accessed October 21, 2018.

45. Rothenberg ME, Mishra A, Brandt EB, et al. Gastrointestinal eosinophils. *Immunol Rev*. 2001;179:139-155. doi:10.1034/j.1398-9995.2001.00005.x.

46. Clouse RE, Alpers DH, Hockenbery DM, et al. Pericrypt eosinophilic enterocolitis and chronic diarrhea. *Gastroenterology*. 1992;103(1):168-176. doi:10.1016/0016-5085(92)91110-P.

47. Hijova E, Chmelaravo A. Short chain fatty acids and colonic health. *Bratisl Lek Listy*. 2007;108(8):354-358. https://www.ncbi.nlm.nih.gov/pubmed/18203540. Accessed October 21, 2018.

48. Canfora EE, Jocken JW, Blaak EE. Short-chain fatty acids in control of body weight and insulin sensitivity. *Nat Rev Endocrinol*. 2015;11(10):577-591. doi:10.1038/nrendo.2015.128.

49. Tuohy KM, Fava F, Viola R. "The way to a man's heart is through his gut microbiota"–dietary pro- and prebiotics for the management of cardiovascular risk. *Proc Nutr Soc*. 2014;73(2):172-185. doi:10.1017/S0029665113003911.

50. Ohira H, Tsutsui W, Fujioka Y. Are short chain fatty acids in gut microbiota defensive players for inflammation and atherosclerosis? *J Atheroscler Thromb*. 2017;24(7):660-672. doi:10.5551/jat.RV17006.

51. Angeloni C, Hrelia S. Quercetin reduces inflammatory responses in LPS-stimulated cardiomyoblasts. *Oxid Med Cell Longev*. 2012;2012. doi:10.1155/2012/837104.

52. Chowdhury R, Nimmanapalli R, Graham T, et al. Curcumin attenuation of lipopolysaccharide induced cardiac hypertrophy in rodents. *ISPN Inflamm*. 2013;2013:539305. doi:10.1155/2013/539305.

53. Qi T, Xu F, Yan X, et al. Sulforaphane exerts anti-inflammatory effects against lipopolysaccharide-induced acute lung injury in mice through the Nrf2/ARE pathway. *Int J Mol Med*. 2016;37(1):182-188. doi:10.3892/ijmm.2015.2396.

54. Sharafkhaneh A, Velamuri S, Badmaev V, et al. The potential role of natural agents in treatment of airway inflammation. *Ther Adv Respir Dis*. 2007;1(2):105-120. doi:10.1177/1753465807086096.

55. Li H, Ruan XZ, Powis SH, et al. EPA and DHA reduce LPS-induced inflammation responses in HK-2 cells: evidence for a PPAR-gamma-dependent mechanism. *Kidney Int*. 2005;67(3):867-874. doi:10.1111/j.1523-1755.2005.00151.x.

56. Riedel CU, Foata F, Philippe D, et al. Anti-inflammatory effects of bifidobacteria by inhibition of LPS-induced NF-kappaB activation. *World J Gastroenterol*. 2006;12(23):3729-3735. https://www.ncbi.nlm.nih.gov/pubmed/16773690. Accessed October, xx, 2018.

57. Morenga LT, Docherty P, Williams S. The effect of a diet moderately high in protein and fiber on insulin sensitivity measured using the dynamic insulin sensitivity and secretion test (DISST). *Nutrients*. 2017;9(12):1291. doi:10.3390/nu9121291.

58. Lam V, Su J, Koprowski S, et al. Intestinal microbiota determine severity of myocardial infarction in rats. *FASEB J*. 2012;26(4):1727-1735. doi:10.1096/fj.11-197921.

59. Moco S, Martin FP, Rezzi S. Metabolomics view on gut microbiome modulation by polyphenol-rich foods. *J Proteome Res*. 2012;11(10):4781-4790. doi:10.1021/pr300581s.

60. *The Precise Reason for the Health Benefits of Dark Chocolate: Mystery Solved [news Release]*. Dallas, TX. American Chemical Society; March 18, 2014. https://www.acs.org/content/acs/en/press-room/newsreleases/2014/march/the-precise-reason-for-the-health-benefits-of-dark-chocolate-mystery-solved.html. Accessed October xx, 2018.

61. Cowan TE, Palmnas MSA, Yang J. Chronic coffee consumption in the diet-induced obese rat: impact on gut microbiota and serum metabolomics. *J Nutr Biol*. 2014;25(4):489-495. doi:10.1016/j.jnutbio.2013.12.009.

28

Periodontal Disease, Inflammation, and Cardiovascular Disease

Douglas Thompson, DDS, FAAMM, ABAAHP and Gregori M. Kurtzman, DDS, MAGD, FPFA, FACD, FADI, DICOI, DADIA, DIDIA

Introduction

Periodontal disease is one of the most prevalent diseases affecting humans and is a chronic inflammatory disease that affects the gum (gingival) tissue and the bone supporting the teeth. If left untreated, periodontal disease can lead to tooth loss due to loss of the supporting bone. Recent studies suggest that one out of every two adults aged 30 years and older has periodontal disease. Research has also shown that periodontal disease is associated with multiple health conditions, including cardiovascular and renal issues, diabetes, osteoporosis, and pulmonary disorders, to name a few.

Data from the 2009 and 2010 National Health and Nutrition Examination Survey (NHANES) reported that over 47% of the sample, representing 64.7 million adults, had periodontitis, distributed as mild (8.7%), moderate (30.0%), and severe periodontitis (8.5%). Adults aged 65 years and older presented with moderate or severe periodontitis 64% of the time.[1] Prevalence was highest in Hispanics (63.5%) and non-Hispanic blacks (59.1%), followed by non-Hispanic Asian Americans (50.0%), and lowest in non-Hispanic whites (40.8%). A twofold increase in prevalence was reported between the lowest and highest levels of socioeconomic status, whether defined by poverty or education.[2] Periodontal disease is also reported to be higher in men (56.4%) than women (38.4%) and positively associated with increasing age. Additionally, we observe a higher prevalence rate with current smokers (64.2%), those living below the federal poverty level (65.4%), and those with less than a high school education (66.9%).

Periodontal Disease and Oral Biofilm

What Is Periodontal Disease and What Causes It?

Periodontal disease is an inflammatory process initiated by oral bacteria, yeast, viruses, their byproducts, and the host immunoinflammatory response to them. This response results in inflammation and ultimately bone loss around the teeth. Every person has a unique host response generated from their combined innate (genetic) and acquired (environmental) risk factors. Innate (genetic) risk factors are things you cannot change such as ethnicity, gender, and age. Acquired (environmental) risk factors are alterable things such as smoking, nutrition, stress management, sleep quantity and quality.

This polymicrobial disease can be slowly progressing or quite aggressive. It is also episodic in nature based on the varying health of the immune system. Therefore, periodontal disease is biofilm induced but host modulated. Our traditional focus has been on controlling this disease to prevent bone loss and ultimately tooth loss. Today, we have additional concerns. Oral bacteria, yeast, and viruses contained in dental plaque were long ignored for any effects outside the oral cavity and the connection to systemic effects have been poorly understood. Recently, research has been strong connecting a link between oral health and systemic disease, with 200 possible connections.[3]

Plaque is a community of microorganisms found on the tooth surface or within the sulcus (periodontal pocket) which are embedded in a matrix of polymers of host and bacterial origin. This is a more complex bio-environment than previously recognized and has been retermed biofilm as a result.[4,5]

Over 700 different species of bacteria naturally reside in the mouth. Most are considered innocuous, but some of these microorganisms have been identified as pathogenic. This aggregation of bacteria work together as a community, producing specific proteins and enzymes utilizing oral fluids as the vector for transmission.[6] It has been long demonstrated that these microbial communities can display enhanced pathogenicity (pathogenic synergism). Additionally, unlike planktonic (free-floating) bacteria those in biofilms restrict penetration of antimicrobial agents and are less susceptible to antimicrobials applied locally or administered systemically.[7,8] To summarize, bacteria in these complex biofilms act and react differently than bacteria that are planktonic in nature, which complicates management and treatment.

Oral Biofilm Formation and Effects

The bacterial community composition in the biofilm is very diverse. Variations in the many species can be detected and may be different from site to site in the same patient. With biofilm maturation, the microbial composition changes from one that is primarily gram-positive and streptococcus-rich to a structure filled with gram-negative anaerobes.[9]

Formation of the biofilm includes a series of steps that begins with the initial colonization of the pellicle through adsorption of bacterial molecules creating an adhesive on the tooth surface. Other diverse bacterial species co-adhere using bacterial receptors creating diversity and have both synergistic and antagonistic biochemical interactions among the inhabitants. The bacteria continue to divide until a three-dimensional mixed-culture biofilm forms that is specially and functionally organized with polymer production leading to development of an extracellular matrix. This matrix is a key structural aspect of the biofilm offering the inhabitants protection from external factors. As the biofilm thickens and becomes more mature, anaerobic bacteria are able to live deeper within the biofilm, further protecting them from the oxygen-rich environment within the oral cavity.

The early biofilm is able to withstand frequent mechanisms on oral bacterial removal such as chewing, swallowing, and salivary fluid flow. Early biofilm colonizers are also able to survive in the high oxygen concentrations present in the oral cavity. This initial biofilm is always present orally, forming immediately after oral cleansing by the patient.

The understanding of how complex oral biofilm and dentists' management of it has evolved as science has demonstrated that "plaque" is not as innocuous as previously thought. We now understand that what is contained in the oral biofilm, and how its components interact, has far reaching (systemic) actions that affect multiple areas including cardiac, pulmonary, renal, diabetes, colon, and a variety of other areas of the body. In fact, periodontal pockets and atheromatous plaques of cardiovascular disease patients can present similarities in the microbial diversity, indicating possible bacterial translocation between periodontal pockets and coronary arteries.[10]

Today, we evaluate, discuss, and treat patients differently than we used to based on a more complete understanding of oral biofilms and its systemic connection. We are now able to improve their dental and periodontal health, prevent oral conditions that may negatively affect systemic health, and aid in improving systemic conditions that may be complicated or worsened by the oral biofilms. Part of that change in care is mutual understanding of oral biofilms and the systemic connection with our medical colleges and involvement by all in managing total patient health care. However, what connection(s) to the systemic system are known and how does that occur?

The Systemic Connection

Harmful strains of bacteria in the oral biofilm can enter the bloodstream during the inflammatory response and can travel to other areas of the body. Increasing evidence indicates patients with periodontal disease have a much higher risk of developing cardiovascular and other systemic issues than those individuals who take preventive measures to eliminate and control the biofilm in their mouths.[11] Below is a review of some of the systemic effects that have been associated with oral biofilm, before examining the cardiovascular connection.

Diabetes

Diabetes is a significant public health problem, affecting 29.1 million patients (9.3% of the US population), with an estimated 8.1 million (27.8%) patients going undiagnosed.[12] Patients with diabetes have twice the risk for periodontal disease than those without the metabolic disorder. In addition, periodontal disease is more prevalent, progresses more rapidly, and is often more severe in patients with type I or type II diabetes.[13,14] Periodontal disease has been classified as the sixth most common complication of diabetes and is a strong, well-established risk factor for severe periodontal disease. Patients with periodontal infections have worse glycemic control over time and thus have greater difficulty managing their diabetes. Much of the dysglycemia is related to inflammation and insulin resistance. Treatment of periodontitis appears to improve glycemic control.[15] Therefore, control of the periodontal infection and associated biofilm should be part of the standard treatment for the diabetic patient.

Pulmonary Disease

Periodontal biofilm is a reservoir of bacteria and a source of lower airway infections, especially in older patients or those who are debilitated. Oral biofilm can inoculate the respiratory tract when aspirated. Severity of the disease is correlated with the pathogenicity of the bacteria in the biofilm. Periodontal pathogens and cariogenic bacteria increase risk factors for aspiration pneumonia.

The highest risk patients for respiratory infection (bronchitis and pneumonia) are medically compromised patients with or without respiratory disease who are unable to perform adequate oral homecare. Patients with removable dental prosthetics (dentures) are particularly prone to aspiration of the oral biofilm accumulating on the prosthesis. Evaluation of 328 articles published over an 11-year period reported linking oral hygiene to oral health care–associated pneumonia or respiratory tract infection in elderly people. The authors reported, "There is sufficient evidence that mechanical oral hygiene practices reduce the progression or occurrence of respiratory diseases in high-risk elderly people in nursing homes or hospitals. Mechanical oral hygiene practices may prevent the death of about 1 in 10 elderly residents of nursing homes from health care–associated pneumonia."[16]

Proper oral homecare is critical in preventing these oral infections by minimizing the potential of aspirating biofilm into the pulmonary system. One author reported, "Oral hygiene intervention significantly reduced occurrence of pneumonia in institutionalized subjects."[17] Frequent tooth brushing and preoperative use of 0.12% chlorhexidine mouthrinse or gel reduced nosocomial respiratory tract infections.[18] It has also been demonstrated that use of low-concentration peroxides in custom trays has a positive effect on oral biofilms, reducing the bacterial load and decreasing pathogenic material that may be aspirated. This may be a more predictable approach in elderly patients who lack manual dexterity to perform oral homecare with a toothbrush. Those patients with removable prosthetics, dentures, also need to keep them clean to keep oral biofilm down on the appliances as this biofilm may be aspirated leading to pulmonary issues as outlined above.[19]

Prostate Disease

Prostate-specific antigen (PSA), an enzyme created in the prostate normally secreted in very small quantities, has been reported to be secreted at much higher levels in men with periodontal disease.[20] Inflammation of the prostate or presence of infection or being affected by cancer demonstrates elevated PSA levels. Elevated PSA levels are a classic indicator of prostate cancer.[21] Research has demonstrated that men with indicators of periodontal disease and prostatitis have higher levels of PSA than men who do not have periodontal disease.[22]

Colon Cancer

Colon cancer is responsible for 50,000 deaths annually in the United States. Yet, the link to an oral connection and periodontal disease via biofilm is just becoming known in recent years. The bacterium *Fusobacterium nucleatum*, found in the mouth and in periodontal biofilm, has a role in periodontal disease. This bacterium has also been shown to colonize the gut and attach to cells in the colon, triggering a sequence that can lead to colon cancer. It has been reported that patients with periodontal disease have much higher levels of *F. nucleatum* then those with normal periodontal status.[23,24] Although a possible association was found between oral infections and colon cancer, a cause-and-effect relationship has not been found. Published studies show how *F. nucleatum* can speed the accumulation of cancer cells.[25,26] Minimizing *F. nucleatum* by controlling the oral biofilm may lower the risk for those who are at increased risk of developing colorectal cancer.

Pancreatic Cancer

Annually 30,000 people die from pancreatic cancer in the United States. Pancreatic cancer risk factors include cigarette smoking and chronic pancreatitis. But the role of inflammation from periodontal disease *may* promote this cancer.[27] The Harvard School of Public Health and Dana-Farber Cancer Institute researchers found that periodontal disease *may* be associated with an increased risk of cancer of the pancreas. Additionally, research shows men with periodontal disease had a 63% higher risk of developing pancreatic cancer compared with those reporting no periodontal disease.[28]

Preterm Pregnancy

Inflammation of the periodontal tissues due to the formation of biofilm increases dramatically during the course of a normal pregnancy.[29] Evidence has linked an association between the presence of periodontitis and preterm delivery and low birth weight infants. Oral bacteria have been identified in fetal membranes. Biofilm inflammatory molecules can enter the circulatory system and cross the placenta to reach the fetal membranes and cause preterm delivery. Lipopolysaccharides from cell walls of periodontal pathogens can trigger production of prostaglandins and a periodontal infection can lead to the release of these prostaglandins into the circulatory system. Translocation of periodontal bacteria to the fetus occurs via the placenta, which stimulates the release of prostaglandins.[30] These prostaglandins stimulate oxytocin production, which can initiate preterm labor and result in lower birth weight babies.

Cardiovascular Disease

Periodontal disease and the cardiovascular connection provides the strongest cause and effect with oral biofilm. Unfortunately, this connection has been ignored or misunderstood by dentists and physicians alike until recent literature has provided evidence of that connection.

CVD, an umbrella term for heart and blood vessel conditions, such as atherosclerosis, coronary heart disease, stroke, and myocardial infarction, is the result of a complex set of genetic and environmental factors.[31] It is commonly accepted that genetic factors including age, lipid metabolism, obesity, hypertension, and diabetes have a direct connection to CVD and its severity. But environmental risk factors also play a key component and include socioeconomic status, exercise, stress, diet, smoking, and chronic infections. Classic risk factors such as hypertension, hypercholesterolemia, and cigarette smoking may only account for one-half to two-thirds of the incidence of CVD.[32] There is increasing evidence linking chronic infection, inflammation, oxidative stress, and immune dysfunction to CVD with the biofilm as a predisposing factor.[33,34] The connection between oral bacteria and cardiac disease is not a recent development in the literature. Oral bacteria, specifically *Streptococcus mutans* (cariogenic) and *Porphyromonas gingivalis* (periodontitis), induce platelet aggregation, leading to thrombus formation.[35]

One or more periodontal pathogens as reported in the literature are found in 42% of atheromas in patients with severe periodontal disease.[36] It has been reported that *P gingivalis* actively can adhere to and invade fetal bovine heart endothelial cells and aortic endothelial cells.[37] Additionally, a 14-year study found periodontal disease patients had a 25% higher risk to develop CVD than their healthy counterparts.[38] Men younger than 50 years with periodontal disease demonstrate 72% more risk to develop CVD. Additionally, periodontal disease increased risk for both fatal and nonfatal strokes twofold.[39] Despite the strong evidence of an association between periodontal disease and CVD, it is unknown if it is a direct or causal relationship.

Periodontal disease releases bacteria that may enter the circulation, invading the heart and vascular tissue, causing harmful effects. People with higher levels of bacteria in their mouths tend to have thicker carotid arteries, an indicator of CVD.[40] Bacteria near diseased gingiva appears to induce clumping of blood platelets, which can then cause the clotting and blockages that can lead to heart attacks or strokes. The body's response to periodontal infection includes production of inflammatory mediators, which travel through the circulatory system and may cause harmful effects on the heart and blood vessels. Inflammatory mediators such as lipoprotein and triglycerides are significantly higher in patients with periodontitis than in control groups.[41] Increased levels of C-reactive protein, a biomarker for inflammation, is associated with periodontitis.[42] Periodontal disease's emergence as a potential risk factor for CVD is leading to a convergence in oral and medical care. Proper management of oral health may very well be key to prevention of cardiac disease or worsening of existing heart conditions.

Atherosclerosis and Periodontal Disease as Inflammatory Processes

The major component of the pathology of cardiovascular disease, particularly atherosclerosis, involves an inflammatory response to the multiple components of the adaptive immune system.[43] Links between atherosclerosis and periodontal disease can be predicted based on the bacterial initiated inflammatory mechanisms associated with periodontal disease both locally and systemically. This has an influence on the initiation and propagation of atherosclerotic lesions, which may be initiated by local or systemic inflammation.

Inflammation produces cytokines and chemotactic agents causing endothelial changes, which include upregulation of adhesion molecules.[44] These endothelial changes promote interactions with leukocytes (monocytes) promoting leukocyte migration into the interior layer of the arteries. Lipid streaks result. Additionally, upregulation of the endothelium releases chemotactic cytokines (monocyte chemotactic protein-1 [MCP-1]), which further attract cells that can transport bacteria into the lesion. Resident dendritic cells (DCs) and monocytes attracted by cytokines become foam cells following ingestion of LDLs releasing inflammatory cytokines and matrix metalloproteinases (MMPs) further enhancing the localized inflammatory response.[45] Thus, initiation and propagation of early atherosclerotic lesions may be enhanced by periodontal disease when periodontal bacteria or their effects on the host immune response such as T-cell responses contribute to endothelial dysfunction. Additionally, attraction of monocytes and enhanced lipid uptake by the cells leads to plaque formation in the vessel wall (Figure 28.1). Excess inflammation mediated by those inflammatory cells can cause plaque cap instability leading to rupture resulting in myocardial infarction or a stroke.[46]

Periodontal disease is generated by microorganisms that can enter the general circulation causing a bacteremia. Some species have been identified as high-risk pathogens. High-risk pathogens are currently understood as Aa, Pg, Tf, Td, and Fn. These high-risk pathogens can adversely influence the atherosclerosis pathogenesis triad in three distinct ways. High-risk periodontal pathogens affect serum lipoprotein concentration, endothelial permeability, and lipoprotein binding in the intima. Also, strong evidence supports periodontal bacteria affect vascular elasticity, lipid concentration, vascular biomarkers, HDL efflux, and endothelial function. Therefore, the dental community has a substantial opportunity to assist in mitigating the number one cause of morbidity and mortality, namely cardiovascular disease, by effective management of periodontal disease due to those high-risk pathogens.[47,48]

Diagnosing Periodontal Disease

Periodontal disease is not strictly a bacterial issue. We now know that yeast and viruses play a role in periodontal disease progression and are part of the complex biofilm. It is the biofilm that initiates a personalized immunoinflammatory process that is host dependent on genetics and environmental influence. It is this unique host response that ultimately determines the individual's sensitivity and reaction to the initiating insult.[49] Chronic stress (an environmental factor) has been shown to increase the severity of the pathological progression of periodontal disease, and lifestyle modification may improve oral health status but also its systemic connections.[50] As with inflammation systemically, patients' response will vary from patient to patient to the same insult. Periodontally, some patients will exhibit high degrees of inflammation with minimal insult from the biofilm present, whereas other patients will present with high levels of biofilm but exhibit minimal or no gingival inflammation. Recognizing the etiology and the inflammatory nature of periodontal disease opens new opportunities for diagnosis, treatment, and

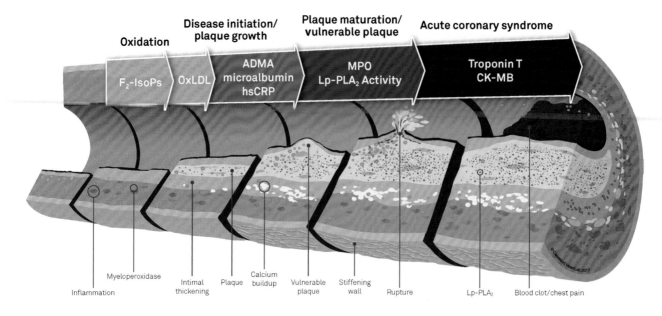

Figure 28.1 *Artery cutaway of various disease stages with related biomarkers. Initiation and propagation of endothelial inflammation leading to plaque formation may be initiated by periodontal inflammation and other risk factors. (Courtesy of the Cleveland Heart Lab. In: Penn MS, Klemes AB. Multimarker approach for identifying and documenting mitigation of cardiovascular risk.* Future Cardiol. *2013;9(4):497-506.)*

long-term management of the disease. Managing the disease can prevent tooth loss and improve cardiovascular and other systemic involvement.

Traditionally, periodontal disease has been diagnosed by increases in pocket depth, bleeding gums, and bone loss around the teeth leading to clinical attachment loss. Today, we are using the same information to determine if the disease is and has been present; however, we are using the presence of gingival bleeding (bleeding on probing) to determine if the disease is active or stable. The presence of a periodontal pocket (4 mm or greater) alone does not indicate active disease, especially when bleeding is not identified on probing. As with radiographic evidence of bone loss associated with the teeth, this may indicate prior disease that is currently not active. When bleeding on probing has been identified, it confirms the presence of inflammation. Recognize that identifying inflammation requires a histological diagnosis and bleeding on probing is a result of that inflammation. All dental practitioners must recognize that bleeding on probing and gingival inflammation can also be initiated by other systemic issues as well such as caries, failing restorative dentistry, some herbals taken in supplement form, and others.

For the purposes of this chapter we are referring to inflammation of the gum complex that is biofilm mediated and host modulated. When periodontal disease is biofilm related, treatment traditionally consisted of mechanical debridement of the supra and subgingival tooth surfaces (scaling and root planning) to remove the oral biofilm (plaque) and any hard deposits (calculus) present. Following a healing period, traditionally of 6 weeks, we expect a favorable host response evidenced by the elimination of bleeding on probing. Observing zero bleeding on probing becomes a surrogate endpoint and a sign that the periodontal disease and its associated inflammation has been arrested.

In addition to the bacteria in the biofilm, numerous studies have demonstrated periodontitis severity in adults is closely linked with increases in local inflammatory mediators due to genetic mutations of genes regulating the production of inflammatory cytokines. One commonly recognized cytokine is interleukin-1(IL-1). A mutation of the IL-1 gene can cause overexpression of IL-1, making it a key player in the inflammatory process and a prime candidate for a genetic association with periodontal disease.[51-53,103] Thirty (30) percent of the population can be identified with IL-1 polymorphisms.[54] Presence of the IL-1 genotype does not confer an expected periodontal disease diagnosis; however, the gene mutation has been implicated as a contributory factor to the host immunoinflammatory response determining the severity of adult periodontitis.[55]

Several unique salivary tests are now available to dentists that are reliable, affordable, and easy requiring only minutes to collect. These tests evaluate bacteria, yeast, viruses, and genetic variations in genes that express inflammatory mediators. Utilizing these tests, or some combination of them, can significantly enhance the practitioner's knowledge about the initiators of the periodontal disease process. An example of one of the most common bacterial tests is the MyPerioPath test from OralDNA Labs, Eden Prairie, MN. This test is utilized to determine both the quality (type) and quantity (bacterial inflammatory burden) of specific pathogenic microorganisms associated with periodontal infections.[56] Another test, Celsus One from OralDNA Labs, is utilized to identify eight genetic polymorphisms that affects the body's immune response. These genetic variations, which affect the production of beta-defensin, CD14, TNF-alpha, IL-1, IL-6, IL-17A, and matrix metallopeptidase 3 are associated with an increased risk for more severe periodontal infections, as well as increased risk for peri-implantitis (periodontal disease associated with dental implants), diabetes, and cardiovascular disease. Both tests are intended as supportive adjuncts to conventional diagnostic methods of recording probing depths, recession, bleeding, mobility, as well as radiographic examination and a personal/family history of periodontal disease. Depending on the test results, the practitioner can make informed decisions on what type of treatment enhancers may be necessary to manage the disease. A hallmark of periodontal disease management is biofilm control involving mechanical debridement and chemotherapeutics including systemic antibiotics when recommended based on disease severity.

Saliva consists of the fluid excreted from the major and minor salivary glands, containing proteins, enzymes, and buffers that are designed to provide protection and buffering and aid in digestion and swallowing. It also contains gingival crevicular fluid. In inflamed tissues, this serum exudate serves as a protective mechanism to cleanse the "pocket" of the bacteria and debris that reside within the sites. Gingival crevicular fluid contains bacteria, viruses, serum, white blood cells, inflammatory mediators, and MMPs. Thus, saliva is an excellent source for bacterial and human cell DNA. Both kinds of DNA can be extracted and analyzed through a laboratory process called polymerase chain reaction (PCR). In molecular biology, PCR is a technique for detection and elongation of DNA strands, an indispensable technique for duplicating DNA so that it can be analyzed for the identification of hereditary diseases, as well as the detection and diagnosis of infectious disease. DNA-PCR also permits identification of mycobacteria, anaerobic bacteria, or viruses from the saliva sample sent for testing. Within 4 to 5 days of receipt of the saliva test sample a comprehensive interpretation of the periodontal pathogens that were detected and the quantity of the detection are sent to the clinician.

These clinical lab reports, as in medicine, serve to help further define risk for disease and/or disease progression allowing management decisions to be made based on objective biological information. Test reports also serve as a persuasive means to instill the need for periodontal therapy and patient compliance in order to achieve the best possible treatment outcome. Furthermore, a "control analysis" post therapy using microbial, yeast, or viral testing also serves to confirm the efficacy of the treatment.

Pathogens identified by the most common microbial tests are classified into two taxa: facultative and anaerobic. These data plus data about their concentration can help determine if antibiotic antimicrobial therapy should be used to help stabilize the disease. Antimicrobial therapy can be used systemically or locally with use of antiseptics and locally applied medications. However, without knowing the virulence and pathogenic properties of the bacteria, there is no organized way to determine which patients are best suited for which antimicrobials. The graphical portion of the report shows the types of pathogens present, and the pathogen load. The report section discusses the risk of each pathogen based on virulence factors. Longitudinal studies

have shown the potential risk for each of these pathogens. This gives the clinician information to "target" pathogens with the goal of elimination or suppression of the pathogens associated with disease. Identification of the pathogens present and their concentration may yield a suggestion of a specific antibiotic regimen that targets the taxa of the pathogens detected. This allows selection of antibiotics based on the actual causative agent(s) rather than the indiscriminate use without objective data.

Without salivary diagnostics dental practitioners have been unable to determine if bacterial levels have changed, pathogenic species have been eliminated, or a microbial shift has taken place. Elimination of bleeding does not confirm an absence of bacteria or offending biofilm. Below is an example of a patient who presents with isolated bleeding on probing during periodontal examination, a history of periodontal disease confirmed by prior bone loss, and increased pocketing. Salivary testing was performed to learn the microbial makeup prior to disinfection treatment. Treatment consisted of traditional scaling and root planning and the recommendation to rinse for 2 weeks with chlorhexidine (a common periodontal disease treatment approach taught in most dental schools) (**Figure 28.2** left). At 6-week recall to evaluate the periodontal healing, probing identified less bleeding and the periodontal chart showed improving pocket depths. Salivary testing was performed to check type and levels of pathogenic bacteria post-treatment. Although clinical evidence of periodontal disease and the associated inflammation was better, the retest report demonstrated no significant changes in the pathogenic bacteria load (**Figure 28.2** right). These retest results confirmed that traditional nonsurgical periodontal treatment methods may not be effective in shifting the oral biofilm to levels that do not encourage long-term periodontal stability.

Treatment and Maintenance of Periodontal Disease

Goals of periodontal treatment are eliminating or reduction of the pathogenic biofilm to levels that do not initiate a host immunoinflammatory response. Squelching the host response prevents the release of cytokines that break down connective tissue, supporting bone, and induces inflammation and ultimately a dysregulation of bone metabolism resulting in more destruction. The goals of periodontal treatment have been to eliminate deep pockets and gingival bleeding inflammation/infection, and provide education to the patient so they can attain adequate plaque control at home. Periodontal disease is a complex disease that ultimately when left untreated, results in significant tissue damage and possible tooth loss. Contemporary periodontal treatment goals should be based on recognizing the multifactorial nature of the disease and the individual variability in how patients manifest the disease. We ultimately want our patients to be free of pathogenic microorganisms and inflammation, to respond to treatment, and to undertake

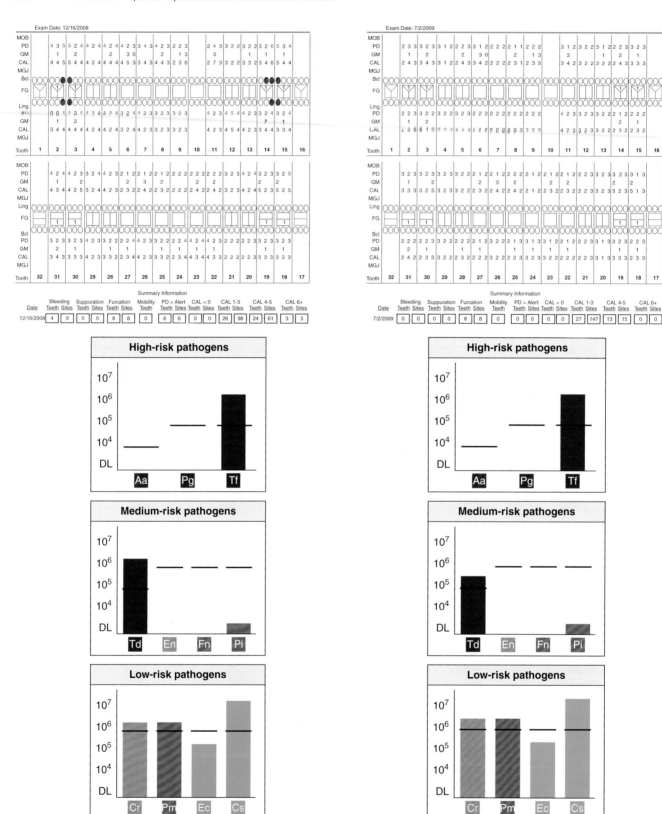

Figure 28.2 *Pretreatment and post-treatment results of a patient with pretreatment clinical signs of active periodontal disease. Testing produced objective information showing unaltered microbial flora after traditional mechanical debridement methods. This revelation resulted in developing the Thompson Disinfection Protocol.*

appropriate homecare regimes based on their ability to control the biofilm. An innovative approach takes into account individual differences in people's genes, environments, and lifestyles or behaviors.[57]

As outlined, periodontal disease is identified with the presence of gingival bleeding, inflammation, and possibly tooth mobility typically during routine examination. Once identified, treatment will consist of mechanical debridement (scaling and root planning, SRP) of the periodontal pockets and associated teeth to remove hard formations (calculus) with the goal to disrupt and remove the sulcular biofilm (plaque) to levels that do not provoke a host response. Additionally, other host modulatory strategies may also be employed to alter the host response and to strengthen the autoimmune system. Salivary testing is performed prior to treatment to identify those patients at risk based on pathogenicity of the bacteria present and their concentrations. This information is a pretreatment baseline to compare to a post-treatment report confirming if the flora has been altered and if additional care is required. Genetic testing can also be obtained to learn information about the possible severity of the innate and acquired host response.

Host Modulation

When we recognize the importance of modulating the inflammatory response, new treatment opportunities arise that may be adjuncts to mechanical debridement. In the future, various methods to modulate the host response will be a significant opportunity to guard against disease progression. These will focus on controlling or resolving inflammation either during the dental appointment or with homecare.[58]

Because the host response is made up of a person's genetics and their acquired risk factors, several opportunities present. Depending on their innate genetic makeup and lifestyle factors that increase the risk of disease severity such as smoking, stress, and nutrition, we have several options. One method of host modulation that has been available for years is the administration of a subantimicrobial dose of doxycycline that acts as a collagenase inhibitor. Others will be explored as well.

Although doxycycline has been used as an antibacterial agent, use in lower doses has proven to help modulate the activities of some host-derived MMPs responsible for tissue breakdown. It also has an inhibitory effect on collagenase. The use of a subantimicrobial dose of doxycycline (Periostat [doxycycline hyclate]) 20 mg BID daily as an adjunct following scaling and root planning provided significantly greater clinical benefits than SRP alone in the treatment of moderate to severe periodontal disease.[59] It can be prescribed for 9 months followed by a 3-month drug holiday and then repeated. Usage beyond 9 months has not been well reported, so continued benefits may be present, but further study is needed to confirm.

Anticytokine therapy is another promising area with regard to host modulation, which targets interleukin-1 and tumor necrosis factor.[60] Etanercept (a tumor

necrosis factor-alpha receptor antagonist) has been reported in a periodontitis animal model to assist in the reduction of inflammation by way of reduced neutrophil infiltration, nitric oxide levels, and decreased apoptosis.[61] However, one of the major problems with anticytokine therapy is that a functional redundancy of cytokines can enable the host to activate alternative pathways of inflammation if only one specific cytokine is targeted.[62]

Two areas of considerable interest are diet and specific synthetic and natural resolvins as adjuncts to periodontal therapy. Biological resolution of inflammation may be enhanced by resolvins, lipoxins, and protectins. Utilization of omega-3 polyunsaturated fatty acids (resolvins precursor) have well-documented anti-inflammatory properties. There is emerging evidence that dietary supplementation with fish oil may be of some benefit.[63] A cost-effective adjunctive therapy to the management of periodontal disease could be dietary supplementation with fish oil.[64] Several studies report the clinical benefit is enhanced when combined with low-dose aspirin.[65,66] Addition of aspirin to the treatment regime is based on its ability to significantly increase the production of stable resolvins.[67] In this context, resolvin E1 has been shown to regulate inflammation at the tissue and cellular level. It has been demonstrated by resolving experimentally induced inflammation and periodontitis, damaged bone is able to regenerate in the absence of any adjunctive antimicrobial or regenerative therapies.[68]

How Can We Better Manage Oral Biofilms?

Professional mechanical debridement no matter the method or the amount of time spent has been shown to leave some of the biofilm on the teeth. Complete biofilm removal with mechanical methods alone is impossible. Despite our best mechanical attempts and our homecare approaches of brushing, flossing, or other in-between the teeth plaque management modalities, we are learning the biofilm is hard to manipulate. Additionally, biofilm live in other areas of the mouth that mechanical debridement does not target such as the cheeks, the tongue, and the pharyngeal spaces.

Therefore, nonsurgical periodontal disease management must begin with debridement of the teeth and follow with methods to target the biofilm in the rest of the mouth. Following biofilm manipulation in the dental office the disease must be maintained with meticulous homecare if therapy is to succeed. Because we cannot mechanically manipulate the other soft tissues of the mouth, we use antimicrobial rinses and other chemotherapeutics to manage these areas. It has become clear to be successful we need mechanical methods of plaque removal in the office and at home. In addition, we also need chemotherapeutic methods of plaque disruption in the office and at home.

Because the office exposure is of such limited time (2-6 appointments each year), homecare is critical. In spite of great diligence, homecare can be compromised with limitations of our cleaning devices. For example, toothbrush bristles are unable to extend more then 3 to 4 mm into the pocket and is unable to mechanically contact the biofilm located at deeper depths. A similar problem presents with oral irrigators not allowing irrigation to the bottom of the pockets. Compliance with regular daily use can also be a challenge. The sulcular environment is difficult for most patients to reach with brushing and flossing, making it impossible to control oral biofilms by mechanical means alone as the bacteria grow and replicate so rapidly. Biofilm redevelopment after cleaning is more rapid and complex, and without great care can exceed precleaning levels within 2 days.[69,70]

Bacteria embedded in the biofilm are up to 1000-fold more resistant to antibiotics compared with planktonic bacteria. Therefore, the use of antibiotics either systemically or in oral rinses are often unable to eliminate or manage the biofilm bacteria adequately.[71,72] This has implications both with natural teeth and with dental implants. Periodontal disease around implants is called peri-implantitis.[73]

Owing to limitations with mechanical homecare methods used alone, the addition of select antimicrobial rinses is critical for long-term biofilm management. An ideal adjunctive rinse would be one with antibacterial, antiviral, and antifungal properties and have no side effects. It would also be accessible and inexpensive if it is to be used in therapy or maintenance of the disease. We will outline some of the most popular adjunctive rinses.

Chlorhexidine has been the gold standard in periodontal disease and caries management. It is antibacterial, antifungal, and antiviral. Chlorhexidine has been reported to have an effect on young biofilms, but the bacteria in mature biofilms and nutrient-limited biofilms have been shown to be more resistant to its effects.[74,75] Numerous studies have confirmed the antiplaque and antigingivitis effects of chlorhexidine.[76] Chlorhexidine has the ability to adhere to the dental pellicle and oral mucosa extending its antiplaque effect and is used in dentistry as a 0.12% to 0.2% mouthwash used twice daily. The cationic chlorhexidine is incompatible with anionic surfactant compounds in toothpastes, which neutralize its antimicrobial action; therefore, chlorhexidine should not be used in conjunction with tooth brushing.[77] Chlorhexidine can affect fibroblast development affecting periodontal healing, has poor taste, and allergic reactions have been reported. Today, there are other options to chlorhexidine.

Sodium hypochlorite (NaOCl) is a highly active cytotoxic oxidant recognized as a potent antiseptic and disinfectant against bacteria, fungi, and viruses. Sodium hypochlorite reacts with proteins, nucleic acids and lipids and inactivates enzymes essential in the energy-yielding metabolism of microorganisms. Hydrolysis occurs when NaOCl contacts water forming hypochlorous acid (HOCl) and the less active hypochlorite ion (OCl). Hypochlorous acid then splits into hydrochloric acid (HCl) and the oxygen atom (O), a strong oxidator, which diffuses through the microbial cell wall, changing the oxidation-reduction potential of the cell. As NaOCl is naturally occurring in human neutrophils, monocytes, and macrophages, an allergic reaction does not occur,

and it is not mutagenic or carcinogenic, with a century-long safety record.[78,104] NaOCl, at concentrations of 5% to 6% as found in household bleach, can cause irritation to the skin, mucous membranes, and the eyes, although the irritant effect is reversible. For periodontal disease management, studies have shown that a very dilute solution 0.2% is highly effective as an antiseptic.

NaOCl has been used as an antiseptic agent in dentistry for more than a century and remains a widely used root canal irrigant at concentrations of 1.0% to 5.25%.[79] Additionally, NaOCl rinsing at lower concentrations exerts broad antimicrobial activity against oral biofilms, with an 80-fold decrease in biofilm endotoxin compared to water alone.[80-82] One study reported that patients who abstained from oral hygiene for 21 days, but performed supervised twice-daily 0.05% sodium hypochlorite oral rinses, had a 48% reduction in Plaque Index score, 52% reduction in Gingival Index score, and 39% reduction in bleeding on probing sites compared with water rinse alone.[83] Another study in college students abstaining from oral hygiene, the clinical effect of rinsing with 0.5% NaOCl (Carrel-Dakin solution) reported similar results and produced a 47% greater reduction in dental plaque amount compared with water-rinsing. Low pretreatment gingivitis scores were maintained around teeth receiving the sodium hypochlorite rinse, whereas the gingivitis score increased by 50% in water-treated sites.[84] Zou et al. reported that NaOCl can also penetrate into and potentially kill cariogenic bacteria within dentinal tubules decreasing potential for dental caries.[85] Histologically, it was found that NaOCl solution applied subgingivally exhibited no detrimental effect on periodontal healing and dilute NaOCl has no contraindications.[86]

Jorgen Slots has reported that dilute NaOCl (household bleach) has a basic pH and does not pose a risk of tooth erosion and does not corrode titanium implant surfaces.[87] The lowest concentration of NaOCl solution found to reliably inactivate bacteria in vitro is 0.01%.[88] But Slots reported that a suitable concentration of NaOCl for periodontal pocket irrigation is 0.5%. Following Slots recommendations this is equivalent to 10 mL (two teaspoonfuls) of 6.0% household bleach in 125 mL (one half-glass) of water. Patients are advised to rinse two-three times weekly for 30 seconds with 8 mL of the solution. The solution may also be used in an oral irrigator (Waterpik) at a low-pressure setting with patients with deeper periodontal pockets to aid in contact with subgingival biofilm.

Hydrogen peroxide solution has little effect on periodontal pathogens; however, hydrogen peroxide gel (H_2O_2) has been documented as a means of both eliminating the biofilm as well as preventing its reformation without bacterial resistance issues found with other site-specific treatment modalities. H_2O_2 gel has been documented used daily up to 6 years with no adverse effects or carcinogenic activity, while showing a decrease in biofilm (plaque), and enhanced wound healing, and improved gingival bleeding.[89] Furthermore, no allergic reactions have been reported and bacterial strains demonstrate no resistance. Functionally it debrides the biofilm slime matrix and bacterial cell walls, essentially peeling the biofilm back layer by layer. This causes irreversible cleaving of the amino acids in the protein chains of the bacteria in the biofilm, acting to break down the protein pellicle attaching the biofilm to the tooth surface, and decreases localized inflammation in the pocket by inhibiting IL-8mRNA.[90]

Oxygen is required for successful wound healing because of increased demand of the reparative processes such as cell proliferation, bacterial defense, angiogenesis, and collagen synthesis.[91] New cell growth requires oxygen, which induces the growth of new blood vessels. This increases flow of oxygenated blood to the wound, beginning the healing process. As healing progresses, new granulation tissue that is exposed to oxygen is better vascularized leading to higher tensile strength collagen being formed, during wound healing. Hyperbaric oxygen has been well documented to be bactericidal for anaerobic bacteria.[92] Hydrogen peroxide gel oxygenates the pocket, changing the environment from anaerobic to aerobic and creating a hyperbaric oxygen chamber in the sulcus to destroy the biofilms occupants. Additionally, neutrophils in the presence of hydrogen peroxide and chloride will produce ozone through the cholesterol ozonolysis process.[93] Ozone has antimicrobial activity by oxidation of biomolecule precursors and microbial toxins that have been implicated in periodontal diseases, which causes healing and tissue regeneration.[94]

Published studies have documented that the ideal concentration of hydrogen peroxide gel is 1.7% as this is effective in breaking down the biofilm and virtually eliminates any irritation issues reported with higher concentrations. It has been determined that a 10-minute exposure to a 1.7% hydrogen peroxide gel penetrates the biofilm slime matrix, debriding the bacterial cell walls within. Maintaining the peroxide in the periodontal pocket releases oxygen and changes the subgingival microenvironment, making survival of the anaerobic bacteria more difficult.[95,96] But, with quick redevelopment of the biofilms, to be effective, peroxide application needs to be part of the daily homecare routine.

Other rinses or gels to consider that may have applications in treatment or maintenance are rinses made from essential oils, biobotanical products, or other ingredients that support properties that are antimicrobial, antiviral, and antifungal. Using microbial testing pretreatment and post-treatment and during maintenance can help determine if a periodontal disease regimen is effective on the biofilm load.

Biofilm Elimination Over the Long-Term

The key to elimination of oral inflammation and long-term alteration of the bacteria in the biofilm relies on treatment in the dental office as well as daily patient homecare. With strict homecare compliance following thorough in-office disinfection, long-term alteration of the bacteria with a shift to nonpathogenic species can be accomplished. Elimination of bleeding on probing is a positive clinical sign but does not guarantee a change in the pathogenicity of the bacteria intraorally, for example, a patient presented with pathogenic bacteria as documented by the MyPerioPath saliva test prior to traditional periodontal treatment (Figure 28.3). Traditional treatment consisted of scaling and root planning and the use of chlorhexidine for 3 weeks and reevaluation at 6 weeks. The microbial test was repeated at 6 weeks post-periodontal treatment with surprising results that showed no alteration in the pathogenic bacteria. The results after conventional SRP produced a reduction of bleeding on probing and pocket depth but affected the pathogen profile very little (Figure 28.3 second image). This highlighted the need to take a more comprehensive approach to disease treatment and employ a total-mouth disinfection methodology.

This method addresses the following areas:
1. Occlusal analysis to identify and remove any fremitus in chewing.
2. Attack the bacteria in the pockets mechanically (using SRP).
3. Attack the bacteria in the pockets chemically by irrigating with a .2% dilute NaOCl rinse (CariFree Treatment Rinse Oral BioTech, www.carifree.com), and depositing a locally applied timed release antibiotic (Arestin OraPharma, Inc., www.orapharma.com) in all pockets ≥5 mm.
4. Attack the bacteria in the bloodstream with the antibiotic regimen suggested on the microbial (OralDNA MyPerioPath) report.
5. Attack the bacteria in the rest of the oral cavity with 0.2% NaOCl rinse (CariFree Treatment Rinse), to control oral microbial load. Use this rinse for 1 minute twice daily.
6. Prescribe homecare adjuncts such as a mechanical toothbrush, water flosser like a Waterpik (Water Pik, Inc., www.waterpik.com) or Hydroflosser (Shazzam Tsunami, Bling Dental Products, www.blingdentalproducts.com), and interproximal aids for enhanced bacteria load control.
7. Maintain tight 2-month reevaluation appointments until zero bleeding on periodontal chart has been achieved. (We refer to this as periodontal stability.)
8. Retest using the same testing method that was used pretreatment to reevaluate the microbial profile.

The patient was kept on a tight 2-month reevaluation schedule until zero bleeding was established. The patient was then retested using MyPerioPath (Figure 28.3 fourth graphic). With the use of a total-mouth disinfection approach utilizing oral rinses with greater microbial killing efficiency, the microbial profile was altered. Our goal is to eradicate, suppress, or alter the bacterial load to a point it does not provoke an immune-inflammatory response. It is important to note this profile was measured when there was zero bleeding, a clinical sign to suggest gingival stability. Following an enhanced disinfection protocol addressing the teeth, the sulcus around the teeth, the rest of the mouth, and placing the patient on a biofilm altering rinse for up to 4 months following scaling and root planning plus meticulous homecare, the 4-month follow-up bacterial test (**Figure 28.3** fourth graphic) shows significant biofilm shift.

The next logical question to ask is: How long can the practitioner and the patient be working together to maintain periodontal stability? Look further at **Figure 28.3**. You can see subsequent reports for up to 9 years. This 9-year follow-up demonstrated that continuation of the recommended

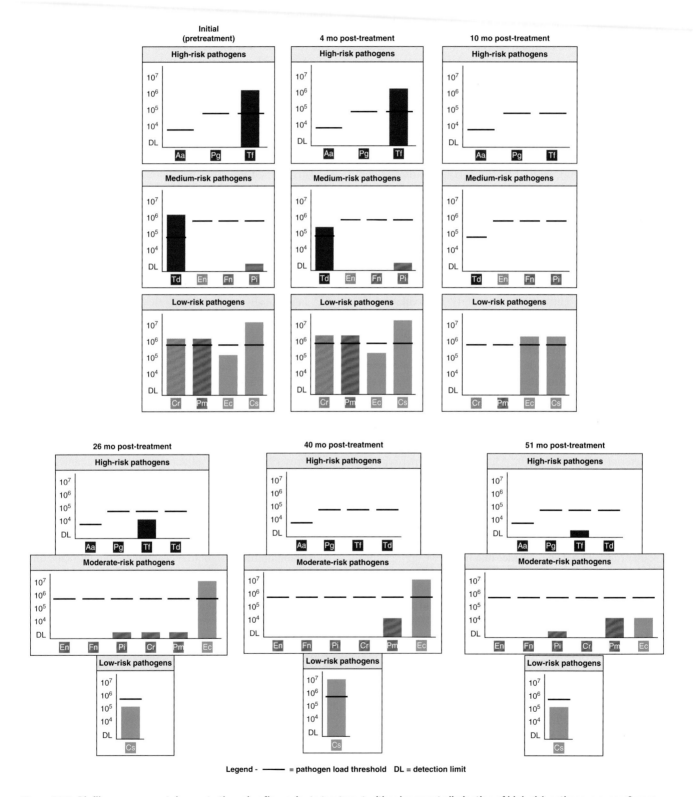

Figure 28.3 *Biofilm management demonstrating microflora prior to treatment with subsequent elimination of high-risk pathogens over a 9-year period without reactivation of the disease.*

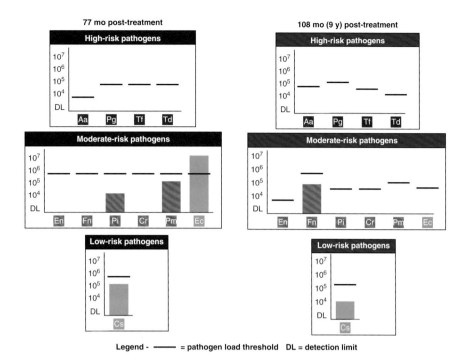

Figure 28.3 *Biofilm management demonstrating microflora prior to treatment with subsequent elimination of high-risk pathogens over a 9-year period without reactivation of the disease. (Continued.)*

homecare plus routine in-office supportive periodontal maintenance appointments maintained the elimination of the high-risk pathogenic bacteria and reduction of moderate-risk pathogenic bacteria. With modification and maintenance of the oral bacteria associated with the biofilm, inflammation can be controlled, and its affect systemically becomes much less of an overall health risk factor.

Collaboration Between the Physician and Dentist

Current research has merged what happens intraorally with the whole body and total health care connects these areas by inflammation. As has been suggested, oral biofilm represented by high and moderate risk pathogens that stimulate the host response resulting in chronic inflammation can be identified and managed and this has a positive outcome on systemic issues especially cardiac and vascular. Considering the 50 plus other associative systemic disease conditions related to periodontal biofilm, dentists will help their patients best by personalizing treatment strategies to eliminate or suppress a pathogenic biofilm load. They will also benefit their patients by providing options to modulate the host response to the biofilm, ultimately reducing exposure to inflammatory byproducts that slowly degrade health. Host modulation will come in the form of products, medicines, or supplements as well as lifestyle factors that alter the immune response. It is becoming clearer and clearer that periodontal disease is a medical condition harbored in the mouth and has been left to dentists to diagnose and treat. Because this disease is polymicrobial, multifactorial, and episodic with a bidirectional relationship

to other systemic diseases (eg, Diabetes), dentists cannot best treat the disease alone. Dentists and physicians need to collaborate to help their patients be as successful as they can be. The result: improving total health care for our mutual patients.

Physicians can screen for some obvious clinical signs of periodontal disease. When the physician is examining the patient, some simple questions may aid in coordination of care. Those include: "When was the last time you saw a dentist for a cleaning and exam?" "Do your gums bleed when you brush and floss?" "Do you floss?" "Do you have bad breath?" and "Have you noticed any teeth shifting or getting loose or sensitive?" Those patients with diagnosed cardiac or vascular issues should be encouraged to see a dentist on a routine basis to help manage the oral biofilm and associated bacteria. Taking it a step further, physicians practicing preventative cardiology may consider utilizing a metric to learn the biofilm makeup to see the level of high-and moderate-risk pathogens that have research behind them implicating them in the vascular disease process. Ultimately, controlling this biofilm may help improve vascular and other systemic issues being treated and managed.

Likewise, dentists should be vigilant when identifying periodontal disease and oral inflammation in those patients with a positive medical history for cardiac, vascular, and other systemic diseases that were outlined and coordinate ongoing care with their physician. Educating the patient as to the connection between oral and systemic health brings the patient into the process and improves overall health care with an understanding of daily maintenance needs.

The key to improving health care is an understanding of the inflammation connection and early diagnosis of periodontal disease. When identified, treatment needs to be directed at the specific causative agents (microbes) and patient lifestyle factors that may be influencing the inflammatory process. Daily homecare maintenance is important to keep oral biofilm and the associated bacteria at low levels so that inflammatory systemic consequences can be minimized, and the patient maintained in a stable state.

Many physicians are taking a much broader root cause approach to disease management. Traditional symptom management or late stage disease management carries a high expense burden of unnecessary hospital experiences, and less than favorable disease outcomes. One example of a medical model (BaleDoneen Method) has been found to be effective in preventing heart attack, stroke, and diabetes. Eight-year outcome data using sequential Carotid Intima Media Thickness reports are suggesting that following a vascular disease management method such as this has positive outcomes on lipids and CIMT thickness. The Bale/Doneen Method is effective in generating a positive effect on the atherosclerotic disease process by achieving regression of disease in the carotid arteries. A big part of this BaleDoneen Method is stressing the importance of oral health in the reduction of inflammation and bacterial burden causing vascular changes.[97-99] This model challenges the current standard of health care, utilizing a preventative, comprehensive, holistic approach focused on a disease/inflammatory treatment paradigm to achieve optimum health.

The BaleDoneen Method comprises six basic elements that should be considered in any vascular disease management program.[100-102] This includes:

1. Education—Each patient is educated about the disease state of atherosclerosis and understands how myocardial infarctions and ischemic strokes occur.

2. Disease—Each patient is evaluated for the presence of atherosclerosis, using noninvasive office-based techniques, to find asymptomatic vascular disease, and is monitored annually with an intima-media thickness (IMT) test to follow the individual trajectory of atherosclerotic disease. In addition, all patients are monitored annually with a carotid IMT test to follow the atherosclerotic disease over time in the individual patient.

3. Inflammation—Biomarkers are used to routinely determine the inflammatory state of the vascular system. Endothelial markers include hs-C-reactive protein, microalbumin/creatinine urine ratio, and fibrinogen. Lipoprotein-associated phospholipase A2 is evaluated for intima activity. Patients are instructed to have these assessed at least biannually.

4. Root causes—The root cause or causes of the atherosclerotic process are determined and managed for each patient. Root causes of atherosclerosis can include insulin resistance, lipo(a), familial hyperlipidemia, and vitamin D deficiency. Appropriate follow-up testing for effective management of a root cause is done on average quarterly to semiannually.

5. Optimal goals—Goals of therapy are set based on peer-reviewed, reliable research and guidelines, with optimal targets to minimize risk and often going beyond the values set for the standard of care. Attainment of goals are evaluated, on average, every 3 to 6 months.

6. Genetics—Genetic information is obtained on patients to aid in the assessment of their cardiovascular risk and to help guide therapy. These tests are never repeated. Their clinical utility never expires, unlike other biomarkers. This makes them arguably the least expensive tests performed.

This method is mentioned and outlined here because a significant source of inflammation can be from the mouth in both periodontal disease and endodontic disease. Therefore, oral health is a major root factor, and in the training of this method it is made clear that anyone practicing preventative cardiology needs a competent oral health care provider to evaluate the mouth for any contributing pathology.

These above basic elements of this prevention strategy are reinforced with abundant patient education. A huge part of this education is on lifestyle modification, the number one way to prevent cardiovascular disease. Lifestyle skills are taught in physical activity, proper diet, adequate sleep, anxiety management, weight control, nicotine cessation, and oral health maintenance. These are all host modulation issues that affect cardiovascular disease. Likewise, many similarities exist between cardiovascular disease and the lifestyle issues that affect periodontal disease. Because of this, there is great opportunity to collaborate on patient education reinforcement between the medicine and dental disciplines. The future is bright for medical/dental collaboration for best overall oral and systemic disease management.

References

1. Eke PI, Dye BA, Wei L, Thornton-Evans GO, Genco RJ. Prevalence of periodontitis in adults in the United States: 2009 and 2010. *J Dent Res.* 2012;91(10):914-920. Epub 2012 August 30.

2. Eke PI, Dye BA, Wei L, et al. Update on prevalence of periodontitis in adults in the United States: NHANES 2009 to 2012. *J Periodontol.* 2015;86(5):611-622. doi:10.1902/jop.2015.140520. Epub 2015 February 17.

3. Loos BG. Systemic effects of periodontitis. *Int J Dent Hyg.* 2006;4(suppl 1):34-38; discussion 50-52.

4. Marsh PD. Dental plaque as a microbial biofilm. *Caries Res.* 2004;38(3):204-211.

5. Socransky SS, Haffajee AD. Dental biofilms: difficult therapeutic targets. *Periodontol 2000.* 2002;28:12-55.

6. Hojo K, Nagaoka S, Ohshima T, Maeda N. Bacterial interactions in dental biofilm development. *J Dent Res.* 2009;88(11):982-990. doi:10.1177/0022034509346811.

7. Kanwar IL, Sah AK, Suresh PK. Biofilm-mediated antibiotic-resistant oral bacterial infections: mechanism and combat strategies. *Curr Pharm Des.* 2017;23(14):2084-2095.

8. van Steenbergen TJ, van Winkelhoff AJ, de Graaff J. Pathogenic synergy: mixed infections in the oral cavity. *Antonie Van Leeuwenhoek.* 1984;50(5-6):789-798.

9. Hua X, Cook GS, Costerton JW, et al. Intergeneric communication in dental plaque biofilms. *J Bacteriol.* 2000;182:7067-7069.

10. Serra e Silva Filho W, Casarin RC, Nicolela EL Jr, Passos HM, Sallum AW, Gonçalves RB: Microbial diversity similarities in periodontal pockets and atheromatous plaques of cardiovascular disease patients. *PLoS One.* 2014;9(10):e109761. doi:10.1371/journal. pone.0109761. eCollection 2014.

11. Párkányi L, Vályi P, Nagy K, Fráter M. Odontogenic foci and systemic diseases. A review. *Orv Hetil.* 2018;159(11):415-422. doi:10.1556/650.2018.31008.

12. National Diabetes Statistics Report, 2014. Centers for Disease Control and Prevention website. www.cdc.gov/diabetes/pubs/statsreport14/national-diabetes-report-web.pdf.

13. Kim EK, Lee SG, Choi YH, et al. Association between diabetes-related factors and clinical periodontal parameters in type-2 diabetes mellitus. *BMC Oral Health.* 2013;13:64. doi:10.1186/1472-6831-13-64.

14. Stanko P, Izakovicova Holla L. Bidirectional association between diabetes mellitus and inflammatory periodontal disease. A review. *Biomed Pap Med Fac Univ Palacky Olomouc Czech Repub.* 2014;158(1):35-38. doi:10.5507/bp.2014.005. Epub 2014 January 27.

15. Taylor GW, Burt BA, Becker MP, et al. Severe periodontitis and risk for poor glycemic control in patients with non-insulin-dependent diabetes mellitus. *J Periodontol.* 1996;67(10 suppl):1085-1093.

16. Rosenblum R Jr. Oral hygiene can reduce the incidence of and death resulting from pneumonia and respiratory tract infection. *J Am Dent Assoc.* 2010;141(9):1117-1118.

17. Scannapieco FA, Bush RB, Paju S. Associations between periodontal disease and risk for nosocomial bacterial pneumonia and chronic obstructive pulmonary disease. A systematic review. *Ann Periodontol.* 2003;8(1):54-69.

18. Sjögren P, Nilsson E, Forsell M, et al. A systemic review of the preventive effect of oral hygiene on pneumonia and respiratory tract infection in elderly people in hospitals and nursing homes: effect estimates and methodological quality of randomized controlled trials. *J Am Geriatr Soc.* 2008;56(11):2124-2130.

19. Pires CW, Fraga S, Beck AC, Braun KO, Peres PE. Chemical methods for cleaning conventional dentures: what is the best antimicrobial option? An in vitro study. *Oral Health Prev Dent.* 2017;15(1):73-77. doi:10.3290/j.ohpd.a37716.

20. https://www.perio.org/consumer/erectile_dysfunction.

21. Seymour RA. Is oral health a risk for malignant disease? *Dent Update.* 2010;37(5):279-280, 282-3.

22. Joshi N, Bissada NF, Bodner D, et al. Association between periodontal disease and prostate specific antigen levels in chronic prostatitis patients. *J Periodontol.* 2010;81(6):864-869. doi:10.1902/jop.2010.090646.

23. Han YW, Wang X. Mobile microbiome: oral bacteria in extra-oral infections and inflammation. *J Dent Res.* 2013;92(6):485-491. doi:10.1177/0022034513487559. Epub 2013 April 26.

24. Han YW. Fusobacterium nucleatum: a commensal-turned pathogen. *Curr Opin Microbiol.* 2015;23:141-147. doi:10.1016/j.mib.2014.11.013. Epub 2015 January 8.

25. Colucci F. An oral commensal associates with disease: chicken, egg, or red herring? *Immunity.* 2015;42(2):208-210. doi:10.1016/j.immuni.2015.01.024.

26. Leung A, Tsoi H, Yu J. Fusobacterium and Escherichia: models of colorectal cancer driven by microbiota and the utility of microbiota incolorectal cancer screening. *Expert Rev Gastroenterol Hepatol.* 2015;9(5):651-657. doi:10.1586/17474124.2015.1001745. Epub 2015 January 12.

27. Periodontal Disease and Pancreatic Cancer. Published online January 19, 2007. Available at www.medicalnewstoday.com.

28. Michaud DS. Role of bacterial infections in pancreatic cancer. *Carcinogenesis.* 2013;34(10):2193-2197. doi:10.1093/carcin/bgt249. Epub 2013 July 10.

29. Silva de Araujo Figueiredo C, Gonçalves Carvalho Rosalem C, Costa Cantanhede AL, et al. Systemic alterations and their oral manifestations in pregnant women. *J Obstet Gynaecol Res.* 2017;43(1):16-22. doi:10.1111/jog.13150.

30. Lux J, Lavigne S. Your mouth – portal to your body. *Probe.* 2004;38(4):155-171.

31. Herzberg MC, Weyer MW. Dental plaque, platelets, and cardiovascular diseases. *Ann Periodontol.* 1998;3(1):151-160.

32. Scannapieco FA. Position paper of The American Academy of Periodontology: periodontal disease as a potential risk factor for systemic diseases. *J Periodontol.* 1998;69(7):841-850.

33. Syrjänen J. Vascular diseases and oral infections. *J Clin Periodontol.* 1990;17(7 pt 2):497-500.

34. Valtonen VV. Infection as a risk factor for infarction and atherosclerosis. *Ann Med.* 1991;23(5):539-543.

35. Nomura R, Otsugu M, Naka S, et al. Contribution of the interaction of Streptococcus mutans serotype k strains with fibrinogen to the pathogenicity of infective endocarditis. *Infect Immun.* 2014;82(12):5223-5234.

36. Haraszthy VI, Zambon JJ, Trevisan M, et al. Identification of pathogens in atheromatous plaques [abstract 273]. *Dent Res.* 1998;77(special issue B):666.

37. Deshpande RG, Khan MB, Genco CA. Invasion of aortic and heart endothelial cells by Porphyromonas gingivalis. *Infect Immun.* 1998;66(11):5337-5343.

38. Dhadse P, Gattani D, Mishra R. The link between periodontal disease and cardiovascular disease: how far we have come in last two decades? *J Indian Soc Periodontol.* 2010;14(3):148-154. doi:10.4103/0972-124X.75908 PMCID: PMC3100856.

39. Persson GR, Imfeld T. Periodontitis and cardiovascular disease. *Ther Umsch.* 2008;65(2):121-126.

40. Desvarieux M, Demmer RT, Rundek T, et al. Periodontal microbiota and carotid intima-media thickness: the Oral Infections and Vascular Disease Epidemiology Study (INVEST). *Circulation.* 2005;111(5):576-582.

41. Loesche WJ, Schork A, Terpenning MS, et al. The relationship between dental disease and cerebral vascular accident in elderly United States veterans. *Ann Periodontol.* 1998;3(1):161-174.

42. Wu T, Trevisan M, Genco RJ, Falkner KL, Dorn JP, Sempos CT. Examination of the relation between periodontal health status and cardiovascular risk factors: serum total and high density lipoprotein cholesterol, C-reactive protein, and plasma fibrinogen. *Am J Epidemiol.* 2000;151(3):273-282.

43. Libby P, Ridker PM, Hansson GK: Inflammation in atherosclerosis: from pathophysiology to practice. *J Am Coll Cardiol.* 2009;54(23):2129-2138. doi:10.1016/j.jacc.2009.09.009

44. Schenkein HA, Loos BG. Inflammatory mechanisms linking periodontal diseases to cardiovascular diseases. *J Periodontol.* 2013;84(4 suppl):S51-S69. doi:10.1902/jop.2013.134006.

45. Cybulsky MI, Jongstra-Bilen J. Resident intimal dendritic cells and the initiation of atherosclerosis. *Curr Opin Lipidol.* 2010;21(5):397-403. doi:10.1097/MOL.0b013e32833ded96.

46. Imanishi T, Akasaka T. Biomarkers associated with vulnerable atheromatous plaque. *Curr Med Chem.* 2012;19(16):2588-2596.

47. Bale B, Doneen A, Vigerust D. High-risk periodontal pathogens contribute to the pathogenesis of atherosclerosis. *Postgrad Med J.* 2016;0:1-6.

48. Kozarov EV, Dorn BR, Shelburne CE, Dunn WA Jr, Progulske-Fox A. Human atherosclerotic plaque contains viable invasive Actinobacillus actinomycetemcomitans and Porphyromonas gingivalis. *Arterioscler Thromb Vasc Biol.* 2005;25(3):e17-e18. Epub 2005 January 20.

49. Socransky SS, Haffajee AD. The bacterial etiology of destructive periodontal disease: current concepts. *J Periodontol.* 1992;63(suppl 4):322-331.

50. Lu H, Xu M, Wang F, Liu S, Gu J, Lin S. Chronic stress enhances progression of periodontitis via α1-adrenergic signaling: a potential target for periodontal disease therapy. *Exp Mol Med.* 2014;46:e118. doi:10.1038/emm.2014.65.

51. Ferreira SB Jr, Trombone AP, Repeke CE, et al. An interleukin-1beta (IL-1beta) single-nucleotide polymorphism at position 3954 and red complex periodontopathogens independently and additively modulate the levels of IL-1beta in diseased periodontal tissues. *Infect Immun.* 2008;76:3725-3734.

52. Socransky SS, Haffajee AD, Smith C, et al. Microbiological parameters associated with IL-1 gene polymorphisms in periodontitis patients. *J Clin Periodontol.* 2000;27:810-818,

53. Havemose-Poulsen A, Sørensen LK, Bendtzen K, et al. Polymorphisms within the IL-1 gene cluster: effects on cytokine profiles in peripheral blood and whole blood cell cultures of patients with aggressive periodontitis, juvenile idiopathic arthritis, and rheumatoid arthritis. *J Periodontol.* 2007;78:475-492.

54. Caffesse RG, de la Rosa MR, de la Rosa MG. Interleukin-1 gene polymorphism in a well-maintained periodontal patient population. *Braz J Oral Sci.* 2002;1:1-6.

55. Laine ML, Leonhardt A, Roos-Jansåker AM, et al. IL-1RN gene polymorphism is associated with periimplantitis. *Clin Oral Implants Res.* 2006;17:380-385.

56. Nabors TW, McGlennen RC, Thompson D. Salivary testing for periodontal disease diagnosis and treatment. *Dent Today.* 2010;29(6):53-54, 56, 58-60; quiz 61.

57. Lang NP, Tonetti MS. Periodontal risk assessment (PRA) for patients in supportive periodontal therapy (SPT). *Oral Health Prev Dent.* 2003;1:7-16.

58. Bartold PM, Van Dyke TE. Host modulation: controlling the inflammation to control the infection. *Periodontol 2000.* 2017;75(1):317-329. doi:10.1111/prd.12169.

59. Novak MJ, Dawson DR III, Magnusson I, et al. Combining host modulation and topical antimicrobial therapy in the management of moderate to severe periodontitis: a randomized multicenter trial. *J Periodontol.* 2008;79(1):33-41. doi:10.1902/jop.2008.070237.

60. Gokhale SR, Padhye AM. Future prospects of systemic host modulatory agents in periodontal therapy. *Br Dent J.* 2013;214:467-471.

61. Di Paola R, Mazzon E, Muià C, et al. Effects of etanercept, a tumour necrosis factor-alpha antagonist, in an experimental model of periodontitis in rats. *Br J Pharmacol.* 2007;150:286-297.

62. Han JY, Reynolds MA. Effect of anti-rheumatic agents on periodontal parameters and biomarkers of inflammation: a systematic review and meta-analysis. *J Periodontal Implant Sci.* 2012;42:3-12.

63. Chee B, Park B, Fitzsimmons T, Coates AM, Bartold PM. Omega-3 fatty acids as an adjunct for periodontal therapy – a review. *Clin Oral Investig.* 2016;20:879-894.

64. El-Sharkawy H, Aboelsaad N, Eliwa M, et al. Adjunctive treatment of chronic periodontitis with daily dietary supplementation with omega-3 fatty acids and low-doseaspirin. *J Periodontol.* 2010;81:1635-1643.

65. Elkhouli AM. The efficacy of host response modulation therapy (omega-3 plus low-dose aspirin) as an adjunctive treatment of chronic periodontitis (clinical and biochemical study). *J Periodontal Res.* 2011;46:261-268.

66. Naqvi AZ, Hasturk H, Mu L, et al. Docosahexaenoic acid and periodontitis in adults: a randomized controlled trial. *J Dent Res.* 2014;93:767-773.

67. Serhan CN, Chiang N, Van Dyke TE. Resolving inflammation: dual anti-inflammatory and pro-resolution lipid mediators. *Nat Rev Immunol.* 2008;8:349-361.

68. Hasturk H, Kantarci A, Goguet-Surmenian E, et al. Resolvin E1 regulates inflammation at the cellular and tissue level and restores tissue homeostasis in vivo. *J Immunol.* 2007;179:7021-7029.

69. Teles FR, Teles RP, Sachdeo A. Comparison of microbial changes in early redeveloping biofilms on natural teeth and dentures. *J Periodontol.* 2012;83(9):1139-1148. doi:10.1902/jop.2012.110506. Epub 2012 March 23.

70. Teles FR, Teles RP, Uzel NG, et al. Early microbial succession in redeveloping dental biofilms in periodontal health and disease. *J Periodontal Res.* 2012;47(1):95-104. doi:10.1111/j.1600-0765.2011.01409.x. Epub 2011 September 5.

71. Kouidhi B, Al Qurashi YM, Chaieb K. Drug resistance of bacterial dental biofilm and the potential use of natural compounds as alternative for prevention and treatment. *Microb Pathog.* 2015;80:39-49. doi:10.1016/j.micpath.2015.02.007. Epub 2015 February 21.

72. Rams TE, Degener JE, van Winkelhoff AJ. Antibiotic resistance in human chronic periodontitis microbiota. *J Periodontol.* 2014;85(1):160-169. doi:10.1902/jop.2013.130142. Epub 2013 May 20.

73. Rams TE, Degener JE, van Winkelhoff AJ. Antibiotic resistance in human peri-implantitis microbiota. *Clin Oral Implants Res.* 2014;25(1):82-90. doi:10.1111/clr.12160. Epub 2013 April 2.

74. Shen Y, Stojicic S, Haapasalo M. Antimicrobial efficacy of chlorhexidine against bacteria in biofilms at different stages of development. *J Endod.* 2011;37(5):657-661. doi:10.1016/j.joen.2011.02.007. Epub 2011 March 23.

75. Guggenheim B, Meier A. In vitro effect of chlorhexidine mouth rinses on polyspecies biofilms. *Schweiz Monatsschr Zahnmed.* 2011;121(5):432-441.

76. Addy M, Moran JM. Clinical indications for the use of chemical adjuncts to plaque control: chlorhexidine formulations. *Periodontol 2000.* 1997;15:52-54.

77. Jones CG. Chlorhexidine: is it still the gold standard? *Periodontol 2000.* 1997;15:55-62.

78. Bruch MK. Toxicity and safety of topical sodium hypochlorite. *Contrib Nephrol.* 2007;154:24-38.

79. Zehnder M. Root canal irrigants. *J Endod.* 2006;32:389-398.

80. Gosau M, Hahnel S, Schwarz F, Gerlach T, Reichert TE, Burgers R. Effect of six different peri-implantitis disinfection methods on in vivo human oral biofilm. *Clin Oral Implants Res.* 2010;21:866-872.

81. Sarbinoff JA, O_Leary TJ, Miller CH. The comparative effectiveness of various agents in detoxifying diseased root surfaces. *J Periodontol.* 1983;54:77-80.

82. Spratt DA, Pratten J, Wilson M, Gulabivala K. An in vitro evaluation of the antimicrobial efficacy of irrigants on biofilms of root canal isolates. *Int Endod J.* 2001;34:300-307.

83. De Nardo R, Chiappe V, Go´mez M, Romanelli H, Slots J. Effect of 0.05% sodium hypochlorite oral rinse on supragingival biofilm and gingival inflammation. *Int Dent J.* 2012;62:208-212.

84. Lobene RR, Soparkar PM, Hein JW, Quigley GA. A study of the effects of antiseptic agents and a pulsating irrigating device on plaque and gingivitis. *J Periodontol.* 1972;43:564-568.

85. Zou L, Shen Y, Li W, Haapasalo M. Penetration of sodium hypochlorite into dentin. *J Endod.* 2010;36:793-796.

86. Kalkwarf KL, Tussing GJ, Davis MJ. Histologic evaluation of gingival curettage facilitated by sodium hypochlorite solution. *J Periodontol.* 1982;53:63-70.

87. Slots J. Low-cost periodontal therapy. *Periodontol 2000.* 2012;60(1):110-137. doi:10.1111/j.1600-0757.2011.00429.x.

88. Rutala WA, Cole EC, Thomann CA, Weber DJ. Stability and bactericidal activity of chlorine solutions. *Infect Control Hosp Epidemiol.* 1998;19:323-327.

89. Marshall MV, Cancro LP, Fischman SL. Hydrogen peroxide: a review of its use in dentistry. *J Periodontol.* 1995;66(9):786-796.

90. Lekstrom-Himes JA, Kuhns DB, Alvord WG, Gallin JI. Inhibition of human neutrophil IL-8 production by hydrogen peroxide and dysregulation in chronic granulomatous disease. *J Immunol.* 2005;174(1):411-417.

91. Schreml S, Szeimies RM, Prantl L, et al. Oxygen in acute and chronic wound healing. *Br J Dermatol.* 2010;163(2):257-268. doi:10.1111/j.1365-2133.2010.09804.x. Epub 2010 April 15.

92. Phillips J. The Wound Care Institute, Inc. for the Advancement of Wound Healing & Diabetic Footcare. *Wound Care Institute Newsletter.* Fall 1996.

93. Tomono S, Miyoshi N, Sato K, et al. Formation of cholesterol ozonolysis products through an ozone-free mechanism mediated by themyeloperoxidase-H2O2-chloride system. *Biochem Biophys Res Commun.* 2009;383(2):222-227. doi:10.1016/j.bbrc.2009.03.155. Epub 2009 April 5.

94. Gupta G, Mansi B. Ozone therapy in periodontics. *J Med Life.* 2012;5(1):59-67. Epub 2012 March 5.

95. Dunlap T, Keller DC, Marshall MV, et al. Subgingival delivery of oral debriding agents: a proof of concept. *J Clin Dent.* 2011;22:149-158.

96. Schaudinn C, et al. Manipulation of the microbial ecology of the periodontal pocket. *World Dental.* 2010;2(1):14-18.

97. Bale B, Doneen A, Collier L. *Beat the Heart Attack Gene: The Revolutionary Plan to Prevent Heart Disease, Stroke, and Diabetes.* New York, NY: Wiley Gen. Trade, Turner Publishing: 2014;135-137.

98. Doneen AL, Bale BF. The BaleDoneen Method (BDM): a disease-inflammation approach to achieve arterial wellness. *Cranio.* 2018;36(4):209-210. doi:10.1080/08869634.2018.1479491.

99. Feng D, Esperat MC, Doneen AL, Bale B, Song H, Green AE. Eight-year outcomes of a program for early prevention of cardiovascular events: a growth-curve analysis. *J Cardiovasc Nurs.* 2015;30(4):281-291. doi:10. 1097/jcn.0000000000000141.

100. Preshaw PM. Host modulation therapy with anti-inflammatory agents. *Periodontol 2000.* 2018;76(1):131-149. doi:10.1111/prd.12148. Epub 2017 November 29.

101. Salvi GE, Lang NP. Host response modulation in the management of periodontal diseases. *J Clin Periodontol.* 2005;32(suppl 6):108-129.

102. Shinwari MS, Tanwir F, Hyder PR, Bin Saeed MH. Host modulation therapeutics in periodontics: role as an adjunctive periodontal therapy. *J Coll Physicians Surg Pak.* 2014;24(9):676-684. doi:08.2014/JCPSP.676684.

103. Parkhill JM, Hennig BJ, Chapple IL, et al. Association of interleukin-1 gene polymorphisms with early-onset periodontitis. *J Clin Periodontol.* 2000;27:682-689.

104. Harrison JE, Schultz J. Studies on the chlorinating activity of myeloperoxidase. *J Biol Chem.* 1976;251:1371-1374.

29

Obesity, Adipokines, Inflammation, and Cardiovascular Disease

Joseph J. Lamb, MD

Introduction

As noted by Hotamisligil,[1] the interactions between immune and metabolic pathways are highly ordered, evolutionary conserved, and are important for tissue and organism health. When this balance is disrupted by maladaptive gene-environment interactions, the result is the development of chronic noncommunicable diseases associated with inflammation and aging including obesity, diabetes, and cardiovascular disease. Complex signaling pathways play an integral role in mediating the interactions between systems designed to provide the best response to physiologic stresses due to environmental change, to provide the balance of nutrient intake both at a micronutrient and macronutrient and informational level, and finally to initiate the complex orchestration of inflammatory responses that lead to the most adaptive response to these environmental challenges.

A significant body of research demonstrates that nutrients and metabolites modulate the inflammatory pathways, the stress pathways, and the energy regulation pathways, resulting in either desired optimal health or the progression to the chronic noncommunicable diseases of aging. An excellent review by Saltiel and Olefsky[2] supports the hypothesis that inflammation is an early response activated during adipose expansion and during the development of chronic obesity. These changes lead to an activation of the immune system and a shift to a pro-inflammatory phenotype. This pro-inflammatory phenotype is not limited to the activation of the innate adaptive immune systems but instead is hallmarked by inflammatory changes within many organ systems including the pancreas, the brain, liver, gut, and muscle. Excessive nutrient intake associated with an overall positive energy balance leads to the accumulation of excessive fat and adipocytes both in the subcutaneous and visceral spaces. The initiation of an inflammatory response is a beneficial physiologic response to the stresses that obesity places on adipocytes. However, long-term activation is maladaptive in the long term.[3] As noted by Scherer et al.,[4] adipocytes to be successful in their role as the major energy storing tissue in the body require an almost unlimited capacity to expand. Thus, adipocytes require the ability to remodel acutely and chronically. This remodeling can be challenged because of the overexpansion of adipocytes and the limit of oxygen due to the failure to develop adequate vascular supply. In this setting, hypoxia becomes an early determinate of the health of the expanding adipose tissue.

Inflammation is characterized by the deterioration of metabolic health that is clearly detrimental to longevity. Caloric excess disrupts healthy metabolic pathways and accelerates aging, while conversely calorie restriction has been associated with restoration of normal function, prevention of chronic diseases, and maintenance of longevity. Using a genetic mouse model lacking FABP4/5 that confers protection against metabolic diseases, Charles et al.[5] demonstrated that FABP4-deficient mice exhibited preserved insulin sensitivity resulting in reduced inflammation, maintenance of adipose tissue integrity, and prevention of fatty liver disease. These mice, however, did not gain an extension of life span. The authors conclude that a complex interplay of environmental signals, divergent metabolic pathways, and functional and dysfunctional physiologic responses dictate the overall response of the organism to its environment.

Obesity and the Link to Inflammation and Cardiovascular Disease

A comparison of the anatomical changes during the evolution from a common fruit fly to the anatomy of a mammal over 600 million years demonstrates the development of unique organ systems replacing what is in the fruit fly, a non-specialized fat body. This fat body is a vascularly supplied collection of the adipocytes, metabolically active cells, and immune cells that would eventually specialize into specialized adipose stores, the metabolically active organs (liver and pancreas), and the innate and adaptive immune systems.[6] A consequence of this shared evolutionary origin for these cell types is the conservation of paracrine (cell to cell transmission) signals (adipokines, cytokines, hormones) into autocrine hormonal signaling and inflammatory signaling (organ to organ signaling at a distance dependent on the neuroendocrine systems). These shared signaling pathways reflect an evolutionary integration of regulatory pathways governing the body's responses to pathogens and nutrition. Zhang et al.[7] postulate that the hypothalamus developed the unique ability to respond to the environment through inflammatory signaling. This pro-inflammatory response which for our ancestors was adaptive and typically activated by pathogenic exposures is now quite detrimental in the setting of repeated responses to nutrient excess provided by our diet of convenience and conspicuous consumption. Toll-like receptors (TLRs) share an important function in this signaling. TLR4-deficient mice were noted to have aggravated fasting hypoglycemia. Overstimulation of TLR4 has been associated with the development of insulin resistance. Pang[8] suggests that TLR4 is thus critical for the maintenance of glucose and lipid metabolism independent of insulin signaling. Although TLR4 is classically recognized as the receptor for lipopolysaccharides, Shi et al.[9] have demonstrated that the obesity-associated increase in nutritional fatty acid levels activate TLR4 signaling and adipocytes and macrophages, resulting in the induction of inflammatory signaling. They demonstrate that mice lacking TLR4 do not develop impaired insulin signaling in muscle or the development of insulin resistance with the infusion of systemic lipids.

Howitz and Sinclair[10] note that the pathways linking inflammation, energy utilization, and stress responses are driven by a collection of signaling molecules and kinases, with AMP kinase playing an important role in the center of the pathway, pro-inflammatory signaling influencing MTOR production, and PGC1α being the link between energy utilization and stress responses. Although the signals and mediators responsible for our autonomic responsiveness (the fight-or-flight response and the Tend-and-Befriend response), and the counterregulatory hormones necessary to maintain homeostasis of glucose and other energy-producing molecules are well understood, the regulation of energy utilization and storage in adipocytes is less well defined. It is clear, however, that adipose tissue, specifically the metabolically active visceral adipose tissue, is a central mediator of paracrine and autocrine signaling.

Prentice et al.[11] note that fatty acid binding protein 4 (FABP4) functions in maintaining glucose homeostasis and is a key regulatory node facilitating communication in life's threatening situations between energy storage systems and distant organs. However, chronic engagement of FABP4 in settings such as obesity or nutrient excess aggravates the chronic noncommunicable diseases of aging including diabetes, asthma, cancer, and atherosclerosis.

The benefits of fasting and calorie restriction have been well documented in yeast, round worms, and several mammalian models. The longevity associated with calorie restriction is mediated through sirtuin regulation.[12] It has been demonstrated that calorie restriction and resulting physiologic changes are associated with activation of cellular stress response elements, improved autophagy, modification of apoptosis, and alteration in hormonal signaling.[12] Sirtuin enzymes, specifically the seven mammalian ones (SIRT1-7), are integral to self-survival, in essence, as key regulators of metabolism and genomic stability.[13] SIRT 1 and SIRT 6 signaling has been implicated in the balance between insulin sensitivity and resistance, resulting in the development of type 2 diabetes, fatty liver disease, and cardiovascular disease. Sirtuins regulate the production of energy matching output from resources to demands. SIRT 1 enhances fat metabolism and modulates mitochondrial respiration to optimize energy harvesting. The AMP kinase/SIRT1/PGC1α-PPAR axis and mitochondrial sirtuins are pivotal to maintaining healthy mitochondrial function. Downregulation of sirtuins with aging may explain much of the pathophysiology that is generally associated with aging.[14] The nuclear sirtuins (SIRT 1, 2, 6, and 7) are all intimately associated with the regulation of inflammatory signaling pathways and play a role to reduce pro-inflammatory signaling.[15]

Adipose tissue with its complex interplay of hormonal and adipocytokine signaling plays a significant role in hormonal regulation of metabolic homeostasis. This regulatory function of the adipose tissue depends on its ability to secrete a large number of hormones, cytokines, extracellular matrix proteins, and growth factors influencing local and systemic metabolism. Barchetta et al.[16] note that in conditions of nutrient excess leading to chronic positive energy balance, the expansion of adipose tissue with resultant hypoxia, apoptosis, and inflammatory changes leads to dysfunction and subsequent delivery of paracrine and autocrine alarm messages, resulting in metabolic derangements. Thus, this nutrient excess, with its resultant mismatch between environmental supply of energy and the requirements of cellular homeostasis, dysregulates appropriate physiologic function of adipose tissue with the subsequent development of signaling incongruent with optimal health. This dysfunction creates a milieu of angry sick fat exacerbated by the presence of lipopolysaccharide in the visceral adipose tissue that is bathed in enterohepatic circulation of the portal system. Visceral adipose tissue is thought to be more metabolically sensitive and active than subcutaneous adipose tissue.

The distinction between visceral and subcutaneous adipose tissue is not the only macroscopically observed difference between adipose tissues. White adipose tissue (WAT) can be differentiated from brown adipose tissue (BAT) on a macroscopic and microscopic level because of the presence of an enriched mitochondrial population in BAT. WAT's primary function is to accumulate surplus energy (predominately in the form of triglycerides), whereas BAT dissipates energy directly as heat and plays critical functions in the maintenance of temperature homeostasis.

Subcutaneous and visceral adipocytes have different progenitor cells with resultant differences in gene expression patterns. Thus, subcutaneous WAT is more responsive to the antilipolytic effects of insulin. It actually secretes more adiponectin and fewer inflammatory cytokines.[17] BAT plays a critical role in the ability of hibernating mammals to sustain their physiologies throughout the winter months and to maintain their temperature regulation. BAT's thermoregulatory properties provide a resource for infants with their high body surface area to mass ratios requiring energy support. Medina Gomez[18] has suggested that strategies targeting adipocyte mitochondrial function in WAT and BAT may play a critical role in the development of therapies fighting obesity and its complications in the near future.[19] Another critical function of sirtuins is the ability of SIRT 5 to influence brown adipocyte differentiation with the results of browning of WAT resulting in what may be regarded as beige adipose tissue as the WAT gains some of the responsiveness of BAT to appropriate environmental signaling.

This browning of adipose tissue requires an adaptive increase in proteasomal activity resulting in responsiveness to nutrient excess and xenohormetic messages such as fasting and cold exposures. Bartelt et al.[20] demonstrated that cold adaptation induces Nrf1 in BAT and is thus crucial for maintaining endoplasmic reticulum (ER) homeostasis and integrity. In a mouse model, deletion of Nrf1 in thermogenic conditions resulted in ER stress, tissue inflammation, decreased mitochondrial functioning, and whitening of BAT.

Obesity and diabetes are certainly the consequences of disordered regulatory signaling in metabolically sensitive tissue. These metabolically sensitive tissues are certainly not limited to white and brown adipose tissues, including hepatocytes, pancreatic beta cells, and myocytes, and also including our immune signaling and our neuro tissues as our previous discussion has suggested. Corkey et al.[21] suggest that our redux metabolome coordinates tissue responses by virtue of a circulating communication system. Branched chain amino acids, lactate, and free fatty acids all generate increases in mitochondrial NADH through their metabolism, influencing the oxidative reductive balance. A possible circulating master metabolic regulator, recognizing the balance between lactate and pyruvate, between beta-hydroxybutyrate and acetoacetate, between reduced and oxidized thiocytosine and the presence of reductive reactive oxygen species, coordinates signaling between the gut and the brain in terms of hunger and satiety, the balance in the liver between glycogen storage and glucose release, the balance in the adipocyte between lipolysis and lipogenesis, and the balance between insulin and glucagon secretion in pancreatic beta cells.

Interestingly, the balance between these oxidative and reductive compounds is maintained through mitochondrial function. Wallace[22] in 2010 notes that "mitochondrial mutations provide heritable and stable adaptation to regional differences while mitochondrially-mediated changes in the epigenome (Nuclear DNA) permit reversible modulation of gene expression in response to fluctuations in the energy environment." Thus, the balance in oxidative reductive

reserves not only dictate the immediate short-term responsiveness but also influence the long-term responsiveness of the system allowing for transgenerational and regional adaptations to changing environmental stimuli.

Lee et al.[23] report that an early change during the consumption of a high-fat diet is the uncoupling of adipocyte respiration, leading to increased oxygen consumption in a state of relative adipocyte hypoxia. Adipose hypoxia defined as a relative oxygen deficiency is a potential contributor to adipose tissue dysfunction. Each 5 pounds of adipose tissue has a vascular supply of approximately one additional mile of capillaries, arterials, and venules, resulting in a vascular bed with increased systemic resistance and consequences for a systemic hypertension and vascular dysfunction. Lempesis[24] suggests that alternations in adipose tissue oxygenation directly impact metabolic homeostasis resulting in adipocyte hypertrophy, impaired adipokine secretion, chronic inflammatory changes, and the development of insulin resistance.

Clearly in our Westernized world, there has been a significant change in the diseases that contribute most dramatically to morbidity and mortality. The burden of infectious diseases has responded to improved hygiene and the development of effective antibiotics. However, for those living in Westernized countries who could be considered to be participating the largest dietary study ever initiated, specifically the industrialization of the diet, resulting in excessive consumption of fat, cholesterol, proteins, carbohydrates, specifically refined sugar and salts as a consequence of the frequent consumption of processed and fast foods and decreased consumption of phytonutrients and fiber, the dietary pattern has created an environment where metabolic, cardiovascular, and autoimmune diseases are almost epidemic.

T cell regulation links the dietary influences of a Western diet to the development of autoimmune pathology and the possible promotion of the chronic noncommunicable diseases of aging.[25] It is well recognized that inflammation is linked with the development of nonalcoholic fatty liver disease, diabetes, and endothelial dysfunction, resulting in coronary artery disease and immune dysregulation. Similar patterns of dysfunction are noted beyond the cardiovascular system. An additional consequence of these inflammatory changes is the increased permeability of the blood-brain barrier. Chronic systemic inflammation induced by obesity and type 2 diabetes promotes the blood-brain barrier breakdown with decreased removal of wastes and increased infiltration of immune cells. These changes result in the development of a pro-inflammatory pattern which has been characterized as a brain on fire with a resultant development of neuroinflammation and its connection to Alzheimer's disease and multiple sclerosis.[26] Similarly, Wang et al.[27] have documented the cross talk between osteoarthritis and obesity resulting in increases in pro-inflammatory adipokines and cytokines driving the localized and systemic pro-inflammatory condition.

For quite some time, the cholesterol hypothesis has been predominant in our understanding of the pathophysiology of coronary artery disease, and certainly the continued profound primacy of the HMG-CoA reductase inhibitors (statins) as one of the most frequently prescribed pharmaceutical agents would suggest that the association of inflammation with both coronary artery disease, obesity, and the chronic noncommunicable diseases of aging has not yet been recognized. Statins obviously possess anti-inflammatory properties, but they are recognized by the public and many prescribers as primarily cholesterol-lowering agents. Ridker et al.[28] demonstrated in 2007 that LDL reduction not associated with the reduction in inflammation as marked by a reduction in HSCRP would not be associated with a reduction in cardiovascular risk. They demonstrated in the Jupiter trial that apparently healthy persons without hyperlipidemia but with HSCRP protein levels noted a significant reduction in the incidence of major cardiovascular event with rosuvastatin treatment. Winer and Winer[29] have noted that chronic inflammation of visceral adipose tissue has gained acceptance as one of our lead promoters of insulin resistance in obesity. The infiltration of the adipose tissue by both B and T lymphocytes, the resultant secretion of cytokines, and macrophage modulation dictate the development of a local inflammatory response with the resultant development of insulin resistance and a systemic inflammatory pattern.[29] The unique role of the visceral adipose tissue is demonstrated by Klein et al.[30] who reported that liposuction did not significantly alter the insulin sensitivity of myocytes, hepatocytes, or adipose tissue despite the removal of 20 pounds of subcutaneous fat. Plasma concentrations of HSCRP, IL-6, tumor necrosis factor-alpha (TNF-α), and adiponectin were not altered and there was no significant impact upon other risk factors for coronary artery disease. Engin[31] notes that novel and highly active molecules are released abundantly by adipocytes including leptin, resistin, adiponectin, and visfatin as well as some of the more classical cytokines. Cytokines that are released by inflammatory cells infiltrating obese adipose tissue include TNF-α, interleukin-6 (IL-6), monocyte chemoattractant protein 1 (MCP-1), and IL-1. These molecules, acting on immune cells, lead to local and generalized inflammation. Stimulation of the TLR-4 modulation of the phosphatidylinositol-3 kinase (PI3K), of protein kinase B (Akt) signaling, of the uncoupling of the unfolded protein response due to ER stress, and finally of activation of the c-Jun N-terminal Kinase (JNK) Activator Protein 1, an inhibitor of nuclear factor kappa-B pathways, plays an important role resulting in vascular endothelial dysfunction by modulating vascular nitric oxide and super oxide release. The development of systemic oxidative stress results in macrophage recruitment, increases in the expression of NOD-like receptor family proteins (NLRP3) in the inflammasome, and adipocyte death, which are predominant determinants in the pathogenesis of obesity-associated adipose tissue inflammation. The infiltrating macrophages produce not only cytokines but also metalloproteinases, reactive oxygen species, and chemokines. These participate in tissue remodeling, cell signaling, and the regulation of immunity with the resultant influence on adjacent tissues and organs. Guzik et al.[32] note that "in blood vessels, perivascular adipose tissue and inflammation leads to vascular remodeling, super oxide production, and endothelial

dysfunction with loss of nitric oxide bioavailability contributing to the development of vascular disease, atherosclerosis and plaque instability." Erridge et al.[33] noted that the postprandial endotoxemia associated with the consumption of a Westernized diet is a potential contributor to endothelial activation and the development of atherosclerosis. Pendyala et al.[34] investigated the connection between a Western style diet and endotoxemia. The Western style diet, inclusive of approximately 100 g of fat intake per day, produced a 71% increase in plasma endotoxin levels, while a prudent style diet reduced the levels by 31%. Cani et al.[35] demonstrated that metabolic endotoxemia initiates obesity and insulin resistance. In a fascinating study, mice were fed a high-fat diet compared with the standard chow diet with the subsequent development of obesity. Endotoxin levels were measured in the mice receiving the high-fat diet compared with a standard chow diet. A second experimental group received an infusion of endotoxin while consuming a standard chow diet. The group receiving endotoxin and the lower caloric diet had metabolic changes resulting in the development of obesity and a pattern similar to the mice fed the high-fat diet. Mehta et al.[36] demonstrated that an infusion of endotoxin in humans produced insulin resistance and activation of the innate adaptive immune systems. Interestingly, the development of acute inflammation and adipose tissue changes were noted in the subcutaneous adipose tissue and not restricted to the visceral adipose tissue. The consequences of excessive nutrient intake (both dietary fats and refined carbohydrates), the increase in lipopolysaccharide absorption and increased environmental toxicities, result in a pattern of physiologic changes of which early signs are fatty acid infiltration in the liver, beta cell apoptosis and dysfunction, and the expansion of visceral adiposity. The early physiologic changes contemporaneous with the development of visceral tissue expansion suggest that obesity is not an etiologic determinant of type 2 diabetes, atherosclerosis, Alzheimer's/dementia and the other chronic noncommunicable diseases of aging but is instead an early sign and symptom of the disordered pathophysiologies associated with our patterns of Western living.

Hormonal Signaling in Obesity: Regulation of Feeding and Satiety

A broad range of neurotransmitters and hormones influence feeding and satiety in the hypothalamus, resulting in the control of nutrient balance. A partial list of those hormones that decrease feeding (anorexigenic) include leptin, serotonin, norepinephrine (NE), cortisol-releasing hormone (CRH), insulin, CCK, peptide YY. A similar list of hormones that increase feeding (orexigenic) include neuropeptide Y (NPY), orexins A and B, endorphins, amino acids (glutamate and γ-aminobutyric acid), cortisol, ghrelin, endocannabinoids, agouti-related protein (AGRP).[37] These hormones act upon two distinct types of neurons in the hypothalamus. The proopiomelanocortin neurons (POMC) upon anorexigenic activation decrease food intake and increase energy expenditure.

NPY/AGRP neurons upon orexigenic activation increase food intake and decrease energy expenditures. POMC neurons secrete α-melanocyte-stimulating hormones (MSH), and defective signaling is associated with the extreme obesity. Mutations of the melanocortin receptors specifically MCR-4 is possibly the most commonly known monogenic cause of human obesity accounting for 5% to 6% of early onset of severe obesity in children.[38,39] Oral receptors including taste receptors mediate food intake as demonstrated by experiments where patent esophageal fistulas leading to the loss of ingested food decrease feeding behaviors.[40] Orexigenic hormone signaling, including ghrelin, increased feeding. Blood ghrelin levels increase during fasting, peak just before eating, and fall rapidly after a meal. Ghrelin is secreted by the stomach. Decreases in blood glucose concentration causes hunger and increases feeding behavior. Similar changes in amino acids and free fatty acids result in the development of hunger as well. Interestingly, the stimulation of POMC neurons by synergistic insulin and leptin signaling leads to the browning of WAT. Stimulation of AGRP neurons by ghrelin, cortisol, and endocannabinoids suppresses WAT browning.[41]

Hormonal Signaling in Obesity: Insulin Signaling

It is generally accepted that the interaction of environmental signals, genetic influences, and food consumption leads to the development of increased visceral adiposity and the reduction in adiponectin levels. These changes result in the development of insulin resistance manifested by hyperlipidemia, diabetes mellitus, hypertension, and the subsequent development of atherosclerosis.[42] Dr Barbara Corkey was awarded the Banting Award for excellence in diabetic research in 2011; in her Banting Lecture, she proposed that an early etiology of insulin resistance is the hyperinsulinemia, which is a consequence of the increased beta cell secretion of insulin. She identified that mono-oleoylglycerols, iron, and saccharin are all common dietary ingredients that are capable of producing this hyperinsulinemia.[43] The hypersecretion of insulin due to mitochondrial toxicity of the beta cells leads to increased circulating insulin levels and may be associated with the downregulation of insulin receptors with the consequence of the development of insulin resistance separate from the role played by glucose and lipid toxicity. It has been noted by Schauer et al.[44] that obese patients with diabetes respond differently to gastric bypass surgery versus intensive medical therapy. They noted that the use of antihypertensive, antidiabetic, and lipid modulating drugs decrease significantly after surgical treatment but increased in patients receiving medical therapies only. The homeostatic model of assessment for insulin resistance score improved significantly only in the bariatric surgery group. It is interesting to note that insulin-requiring diabetics undergoing bariatric surgery have an almost immediate reduction in the amount of insulin required during the postoperative period. Individuals who are NPO for other major abdominal surgeries, including

cholecystectomies and colectomies, do not have a reduction in their requirements for insulin. This reduction in insulin dosing takes place well before associated weight loss. This effect is seen in individuals undergoing the Roux-en-y procedure and is not seen in patients with gastric reduction or gastric sleeves. The Roux-en-y procedure results in anatomical changes that result in the food stream bypassing the duodenum and the proximal jejunum. G-protein–coupled receptor signaling is modified by the changes in the food stream present after the Roux-en-y procedure. G-coupled protein receptors and kinase signaling are closely linked with the regulation of energy utilization as well as inflammatory signaling. Stimulation of the G-coupled protein receptor 120 leads to secretion of glucagon-like peptide-1 (GLP-1). Food has a dramatic influence on GLP-1 secretion. GLP-1 increases insulin sensitivity and reduces inflammation. Lockie et al.[45] note that activation of central nervous system GLP-1 receptors and additional g-coupled protein receptors actually stimulate brown adipose activity through the sympathetic nervous system. Stimulation of g-coupled protein receptor by omega-3 fatty acids (DHA) lead to GLP-1 secretion with improved glucose stimulated insulin secretion and reductions in inflammation and insulin resistance.[46]

Traditionally, we recognize four different primary tastes that can be distinguished by the taste receptors on the tongue. These include sweet, sour, salty, and bitter. An additional taste that has been identified which is umami, a savory taste that is signaled by receptors responsive to glutamates. A sixth receptor is postulated that senses fat in foods and this receptor may be linked to the bitter taste receptors. Traditionally, bitter agents have been used for their influences upon digestion as both aperitifs and digestifs. Herbal and botanical medicine has also recognized the value of bitter plants for their effects on inflammation and metabolism. Specific bitter phytonutrients have been identified to communicate through selective kinase response modulators and L-cells in the gut to regulate inflammation and insulin signaling through GLP-1 secretion. Rozengurt and Sternini[47] note that molecular sensing by gastrointestinal cells mediated through G-coupled protein receptors results in gastrointestinal peptide release that modulate food intake, that regulate cell proliferation, and that contribute to gastric emptying, gall bladder contraction, small intestinal mobility, and afferent vagal responses.

Feeney et al.[48] noticed that genetic variation in taste perception was associated with BMI in women. Nontasters had a higher mean BMI than tasters or super tasters. Super tasters had a nutrient intake pattern indicated of healthy eating.[49]

Exposure of cultured GI endocrine cells to bitter tastes has been demonstrated to release GLP-1. A derivative of a hops iso-humulone with antidiabetic properties was found to signal through Tas2rs, stimulating GLP-1 secretion with enhanced glucose tolerance.[50] This work suggests that targeting extra oral bitter receptors may be useful in metabolic diseases. Interestingly, ovaries also express Tas2rs108 and it has been found that oral administration of the same hops isohumulone ligand resulted in the resolution of PCOS in a mouse model induced by chronic feeding with a high-fat diet.[51]

Wiener et al.[52] note that green tea catechins, soy isoflavones, caffeine, bitter melon, berberine, fenugreek, and luteolin are associated with improved insulin signaling.

It has been noted that the intestinal immune system has been implicated as an important contributor to metabolic diseases. Increased fat consumption associated with obesity predisposes to changes in intestinal immunity and gut permeability associated with endotoxic levels. These changes are associated with changes in the gut microbiota, intestinal barrier function, and modulation of the gut residing in adaptive immune cells as well as oral tolerance to luminal antigens.[53] Luck et al.[54] demonstrated that the gut immune system is altered during the consumption of a high-fat diet and is a regulator of insulin resistance. They demonstrated in a mouse model that treatment with the local gut anti-inflammatory 5-aminosalicylic acid (5-ASA) reverses bowel inflammation and improves metabolic parameters. These changes were dependent on adaptive gut immune function and were associated with reduced intestinal permeability of endotoxin.

Neurotensin is an amino acid peptide located in the neuroendocrine cells of the small intestine. Its action is to increase fat absorption and fatty acid translocation in response to lipid ingestion.

Barchetta et al.[55] investigated the relationship between plasma pro-NT levels and the presence of visceral adipose tissue inflammation in 40 obese subjects undergoing bariatric surgery. Higher pro-NT levels were significantly associated with greater macrophage infiltration.

Hormonal Signaling in Obesity: Leptin Signaling

Our bodies store energy predominately as fat, the amount of which can vary considerably between individuals. Hall notes that the regulation of this energy reserve and its variability among individuals is regulated by leptin.[56] Increasing stores of fat resulting in expansion of adipose tissue produce increased amounts of leptin. Leptin is sensed by the POMC neuron of the paraventricular nuclei. Stimulation of leptin receptors decreases fat storage through decreased production of appetite stimulators, activation of POMC neurons with secretion of alpha-melanocytes stimulating hormone, increased production of hypothalamic secreted corticotropin-releasing hormone, increased sympathetic nervous system activity, and decreased insulin secretion by pancreatic beta cells. Analogous to the pattern of insulin resistance and thyroid hormone resistance, leptin resistance can develop resulting in marked increases in appetite and the development of morbid obesity. It is believed that resistant leptin receptors or modification of postreceptor signaling pathways normally activated by leptin are active mechanisms in obese people who continue to eat despite having very high levels of leptin.[56]

Fruhwürth et al.[57] noted that several hypotheses have been proposed to explain impaired central responsiveness to the effects of leptin obesity including ineffective transport across the blood-brain barrier, hypothalamic ER stress, and

the development of neuroinflammation. They also propose a new explanation based upon a discovery of a signaling pathway identified as "NSAPP." The pathway consists of an oxide transport chain with the ability to modulate redox sensitive members of the protein tyrosine phosphatase family. It is noted that leptin and insulin signaling require the NSAPP oxide transport chain, suggesting a defect in this pathway explains the resistance to the appetite suppressing effects of insulin and leptin.

Ye et al.[58] note that obesity may be associated with the development of ER stress and that one of its stress responses (the unfolded protein response) is the mechanism associated with the development of obesity-associated leptin resistance. Boden et al.[59] note that excess nutrient intake produces as an early consequence ER stress, which is likely to be the cause for insulin resistance and inflammation.

NRF-1 ER bound transcription factor is an important mediator against cholesterol excess in the ER.[60] In NRF-1 deficiency, cholesterol challenge induces hepatic cholesterol accumulation and damage. Petremand et al.[61] demonstrated that pancreatic beta cells treated with thapsigargin, cyclopiazonic acid, palmitate, or exposed to insulin overexpression and high glucose concentrations demonstrate ER stress. They found that high-density lipoproteins (HDLs) can restore ER homeostasis promoting beta cell survival. Lee et al.[62] have demonstrated that HDL inhibits M1 macrophage polarization which would result in pro-inflammatory signaling. The protective effects of HDL in reducing inflammation as suggested by these two studies highlight the need for identifying functional versus dysfunctional HDL activity, which at present can only be inferred through measurement of myeloperoxidase.

Hormonal Signaling in Obesity: Interleukin Signaling

Ghazarian[63] notes that one of the key events in the development of adipose tissue inflammation is the switching of macrophages toward the pro-inflammatory M1 phenotype. The interleukin-1 superfamily of cytokines that consist of IL-1β, IL-18, and IL-33 are critical to the regulation of the low-grade inflammation associated with obesity and metabolic disorders. IL-1β is a well-known inflammatory mediator, while IL-18 predominately opposes metabolic dysregulation.[64] IL-18 functions in an apoptogenic fashion depending upon the presence of IL-12. It can either be a pro-inflammatory cytokine that facilitates type 1 immune responses or in the presence of IL-2 stimulates a type 2 response.[65] The NLRP family of receptors and the accompanied inflammasomes play an important role in the intracellular sensing of endogenous damage associated molecular patterns (DAMPs). These DAMPs play a key role in the induction and stimulation of chronic inflammation in type 2 diabetes through the release of interleukin-1β and IL-18.[66]

Murphy et al.[67] noted that mice lacking NLRP-1 resulting in lower IL-18 levels had spontaneous obesity because of intrinsic lipid accumulation. This was exacerbated when mice were fed either a high-fat diet or a high-protein diet but not when the mice were fed a high-fat diet with a high-fiber intake resulting in a low energy density. Mice with an activating mutation in the NLRP-1 with increased interleukin-18 production have decreased adiposity and are resistant to diet-induced obesity. Additionally, alterations in NLRP3 expression in adipose tissue are associated with the development of chronic inflammation characteristic of obesity and insulin resistance. Increased activation of NLRP3 inflammasome leads to the maturation of interleukin-1β and interleukin-18. In murine models, high-fat diets increased NLRP3 expression, whereas calorie-restricted diets decreased its expression. NLRP3 blockade in mice has protected against diet-induced obesity and insulin resistance. A SNIP associated with increased NLRP3 activity is associated with an increased risk for type 2 diabetes in Chinese populations.[68]

Ghazarian et al.[69] note that in nonalcoholic fatty liver disease activation of NLRP results in the accumulation of pathogenic CD8+ T cells subsets, which negatively influence hepatic insulin sensitivity in gluconeogenesis during diet-induced obesity in mice. Complicating our understanding of the impact of interleukins and adipokines and their activity is the tissue specificity resulting in differential responses. Several inflammatory cytokines including tumor necrosis factor-α, interleukin-6, interleukin-1β have been associated with anorexia and cachexia in the setting of cancer. This effect seems to be mediated by activation of the melanocortin system in the hypothalamus.[70]

Hormonal Signaling in Obesity: Other Cytokine and Adipokine Signaling

Böstrom et al.[71] demonstrated that PGC1-α expression in muscles led to an increase in a newly identified hormone irisin. Irisin acts on white adipose cells in culture and stimulates UCP-1 expression and the movement toward the development of beige fat or a browned WAT. One of the strongest influences on PGC1-α expression is exercise. Boss et al.[72] note that resistance to obesity and associated disorders in various rodent models is due to increased BAT mass, the number of brown adipocytes, and UCP-1 expression. It is interesting to note that AMP kinase agonists including metformin in the periphery enhance insulin sensitivity. However, in the hypothalamus, AMPK-activated protein kinase activity leads to weight gain and insulin resistance. Administration of liothyronine (T3) decreases hypothalamic AMPK activity and upregulates thermogenesis in BAT. Thus, thyroid hormone–induced modulation of AMPK activity in lipid metabolism is a major regulator of whole-body energy homeostasis.[73]

The classical actions of natriuretic peptides are to promote natriuresis, diuresis, and vasodilation. However, these metabolic regulators can stimulate lipolysis in a manner similar to catecholamines. In mouse studies, B-type natriuretic peptide is protected against weight gain and glucose intolerance. Weight loss, exercise, and cold exposure stimulate natriuretic peptide release.[74]

The Interconnected Web: Signaling-Driven Pathophysiologic Expressions of Obesity

A response to a threatening environment is mediated by endocrine signaling and mitochondrial responsiveness. Corkey's model[21] of oxidative reductive potential and global regulation of energy demands, insulin signaling, inflammatory response, and stress responses is an effective model for predicting physiologic responses. Nunn et al.[75] suggest "that fine tuning of redox-thriftiness is achieved by hermetic (mild stress) signals that stimulate mitochondrial biogenesis and resistance to oxidative stress, which improved metabolic flexibility." However, in a setting of environmental stresses and internal alarm signaling, adaptive responses driven by fine changes in the oxidative reductive potential may lead to increased insulin resistance and increased oxidative stress owing to an increasing inflexibility due to mitochondrial overload. Epigenetic book marking of mitochondrial and nuclear DNA allow for an adaptiveness to environmental responses. Once a tipping point has been reached, protective insulin resistance becomes maladaptive inflammatory resistance. As demonstrated by Larsen et al.[76] in the DIOGENES Study of 742 participants losing on average ≥8% of their initial total body weight loss, their responsiveness to one of five different dietary programs differentiated by varied glycemic indexes and amount percentage of dietary protein suggests that genetic variation and nutrient-sensitive genes can modify the responsiveness to dietary programs.

The increasing prevalence of asthma and obesity in children has been globally noted in recent years. The link is believed to be one between the mechanical effects of obesity such as gastroesophageal reflux disease (GERD) and sleep disorder breathing as well as an inflammatory link driving the development of asthma.[77] In our personal experience during the Weight Loss Management 1 trial at the Functional Medicine Research Center, we noted that a significant number of the participating individuals were able to discontinue their use of inhaled cortical steroids and inhaled rescue albuterol during the course of a 66-week trial in which the average participant lost approximately 11% of their total body weight loss.

There is a clear association between obesity and the development of osteoarthritis. Osteoarthritis is generally considered a nonsystemic process with markers of only localized inflammatory responses. However, this wear and tear arthritis can certainly be exacerbated by the mechanical stresses related to increased body weight. With each step an individual takes, they experience across the knee joint a force that is seven times greater than their body weight. An additional 40 to 50 pounds would thereby generate 280 to 350 pounds of additional force with each step. Rios et al.[78] have demonstrated the beneficial effects of a prebiotic and exercise intervention in a rat model of diet-induced obesity. They found that prebiotic fiber supplementation and aerobic exercise and the combination of the two interventions completely prevented knee joint damage that is otherwise observed in this model of rat obesity.

Bakirci[79] notes the correlation between the systemic inflammation related to obesity and the development spondyloarthritis. Rosen et al.[80] have suggested in a 2006 paper in *Rheumatology* that osteoporosis may indeed represent obesity of the bone. Bone marrow composition shifts with aging to favor the presence of adipocytes, while osteoclast activity increases and osteoblast function declines, resulting in osteoporosis. Diabetes mellitus, glucocorticoid administration, and immobility as secondary causes of osteoporosis are associated with bone-marrow adiposity. In a mouse model of obesity and osteoporosis, Whitfield et al.[81] noted that low-levels of bone morphogenic protein 2 (BMP-2) in the setting of activation of PKC, a kinase dysregulated in insulin resistance, promote pluripotent bone marrow mesenchymal stem cells to differentiate into adipocytes as opposed to osteoblasts.

In mouse and human studies, it has been demonstrated that the product of the ESP gene which encodes a protein tyrosine phosphatase present in osteoblasts and increased levels of vitamin D lead to increased osteocalcin calcium levels.[82] Osteocalcin, traditionally considered a marker of bone formation, is perhaps better considered a marker of bone turnover as its levels are increased by both production by osteoblasts and by liberation by osteoclasts in mismatched bone turnover. In the presence of vitamin K, osteocalcin is carboxylated and becomes the anchor for mineralization of the bone matrix. Interestingly, carboxylated osteocalcin through interactions with pancreatic beta cells directly stimulates beta cell proliferation with increases in insulin sensitivity, energy expenditure, adiponectin levels, and decreased adiposity.[83] As such, the mechanoreceptors in osteocytes coordinating bone remodeling and the production of osteocalcin transduce a mechanical message of activity and resultant wear and tear on the bones into a message stimulating energy expenditures consistent with a more active lifestyle.

Similarly, Barchetta et al.[84] reported in a study of type 2 diabetic patients, with age- and sex-matched nondiabetic subjects as a controlled group, that osteopontin and osteoprotegerin levels correlated with elevated systolic blood pressures, abnormal HOMA-IR scores, and the presence of dyslipidemia and carotid atherosclerosis.

More directly correlated to cardiovascular diseases, Vilahur et al.[85] report that adipokines have been linked to platelet activation and induction of the coagulation cascade. Obesity impairs platelets sensitivity to insulin signaling and it enhances the production of bioactive isoprostanes (oxidative stress products), resulting in platelet reactivity. Also noted, obese subjects have elevated circulating levels of von Willebrand factor coagulation factors (VII and VIII) and fibrinogen as well as increased secretion of plasminogen activator inhibitor and thrombin activatable fibrinolysis inhibitor.

Dysfunctional adipose tissue signaling promotes endothelial damage, platelet reactivity, enhanced coagulation, and impaired fibrinolysis in obese subjects. Ruscica et al.[86] note that although the link in animal models between obesity, low-grade inflammation, and the development of cardiovascular diseases is well established, the links are less clear in humans. However, an increasing body of work supports this connection in human studies. In a study of 65 patients with premature coronary artery disease compared with a controlled group of normal individuals and a controlled group with metabolic syndrome, three adipokines, omentin-1, visfatin, and ZAG2, were demonstrated to differentiate between groups.[87]

The physiology of epicardial fat has been a focus of research interest. This unique adipose tissue is located between the myocardium and the visceral layer of the pericardium and is characterized by active fatty acid metabolism and highly expressed thermogenic genes. Clinical studies have demonstrated the significant association between increased amounts of epicardial fat and coronary artery disease. In a pattern analogous to the activation of visceral adiposity, the development of a pro-inflammatory state in epicardial fat and the subsequent release of pro-inflammatory cytokines and adipokines is associated with an increased risk for cardiovascular disease.[88]

Nakajima et al.[89] in a study of mitochondrial function in epicardial adipose tissue demonstrated impaired mitochondrial function in the epicardial fat of subjects with coronary artery disease. This reduced mitochondrial oxidative phosphorylation capacity was closely linked to decreased concentration of adiponectin and increased severity of coronary atherosclerosis. Souza et al. in 2017[90] demonstrated that lower serum adiponectin levels were associated with an increased risk for obstructive coronary artery disease.

Laboratory Evaluation

Despite the increasing availability of testing for both inflammatory cytokines and adipokines as well as advanced cardiovascular testing, it is important to remember that the clinical interpretation of this testing must be viewed with a few caveats in mind. The total laboratory variation including day to day biological variation in an individual coupled with variation in laboratory testing can lead to significant day to day variations in results. For example, it has been demonstrated that calculated LDL cholesterol levels can vary as much 15% per day. Thus, a level of 100 at the top end of the optimal guidelines for LDL cholesterol in individuals without established coronary artery disease could be as low as 85 and as high as 115 the next day. Similarly, an elevated level of LDL cholesterol calculated at 150, which would represent a possible indication for treatment with an HMG CO-A reductase inhibitor, when repeated the next day may be as low as 128 or as high as 172. The 128 level would be consistent achieving goals for individuals with two risk factors, and thus could be considered an indication for successful treatment. As such, for tests with high day to day variation, it is important to recognize that repeat sampling over time is important. Establishing a baseline with 1 to 2 baseline levels and following trends over time with treatment as opposed to a few limited data points is important. It is also important to recognize that analytes established in animal studies as markers of conditions may not have been validated as yet in human studies.

One of the great values of a clinical trial is the statistical power to see differences with treatment in laboratory testing as the number of individuals participating in a trial increase. Thus, differences that would be masked in an individual can be noted in groups of 10, 100, or 1000 individuals. Although a clinical trial may report that a certain biomarker, adipokine or inflammatory cytokine is different between groups in their study, discerning the value of baseline and treatment in a specific patient. For example, Ndrepepa et al.[91] reported that myeloperoxidase was a more accurate predictor of acute coronary syndrome than high sensitivity c-reactive protein. In their study, they demonstrated that the average value of MPO in stable coronary artery disease was 61.2 µg/L, that the average value in acute coronary syndrome was 99.2 µg/L, and that the average level in acute myocardial infarction was 129.5 µg/L. These findings were statistically significant with a $P < .001$. However, in this study with over 600 individuals, it is important to note that a level of 80 µg/L as a one-time measurement could indeed put someone within the standard deviation from the mean for all three diagnostic categories.

At present, the data accumulating regarding inflammatory signaling by cytokines, adipokines, and hormones in obesity and its connection with chronic noncommunicable diseases of aging are best utilized to understand mechanisms as opposed to diagnose and/or prognosticate specific conditions in individuals.

Implication for Therapeutics: How an Expanding Understanding of Physiology Influences Selection of Therapeutic Interventions

In an excellent review paper, Martel et al.[92] note that defensive cellular responses such as autophagy, DNA repair, and the induction of antioxidant enzymes systems are induced by caloric restriction, intermittent fasting, and exercise. It has been demonstrated that phytochemicals such as alkaloids, polyphenols, and terpenoids activate the same cellular defense mechanism and improve health and longevity by protecting cells and organs against damaged DNA mutation and oxidative stress.

Koch[93] has coined a new word, meta-inflammation, to describe the subclinical permanent inflammation associated with the chronic noncommunicable diseases of aging. The resultant metabolic cascade of dysfunctional oxidative reductive balance, early atherosclerosis, and the development of insulin resistance links to the development of diseases and conditions associated with inflammation. Polyphenols, as a major group of nonnutrient phytonutrients, play an important role in the modulation of physiology and the reduction of cardiovascular risk.

Amano et al.[94] have demonstrated that telomere shortening, associated with stem cell decline, fibrotic disorders, and premature aging, is associated with downregulation of sirtuin gene expression with the resultant impairment of their antiaging effects. The administration of nicotinamide

mononucleotide NAD (+) maintains telomere length and improves mitochondrial function.

An area of emerging interest is the close relationship between the intestinal microbiome and our systemic physiologic function. Possemiers et al.[95] note that the intestinal microbiome is closely involved in the first pass metabolism of dietary compounds being especially true for botanical supplements. The interplay of the microbiome metabolism with translocation, absorption, and the subsequent metabolism of these phytonutrients is crucial for the proper interpretation of the biological response to ingested phytonutrients. Indeed, Kang, et al.[96] note that the gut microbiota has been demonstrated to mediate the protective effects of the intake of capsaicin against low-grade inflammation and associated obesity induced by a high-fat diet; they report that dietary capsaicin increased levels of butyrate-producing microbiota while reducing levels of gram-negative bacteria–producing lipopolysaccharide. Interestingly, they identified that inhibition of cannabinoid receptor type 1 by capsaicin contributed to the prevention of a high-fat diet–induced gut barrier. They found that reduction of colonic microbiota through antibiotic treatments could block these protective effects of dietary capsaicin. González-Castejón et al.[97] in an informative review identified a broad range of dietary phytochemicals that would be beneficial for the nutritional support of individuals with obesity. Examples include the polyphenols: caffeic acid, chlorogenic acid; the stilbenes: resveratrol; curcuminoids, lignans, flavonoids: quercetin, proanthocyanidins, catechins, luteolin; isoflavones; carotenoids; organosulfurs: allicin; and phytosterols: diosgenin (fenugreek, wild yam), guggulsterone. Our experience at the Functional Medicine Research Center demonstrated that acacia and the reduced iso-alpha acids from hops are active in this regard as well.

Nonbotanical dietary ingredients including fish oils and their metabolites, the pro-resolving mediators, have been linked to a reduction in inflammation. Izaola et al.[98] report that these pro-resolving mediators are possible therapeutic targets in the treatment of obesity. Fish oil fractions rich in special pro-resolving molecules are now commercially available for supplementation in patients.

Certainly, in this chapter, we have demonstrated the relationship between altered inflammatory signaling by adipokines and the development of systemic diseases. Cimini et al.[99] demonstrate the relationship between adipose dysfunction and the development of nonalcoholic fatty liver disease (NAFLD). They note that low vitamin D levels are associated with a pro-inflammatory state that heightens the progression to the development of NAFLD. This highlights that vitamin D should be considered an anti-inflammatory agent with target levels for supplementation between 50 and 70 ng/mL.

Szewcyk-Golec et al.[100] have demonstrated that melatonin supplementation lowers oxidative stress and regulates adipokines in obese patients on calorie-restricted diets. Supplementation with 10 mg of melatonin increased adiponectin and omentin-1 levels and glutathione peroxidase activity while reducing malondialdehyde levels, a marker for oxidative stress. In a very recent paper from April 2019, Silva et al.[101]

demonstrated the beneficial effects of a Mediterranean diet compared with a fast-food diet on exercise-induced adipokine levels. They demonstrated that a preexercise Mediterranean meal potentiated the increase of adipsin after acute exercise. Adipsin is a potent insulin secretagogue stimulating glucose-stimulated insulin secretion. This is confirmation that pre-exercise diet composition influences the body's response to exercise. Lo et al.[102] note that β cell function is improved by the administration of adipsin in type 2 diabetics. This physiologic link between circulating adipokine levels, specifically adipsin, and exercise suggests the benefits of a structured exercise program for individuals with insulin resistance prediabetes and established diabetes as well as the other chronic noncommunicable diseases of aging. In a randomized crossover clinical trial of 30 overweight women with metabolic syndrome, the replacement of carbohydrates with unsaturated fats reduced levels of serum amyloid A and increased levels of adiponectin.[103] In an interesting study by Deibert et al.[104] of individuals with nonalcoholic steatohepatitis (NASH), a comprehensive lifestyle intervention was compared with a soy protein–based meal replacement. Interestingly, similar benefits of significant weight reduction and reduction in hepatic lipid content were noted in both groups. There was a strong correlation between the reduction in liver fat and a decrease in ALT with both groups also showing improvements in glycemic control and lipid profile. Changes in adipokines, particularly in adiponectin and leptin, were closely related to fatty changes in the liver.

In a 6-week study by Markova et al.,[105] a Mediterranean-style low-glycemic load food plan with approximately 30% of caloric intake from protein, 40% from carbohydrates, and 30% from fats, either featuring predominately animal proteins or plant proteins similarly reduced pro-inflammatory adipokines, chemerin, and progranulin. The effects of animal and plant protein were not consistent for transforming growth factor β1 and calprotectin. No statistically significant differences were noted in concentrations of interleukin-6, TNF-α, and lactoferrin. Further work exploring the differential effects of diet on physiology was done by Asle Mohammadi Zadeh et al.[106] who evaluated the benefits of an interval training program with different dietary programs for individuals with obesity and type 2 diabetes. The four dietary programs consisted of a control diet, a low-carbohydrate diet, a low-fat diet, and a high-fat diet. After 24 weeks, it was demonstrated that high-intensity interval training combined with a low-carbohydrate food plan overall improved cardiovascular parameters including glucose levels, cholesterol levels, HDL levels, triglycerides levels,

and weight with beneficial changes in interleukin-6 (IL-6), resistin, and leptin levels. It is clear that a body of evidence suggests that one food plan does not fit all subjects and a truly personalized lifestyle medicine approach evaluates an individual's physiology, psychology, and desires before prescription.

Paoli et al.[107] note that individuals following a staged diet protocol of a Mediterranean normocaloric diet, followed by a low-carbohydrate nonketogenic diet and a ketogenic Mediterranean ketogenic a Mediterranean diet enhanced with phytoextracts experienced a led to significant weight loss and reduction in body fat followed by successful maintenance without weight regain. The benefits of a phytonutrient-enhanced dietary program and the benefits of a phytonutrient-rich Mediterranean diet as well as the benefits of a high-quality meal replacements with phytonutrient-enhanced profiles have been well demonstrated. Peluso et al.[108] note that the beneficial effects of compliance with the broadly defined Mediterranean diet can perhaps be gained through attention to four specific dietary components. These four components are the four P's: probiotics, prebiotics, omega-3 polyunsaturated fatty acids, and polyphenols. One can conclude that supplementation with thoughtful combinations of omega-3 polyunsaturated fats, prebiotics, probiotics, and antioxidant rich polyphenols would be of benefit in the metabolic syndrome prevention and treatment and also applicable.

Conclusions

Dysregulated adipokine and cytokine signaling, a consequence of obesity, precipitates a feed forward cycle of inflammation, endothelial dysfunction, and pathophysiological phenotypic expression, which we recognize as the chronic noncommunicable diseases of aging. This highly ordered, evolutionarily conserved hormonal signaling and the distinctive physiologies, of visceral, epicardial and subcutaneous adipose tissue, and white and brown adipose tissues, mediate the interactions between a potentially threatening, potentially toxic external environment, our genotype, and our currently expressed phenotype. Defensive cellular responses such as autophagy, DNA repair, and the induction of antioxidant enzymes systems are induced by caloric restriction, intermittent fasting, and exercise. Personalized lifestyle medicine and an understanding of obesity signaling offer the clinician a unique opportunity to optimize prevention and lifestyle-related treatment for the chronic, noncommunicable diseases of aging.

References

1. Hotamisligil GS. Foundations of immunometabolism and implications for metabolic health and disease. *Immunity*. 2017;47(3):406-420.
2. Saltiel AR, Olefsky JM. Inflammatory mechanisms linking obesity and metabolic disease. *J Clin Invest*. 2017;127(1):1-4.
3. Reilly SM, Saltiel AR. Adapting to obesity with adipose tissue inflammation. *Nat Rev Endocrinol*. 2017;13(11):633-643.
4. Sun K, Kusminski CM, Scherer PE. Adipose tissue remodeling and obesity. *J Clin Invest*. 2011;121(6):2094-2101.
5. Charles KN, Li MD, Engin F, Arruda AP, Inouye K, Hotamisligil GS. Uncoupling of metabolic health from longevity through genetic alteration of adipose tissue lipid-binding proteins. *Cell Rep*. 2017;21(2):393-402.
6. Hotamisligil GS. Inflammation and metabolic disorders. *Nature*. 2006;444:860-867.
7. Zhang X, Zhang G, Zhang H, Karin M, Bai H, Cai D. Hypothalamic IKKβ/NF-κB and ER stress link overnutrition to energy imbalance and obesity. *Cell*. 2008;135:61-73.

8. Pang S, Tang H, Zhuo S, Zang YQ, Le Y. Regulation of fasting fuel metabolism by toll-like receptor 4. *Diabetes*. 2010;59(12):3041-3048.

9. Shi H, Kokoeva MV, Inouye K, Tzameli I, Yin H, Flier JS. TLR4 links innate immunity and fatty acid-induced insulin resistance. *J Clin Invest*. 2006;116(11):3015-3025.

10. Howitz KT, Sinclair DA. Xenohormesis: sensing the chemical cues of other species. *Cell*. 2008;133(3):387-391.

11. Prentice KJ, Saksi J, Hotamisligil GS. Adipokine FABP4 integrates energy stores and counterregulatory metabolic responses. *J Lipid Res*. 2019;60(4):734-740.

12. Golbidi S, Daiber A, Korac B, Li H, Essop MF, Laher I. Health benefits of fasting and caloric restriction. *Curr Diab Rep*. 2017;17(12):123.

13. Zhou S, Tang X, Chen HZ. Sirtuins and insulin resistance. *Front Endocrinol (Lausanne)*. 2018;9:748.

14. Morris BJ. Seven sirtuins for seven deadly diseases of aging. *Free Radic Biol Med*. 2013;56:133-171.

15. Mendes KL, Lelis DF, Santos SHS. Nuclear sirtuins and inflammatory signaling pathways. *Cytokine Growth Factor Rev*. 2017;38:98-105.

16. Barchetta I, Cimini FA, Ciccarelli G, Baroni MG, Cavallo MG. Sick fat: the good and the bad of old and new circulating markers of adipose tissue inflammation. *J Endocrinol Invest*. May 9, 2019. doi:10.1007/s40618-019-01052-3. [Epub ahead of print].

17. Gil A, Olza J, Gil-Campos M, Gomez-Llorente C, Aguilera CM. Is adipose tissue metabolically different at different sites? *Int J Pediatr Obes*. 2011;6(suppl 1):13-20.

18. Medina-Gómez G. Mitochondria and endocrine function of adipose tissue. *Best Pract Res Clin Endocrinol Metab*. 2012;26(6):791-804.

19. Shuai L, Zhang LN, Li BH, et al. SIRT5 regulates brown adipocyte differentiation and browning of subcutaneous white adipose tissue. *Diabetes*. April 22, 2019. pii:db181103. doi:10.2337/db18-1103. [Epub ahead of print].

20. Bartelt A, Widenmaier SB, Schlein C, et al. Brown adipose tissue thermogenic adaptation requires Nrf1-mediated proteasomal activity. *Nat Med*. 2018;24(3):292-303.

21. Corkey BE, Shirihai O. Lactate and free fatty acids all generate increases in mitochondrial NADH through their metabolism. *Trends Endocrinol Metab*. 2012;23(12):594-601.

22. Wallace DC. Bioenergetics and the epigenome: interface between the environment and genes in common diseases. *Dev Disabil Res Rev*. 2010;16(2):114-119.

23. Lee YS, Kim JW, Osborne O, et al. Increased adipocyte O2 consumption triggers HIF-1α, causing inflammation and insulin resistance in obesity. *Cell*. 2014;157(6):1339-1352.

24. Lempesis IG, van Meijel RLJ, Manolopoulos KN, Goossens GH. Oxygenation of adipose tissue: a human perspective. *Acta Physiol (Oxf)*. 2019:e13298. doi:10.1111/apha.13298. [Epub ahead of print].

25. Manzel A, Muller DN, Hafler DA, Erdman SE, Linker RA, Kleinewietfeld M. Role of "Western diet" in inflammatory autoimmune diseases. *Curr Allergy Asthma Rep*. 2014;14(1):404.

26. Van Dyken P, Lacoste B. Impact of metabolic syndrome on neuroinflammation and the blood-brain barrier. *Front Neurosci*. 2018;12:930.

27. Wang T, He C. Pro-inflammatory cytokines: the link between obesity and osteoarthritis. *Cytokine Growth Factor Rev*. 2018;44:38-50.

28. Ridker PM, Danielson E, Fonseca FAH, et al. for the JUPITER Study Group. Rosuvastatin to prevent vascular events in men and women with elevated C-reactive protein. *N Engl J Med*. 2008;359:2195-2207.

29. Winer S, Winer DA. The adaptive immune system as a fundamental regulator of adipose tissue inflammation and insulin resistance. *Immunol Cell Biol*. 2012;90(8):755-762.

30. Klein S, Fontana L, Young L, et al. Absence of an effect of liposuction on insulin action and risk factors for coronary artery disease. *N Engl J Med*. 2004;350(25):2549-2557.

31. Engin A. The pathogenesis of obesity-associated adipose tissue inflammation. *Adv Exp Med Biol*. 2017;960:221-245.

32. Guzik TJ, Skiba DS, Touyz RM, Harrison DG. The role of infiltrating immune cells in dysfunctional adipose tissue. *Cardiovasc Res*. 2017;113(9):1009-1023.

33. Erridge C, Attina T, Spickett CM, Webb DJ. A high-fat meal induces low-grade endotoxemia: evidence of a novel mechanism of postprandial inflammation. *Am J Clin Nutr*. 2007;86(5):1286-1292.

34. Pendyala S, Walker JM, Holt PR. A high-fat diet is associated with endotoxemia that originates from the gut. *Gastroenterol*. 2012;142:1100-1101.

35. Cani PD, Amar J, Iglesias MA, et al. Metabolic endotoxemia initiates obesity and insulin resistance. *Diabetes*. 2007;56:1761-1772.

36. Mehta NN, McGillicuddy FC, Anderson PD, et al. Experimental endotoxemia induces adipose inflammation and insulin resistance in humans. *Diabetes*. 2010;59(1):172-181.

37. Hall JE. *Guyton and Hall Textbook of Medical Physiology (Guyton Physiology)*. 13th ed. Kindle. Philadelphia, PA: Elsevier Health Sciences; 2016:890.

38. Doulla M, McIntyre AD, Hegele RA, Gallego PH. A novel MC4R mutation associated with childhood-onset obesity: a case report. *Paediatr Child Health*. 2014;19(10):515-518.

39. Hall JE. *Guyton and Hall Textbook of Medical Physiology (Guyton Physiology)*. 13th ed. Kindle. Philadelphia, PA: Elsevier Health Sciences; 2016:891.

40. Hall JE. *Guyton and Hall Textbook of Medical Physiology (Guyton Physiology)*. 13th ed. Kindle. Philadelphia, PA: Elsevier Health Sciences; 2016:892.

41. Rodrigues KCDC, Pereira RM, de Campos TDP, et al. The role of physical exercise to improve the browning of white adipose tissue via POMC neurons. *Front Cell Neurosci*. 2018;12:88.

42. Matsuzawa Y, Funahashi T, Kihara S, Shimomura I. Adiponectin and metabolic syndrome. *Arterioscler Thromb Vasc Biol*. 2004;24:29-33.

43. Corkey BE. Banting Lecture 2011. Hyperinsulinemia: cause or consequence? *Diabetes*. 2012;61(1):4-13.

44. Schauer PR, Kashyap SR, Wolski K, et al. Bariatric surgery versus intensive medical therapy in obese patients with diabetes. *N Engl J Med*. 2012;366(17):1567-1576.

45. Lockie SH, Heppner KM, Chaudhary N, et al. Direct control of brown adipose tissue thermogenesis by central nervous system glucagon-like peptide-1 receptor signaling. *Diabetes*. 2012;61(11):2753-2762.

46. Saltiel AR. Fishing out a sensor for anti-inflammatory oils. *Cell*. 2010;142(5):672-674.

47. Rozengurt E, Sternini C. Taste receptor signaling in the mammalian gut. *Curr Opin Pharmacol*. 2007;7(6):557-562.

48. Feeney E, O'Brien S, Scannell A, Markey A, Gibney ER. Genetic variation in taste perception: does it have a role in healthy eating? *Proc Nutr Soc*. 2011;70(1):135-143.

49. Goldstein GL, Daun H, Tepper BJ. Adiposity in middle-aged women is associated with genetic taste blindness to 6-n-propylthiouracil. *Obes Res*. 2005;13:1017-1023.

50. Kok BP, Galmozzi A, Littlejohn NK, et al. Intestinal bitter taste receptor activation alters hormone secretion and imparts metabolic benefits. *Mol Metab*. 2018;16:76-87.

51. Wu S, Xue P, Grayson N, Bland JS, Wolfe A. Bitter taste receptor ligand improves metabolic and reproductive functions in a murine model of PCOS. *J Endocrinol*. 2019;160(1):143-155.

52. Wiener A, Shudler M, Levit A, Niv MY. BitterDB: a database of bitter compounds. *Nucleic Acids Res*. 2012;40(Database Issue):D413-D419.

53. Winer DA, Luck H, Tsai S, Winer S. The intestinal immune system in obesity and insulin resistance. *Cell Metab*. 2016;23(3):413-426.

54. Luck H, Tsai S, Chung J, et al. Regulation of obesity-related insulin resistance with gut anti-inflammatory agents. *Cell Metab*. 2015;21(4):527-542.

55. Barchetta I, Cimini FA, Capoccia D, et al. Neurotensin is a lipid-induced gastrointestinal peptide associated with visceral adipose tissue inflammation in obesity. *Nutrients* 2018;10(4). pii:E526.

56. Hall JE. *Guyton and Hall Textbook of Medical Physiology (Guyton Physiology)*. 13th ed. Kindle. Philadelphia, PA: Elsevier Health Sciences; 2016:893.

57. Fruhwürth S, Vogel H, Schürmann A, Williams KJ. Novel insights into how overnutrition disrupts the hypothalamic actions of leptin. *Front Endocrinol (Lausanne)*. 2018;9:89.

58. Ye Z, Liu G, Guo J, Su Z. Hypothalamic endoplasmic reticulum stress as a key mediator of obesity-induced leptin resistance. *Obes Rev*. 2018;19(6):770-785.

59. Boden G. Endoplasmic reticulum stress: another link between obesity and insulin resistance/inflammation? *Diabetes*. 2009;58:518-519.

60. Widenmaier SB, Snyder NA, Nguyen TB, et al. NRF1 is an ER membrane sensor that is central to cholesterol homeostasis. *Cell.* 2017;171(5):1094-1109.

61. Pétremand J, Puyal J, Chatton JY, et al. HDLs protect pancreatic β-cells against ER stress by restoring protein folding and trafficking. *Diabetes.* 2012;61(5):1100-1111.

62. Lee MK, Moore XL, Fu Y, et al. High-density lipoprotein inhibits human M1 macrophage polarization through redistribution of caveolin-1. *Br J Pharmacol.* 2016;173(4):741-751.

63. Ghazarian M, Luck H, Revelo XS, Winer S, Winer DA. Immunopathology of adipose tissue during metabolic syndrome. *Turk Patoloji Derg.* 2015;31(suppl 1):172-180.

64. Lee MK, Yvan-Charvet L, Masters SL, Murphy AJ. The modern interleukin-1 superfamily: divergent roles in obesity. *Semin Immunol.* 2016;28(5):441-449.

65. Yasuda K, Nakanishi K, Tsutsui H. Interleukin-18 in health and disease. *Int J Mol Sci.* 2019;20(3).

66. Sepehri Z, Kiani Z, Afshari M, Kohan F, Dalvand A, Ghavami S. Inflammasomes and type 2 diabetes: an updated systematic review. *Immunol Lett.* 2017;192:97-103.

67. Murphy AJ, Kraakman MJ, Kammoun HL, et al. IL-18 production from the NLRP1 inflammasome prevents obesity and metabolic syndrome. *Cell Metab.* 2016;23(1):155-164.

68. Rheinheimer J, de Souza BM, Cardoso NS, Bauer AC, Crispim D. Current role of the NLRP3 inflammasome on obesity and insulin resistance: a systematic review. *Metabolism.* 2017;74:1-9.

69. Ghazarian M, Revelo XS, Nøhr MK, et al. Type I interferon responses drive intrahepatic t cells to promote metabolic syndrome. *Sci Immunol.* 2017;2(10). pii:eaai7616.

70. Hall JE. *Guyton and Hall Textbook of Medical Physiology (Guyton Physiology).* 13th ed. Kindle. Philadelphia, PA: Elsevier Health Sciences; 2016:896.

71. Boström P, Wu J, Jedrychowski MP, et al. A PGC1-α-dependent myokine that drives brown-fat-like development of white fat and thermogenesis. *Nature.* 2012;481(7382):463-468.

72. Boss O, Farmer SR. Recruitment of brown adipose tissue as a therapy for obesity-associated diseases. *Front Endocrinol (Lausanne).* 2012;3:14.

73. Cannon B, Nedergaard J. Thyroid hormones: igniting brown fat via the brain. *Nat Med.* 2010;16(9):965-967.

74. Wang TJ. The natriuretic peptides and fat metabolism. *NEJM.* 2012;367(4):377-378.

75. Av N, Bell JD, Guy GW. Lifestyle-induced metabolic inflexibility and accelerated ageing syndrome: insulin resistance, friend or foe? *Nutr Metab (Lond).* 2009;6:16.

76. Larsen LH, Angquist L, Vimaleswaran KS, et al. Analyses of single nucleotide polymorphisms in selected nutrient-sensitive genes in weight-regain prevention: the DIOGENES study *A JCN.* 2012;95(5):1254-1260.

77. Gupta S, Lodha R, Kabra SK. Asthma, GERD and obesity: triangle of inflammation. *Indian J Pediatr.* 2018;85(10):887-892.

78. Rios JL, Bomhof MR, Reimer RA, Hart DA, Collins KH, Herzog W. Protective effect of prebiotic and exercise intervention on knee health in a rat model of diet-induced obesity. *Sci Rep.* 2019;9(1):3893.

79. Bakirci S, Dabague J, Eder L, McGonagle D, Aydin SZ. The role of obesity on inflammation and damage in spondyloarthritis: a systematic literature review on body mass index and imaging. *Exp Rheumatol.* April 29, 2019. [Epub ahead of print].

80. Rosen CJ, Bouxsein ML. Mechanisms of disease: is osteoporosis the obesity of bone?. *Nat Clin Pract – Rheumatol.* 2006;2(1):35-43.

81. Whitfield JF. Polishing the Anabolic Holy Grail – PTH at the 22nd Annual Meeting of ASBMR. http://www.medscape.com/viewarticle/419250.

82. Semenkovich CF, Teitelbaum SL. Bone weighs in on obesity. *Cell.* 2007;130(3):409-411.

83. Lee NK, Sowa H, Hinoi E, et al. Endocrine regulation of energy metabolism by the skeleton. *Cell.* 2007;130(3):456-469.

84. Barchetta I, Ceccarelli V, Cimini FA, et al. Impaired bone matrix glycoprotein pattern is associated with increased cardio-metabolic risk profile in patients with type 2 diabetes mellitus. *J Endocrinol Invest.* 2019;42(5):513-520.

85. Vilahur G, Ben-Aicha S, Badimon L. New insights into the role of adipose tissue in thrombosis. *Cardiovasc Res.* 2017;113(9):1046-1054.

86. Ruscica M, Baragetti A, Catapano AL, Norata GD. Translating the biology of adipokines in atherosclerosis and cardiovascular diseases: gaps and open questions. *Nutr Metab Cardiovasc Dis.* 2017;27(5):379-395.

87. Smékal A, Václavík J, Stejskal D, et al. Plasma levels and leucocyte RNA expression of adipokines in young patients with coronary artery disease, in metabolic syndrome and healthy controls. *Cytokine.* 2017. pii:S1043-4666(17)30082-0. [Epub ahead of print].

88. Wu Y, Zhang A, Hamilton DJ, Deng T. Epicardial fat in the maintenance of cardiovascular health. *Methodist Debakey Cardiovasc J.* 2017;13(1):20-24.

89. Nakajima T, Yokota T, Shingu Y, et al. Impaired mitochondrial oxidative phosphorylation capacity in epicardial adipose tissue is associated with decreased concentration of adiponectin and severity of coronary atherosclerosis. *Sci Rep.* 2019;9(1):3535.

90. Souza RA, Alves CMR, de Oliveira CSV, Reis AF, Carvalho AC. Circulating levels of adiponectin and extent of coronary artery disease in patients undergoing elective coronary angiography. *Braz J Med Biol Res.* 2017;51(2):e6738.

91. Ndrepepa G, Braun S, Mehilli J, Von Beckerath N, Schömig A, Kastrati A. Myeloperoxidase level in patients with stable coronary artery disease and acute coronary syndromes. *Eur J Clin Invest.* 2008;38:90-96.

92. Martel J, Ojcius DM, Ko YF, et al. Hormetic effects of phytochemicals on health and longevity. *Trends Endocrinol Metab.* May 3, 2019. pii:S1043-2760(19)30063-3. [Epub ahead of print].

93. Koch W. Dietary polyphenols-important non-nutrients in the prevention of chronic noncommunicable diseases. *A Syst Rev Nutrients.* 2019;11(5). pii:E1039. doi:10.3390/nu11051039.

94. Amano H, Chaudhury A, Rodriguez-Aguayo C, et al. Telomere dysfunction induces sirtuin repression that drives telomere-dependent disease. *Cell Metab.* March 20, 2019. pii:S1550-4131(19)30129-9. [Epub ahead of print].

95. Possemiers S, Bolca S, Verstraete W, Heyerick A. The intestinal microbiome: a separate organ inside the body with the metabolic potential to influence the bioactivity of botanicals. *Fitoterapia.* 2011;82(1):53-66.

96. Kang C, Wang B, Kaliannan K, et al. Gut microbiota mediates the protective effects of dietary capsaicin against chronic low-grade inflammation and associated obesity induced by high-fat diet. *MBio.* 2017;8(3). pii:e00470-17. doi:10.1128/mBio.00470-17.

97. González-Castejón M, Rodriguez-Casado A. Dietary phytochemicals and their potential effects on obesity: a review. *Pharmacol Res.* 2011;64(5):438-455.

98. Izaola O, de Luis D, Sajoux I, Domingo JC, Vidal M. Inflammation and obesity (lipoinflammation). [Article in Spanish] *Nutr Hosp.* 2015;31(6):2352-2358.

99. Cimini FA, Barchetta I, Carotti S, et al. Relationship between adipose tissue dysfunction, vitamin D deficiency and the pathogenesis of non-alcoholic fatty liver disease. *World J Gastroenterol.* 2017;23(19):3407-3417.

100. Szewczyk-Golec K, Rajewski P, Gackowski M, et al. Melatonin supplementation lowers oxidative stress and regulates adipokines in obese patients on a calorie-restricted diet. *Oxid Med Cell Longev.* 2017;2017:8494107. doi:10.1155/2017/8494107. Epub 2017 Sep 21.

101. Silva D, Moreira R, Beltrão M, et al. What is the effect of a Mediterranean compared with a Fast Food meal on the exercise induced adipokine changes? A randomized cross-over clinical trial. *PLoS One.* 2019;14(4):e0215475.

102. Lo JC, Ljubicic S, Leibiger B, et al. Adipsin is an adipokine that improves β cell function in diabetes. *Cell.* 2014;158(1):41-53.

103. Rajaie S, Azadbakht L, Saneei P, Khazaei M, Esmaillzadeh A. Comparative effects of carbohydrate versus fat restriction on serum levels of adipocytokines, markers of inflammation, and endothelial function among women with the metabolic syndrome: a randomized cross-over clinical trial. *Ann Nutr Metab.* 2013;63(1-2):159-167.

104. Deibert P, Lazaro A, Schaffner D, et al. Comprehensive lifestyle intervention vs soy protein-based meal regimen in non-alcoholic steatohepatitis. *World J Gastroenterol.* 2019;25(9):1116-1131.

105. Markova M, Koelman L, Hornemann S, et al. Effects of plant and animal high protein diets on immune-inflammatory biomarkers: a 6-week intervention trial. *Clin Nutr.* March 27, 2019. pii:S0261-5614(19)30132-3. doi:10.1016/j.clnu.2019.03.019. [Epub ahead of print].

106. Asle Mohammadi Zadeh M, Kargarfard M, Marandi SM, Habibi A. Diets along with interval training regimes improves inflammatory & anti-inflammatory condition in obesity with type 2 diabetes subjects. *J Diabetes Metab Disord.* 2018;17(2):253-267.

107. Paoli A, Bianco A, Grimaldi KA, Lodi A, Bosco G. Long term successful weight loss with a combination biphasic ketogenic mediterranean diet and mediterranean diet maintenance protocol. *Nutrients.* 2013;5(12):5205-5217.

108. Peluso I, Romanelli L, Palmery M. Interactions between prebiotics, probiotics, polyunsaturated fatty acids and polyphenols: diet or supplementation for metabolic syndrome prevention? *Int J Food Sci Nutr.* 2014;65(3):259-267.

30

Cerebrovascular Disease, Vascular Dementia, Carotid Artery Disease, and CVA: Diagnosis, Prevention, and Treatment

Alfred S. Callahan III, MD

Cerebrovascular disease or stroke can be separated into ischemic or hemorrhagic with ischemic events predominating often 3:1. Despite the importance of hemorrhagic stroke, this section is devoted to ischemic stroke.

Acute Ischemic Stroke

Rescue

The treatment era of acute ischemic stroke began in December 1995 with the proof of benefit when intravenous thrombolysis was administered within 3 hours of onset (NINDS) in selected subjects.[1] Despite the scientific advance peripheral thrombolysis provided, translation of this benefit to stroke populations in the United States was slow. The next step in treatment was the demonstration of benefit in catheter directed thrombolysis in the middle cerebral artery within 6 hours.[2] However, intra-arterial thrombolysis required cath lab availability, which was limited in the late 1990s. Even extension of the peripheral thrombolysis benefit from 3 to 4.5 hours due to the results of ECASS3 did not increase the number of treated patients.[3] The next step in treatment had to await the development of stent retrievers for clot extraction. In December 2014, mechanical thrombectomy was shown to provide benefit beyond peripheral thrombolysis (MR CLEAN). And, by February 2015 multiple trials showed benefit with mechanical thrombectomy in the anterior circulation compared with peripheral thrombolysis (REVASCAT, Swift Prime, Extend IA, Escape). With the advent of advanced imaging identification of reversibly ischemic brain, the time window for treatments was extended up to 24 hours in selected cases (Defuse 3, DAWN). At last the tissue clock eclipsed the time clock for identification of those who might benefit from rescue treatment.

With these advancements more emphasis has been placed on systems of care beginning with public recognition of transient ischemic attack (TIA)/stroke, prehospital packaging, and development of comprehensive stroke centers with endovascular treatment expertise. Now more than ever where you go for health care can make a certain difference given rescue's proven scientific benefit.

Secondary Stroke Prevention

Concepts

But it was another trial that provided a quantum leap in terms of concepts of secondary stroke prevention. Heretofore, stroke was felt to be a heterogeneous group of etiologies, eg, embolism from a distance without atherosclerosis in atrial fibrillation, large vessel disease with local occlusion and distal flow failure or arterial to arterial embolism from activated plaque(precerebral or intracerebral), small vessel disease or lipohyalinosis, embolism from genetic thrombophilias, or dissection of a prior normal artery. And population-based studies had shown no association of cholesterol levels with risk of ischemic stroke (Figure 30.1).[4] Stroke was an outlier compared with the rest of vascular pathology because of its diverse etiologies. A further example of the unique vascular bed hypothesis was that neurologists used warfarin rather than aspirin, aspirin when used was 4 5-gr tablets per day (1300 mg), blood pressures were not reduced acutely in stroke, heparin was utilized rather than the endovascular means for urgent reperfusion, lipids were rarely measured or treated, and until 1996 reperfusion strategies were deemed experimental.

The next leap forward in care occurred with a single secondary prevention study.

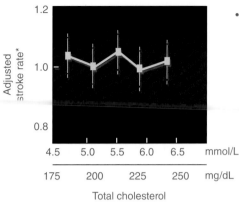

- Prospective studies collaboration
  - 45 prospective observational cohorts
  - Total of 450,000 individuals
  - Mean follow-up of 16 years
  - 13,397 strokes recorded

*Adjusted for study, age, sex, diastolic BP, CAD history, and ethnicity.

Figure 30.1 *Observational studies: association of serum cholesterol and stroke rates. (Adapted from Prospective Studies Collaboration. Cholesterol, diastolic blood pressure, and stroke: 13,000 strokes in 450,000 people in 45 prospective cohorts.* Lancet. *1995;346:1647-1653.)*

The Stroke Prevention by Aggressive Reduction of Cholesterol Levels (SPARCL) study enrolled subjects with recent stroke or TIA and no known heart disease. Atorvastatin 80 mg daily or placebo was given to 4732 subjects. Subjects with cardiocerebral embolism were not enrolled because oral anticoagulation provided for reduction of stroke risk to 1% annually. When published in August 2006 (NEJM), intensive lipid lowering was shown to provide a statistically significant benefit for secondary stroke prevention.[5] And, such treatment also reduced the risk of coronary artery disease as well as carotid revascularization. There was neuroprotection as strokes that occurred in the treated group were smaller and less disabling and renoprotection as well. Three years into the study, subjects were more likely to have their first myocardial infarction rather than their second stroke. Seen from this perspective, SPARCL showed the issue was not disease in a specific vascular bed but vascular disease without regard to its geography. The issue became diseases of blood vessels rather than the organ in which the blood vessels were located.

Intensive lipid lowering after ischemic stroke or TIA was established by this single study and accepted on a worldwide basis in all treatment guidelines.

Studies in stroke showing the lack of benefit of warfarin beyond aspirin in symptomatic intracranial disease[6] and the benefit of immediate endovascular reperfusion (MR CLEAN, Swift prime, Escape, Extend IA) all served to reinforce the notion that there could be a unified approach to vascular disease. Rather than organ-specific care there could be angiologists.

Falk had already shown that severe coronary stenosis was not the most common cause of death in acute coronary syndrome.[7] His studies showed it was a nonstenotic lipid-rich plaque with inflammation and a thin cap that was the culprit lesion. Further evidence that the issue was not severely narrow arteries was shown in COURAGE[8] where cardiologists performing PCI (percutaneous coronary intervention) in chronic stable angina subjects with severe coronary narrowing did not extend life or prevent acute coronary syndrome.

Endovascular treatments for peripheral arterial disease did not result in any improvement in walking distance compared to intensive lipid lowering. Rather than severe vascular stenosis, the issue was now framed as the arterial wall contents and inflammation.

Because WHO estimates vascular disease will affect at least 45% of all the world's inhabitants (lifetime risk), the most prevalent preventable disease is vascular disease. The stage was now set to propose not primary prevention of vascular disease, but primordial prevention. Although vascular disease is a time-dependent process, there was no reason to wait for the development of risk factors to modify future vascular risk. The ability to image subclinical atherosclerosis selects patients for treatment sooner than age-dependent risk factor algorithms. And, systems of care could be planned to translate benefit to populations at risk by addressing personalized communication to change behavior in novel settings/locations for care delivery that had enhanced social capital.

Prevention (Primordial/Primary/Secondary)

Risk

With the publication of NASCET in 1991, it was clear that activated carotid plaque with at least 70% stenosis was best managed by surgical removal (carotid endarterectomy). Subjects with 50% to 69% stenosis were the subject of another publication by the NASCET group in 1998. This group with moderate to severe stenosis had subgroups who were benefited with surgical revascularization. But included in the publication was a figure of the original NASCET cohort since 1991.[9] The group with severe stenosis had ipsilateral strokes for 3 years, and then for the next 5 years had a stroke rate equal to those who had their carotid plaques removed. Only 25% of the group randomized to medical care had a subsequent stroke, but 75% did not. This graph suggested that despite severe symptomatic stenosis in a large capacitance precerebral artery active plaques might become stable over time. But, the article did not indicate why or how this might have occurred.

Another example of the change in risk over time can be shown with the placebo groups in peripheral thrombolysis studies of acute ischemic stroke. The initial NINDS publication in 1995 had a placebo death rate of >20%.[10] By 2008 (13 years later) in the extended time window study,[11] the placebo death rate was 8.2%. When death is less, the relative benefit from treatment is also less against the comparator. Trialists have experienced changing risk when vascular event rates were lower than predicted requiring expansion of their study population to retain statistical power.

The change (decrease) over time in levels of risk has been influenced by the advent of better antihypertensives, intensive lipid-lowering medications, and better access to cath labs for urgent reperfusion. And it may also be that the sickest have fallen first and earlier from the present (Darwinian selection). Historic risk may not be a guide to present or future risks as contemporary treatment(s) may have made a difference.

Stroke Type/Mechanism

Large Vessel Disease/Occlusion

LOW HANGING FRUIT—ATRIAL FIBRILLATION

Atrial fibrillation accounts for about 15% of all acute ischemic strokes and the majority of disabling strokes. As the most common adult arrhythmia ensuring a high prevalence and the left atrial appendage being able to produce large volume clots, it is not surprising that devastating strokes occur since the first two vessels off the aortic arch provide the anterior circulation of the brain.

Cardiocerebral embolism is more apt to produce death, hemorrhagic conversion, nursing home placement, dependency than other etiologies of ischemic stroke (Lisbon #24). And because the affected population is older, it is no surprise that women are the majority of patients.

Adjusted dose warfarin has been known since the 1960s to reduce the absolute ischemic stroke rate by 4% and provide for relative risk reduction of 75+%. Despite the known benefit of such treatment, a large untreated population exists worldwide (Figure 30.2). The difficulty of dosing with a narrow therapeutic index agent, interactions with diet requiring careful patient adherence to choice of foods, slow onset of effectiveness, frequent interaction with other medications, high protein binding, and the concern of causing brain hemorrhage have all limited the use of effective treatment with warfarin.

Effective alternatives to adjusted dose warfarin were introduced into clinical practice in 2008 with dabigatran an oral direct thrombin inhibitor. By 2011 the first of the anti-Xa agents was approved for the reduction of risk in atrial fibrillation (rivaroxaban) and by the end of 2012 a second (apixaban) was approved for the same indication. There are currently three anti-Xa agents available. These new classes of agents do not require dietary modification or routine monitoring. They are fully active within 3 hours and have short half-lives. Antidotes to oral direct thrombin inhibitors and anti-Xa agents are now available.

Algorithms to stratify risk in atrial fibrillation have been modified to provide an extra point for female gender and two additional points for age (>65 and >75 years). Using CHA2DS2-VASc helps identify more subjects at risk who would be benefited by oral anticoagulation.[12,13]

Bleeding algorithms are not as well prospectively validated but are available (Figure 30.3). Bleeding remains the largest safety issue with oral anticoagulation, especially

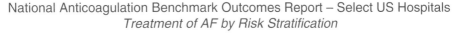
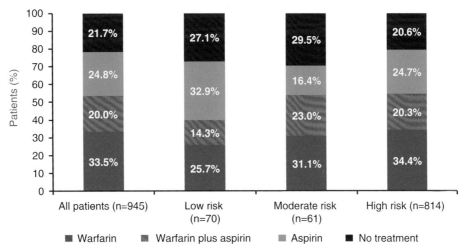

National Anticoagulation Benchmark Outcomes Report – Select US Hospitals
Treatment of AF by Risk Stratification

Figure 30.2 *Underuse of oral anticoagulation in atrial fibrillation patients. (Reproduced from Waldo AL, et al. Hospitalized patients with atrial fibrillation and a high risk of stroke are not being provided with adequate anticoagulation.* J Am Coll Cardiol. *2005;46:1729-1736, with permission from Elsevier.)*

HAS-BLED Score

Risk Factor	Score
Hypertension, SBP >160 mm Hg	1
Abnormal renal or liver function	1 each
Stroke	I
Bleeding history or predisposition	1
Labile INRs	1
Elderly: age ≥65 years	1
Drugs or alcohol --antiplatelets or NSAIDs --alcohol use >8 servings/wk	1 1
MAXIMUM	9

Incidence of Major Bleeds in European Heart Study

HAS-BLED Score	N (Bleeds)	Bleeds/ 100 patient-years
0	798 (9)	1.13
1	1,286 (13)	1.02
2	744 (14)	1.88
3	187 (7)	3.74
4	46 (4)	8.70
5	8 (1)	12.50
6	2 (0)	0.0
7	0	…
8	0	…
9	0	…

Figure 30.3 *Balancing stroke and bleeding risk tools for assessing bleeding risk. (Reproduced from Pisters R, et al. A novel user-friendly score (HAS-BLED) to assess 1-year risk of major bleeding in patients with atrial fibrillation: the Euro Heart Survey. Chest. 2010;138:1093-1100, with permission from Elsevier.)*

intracranial hemorrhage. Some of the newer agents have a safety profile improved over warfarin (Aristotle) and have rearranged the landscape or geography of complicating hemorrhage. GI hemorrhage remains the last frontier to be addressed and modified with the newer agents.

It is hoped that these pharmacologic advances will be translated into reduction in stroke risk worldwide for the millions of patients at risk of stroke with atrial fibrillation.

Despite the advances with oral anticoagulation, there are some patients who are not candidates for medical treatment. Alternative options exist and include surgical extirpation of the left auricular appendage or endovascular occlusion. Studies of efficacy of such alternatives have had a difficult time proving benefit since medical therapy is so effective. Surgical extirpation of the left auricular appendage has been known since the 1930s and is less commonly performed currently. With recent endovascular technology advances, randomized clinical trials have compared percutaneously delivered devices with medical therapy. A lower than expected stroke event rate in the medical arm was a factor in PREVAIL's results.[14] And in PROTECT-AF there was a reduced risk of stroke with confidence intervals that spanned unity.[15] But, for the patient who cannot be given oral anticoagulation, there are now options.

Carotid Disease: Symptomatic/Asymptomatic

C. Miller Fisher noted carotid stenosis produced stroke in the early 1950s and proposed that removal of the plaques by surgical means might be effective. In 1954 Dr Debakey performed the first carotid endarterectomy. By 1991 the NASCET randomized clinical trial confirmed the effectiveness of surgical endarterectomy with an absolute reduction of risk of 17% and a number needed to treat (NNT) of 6.

Development of PCI for the coronary arteries led to stents sized for the larger carotid bifurcation. A comparison of surgical endarterectomy versus carotid angioplasty and stenting showed comparable results when a distal protection device was utilized in the endovascular treatment arm (CREST).

Current guidelines recommend revascularization in symptomatic severe carotid stenosis (>70%) by surgical or endovascular means.

An early study of asymptomatic carotid disease in 1995 showed benefit in selected populations (ACAS) versus medical management with 60% stenosis.[16] Men were benefitted more than women and women had a higher rate of postoperative complications (reperfusion syndrome). Given the subsequent improvement in antihypertensives and intensive lipid-lowering agents, a new study is underway (CREST 2) to provide contemporary clarity. Crest 2 has three treatment arms: medical, surgical, or endovascular. At least 70% stenosis is required at baseline before randomization of asymptomatic subjects. Because the study design did not require subjects with progressive plaque despite best medical therapy, eventual results will provide a measure of maximum risk reduction by current medication(s) in the medical arm. If there are enough subjects randomized to medical care who are nonresponders to medication, then surgery or endovascular treatment may be able to show benefit. But if the medical nonresponders are fewer than 30% it is unlikely that the study will be powered to show benefit in the intervention arms since n = 2480. The more responders in the medical treatment arm, the higher the NNT will be in the endovascular and surgical treatment arms. Results are not expected for several years (date).

Medical management of severe carotid stenosis can produce plaque regression. A patient who is a treatment responder is presented. This patient was a lifelong runner, never smoked, baseline LDL of 107 mg/dL, CAC of 4, and had neither hypertension nor type 2 diabetes. Serial B-mode ultrasounds show progressive plaque regression resulting in elimination of severe stenosis over an observation period of several years (**Figure 30.4**, with tabulation of near/far wall max IMT).

Carotid plaque regression with intensive lipid lowering

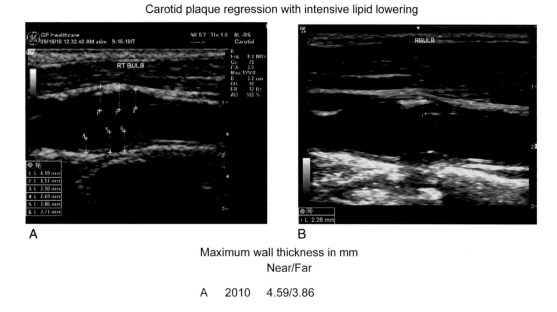

Maximum wall thickness in mm
Near/Far

A   2010   4.59/3.86

B   2018   2.28/2.04

Figure 30.4 *A 61-year-old man without risk factors, LDL 107 mg/dL, CAC 4. Given rosuvastatin 29 mg daily after image A. Image B is nearly 8 years later.*

Not all patients treated with intensive LDL reduction by statins will respond with lipid unloading or plaque stabilization. It remains to be seen if more dramatic reductions in LDL by the PCSK9 agents producing LDL levels <20 mg/dL can reduce the number of nonresponders. These agents will also provide data about safety of such very low LDL levels as well. Presumably at some point supplementation of fat-soluble vitamins might become an issue as well as how certain drugs (eg, cyclosporine) are dosed when buffered by circulating lipids. There is the potential for delirium if insufficient medication is buffered peripherally as the brain provides a vast reservoir for lipid-soluble drugs.

Intracranial Disease

Symptomatic intracranial disease is a less common cause of stroke and is more common in certain racial subgroups. An early study looking at the use of warfarin in such subjects (WASID) showed that warfarin did not provide any advantage over aspirin for secondary stroke reduction. The aspirin dose in WASID was 1300 mg daily. In the endovascular treatment era a study of symptomatic intracranial disease that compared angioplasty and stenting with medical treatment (SAMMPRIS) failed to show benefit compared to medical care.[17] The study was stopped early because of hazard in the endovascular group. Both groups received the same medical care including dual antiplatelet therapy, intensive lipid lowering (rosuvastatin), and blood pressure control (target <140 mm Hg).

Medical treatment seems favored based upon studies completed to date. Whether angioplasty without stenting might provide benefit over medication is unknown.

Small Vessel Disease

Small vessel disease is the most frequent form of acute ischemic stroke. In the NINDS trial, the placebo group with small vessel disease had a 50% chance of being normal at 90 days. Often patients with small strokes even in classic lacunar stroke locations can have near or full recoveries. Hypertension is considered the cause of such strokes though Dr. Fisher did suggest that other less common causes can occur (microemboli). Blood pressure control remains the mainstay for secondary stroke prevention, and blood pressure control has been shown effective for primary stroke prevention as well.

In SPS3 a secondary stroke prevention study with MRI documentation of lacunar type stroke more intense reduction in blood pressure (target < 130 systolic) resulted in a nonsignificant 19% reduction of recurrent ischemic stroke but a 63% reduction in intracerebral hemorrhage.[18] However, intracerebral hemorrhages occurred an order of magnitude less than ischemic strokes during follow-up. And 71% of incident ischemic strokes were lacunar infarctions. This study also confirmed that aspirin monotherapy was superior to dual antiplatelet treatment for secondary prevention in lacunar stroke.

Cryptogenic Stroke

Despite advances in imaging and laboratory testing, there remain groups of individuals with stroke for whom a cause cannot be identified.[19] This group is called cryptogenic stroke. Often advanced imaging is compatible with embolization because there is predominant cortical involvement.

The etiology of cryptogenic stroke is most often framed as determining the source of embolism.

Serologic studies are utilized to identify those subjects with cryptogenic stroke who have a genetic thrombophilia. Sometimes these individuals will have cerebral venous thrombosis as the cause of stroke. For younger patients, full body CT scans are often utilized to identify an unknown malignancy which may have contributed to embolic stroke risk.

Patent foramen ovale (PFO) is commonly identified on echocardiography in stroke patients, which is not unexpected given its prevalence in the general population. But, the frequency of PFO identification is reported higher in the cryptogenic stroke population (Stroke update 2018 slide 82). In an older study of warfarin versus aspirin for recurrent stroke (WARS), the presence of PFO or its size was not associated with a higher subsequent stroke risk. And, warfarin did not provide a benefit over aspirin in those subjects without or with PFO.

The development of PFO closure devices has led to trials of PFO closure for secondary stroke prevention. The more recent trials have been able to show benefit for populations that are younger than 60 years (stroke update 2018 slide 84, which came from JAMA neurology).

The placement of subcutaneous devices to monitor for paroxysmal atrial fibrillation as a cause for such strokes has become common. Studies have shown implantable subcutaneous devices improve detection of atrial fibrillation over external monitors (CRYSTAL AF and EMBRACE). But, it is not known how much paroxysmal atrial fibrillation is needed to assign arrhythmia as the cause of the stroke. Furthermore, the implantable device algorithm is less sensitive than pacemakers in identifying atrial fibrillation. Newer wearable devices may become an alternative to invasive devices. If so, then the clinical question of whether the identified arrhythmia should change treatment to oral anticoagulation remains to be answered, ie, how little a fib is dangerous?

A recent study of anti-Xa inhibitors (rivaroxaban) in cryptogenic stroke failed to reduce recurrent stroke risk over aspirin and resulted in a higher rate of bleeding.[20]

Vascular Dementia (Can There Be?)

Amnesia can be produced by bilateral infarctions of the medial temporal lobes or the medial dorsal thalamus. The former is most often embolic disease in the posterior cerebral arteries or top of the basilar embolic occlusion while the latter can occur with cerebral venous thrombosis. Global low flow can also produce a permanent amnesia with bilateral border zone infarctions. Rare cases of hypoxic ischemic encephalopathy may be indistinguishable from Korsakoff's.

Multiple small vessel strokes can produce a typical gait called petit-pas from involvement of the upper motor neurons bilaterally. Generally any disturbance of executive functioning from small vessel disease occurs in the setting of a gait disturbance.

Most commonly dementia is a degenerative neurologic process which may be associated with other neurodegenerative syndromes such as Parkinson disease or amyotrophic lateral sclerosis. The hallmark of dementia is the progressive decline of functioning (especially memory) whereas stroke is more ictal with subsequent improvement or stabilization. The degenerative dementias are characterized by inexorable clinical progression and eventually encompass executive brain function as well as memory declines.

In order to have sufficient memory storage, there must be connections other than axonal to neuronal ones. There do not appear to be sufficient neurons to account for memory's phenomenology. The dendritic field tree has sufficient arborization for dendrodendritic synapses to provide sufficient storage of memories and be remodeled as a function of experience(s). It is only this vast number of synapses that can be envisioned to be an n-dimensional space of what computation specialists might liken to "mother boards."

Although proteinopathies can clearly produce neuronal depopulation, it may be that dementia is a failure of maintenance of the dendrodentritic synapses rather than neuronal cell loss. Stroke is too broad a brush to prune memory's synaptic substrate.

It is unlikely that widespread effective vascular risk reduction will reduce the number of patients with dementia.

Aspirin

Antiplatelet therapy with aspirin has been shown to be effective in reducing the risk of first stroke when taken by women in low dose (100 mg) every other day.[21] It has been harder to demonstrate such protection in men though presumably the antiplatelet effect of aspirin is not gender specific.[22] Although NASCET had suggested that high-dose aspirin (1300 mg daily) was preferable, a subsequent study of varying aspirin doses in subjects undergoing carotid endarterectomy failed to show benefit from the higher dose. There was no reduction in ischemic complications with the high-dose over low-dose aspirin in ACE trial.[23] This study was a surgical one and limited to 90 days of follow-up, but the use of 81 mg aspirin for low dose has become popular in other populations as well.

The addition of P2Y12 inhibitors to aspirin has been utilized in subjects receiving endoprotheses and for 90 days in subjects with symptomatic intracranial stenosis treated medically. In SPS 3 the use of aspirin and clopidogrel in lacunar infarctions did not reduce recurrent ischemic events compared with aspirin alone. The combination antiplatelet program was associated with an increase in all-cause mortality and a near doubled rate of complicating hemorrhage.

Although there appears to be benefit with dual antiplatelet therapy for 90 days,[24] in a more recent study the benefit was accompanied by an increase in complicating hemorrhage.[25] In POINT, recurrent events were more common within 7 days of the initial stroke suggesting that benefit's time window with dual antiplatelet therapy may be as short as 7 days.

The optimal dose of aspirin will likely never be known because most clinical trials focus on more costly interventions. But, there has been a gradual trend for reduction in dose without loss of efficacy and a gain in safety (from bleeding). An initial higher dose of aspirin for the first 5 to 7 days, followed by a reduction to 81 mg daily is in widespread use for secondary prevention.

Controversies

Incident Diabetes

The reporting of an association of incident diabetes in SPARCL[26] led to widespread Internet controversy, which was especially befuddling to patients. Any program of risk reduction depends upon adherence, and any influence that reduces adherence is expected to translate to unmitigated risk. The negative influence of Internet reporting appears to be quite potent to patients who fail to appreciate its uniform lack of judgment.

In SPARCL the diabetic subgroup at enrollment was especially benefited by treatment with 80 mg of atorvastatin daily. At enrollment subjects with only two factors for metabolic syndrome did not have an increase in incident diabetes during study time. However, those subjects with three or more such risk factors did have an increase in incident diabetes. There were 50 more of these subjects with incident diabetes randomized to treatment over placebo. None of these subjects had a vascular endpoint during study time though since treatment had protected them. Compared with placebo there were 157 patients on treatment who did not have any cardiovascular event emphasizing the preponderance of treatment's benefit.

The net benefit from treatment with 80 mg atorvastatin daily is very certain in SPARCL thought obscured on Internet postings. The signal of incident diabetes has been seen with other statins though the mechanism is not known. Having protected the diabetic patients we "made" from statin use may be the central theme.

Cerebral Hemorrhage

In an early observational study, MR FIT, lower cholesterol levels were associated with cerebral hemorrhage. This risk was most among male hypertensives. In SPARCL there was also a signal of cerebral hemorrhage. There were 88 incident hemorrhages with 55 in the treatment arm and 33 in placebo. SPARCL permitted enrollment at the investigator's discretion of subjects with cerebral hemorrhage as their enrolling event. The rationale in the study design was that such subjects might have an increased risk of ischemic events for whom intensive lipid lowering might provide benefit. There were 92 subjects whose prerandomization event was cerebral hemorrhage. These had nine primary endpoints during study time which were all repeat cerebral hemorrhage. This 10% recurrent event rate is similar to the 12% overall primary event rate in the trial. However, seven of those with recurrent

hemorrhage had been randomized to atorvastatin 80 mg daily and two to placebo.

Had subjects with hemorrhage at enrollment been excluded, then the net increase in hemorrhage would have been 17. In the Heart Protection Study there were 15 such subjects with incident hemorrhage in those randomized to simvastatin 40 mg daily versus placebo. In HPS this difference in incident cerebral hemorrhage was thought to be chance.

In SPARCL the subjects with incident hemorrhage were most likely men, hypertensive at their last study visit prior to the incident hemorrhage (systolic > 160 mm Hg) and their LDLs at that study visit were unchanged from baseline despite being randomized to atorvastatin 80 mg daily. Furthermore, all subjects with the lowest levels of LDL (<40 mg/dL) during study time had no increase in risk of cerebral hemorrhage from treatment.[27]

The small number of subjects with hemorrhage at enrollment did not permit measurement of any signal of increased ischemic risk for this cohort. Whether intensive lipid-lowering treatment is of benefit to this group is not known.

Future Directions

Primordial Prevention

The secondary prevention population has been determined by their experience of a clinical endpoint. This group has increased short-term risk of another event and a persisting high residual risk of a vascular event in another territory. Owing to increased risk, therapies of risk reduction have been shown to be effective in terms of NNTs. The primary prevention population is much larger than the secondary prevention one and is typically characterized or stratified by risk factors. The addition of measures of subclinical atherosclerosis has been shown to increase the numbers needing treatment (see chapter 19) in primary prevention populations. Such measures can identify subjects at earlier ages than is typical for primary prevention strategies.

Primordial prevention focuses on subjects with increased lifetime vascular risk prior to the development of risk factors and prior to the time when risk algorithms would suggest near-term risk (over the next 10 years). The primordial population is much larger than the primary prevention one, although it is the feeder or funnel from which the primary prevention population will flow from. This group could participate in a long-term strategy of risk reduction. Although we expect those treated in the primordial population of risk to be potential members of the secondary prevention group, effective treatment would reduce their risk of such membership. And, because we are going to treat a larger population much longer, any treatments would have to be cost-effective. With most classes of antihypertensives and intensive lowering statins becoming generic, medication cost should make such programs affordable.

But in order to save lives cheaply, which is the goal of primordial prevention, medication cost is not the only issue.

Systems of care would have to be developed to gain access to the entire population for risk stratification. Once the primordial risk population has been identified, then vascular risk has to be communicated in a way that changes behavior. Personalized communication may be an important variable for behavioral change. The images of plaque from ultrasound screenings may be a way to personalize the communication. To reach communities at risk, novel sites of care may prove useful such as barbershops[28] and could include "care there" rather than serving as conduits to traditional medical sites. Nontraditional medical sites might be selected by examining their social capital in the targeted communities.

Finally, a care paradigm that delivers success is at the scientific center of a primordial prevention program. If the blood pressure target is <120/80 mm Hg, then subjects with systolic blood pressures >160 mm Hg will not achieve goal by dietary change or a single antihypertensive. If the LDL goal is a 50% reduction (intensive lipid lowering), then low doses of modest lipid-lowering agents will not achieve the goal. Often in communities of risk, patients have never heard the proposed program is working. Most often they have heard "it's not working," which is interpreted by them as personal failure ("what's wrong with you?") rather than the advice proffered was not destined to achieve goal. Achieving targets at the next patient encounter can be very empowering to patients and ensure clinical traction. As Surgeon Koop used to say "pills don't work in the bottle."

Although rescue medicine and secondary prevention are important and fill the medical literature landscapes, it may be that programs of primordial prevention have the ability to reduce the inexorable rise in medical costs. A program of cost containment that does not include rationing in disguise should be a suitable advance. Perhaps primordial prevention will be shown to provide such a function.

Summary

Acute stroke treatment by endovascular means for selected patients by advanced imaging has been shown to be effective in large vessel occlusion with expanded time (now tissue) windows. Oral anticoagulation with newer agents is effective for reduction of risk of stroke and systemic embolism in atrial fibrillation with benefits beyond adjusted dose warfarin. In small vessel disease, controlling blood pressure remains the mainstay of treatment. Aspirin in low dose and judicious use of short time frame dual antiplatelet treatment has replaced warfarin. Optimal medical treatment includes intensive lipid lowering and blood pressure control with blood pressure targets still controversial. The stage is now set for vascular risk reduction to groups at risk lowering annual medical expenditures to permit saving lives cheaply.

References

1. National Institute of Neurological Disorders and Stroke rt-PA Stroke Study Group. Tissue plasminogen activator for acute ischemic stroke. *N Engl J Med*. 1995;333(24):1581-1587.

2. Furlan A, Higashida R, Wechsler L, et al. Intra-arterial prourokinase for acute ischemic stroke. The PROACT II study: a randomized controlled trial. Prolyse in Acute Cerebral Thromboembolism. *JAMA*. 1999;282(21):2003-2011.

3. Hacke W, Kaste M, Bluhmki E, et al. Thrombolysis with alteplase 3 to 4.5 hours after acute ischemic stroke. *N Engl J Med*. 2008;359(13):1317-1329. doi: 10.1056/NEJMoa0804656.

4. Prospective Studies Collaboration. Cholesterol, diastolic blood pressure, and stroke: 13,000 strokes in 450,000 people in 45 prospective cohorts. *Lancet*. 1995;346(8991-8992):1647-1653.

5. Amarenco P, Bogousslavsky J, Callahan A III, et al. High-dose atorvastatin after stroke or transient ischemic attack. *N Engl J Med*. 2006;355(6):549-559.

6. Chimowitz M, Lynn MJ, Howlett-Smith H, et al. Comparison of warfarin and aspirin for symptomatic intracranial arterial stenosis. *N Engl J Med*. 2005;352(13):1305-1316.

7. Falk E, Shah PK, Fuster V. Coronary plaque disruption. *Circulation*. 1995;92(3):657-671.

8. Boden WE, O'Rourke RA, Teo KK, et al. Optimal medical therapy with or without PCI for stable coronary disease. *N Engl J Med*. 2007;356(15):1503-1516. Epub 2007 March 26.

9. Barnett HJ, Taylor DW, Eliasziw M, et al. Benefit of carotid endarterectomy in patients with symptomatic moderate or severe stenosis. North American Symptomatic Carotid Endarterectomy Trial Collaborators. *N Engl J Med*. 1998;339(20):1415-1425.

10. NINDS rt-PAStroke Study Group. Tissue plasminogen activator for acute ischemic stroke. *N Engl J Med*. 1995;333:1581-1587.

11. Hacke W, Kaste M, Bluhmki E, et al. Thrombolysis with alteplase 3 to 4.5 hours after acute ischemic stroke. *N Engl J Med*. 2008;359:1317-1329.

12. Gage BF, Waterman AD, Shannon W, Boechler M, Rich MW, Radford MJ. Validation of clinical classification schemes for predicting stroke: results from the National Registry of Atrial Fibrillation. *JAMA*. 2001;285(22):2864-2870.

13. European Heart Rhythm Association; European Association for Cardio-Thoracic Surgery; Camm AJ, Kirchhof P, Lip GY, et al. Guidelines for the management of atrial fibrillation: the Task Force for the Management of Atrial Fibrillation of the European Society of Cardiology (ESC). *Eur Heart J*. 2010;31(19):2369-2429. doi:10.1093/eurheartj/ehq278. Epub 2010 August 29.

14. Holmes DR Jr, Kar S, Price MJ, et al. Prospective randomized evaluation of the Watchman Left Atrial Appendage Closure device in patients with atrial fibrillation versus long-term warfarin therapy: the PREVAIL trial. *J Am Coll Cardiol*. 2014;64(1):1-12. doi:10.1016/j.jacc.2014.04.029.

15. Reddy VY, Sievert H, Halperin J, et al. Percutaneous left atrial appendage closure versus. warfarin for atrial fibrillation: a randomized clinical trial. *JAMA*. 2014;312(19):1988-1998. doi:10.1001/jama.2014.15192.

16. Executive Committee for the Asymptomatic Carotid Atherosclerosis Study. Endarterectomy for asymptomatic carotid artery stenosis. *JAMA*. 1995;273(18):1421-1428.

17. Chimowitz MI, Lynn MJ, Derdeyn CP, et al. Stenting versus aggressive medical therapy for intracranial arterial stenosis. *N Engl J Med*. 2011;365(11):993-1003. doi:10.1056/NEJMoa1105335. Epub 2011 September 7.

18. SPS3 Investigators, Benavente OR, Hart RG, McClure LA, et al. Effects of clopidogrel added to aspirin in patients with recent lacunar stroke. *N Engl J Med*. 2012;367(9):817-825. doi:10.1056/NEJMoa1204133.

19. Strum WB. Colorectal adenomas. *N Engl J Med*. 2016;374:1065-1075.

20. Hart RG, Sharma M, Mundl H, et al. Rivaroxaban for stroke prevention after embolic stroke of undetermined source. *N Engl J Med*. 2018;378(23):2191-2201. doi:10.1056/NEJMoa1802686. Epub 2018 May 16.

21. Ridker PM, Cook NR, Lee IM, et al. A randomized trial of low-dose aspirin in the primary prevention of cardiovascular disease in women. *N Engl J Med.* 2005;352(13):1293-1304. Epub 2005 March 7.

22. Berger JS, Roncaglioni MC, Avanzini F, Pangrazzi I, Tognoni G, Brown DL. Aspirin for the primary prevention of cardiovascular events in women and men: a sex-specific meta-analysis of randomized controlled trials. *JAMA.* 2006;295(3):306-313.

23. ASA and Carotid Endarterectomy (ACE) Trial Collaborators; Taylor DW, Barnett HJ, Haynes RB, et al. Low-dose and high-dose acetylsalicylic acid for patients undergoing carotid endarterectomy: a randomized controlled trial. *Lancet.* 1999;353(9171):2179-2184.

24. Wang Y1, Wang Y, Zhao X, et al. Clopidogrel with aspirin in acute minor stroke or transient ischemic attack. *N Engl J Med.* 2013;369(1):11-19. doi:10.1056/NEJMoa1215340. Epub 2013 June 26.

25. Johnston SC, Easton JD, Farrant M, et al. Clopidogrel and aspirin in acute ischemic stroke and high-risk TIA. *N Engl J Med.* 2018;379(3):215-225. doi:10.1056/NEJMoa1800410. Epub 2018 May 16.

26. Waters DD1, Ho JE, DeMicco DA, et al. Predictors of new-onset diabetes in patients treated with atorvastatin: results from 3 large randomized clinical trials. *J Am Coll Cardiol.* 2011;57(14):1535-1545. doi:10.1016/j.jacc.2010.10.047.

27. Goldstein LB, Amarenco P, Szarek M, et al. Hemorrhagic stroke in the stroke prevention by aggressive reduction in cholesterol levels study. *Neurology.* 2008;70(24 pt 2):2364-2370. Epub 2007 December 12.

28. Victor RG, Lynch K, Li N, et al. A cluster-randomized trial of blood-pressure reduction in black barbershops. *N Engl J Med.* 2018;378(14):1291-1301. doi:10.1056/NEJMoa1717250. Epub 2018 March 12.

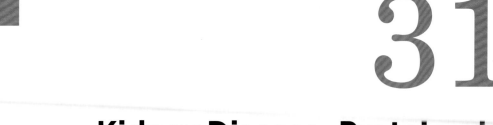

Kidney Disease, Proteinuria: Implications for Cardiovascular Risk

Hillel Sternlicht, MD and George L. Bakris, MD

Introduction

Albumin is a protein produced by the liver with a half-life of 28 days and reflects our nutritional status. It is also responsible for maintaining our plasma oncotic pressure to prevent peripheral edema. In healthy people, the filtering head of the nephron, the glomerulus, is impermeable to albumin (molecular weight: 65,000 Da) and therefore, only present in minute quantities. Hence, high levels of albumin in the urine, ie, albuminuria, signify some underlying pathophysiologic problem associated with an inflammatory process in almost all cases.

Although the terms proteinuria and albuminuria are often employed interchangeably, this is not correct. Albumin is but one of several proteins that may be found in the urine. The most frequently encountered and largest is uromodulin (Tamm-Horsfall proteins), a mucinous, glycosylated urinary protein. Because uromodulin weighs 80,000 Da and the glomerulus only allows proteins less than 40,000 Da in mass to traverse the basement membrane, it does not enter the urine by filtration but rather is secreted by the distal tubule (ie, tubular proteinuria).[1] "Low-molecular-weight" proteins (<25,000 Da) such as immunoglobulins, beta-2 microglobulin, and light chains are freely filtered but subsequently reabsorbed by the proximal tubule.[2]

Levels of albuminuria between 30 and 300 mg/d are defined as high albuminuria (formerly microalbuminuria) and levels above 300 mg/d designated as very high albuminuria (previously macroalbuminuria).[3] Levels at 30 mg/d or higher signify underlying inflammation that can be from a variety of causes (**Figure 31.1**). Albuminuria levels above 300 mg/d signify the presence of kidney disease and an even higher inflammatory burden. Because albuminuria has been extensively investigated concerning cardiovascular and renal outcomes, albuminuria and its integration into cardiorenal risk stratification is the focus of this chapter.[3]

Pathophysiology

The glomerulus and the proximal tubule of the nephron are responsible for plasma filtration and albumin retention. A nearly albumin-free ultrafiltrate (ie, urine) is assured through glomerular pores with size- and charge-selective restrictions; the proximal tubule reabsorbs albumin that does pass into the urinary space.[2] Cytoarchitectural distortions resulting in a loss of glomerular sieving capacity may be the result of mutations in the gene *NPHS1*, which encodes the protein nephrin; abnormalities in the proximal tubule protein cubilin would result in defects in albumin reabsorption.[4,5]

Among those with diabetes, glycosylation of albumin is associated with the generation of reactive oxygen species, a potential agent of vascular damage.[6] This injury can be further exacerbated by angiotensin II, which generates a vascular "leakiness" that predisposes to extravasation of albumin into the extravascular space.[7] Impaired vasodilation in response to nitric oxide release by the endothelium among those with albuminuria, particularly those with diabetes, further suggests an element of vascular dysfunction.[8,9] Finally, circulating levels of von Willebrand Factor antigen (vWF), a glycoprotein secreted in greater amounts when the vascular endothelium is damaged, has been identified as being proportionate to the severity of albuminuria among hypertensives such that those with greater degrees of albuminuria have higher serum levels of von Willebrand Factor.[10]

Despite the well-established association between albuminuria levels and cardiovascular and kidney disease, alterations within the kidney that result in the loss of albumin in the urine are incompletely understood. Moreover, while injury to the nephrons leads to albuminuria, this final "common pathway" obfuscates the diverse number of disease states that can serve as the upstream precipitant (**Figure 31.1**). The precise pathways whereby atherosclerotic disease precipitates albuminuria have yet to be identified. As such, the

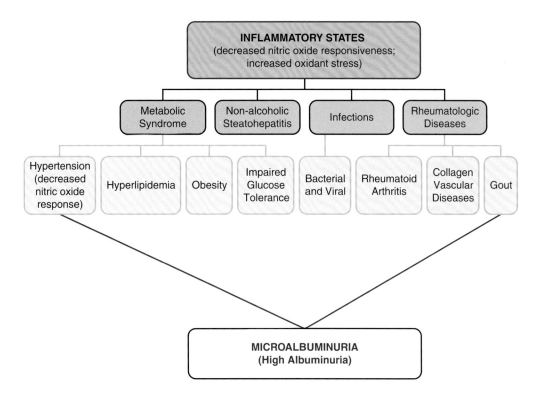

Figure 31.1 *An overview of inflammatory conditions that contribute to the development of high albuminuria. (From Bakris GL, Molitch M.* Microalbuminuria as a risk predictor in diabetes: the continuing saga. **Diabetes Care.** *2014;37:867-875.)*

concepts herein represent only a partial understanding of these processes with underlying inflammation being a unifying hypothesis (**Figure 31.1**).

An emerging theory is that the presence of albuminuria may also promote hypertension. Causality is possible because albuminuria can precede elevations in blood pressure and cardiovascular disease. A putative mechanism for the relationship of albuminuria antedating hypertension has yet to be described. Some have proposed that proteinuria, more broadly, can activate the epithelial sodium channel in the distal tubule of the kidney. By promoting sodium retention, blood pressure is thus increased.[11]

Measurement of Albuminuria

The urinary dipstick can detect albumin, but determination of the severity of urinary albumin loss is imprecise because of grading (eg, 1+, 2+, etc), and currently this is not a recommended screening test by the American Diabetes Association[12]. Quantitative assays of daily urinary albumin excretion using a 24-hour collection or single void ("spot urine") are preferable. A 24-hour urine sample is ideal but often difficult for patients to execute correctly. Therefore, a total urine creatinine is mandated to ensure accuracy with this type of collection. A spot urine sample collected upon awakening is an endorsed alternative but should be repeated at least once because there is as much as a 20% daily variance in albumin excretion.[13] Single void proteinuria quantification is reported in the unit "mg/g" and approximates an individual's daily urine albumin loss.

There is no unified national guideline concerning screening for albuminuria such as those made by the United States Preventive Services Task Force (USPSTF).[14] Subspecialty and disease-specific guidelines such as those issued by the American Diabetes Association recommend screening at the time of diagnosis of type 2 diabetes (DM2) or 5 years after the onset of diabetes in those with type 1 diabetes (DM1). The American Heart Association categorizes urinary albumin testing as optional among those with newly diagnosed hypertension but states it should be considered if (renal) end-organ damage is suspected.[15] The Kidney Disease Improving Global Outcomes (KDIGO) guidelines recommend annual screening for albuminuria among those with chronic kidney disease (CKD), ie, estimated glomerular filtration rate (eGFR) < 60 mL/min per 1.73 m^2.[3] Despite these specialty society recommendations, the USPSTF has concluded there is insufficient evidence to recommend screening for all people without risk factors such as hypertension or diabetes.[16] Cost-effectiveness analysis only supports screening among those with these or other risk factors for kidney or cardiovascular (CV) disease.[17] Thus, all people with hypertension and Stage 2 or higher kidney disease should be evaluated annually for albuminuria. If levels are >300 mg/d, then reassessment should occur every 6 months with reductions of 30% sought.[18] This will be discussed later in the chapter. Quantitative screening through a 24-hour urine collection or spot urine albumin:creatinine ratio (ACR) is acceptable but should be repeated within 2 to 3 months in order to exclude transient causes of albuminuria.[19] Confirmation of elevated levels of albuminuria are necessary because daily fluctuations of 20% can occur as a result of infection, sodium intake, or rheumatologic disease.[20-22]

Link Between Albuminuria, Kidney Disease, and Cardiovascular Disease

The formal staging of chronic kidney disease was introduced in 2002 and subsequently updated in 2011 to incorporate albuminuria, reflecting not only a poor kidney prognosis but also the presence of higher CV risk (**Figure 31.2**).[23] The incorporation of albuminuria into the staging of CKD was based on studies demonstrating that increased levels were a potent and reproducible predictor of a wide range of CV events from heart failure to stroke and from cardiovascular to all-cause mortality.[3] A meta-analysis of 21 community-based studies of more than 100,000 individuals analyzing the effects of GFR or albuminuria on mortality supports this assertion. The authors found that the hazard ratio for CV and all-cause mortality over 8 years rose once the eGFR fell below 60 mL/min per 1.73 m^2 in the absence of albuminuria. Among those with preserved GFR (ie, 90-105 mL/min per 1.73 m^2), similar endpoints were encountered more frequently once daily albuminuria exceeded 10 mg (**Figure 31.3**).[24] These results have been configured in the form of "heat-maps" in order to demonstrate the relative risk of various outcomes of interest as a function of a variety of levels of kidney disease and albuminuria (**Figure 31.2**).[23]

Shortly after the initial staging of CKD in 2002, an epidemiological study of over one million people in a large health network defined CV event rates by stages of kidney disease.[25] This study demonstrated that those with an eGFR <45 mL/min per 1.73 m^2 have a significantly higher risk of dying from CV events compared with people with preserved kidney function. In a separate study, individuals older than 65 years with CKD had all-cause mortality rates 2.5-fold higher than the general population, even when adjusted for comorbid conditions (**Figure 31.4**).[26] Because this high fatality rate is primarily driven by atherosclerotic sequelae and the event rates among those with kidney disease are comparable to those of persons with an established history of CV disease, cardiac and renal specialty societies have designated CKD as a coronary heart disease risk equivalent.[27] However, it is very difficult to truly establish the presence of CKD as a CV risk factor (versus a risk marker) because in most cases the preexisting atherosclerotic disease is present.

Defining an Elevated Risk for CKD Progression and CV Events

In order to understand the relationship between albuminuria, the stage of kidney disease, and cardiovascular outcomes, one needs to understand the epidemiology surrounding the level of kidney disease in the context of albuminuria and CV outcomes. The 2015 to 2016 National Health and Nutrition Examination Survey (NHANES)

Composite ranking for relative risks by GFR and albuminuria (KDIGO 2009)				Albuminuria stages, description and range (mg/g)				
				A1		A2	A3	
				Optimal and high-normal		High	Very high and nephrotic	
				<10	10–29	30–299	300–1999	≥2000
GFR stages, description and range (ml/min per 1.73 m^2)	G1	High and optimal	>105					
			90–104					
	G2	Mild	75–89					
			60–74					
	G3a	Mild-moderate	45–59					
	G3b	Moderate-severe	30–44					
	G4	Severe	15–29					
	G5	Kidney failure	<15					

Figure 31.2 *Composite Ranking for Relative Risks by glomerular filtration rate (GFR) and Albuminuria. Green = no risk for CV/CKD events, yellow = very low risk for CKD/CV, orange = moderate risk for CKD/CV events, red = high risk for both CKD/CV events, and striped red = very high risk for CKD/CV events. (From Levey AS, de Jong PE, Coresh J, et al. The definition, classification, and prognosis of chronic kidney disease: a KDIGO Controversies Conference report.* **Kidney Int.** *2011;80:17-28.)*

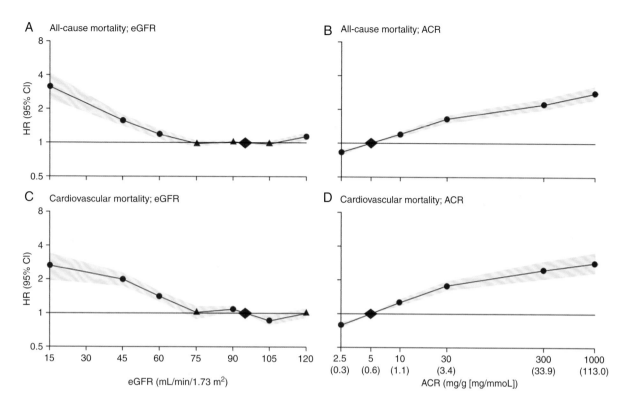

Figure 31.3 *Hazard ratios and 95% CIs for cardiovascular (CV) and all-cause mortality events according to spline estimated glomerular filtration rate (eGFR) and albumin:creatinine ratios (ACR). A, All-cause mortality, eGFR; B, all-cause mortality, ACR; C, cardiovascular mortality, eGFR; D, cardiovascular mortality, ACR. Hazard ratios and 95% CIs (shaded areas) according to eGFR (A, C) and ACR (B, D) adjusted for each other, age, sex, ethnic origin, history of cardiovascular disease, systolic blood pressure, diabetes, smoking, and total cholesterol. The reference (diamond) was eGFR 95 mL/min per 1.73 m² and ACR 5 mg/g (0.6 mg/mmol), respectively. Circles represent statistically significant and triangles represent not significant. ACR plotted in mg/g. To convert ACR in mg/g to mg/mmol multiply by 0.113. Approximate conversions to mg/mmol are shown in parentheses. (From Matsushita K, van der Velde M, Astor BC, et al. Association of estimated glomerular filtration rate and albuminuria with all-cause and cardiovascular mortality in general population cohorts: a collaborative meta-analysis.* Lancet. *2010;375:2073-2081.)*

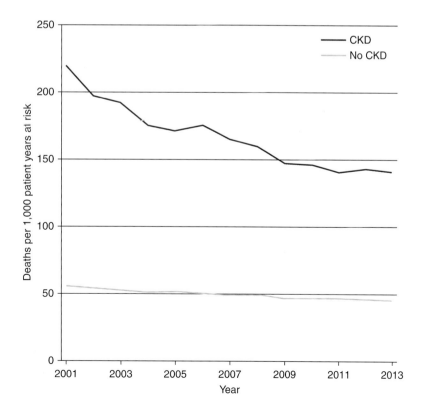

Figure 31.4 *All-Cause mortality rates (per 1000 patient-years at risk) for Medicare patients older than 66 years, by chronic kidney disease (CKD) status and year, 2001-2013 (adjusted). (From National Institutes of Diabetes Digestive and Kidney Disease Statistics for the United States. 2016.)*

Table 31.1

CRUDE INCIDENCE RATES PER 1000 PERSON-YEARS (AND 95% CIS) FOR ALL-CAUSE, CV, AND NON-CV MORTALITY BY UAC

UAC	Mortality Status, Rate (95% CI)		
	Total Population	CV Death	Non-CV Death
0-10 mg/L	3.5 (3.1-3.9)	1.2 (1.0-1.5)	2.3 (2.0-2.8)
10-20 mg/L	4.5 (3.6-5.5)	1.3 (0.8-2.0)	3.2 (2.4-4.2)
20-200 mg/L	11.2 (9.1-13.7)	4.7 (3.2-6.6)	6.5 (4.8-8.7)
>200 mg/L	29.1 (19.3-43.7)	16.6 (8.9-29.1)	12.5 (5.9-24.7)
P for trend	<.001	<.001	<.001

From Hillege HL, Fidler V, Diercks GF, et al. Urinary albumin excretion predicts cardiovascular and noncardiovascular mortality in general population. *Circulation.* 2002;106:1777-1782.
CV, cardiovascular.

found an 8.4% prevalence of high albuminuria and 1.7% prevalence of very high albuminuria among the US population. One-third of those with an eGFR of 30 to 60 mL/min per 1.73 m^2 (CKD stage 3) and over half of those with an eGFR of 15 to 30 mL/min per 1.73 m^2 (CKD 4) had some level of albuminuria.[28] According to NHANES data, the prevalence of CKD stages 1 to 5 was 15% in the 2011 to 2014 period (approximately 45 million Americans), with nearly 80% of these individuals with stages 1 to 3. The rate of stage 3 CKD or higher among those greater than 60 years of age was 33%.[28] In 2016, there were 500,000 individuals on dialysis and 200,000 living with a kidney transplant.[29]

There is a proportionate, graded relationship between levels of albuminuria and CV event rates with heightened risks beginning with even subclinical levels of albuminuria. This is exemplified in a community-based Scandinavian cohort of 40,000, where rates of death from CV disease after 2.5 years of follow-up were proportionate to the severity of albuminuria (Table 31.1). This relationship remained intact even when comorbid conditions such as diabetes, hypertension, and dyslipidemia were taken into account.[30] A comparable study of 2700 Scandinavians followed up for 7 to 9 years confirmed this observation and found nearly twice as many deaths among those with as little as 7 mg/d of albuminuria, well below the 30 mg/d threshold for high albuminuria.[31] Meta-analyses confirm this "dose-response" relationship among individuals with high albuminuria and very high albuminuria demonstrating a 50% and 100% greater risk of suffering an atherosclerotic event, respectively, than matched populations without albuminuria.[32] This additive morbidity associated with albuminuria persists in high-risk populations as well suggesting that albuminuria serves as a marker for enhanced atherosclerotic sequelae irrespective of baseline risk status.

A systematic review among people with type 2 diabetes found high albuminuria was associated with a twofold increase in death over 6 years of follow-up compared with those who had diabetes without albuminuria[33] A similar doubling of morbidity was observed among hypertensives with albuminuria when compared with nonalbuminuric hypertensives over 10 years of surveillance.[34] It is therefore not surprising that it is more predictive of future atherosclerotic events than C-reactive protein.[35,36] However, CV risk profiling through the use of multivariate models ("risk calculators") for primary prevention remains superior to the use of albuminuria alone for determining atherosclerotic event rates, and the predictive value of these models does not improve with the inclusion of albuminuria. Therefore, recent risk profiling tools such as the 2017 American College of Cardiology/American Heart Association Guidelines do not include urinary albumin.[37] Data published since this guideline's release suggest that albuminuria, but not eGFR, may be of predictive value with respect to heart failure but not stroke.[38]

Incorporating Albuminuria, CKD, and CV Risk

A recurrent hypothesis is that the presence of CKD itself reflects heightened inflammation which in advanced stages contributes to diffuse endovascular injury. Evidence for this hypothesis comes from post hoc analyses of the Modification of Diet in Renal Disease (MDRD) study. Asymmetric dimethylarginine (ADMA) is a protein responsible for inhibiting nitric oxide production and as a result, reduces free radical scavenging. In the MDRD (mean eGFR 32 mL/min per 1.73 m^2), increasing ADMA concentrations at the time of randomization were associated with higher baseline levels of CV disease. Upon surveillance termination 10 years later, those with the highest entry ADMA levels had the highest incidence of CV mortality.[39] In this study, there was also a similar relationship with CV mortality related to elevations in C-reactive protein.[40] By contrast, analysis of a potential association between homocysteine and CVD was not significant when adjusted for hypertension, diabetes, and dyslipidemia.[41] This would imply that these medical conditions are responsible for the generation of an inflammatory milieu rather than CKD itself.

Additional contributors to this atherosclerotic disease burden include hyperphosphatemia, a disorder linked to vascular calcification and fibrosis and seen in advanced stage 4 CKD.[42] It does appear that the uremic state, and perhaps anemia, contribute to endothelial abnormalities but these too remain poorly understood.[43] Taken together, there is a consensus that long-standing kidney failure embodies a unique pathologic entity that cannot be explained by the sum of its risk factors.

CKD and Cardiovascular Outcomes— Prognostic Implications

Over the past 40 years, there has been progress in slowing CKD progression and reducing CV mortality. An analysis of two very large follow-up studies of over 40 years' duration in patients with type 1 diabetes demonstrated a 40% reduction in the likelihood of requiring dialysis among those born after 1980. Moreover, even if dialysis is required, it is initiated at a more advanced age, that of 69, compared to 59 (as was the case in 1985).[44]

The importance of albuminuria in predicting progression of CKD was clearly shown in a recent meta-analysis evaluating changes in albuminuria over time and CKD outcomes. After the analysis of 28 cohorts including 693,816 individuals and 7461 end-stage kidney disease (ESKD) events, the

authors found an adjusted hazard ratio of ESKD following a 30% decrease in ACR during a 2-year baseline period to be 0.83 (95% CI 0.74-0.94). After further adjustment for regression dilution, it was 0.78 (95% CI 0.66-0.92). Adjusted hazard ratios were somewhat stronger at higher ACR. Among persons with ACR >30 mg/g, a true reduction in ACR of 30% over 2-years was estimated to confer >1% absolute reduction in 10-year ESKD risk even at earlier stages of CKD.[45]

Perhaps the best outcome studies to exemplify reduction in cardiovascular disease with slowed CKD progression among people with high and very high albuminuria are the recent trials with sodium-glucose cotransporter-2 inhibitors (SGLT2i)—Empagliflozin, Cardiovascular Outcomes, and Mortality in Type 2 Diabetes (EMPA-REG),[46] Canagliflozin and Cardiovascular and Renal Events in Type 2 Diabetes (CANVAS),[47] and Dapagliflozin and Cardiovascular Outcomes in Type 2 Diabetes (DECLARE).[48] A meta-analysis including data from these three trials (N = 34,322 patients, 60% with established atherosclerotic cardiovascular disease, 3342 major adverse cardiovascular events, 2028 cardiovascular deaths or hospitalization for heart failure events, and 766 renal composite outcomes) demonstrated that SGLT2i reduced major adverse cardiovascular events by 11% (Figure 31.5). The benefit was only seen in patients with atherosclerotic cardiovascular disease. SGLT2i reduced the risk of cardiovascular death or hospitalization for heart failure by 23%, with a similar benefit in patients with and without atherosclerotic cardiovascular disease and with and without a history of heart failure. SGLT2i also reduced the risk of renal disease progression by 45%, with a similar benefit in those with and without atherosclerotic cardiovascular disease. The magnitude of benefit of SGLT2i varied with baseline renal function, with greater reductions in hospitalizations for heart failure and lesser reductions in CKD progression in patients with more severe kidney disease at

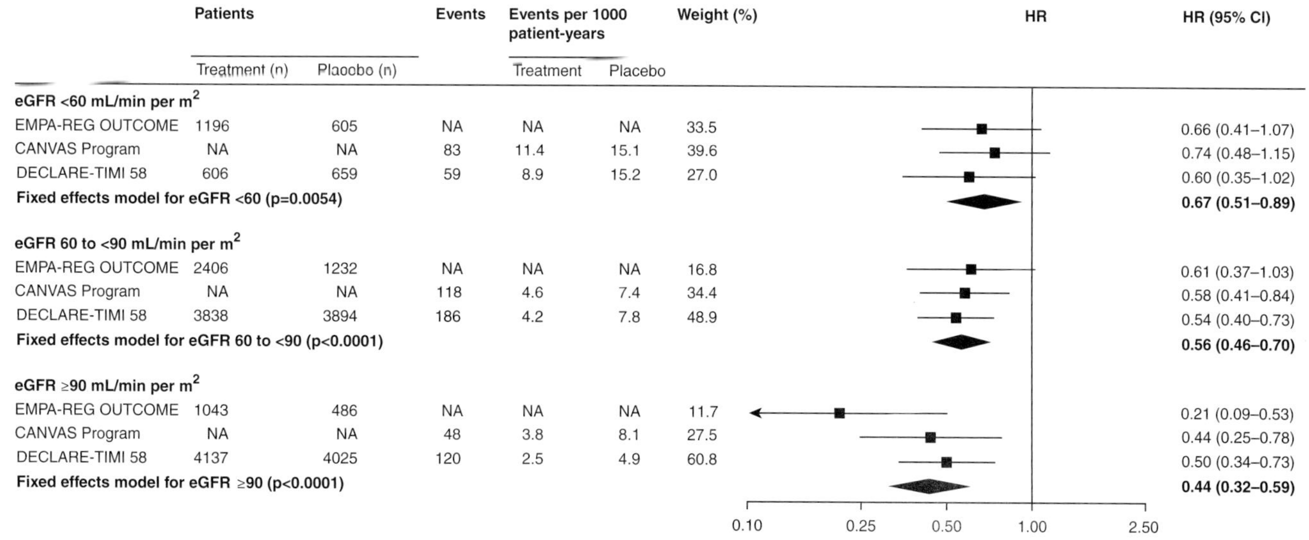

	Patients		Events	Events per 1000 patient-years		Weight (%)	HR	HR (95% CI)
	Treatment (n)	Placebo (n)		Treatment	Placebo			
eGFR <60 mL/min per m^2								
EMPA-REG OUTCOME	1196	605	NA	NA	NA	33.5		0.66 (0.41–1.07)
CANVAS Program	NA	NA	83	11.4	15.1	39.6		0.74 (0.48–1.15)
DECLARE-TIMI 58	606	659	59	8.9	15.2	27.0		0.60 (0.35–1.02)
Fixed effects model for eGFR <60 (p=0.0054)								**0.67 (0.51–0.89)**
eGFR 60 to <90 mL/min per m^2								
EMPA-REG OUTCOME	2406	1232	NA	NA	NA	16.8		0.61 (0.37–1.03)
CANVAS Program	NA	NA	118	4.6	7.4	34.4		0.58 (0.41–0.84)
DECLARE-TIMI 58	3838	3894	186	4.2	7.8	48.9		0.54 (0.40–0.73)
Fixed effects model for eGFR 60 to <90 (p<0.0001)								**0.56 (0.46–0.70)**
eGFR ≥90 mL/min per m^2								
EMPA-REG OUTCOME	1043	486	NA	NA	NA	11.7		0.21 (0.09–0.53)
CANVAS Program	NA	NA	48	3.8	8.1	27.5		0.44 (0.25–0.78)
DECLARE-TIMI 58	4137	4025	120	2.5	4.9	60.8		0.50 (0.34–0.73)
Fixed effects model for eGFR ≥90 (p<0.0001)								**0.44 (0.32–0.59)**

0.10   0.25   0.50   1.00   2.50

Figure 31.5 *Meta-analysis of SGLT2i trials on the composite outcomes of worsening renal function, end-stage renal disease, or renal death. (From Zelniker TA, Wiviott SD, Raz I, et al. SGLT2 inhibitors for primary and secondary prevention of cardiovascular and renal outcomes in type 2 diabetes: a systematic review and meta-analysis of cardiovascular outcome trials.* Lancet. *2019;393:31-39.)*

baseline. In all three trials evaluated in this meta-analysis, progression to very high albuminuria was further retarded.[49] The first statistically powered renal outcome trial with the SGLT2-inhibitor canagliflozin, the Evaluation of the Effects of Canagliflozin on Renal and Cardiovascular Outcomes in Participants With Diabetic Nephropathy (CREDENCE) will be published in mid-2019. The baseline data are currently available.[50] CREDENCE is a double-blind, placebo-controlled trial of 4401 patients with a baseline albuminuria of over 900 mg/d and an eGFR of 56 mL/min per 1.73 m². The results of this study will hopefully further support the concept of albuminuria reduction and renal preservation. An addition trial of interest is the Efficacy and Safety of Finerenone in Subjects with Type 2 Diabetes Mellitus and Diabetic Kidney Disease (FIDELIO-DKD). It is a double-blind, placebo-controlled trial of finerenone, a novel non-steroidal mineralocorticoid receptor antagonist, involving 5500 individuals with type 2 diabetes and kidney disease at high CV risk. The coprimary endpoints include CV events and renal outcomes such as time to dialysis. It will be completed in 2020.

Summary and Take-Home Points

- Presence and magnitude of albuminuria indicates level of inflammation and at levels above 300 mg/d clear presence of kidney disease. Reduction of greater than 30% in albuminuria after a few months of treatment indicates

reduction in kidney disease progression and should be a goal of therapy not just adding a blocker of the renin angiotensin system (RAS). Additionally, high albuminuria 30 to 299 mg/d indicates increased cardiovascular risk; thus, to help assess both cardiovascular and renal risk spot or 24 hour urine albumin:creatinine should be checked annually among all those with diabetes and/or heart or kidney disease. Measuring albumin creatinine among those with hypertension in the absence of diabetes has not been shown to be cost-effective. Moreover, presence of high albuminuria with normotension does not indicate diabetic kidney disease among those with diabetes.

Take-Home Points

- Very high albuminuria (30-299 mg/d) indicates an underlying inflammatory process and should be viewed as a risk marker similar to CRP.
- Presence of very high albuminuria 300 mg/d or greater indicates presence of kidney disease regardless of etiology and should be managed with RAS blockers to try and reduce the level by at least 30% within 3 months. This magnitude of albuminuria reduction is an indicator of a better renal prognosis.
- Other major CV risk factors that should be managed aggressively in the presence of albuminuria include blood pressure, lipid abnormalities, and glycemic control.

References

1. Devuyst O, Olinger E, Rampoldi L. Uromodulin: from physiology to rare and complex kidney disorders. *Nat Rev Nephrol.* 2017;13:525-544.
2. D'Amico G, Bazzi C. Pathophysiology of proteinuria. *Kidney Int.* 2003;63:809-825.
3. Kidney disease: improving global outcomes (KDIGO) CKD Work Group. KDIGO 2012 clinical practice guideline for the evaluation and management of chronic kidney disease. *Kidney Int Suppl.* 2013;3:1-150.
4. Brinkkoetter PT, Ising C, Benzing T. The role of the podocyte in albumin filtration. *Nat Rev Nephrol.* 2013;9:328-336.
5. Böger CA, Chen MH, Tin A, et al. CUBN is a gene locus for albuminuria. *J Am Soc Nephrol.* 2011;22:555-570.
6. Nannipieri M, Penno G, Rizzo L, et al. Transcapillary escape rate of albumin in type II diabetic patients. The relationship with microalbuminuria and hypertension. *Diabetes Care.* 1997;20:1019-1026.
7. Jensen JS, Borch-Johnsen K, Jensen G, Feldt-Rasmussen B. Microalbuminuria reflects a generalized transvascular albumin leakiness in clinically healthy subjects. *Clin Sci (Lond).* 1995;88:629-633.
8. Clausen P, Jensen JS, Jensen G, Borch-Johnsen K, Feldt-Rasmussen B. Elevated urinary albumin excretion is associated with impaired arterial dilatory capacity in clinically healthy subjects. *Circulation.* 2001;103:1869-1874.
9. Cosson E, Pham I, Valensi P, Pariès J, Attali JR, Nitenberg A. Impaired coronary endothelium-dependent vasodilation is associated with microalbuminuria in patients with type 2 diabetes and angiographically normal coronary arteries. *Diabetes Care.* 2006;29:107-112.
10. Pedrinelli R, Giampietro O, Carmassi F, et al. Microalbuminuria and endothelial dysfunction in essential hypertension. *Lancet.* 1994;344:14-18.
11. Gansevoort RT, Snieder H. Albuminuria as a cause of hypertension. *Nat Rev Nephrol.* 2019;15:6-8.
12. Sacks DB, Arnold M, Bakris GL, et al. Guidelines and recommendations for laboratory analysis in the diagnosis and management of diabetes mellitus. *Diabetes Care.* 2011;34:e61-e99.
13. Naresh CN, Hayen A, Craig JC, Chadban SJ. Day-to-day variability in spot urine protein-creatinine ratio measurements. *Am J Kidney Dis.* 2012;60:561-566.
14. Published Recommendations. US Preventive Services Task Force. https://www.uspreventiveservicestaskforce.org/BrowseRec/Index/browse-recommendations.
15. Whelton PK, Carey RM, Aronow WS, et al. 2017 ACC/AHA/AAPA/ABC/ACPM/AGS/APhA/ASH/ASPC/NMA/PCNA guideline for the prevention, detection, evaluation, and management of high blood pressure in adults: a report of the American College of Cardiology/American Heart Association task force on clinical practice guidelines. *Circulation.* 2018;138:e484-e594.
16. Moyer VA; Force USPST. Screening for chronic kidney disease: U.S. Preventive Services Task Force recommendation statement. *Ann Intern Med.* 2012;157:567-570.
17. Komenda P, Ferguson TW, Macdonald K, et al. Cost-effectiveness of primary screening for CKD: a systematic review. *Am J Kidney Dis.* 2014;63:789-797.
18. Lea J, Greene T, Hebert L, et al. The relationship between magnitude of proteinuria reduction and risk of end-stage renal disease: results of the African American study of kidney disease and hypertension. *Arch Intern Med.* 2005;165:947-953.
19. Mellitus ECotDaCoD. American Diabetes Association: clinical practice recommendations 2002. *Diabetes Care.* 2002;25(suppl 1):S1-S147.
20. Bakris GL, Molitch M. Microalbuminuria as a risk predictor in diabetes: the continuing saga. *Diabetes Care.* 2014;37:867-875.

21. D'Elia L, Rossi G, Schiano di Cola M, Savino I, Galletti F, Strazzullo P. Meta-analysis of the effect of dietary sodium restriction with or without concomitant renin-angiotensin-aldosterone system-inhibiting treatment on albuminuria. *Clin J Am Soc Nephrol.* 2015;10:1542-1552.

22. Oh SW, Koo HS, Han KH, Han SY, Chin HJ. Associations of sodium intake with obesity, metabolic disorder, and albuminuria according to age. *PLoS One.* 2017;12:e0188770.

23. Levey AS, de Jong PE, Coresh J, et al. The definition, classification, and prognosis of chronic kidney disease: a KDIGO Controversies Conference report. *Kidney Int.* 2011;80:17-28.

24. Matsushita K, van der Velde M, Astor BC, et al. Association of estimated glomerular filtration rate and albuminuria with all-cause and cardiovascular mortality in general population cohorts: a collaborative meta-analysis. *Lancet.* 2010;375:2073-2081.

25. Go AS, Chertow GM, Fan D, McCulloch CE, Hsu CY. Chronic kidney disease and the risks of death, cardiovascular events, and hospitalization. *N Engl J Med.* 2004;351:1296-1305.

26. National Institutes of Diabetes Digestive and Kidney Disease Statistics for the United States. 2016. https://www.niddk.nih.gov/health-information/health-statistics/kidney-disease. Accessed January 19, 2019.

27. Tonelli M, Muntner P, Lloyd A, et al. Risk of coronary events in people with chronic kidney disease compared with those with diabetes: a population-level cohort study. *Lancet.* 2012;380:807-814.

28. Centers for Disease Control and Prevention. Chronic Kidney Disease Surveillance System—United States. https://nccd.cdc.gov/ckd/default.aspx.

29. Saran R, Robinson B, Abbott KC, et al. US Renal Data System 2017 Annual Data Report: epidemiology of kidney disease in the United States. *Am J Kidney Dis.* 2018;71:A7.

30. Hillege HL, Fidler V, Diercks GF, et al. Urinary albumin excretion predicts cardiovascular and noncardiovascular mortality in general population. *Circulation.* 2002;106:1777-1782.

31. Klausen K, Borch-Johnsen K, Feldt-Rasmussen B, et al. Very low levels of microalbuminuria are associated with increased risk of coronary heart disease and death independently of renal function, hypertension, and diabetes. *Circulation.* 2004;110:32-35.

32. Perkovic V, Verdon C, Ninomiya T, et al. The relationship between proteinuria and coronary risk: a systematic review and meta-analysis. *PLoS Med.* 2008;5:e207.

33. Dinneen SF, Gerstein HC. The association of microalbuminuria and mortality in non-insulin-dependent diabetes mellitus. A systematic overview of the literature. *Arch Intern Med.* 1997;157:1413-1418.

34. Borch-Johnsen K, Feldt-Rasmussen B, Strandgaard S, Schroll M, Jensen JS. Urinary albumin excretion. An independent predictor of ischemic heart disease. *Arterioscler Thromb Vasc Biol.* 1999;19:1992-1997.

35. Gerstein HC, Mann JF, Yi Q, et al. Albuminuria and risk of cardiovascular events, death, and heart failure in diabetic and nondiabetic individuals. *JAMA.* 2001;286:421-426.

36. Kistorp C, Raymond I, Pedersen F, Gustafsson F, Faber J, Hildebrandt P. N-terminal pro-brain natriuretic peptide, C-reactive protein, and urinary albumin levels as predictors of mortality and cardiovascular events in older adults. *JAMA.* 2005;293:1609-1616.

37. Stone NJ, Robinson JG, Lichtenstein AH, et al. 2013 ACC/AHA guideline on the treatment of blood cholesterol to reduce atherosclerotic cardiovascular risk in adults: a report of the American College of Cardiology/American Heart Association Task Force on Practice Guidelines. *Circulation.* 2014;129:S1-S45.

38. Matsushita K, Coresh J, Sang Y, et al. Estimated glomerular filtration rate and albuminuria for prediction of cardiovascular outcomes: a collaborative meta-analysis of individual participant data. *Lancet Diabetes Endocrinol.* 2015;3:514-525.

39. Young JM, Terrin N, Wang X, et al. Asymmetric dimethylarginine and mortality in stages 3 to 4 chronic kidney disease. *Clin J Am Soc Nephrol.* 2009;4:1115-1120.

40. Menon V, Greene T, Wang X, et al. C-reactive protein and albumin as predictors of all-cause and cardiovascular mortality in chronic kidney disease. *Kidney Int.* 2005;68:766-772.

41. Menon V, Sarnak MJ, Greene T, et al. Relationship between homocysteine and mortality in chronic kidney disease. *Circulation.* 2006;113:1572-1577.

42. Da J, Xie X, Wolf M, et al. Serum phosphorus and progression of CKD and mortality: a meta-analysis of cohort studies. *Am J Kidney Dis.* 2015;66:258-265.

43. Thuraisingham RC, Yaqoob MM. Oxidative consumption of nitric oxide: a potential mediator of uremic vascular disease. *Kidney Int Suppl.* 2003;(84):S29-S32.

44. Bakris GL, Molitch M. Are all patients with type 1 diabetes destined for dialysis if they live long enough? Probably not. *Diabetes Care.* 2018;41:389-390.

45. Coresh J, Heerspink HJL, Sang Y, et al. Change in albuminuria and subsequent risk of end-stage kidney disease: an individual participant-level consortium meta-analysis of observational studies. *Lancet Diabetes Endocrinol.* 2019;7:115-127.

46. Zinman B, Wanner C, Lachin JM, et al. Empagliflozin, cardiovascular outcomes, and mortality in type 2 diabetes. *N Engl J Med.* 2015;373:2117-2128.

47. Neal B, Perkovic V, Mahaffey KW, et al. Canagliflozin and cardiovascular and renal events in type 2 diabetes. *N Engl J Med.* 2017;377:644-657.

48. Wiviott SD, Raz I, Bonaca MP, et al. Dapagliflozin and cardiovascular outcomes in type 2 diabetes. *N Engl J Med.* 2019;380:347-357.

49. Zelniker TA, Wiviott SD, Raz I, et al. SGLT2 inhibitors for primary and secondary prevention of cardiovascular and renal outcomes in type 2 diabetes: a systematic review and meta-analysis of cardiovascular outcome trials. *Lancet.* 2019;393:31-39.

50. Jardine MJ, Mahaffey KW, Neal B, et al. The canagliflozin and renal endpoints in diabetes with established nephropathy clinical evaluation (CREDENCE) study rationale, design, and baseline characteristics. *Am J Nephrol.* 2017;46:462-472.

Grounding and the Cardiovascular System

Steve Sinatra, MD

In 1977, I became a board-certified cardiologist. After writing dozens of peer review articles, books, and chapters in medical text books over the past 40 years, I thought about my greatest discoveries as a physician. Indeed, it was the utilization of coenzyme Q10 in my patients as well as the cardiovascular implications of grounding, also known as Earthing the body. This chapter is a testimony to the incredible discovery of grounding to the natural electric charge of the planet.

It was almost 15 years ago at an American College of Cardiology conference that I met Clint Ober in San Diego. He introduced to me the theory of grounding, and it made a lot of sense to me. I was excited about the entire concept, as well as trying to take it to a higher level. However, like anything else in medicine, the theory behind grounding needed intensive research. Ever since that encounter with Clint, more than 20 peer reviewed articles on the benefits of grounding have become available to mainstream medicine.

Over the past 4 decades, I have treated hundreds of patients with acute coronary syndrome and unstable angina, as well as acute myocardial infarction. Although the utilization of thrombolytic therapies, percutaneous transluminal coronary angioplasty, stents, and statin medications are crucial in the care of these patients, the grounding phenomena also needed to be recognized. This chapter will discuss the cardiovascular implications such as blood pressure control, improving heart rate variability, and blood thinning. All these crucial elements reduce cardiovascular risk.

Blood Pressure Considerations

Although most doctors are privy to pathological situations in raising blood pressure such as coarctation of the aorta, adrenal tumors, thyroid storm, and acute renal shutdown, to name a few, most hypertensive situations are of an idiopathic nature requiring pharmaceutical and lifestyle changes for appropriate control.

Over the years, I have used a nonpharmaceutical approach in many of my patients utilizing Mediterranean-type diets, mind/body techniques, targeted nutritional supplements, detoxification, and low-level exercise programs. Fortunately, high blood pressure in most cases is an easy situation to control without pharmaceutical support. However, in any patient with moderate to severe hypertension with any involvement of renal insufficiency, aggressive pharmaceutical therapy needs to be considered. In many patients, simple weight loss of a mere 5 to 10 pounds can be therapeutic, especially when taking targeted nutraceutical supplements.

Over the last decade or so, our research group has encountered multiple anecdotal reports of patients sleeping grounded or walking barefoot on the earth who appreciated subsequent blood pressure lowering. In many of my own patients who were borderline hypertensives, sleeping grounded assuaged higher blood pressure numbers. Other doctors reported similar results with their own patients. Although my colleagues were seeing anecdotal results, a clinical investigation needed to be done.

A small pilot study was performed by one of my cardiovascular colleagues, and all 10 patients in the study had remarkable blood pressure lowering at the end of the trial period and several were able to discontinue their pharmaceutical medications.[1] Systolic levels decreased over this time, ranging individually from 8.6% to 22.7%, with an average decrease of 14.3%.

The reasons why earthing can have such a profound impact on blood pressure lowering is that it reduces inflammation and pain,[2] calms and attenuates an overactive sympathetic nervous system,[3] while improving the electrodynamics of blood viscosity at the same time.[4] Earthing perhaps may be the easiest possible way to lower blood pressure. The most recent pilot study combined with my own clinical experience demonstrates that people with mild to moderate hypertension can normalize with grounding interventions. In patients with moderate to severe hypertension, the reduction in pharmaceutical support has also been realized when grounding the patient. In addition to blood pressure lowering, many of my patients commented that arrhythmia awareness was attenuated as well.

Premature ventricular ectopic activity (PVC) may be seen in the hypertensive individual as well as in patients who consume too much caffeine, alcohol, and even sugar. Although PVCs are generally harmless in patients with normal left ventricular function, they can create undo stress and worry for many. Several of my patients who slept grounded who also had PVCs reported sleeping better with life-changing attitudes. Perhaps that improvement in PVC awareness was related to a reduction in sympathetic tone and attenuation of the "stress response."

In a study of 27 patients, grounded participants had improvements in heart rate variability (HRV) that went beyond basic relaxation[3] (**Figure 32 1**). HRV refers to beat-to-beat alterations in heart rate. During resting conditions, the electrocardiogram (ECG) in normal individuals demonstrates periodic variation in R-R intervals (the R peak is the most visually obvious peak of the ECG). To simplify, "fixed" heart rates without any variation are detrimental to the cardiovascular system. Variable heart rates provide reliable, noninvasive information on the autonomic nervous system (ANS), including its sympathetic and parasympathetic components. HRV is an important indicator of the status of autonomic balance as well as stress on the cardiovascular system.[5] A decrease in HRV indicates autonomic dysfunction and is a predictor of not only stress on the cardiovascular system but also sudden cardiac death and progression of coronary artery disease as well. The positive effects of grounding on HRV suggest that simple grounding supports the cardiovascular system. Excessive sympathetic stimulation and/or diminished vagal tone are markers of a stressed cardiovascular

Table 32.1

FACTORS CONTRIBUTING TO CHRONIC SYMPATHETIC ACTIVATION

Environmental Conditions

Air pollution: Ambient particulate matter <10 µm [PM (10)]

Health conditions

Obesity

Insulin resistance, diabetes, or metabolic syndrome

Hypertension

Depression, anxiety

Congestive heart failure

Sleep apnea

Psychosocial and behavioral conditions

Chronic stress

Social isolation and loneliness

Hostility, anger, or rage

Smoking

Sleep deprivation

Sugar-laden diet

Sedentary lifestyle

Abuse of stimulants

Pharmaceutical drugs

Short-acting calcium channel blockers

B-agonist bronchodilators

Peripheral alpha-blockers

system. There are multiple situations that contribute to sympathetic activities including physical, emotional, behavioral, and pharmaceutical factors (see **Table 32 1**).

Simply stated, when one grounds to the electron-enriched earth, an improved balance of the ANS occurs. Improvements in HRV can support patients with emotional stress, anxiety, fear, and any other symptoms of autonomic dystonia.

Negative emotions such as anxiety,[6] depression,[7] hostility,[8] and panic[9] have all been demonstrated to reduce HRV. Grounding has the potential to support HRV, reduce excessive sympathetic overdrive, balance the ANS, and thus attenuate the stress response. This has important prognostic considerations, especially because an association between depression and increased risk of cardiovascular events has repeatedly been observed in both the healthy population and those with established cardiovascular disease (CVD).[7] The premature infant can also benefit from earthing.

A 2017 study performed at the Pennsylvania State University Children's Hospital Neonatal Intensive Care Unit in Hershey revealed that grounding premature infants produced

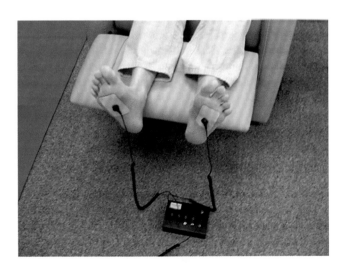

Figure 32.1 *Grounding system showing patches, wires, and box connecting to a ground rod planted outside through a switch (not shown) and a fuse (not shown). Similar patches and wires from the hands were also connected to the box to ground the hands.*

immediate and significant improvements in measurements of the ANS.[10] Grounding improves vagal tone and may support resilience to stress, which could lower the risk of neonatal mortality in preterm infants.

Grounding the babies, from 5 to 60 days of age, increased HRV, indicating improved vagal tone. Grounding was achieved by adhering a grounding patch on the skin of the babies, while in their incubators or cribs, and connecting the patch wire to the hospital's grounding system. Among the babies tested, grounding raised parasympathetic tone, which may enhance vagus nerve transmission and thereby improve the stress and inflammatory regulatory mechanisms in the preterm infants.

Recent research has revealed that the vagus nerve plays a major role in the so-called anti-inflammatory reflex, a mechanism controlling basic immune responses and inflammation during pathogen invasion and tissue injury. Among other things, the nerve's actions help to inhibit excessive production of proinflammatory chemicals.[11,12]

Grounding, indeed, has tremendous therapeutic potential to support those in need. In fact, it is perhaps the most common intervention to improve autonomic function (Tables 32 2). But how do we explain this healing, energetic phenomenon? It is well known that the earth possesses a slightly negative charge, the result of countless lightning strikes as well as solar radiation. This planetary attribute is based on a limitless, renewable reservoir of free-electrons, which are negatively charged subatomic particles.[13,14]

Table 32.2

INTERVENTIONS TO IMPROVE AUTONOMIC FUNCTION

Modalities

Grounding to the Earth

Alternative nostril breathing

Lifestyle modifications

  Exercise

  Social support

  Religiosity or faith

  Meditation, yoga, tai chi, and/or qi gong

  Restoration of normal sleep

  Weight loss

  Smoking cessation

  Stress reduction, biofeedback

Medications

  Beta-blockers

  Angiotensin-converting enzyme inhibitors

  Omega-3 fatty acids

The earth's charge and storehouse of electrons represent a major natural resource for health and healing. Research on biological grounding suggests that this very same electric charge on the planet's surface plays a nurturing role for both the animal and plant kingdoms. This form of electric nutrition appears to have the potential to restore and stabilize the internal environment of the human body's bioelectric systems that supervise the functions of organs, tissues, cells, and biological rhythms.[15,16]

The Schumann response, 7.83 Hz is the "vibration" or a "humming" of the energetic surface of the earth. Whenever we are in contact with the earth's electron-enriched field, a transfer of electrons results in an instant and significant physiological change in the body. This Schumann resonance or the electric field of the earth is not uniform but varies from moment to moment in a rhythm. Thus, the surface of the earth is electronically active and dynamic.

Behind the world that we can see and feel with our senses lies a powerful web of invisible energies and forces that affect us continuously that can be referred to as *geophysical fields*.[17] These invisible energies of the earth's gravity, electricity, and electromagnetism have consumed centuries of human knowledge in the scientific fields of biology, physics, astronomy, astrophysics, and cosmology.

Relationships with these geophysical rhythms are vital for health. Human physiology has more than 100 biological rhythms that are timed and coordinated with rhythms in the environment.[18]

The Schumann resonance, the key frequency in the grounding phenomenon is a standing wave made of electromagnetic fields, vibrating at 7.83 Hz, vibrating eight times per second. Higher frequencies, produced by lightning strikes throughout the world, have also been determined by physicists and astrophysicists as well.

Cloud to earth lightning bolts pump energy into the atmosphere, creating electromagnetic waves that travel around the earth at the speed of light. The frequency of the Schumann resonance varies as the ionosphere "breathes" in and out owing to atmospheric tides. Scientists have also recognized the similarity of the Schumann signal and the alpha brain wave measured with an electroencephalogram. It has been suggested that the Schumann resonance has been engrained into all life. Biologists have concluded that the frequency overlap of such resonances and biological fields is not an accidental phenomenon.[17]

Grounding and the Immune System

Scientists believe that our immune system evolved in the course of millions of years of barefoot contact with the surface of the Earth. One can assume that protective antioxidant and anti-inflammatory electrons from Earth were readily obtained by previous cultures during this vast stretch of time as a result of ordinary existence. Life involved direct contact with Earth, which is no longer the case. Something changed in our environment, which disconnected us from the natural healing energy of the earth's surface.

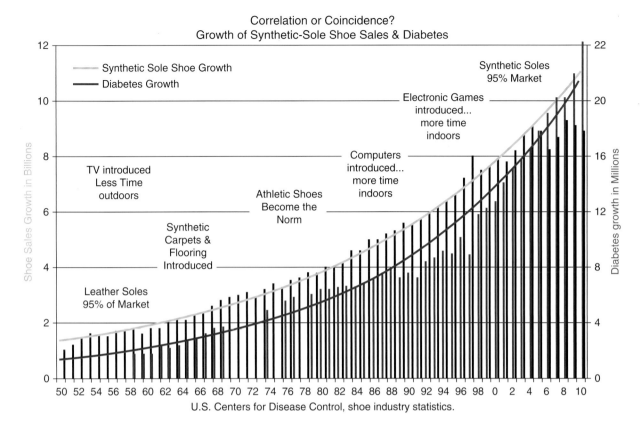

Figure 32.2 *Possible relationship between a shoe-driven disconnection from earth's natural electric charge and diabetes, an inflammatory-related disease.*

An interesting phenomenon has occurred over the last 60 or so years with the parabolic growth of synthetic sole shoes and the growth of diabetes.[17] **Figure 32 2** demonstrates a relationship between the shoe-driven disconnection from earth's natural electric charge and the inflammatory-related disease, diabetes. It is an interesting phenomenon in which sales of shoes with synthetic soles have increased in the United States since the 1950s. The curve of walking on synthetic shoes is similar to the curve of diabetes mellitus. As an antidote, I can remember when I was 8 years old walking to third grade elementary school on leather shoes. That was approximately 64 years ago. Before the mid-1950s, 95% of the shoes were made with leather soles, many of which were conducted to the Schumann resonance. Currently, 95% or more of shoes have synthetic, nonconductive, mostly rubber-like soles. The interesting question, observation, or perhaps coincidence arises. Is there a connection of us being ungrounded walking on nonconductive shoes and the alarming increase in the rise of diabetes as well as other inflammatory situations? Could the combination of foods that are laden with sugar and other high-fructose corn syrup sweeteners in combination with a lack of exercise and being ungrounded, perhaps create the perfect storm for diabetes to emerge? Obviously as a cardiologist, the connection of heart disease and diabetes is significant to say the least. Although diabetes with high blood sugar concentrations is a significant risk factor for CVD, perhaps the diabetic connection of a less optimal blood viscosity is even a more meaningful risk factor to consider.

The electrophoretic activity of red blood cells (RBCs) is a function of net negative charge or zeta potential. In other words, the more the RBCs repel each other, a more robust zeta potential is realized.[4]

In a study of 50 patients with occlusive arterial disease and 50 control counterparts ($N = 100$), the migration time of red cells (seconds) was longer and the electrophoretic mobility (µsec/V/cm) was less in the patients with occlusive disease than in the healthy controls. This study on electrophoretic mobility suggested differences in RBC surface charge (zeta potential). The researchers concluded that patients with occlusive arterial disease have one or more factors in their plasma and RBCs that reduce the net negative charge (zeta potential) of the cells, thereby facilitating RBC aggregation.[19] This finding supports the notion that there are definitely many factors that can reduce zeta potential, and thereby increase blood viscosity and increase RBC aggregation, both of which play a major role in the pathogenesis of arteriosclerosis.

A meta-analysis evaluating the connection between blood viscosity and CVD demonstrates clearly that the risk of major cardiovascular events increase with higher blood viscosity levels.[20] In the Edinburgh Artery Study, a population of 4860 men 45 to 59 years of age was observed for 5 years. The 20% of the men with the highest blood viscosity had a 3.2 times greater risk for cardiac events, compared with the 20% of men with the lowest blood viscosity. About 55% of major cardiovascular events occurred in the highest blood viscosity group versus only 4% in the lowest blood viscosity group.[21]

The role of increased blood viscosity in the pathogenesis of occlusive arterial disease was clearly and succinctly described by Kensey.[22] Endothelial dysfunction, mechanical shear forces, and alterations in blood flow mechanics at arterial bifurcations and areas of low blood flow eddies are correlated with plaque progression in the coronary vasculature. Similarly, blood viscosity is known to increase in a number of clinical situations, such as hypertension, smoking, lipid disorders, advancing age, and diabetes mellitus.

A 2008 study was the first to report on the zeta potential of RBCs in patients with diabetes.[23] Researchers from the University of Calcutta described a "remarkable alteration" in the electrodynamics of RBCs, a progressive deterioration of the zeta potential and hypercoagulability among patients with diabetes, which was even worse among those who also had CVD. The researchers also indicated that high blood sugar levels are associated with significant alterations in the electrodynamics of an RBC's outer membrane and may increase the potential for RBC clumping. It was concluded that zeta potential could and should be used as an indicator of CVD in patients who have diabetes.[23]

Based on a randomized placebo-controlled primary prevention trial (the West of Scotland Coronary Prevention Study), researchers suggested that pravastatin therapy may lower the risk for coronary heart disease and mortality partially by lowering both plasma viscosity and blood viscosity.[24] Many subsequent investigations have demonstrated the pleiotropic effects of statins on blood rheology, including reductions in plasma viscosity,[25] whole-blood viscosity, RBC deformities, and RBC aggregation.[26]

Attenuating inflammation and reducing blood viscosity will help physicians address primary and secondary prevention issues. Blood viscosity can be modified through a number of recognized primary prevention strategies. Moderate exercise, dietary adjustments (low sodium and sugar intake, and no trans fats), smoking cessation, and blood donation all have a positive impact on viscosity as do specific blood viscosity–modifying supplements, such as omega-3 essential fatty acids and pharmaceutical drugs (statins).

Grounding to the earth represents yet another invention that lowers blood viscosity by raising zeta potential, which results in a decrease in RBC aggregation.[4] The Earth's surface is electrically conductive and is maintained at a negative potential by a global electrical circuit. This circuit has three main generators: the solar wind entering the magnetosphere; the ionospheric wind; and thunderstorms. An estimated 1000 to 2000 thunderstorms are continually active around the globe, emitting thousands of lightning strikes per minute. This creates a constant current of thousands of amperes transferring positive charge to the upper atmosphere and negative charge to the surface of the Earth.[27] The Earth's surface is therefore an abundant source of free electrons. As soil electrons are conducted to the human body, the grounded body assumes favorable physiologic and electrophysiologic changes. Attenuation of the inflammatory response and a

favorable impact on blood viscosity and RBC aggregation have been the most significant findings.

Increased blood viscosity in the general population may be a predictor of cardiovascular events because of its influences on hypertension, thrombogenesis, ischemia, and arthrogenesis. Unfortunately, blood viscosity has become a forgotten risk factor and is rarely measured in clinical practice.[28] Interventions that reduce blood viscosity and RBC aggregation are important. Statins appear to be effective for modulating blood viscosity but can have serious side effects, including death. Moreover, many patients have some degree of statin intolerance.[29]

Grounding and Energy

The search for evidence-based improvements without significant risk will continue in the healing arts. It has been suggested that a system-wide network or electronic living matrix, a semiconductor network capable of rapid charge transfer throughout the body, will someday be recognized in the healing profession.[30]

Connective tissues, myofascial, tendons, cell membranes, and cellular cytoskeletal networks belong to this electronic infrastructure. The multiple pathways of this living matrix facilitate the influx of free electrons to reach and neutralize free radicals that are the hallmark of chronic inflammation. Not only that, this arrangement also helps explain why many grounded individuals feel better and more energized. It seems logical to suggest that the influx of electrons from the Earth saturates their mitochondrial electron transport chains that generate adenosine triphosphate (ATP), the energy molecule that powers all of life's activities.

I have always believed in the energetic nature of the contribution of ATP providing the vital energy source for life. As a cardiologist, I have utilized ATP-supporting ingredients such as D-ribose, coenzyme Q10, L-carnitine, and magnesium as a way of biochemically driving ATP in a preferential direction. It is a simple concept, whenever you promote the body's energy source (ATP), you are optimizing the energy production in the heart as well as the body. Although the nutritional approach to improve the bioenergetics of the nutrient-starved heart has been life saving for many of my patients, the concept of grounding also has provided relief as well. Let me explain.

Earthing provides another primary source of cellular restoration and energy. As I mentioned in my previous chapter on Metabolic Cardiology, the mitochondria or microscopic power plants literally provide the energy to the cell.

Inside the mitochondrial complex, electrons are passed along through an assembly line of enzymes creating ATP. When the body comes in contact with the electrons from Mother Earth, the limitless supply of energy is absorbed into the body. Earthing may perhaps be a way to transfer electrons and fortify mitochondria thus contributing to optimum levels of ATP production in all our cells. As I stated in the previous chapter, it has taken most of my cardiology career to discover that the heart is all about ATP and effective healing in any form of CVD requires the restoration of the heart's ATP production. As I mentioned before, sick hearts leak out and lose vital ATP. Any cardiac condition such as angina, heart failure, silent ischemia, mitral valve prolapse, and diastolic dysfunction can also result in some form of ATP deficit. Mother Earth's energy may indeed come to the rescue of vulnerable heart cells.

Grounding or Earthing is virtually harmless while having incredible health implications at the same time. Blood pressure lowering, supportive HRV, and thinning the blood are significant contributions in reducing cardiovascular risk, including myocardial infarction and even sudden cardiac death. One caveat of grounding is to exercise caution in anyone taking Coumadin-like blood thinners as the combination of pharmaceutical blood thinning and grounding can virtually make the blood too thin. Cardiologist's like myself have seen such cases of excessive blood thinning in their patients. It is imperative that patients taking Coumadin-like derivatives discuss earthing or grounding with their doctor to avoid the possibility of any complications.[4]

Summary

New research indicates that grounding the body generates broad, beneficial, and significant physiological changes. The source of these effects is believed to be the mobile electrons omnipresent on the surface of the Earth, which are responsible for the planet's negative charge. Lifestyle changes have disconnected most humans from this primordial health and healing resource, creating what may be an unrecognized electron deficiency in the body, an overlooked cause or contributor to chronic inflammation and common chronic and degenerative diseases. High blood pressure, disturbed HRV, and hyperviscosity are cardiovascular situations that can be improved with grounding.

When Earth connection is restored through grounding, electrons flood throughout the body, reducing inflammation and oxidative stress while also reinforcing the body's own defense mechanisms. Electron transfers are the basis of virtually all antioxidant and anti-inflammatory activity. And Earth may very well be the ultimate supplier! When the supply is restored, humans have the potential to thrive.[4]

Earthing or grounding may someday become one of the everyday tools of the conventional cardiologist. In 2019, it is still in its infancy and more research is presently being done. When we physicians recommend evidence-based, harmless, and simple therapeutic natural interventions to reduce human suffering and improve quality of life, we have done our job in the interest of the patient. After all, as Dr Peabody stated almost a century ago, "The most important aspect in the care of the patient is the care of the patient."[31]

References

1. Elkin H, Winter A. Grounding patients with hypertension improves blood pressure: a case history series study. *Altern Therapies*. 2019. In press.
2. Ghaly M, Teplitz D. The biological effects of grounding the human body during sleep, as measured by cortisol levels and subjective reporting of sleep, pain, and stress. *J Altern Complement Med*. 2004;10(5):767-776.
3. Chavalier G, Sinatra ST. Emotional stress, heart rate variability, grounding and improved autonomic tone: clinical applications. *Integ Med*. 2011;10(3):16-21.
4. Chevalier G, Sinatra ST, Oschman JL, et al. Earthing (grounding) the human body reduces blood viscosity – a major factor in cardiovascular disease. *J Altern Complement Med*. 2013;19(2):102-110.
5. Kleiger RE, Bigger JT, Bosner MS, et al. Stability over time of variables measuring heart rate variability in normal subjects. *Am J Cardiol*. 1991;68(6):626-630.
6. Kawachi I, Colditz GA, Asherio A, et al. Prospective study of phobic anxiety and risk of coronary heart disease in men. *Circulation*. 1994;89(5):1992-1997.
7. Carney RM, Freedland KE. Depression and heart rate variability in patients with coronary heart disease. *Cleve Clin J Med*. 2009;76(suppl 2):S13-S17.
8. Sloan RP, Shapiro PA, Bigger JT Jr, et al. Cardiac autonomic control and hostility in healthy subjects. *Am J Cardiol*. 1994;74(3):298-300.
9. Yeragani VK, Pohl R, Berger R. Decreased heart rate variability in panic disorder patients: a study of power-spectral analysis of heart rate. *Psychiatry Res*. 1993;46(1):89-103.
10. Passi R, Doheny KK, Gordin Y, et al. Electrical grounding improves vagal tone in preterm infants. *Neonatology*. 2017;112(2):187-192.
11. Thayer J. Vagal tone and the inflammatory reflex. *Cleve Clin J Med*. 2009;76(suppl 2):S23-S26.
12. Schoemaker R, Eisel U. Chapter 5: cross talk between the brain and inflammation. In: Blankesteijn M, Altara R, eds. *Inflammation in Heart Failure*. Boston: Academic Press;2015:81-91.
13. Sokal K, Sokal P. Earthing the human body influences physiologic processes. *J Altern Complement Med*. 2011;17(4):301-308.
14. Williams E, Heckman S. The local diurnal variation of cloud electrification and the global diurnal variation of negative charge on the Earth. *J Geophys Res*. 1993;98(D3):5221-5234.
15. Anisimov S, Mareev E, Bakastov S. On the generation and evolution of aeroelectric structures in the surface layer. *J Geophy Res*. 1999;104(D12):14359-14367.
16. Oschman J. Perspective: assume a spherical cow: the role of free or mobile electrons in bodywork, energetic and movement therapies. *J Bodywork Movement Ther*. 2008;12:40-57.
17. Sinatra ST, Oschman JL, Chevelier G, Sinatra D. Electric nutrition: the surprising health and healing benefits of biological grounding (earthing). *Altern Ther*. 2017;23(5):8-16.
18. Palmer JD. *The Living Clock: The Orchestrator of Biological Rhythms*. Oxford, United Kingdom: Oxford University Press; 2002.
19. Begg TB, Wade IM, Bronte-Stewart B. The red cell electrophoretic mobility in atherosclerotic and other individuals. *J Atheroscler Res*. 1966;6:303-312.
20. Danesh J, Collins R, Peto R, et al. Haematocrit, viscosity, erythrocyte sedimentation rate: meta-analysis of prospective studies of coronary heart disease. *Eur Heart J*. 2000;21:515-520. Comment in *Eur Heart J*. 2000;21:513-514.
21. Lowe GD, Lee AJ, Rumley A, et al. Blood viscosity and risk of cardiovascular events: the Edinburgh Artery Study. *Br J Haematol*. 1997;96:168-173.
22. Kensey KR. Rheology: an overlooked component of vascular disease. *Clin Appl Thromb/hemostasis*. 2003;9:93-99.
23. Adak S, Chowdhury S, Bhattacharyya M. Dynamic and electrokinetic behavior of erythrocyte membrane in diabetes mellitus and diabetic cardiovascular disease. *Biochim Biophys Acta*. 2008;1780:108-115.
24. Lowe G, Rumley A, Norrie J, et al. Blood rheology, cardiovascular risk factors, and cardiovascular disease: the West of Scotland Coronary Prevention Study. *Thromb Haemost*. 2001;85:946.

25. Doncheva NI, Nikolov KV, Vassileva DP. Lipid-modifying and pleiotropic effects of gemfibrozil, simvastatin, and pravastatin in patient in patients with dyslipidemia. *Folia Med (Plodiv)*. 2006;48(3-4):56-61.

26. Muravyov AV, Yakusevick VV, Surovaya L, et al. The effect of simvastatin therapy on hemorheological profile in coronary heart disease (CHD) patients. *Clin Hemorheol Microcirc*. 2004;31:251-256.

27. Volland H. Atmospheric electrodynamics. In: Lanzerotti LJ, ed. *Physics and Chemistry in Space*. Vol 11. Berlin & New York: Springer-Verlag; 1984.

28. Kesmarky G, Kenyeres P, Rabai M, et al. Plasma viscosity: a forgotten variable. *Clin Hemorheol Micro*. 2008;39(1-4):243-246.

29. Golomb BA, Evans MA. Statin adverse effects: a review of the literature and evidence for a mitochondrial mechanism. *Am J Cardiovasc Drugs*. 2008;8:373-418.

30. Oschman J. Charge transfer in the living matrix. *J Bodywork Movement Ther*. 2009;13:215-228.

31. Peabody FW. The care of the patient. *JAMA*. 1927;88(12):877-882.

33

Depression, Anxiety, Stress, and Spirituality in Cardiovascular Disease

Mimi Guarneri, MD, FACC and Shyamia Stone, ND, MPH

Introduction

The human heart is notoriously understood as the life-giving organ of the body. With each contraction, it sends blood and nourishment to every organ and every cell of the body. As medical professionals, we are taught about the structure and function of the heart, its capacity for disease, and its centrality to life. However, across medical and cultural traditions, the heart is given many connotations outside of its cardiovascular functions. The heart is seen as the seat of the soul, of love, pain, and general emotion. Colloquialisms such as "follow your heart" and "brokenhearted" call to mind reminiscences of intuition and emotion, evoking memories and feelings in those who hear these phrases.

It is easy for medical professionals to discount the emotional connotations of the heart as mutually exclusive concepts or social folklore, but this interconnectedness of heart, body, mind, and soul has been described by medical practitioners for hundreds of years. Traditional Chinese Medicine (TCM) discusses a connection between diseases of the heart and excess stimulation; however, it is known in TCM that all emotions affect the heart, including sadness, grief, worry, fear, pensiveness, and anger.[1] Ancient Grecian physicians saw cardiovascular disease (CVD) as a manifestation of emotion and psychological disorder, and in 1937 there was a scientific correlation noted between CVD outcomes and psychological pathology, noting an increase in cardiovascular-related deaths in those with depression.[2,3]

Medical knowledge and literature have illustrated many structural, biochemical, and genetic etiological mechanisms of CVD. Although these are important, it is necessary to look past each of these segregated components at the whole person when attempting to paint a complete picture of underlying risk factors and comorbidities. An individual's biology does not exist in isolation of his or her surroundings, but rather within an internal and external milieu. From a public health perspective, it is possible to see the numerous ways that environment and lifestyle factors play a role in health outcomes. We see components such as toxic exposures,[4,5] nutrition, and exercise[6,7] as impacting physiology and being linked to CVD risk, although an often-overlooked part of one's environment is external stressors and internal responses, along with other mental emotional states.

Although the connections between mind and body can be seen anecdotally, we also now know that mental-emotional and psychological states contribute to physiology through very real neurotransmitter and biochemical pathways that impact pathology and/or resilience. Depression and anxiety are emotional and physiological results of various types of stress that span from the biochemical to environmental.

Purpose of the Chapter

This chapter will outline what is known about depression, anxiety, and stress as pathological states and their connection with CVD. We will then present integrative medicine treatments including conventional therapies, nutrition, lifestyle, herbal, and mind-body mechanisms. It will show the ways in which it is imperative to address depression, anxiety, stress, and CVD both symptomatically and through identifying the root cause on the levels of mind, body, and spirit.

Depression

Depression in its broadest reach may be understood as a state of being that spans from a fleeting emotional experience or mood to that of a more long-term pathological state. People often experience depressed mood as feelings of sadness, despair, emptiness, or discouragement with associated rumination and fixation on the past. When sadness is experienced as an emotion, it is important that it is acknowledged as a normal part of the human experience, allowed to be expressed and not suppressed. However, if this state continues and is accompanied by other features, it is possible for depression to cross over into a state of pathology.

According to the Diagnostic and Statistical Manual of Mental Disorders (DSM-5), depression as a disorder may be classified as Disruptive Mood Dysregulation Disorder, Major Depressive Disorder, Persistent Depressive Disorder (Dysthymia), or Depressive Disorder Due to Another Medical Condition.[8] The most commonly studied clinical diagnosis of depression related to CVD is Major Depressive Disorder (MDD). Although the DSM-5[8] is the gold standard in diagnosis of depressive disorders and is utilized extensively by mental health professionals, depression is often identified in medical offices through a variety of self-report measures (Table 33.1). These instruments provide information about the severity of depressive symptoms based on the frequency, severity, and impact on quality of life. Each of these measures simplify DSM criteria for self-report format and provide an estimated guideline of level of depression that may include categories such as normal/not depressed, mild, borderline, moderate, or severe depression.[9-12] A measure specifically for cardiac patients has been developed that also assesses specific presentations of depression that may occur after a cardiovascular incident, including concern about health and recovery, feeling as if one is changed after their incident, fear or dread of impending health issues or dying, and loss of independence or function.[13]

The fact that a measure has been created for patients who have cardiac concerns shows that the presentation of depression may vary between patients and comorbidities. It is important to recognize symptoms of depression in patients even if they do not fit the criteria for diagnosis of MDD. It is not necessary for a patient to have MDD to be at risk for depressive symptoms contributing to CVD, as depressive symptoms in themselves have been correlated with adverse cardiac outcomes.[14,15]

From an etiological standpoint, studies have determined that patients with depression have twice the risk of developing new-onset CVD.[16] Depression is also correlated with greater mortality in patients with a history of acute myocardial infarction (MI), with depressed patients having three times increased incidence of mortality post-MI than patients who are not depressed.[16] These outcomes are not related only to the presence or absence of depression, as the 5-year mortality rate has been correlated with the severity of depression.[17] Interestingly, MDD is noted as the second leading cause of disability in America, behind ischemic heart disease, which ranks number one,[18] although arguably, these could be varying manifestations of related disease processes, which will be discussed in the pathophysiology section.

As depression exists on a continuum from normal emotion to pathology, with variations in clinical presentation, the etiology of depression is still being discovered with potential for differing mechanisms at work in each of the presenting criteria.[19] Perhaps the most comprehensive integrative view is the biopsychosocial model of depression, which shows a multifactorial etiology including genetics,[19] biochemistry, cognition, personality traits, environmental factors, trauma,[20] and social interactions.[21] Pathophysiological features of depression can include structural and functional brain changes as witnessed through neuroimaging studies,[22,23] specifically showing reduction of dopamine network responses in the brain.[22] Overall, MDD is thought to be due to deficiencies of dopamine, serotonin, and/or norepinephrine, which may occur concurrently or may lead into one another.[24]

Anxiety

Overlap Between Anxiety and Depression

When discussing anxiety and depression, it is difficult to draw a clear line where one ends and the other begins. There is a high level of comorbidity between depression and anxiety, even in their clinical forms of MDD and Generalized Anxiety Disorder (GAD). In fact, it has been hypothesized that MDD and GAD may be different presentations of the same disorder.[25] Comorbidity rates between MDD and GAD range from 40% to 98%, with 67% of individuals with GAD reporting MDD at some point in their lives and 20% of individuals with MDD reporting GAD in the past.[26] A common component between the disorders is that of general distress, yet uniquely differentiating components are that of excessive worry in GAD and anhedonia in MDD.[26] In addition to common features, there also appears to be shared etiological factors, including similar genetics,[27] and the trait of neuroticism that predisposes for both depression and anxiety.[26] Appearance of comorbidity may also be due to overlap in the diagnostic criteria for disorders such as MDD and GAD.[28] Regardless, both depression and anxiety have been shown to be correlated with CVD.

Table 33.1

SCREENING MEASURES FOR DEPRESSION AND ANXIETY

Depression	Patient Health Questionnaire (PHQ-9)[9]
	Beck Depression Inventory (BDI)[11]
	Hospital Anxiety Depression Scale (HADS)
	Center for Epidemiologic Studies Depression Scale-10 (CES-10)[10]
	Cardiac Depression Scale[13]
Anxiety	Generalized Anxiety Disorder (GAD-7) questionnaire[31]
Depression and Anxiety	Patient Health Questionnaire Anxiety and Depression Scale (PHQ-ADS)[32]

Defining Anxiety

As with depression, anxiety exists on a spectrum from that of a mental-emotional state, or a trait, to that of a psychological disorder.[29] A *state* of anxiety is fleeting and is experienced as a momentary fear of a potential threat.[30] This heightened emotional state can be a healthy part of the human experience, leading to motivation and vigilance when situationally necessary. Anxiety can also be in response to a positive event, manifesting as the stimulation of excitement. An individual with *trait* anxiety is predisposed to experience an anxious state of fear and/or apprehension about distant and potential threats as opposed to real ones.[30] When this experience transcends into inappropriate situations and adopts a state of chronicity, anxiety can become a psychological *disorder* with an impact on daily functioning.

Anxiety Disorders as outlined in the DSM-5 include Separation Anxiety Disorder, Phobias, Social Anxiety Disorder, Panic Disorder, Agoraphobia, and Generalized Anxiety Disorder. The two disorders that have been the most extensively studied in conjunction with CVD are GAD and Panic Disorder (PD).[8]

Trait forms of anxiety may be screened in a clinical setting through use of self-report measures, which has primarily consisted of the Generalized Anxiety Disorder (GAD-7) questionnaire.[31] However, recently, a combined measure called the Patient Health Questionnaire Anxiety and Depression Scale (PHQ-ADS) has been created to combine PHQ-9 and GAD-7 into one measure.[32] Although the PHQ-ADS is still in its initial validation phase, it shows promise as an initial screening tool because of the overlap between anxiety and depression.

The etiology of anxiety appears to be multifactorial including inheritance, biological processes, and environmental risk factors. Some individuals with anxiety show genetic predisposition for dysregulation of serotonin[33] and glutamic acid decarboxylase.[34] Disturbances of neurotransmitters norepinephrine, serotonin, and gamma aminobutyric acid (GABA) have also been associated with GAD.[22] Although there are widely varying experiences of anxiety that are reflected in the spectrum of state, trait, or disorder, functional magnetic resonance imaging data have shown similar neurological networks in the brain that are activated across all forms of anxiety.[30] Areas of activation correspond with heightened amygdala responses and overall greater emotional responsiveness.[35] Additional environmental risk factors associated with development of GAD include a greater incidence of trauma throughout life and adverse childhood events.[36]

Clinical presentation of anxiety may appear through emotional complaints that can be assessed through the above-mentioned DSM-5 criteria or GAD-7 assessment. However, anxiety may also present as physical symptoms such as sleep disturbance, fatigue, difficulty relaxing, muscle tension (especially in the neck, shoulders, and back), and recurrent headaches.[37] It is important as a practitioner to keep anxiety in the differential diagnosis when these physical symptoms present.

Stress

Psychological stress is defined as a perceived tension or worry that impacts an individual's behaviors and ability to traverse life events.[38] In many ways, depression and anxiety are both manifestations of chronic stress and occur either as a result of the interplay of stress with the above-mentioned etiological factors or lead to a physiological state that simulates chronic stress in the body.[38]

Stressors

The term "stress" has also been used to describe stressors themselves, those things that one encounters that incite a stressful response. Humans exist in a context of a complex interplay of factors including internal environment, social environment, and physical environment. Stressors may exist in any of these arenas, thereby increasing the strain put on the body's systems to come back to a point of balance, which has been termed "allostasis."[39] The concept of allostasis illustrates the way in which the body has an active regulatory process to maintain physiological balance and adapt to changing needs utilizing physiological responses such as hormones, temperature changes, and blood pressure.[40] Therefore, it is possible to see that stressors have a direct impact on physiology through the body's mechanisms to perceive these events, react, and then compensate in attempt to preserve balance. There are times when balance is unable to be achieved, and this is referred to as "allostatic load," a state wherein the normal balancing processes are overtaxed or fail to act, leading to a lack of adaptation and dysregulation of the physiological systems that are in flux in response to stressors.[41] These systems include the autonomic nervous system, hypothalamic-pituitary-adrenal (HPA) axis, sympathetic nervous system, and immune system.[41]

Stressors may be acute or chronic and may vary between individuals based on their perceptions of what is and is not stress. Acute stressors are encountered on a daily basis in small doses, such as having to complete tasks of daily living. They may also come in response to unexpected life changes in health, family, home, or livelihood. Acute stressors can negatively impact individuals, although chronic stressors appear to have a greater cumulative burden on the body's ability to allostatically adjust. Chronic stressors have been shown to include low social support, low socioeconomic status, occupational stress, marital or relationship stress, and caregiver strain.[15]

Pathophysiology

As there is considerable overlap in the underlying processes of depression, anxiety, and stress, it makes sense that the mechanisms that correlate these emotional states/pathologies to CVD also share similarities. There is a two-fold interaction between the mental-emotional states of depression, anxiety, and stress and the physical manifestation of CVD, including both biological and behavioral mechanisms. Much of the literature regarding depression, anxiety, and chronic stress are unable to control for comorbidities, and thus mechanisms of interaction with the cardiovascular system appear to be mostly similar across these mental emotional states, although exceptions are elucidated in the following text.

Biological Mechanisms

INFLAMMATION

Inflammation is a complex process that involves the immune system's response to potentially harmful stimuli, which triggers the signaling of various cytokines and chemokines to create a variety of protective responses within the body.[42] However, when inflammatory processes are systemic, the attempt at homeostasis can lead to an increased risk of CVD. Inflammation is a common thread that appears to connect depression, anxiety, and CVD.

Various reviews have shown inflammation as a major underlying causal factor for depression,[43,44] anxiety,[45] and CVD.[46] Xiong and colleagues found that patients with MDD and congestive heart failure (CHF) had statistically significant higher levels of inflammatory markers than patients without MDD and CHF. Elevated serum markers in depression included cytokines interleukin (IL)-1, IL-4, IL-6, IL-17, interferon (IFN)-gamma, macrophage inflammatory protein (MIP)-1, and tumor necrosis factor (TNF)-alpha.[44] The Third National Health and Nutrition Examination Study had also revealed a higher serum C-reactive protein (CRP) in patients with MDD,[47] a marker that is highly correlated with CVD risk.[48] Elevated proinflammatory cytokines have also been found in patients with anxiety, as Godbout and Glaser[38] found increased levels of IL-6 and CRP in patients who were experiencing chronic stress. Inflammatory cytokines have been found to increase autonomic imbalance, stimulate the sympathetic nervous system, cause electrical instability in the myocardium, depress cardiac function, lead to endothelial dysfunction, cause vasoconstriction, and generate atherosclerosis.[46]

Interestingly, Steenkamp and colleagues[49] evaluated oxidative stress levels (measured by F2-isoprostanes and oxidized glutathione) in patients with MDD and found that the symptoms of *anxiety* that the patients experienced were more closely correlated with oxidative stress than the symptoms of depression. Oxidative stress negatively impacts cell membranes, proteins, nucleic acids, and lipids[49] and has also been correlated with exacerbation of symptoms of anxiety and hypertension.[45] This again shows the difficulty in disambiguating between the influence of anxiety and depression in pathogenesis of CVD, as outcomes may be symptom related as opposed to diagnosis related, and multidirectional.

PLATELET ACTIVATION

Increased inflammation may also be correlated with greater platelet activation that is found in depressed patients with CVD, leading to an increased risk of coronary artery occlusion.[50] Depression has been associated with a hyperactive platelet 5-HT2A receptor signal transduction system, which

leads to increased thrombosis.[29] Pronounced platelet activation has been associated not only with depression but also chronic stress and anxiety symptoms.[51]

AUTONOMIC DYSFUNCTION

Depression and anxiety may also be correlated with CVD through their influence on altering autonomic vascular tone. This has been most directly studied through the concept of heart rate variability (HRV). HRV is a measurement of R-R intervals and the cyclic variation that reflects autonomic balance between sympathetic and parasympathetic nervous system activity.[52] Autonomic nervous system imbalance comprising increased sympathetic nervous system activation with decreased vagal tone has been correlated with CVD and risk of adverse cardiac events,[52] through such mechanisms as triggering atherosclerosis and/or platelet aggregation and leading to changes in lipid metabolism.[53] Low HRV is related to poor cardiac outcomes and an increased risk of post-MI mortality[54] and is correlated with sudden cardiac death even in those who have not been diagnosed with CVD.[55] But what causes lower HRV? Mental emotional states have been shown to have a large impact on HRV, with lower HRV in patients with coronary artery disease who are depressed,[54] as well as patients who present with anxiety.[55]

HPA AXIS DYSFUNCTION

Because HRV is a description of the sympathetic and parasympathetic nervous system balance, it is no surprise that we would see a connection between depression, anxiety, and the HPA axis. Various studies have shown increased levels of cortisol in individuals with both depression[53,55,56] and anxiety,[38] illustrating a correlation between HPA axis activation and emotional disorders.

Elevated cortisol leads to an increased risk of insulin resistance, central obesity, and hyperlipidemia, which are well known risk factors for CVD.[29,53] Other catecholamines such as norepinephrine have also been shown to be increased in depression[57,58] and chronic stress.[51] Increased catecholamine levels have been found to cause damage to cardiac myocytes[59] and lead to apoptosis of ventricular myocytes,[60] thereby increasing the risk of adverse cardiac outcomes.[57] Chronic HPA axis activation has been shown to decrease immune function and impact susceptibility to infection, as well as increase proinflammatory cytokines, feeding back into the inflammatory cycle.[29]

ENDOTHELIAL DYSFUNCTION

Endothelial dysfunction is the earliest indicator of vascular disease leading to atherosclerosis and adverse cardiac events including aneurysm, ischemia, and infarction. A study by van Sloten and colleagues[61] illustrates a much greater level of endothelial dysfunction in elderly individuals with depression even after adjusting for those with CVD, whereas a study by Stillman and colleagues[62] showed that anxiety decreased endothelial function and vascular smooth muscle function in individuals with atherosclerosis, even in the absence of depression. Endothelial dysfunction caused by depression and anxiety may lead to even worse prognostic outcomes in CVD.

CARDIOVASCULAR REACTIVITY

On encountering stressors, the cardiovascular system has various compensatory mechanisms to increase perceived need. Anxiety and chronic stress have been hypothesized to increase cardiac reactivity resulting in alteration of cardiovascular mechanisms. For example, individuals with anxiety have increases in resting heart rate, dysfunction in the baroreflex, and variability in ventricular repolarization.[29] All of these mechanisms increase the risk of cardiovascular events.

ACUTE EMOTIONAL EFFECTS

Although chronic depression, anxiety, and stress are shown to impact CVD through the various mechanisms described earlier, it is also possible for there to be acute effects in response to sudden emotional stress. Individuals with underlying coronary artery disease may experience adverse effects from hemodynamic stress including disrupting an atherosclerotic plaque that leads to thrombus,[29] whereas another phenomenon that may occur in patients without known CVD is intense, sudden emotional stress triggering the onset of myocardial stunning.[63,64] This phenomenon has been thought to be related to increased activation of the sympathoneural and adrenomedullary systems and has been termed acute myocardial stunning, left ventricular apical ballooning syndrome, takotsubo cardiomyopathy, or broken heart syndrome.[64] An increase in cardiac events was seen following the terrorist attack on the World Trade Center on September 11, 2001. On the date of this event, intakes at the New York Methodist Hospital Telemetry and Coronary Care units reported significantly higher rates of acute MI (4.3% elevation) and tachyarrhythmia (6.3% elevation).[65] Natural disasters such as earthquakes are associated with an increased incidence of MI and cardiac mortality. A review by Bazoukis and colleagues[66] also demonstrated an increase in acute coronary syndrome after several large scale earthquakes, including Christchurch, Great East Japan, Niigata-Chuetsu, Northridge, Great Hanshin-Awaji, Sichuan, Athens, Armenia, and Noto Peninsula.

Behavioral Mechanisms

Although there are known biological correlates between depression, anxiety, chronic stress, and CVD, these emotional states have many effects on behaviors. In depression, this occurs primarily through neglect of self-care and difficulty adhering to treatment protocols, including medication adherence and lifestyle recommendations. In a study performed by Ziegelstein and colleagues,[67] within a hospital setting, patients who were found to have depression (spanning from mild depression to MDD or dysthymia) showed lower adherence to treatment protocols, including low-fat diet, exercise, stress reduction, and increasing social support. Additionally, those patients who had MDD took all prescribed medications less consistently.[67]

In patients with anxiety, there is also neglect of self-care, including tendencies toward lower physical activity and unhealthy eating.[29] In depression, these behaviors are related to neglect and apathy, whereas in persons with anxiety they appear to be primarily due to avoidance of situations that cause worry.[29] There are also additive behaviors of self-medication that serve as risk factors for CVD, such as cigarette smoking, excess alcohol consumption,[68] and overeating.[69]

Prevention and Screening

In patients with known CVD, it is important to perform screenings for emotional disorders of depression, anxiety, and chronic stress. It is possible to utilize the self-report screening measures mentioned previously (**Table 33.1**) or work in collaboration with a mental health professional to determine patient risk. Although these measures may provide information regarding a patient's emotional state, they can be impersonal, and owing to the stigma of mental health concerns, patients are not always forthcoming in this format. It is important to develop a positive relationship with the patient to facilitate trust and openness, while allowing the practitioner to attend to underlying emotional concerns.

Conversely, there is controversy regarding whether all patients with CVD should be screened for depression and anxiety, owing to potential for overdiagnosis and overtreatment in a clinical setting. It is debatable whether psychotherapy and pharmacotherapy for depression and anxiety help to mitigate CVD risk, and overtreatment may result in adverse cardiovascular side effects.[70,71] It is therefore important to aim for prevention through integrative therapies, which are described in detail later.

Because the connections between depression, anxiety, chronic stress, and CVD are multidimensional and multidirectional, there are many treatment approaches that can be taken. We will begin by discussing the conventional mitigation of comorbid mental health disorders and CVD and then expand to discuss less invasive, integrative modalities to target the underlying factors that lead to these states.

Treatment

Conventional Treatment

For many patients with CVD, signs of depression and anxiety go unnoticed until after they have experienced a cardiac event. Therefore, mitigation of this comorbidity and interplay has been studied in hospital settings and specialized cardiology care. One method of treatment of depression and anxiety in CVD involves planned collaborative care, which includes screening for mental health disorders in cardiac patients, and subsequent provision of adjunctive care between cardiologists and mental health professionals or nurses.[72,73] Several trials of this method have shown significant reductions in depression, as well as other cardiac risk factors (eg, low-density lipoprotein [LDL] cholesterol, blood pressure).[72-74] Most of the studies done in this setting have focused on depression as it is the most highly correlated with adverse cardiac outcomes, but very few have looked specifically at anxiety or chronic stress. There are potential barriers to screening anxiety in an acute care setting because many anxiety symptoms can be cardiac in nature, such as heart palpitations, tachycardia, and chest pressure.[29] Some patients having panic attacks may also perceive that they are having a MI, as it is suspected that up to 25% of patients presenting to the emergency department for symptoms of MI may be experiencing a panic attack, although it is rarely diagnosed.[75]

Conventional mental health treatment that is used in the collaborative care setting is a combination of psychotherapy and pharmacotherapy. Psychotherapy generally takes place in the form of Cognitive Behavioral Therapy (CBT) performed by a mental health professional, which focuses on identifying and altering thoughts and behaviors that lead to depression and/or anxiety,[58] or Interpersonal Therapy, which involves identifying problematic social situations and developing increased social skills to mitigate depression or anxiety.[76] Although these are considered safe and effective, there is a risk that symptoms may increase through increasing awareness of negative thoughts,[58] but this form of therapy is still considered standard of care in the treatment of depression and anxiety and safe for those with comorbid CVD.

It has been recommended that pharmacotherapy for individuals with CVD should start with first-line selective serotonin reuptake inhibitors (SSRIs) such as citalopram or sertraline.[58] Although effectiveness of SSRIs is similar across types, citalopram and sertraline have fewer interactions with cytochrome p450 and subsequently are less likely to cause pharmacokinetic interactions with cardiac medication.[58] However, SSRIs are contraindicated when used in conjunction with other medications that lead to QT interval prolongation.[77] In a review by Von Ruden and colleagues[78] evaluating the association between SSRIs and cardiovascular risk, of 13 studies evaluated, 5 showed decreased cardiovascular morbidity or mortality with use of SSRIs, 2 showed worsened prognosis, and 6 found no association. One of the few positive and well-known studies, Sertraline Against Depression and Heart Disease in Chronic Heart Failure (SADHART) specifically evaluated the use of sertraline as an antidepressant agent and its impact on CHF. Results ultimately found that, of the 44.3% of patients with remittance of depression, there were significantly fewer cardiovascular events in comparison with the 41.4% that did not achieve remission, although the latter group was determined to have a greater severity of depression at baseline.[79] Therefore, it appears that remission of depression is most strongly associated with improved cardiovascular outcomes, and although SSRIs can assist in some cases, there is room for alternative therapies.

Other pharmaceutical agents may also be employed; for example, bupropion may be an effective alternative in patients who are sensitive to side effects of SSRIs or who are attempting smoking cessation.[58] However, tricyclic antidepressants have been associated with adverse cardiac events and should be avoided in patients with CVD.[58] Although

there are many alternatives to pharmaceuticals as outlined subsequently, if there is a need to treat with psychopharmacological agents, there are tools that have been developed to assist in mitigating adverse reactions. Pharmacogenetic testing sequences a patient's DNA in regards to specific drug metabolism and adverse effects, helping to select safe and effective pharmacological treatment of an individual patient, avoiding both undesirable side effects and the need for multidrug therapies.[80]

Integrative Treatment

Although conventional treatment may be helpful for some individuals to manage symptoms and progression of risk associated with depression and CVD, integrative medical modalities should be employed to target underlying causes of pathology. There are myriad options to target common etiological factors of depression, anxiety, and CVD as well as interventions to prevent progression of CVD due to depression, anxiety, or chronic stress. These range from nutrition to supplements and herbs and lifestyle alterations.

DIET

One of the behavioral factors underlying depression, anxiety, and impact on CVD involves the difficulty of adhering to self-care and dietary changes. Depression has been specifically correlated with anhedonia, or the inability to experience pleasure. Subsequently, the dopaminergic reward pathways that are often associated with changing behaviors are not activated, resulting in much lower motivation to exert extra effort for little-to-no feeling of reward.[22] Despite this inability to feel pleasure, when given sucrose solutions, depressed patients show enjoyment and preference for sweet solutions, indicating that the pleasure response is still possible.[22] Because depressed patients have very little motivation or ability to experience reward, yet still experience pleasure from consumption of sugar, it is certainly difficult to impact positive dietary changes.

Correspondingly, anxiety processes also impact reward processing through different mechanisms. Individuals with anxiety who are experiencing acute stress or feelings of threat show blunted responses to reward.[22] Brain imaging studies have shown that acute stress causes a reduction in neural reward responses, thus altering reward circuitry.[22]

Although dietary changes are difficult to enact for patients with depression and anxiety, they are important to mitigate the progression of these disorders and CVD. It may not come as a surprise that the Western diet consisting of processed/fried foods, refined grains, and sugary products has been shown to increase the risk of depression and anxiety.[81-83] Hypoglycemia and poor blood sugar control has also been linked with increased cortisol in anxiety disorders,[84] and the very-low-carbohydrate diet in certain individuals may potentiate depression.[85]

Most studies show that the diet that mitigates depression risk most is characteristically anti-inflammatory, with an emphasis on whole foods, specifically vegetables rich in folate, olive oil, fish, nuts, and legumes.[81,86] This is essentially the Mediterranean Diet, a diet that has been touted for cardiovascular health for many years.[87,88] The idea behind the Mediterranean Diet is that it contains foods with anti-inflammatory properties, making it fairly similar to the Anti-Inflammatory Diet. The Anti-Inflammatory Diet emphasizes finding the forms of macronutrients that are the least inflammatory: increasing omega-3 fatty acids and decreasing omega-6 fatty acids and saturated fats, having lower amounts of high-glycemic carbohydrates in the diet to avoid excess insulin production, and overall consumption of fewer calories.[89] Based on the common mechanism of inflammation underlying depression, anxiety, chronic stress, and CVD, it would follow that focusing on reduction of inflammation is a large component of reducing cardiac risk.

However, the more we learn about individual processing of foods, the more it is clear that diets are not one-size-fits-all, or even specific to a particular health concern. It is possible for the body to develop an immunological response to foods, leading to food intolerances and food sensitivities. These reactions have been found to increase inflammation[90] and activate immune cells, such as mast cells.[91] Food sensitivities and intolerances have been linked with a variety of health issues and symptoms that include depression and anxiety.[70,92] Although randomized control trials performed regarding food intolerances or sensitivities as correlated with anxiety and depression are limited, clinical experience suggests that an elimination diet impacts symptoms owing to a reduction in inflammation. However, with any restrictive diet, it is important to monitor patient anxiety levels, as it is possible that prescribing a restrictive diet may actually exacerbate anxiety symptoms.

Because dietary changes are so difficult for depressed individuals to undertake, there are solutions that the practitioner can employ to help make these changes more tangible. Dietary recommendations should be individualized for patients based on their level of functioning and motivation and accompanied by easy recipes, lists of healthful prepared foods from local stores and restaurants, and use of medical food or meal replacement powders to assist in lowering the threshold of effort required for patients to be successful. Patient buy-in is extremely important; allowing them to be a part of creating their plan has been shown to increase outcomes.[73]

An underutilized resource to assist patients with CVD in making behavioral changes is secondary prevention programs such as cardiac rehabilitation. Most cardiac rehabilitation programs focus on nutritional education, physician-supervised exercise, stress management, and group support,[93,94] although traditional cardiac rehabilitation programs have the greatest emphasis on exercise. Intensive cardiac rehabilitation programs, such as the Ornish Lifestyle Medicine program and the Pritikin program, provide greater focus on all of the components listed earlier and have been shown to influence favorable outcomes such as reducing angina, body mass index, systolic blood pressure, total cholesterol, LDL cholesterol, and blood glucose.[93]

The Ornish program has also been shown to reverse coronary artery disease, showing the tremendous impact of lifestyle medicine on cardiac rehabilitation.[93-95] Programs such as this could be especially impactful for individuals with depression and anxiety that can benefit from the additional support to implement lifestyle changes accompanied by a social support system.

GUT HEALTH

Research on the "gut brain axis" is shedding light on the role of the microbiome in health. Changes in the gut microbiome have been linked to metabolic disorders such as obesity, diabetes,[96] depression, and anxiety.[97] The composition of the microbiome is dependent on many factors such as inoculation of bacteria at birth, hormone levels, and exposure to various strains of bacteria throughout one's life. However, the gut microbiome is also closely linked with diet and responds quickly to dietary changes.[97] Animal studies have shown that inoculation with Western diets and certain dietary carbohydrates can alter the microbiome within the first 24 hours after consumption.[96] Although this emphasizes the need for a balanced diet high in plant foods that serve as prebiotics, it also emphasizes the potential benefit of analyzing an individual's gut microbiome to determine areas of overgrowth or depletion. Stool testing allows for sequencing of the microbiome and identification of pathogenic bacterial strains, as well as showing inflammation and digestive by-products, thereby determining if patients are absorbing the nutrients that they are consuming. In functional medicine, there is a gut repair protocol called the "5 R Framework for Gut Restoration," which follows a sequence of steps including remove, replace, repair, reinoculate, and rebalance, to heal the gut and the microbiome.[98]

NUTRIENT THERAPY

Because depression and anxiety are frequently linked to poor food choices and microbiome imbalance, it is not uncommon to find significant nutrient deficiencies. In cases of malabsorption, practitioners may consider short-term implementation of intravenous nutrient therapy to bypass the gastrointestinal tract and deliver nutrients to achieve therapeutic dosages. Nutrient deficiencies should also be monitored to determine if they are impacting depression or anxiety. Depression has been associated with a multitude of nutrient deficiencies, including thiamine, riboflavin, niacin, biotin, pantothenic acid, vitamin B6, folic acid, vitamin B12, vitamin C,[70] and vitamin D.[99] Both depression and anxiety have also been correlated with iron-deficiency anemia.[100,101] Subsequently, a general nutrient evaluation should be included in the evaluation of patients with depression and/or anxiety and CVD. In addition to any nutrients that may be deficient, there are important nutrients that have been shown to work therapeutically to impact depression and anxiety; these are highlighted in the following text.

Fatty Acids

Omega-3 fatty acids in concentrations up to 9.6 g/d have been found to reduce symptoms of depression.[102,103] It appears that the eicosapentaenoic acid concentration correlates more with mitigation of depression than docosahexaenoic acid.[104] Smaller doses of omega-3 fatty acids do not appear to have the same benefit for depression, but decreased CVD risk has been associated with doses of 3 to 4 g/d.[105,106] Just 2 g/d of omega-3 fatty acids significantly reduced symptoms of anxiety.[107] It is often difficult to gain compliance with such a high dose of omega-3 fatty acids, and subsequently, it may be pertinent to look for high-dose formulations. It is also important to prescribe high quality of sources of omega-3 fatty acids to ensure that they are low in mercury and other toxins. Mercury may exacerbate autonomic nervous system dysfunction,[70,108] further contributing to depression, anxiety, and CVD.

Vitamin D

A fat-soluble vitamin, vitamin D is synthesized by exposure to the sun; however, it can also be consumed with benefit orally. Vitamin D is crucial for brain function, and a deficiency of vitamin D is associated with an 8% to 14% increase in depression and a 50% increase in suicide.[109] Even outside of laboratory-defined deficiency, serum concentration of vitamin D had an inverse correlation with depressive symptoms.[110] Ideal functional laboratory ranges find that levels closer to the middle of the laboratory reference range are protective for a variety of conditions, lower oxidative stress, and decrease LDL levels.[109] The connection between vitamin D and depression may be further elucidated through the vitamin D receptor genetic mutation, which predisposes one to having lower levels of vitamin D as well as higher rates of depression.[111]

Minerals

Minerals serve as cofactors for a variety of processes that ultimately may contribute to depression. Zinc has been shown to be an antagonist of the N-methyl-D-aspartate glutamate receptor, and levels have been found to be decreased in depressed patients.[112] In a study of patients with MDD, 25 mg of zinc supplementation reduced depressive symptoms in conjunction with SSRIs, in comparison with placebo.[112] Additionally, selenium has been found to be reduced in patients with depression, particularly those with comorbid alcoholism, and in higher concentrations has been shown to improve mood.[113] Chromium picolinate at 400 μg has been found to impact differential outcomes for atypical depression[114] by altering brain serotonin levels[115] and is also correlated with reducing insulin resistance,[116] an outcome that benefits both depression and CVD risk.

Magnesium is an essential cofactor in many biochemical reactions in the body.[117] It has been studied for its relationship to stress. Stress hormones trigger extracellular shunting of magnesium, leading to a decrease in serum magnesium concentration.[117] Low serum magnesium has in turn been shown to increase stress hormones such as catecholamines and cortisol, which perpetuates a cycle of stress and hypomagnesemia.[117] Mitral valve prolapse has been strongly correlated with hypomagnesemia, and symptoms of anxiety, chest pain, weakness, dyspnea, and palpitations can be significantly diminished after supplementation with magnesium.[118] Existing evidence shows a correlation between magnesium supplementation and reduction in anxiety-related symptoms such as perceived stress and insomnia.[117] Although there are not many studies on magnesium as a monotherapy for anxiety as a disorder, there are numerous studies that show benefits of magnesium for anxiety symptoms in combination with other nutrients such as vitamin B6 and anxiolytic herbs.[117,119]

B Vitamins

Several B-vitamin deficiencies have been correlated with depression, including thiamine, riboflavin, niacin, biotin, pantothenic acid, B6, folic acid, and B12.[70] A well-rounded, high-quality B-complex vitamin may serve to assist in mitigating these deficiencies. However, several of these have been studied for their effects at higher therapeutic doses.

Vitamin B6 (pyridoxine) has been proposed to exert a modulatory effect on serotonin and GABA and has also been shown to reduce blood pressure, reduce homocysteine levels, and downregulate glucocorticoid receptors.[120] It may be used therapeutically in doses of 100 to 300 mg daily to incite these effects, decreasing anxiety and depression, and leading to greater overall cardiovascular health.[120] It can also be combined with magnesium for a synergistic effect on anxiety.[117]

Folic acid in doses of 500 μg has been found to improve depression symptoms when added to a protocol with an SSRI.[121] Folic acid supplementation has been the subject of much nutritional research owing to its varying bioavailability in certain forms based on genetic polymorphisms. If an individual has a heterozygous or homozygous mutation at the methylenetetrahydrofolate reductase (MTHFR) gene, it suggests an inability to methylate B vitamins, thus requiring supplementation with forms of B vitamins that are already methylated, specifically L-methylfolate and methylcobalamin.[122] The MTHFR C677T polymorphism has also been associated with an increased risk of depression,[122,123] as well as cardiovascular risk factors such as increased blood pressure.[124] Currently, there are no studies linking MTHFR polymorphism to anxiety; however, there are other related polymorphisms that should be taken into consideration, such as COMT. A COMT polymorphism, especially at the met158 allele, is linked to higher anxiety levels,[125,126] indicating an overactive methylation pathway. In patients with this polymorphism, supplementation with B vitamins, particularly methylfolate, may cause anxiety. Subsequently, it is recommended that patients' MTHFR polymorphisms are tested and they are supplemented according to their need for 5-methyltetrahydrofolate (L-methylfolate or 5-MTHF) or unmethylated folinic acid.

S-adenosyl-L-methionine (SAMe) has also been studied in the treatment of depression. One mechanism of its action may be linked to the MTHFR polymorphism as it is a universal methyl donor. SAMe in doses of 150 mg/d to 400 mg three times per day have been found to be equally or more effective than tricyclic antidepressants for the treatment of MDD.[127] SAMe should be avoided in individuals with anxiety or bipolar disorder, as it may contribute to mania and anxiety. SAMe also may enhance SSRI effects[128] and should be avoided in individuals with a homozygous COMT polymorphism as this may increase the risk of anxiety.

Amino Acids

L-Tryptophan and *5-hydroxytryptamine (5-HTP)* have been used to increase levels of serotonin, in lieu of SSRI medication for both depression and anxiety. L-Tryptophan intake at a dose of 2 g three times per day was studied in the 1970s and found to have equivalent outcomes with tricyclic antidepressants (TCAs).[129] Since this time, it has become more controversial because of its potential interaction with SSRIs and development of serotonin syndrome. However, if no serotonin-producing drugs are being utilized, tryptophan and 5-HTP can serve to potentiate serotonin and decrease depressive or anxious symptoms. A study performed by Lu and colleagues found that, in an animal model, a post-MI population had lower 5-HTP levels in the hippocampus, suggesting this as a potential mechanism of post-cardiac event depression.[130] A proposed mechanism of low tryptophan in depression is based on HPA axis regulation of tryptophan.[131] Because HPA axis dysregulation in itself is a mechanism of correlation between depression and CVD, targeting HPA axis regulation is a related area of treatment.

L-Lysine and *L-Arginine* are additional amino acids that serve to impact stress and anxiety. L-Lysine has been shown to act as a partial serotonin receptor 4 antagonist and a partial benzodiazepine agonist.[132] Although there is not much research available for the use of L-lysine as a monotherapy, when L-lysine is used in combination with L-arginine, they reduce subjective trait and stress-induced state anxiety, as well as levels of stress hormones such as cortisol.[119,132]

HERBAL THERAPIES

Herbal traditions span over thousands of years and have been used to treat a multitude of ailments. Many herbal therapies exist that can serve to mimic actions of pharmaceuticals or mitigate underlying mechanisms that link depression, anxiety, and CVD.

Perhaps one of the most widely used herbal antidepressants and anxiolytics is *Hypericum perforatum* or St. John's wort. This is an acceptable treatment of depression or anxiety to reduce CVD risk; however, it is also a strong inducer of cytochrome P450 3A4 (CYP3A4) enzyme, thereby reducing plasma concentrations of drugs metabolized in this pathway.[133] Because many patients with CVD are on a polypharmacy regimen, *H perforatum* is not recommended unless close consideration of herb-drug interactions has taken place.

Herbal Anxiolytics

Several herbs have been well studied for their anxiolytic properties and used across various cultures to treat anxiety.

Passiflora incarnata (passionflower) has been used for hundreds of years and considered an acceptable treatment of restlessness and nervousness. It has been studied in comparison with benzodiazepines for the treatment of chronic anxiety, and one study showed passionflower to be as effective as benzodiazepines in managing symptoms of anxiety.[134]

Perhaps the greatest differences noted were that benzodiazepines had a faster onset and passionflower did not incite the adverse effect of performance impairment found with benzodiazepines.[134] There are few rarely experienced adverse effects with the use of passionflower that may include minor dizziness, drowsiness, or confusion.[119]

Piper methysticum is commonly known as kava and has been used for centuries as a drink to decrease anxiety, restlessness, and insomnia.[119] Kava has been found to inhibit norepinephrine and dopamine reuptake as well as monoamine oxidase B (MAOB) and enhance GABA binding.[119] This combination of actions allows kava to have unique properties in that it is anxiolytic but not sedative like benzodiazepines. There have been controversies about the safety of kava in the past owing to reports of hepatotoxicity; however, the rarity of these claims suggest potential poor supplement quality or overdose due to irresponsible consumption as it has also been used as a recreational beverage.[119]

Herbal Adaptogens

Herbal adaptogens serve to mitigate adaptation to stress and normalize HPA axis function.[135] Deviations from the normal cortisol rhythm throughout the day can cause symptoms of depression and anxiety, and normalization of this rhythm can be accomplished through the utilization of herbal adaptogens. Salivary and urine metabolite testing can offer a snapshot of a patient's HPA axis functioning to assess the appropriate type of treatment required. When cortisol is lower than the norm, it is helpful to utilize stimulating adaptogenic herbs such as *Eleutherococcus senticosus* and *Rhodiola rosea*.[135] *R rosea* has also been studied for its antidepressant properties.[76] *Ginkgo biloba* is particularly beneficial in elderly patients through increasing cerebrovascular blood flow[136] and has been used as an herb to support cardiovascular health as its actions include antioxidant activity, free-radical scavenging, vasodilation, vascular protection, membrane stabilization, inhibition of platelet-activating factor, and regulation of metabolism.[136] Of course, the use of *G biloba* in combination with other blood thinners is not recommended.

Some adaptogenic herbs can have a more equalizing effect on the cortisol rhythm and are good to consider when a patient's cortisol rhythm is unknown. These modulating adaptogens include *Schisandra chinensis* and *Withania somnifera* (ashwagandha). Ashwagandha has been researched as an anxiety treatment and has shown significant improvements in subjective anxiety and stress.[137] One study demonstrated better outcomes with use of ashwagandha and naturopathic care versus psychotherapy in the form of CBT and placebo.[138] Ashwagandha has also been shown to decrease oxidative stress and offers neuroprotection when under chronic stress.[139]

LIGHT THERAPY

It is commonly known that depression can be impacted by lack of sunlight exposure, leading to a diagnosis of seasonal affective disorder (SAD). This has led to research exploring the impact of light on depression and serotonin synthesis,[140] which has implications for all types of depression. Although light therapy is a highly accepted form of treatment of SAD, it also has been studied as a noninvasive modality to treat non-seasonal depression.[141-143] A review by Zhao and colleagues[144] illustrates the efficacy of utilizing bright light therapy in the morning, within 30 minutes of waking, to combat depression in various populations, including geriatric populations, individuals with MDD, and those with minor depression. Significant decrease in depressive symptoms was found across various treatment conditions, although the greatest results were found when white or pale blue light is administered at an intensity of 5000 lux for 50 minutes within 30 minutes of waking for a duration of 2 to 4 weeks.[144] Light therapy is noninvasive, with no reported adverse effects, and additional benefits of increasing sleep efficacy and evening melatonin production.[145] Where possible, light therapy could also be incorporated with exercise by encouraging patients to go for a 50- to 60-minute walk in the sun every morning upon waking.

MIND-BODY TECHNIQUES

Heart Rate Variability

As previously discussed, autonomic dysfunction is a risk factor for CVD that is perpetuated through states of depression and anxiety and is measured through the construct of HRV. Low HRV is associated with poorer health outcomes, whereas higher HRV is protective for cardiovascular health. HRV is something that can be measured in patients and utilized to help foster self-awareness and facilitate control of physiological processes such as heart rate and breathing.[146] Performing HRV training assists in increasing resting HRV[146] as well as increasing parasympathetic tone in the face of stressors,[147] thus leading to lower anxiety and lower risk of CVD. HRV training may be performed with comprehensive biofeedback software, or with HRV-specific software, which is also available for home use.[147,148]

Breathing

There are many mind-body techniques that impact the autonomic nervous system and overall health. Breathing exercises are among the simplest. Making exhalation a few seconds longer than inhalation stimulates the parasympathetic nervous system and promotes relaxation. This has been shown to decrease perceived stress and lower blood pressure. Breathing exercises can easily be given to patients after illustrating the practice in office and should be encouraged during stressful periods, before bed, or several times a day to promote the relaxation response.

Meditation

Mindfulness and meditation techniques have been found to impact CVD through modulation of the autonomic and parasympathetic nervous systems.[93] Transcendental meditation (TM) is a practice that focuses the mind on silent repetition of a mantra in the form of a word or phrase until the mind is free of thought and no longer requires the repetition.[149] The practice of TM has been shown to decrease anxiety and

posttraumatic stress disorder (PTSD) symptoms,[149] and when practiced twice daily for 20 minutes TM has been shown to contribute to a 48% decrease in major adverse cardiac events over a period of 5 years in African-American patients with hypertension.[93,150] Mindfulness Based Stress Reduction, based on the Buddhist form of meditation, has been shown to improve telomerase activity.[131] Both forms of meditation are easy to learn, and training is readily available. Some patients may prefer guided meditation, and there are many mobile phone applications, recordings, and programs that can be utilized to help patients develop a meditation practice.

LIFESTYLE

Although behavioral change is one of the most difficult treatments when it comes to comorbid depression and CVD, it can also be the most impactful. Eliminating tobacco use and alcohol consumption is necessary for both cardiovascular health and depression. Nicotine increases adrenal hormone secretion, raising cortisol levels and leading to the HPA axis dysfunction that underlies depression and CVD.[70] Cortisol elevation decreases levels of tryptophan, serotonin, and melatonin in the brain and also desensitizes serotonin receptors.[70] Cigarette smoking generates an abundance of free radicals, causes oxidative stress, and reduces levels of antioxidants in the body that are protective against both depression and CVD.[70] Alcohol is a well-known chemical depressant, which also increases adrenal hormone secretion, alters brain function, disrupts sleep cycles, leads to reactive hypoglycemia, and depletes nutrients that are necessary for mood stabilization.[70] Addictions such as nicotine, alcohol, and food addiction may serve to perpetuate difficulties in behavior change. Patients should be strongly encouraged to undergo concurrent addiction treatment to remove these barriers to health.

Exercise

Exercise is perhaps the most beneficial treatment of both depression and cardiovascular health.[152] Regular exercise works to prevent obesity, a risk factor for both depression and CVD, and to lower systemic inflammation.[70] Exercise has been shown to decrease cortisol levels and increase levels of mood-boosting beta-endorphins.[153] Recent research on exercise has elucidated the ability of exercise to increase brain-derived neurotrophic factor (BDNF), a growth factor responsible for cell growth and regeneration, and synaptic remodeling and plasticity, while also impacting hypothalamic pathways of homeostasis, central metabolism, and regulation of angiogenesis and muscle regeneration.[154] A study performed by Zembron-Lacny and colleagues[154] showed that individuals who were more active had higher BDNF and better lipoprotein profiles with less oxidative stress and inflammation. This relationship through BDNF helps to illustrate the way in which exercise positively impacts brain health as well as cardiovascular risk.

Yoga

Yoga is a practice that literally means "union," as its purpose is to unite the body and mind. It is a practice that incorporates both breathing techniques and physical exercise. Yoga has been shown to impact stress levels positively, leading to greater resilience of both body and mind. It is a form of meditation in movement, and a gentle form of exercise that can be particularly useful for patients with anxiety and chronic stress. The practice of yoga has also been shown to decrease episodes of angina and atrial fibrillation,[93] as well as cardiovascular risk factors, including lowering blood pressure,[155] decreasing cortisol and inflammatory markers,[93] decreasing LDL and triglycerides, and increasing HDL cholesterol.[156] Additionally, yoga may help to mitigate some of the connections between depression/anxiety/stress and CVD through increasing HRV[157] and normalizing autonomic function.[158] The Ornish program for reversing heart disease combined yoga and meditation with vegetarian diet, group support, and exercise. The result of this integrative health approach in the secondary prevention of CVD was a 91% reduction in angina and evidence of coronary disease reversal.[93-95]

Social Support

Social support, which aids in compliance, can have a profound impact on depression and CVD. One path to success includes developing a collaborative treatment plan with the patient, meeting them where they are, and allowing them to have some control over what therapies are included in their treatment regimen. Patients are often disempowered in the medical system, which in itself can lead to feelings of learned helplessness after an acute cardiovascular event. Working with a patient to determine what is reasonable for them gives them back the power to make health care decisions and solicits greater investment from the patient. Motivational interviewing can be helpful in this process.

It is also exceedingly helpful for a patient to have a social support system. Humans are social creatures who thrive when surrounded by supportive groups of people. Patients with chronic disease are much more likely to practice self-care with support from friends and family to assist them in making the necessary lifestyle changes and taking the medications and/or supplements prescribed.[159] Although a therapist should certainly be a part of the team, it is also important for a depressed or anxious patient to have regular social interactions. Cardiac rehabilitation, for example, provides an excellent and safe social support network.

In our modern society, we are often physically isolated from one another, which some may attribute to an increased use of technology; however, technology has provided novel ways to help patients who are depressed. There are online communities of individuals who have experienced similar health concerns, and people can gain validation through reading about these experiences on message boards, from telling their stories, and from being heard. There are also several mobile phone applications that may serve to fill in the gaps for some people with mental-emotional concerns. There are apps with daily reminders to eat, drink water, take medications, shower, and seek social interaction, all things that are difficult for depressed or anxious individuals.[160] There are mindfulness and meditation apps to help individuals relax and cope with stress through guided imagery or progressive relaxation. There is even an automated messaging system that employs methods from CBT to provide guidance to patients through a text message conversation, allowing for on-demand support.[161] Although lifestyle changes may be difficult, there are many ways to make them more accessible and achievable for patients. As practitioners, we just have to be willing to think outside the box. Where possible, cardiac rehabilitation is the preferred environment for individuals to learn lifestyle change and connect with others having similar health challenges, although it is important to keep these additional tools in mind.[93]

SPIRITUALITY

An integrative view of health must consider the full person: mind, body, and spirit. Spirituality is often used as a term to encompass many matters of belief including religion, secular belief systems, and a general sense of meaning.[162] This broad understanding of the term creates a situation wherein patients are able to define spirituality for themselves. Some individuals may adopt spiritual practices that are in line with an existing doctrine, whereas others may find a unique connection with something such as a higher power or even nature.[21]

Spirituality has been found to be associated with positive health outcomes, including decreased physical symptoms such as pain and fatigue, increased quality of life,[163] and even greater longevity.[164] Patients with religious involvement or spiritual practices have better coping skills and less anxiety and depression.[164] A review by Lucchese and colleagues[162] analyzed the relationship between religion, spirituality, and CVD, concluding that religion and spirituality have a multifaceted impact on CVD through manifesting positive emotions, decreasing depression/anxiety/substance abuse, leading to healthier lifestyle, and creating situations to manifest supportive social relationships. Several studies have found much better cardiovascular outcomes in individuals with a religious practice,[165-167] including decreased odds of MI[165] and decreased risk of mortality from coronary heart disease[166] or elective cardiovascular surgery.[167]

Spirituality can cause a large difference in patient outcomes and may help to create resilience both physically and psychologically, to mitigate the impact of chronic stress, depression, and anxiety on cardiovascular health. Subsequently, it is important for practitioners to be willing to engage in discussions with patients about spiritual practices and encourage patients' agency in finding the spiritual practice that works for them. Spirituality may include religious practices or practices such as meditation, mindfulness, prayer, and gratitude.[168]

Summary

CVD is not just a disease of the cardiovascular system but perhaps should be seen as a disease of the heart in all of its meanings. It is a reflection of the health of the whole human being, including biochemical states, emotional states, social connectedness, stress, and spirituality. If practitioners focus solely on the classic CVD risk factors such as tobacco use and hypertension, they will miss not only the important comorbidities of depression, stress, and anxiety but also the opportunity to treat these root causes.

Depression, perceived stress, and anxiety have direct physiological impacts on cardiovascular health, through mechanisms such as inflammation, autonomic dysfunction, HRV, platelet activation, and cardiac reactivity. It is no mystery that depression, stress, and anxiety have biochemical impacts on various body systems, both directly and through alteration of behavioral practices. Subsequently, treatment of an individual with CVD must not only address the structural and physiological pathology but also look beyond that pathology for triggers that are psychological. Utilizing integrative therapies such as nutrition, botanicals, mind-body medicine, spirituality, and lifestyle counseling assists patients with CVD to truly heal their hearts and develop resilience.

- Mental-emotional states such as depression, anxiety, and stress negatively impact cardiovascular health and outcomes.
- Extensive research has shown the correlation between depression and CVD as well as post-MI mortality rates. However, the overlap between depression and anxiety shows that there are likely many of the same pathways at work.
- Depression, anxiety, and CVD are connected through a variety of mechanisms, including inflammation, oxidative stress, platelet activation, autonomic dysfunction, HPA axis dysfunction, endothelial dysfunction, cardiovascular reactivity, and behavioral mechanisms. Although these connections exist, it is difficult to determine the directionality of causation, and thus there is room for intervention on all sides through prevention of CVD, prevention of depression/anxiety, lowering of stress, and mitigating every stage of the pathogenesis by focusing on the mechanisms listed earlier.
- Patients with CVD should be screened for depression and anxiety to allow for secondary prevention of adverse cardiac events and outcomes.
- Treatment should be individualized, collaborative, and integrative. Patients have different vulnerabilities based on factors such as comorbidities, mental-emotional health, genetics, gut health, and nutritional status. Patients should be tested for any root cause risk factors and treated for these using appropriate treatment modalities.
- Treatments should include an appropriate combination of psychotherapy or counseling, mind-body modalities, lifestyle changes, herbal or nutritional antidepressants/anxiolytics, and/or pharmaceuticals such as SSRIs when indicated.
- Patients have a difficult time implementing lifestyle and behavioral change, and practitioners should strongly consider comprehensive programs such as cardiac rehabilitation. It is also possible to use patient social support systems, technology, and spirituality to assist in patient motivation and compliance.

Challenges

The research presented within this chapter shows the breadth of exploration that has been done in correlating depression, anxiety, stress, and CVD. Presently, standard of care of CVD does not provide any screening or treatment recommendations for this prominent comorbidity. It has been argued that screening may lead to overtreatment with pharmaceutical therapy for patients that show signs of depression and anxiety. However, if the tools presented within this chapter are utilized to mitigate depression, anxiety, and stress in patients with CVD in lieu of overmedicalization of the mental-emotional concerns, it is possible to treat the underlying causes of the comorbidity. There are opportunities to explore these connections further, to evaluate outcomes of patients who are treated with an integrative approach that involves prevention, nutritional therapies, lifestyle change, counseling, and spirituality. At a minimum, it is exceptionally important to listen to patients with CVD, provide heart-centered care, and normalize the emotions of sadness, stress, and anxiety.

Acknowledgments

We would like to thank the following supporters: Don and Ruth Taylor, The Taylor Family Foundation, and Miraglo Foundation.

References

1. Maciocia G. *The Foundations of Chinese Medicine*. 3rd ed. London, UK: Elsevier Health Sciences; 2015.
2. Davidson KW, Alcántara C, Miller GE. Selected psychological comorbidities in coronary heart disease: challenges and grand opportunities. *Am Psychol*. 2018;73(8):1019-1030.
3. Malzberg B. Mortality among patients with involution melancholia. *Am J Psychiatry*. 1937;93:1231-1238.
4. Bulka CM, Daviglus ML, Persky VW, et al. Association of occupational exposures with cardiovascular disease among US Hispanics/Latinos. *Heart*. 2019;105(6):439-448.
5. Alissa EM, Ferns GA. Heavy metal poisoning and cardiovascular disease. *J Toxicol*. 2011;2011:870125.
6. Ignarro LJ, Balestrieri ML, Napoli C. Nutrition, physical activity, and cardiovascular disease: an update. *Cardiovasc Research*. 2007;73:326-340.
7. Joseph MS, Konerman MA, Zhang M, et al. Long-term outcomes following completion of a structured nutrition and exercise lifestyle intervention program for patients with metabolic syndrome. *Diabetes Metab Syndr Obes Targets Ther*. 2018;11:753-759.
8. American Psychiatric Association. *Diagnostic and Statistical Manual of Mental Disorders*. 5th ed. Washington, DC: American Psychiatric Association; 2013.
9. Kroenke K, Spitzer RL. The PHQ-9: a new depression diagnostic and severity measure. *Psychiatr Ann*. 2002;32(9):509-515.

10. Radloff LS. The CES-D scale: a self-report depression scale for research in the general population. *Appl Psychol Meas*. 1977;1(3):385-401.

11. Beck AT, Steer RA, Brown GK. Beck depression inventory-II. *San Antonio*. 1996;78(2):490-498.

12. Steer RA, Brown GK, Beck AT, Sanderson WC. Mean Beck Depression Inventory-II scores by severity of major depressive episode. *Psychol Rep*. 2001;88(3 pt 2):1075-1076.

13. Hare DL, Davis CR. Cardiac depression scale: validation of a new depression scale for cardiac patients. *J Psychosom Res*. 1996;40(4):379-386.

14. Nicholson A, Kuper H, Hemingway H. Depression as an aetiologic and prognostic factor in coronary heart disease: a meta-analysis of 6362 events among 146 538 participants in 54 observational studies. *Eur Heart J*. 2006;27(23):2763-2774.

15. Rozanski A, Blumenthal JA, Davidson KW, Saab PG, Kubzansky L. The epidemiology, pathophysiology, and management of psychosocial risk factors in cardiac practice: the emerging field of behavioral cardiology. *J Am Coll Cardiol*. 2005;45:637-651.

16. Hare DL, Toukhsati SR, Johansson P, Jaarsma T. Depression and cardiovascular disease: a clinical review. *Eur Heart J*. 2014;35(21):1365-1372.

17. Lesperance F, Frasure-Smith N, Talajic M, Bourassa MG. Five-year risk of cardiac mortality in relation to initial severity and one-year changes in depression symptoms after myocardial infarction. *Circulation*. 2002;105:1049-1053.

18. Montgomery SA. The under-recognized role of dopamine in the treatment of major depressive disorder. *Int Clin Psychopharmacol*. 2008;23(2):63-69.

19. Hasler G. Pathophysiology of depression: do we have any solid evidence of interest to clinicians? *World Psychiatry*. 2010;9(3):155-161.

20. Heim C, Newport DJ, Mletzko T, Miller AH, Nemeroff CB. The link between childhood trauma and depression: insights from HPA axis studies in humans. *Psychoneuroendocrinology*. 2008;33(6):693-710.

21. Oberg E. Wellness, lifestyle and preventive medicine. In: Wardle J, Sarris J, eds. *Clinical Naturopathy: An Evidence-Based Guide to Practice*. 2nd ed. Chatswood, NSW, Australia: Elsevier Health Sciences; 2014.

22. Dillon DG, Rosso IM, Pechtel P, Killgore WD, Rauch SL, Pizzagalli DA. Peril and pleasure: an rdoc-inspired examination of threat responses and reward processing in anxiety and depression. *Depress Anxiety*. 2014;31(3):233-249.

23. Singh MK, Gotlib IH. The neuroscience of depression: implications for assessment and intervention. *Behav Res Ther*. 2014;62:60-73.

24. Dunlop BW, Nemeroff CB. The role of dopamine in the pathophysiology of depression. *Arch Gen Psychiatry*. 2007;64(3):327-337.

25. Blanco C, Rubio JM, Wall M, Secades-villa R, Beesdo-baum K, Wang S. The latent structure and comorbidity patterns of generalized anxiety disorder and major depressive disorder: a national study. *Depress Anxiety*. 2014;31(3):214-222.

26. Zbozinek TD, Rose RD, Wolitzky-taylor KB, et al. Diagnostic overlap of generalized anxiety disorder and major depressive disorder in a primary care sample. *Depress Anxiety*. 2012;29(12):1065-1071.

27. Roy MA, Neale MC, Pedersen NL, Mathé AA, Kendler KS. A twin study of generalized anxiety disorder and major depression. *Psychol Med*. 1995;25(5):1037-1049.

28. Sunderland M, Mewton L, Slade T, Baillie AJ. Investigating differential symptom profiles in major depressive episode with and without generalized anxiety disorder: true co-morbidity or symptom similarity? *Psychol Med*. 2010;40(7):1113-1123.

29. Thurston RC, Rewak M, Kubzansky LD. An anxious heart: anxiety and the onset of cardiovascular diseases. *Prog Cardiovasc Dis*. 2013;55(6):524-537.

30. Takagi Y, Sakai Y, Abe Y, et al. A common brain network among state, trait, and pathological anxiety from whole-brain functional connectivity. *Neuroimage*. 2018;172:506-516.

31. Spitzer RL, Kroenke K, Williams JB, Löwe B. A brief measure for assessing generalized anxiety disorder: the GAD-7. *Arch Intern Med*. 2006;166(10):1092-1097.

32. Chilcot J, Hudson JL, Moss-morris R, et al. Screening for psychological distress using the Patient Health Questionnaire Anxiety and Depression Scale (PHQ-ADS): initial validation of structural validity in dialysis patients. *Gen Hosp Psychiatry*. 2018;50:15-19.

33. You JS, Hu SY, Chen B, Zhang HG. Serotonin transporter and tryptophan hydroxylase gene polymorphisms in Chinese patients with generalized anxiety disorder. *Psychiatr Genet*. 2005;15(1):7-11.

34. Unschuld PG, Ising M, Specht M, et al. Polymorphisms in the GAD2 gene-region are associated with susceptibility for unipolar depression and with a risk factor for anxiety disorders. *Am J Med Genet B Neuropsychiatr Genet*. 2009;150B(8):1100-1109.

35. Nitschke JB, Sarinopoulos I, Oathes DJ, et al. Anticipatory activation in the amygdala and anterior cingulate in generalized anxiety disorder and prediction of treatment response. *Am J Psychiatry*. 2009;166(3):302-310.

36. Safren SA, Gershuny BS, Marzol P, Otto MW, Pollack MH. History of childhood abuse in panic disorder, social phobia, and generalized anxiety disorder. *J Nerv Ment Dis*. 2002;190(7):453-456.

37. Baldwin D. Generalized anxiety disorder in adults: epidemiology, pathogenesis, clinical manifestations, course, assessment, and diagnosis. In: Stein MB, Hermann R, eds. *UpToDate*. Waltham, MA: UpToDate; 2018. www.uptodate.com. Accessed October 10, 2018.

38. Godbout JP, Glaser R. Stress-induced immune dysregulation: implications for wound healing, infectious disease and cancer. *J Neuroimmune Pharmacol*. 2006;1:421-427.

39. Sterling P, Eyer J. Allostasis: a new paradigm to explain arousal pathology. In: Fisher S, Reason J, eds. *Handbook of Life Stress, Cognition, and Health*. New York: John Wiley & Sons; 1988:629-649.

40. Logan JG, Barksdale DJ. Allostasis and allostatic load: expanding the discourse on stress and cardiovascular disease. *J Clin Nurs*. 2008;17(7B):201-208.

41. Schulkin J. *Allostasis, Homeostasis, and the Costs Of Physiological Adaptation*. New York: Cambridge University Press; 2004.

42. Antonelli M, Kushner I. It's time to redefine inflammation. *FASEB J*. 2017;31(5):1787-1791.

43. Zuzarte P, Duong A, Figueira ML, Costa-vitali A, Scola G. Current therapeutic approaches for targeting inflammation in depression and cardiovascular disease. *Curr Drug Metab*. 2018;19(8):674-687.

44. Xiong GL, Prybol K, Boyle SH, et al. Inflammation markers and major depressive disorder in patients with chronic heart failure: results from the sertraline against depression and heart disease in chronic heart failure study. *Psychosom Med*. 2015;77(7):808-815.

45. Salim S, Asghar M, Taneja M, et al. Potential contribution of oxidative stress and inflammation to anxiety and hypertension. *Brain Res*. 2011;1404:63-71.

46. Smykiewicz P, Segiet A, Keag M, Żera T. Proinflammatory cytokines and ageing of the cardiovascular-renal system. *Mech Ageing Dev*. 2018;175:35-45.

47. Ford DE, Erlinger TP. Depression and C-reactive protein in US adults: data from the Third National Health and Nutrition Examination Survey. *Arch Intern Med*. 2004;164:1010-1014.

48. Dong Y, Wang X, Zhang L, et al. High-sensitivity C reactive protein and risk of cardiovascular disease in China-CVD study. *J Epidemiol Community Health*. 2019;73(2):188-192.

49. Steenkamp LR, Hough CM, Reus VI, et al. Severity of anxiety- but not depression- is associated with oxidative stress in Major Depressive Disorder. *J Affect Disord*. 2017;219:193-200.

50. Serebruany VL, Glassman AH, Malinin AI, et al. Enhanced platelet/endothelial activation in depressed patients with acute coronary syndromes: evidence from recent clinical trials. *Blood Coagul Fibrinolysis*. 2003;14(6):563-567.

51. Aschbacher K, Mills PJ, Von känel R, et al. Effects of depressive and anxious symptoms on norepinephrine and platelet P-selectin responses to acute psychological stress among elderly caregivers. *Brain Behav Immun*. 2008;22(4):493-502.

52. Cygankiewicz I, Zareba W. Heart rate variability. In: Buijs RM, Swaab DF, eds. *Autonomic Nervous System*. Vol 117. Edinburgh: Elsevier; 2013.

53. Zhang Y, Chen Y, Ma L. Depression and cardiovascular disease in elderly: current understanding. *J Clin Neurosci*. 2018;47:1-5.

54. Carney RM, Blumenthal JA, Stein PK, et al. Depression, heart rate variability, and acute myocardial infarction. *Circulation*. 2001;104(17):2024-2028.

55. Kubzansky LD, Kawachi I, Weiss ST, Sparrow D. Anxiety and coronary heart disease: a synthesis of epidemiological, psychological, and experimental evidence. *Ann Behav Med*. 1998;20(2):47-58.

56. Otte C, Marmar CR, Pipkin SS, Moos R, Browner WS, Whooley MA. Depression and 24-hour urinary cortisol in medical outpatients with coronary heart disease: the Heart and Soul Study. *Biol Psychiatry*. 2004;56(4):241-247.

57. Otte C, Neylan TC, Pipkin SS, Browner WS, Whooley MA. Depressive symptoms and 24-hour urinary norepinephrine excretion levels in patients with coronary disease: findings from the Heart and Soul Study. *Am J Psychiatry*. 2005;162(11):2139-2145.

58. Whooley MA. Depression and cardiovascular disease: healing the broken-hearted. *JAMA*. 2006;295(24):2874-2881.

59. Mann DL, Kent RL, Parsons B, Cooper G. Adrenergic effects on the biology of the adult mammalian cardiocyte. *Circulation*. 1992;85(2):790-804.

60. Communal C, Singh K, Pimentel DR, Colucci WS. Norepinephrine stimulates apoptosis in adult rat ventricular myocytes by activation of the beta-adrenergic pathway. *Circulation*. 1998;98(13):1329-1334.

61. Van sloten TT, Schram MT, Adriaanse MC, et al. Endothelial dysfunction is associated with a greater depressive symptom score in a general elderly population: the Hoorn Study. *Psychol Med*. 2014;44(7):1403-1416.

62. Stillman AN, Moser DJ, Fiedorowicz J, Robinson HM, Haynes WG. Association of anxiety with resistance vessel dysfunction in human atherosclerosis. *Psychosom Med*. 2013;75(6):537-544.

63. Wittstein IS, Thiemann DR, Lima JAC, et al. Neurohumoral features of myocardial stunning due to sudden emotional stress. *N Engl J Med*. 2005;352:539-548.

64. Wittstein IS. The broken heart syndrome. *Cleve Clin J Med*. 2007;74:S17-S22.

65. Feng J, Lenihan DJ, Johnson MM, Karri V, Reddy CV. Cardiac sequelae in Brooklyn after the September 11 terrorist attacks. *Clin Cardiol*. 2006;29(1):13-17.

66. Bazoukis G, Tse G, Naka KK, et al. Impact of major earthquakes on the incidence of acute coronary syndromes – a systematic review of the literature. *Hellenic J Cardiol*. 2018;59(5):262-267.

67. Ziegelstein RC, Fauerbach JA, Stevens SS, et al. Patients with depression are less likely to follow recommendations to reduce cardiac risk during recovery from a myocardial infarction. *Arch Intern Med*. 2000;160:1818-1823.

68. Antonogeorgos G, Panagiotakos DB, Pitsavos C, et al. Understanding the role of depression and anxiety on cardiovascular disease risk, using structural equation modeling; the mediating effect of the Mediterranean diet and physical activity: the ATTICA study. *Ann Epidemiol*. 2012;22:630-637.

69. Goossens L, Braet C, Bosmans G. Relations of dietary restraint and depressive symptomatology to loss of control over eating in overweight youngsters. *Eur Child Adolesc Psychiatry*. 2010;19(7):587-596.

70. Bongiorno P, Murray M. Affective disorders. In: Pizzorno J, Murray M, eds. *Textbook of Natural Medicine*. 4th ed. St. Louis, MS: Elsevier; 2013:1162-1177.

71. Hansen RA, Khodneva Y, Glasser SP, Qian J, Redmond N, Safford MM. Antidepressant medication use and its association with cardiovascular disease and all-cause mortality in the reasons for geographic and racial differences in Stroke (REGARDS) study. *Ann Pharmacother*. 2016;50(4):253-261.

72. Huffman JC, Mastromauro CA, Beach SR, et al. Collaborative care for depression and anxiety disorders in patients with recent cardiac events: the Management of Sadness and Anxiety in Cardiology (MOSAIC) randomized clinical trial. *JAMA Intern Med*. 2014;174(6):927-935.

73. Katon WJ, Lin EH, Von Korff M, et al. Collaborative care for patients with depression and chronic illnesses. *N Engl J Med*. 2010;363:2611-2620.

74. Katon W, Russo J, Lin EH, et al. Cost-effectiveness of a multicondition collaborative care intervention: a randomized controlled trial. *Arch Gen Psychiatry*. 2012;69:506-514.

75. Katon WJ, Von Korff M, Lin E. Panic disorder: relationship to high medical utilization. *Am J Med*. 1992;92:S7-S11.

76. Sarris J. Depression. In: Wardle J, Sarris J, eds. *Clinical Naturopathy: An Evidence-Based Guide to Practice*. 2nd ed. Elsevier Health Sciences; 2014.

77. Angermann CE, Ertl G. Depression, anxiety, and cognitive impairment: comorbid mental health disorders in heart failure. *Curr Heart Fail Rep*. 2018;15(6):398-410.

78. Von ruden AE, Adson DE, Kotlyar M. Effect of selective serotonin reuptake inhibitors on cardiovascular morbidity and mortality. *J Cardiovasc Pharmacol Ther*. 2008;13(1):32-40.

79. Jiang W, Krishnan R, Kuchibhatla M, et al. Characteristics of depression remission and its relation with cardiovascular outcome among patients with chronic heart failure (from the SADHART-CHF Study). *Am J Cardiol*. 2011;107(4):545-551.

80. Perlis RH, Mehta R, Edwards AM, Tiwari A, Imbens GW. Pharmacogenetic testing among patients with mood and anxiety disorders is associated with decreased utilization and cost: a propensity-score matched study. *Depress Anxiety*. 2018;35(10):946-952.

81. Jacka FN, Pasco JA, Mykletun A, et al. Association of Western and traditional diets with depression and anxiety in women. *Am J Psychiatry*. 2010;167(3):305-311.

82. Bakhtiyari M, Ehrampoush E, Enayati N, et al. Anxiety as a consequence of modern dietary pattern in adults in Tehran–Iran. *Eat Behav*. 2013;14(2):107-112.

83. Yannakoulia M, Panagiotakos DB, Pitsavos C, et al. Eating habits in relations to anxiety symptoms among apparently healthy adults. A pattern analysis from the ATTICA Study. *Appetite*. 2008;51(3):519-525.

84. Jezova D, Vigas M, Hlavacova N, Kukumberg P. Attenuated neuroendocrine response to hypoglycemic stress in patients with panic disorder. *Neuroendocrinology*. 2010;92(2):112-119.

85. Brinkworth GD, Buckley JD, Noakes M, Clifton PM, Wilson CJ. Long-term effects of a very low-carbohydrate diet and a low-fat diet on mood and cognitive function. *Arch Intern Med*. 2009;169(20):1873-1880.

86. Sanhueza C, Ryan L, Foxcroft DR. Diet and the risk of unipolar depression in adults: systematic review of cohort studies. *J Hum Nutr Diet*. 2013;26(1):56-70.

87. Estruch R, Ros E, Salas-salvadó J, et al. Primary prevention of cardiovascular disease with a mediterranean diet supplemented with extra-virgin olive oil or nuts. *N Engl J Med*. 2018;378(25):e34.

88. Ros E, Martínez-González MA, Estruch R, et al. Mediterranean diet and cardiovascular health: teachings of the PREDIMED study. *Adv Nutr*. 2014;5(3):330S-6S.

89. Sears B. Anti-inflammatory diets. *J Am Coll Nutr*. 2015;34(suppl 1):14-21.

90. Ohtsuka Y. Food intolerance and mucosal inflammation. *Pediatr Int*. 2015;57(1):22-29.

91. Theoharides TC, Tsilioni I, Patel AB, Doyle R. Atopic diseases and inflammation of the brain in the pathogenesis of autism spectrum disorders. *Transl Psychiatry*. 2016;6(6):e844.

92. Brostoff J, Gamlin L. *Food Allergies and Food Intolerance: The Complete Guide to Their Identification and Treatment*. Rochester, VT: Healing Arts Press; 2000.

93. Freeman AM, Taub PR, Lo HC, Ornish D. Intensive cardiac rehabilitation: an underutilized resource. *Curr Cardiol Rep*. 2019;21(4):19.

94. Silberman A, Banthia R, Estay IS, et al. The effectiveness and efficacy of an intensive cardiac rehabilitation program in 24 sites. *Am J Health Promot*. 2010;24(4):260-266.

95. Ventegodt S, Merrick E, Merrick J. Clinical holistic medicine: the Dean Ornish program ("opening the heart") in cardiovascular disease. *ScientificWorldJournal*. 2006;6:1977-1984.

96. Delzenne NM, Neyrinck AM, Bäckhed F, Cani PD. Targeting gut microbiota in obesity: effects of prebiotics and probiotics. *Nat Rev Endocrinol*. 2011;7(11):639-646.

97. Luna RA, Foster JA. Gut brain axis: diet microbiota interactions and implications for modulation of anxiety and depression. *Curr Opin Biotechnol*. 2015;32:35-41.

98. Institute of Functional Medicine. *The 5R Framework for Gut Restoration. Presented at: Applying Functional Medicine in Clinical Practice*. Baltimore, MD; September 2016.

99. Spedding S. Vitamin D and depression: a systematic review and meta-analysis comparing studies with and without biological flaws. *Nutrients.* 2014;6(4):1501-1518.

100. Peuranpää P, Heliövaara-Peippo S, Fraser I, Paavonen J, Hurskainen R. Effects of anemia and iron deficiency on quality of life in women with heavy menstrual bleeding. *Acta Obstet Gynecol Scand.* 2014;93(7):654-660.

101. Benton D, Donohoe RT. The effects of nutrients on mood. *Public Health Nutr.* 1999;2(3A):403-409.

102. Su KP, Huang SY, Chiu CC, Shen WW. Omega-3 fatty acids in major depressive disorder: a preliminary double-blind, placebo-controlled trial. *Eur Neuropsychopharmacol.* 2003;13(4):267-271.

103. Jazayeri S, Tehrani-doost M, Keshavarz SA, et al. Comparison of therapeutic effects of omega-3 fatty acid eicosapentaenoic acid and fluoxetine, separately and in combination, in major depressive disorder. *Aust N Z J Psychiatry.* 2008;42(3):192-198.

104. Martins JG. EPA but not DHA appears to be responsible for the efficacy of omega-3 long chain polyunsaturated fatty acid supplementation in depression: evidence from a meta-analysis of randomized controlled trials. *J Am Coll Nutr.* 2009;28(5):525-542.

105. Mozaffarian D, Wu JH. Omega-3 fatty acids and cardiovascular disease: effects on risk factors, molecular pathways, and clinical events. *J Am Coll Cardiol.* 2011;58(20):2047-2067.

106. *REDUCE-IT™ Cardiovascular Outcomes Study of Vascepa® (Icosapent Ethyl) Capsules Met Primary Endpoint [Press Release].* Bedminster, NJ: Amarin Corporation; September 24, 2018. https://investor.amarincorp.com/node/15741/pdf. Accessed October 8, 2018.

107. Su KP, Tseng PT, Lin PY, et al. Association of use of omega-3 polyunsaturated fatty acids with changes in severity of anxiety symptoms: a systematic review and meta-analysis. *JAMA Netw Open.* 2018;1(5):e182327.

108. Milioni ALV, Nagy BV, Moura ALA, Zachi EC, Barboni MTS, Ventura DF. Neurotoxic impact of mercury on the central nervous system evaluated by neuropsychological tests and on the autonomic nervous system evaluated by dynamic pupillometry. *Neurotoxicology.* 2017;59:263-269.

109. Sepehrmanesh Z, Kolahdooz F, Abedi F, et al. Vitamin D supplementation affects the beck depression inventory, insulin resistance, and biomarkers of oxidative stress in patients with major depressive disorder: a randomized, controlled clinical trial. *J Nutr.* 2016;146(2):243-248.

110. Hoogendijk WJ, Lips P, Dik MG, Deeg DJ, Beekman AT, Penninx BW. Depression is associated with decreased 25-hydroxyvitamin D and increased parathyroid hormone levels in older adults. *Arch Gen Psychiatry.* 2008;65(5):508-512.

111. Minasyan A, Keisala T, Lou YR, Kalueff AV, Tuohimaa P. Neophobia, sensory and cognitive functions, and hedonic responses in vitamin D receptor mutant mice. *J Steroid Biochem Mol Biol.* 2007;104(3-5):274-280.

112. Nowak G, Szewczyk B. Mechanisms contributing to antidepressant zinc actions. *Pol J Pharmacol.* 2002;54(6):587-592.

113. Finley JW, Penland JG. Adequacy or deprivation of dietary selenium in healthy men: clinical and psychological findings. *J Trace Elem Exp Med.* 1998;11:11-27.

114. Davidson JR, Abraham K, Connor KM, Mcleod MN. Effectiveness of chromium in atypical depression: a placebo-controlled trial. *Biol Psychiatry.* 2003;53(3):261-264.

115. Attenburrow MJ, Odontiadis J, Murray BJ, et al. Chromium treatment decreases the sensitivity of 5HT2A receptors. *Psychopharmacology.* 2002;159:432-436.

116. Anderson RA. Chromium, glucose intolerance and diabetes. *J Am Coll Nutr.* 1998;17:548-555.

117. Pouteau E, Kabir-ahmadi M, Noah L, et al. Superiority of magnesium and vitamin B6 over magnesium alone on severe stress in healthy adults with low magnesemia: a randomized, single-blind clinical trial. *PLoS ONE.* 2018;13(12):e0208454.

118. Lichodziejewska B, Kłos J, Rezler J, et al. Clinical symptoms of mitral valve prolapse are related to hypomagnesemia and attenuated by magnesium supplementation. *Am J Cardiol.* 1997;79(6):768-772.

119. Lakhan SE, Vieira KF. Nutritional and herbal supplements for anxiety and anxiety-related disorders: systematic review. *Nutr J.* 2010;9:42.

120. Mccarty MF. High-dose pyridoxine as an 'anti-stress' strategy. *Med Hypotheses.* 2000;54(5):803-807.

121. Coppen A, Bailey J. Enhancement of the antidepressant action of fluoxetine by folic acid: a randomised, placebo controlled trial. *J Affect Disord.* 2000;60(2):121-130.

122. Jha S, Kumar P, Kumar R, Das A. Effectiveness of add-on l-methylfolate therapy in a complex psychiatric illness with MTHFR C677 T genetic polymorphism. *Asian J Psychiatr.* 2016 Aug 1;22:74-75.

123. Rai V. Genetic polymorphisms of methylenetetrahydrofolate reductase (MTHFR) gene and susceptibility to depression in Asian population: a systematic meta-analysis. *Cell Mol Biol (Noisy-le-grand).* 2014;60(3):29-36.

124. Rashed L, Abdel hay R, Alkaffas M, Ali S, Kadry D, Abdallah S. Studying the association between methylenetetrahydrofolate reductase (MTHFR) 677 gene polymorphism, cardiovascular risk and lichen planus. *J Oral Pathol Med.* 2017;46(10):1023-1029.

125. Woo JM, Yoon KS, Yu BH. Catechol O-methyltransferase genetic polymorphism in panic disorder. *Am J Psychiatry.* 2002;159(10):1785-1787.

126. Pooley EC, Fineberg N, Harrison PJ. The met(158) allele of catechol-O-methyltransferase (COMT) is associated with obsessive-compulsive disorder in men: case-control study and meta-analysis. *Mol Psychiatry.* 2007;12(6):556-561.

127. Papakostas GI, Cassiello CF, Iovieno N. Folates and S-adenosylmethionine for major depressive disorder. *Can J Psychiat.* 2012 Jul;57(7):406-413.

128. Abeysundera H, Gill R. Possible SAMe-induced mania. *BMJ Case Rep.* 2018;2018:bcr-2018-224338. https://casereports.bmj.com/content/2018/bcr-2018-224338.info.

129. Lindberg D, Ahlfors UG, Dencker SJ, et al. Symptom reduction in depression after treatment with L-tryptophan or imipramine. Item analysis of Hamilton rating scale for depression. *Acta Psychiatr Scand.* 1979;60(3):287-294.

130. Lu X, Wang Y, Liu C, Wang Y. Depressive disorder and gastrointestinal dysfunction after myocardial infarct are associated with abnormal tryptophan-5-hydroxytryptamine metabolism in rats. *PLoS One.* 2017;12(2):e0172339.

131. Sorgdrager FJH, Doornbos B, Penninx BWJH, De jonge P, Kema IP. The association between the hypothalamic pituitary adrenal axis and tryptophan metabolism in persons with recurrent major depressive disorder and healthy controls. *J Affect Disord.* 2017;222:32-39.

132. Smriga M, Torii K. L-Lysine acts like a partial serotonin receptor 4 antagonist and inhibits serotonin-mediated intestinal pathologies and anxiety in rats. *Proc Natl Acad Sci USA.* 2003;100(26):15370-15375.

133. Komoroski BJ, Zhang S, Cai H, et al. Induction and inhibition of cytochromes P450 by the St. John's wort constituent hyperforin in human hepatocyte cultures. *Drug Metab Dispos.* 2004;32(5):512-518.

134. Akhondzadeh S, Naghavi HR, Vazirian M, Shayeganpour A, Rashidi H, Khani M. Passionflower in the treatment of generalized anxiety: a pilot double-blind randomized controlled trial with oxazepam. *J Clin Pharm Ther.* 2001;26(5):363-367.

135. Panossian A. Stimulating effect of adaptogens: an overview with particular reference to their efficacy following single dose administration. *Phytother Res.* 2005;19:819-838.

136. Tian J, Liu Y, Chen K. Ginkgo biloba extract in vascular protection: molecular mechanisms and clinical applications. *Curr Vasc Pharmacol.* 2017;15:532-548.

137. Pratte MA, Nanavati KB, Young V, Morley CP. An alternative treatment for anxiety: a systematic review of human trial results reported for the Ayurvedic herb ashwagandha (Withania somnifera). *J Altern Complement Med.* 2014;20(12):901-908.

138. Cooley K, Szczurko O, Perri D, et al. Naturopathic care for anxiety: a randomized controlled trial ISRCTN78958974. *PLoS One.* 2009;4(8):e6628.

139. Durg S, Dhadde SB, Vandal R, Shivakumar BS, Charan CS. Withania somnifera (Ashwagandha) in neurobehavioural disorders induced by brain oxidative stress in rodents: a systematic review and meta-analysis. *J Pharm Pharmacol.* 2015;67(7):879-899.

140. Lambert GW, Reid C, Kaye DM, Jennings GL, Esler MD. Effect of sunlight and season on serotonin turnover in the brain. *Lancet.* 2002;360(9348):1840-1842.

141. Martiny K. Novel augmentation strategies in major depression. *Dan Med J.* 2017;64(4).

142. Mårtensson B, Pettersson A, Berglund L, Ekselius L. Bright white light therapy in depression: a critical review of the evidence. *J Affect Disord.* 2015;182:1-7.

143. Wirz-justice A, Bader A, Frisch U, et al. A randomized, double-blind, placebo-controlled study of light therapy for antepartum depression. *J Clin Psychiatry.* 2011;72(7):986-993.

144. Zhao X, Ma J, Wu S, Chi I, Bai Z. Light therapy for older patients with non-seasonal depression: a systematic review and meta-analysis. *J Affect Disord.* 2018;232:291-299.

145. Lieverse R, Van someren EJ, Nielen MM, Uitdehaag BM, Smit JH, Hoogendijk WJ. Bright light treatment in elderly patients with non-seasonal major depressive disorder: a randomized placebo-controlled trial. *Arch Gen Psychiatry.* 2011;68(1):61-70.

146. Goessl VC, Curtiss JE, Hofmann SG. The effect of heart rate variability biofeedback training on stress and anxiety: a meta-analysis. *Psychol Med.* 2017;47(15):2578-2586.

147. Whited A, Larkin KT, Whited M. Effectiveness of emWave biofeedback in improving heart rate variability reactivity to and recovery from stress. *Appl Psychophysiol Biofeedback.* 2014;39(2):75-88.

148. McCraty R, Atkinson M, Tomasino D, Bradley RT. *The Coherent Heart: Heart-Brain Interactions, Psychophysiological Coherence, and the Emergence of System-wide Order;* 2006. Available at http://www.heartmath.org/research/publications.html.

149. Lang AJ, Strauss JL, Bomyea J, et al. The theoretical and empirical basis for meditation as an intervention for PTSD. *Behav Modif.* 2012;36(6):759-786.

150. Schneider RH, Grim CE, Rainforth MV, et al. Stress reduction in the secondary prevention of cardiovascular disease: randomized, controlled trial of transcendental meditation and health education in Blacks. *Circ Cardiovasc Qual Outcomes.* 2012;5(6):750-758.

151. Lengacher CA, Reich RR, Kip KE, et al. Influence of mindfulness-based stress reduction (MBSR) on telomerase activity in women with breast cancer (BC). *Biol Res Nurs.* 2014;16(4):438-447.

152. Summers KM, Martin KE, Watson K. Impact and clinical management of depression in patients with coronary artery disease. *Pharmacotherapy.* 2010;30(3):304-322.

153. Lobstein DD, Rasmussen CL, Dunphy GE, Dunphy MJ. Beta-endorphin and components of depression as powerful discriminators between joggers and sedentary middle-aged men. *J Psychosom Res.* 1989;33(3):293-305.

154. Zembron-lacny A, Dziubek W, Rynkiewicz M, Morawin B, Woźniewski M. Peripheral brain-derived neurotrophic factor is related to cardiovascular risk factors in active and inactive elderly men. *Braz J Med Biol Res.* 2016;49(7). doi:10.1590/1414-431X20165253.

155. Patel C, North WR. Randomised controlled trial of yoga and bio-feedback in management of hypertension. *Lancet.* 1975;2(7925):93-95.

156. Bijlani RL, Vempati RP, Yadav RK, et al. A brief but comprehensive lifestyle education program based on yoga reduces risk factors for cardiovascular disease and diabetes mellitus. *J Altern Complement Med.* 2005;11(2):267-274.

157. Satyapriya M, Nagendra HR, Nagarathna R, Padmalatha V. Effect of integrated yoga on stress and heart rate variability in pregnant women. *Int J Gynaecol Obstet.* 2009;104(3):218-222.

158. Bernardi L, Sleight P, Bandinelli G, et al. Effect of rosary prayer and yoga mantras on autonomic cardiovascular rhythms: comparative study. *BMJ.* 2001;323(7327):1446-1449.

159. Won MH, Son YJ. Perceived social support and physical activity among patients with coronary artery disease. *West J Nurs Res.* 2017;39(12):1606-1623.

160. Aloe Bud - self-care companion. Aloebud.com. https://aloebud.com/. Published 2018. Accessed October 10, 2018.

161. Woebot - Your charming robot friend who is here for you, 24/7. Woebot.io. https://woebot.io/. Published 2018. Accessed October 10, 2018.

162. Lucchese FA, Koenig HG. Religion, spirituality and cardiovascular disease: research, clinical implications, and opportunities in Brazil. *Rev Bras Cir Cardiovasc.* 2013;28(1):103-128.

163. Boudreaux ED, O'Hea E, Chasuk R. Spiritual role in healing. An alternative way of thinking. *Prim Care.* 2002;29:439-454, viii.

164. Mueller PS, Plevak DJ, Rummans TA. Religious involvement, spirituality, and medicine: implications for clinical practice. *Mayo Clin Proc.* 2001;76(12):1225-1235.

165. Friedlander Y, Kark JD, Stein Y. Religious orthodoxy and myocardial infarction in Jerusalem–a case control study. *Int J Cardiol.* 1986;10(1):33-41.

166. Goldbourt U, Yaari S, Medalie JH. Factors predictive of long-term coronary heart disease mortality among 10,059 male Israeli civil servants and municipal employees. A 23-year mortality follow-up in the Israeli Ischemic Heart Disease Study. *Cardiology.* 1993;82(2-3):100-121.

167. Oxman TE, Freeman DH, Manheimer ED. Lack of social participation or religious strength and comfort as risk factors for death after cardiac surgery in the elderly. *Psychosom Med.* 1995;57(1):5-15.

168. Guarneri M, Bradley R. Be the willow: stress, resiliency, and diseases of the heart. In: Sinatra S, Houston MC, eds. *Nutritional and Integrative Strategies in Cardiovascular Medicine.* Boca Raton: CRC Press; 2015:318-337.

34

Environmental Toxins and Cardiovascular Disease

Joseph Pizzorno, ND

Introduction

The incidence of virtually every chronic disease in almost every age group has increased relentlessly the past half century. A growing body of research has now documented that much, if not most, of this increase is due to the increasing levels of toxic metals and chemicals in the environment. Heavy metals (eg, cadmium, lead, and mercury), meta-metals (eg, arsenic), nonpersistent chemical toxins (eg, PAHs [polyaromatic hydrocarbons], VOCs [volatile organic compounds], glyphosate, organophosphate pesticides), persistent chemical toxins (DDT [dichlorodiphenyltrichloroethane], PCBs [polychlorinated biphenyls], air pollutants (particulate matter, ozone, sulfur, and nitrogen oxides), and several other less pervasive, but still important, classes of toxicants, have all been shown to increase cardiovascular disease (CVD) and many other diseases as well as risk of death. These toxicants contaminate air, water, health and beauty aids, food, packaging, pharmaceuticals, house and yard chemicals—in other words every human contact with the environment.

Everyday exposure to many of these is common, but making the problem far more challenging is that many of them have very long half-lives in humans. Although simple avoidance is critical, substantial skill and effort are needed to help facilitate excretion of the persistent organic pollutants (POPs). The long lifetimes of lead in the body is well known. But far less recognized is that many of these new-to-nature molecules were specifically designed to be difficult to detoxify by biological systems. Particularly problematic for humans are the halogenated compounds. Without intervention, molecules like DDT and PCBs have half-lives measured in years to even decades, causing continuous, unrelenting, cumulative damage. A key reason so much disease occurs later in life is that these long half-lives result in progressively higher body levels as age increases.

This chapter focuses on the worst of the toxicants shown to induce CVD, where they come from, how their body load

is assessed, and key strategies for increasing excretion from the body. Well recognized toxins like smoking are addressed elsewhere. Those who want to dive more deeply into the huge role of environmental toxins in chronic disease are encouraged to read Crinnion and Pizzorno, *Clinical Environmental Medicine*, Elsevier, 2018.

Cardiovascular Diseases Caused or Aggravated by Environmental Toxicants

The key toxicants for each cardiovascular dysfunction/disease are listed alphabetically to avoid misplaced concreteness. Although some toxicants are clearly worse than others, there is huge variability according to each person's biochemical individuality, nutritional status, and exposure to other toxicants. Another challenge is that research on chronic, low level exposure to toxicants and disease risk as well as mechanisms of damage is still at an early stage. Some toxicants may appear worse simply because they have been subjected to more research or, like lead, have been damaging humans for much longer. This list includes those toxicants that increase disease risk at least 20% and have substantial research support. Also, of substantial significance is the fact that people are rarely exposed to a single toxicant. Because the average person is exposed to multiple toxins, their damaging effects are amplified (Table 34.1).

The Worst Cardiotoxins

Air Pollution (Indoor and Outdoor)

Inexplicably, the American Heart Association (AHA) website does not list air pollution as a significant modifiable cause of heart disease. An AHA expert panel published in 2004 the following[1]:

Table 34.1

DAMAGING EFFECTS OF MULTIPLE TOXINS

Cardiovascular Mortality

- Air pollution
- Lead
- $PM_{2.5}$
- PM_{10}

Coronary Heart Disease/Atherosclerosis

- Arsenic
- Bisphenol A (BPA)
- Methyl mercury
- Polychlorinated biphenyls (PCBs)
- $PM_{2.5}$
- PM_{10}

Hypertension

- Arsenic
- BPA
- Lead
- PCBs

Myocardial Infarct Risk

- BPA
- Methyl mercury
- Polyaromatic hydrocarbons (PAHs)
- PCBs
- PM_{10}
- $PM_{2.5}$
- Traffic exhaust

Stroke

- Arsenic
- Cadmium
- PCBs
- $PM_{2.5}$
- PM_{10}

- Short-term exposure to elevated particular matter (PM) significantly contributes to increased acute cardiovascular mortality, particularly in certain at-risk subsets of the population.
- Hospital admissions for several cardiovascular and pulmonary diseases acutely increase in response to higher ambient PM concentrations.
- Prolonged exposure to elevated levels of PM reduces overall life expectancy by a few years.

A more recent expert panel report in 2015 added further support to the problem of air pollution and CVD[2]:

"There is now abundant evidence that air pollution contributes to the risk of cardiovascular disease and associated mortality, underpinned by credible evidence of multiple mechanisms that may drive this association. In light of this evidence, efforts to reduce exposure to air pollution should urgently be intensified and supported by appropriate and effective legislation."

Another significant risk factor for CVD is solvent exposure such as found in beauty salons. The regular exposure experienced by salon workers causes an elevation in C-reactive protein (CRP) and 8-hydroxy deoxyguanosine (8-OHdG), indicating both inflammation and oxidative stress.[3] These are nonpersistent toxicants as demonstrated by dramatic decreases in these measures on days when the salons were not working. CRP levels average 10.9 mg/dL when working but only 1.1 mg/dL when not working. 8-OHdG shows the same results, dropping from 4.5 to 0.6 ng/mL. This benefit from decreasing solvent exposure was significant, although VOC levels in the air dropped only from 75 to 44 ppb. Of concern is that their exposure was still significant away from their salon exposure.

This may be explained by the research on home use of indoor freshening sprays. Their use showed loss of heart rate variability proportionate to the frequency of use, with damage showing up at just one use a week.[4] The same loss of heart rate variability was found with use of cleaning sprays and other home scented products.

Arsenic

According to the latest Centers for Disease Control and Prevention report, arsenic levels in the general US population are well into the toxic damage range (Fourth National Report on Human Exposure to Environmental Chemicals, Updated Tables, January 2019 https://www.cdc.gov/exposurereport/index.html). In general, the threshold for toxic effects is considered 10 µg/L of urine. As can be seen in Table 34.2, approximately 40% of the population exceeds this threshold.

Although most arsenic research is based on urinary levels, toenail arsenic is a better reflection of long-term exposure because of its short (2-4 days) half-life. Several studies have clearly demonstrated that blood pressure increases in proportion to arsenic levels.[5] The STRONG heart study of Native Americans found a strong association between urinary arsenic and heart disease. Urinary arsenic levels of 15.7 µg/g creatinine compared with 5.8 µg/g creatinine had a 65% increased risk of CVD, 71% increased risk of coronary heart disease, and over threefold increased risk of stroke.[6]

Bisphenol A

BPA levels increase dramatically simply by eating food or drinking soy milk stored in cans. This is well demonstrated by the following figure. Compared with fresh lentil soup, one

Table 34.2

URINARY TOTAL ARSENIC (2009-2010), CAS NUMBER 7740-38-2, GEOMETRIC MEAN AND SELECTED PERCENTILES OF URINE CONCENTRATIONS (IN μG/L) FOR THE US POPULATION FROM THE NATIONAL HEALTH AND NUTRITION EXAMINATION SURVEY

Categories (Survey Years)	Geometric Mean (95% Confidence Interval)	50th Percentile (95% Confidence Interval)	75th Percentile (95% Confidence Interval)	90th Percentile (95% Confidence Interval)	95th Percentile (95% Confidence Interval)	Sample Size
Total population (2009-2010)	9.28 (8.47-10.2)	8.15 (7.20-8.98)	18.0 (15.3-20.8)	44.6 (39.0-55.1)	85.6 (64.7-114)	2860

12-oz serving daily for 1 week increases BPA levels 12-fold.[7] Drinking just 6 oz of soy milk from cans rather than glass increases BPA levels by 16-fold and was shown to increase systolic blood pressure by approximately 4.5 mm Hg[8] (Figure 34.1). Bisphenols are ubiquitous and damaging in many ways. Unfortunately, even just maternal exposure to BPA increases a child's future risk for hypertension.[9]

NHANES PBA levels between 2003 and 2006 was used to compare self-reporting of CVDs with urinary BPA levels showed statistically significant risk.[10] Table 34.3 shows the odds ratio per standard deviation for various CVDs, **after** adjusting for all other CVD risk factors. One of the problems with statistically eliminating standard risk factors is that many of these are actually also caused by BPA as well as other common toxicants. Nonetheless, the results are clear (Table 34.4).

Utilizing these data, the 25% of the population with a urinary BPA level of 3.70 to 5.50 were 34% more likely to have some form of CVD. Those in the 95th percentile would have doubled risk. A study in the United Kingdom compared adults without coronary artery disease with those with severe coronary artery disease and found a mean urinary BPA of 1.28 ng/mL in the former and 1.53 ng/mL in the latter.[11] Those with higher urinary BPA are 43% more likely to have severe CAD. However, I cannot help but wonder if the latter group spent more time receiving medical procedures that entailed fluids from PBA-contaminated medical tubing. At this time, such medical BPA exposure has only been documented as problematic in neonates. Risk of developing CAD over 10 years was shown in a large European study to correlate with BPA levels.[12] A study in Swedish showed a similar positive association between BPA and carotid atherosclerosis.[13]

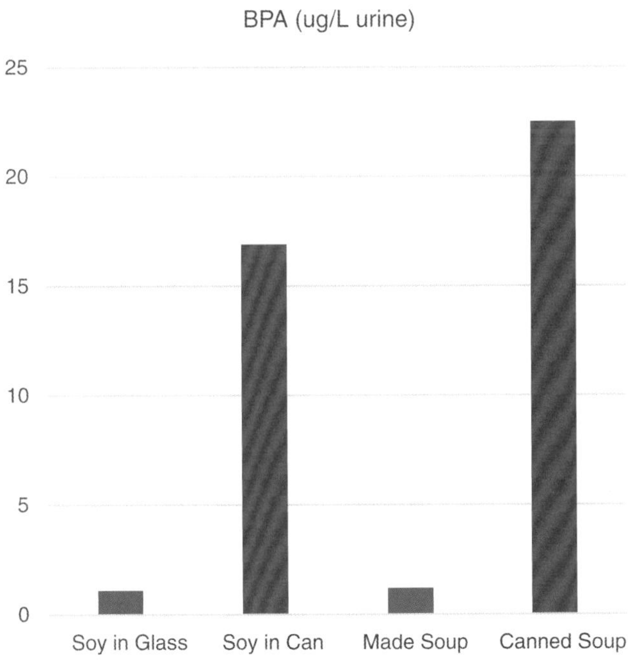

Cadmium

Cadmium is a serious persistent metal toxin that concentrates in the kidneys. Primary sources are cigarette smoking and nonorganic soy products. The threshold for increased disease risk is 0.40 μg/g. As can be seen from the following table, greater than 30% of population exceeds this level (Table 34.5).

Figure 34.1 *Storing food in cans greatly increases bisphenol A levels.*

Table 34.3

INCREASED RISK OF CARDIOVASCULAR DISEASE BY STANDARD DEVIATION OF BPA

Fully Adjusted Odds Ratio per Each Standard Deviation Increase in Urinary BPA

Condition	Pooled NHANES – 03-06
Coronary heart disease	1.42
Myocardial infarction	1.32
Angina	1.24

BPA, bisphenol A; NHANES, National Health and Nutrition Examination Survey.

Table 34.4

URINARY LEVELS OF BISPHENOL A (BPA) IN NHANES 2002-2006 (IN NG/ML)

NHANES BPA	50th Percentile	75th Percentile	95th Percentile
2003-2004	2.80	5.50	16.0
2005-2006	2.00	3.70	11.5
2007-2008	2.10	4.10	13.0
2009-2010	1.90	3.50	9.60

From the Fourth National Report on Human Exposure to Environmental Chemicals. *U.S. Department of Human Health and Human Services Center for Disease Control and Prevention.* Updated September 2013.

The 1999 to 2006 NHANES showed a clear association between blood cadmium levels and stroke and heart failure.[14] Another study found an increased risk of cardiovascular and cerebrovascular diseases.[15]

Lead

The good news is that lead levels are going down as shown in the following table (Table 34.6). Public health measures to decrease environmental toxins have clearly worked. The bad news is that there is still enough lead in the general population to increase the risk of many diseases, especially cardiovascular. And because lead is stored primarily in bone, older people losing bone are at increased risk of toxicity.

Lead causes cardiovascular damage in many ways. This is also covered in standard medical textbooks. Typical examples are elevation of blood pressure by causing renal damage, reduction of available nitric oxide, oxidative damage, increase in circulating vasoconstrictive prostaglandins, and alterations to the renin-angiotensin system.[16]

As the general population levels have decreased, so has the ratio of increased risk of those in the highest quartiles. For example, women in the top quartile of NHANES 1988 to 1994 had an 8.1 OR of both systolic and diastolic hypertension.[17] But NHANES 2003 to 2010 analysis found only a slight nonsignificant association between hypertension and blood lead.[18]

In the Normative Aging Study, a strong correlation was found between blood and tibial lead levels and the risk of ischemic heart disease.[19] Blood lead >3.62 µg/dL was shown in a 12-year prospective study to increase the risk of death from CVD by 55%.[20]

Methyl Mercury

All forms of mercury are toxic, and humans are regularly exposed to many of them. The methyl form may be the most damaging, but the other forms are toxic in many ways as well (Table 34.7).

Because the intake of high-omega-3 fish has been shown to decrease CVD, fish is now a commonly recommended dietary intervention.[21] Unfortunately, some of these fish are also heavily contaminated with the very toxic methyl mercury, which negates many of the benefits.[22] NHANES 1999 to 2000 showed that, for each 1.3 µg/L increase in mercury, the systolic blood pressure increased almost two points.[23] One of the earliest manifestations is elevation of blood pressure.[24]

Table 34.5

BLOOD CADMIUM (2009-2010), CAS NUMBER 81271-94-5, GEOMETRIC MEAN AND SELECTED PERCENTILES OF BLOOD CONCENTRATIONS (IN µG/L) FOR THE US POPULATION FROM THE NATIONAL HEALTH AND NUTRITION EXAMINATION SURVEY

Categories (Survey Years)	Geometric Mean (95% Confidence Interval)	50th Percentile (95% Confidence Interval)	75th Percentile (95% Confidence Interval)	90th Percentile (95% Confidence Interval)	95th Percentile (95% Confidence Interval)	Sample Size
Total population (2009-2010)	.302 (.293-.311)	.260 (.250-.270)	.480 (.460-.510)	.960 (.880-1.01)	1.40 (1.29-1.53)	8793

Table 34.6

BLOOD LEAD (1999-2010), CAS NUMBER 7439-92-1, GEOMETRIC MEAN AND SELECTED PERCENTILES OF BLOOD CONCENTRATIONS (IN µG/DL) FOR THE US POPULATION FROM THE NATIONAL HEALTH AND NUTRITION EXAMINATION SURVEY

Categories (Survey Years)	Geometric Mean (95% Confidence Interval)	50th Percentile (95% Confidence Interval)	75th Percentile (95% Confidence Interval)	90th Percentile (95% Confidence Interval)	95th Percentile (95% Confidence Interval)	Sample Size
Total population (1999-2000)	1.66 (1.60-1.72)	1.60 (1.60-1.70)	2.50 (2.40-2.60)	3.80 (3.60-4.00)	5.00 (4.70-5.50)	7970
Total population (2001-2002)	1.45 (1.39-1.51)	1.40 (1.40-1.50)	2.20 (2.10-2.30)	3.40 (3.20-3.60)	4.50 (4.20-4.70)	8945
Total population (2003-2004)	1.43 (1.36-1.50)	1.40 (1.30-1.50)	2.10 (2.10-2.20)	3.20 (3.10-3.30)	4.20 (3.90-4.40)	8373
Total population (2005-2006)	1.29 (1.23-1.36)	1.27 (1.20-1.34)	2.01 (1.91-2.11)	3.05 (2.86-3.22)	3.91 (3.64-4.18)	8407
Total population (2007-2008)	1.27 (1.21-1.34)	1.22 (1.18-1.30)	1.90 (1.80-2.00)	2.80 (2.67-2.96)	3.70 (3.50-3.90)	8266
Total population (2009-2010)	1.12 (1.08-1.16)	1.07 (1.03-1.12)	1.70 (1.62-1.77)	2.58 (2.45-2.71)	3.34 (3.14-3.57)	8793

Table 34.7

BLOOD METHYL MERCURY (2011-2016), CAS NUMBER 92786-62-4, GEOMETRIC MEAN AND SELECTED PERCENTILES OF BLOOD CONCENTRATIONS (IN µG/L) FOR THE US POPULATION FROM THE NATIONAL HEALTH AND NUTRITION EXAMINATION SURVEY

Categories (Survey Years)	Geometric Mean (95% Confidence Interval)	50th Percentile (95% Confidence Interval)	75th Percentile (95% Confidence Interval)	90th Percentile (95% Confidence Interval)	95th Percentile (95% Confidence Interval)	Sample Size
Total population (2011-2012)	.498 (.423-.587)	.480 (.400-.570)	1.25 (.950-1.61)	2.81 (2.29-3.55)	4.43 (3.46-5.49)	7841
Total population (2013-2014)	.434 (.381-.495)	.420 (.340-.510)	1.09 (.940-1.27)	2.62 (2.18-3.04)	4.28 (3.74-4.93)	5175
Total population (2015-2016)	.413 (.361-.472)	.380 (.320-.490)	1.02 (.860-1.22)	2.30 (1.92-2.78)	3.92 (3.35-4.81)	4938

Hair mercury is a good measure of methyl mercury, although not other forms of mercury. The carotid intima thickness increases in proportion to hair mercury.[25] Elevated hair mercury also strongly correlates with a 60% increase in an acute myocardial infarction (MI), a 68% greater likelihood of having CVD, and a 56% greater risk of having coronary heart disease.[26]

Particulate Matter (PM$_{2.5}$ and PM$_{10}$) and Polyaromatic Hydrocarbons

Particulate matter causes significant damage to tissues and organs,[27-29] and exposure correlates with increased mortality from cardiovascular,[30,31] respiratory,[32] and neoplastic diseases.[33] Much of this damage is mediated by the highly toxic polycyclic aromatic hydrocarbons and volatile organic compounds bound to their surface.[34] Aromatic hydrocarbons are produced from combustion of wood, tobacco, gasoline and diesel. People who suffering an acute MI have higher levels of a major PAH metabolite, 1-hydroxypyrene (1-OHP), than in those who have not had a heart attack.[35]

As levels of both PM$_{2.5}$ and PM$_{10}$ increase, so does the rate of mortality. Living in larger cities increases the risk of premature death by 15% to 17% compared with living in cities with cleaner air.[36] This increase in PM$_{2.5}$, PM$_{10}$, elemental carbon (ultrafine), and other air pollutants (CO, NO$_2$, SO$_2$) increases the incidence of CVD in older adults.[37,38] Increasing a person's air toxin exposure from the bottom 10th to the top 90th percentile increases all-cause mortality by 2.63% for total PM, 2.04% for ozone, and 2.66% for NO$_2$. Cardiovascular mortality increased 2.68% for total PM, 2.52% for ozone, and 2.34% for NO$_2$. Respiratory mortality also increased by 3.24% for PM and 7.71% for NO$_2$. Each 10 µg/m^3 increase of PM$_{2.5}$ results in a 22% increase in nonaccidental death risk.[39]

Simply living close to a major roadway significantly increases the risk of dying from an acute MI. Compared with people living more than 1000 m from a major roadway, those living between 200 and 1000 m away were 13% more likely to have a fatal MI, those living 100 to 200 m away were 19% more likely to die of their MI, and those who lived the closest (within 100 m) had a 27% increased risk of dying of an MI.[40]

In addition to overt disease and death, particulate matter damages the cardiovascular system in many ways. For example, PM exposure increases platelets, fibrinogen, and CRP; increases heart rate; decreases heart rate variability; and increases arrhythmias.[41,42]

The Los Angeles area suffers one of the highest PM$_{2.5}$ exposure in the nation, with an average between 13.4 and 27.1 µg/m^3. Such levels of exposure correlate with increased carotid intima-media thickness (CIMT).[43] Each 10 µg/m^3 increases CIMT by 5.9%. Interestingly, this effect is almost tripled in those taking lipid-lowering agents.

Exposure to high levels of vehicular pollution increases coronary artery calcification.[44] People living within 101 to 200 m from a major roadway were 8% more likely to have a high coronary artery calcification (CAC), those living 51 to 100 m away were 34% more likely to have a high CAC, and those living within 50 m had a 63% greater risk of having high CAC.

Polychlorinated Biphenyls

Virtually all humans have some level of body load of PCBs. Although PCBs were banned in the United States over 4 decades ago, as POPs they are very resistant to environmental degradation and once in the human body have half-lives of excretion of 3 to 25 years. Persistent pollutants indeed. As the body load increases, so does the incidence of CVD. Inexplicably, women appear to suffer more damage by PCBs than men. Table 34.8, extracted from 1999 to 2002 National Health and Nutrition Examination Survey (NHANES), shows the worrisome cardiovascular risk caused by several of the hundreds of PCBs that have polluted our environment.[45] As can be seen, women in the top quartile of PCB body load suffer a huge increased risk for CVD. In other words, one of every four women in the United States has a 4.5 to 13.4-fold increased risk of CVD. This is clearly a huge problem.

Most of PCBs 118, 138, 153, and 180 come from farmed salmon and sardines, with a lesser amount from hamburgers.[46] Although salmon, owing to its high omega-3 content, is a heart protective, the biggest salmon and farmed salmon are likely the opposite.

The damaging effects of PCBs show up in many ways. For example, Swedish seniors with higher levels of several PCBs had more carotid artery atherosclerosis than those with lower levels.[47] Simply living near a Monsanto plant that manufactured PCBs resulted in increased PCB levels, which correlated with elevated blood pressure.[48] PCB levels also correlate with increased systolic and diastolic blood pressure as well as reduced left ventricular ejection fraction.[49]

Tobacco Smoke Exposure

The heart-damaging effects of tobacco use and exposure to its smoke have been well documented for decades. State laws banning workplace tobacco smoke exposure have demonstrated significant population benefits, especially for heart disease. In one state, acute MI was decreased 33% after only 18 months when smoking was forbidden in workplaces, restaurants, and bars.[50] The substantial body of research is readily found in standard medical textbooks and is not duplicated here.

Assessment

Basically, there are four ways to assess toxic load: (1) directly measuring specific toxins in tissues—the best but impractical, painful, and extremely expensive; (2) measuring toxicant levels in blood, urine, or hair, which by the current clinical standard is a better measure of exposure rather than body load and may miss patients unable to excrete a toxicant via the medium tested; (3) challenge testing, whereby a chelating agent is administered to bind to

Table 34.8

CARDIOVASCULAR RISK FOR FEMALES IN 1999-2002 NHANES FROM DETECTABLE LEVELS OF PCBS

Odds Ratio of Women Self Reporting Cardiovascular Disease by Quartile of PCB

PCB	<25th Percentile	25-50th Percentile	50-75th Percentile	>75th Percentile
118 (DL)	1.8	0.6	1.3	4.5
156 (DL)	2.0	2.6	9.2	10.4
138 (NDL)	6.8	1.6	3.6	13.4
153 (NDL)	3.7	3.0	3.6	10.4
170 (NDL)	2.5	3.8	3.5	9.2
180 (NDL)	1.8	2.0	2.0	4.5
187 (NDL)	5.0	3.5	5.8	7.4

DL, dioxin-like; NDL, non-dioxin-like; NHANES, National Health and Nutrition Examination Survey; PCB, polychlorinated biphenyl.
From Ha MH, Lee DH, Jacobs DR. Association between serum concentrations of persistent organic pollutants and self-reported cardiovascular disease prevalence: results from the National Health and Nutrition Examination Survey, 1999-2002. *Environ Health Perspect.* 2007;115(8):1204-1209.

toxicants in the tissues and facilitate their excretion for measurement—but highly controversial with limited research; and (4) indirect measures that indicate which patients likely have a significant toxic load—but does not tell the clinician exactly which toxicants are elevated. Although some toxicants are easily measured, most are challenging. In the ideal world, the level of toxicants should be measured in cells. A reasonably close second is blood. However, most clinically available tests of chemical toxicant exposure utilize urine, which technically only measures what the body is excreting.

Full discussion of how to assess body load of toxicants is beyond the scope and space availability of this chapter. Those wanting to more deeply understand this important topic will find Clinical Environmental Medicine a useful resource and are encouraged to attend the excellent Environmental Health Symposium.

Intervention

Key to understanding how to address a patient's toxin load is to realize that the strategies for persistent and nonpersistent toxicants are different. First, there is, of course, no substitute for avoidance. Once an elevated load of a particular toxin is found, its source must be identified and strategies to avoid developed in collaboration with the patient. This is usually should be adequate approach for nonpersistent toxicants. The earlier discussion of the substantial drop in solvent levels in beauty solon workers on days off is a good example. But notice they still had a high body load. Avoidance is quite challenging, as these toxicants are everywhere: air, water, food, food packaging, health and beauty aids, household cleaning products, yard convenience chemicals, and so on.

Far more challenging is the elimination of persistent toxicants. Although they should, of course, be avoided, their half-lives are measured in months to decades. Active, sophisticated strategies to facilitate their excretion are critically important and require patience.

A full discussion of the many toxin elimination strategies is beyond the scope of this chapter. The following are a few examples of research showing that reducing exposure and body load of toxicants clearly improves cardiovascular health.

Avoidance

Reducing particulate matter and air toxicant exposure is readily achievable and produces significant clinical benefit. This can be achieved with good air filters. If the home has forced air heating/conditioning, the best strategy is to install a MERV 8 or better filter. Figure 34.2 is a MERV 16 filter (99% clearance rate of particulate matter, including the worst—$PM_{2.5}$) installed in the author's home after 9 months. This is not from a dirty or poorly maintained house as we vacuum almost daily, and our white carpets are still white after 20 years. This is all from air pollution in Seattle.

If a whole house air filter is not possible, high efficiency particulate air (HEPA) filters and even face masks can be used. A study in Chinese adults with coronary heart disease showed that utilizing a HEPA face mask while walking outside reduced $PM_{2.5}$ exposure and improved cardiac function.[51] The mask effectively dropped the inhaled $PM_{2.5}$ from 74 to 2 µg/m³ and resulted in a reduction in cardiac symptoms, less ST-segment depression, lower median blood pressure, and improved heart rate variability.

Even lower-quality indoor air purifiers that were only able to reduce PM in the home air 60% still showed a 9.4% improvement in endothelial function and a 32.6% reduction in inflammatory CRP.[52]

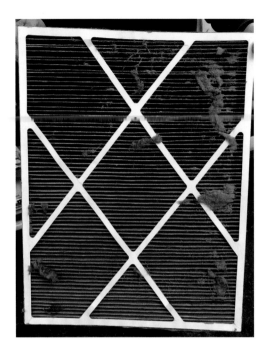

Figure 34.2 *MERV 16 filter after 9 months in author's home.*

Pharmaceuticals

Interestingly, bile sequestrants increase the excretion of the very-difficult-to-excrete PCBs. Although their standard use to reduce cholesterol has shown modest benefit in CVD, none of the research differentiated between those with high versus low PCB levels. And, of course, none of the studies tried to control toxin intake. Nonetheless, as can be seen in **Figure 34.3**, olestra increases PCB excretion. This intervention decreases PCB half-life about 50%. Better results would likely have been produced if PCB sources had been carefully avoided as well. However, at the dosage used (15 g/d), 25% experienced loose stools.

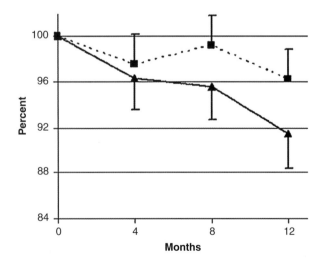

Figure 34.3 *Olestra increases excretion of polychlorinated biphenyls. (From Jandacek RJ, Heubi JE, Buckley DB, et al. Reduction of the body burden of PCBs and DDE by dietary intervention in a randomized trial.* J Nutr Biochem. *2014;25:483-488.)*

Chelation

Although chelation therapy has been shown to be effective in lowering heavy metal levels in industrially exposed populations, its use in nonindustrially exposed populations is controversial. Intravenous calcium-EDTA (edetate calcium disodium) has long been shown in several studies to increase the excretion of lead and nitric oxide levels, resulting in a temporary reduction of elevated blood pressure.[53] However, adverse drug reactions (ADRs) limit its use. In people with a previous MI, weekly infusions of EDTA and nutrients for 30 weeks resulted in a 27% decreased risk of another MI or a stroke and 28% reduction in hospitalization for angina.[54] The protocol for this author for safely increasing the excretion of both lead and mercury is 250 mg of DMSA (2,3-dimercaptosuccinic acid) every third night, 5 extra grams of fiber per day, and NAC (*N*-acetylcysteine) 500 mg/d to increase glutathione levels as well as increase excretion of methyl mercury.[55,56] Unpublished research from my clinical work shows a 40% reduction of lead and mercury after 1 year with no ADRs.

Supplementation

Many nutritional and herbal supplements have been shown to either protect the body from the damage induced by toxicants or facilitate their excretion. For example, fish oil supplements have been shown to reduce the adverse cardiac effects of particulate matter. In one study, 4 weeks of 3 g/d of fish oil prevented PM-induced abnormalities in cardiac rhythm.[57]

A good-quality multivitamin and minerals will normally provide the needed nutrients to support normal detoxification processes. However, a particularly important strategy is to increase glutathione levels. It is almost impossible to overstate the importance of glutathione in protecting tissues from the oxidative damage induced by almost every toxicant and to increase their excretion, particularly mercury and the chemicals detoxified through liver phase II glutathione conjugation. Oral glutathione is controversial because of concerns about it being metabolized to cysteine by gut microflora. Liposomal glutathione and oral NAC have been shown to increase RBC glutathione.[58]

Saunas

Modest-temperature sauna are effective for reducing the total toxicant burden and has been shown to reduce the risk of fatal CVD, sudden cardiac death, and coronary heart disease in many studies.[59,60] Saunas have been shown to increase the excretion of most environmental toxicants.[61,62] Genuis and his team have now published several studies showing that profuse sweating is effective in increasing the excretion of heavy metals, organochlorine pesticides, phthalates, BPA, and so on. Of particular interest, a number of the POPs they found excreted in the sweat were undetectable in blood or urine, suggesting they were sequestered in tissues—but not actually inert.

Conclusion

Environmental toxicants have become a primary driver of chronic disease. Contaminated air, water, and food; health and beauty aids; household cleaning products; and yard chemicals constantly bombard our patients with multiple metals and chemicals that disrupt metabolism, increase oxidative stress, and greatly increase CVD. The astute clinician will help his/her patients understand which toxins are damaging them, where they are coming from, and how to increase the excretion.

References

1. Brook RD, Franklin B, Cascio W, et al. Air pollution and cardiovascular disease: a statement for healthcare professionals from the Expert Panel on Population and Prevention Science of the American Heart Association. *Circulation*. 2004;109(21):2655-2671. PubMed PMID:15173049.
2. Newby DE, Mannucci PM, Tell GS, et al. Expert position paper on air pollution and cardiovascular disease. *Eur Heart J*. 2015;36(2):83-93b. PubMed PMID:25492627.
3. Ma CM, Lin LY, Chen HW, Huang LC, Li JF, Chuang KJ. Volatile organic compounds exposure and cardiovascular effects in hair salons. *Occup Med (Lond)*. 2010;60(8):624-630. PubMed PMID:20819803.
4. Mehta AJ, Adam M, Schaffner E, et al. Heart rate variability in association with frequent use of household sprays and scented products in SAPALDIA. *Environ Health Perspect*. 2012;120(7):958-964.
5. Mordukhovich I, Wright RO, Hu H, et al. Associations of toenail arsenic, cadmium, mercury, manganese, and lead with blood pressure in the normative aging study. *Environ Health Perspect*. 2012;120(1):98-104. PubMed PMID:21878420.
6. Moon KA, Guallar E, Umans JG, et al. Association between exposure to low to moderate arsenic levels and incident cardiovascular disease: a prospective cohort study. *Ann Intern Med*. 2013;159: PubMed PMID:24061511.
7. Carwile JL, Ye X, Zhou X, et al. Canned soup consumption and urinary bisphenol A: a randomized crossover trial. *JAMA*. 2011;306(20):2218-2220.
8. Bae S, Hong YC. Exposure to bisphenol A from drinking canned beverages increases blood pressure: randomized crossover trial. *Hypertension*. 2015;65(2):313-319. PubMed PMID:25489056.
9. Bae S, Lim YH, Lee YA, Shin CH, Oh SY, Hong YC. Maternal urinary bisphenol a concentration during midterm pregnancy and children's blood pressure at age 4. *Hypertension*. 2017;69(2):367-374. PubMed PMID:27920131.
10. Melzer D, Rice NE, Lewis C, Henley WE, Galloway TS. Association of urinary bisphenol a concentration with heart disease: evidence from NHANES 2003/06. *PLoS One*. 2010;5(1):e8673. PMID:20084273.
11. Melzer D, Gates P, Osborne NJ, et al. Urinary bisphenol a concentration and angiography-defined coronary artery stenosis. *PLoS One*. 2012;7(8):e43378. PubMed PMID:22916252.
12. Melzer D, Osborne NJ, Henley WE, et al. Urinary bisphenol A concentration and risk of future coronary artery disease in apparently healthy men and women. *Circulation*. 2012;125(12):1482-1490. PubMed PMID:22354940.
13. Lind PM, Lind L. Circulating levels of bisphenol A and phthalates are related to carotid atherosclerosis in the elderly. *Atherosclerosis*. 2011;218(1):207-213. PubMed PMID:21621210.
14. Peters JL, Perlstein TS, Perry MJ, McNeely E, Weuve J. Cadmium exposure in association with history of stroke and heart failure. *Environ Res*. 2010;110(2):199-206. PubMed PMID:20060521.
15. Agarwal S, Zaman T, Tuzcu EM, Kapadia SR. Heavy metals and cardiovascular disease: results from the National Health and Nutrition Examination Survey (NHANES) 1999-2006. *Angiology*. 2011;62(5):422-429. PubMed PMID:21421632.
16. Vaziri ND. Mechanisms of lead-induced hypertension and cardiovascular disease. *Am J Physiol Heart Circ Physiol*. 2008;295(2):H454-H465. PubMed PMID:18567711.
17. Nash D, Magder L, Lustberg M, et al. Blood lead, blood pressure, and hypertension in perimenopausal and postmenopausal women. *JAMA*. 2003;289(12):1523-1532. PubMed PMID:12672769.
18. Hara A, Thijs L, Asayama K, et al. Blood pressure in relation to environmental lead exposure in the national health and nutrition examination survey 2003 to 2010. *Hypertension*. 2015;65(1):62-69. PubMed PMID:25287397.
19. Jain NB, Potula V, Schwartz J, et al. Lead levels and ischemic heart disease in a prospective study of middle-aged and elderly men: the VA Normative Aging Study. *Environ Health Perspect*. 2007;115(6):871-875. PubMed PMID:17589593.
20. Menke A, Muntner P, Batuman V, Silbergeld EK, Guallar E. Blood lead below 0.48 micromol/L (10 microg/dL) and mortality among US adults. *Circulation*. 2006;114(13):1388-1394. PubMed PMID:16982939.
21. Kromhout D, Bosschieter EB, de Lezenne Coulander C. The inverse relation between fish consumption and 20-year mortality from coronary heart disease. *N Engl J Med*. 1985;312(19):1205-1209. PubMed PMID:3990713.
22. Wennberg M, Strömberg U, Bergdahl IA, et al. Myocardial infarction in relation to mercury and fatty acids from fish: a risk-benefit analysis based on pooled Finnish and Swedish data in men. *Am J Clin Nutr*. 2012;96(4):706-713. PubMed PMID:22894940.
23. Vupputuri S, Longnecker MP, Daniels JL, Guo X, Sandler DP. Blood mercury level and blood pressure among US women: results from the National Health and Nutrition Examination Survey 1999-2000. *Environ Res*. 2005;97(2):195-200. PubMed PMID:15533335.
24. Inoue S, Yorifuji T, Tsuda T, Doi H. Short-term effect of severe exposure to methylmercury on atherosclerotic heart disease and hypertension mortality in Minamata. *Sci Total Environ*. 2012;417-418:291-293. PubMed PMID:22277149.
25. Salonen JT, Seppänen K, Lakka TA, Salonen R, Kaplan GA. Mercury accumulation and accelerated progression of carotid atherosclerosis: a population-based prospective 4-year follow-up study in men in eastern Finland. *Atherosclerosis*. 2000;148(2):265-273. PubMed PMID:10657561.
26. Virtanen JK, Voutilainen S, Rissanen TH, et al. Mercury, fish oils, and risk, of acute coronary events and cardiovascular disease, coronary heart disease, and all-cause mortality in men in eastern Finland. *Arterioscler Thromb Vasc Biol*. 2005;25(1):228-233. PubMed PMID:15539625.
27. Oh SM, Kim HR, Park YJ, Lee SY, Chung KH. Organic extracts of urban air pollution particulate matter (PM2.5)-induced genotoxicity and oxidative stress in human lung bronchial epithelial cells (BEAS-2B cells). *Mutat Res*. 2011;723(2):142-151. PubMed PMID:21524716.
28. Frikke-Schmidt H, Roursgaard M, Lykkesfeldt J, Loft S, Nøjgaard JK, Møller P. Effect of vitamin C and iron chelation on diesel exhaust particle and carbon black induced oxidative damage and cell adhesion molecule expression in human endothelial cells. *Toxicol Lett*. 2011;203(3):181-189. PubMed PMID:21421028.
29. Harrison CM, Pompilius M, Pinkerton KE, Ballinger SW. Mitochondrial oxidative stress significantly influences atherogenic risk and cytokine-induced oxidant production. *Environ Health Perspect*. 2011;119(5):676-681. PubMed PMID:21169125.
30. Zhang P, Dong G, Sun B, et al. Long-term exposure to ambient air pollution and mortality due to cardiovascular disease and cerebrovascular disease in Shenyang, China. *PLoS One*. 2011;6(6):e20827. PubMed PMID:21695220.
31. Ito K, Mathes R, Ross Z, Nadas A, Thurston G, Matte T. Fine particulate matter constituents associated with cardiovascular hospitalizations and mortality in New York City. *Environ Health Perspect*. 2011;119:467-473. PubMed PMID:21463978.

32. Guaita R, Pichiule M, Maté T, Linares C, Díaz J. Short-term impact of particulate matter (PM(2.5)) on respiratory mortality in Madrid. *Int J Environ Health Res*. 2011;21(4):260-274. PubMed PMID:21644129.

33. Katanoda K, Sobue T, Satoh H, et al. An association between long-term exposure to ambient air pollution and mortality from lung cancer and respiratory diseases in Japan. *J Epidemiol*. 2011;21(2):132-143. PubMed PMID:21325732.

34. Yu JZ, Huang XH, Ho SS, Bian Q. Nonpolar organic compounds in fine particles: quantification by thermal desorption-GC/MS and evidence for their significant oxidation in ambient aerosols in Hong Kong. *Anal Bioanal Chem*. 2011;401(10):3125-3139. PubMed PMID:21983947.

35. Brucker N, Moro AM, Charão MF, et al. Biomarkers of occupational exposure to air pollution, inflammation and oxidative damage in taxi drivers. *Sci Total Environ*. 2013;463-464:884-893. PubMed PMID:23872245.

36. Peters A, Skorkovsky J, Kotesovec F, et al. Associations between mortality and air pollution in Central Europe. *Environ Health Perspect*. 2000;108(4):282-287. PubMed PMID:10753084.

37. Mar TF, Norris GA, Koenig JQ, Larson TV. Associations between air pollution and mortality in Phoenix, 1995-1997. *Environ. Health Perspect*. 2000;108(4):347-353. PubMed PMID:10753094.

38. Morgan G, Corbett S, Wlodarczyk J, Lewis P. Air pollution and daily mortality in Sydney, Australia, 1989 through 1993. *Am J Pub Health*. 1998;88:759-764. PubMed PMID:9585741. PubMed PMID:9585741.

39. Chen H, Burnett RT, Copes R, et al. Ambient fine particulate matter and mortality among survivors of myocardial infarction: population-based cohort study. *Environ Health Perspect*. 2016;124(9):1421-1428. PubMed PMID:27152932.

40. Rosenbloom JI, Wilker EH, Mukamal KJ, Schwartz J, Mittleman MA. Residential proximity to major roadway and 10-year all-cause mortality after myocardial, infarction. *Circulation*. 2012;125(18):2197-2203. PubMed PMID:22566348.

41. Schwartz J. Air pollution and blood markers of cardiovascular risk. *Environ Health Perspect*. 2001;109 (suppl 3):405-409. PubMed PMID:11427390.

42. Donaldson K, Stone V, Seaton A, MacNee W. Ambient particle inhalation and cardiovascular system: potential mechanisms. *Environ Health Perspect*. 2001;109(suppl 4):523-527. PubMed PMID:11544157.

43. Künzli N, Jerrett M, Mack WJ, et al. Ambient air pollution and atherosclerosis in Los Angeles. *Environ Health Perspect*. 2005;113(2):201-206. PubMed PMID:15687058.

44. Hoffmann B, Moebus S, Möhlenkamp S, et al. Residential exposure to traffic is associated with coronary atherosclerosis. *Circulation*. 2007;116(5):489-496.PubMed PMID:17638927.

45. Ha MH, Lee DH, Jacobs DR. Association between serum concentrations of persistent organic pollutants and self-reported cardiovascular disease prevalence: results from the National Health and Nutrition Examination Survey, 1999-2002. *Environ Health Perspect*. 2007;115(8):1204-1209. PubMed PMID:17687448.

46. Schecter A, Colacino J, Haffner D, et al. Perfluorinated compounds, polychlorinated biphenyls, and organochlorine pesticide, contamination in composite food samples from Dallas, Texas, *USA*. *Environ Health Perspect*. 2010;118(6):796-802. PubMed PMID:20146964.

47. Lind PM, van Bavel B, Salihovic S, Lind L. Circulating levels of persistent organic pollutants (POPs) and carotid atherosclerosis in the elderly. *Environ Health Perspect*. 2012;120(1):38-43. PubMed PMID:22222676.

48. Goncharov A, Pavuk M, Foushee HR, Carpenter DO. Blood pressure in relation to concentrations of PCB congeners and chlorinated pesticides. *Environ Health Perspect*. 2011;119(3):319-325. PubMed PMID:21362590.

49. Sjöberg Lind Y, Lind PM, Salihovic S, van Bavel B, Lind L. Circulating levels of persistent organic pollutants (POPs) are associated with left ventricular systolic and diastolic dysfunction in the elderly. *Environ Res*. 2013;123:39-45. PubMed PMID:23562393.

50. Hurt RD, Weston SA, Ebbert JO, et al. Myocardial infarction and sudden cardiac death in Olmsted County, Minnesota, before and after smoke-free workplace laws. *Arch Intern Med*. 2012;172(21):1635-1641. PubMed PMID:23108571.

51. Langrish JP, Li X, Wang S, et al. Reducing personal exposure to particulate air pollution improves cardiovascular health in patients with coronary heart disease. *Environ Health Perspect*. 2012;120(3):367-372. PubMed PMID:22389220.

52. Allen RW, Carlsten C, Karlen B, et al. An air filter intervention study of endothelial function among healthy adults in a woodsmoke-impacted community. *Am J Respir Crit Care Med*. 2011;183(9):1222-1230. PubMed PMID:21257787.

53. Foglieni C, Fulgenzi A, Ticozzi P, et al. Protective effect of EDTA preadministration on renal ischemia. *BMC Nephrol*. 2006;7:5. PubMed PMID:16536881.

54. Lamas GA, Goertz C, Boineau R, et al. Effect of disodium EDTA chelation regimen on cardiovascular events in patients with previous myocardial infarction: the TACT randomized trial. *JAMA*. 2013;309(12):1241-1250. PubMed PMID:23532240.

55. Ruha AM, Curry SC, Gerkin RD, et al. Urine mercury excretion following meso-dimercaptosuccinic acid challenge in fish eaters. *Arch Pathol Lab Med*. 2009;133(1):87-92.

56. Graziano JH, Siris ES, LoIacono N, et al. 2,3-Dimercaptosuccinic acid as an antidote for lead intoxication. *Clin Pharmacol Ther*. 1985;37(4):431-438.

57. Tong H, Rappold AG, Diaz-Sanchez D, et al. Omega-3 fatty acid supplementation appears to attenuate particulate air pollution-induced cardiac effects and lipid changes in healthy middle-aged adults. *Environ Health Perspect*. 2012;120(7):952-957. PubMed PMID:22514211.

58. Dodd S, Dean O, Copolov DL, Malhi GS, Berk M. N-acetylcysteine for antioxidant therapy: pharmacology and clinical utility. *Expert Opin Biol Ther*. 2008;8(12):1955-1962.

59. Laukkanen T, Khan H, Zaccardi F, Laukkanen JA. Association between sauna bathing and fatal cardiovascular and all-cause mortality events. *JAMA Intern Med*. 2015;175(4):542-548. PubMed PMID:25705824.

60. Haseba S, Sakakima H, Kubozono T, Nakao S, Ikeda S. Combined effects of repeated sauna therapy and exercise training on cardiac function and physical activity in patients with chronic heart failure. *Disabil Rehabil*. 2016;38(5):409-415. PubMed PMID:25941983.

61. Genuis SJ, Birkholz D, Rodushkin I, Beesoon S. Blood, urine, and sweat (BUS) study: monitoring and elimination of bioaccumulated toxic elements. *Arch Environ Contam Toxicol*. 2011;61(2):344-357.

62. Genuis SJ, Lane K, Birkholz D. Human elimination of organochlorine pesticides: blood, urine, and sweat study. *Biomed Res Int*. 2016;2016:1624643.

35

The Role of Chelation Therapy in Cardiovascular Disease, Diabetes Mellitus, and Heavy Metal Detoxification: The TACT Trials

Jeanne Drisko, MD, CNS, FACN

Introduction

The identification of chelation as a chemical reaction originated in the late nineteenth and early twentieth centuries after discoveries by German and American chemists.[1,2] The word chelation is derived from the Greek word, CHELE, to describe the grabbing by crab or lobster claws. The pinching mechanism of the chemical chelator can effectively grab and bind metals and minerals. This led to attaching the term chelation to the chemical reaction to describe incorporation of a metal ion into a heterocyclic ring structure.

Chelation used in clinical medical practice as a therapeutic intervention usually involves pharmaceutically derived compounds. It is important to understand that the term chelation is a general nonspecific term that defines a chemical equilibrium reaction between a charged metal ion and a complexing agent that results in a chemical bond between the two. The metal is said to be chelated and the complexing agent is the chelator, whether this is from a plant-derived source or any administered pharmaceutical agent. There are many types of chelators, both pharmaceutical and natural products, with wide-ranging chemical structures and differing affinities for metals and minerals. Biological systems in both plants and animals show many types of metal-binding proteins, such as metallothionein.[3] These well-known chelators are central to the natural response of biological systems to toxic chemicals and, in humans, lead to inactivation of heavy metals and their eventual excretion by renal or biliary mechanisms.

Chelation is not a term that is specific to any one form of chelation therapy, although in some groups it has become synonymous with cardiovascular disease (CVD) treatment. To ascribe chelation therapy so narrowly to CVD is

to misunderstand the broad views and rich variety of chelators. That said, this chapter will focus on ethylenediaminetetraacetic acid (EDTA) chelation therapy for CVD practiced for decades by integrative practitioners and currently under investigation in the TACT trials. For readers interested in understanding the use of chelation in other disorders and the widely available chelators, references are provided for more in-depth review.[1,3-6]

History of EDTA Chelation Therapy

In the twentieth century, therapeutic applications of chelation to remove heavy metals in humans was discovered.[2,5,7,8] This was particularly valuable during World War II when chelation therapy was introduced as an antidote for arsenic-based poisonous gas exposures. This led to interest in chelation as a treatment of heavy metal poisoning, and chelation therapy has enjoyed basic science and clinical research through the ensuing years for treating heavy metal toxification. Chelation therapy for heavy metal intoxication has remained a mainstay in conventional toxicology when heavy metal poisoning is documented.[7,9-12] However, conventional toxicologists have not supported the use of chelation therapy by integrative medicine practitioners in the treatment of CVD and heavy metal poisoning.[2,13,14] Yet chelation therapy remains an important tool in integrative medicine when symptomatic patients with positive biological markers for heavy metal toxicity have positive test results with laboratory analysis.

EDTA is a pharmaceutically produced chelator first used in the 1930s in the German textile industry. EDTA was found to be helpful as a chelating agent to remove calcium during dye processing. In the 1940s, Martin Rubin, PhD, along with chemist, Frederick Bersworth, discovered the biological effects of EDTA on calcium homeostasis, leading to its use in the laboratory as an anticoagulant.[15] Rubin subsequently gained approval from the Food and Drug Administration (FDA) for EDTA use in humans with lead poisoning (CaEDTA) and hypercalcemia (disodium EDTA). Abbott Laboratories manufactured disodium EDTA under the tradename Endrate. It is this form of EDTA that is intravenously administered as chelation therapy that has become synonymous with the practice of chelation therapy for CVD.

Chelation therapy for the treatment of CVD dates to the 1950s. Two physicians, Albert Boyle and Norman E. Clarke Sr., separately published case reports that showed improvement in CVD status in patients who were receiving disodium EDTA during treatment of lead poisoning.[2,16] The literature through this period is replete with numerous articles that include case reports, small clinical trials, mechanistic studies, observational studies, and anecdotal reports of benefits when disodium EDTA was administered in patients with atherosclerotic vascular disease (ASVD).[2,17,18] This led to the historical hypothesis that disodium EDTA chelation in CVD decalcified diseased atherosclerotic vascular structures.

Clarke and colleagues treated a small number of patients with severe angina with disodium EDTA and found improved outcomes in 19 of 20 patients.[16] Other small unblinded studies with limited assessment followed but seem to have less dramatic results.[19,20] Because of increasing controversy and variation in outcomes, conventional practitioners abandoned EDTA chelation.[18] Chelation practitioners banded together to form medical organizations with the benefit of standardizing the infusions, doses administered, and rates of administration of disodium EDTA chelation.[2,21-26] Standardizing the administration of EDTA chelation succeeded over the ensuing years to provide a safe in-office practice, and it has been estimated that there have been millions of chelation infusions administered. Chelation practitioners develop protocols to make this therapy exceptionally safe.[2] For example, when EDTA chelation is infused rapidly, hypocalcemia may result. Of interest, there have been only 11 deaths attributed to EDTA chelation reported to the FDA, with 7 of those 11 deaths from prescription or pharmacy errors resulting in infusion of the incorrect form of EDTA.[27]

Conventional physicians and cardiologists exhibited growing skepticism and hostility toward the practice of chelation therapy for CVD, but the practice continued to grow in the hands of integrative medicine practitioners. In 1963, disodium EDTA for CVD came under additional scrutiny when data published from a study with 10 male patients was combined with another trial with 81 patients, all with ASVD.[28] The conclusion of the paper was a recommendation for disodium EDTA chelation therapy to be discontinued as a treatment of CVD because of poor outcomes. Of note, across the 2 years of the study, the authors infused EDTA chelation therapy at a dose of 3 g for 2.5 to 3 hours in 2000 consecutive infusions without a reported adverse event. However, the report by Metzler et al. sparked debate on the part of the practicing chelation physicians calling into question the

merits and pointing out problems with the report. The result of the Metzler et al. paper was to drive the practice of disodium EDTA for CVD underground, becoming the purview of integrative physicians only. As cardiologists warned patients against the practice because of the poor evidence base, integrative physicians continued EDTA chelation therapy for vascular disease to the present time. Case reports continued to be published in non–peer reviewed journals describing reversal of atherosclerotic plaques and reduction in symptomatic complaints of angina or claudication while receiving EDTA chelation. Conventional toxicologic research continued to focus on the use of EDTA for lead toxicity foregoing further research of chelation for CVD.[4,6,7,29-32]

In 2002, the Cochrane Collaboration reviewed EDTA chelation therapy used in ASVD.[17] The report included that there were no trials demonstrating the effectiveness of chelation therapy for coronary or cerebrovascular disease. The majority of trials to the time of the review focused on peripheral vascular disease, specifically investigating EDTA chelation as a treatment of intermittent claudication. The analysis proposed conducting randomized controlled trials in coronary and cerebrovascular disease because of the widespread ongoing use of the therapy. Subsequently, a small randomized trial (PATCH) was conducted in rolling 84 participants with known ischemic heart disease and angina, concluding that there was no evidence to support a beneficial effect of disodium EDTA chelation in CVD in this cohort.[33] The authors acknowledged that the trial was underpowered and therefore unlikely to show effect. Another confounding factor was that the placebo infusions contained IV vitamin C and this could not be excluded from having a beneficial effect.[34] Chelation therapy for CVD was about to enter into its next phase.

Trial to Assess Chelation Therapy (TACT1)

In 2002, the National Institutes of Health, National Center for Complementary and Integrative Health (formerly National Center for Complementary and Alternative Medicine), in partnership with the National Heart Lung and Blood Institute, funded the largest randomized controlled trial investigating disodium EDTA chelation therapy for CVD. The trial was known as the Trial to Assess Chelation Therapy (TACT).[35] TACT was the largest multicenter trial to study disodium EDTA chelation in a randomized placebo-controlled fashion, enrolling 1708 participants with a history of prior myocardial infarction (MI).[35,36] The participants were enrolled to either the placebo arm or the active EDTA chelation arm to receive 40 infusions with the use of low-dose versus high-dose multivitamin regimen.[37] Lamas et al. reported at the conclusion of the TACT trial that disodium EDTA infusions compared with placebo reduced the risk for adverse cardiovascular outcomes.[36] The TACT trial showed a statistically significant effect in decreasing all-cause mortality in the treatment arm.[36] An unexpected finding was a surprising highly significant benefit of disodium EDTA chelation therapy in type II diabetic patients.[38] When the diabetic subgroup was removed from the active treatment arm analysis, no benefit was identified in the remaining participants randomized to the treatment arm.

The treatment arm with disodium EDTA chelation therapy in the diabetic cohort demonstrated remarkable results.[39] Almost 40% of the 633 participants randomized to receive the active chelation solution met the standard definition of diabetes. The authors noted they chose to study diabetic patients as a subgroup not because of anticipated benefits, but rather as a precaution for elevated risk in this group. As expected, the diabetic participants had a higher prevalence of congestive heart failure, stroke, peripheral artery disease, hypertension, and hypercholesterolemia when compared with the nondiabetic participants consistent with elevated risk in this group.

The primary end point of evaluating cardiovascular events was significantly reduced compared with the placebo arm (hazard ratio [HR] 0.59 [0.44, 0.79], $P < .001$) with a 15% absolute decrease in the 5-year primary event rate and a relative reduction of 41%.[39] The secondary end points of cardiovascular death, MI, or stroke were also lower for diabetic participants receiving the active EDTA chelation infusion (HR 0.60 [0.39, 0.91], $P = .017$). Diabetic participants receiving the active disodium EDTA infusion had a significant reduction in all-cause mortality (HR 0.57 [0.36, 0.88], $P = .011$) in recurrent MI (HR 0.48 [0.26, 0.88], $P = .015$) and in coronary revascularization (HR 0.68 [0.47, 0.99], $P = .042$).

With the language of the therapy historically identified as chelation, it is important to highlight that the active EDTA chelation solution contains many ingredients. The infusate contains 3 g of disodium EDTA, 7 g of ascorbic acid, 2 g of magnesium chloride, 100 mg of procaine hydrochloride, 2500 U of unfractionated heparin, 2 mEq of potassium chloride, 840 mg of sodium bicarbonate, 250 mg of pantothenic acid, 100 mg of thiamine, 100 mg of pyridoxine, and sterile water to make up 500 mL of solution.[35] Because these components are administered intravenously and bypass usual metabolic absorption and excretion pathways, it can be said that they are pharmacologic agents with presumed unexpected and unpredicted biologic activity. The TACT trial was not designed to tease out the effects of each of these components or their contribution to the outcome, nor was it designed to determine a plausible mechanism of action. In addition, the trial did not seek to determine whether there was heavy metal toxicity in the participants. It was designed to mimic the real-world administration of EDTA chelation therapy as practiced by integrative medicine practitioners and determine if there was an effect to point the way for further trials or to advocate stopping the therapy entirely. But the way forward must include a broad view of mechanisms, whether they point to the chelating effects alone or include other unanticipated mechanisms related to the components of the infusate.

There are concerns regarding the conclusions and the singular focus on chelation in TACT1. First, the combination of vitamins, minerals, and other components of the intravenous infusion solution have biologic activity that have not been

acknowledged. Second, the focus solely on EDTA chelation and removal of heavy metals as the sole hypothesis of benefit does not adequately explain why only diabetic participants benefited from heavy metal removal. Third, there is no explanation why nondiabetic participants with advanced CVD enrolled in the TACT trial did not benefit from heavy metal removal because it is known that they are also highly exposed to heavy metals. Although heavy metals were not measured in TACT1, this is being remedied as discussed in the following text.

It is plausible that the majority of the effect of the chelation solution was related to EDTA as CVD is associated with heavy metal toxicity.[40,41] Yet it is curious that the effect was seen in diabetic patients only. One could also argue that heavy metal toxicity in individuals could predispose them to type 2 diabetes as there is evidence of this adverse outcome, making EDTA chelation a beneficial therapy.[42,43] It is known that diabetic patients have an increased oxidative burden with increased reactive oxygen species; therefore, any extra heavy metal burden would drive this adverse process.[44] It has been noted as well that some of the antidiabetic medications have in vitro metal-chelating properties.[39] Of interest, Lamas and colleagues describe the effects of oxidative damage and the effects on vitamin C, an important component of redox chemistry. Yet, they do not recognize that vitamin C is an important component of the chelation solution. Although they do provide some explanation regarding prevention of oxidation of vitamin C by the use of conventional cardiology medications, they do not take the extra step to consider its importance as part of the chelation infusate. To their benefit, Lamas and colleagues do acknowledge that the materials cited to support their hypothesis regarding the benefits of chelation therapy observed in "diabetic patients are speculative in nature, and by no means can be viewed as conclusive. They do serve, however, to emphasize the double-edged nature of metals, even essential metals, in biological systems." However, no explanation is given about how nondiabetic patients with CVD and heavy metal overload might escape this destructive damage to the vascular system.

In fact, to prepare for the follow-up TACT trial, Lamas and colleagues point to a trial that collected 24-hour urine specimens, before and after EDTA infusions, to evaluate for the amount of excreted heavy metal and essential minerals.[45] Urinary lead and cadmium excretion rose by 3830% and 514%, respectively, over 2 days post edetate disodium infusion. This, however, was collected solely in diabetic patients, ignoring the nondiabetic patients with CVD who also most certainly have heavy metal burden. But as the authors note, "Whether such an action has any therapeutic value depends, of course, on whether accumulation of higher levels of these metals in the body really has adverse vascular consequences."[39]

Finally, the authors asked whether they had simply improved diabetes management with the caveat that such a significant improvement in diabetes management has never demonstrated such a magnitude in cardiovascular event reduction.[39] Remarkably, diabetic participants receiving the active disodium EDTA treatment had no difference in fasting blood glucose from baseline to the last infusion requiring a blood draw ($P = .64$). Simple diabetic control is an unlikely reason for the remarkable effects seen in the diabetic subgroup. The logical next step would be to repeat the trial in a diabetic cohort with known CVD, which indeed was done and led to TACT2.

Trial to Assess Chelation Therapy 2 (TACT2)

TACT2 is underway to replicate the findings of TACT1 but enrolling diabetic patients with a history of prior myocardial event. As noted, TACT1 found a reduction of recurrent cardiovascular events in post-MI diabetic patients who received the active EDTA solution.[39,40] TACT2 is targeting enrollment of approximately 1200 diabetic patients 50 years or older with a prior MI. Infusions will be administered on a weekly basis for 40 weeks through a peripheral intravenous line over at least 3 hours, as in TACT1. The primary objective of TACT2 is to determine if the chelation-based strategy increases the time to the first occurrence of any of the components of the TACT2 primary end point: all-cause mortality, MI, stroke, coronary revascularization, or hospitalization for unstable angina compared with the placebo chelation strategy.

TACT2 plans to focus primarily on lead and cadmium as factors in diabetic CVD. Heavy metals have been a source of human toxicity since the beginning of time, with many heavy metals such as arsenic and cadmium ubiquitous in the earth's crust and in the water supply. Industrialization and manufacturing have accelerated the universal exposure of many heavy metals such as lead and mercury in humans, making these toxicants part of the air, soil, and water. It is beyond the scope of this chapter to discuss the many types and varieties of heavy metals humankind is exposed to, and references are provided for further reading.[32,46-54] It is sufficient to say that, through disruption of biochemical pathways and acceleration of inflammation, there are untoward effects throughout the body, including the vascular and endocrine systems and these are well documented.

Concerns have been raised regarding administering chelation infusions in diabetic participants who might have impaired renal function. In TACT1, 95 serious, adverse events were reported in the diabetes subgroup, with 56 occurring in patients receiving placebo infusions and 39 in patients receiving active chelation infusions. Drug-related adverse events resulted in 5.7% withdrawal from the trial: 20 subjects in the placebo group and 16 in the active chelation group. Renal function was not further compromised by receiving the chelation infusions. Concerns about safety in diabetic patients were lessened, but careful monitoring of physical and laboratory findings will be conducted as in TACT1.

The TACT2 trialist state reduction in clinical events was enhanced in diabetic patients, to a point not heretofore seen with glycemic control alone.[55] These data point to benefits

related to alternative, new mechanisms that current drug therapies do not address. The researchers hypothesize that the active TACT infusion removes ionic metal catalysts that can promote oxidative stress that catalyzes upstream biochemical pathways that may result in conditions conducive to atherosclerotic plaque formation. In other words, the EDTA chelation effect in diabetic patients is hypothesized to be related to heavy metal binding and removal that mitigates the damaging effects of reactive oxygen species formed leading to atherosclerotic plaque formation.

An added benefit in TACT2 is the analyses of blood and urine lead and cadmium levels to compare the change from baseline to the 40th infusion or in 1 year in the active versus placebo infusion arms. Metal collections and the biorepository were designed to support analyses to determine whether preinfusion metal measurements compared with postinfusion urine metal measurements have clinical prognostic significance for predicting outcomes and clinical benefit of chelation in TACT2.[40,55]

Future Directions

What is known from TACT1 is a significantly beneficial effect of the infusion containing multiple components that has been referred to as chelation therapy, and this effect seems to be primarily confined to diabetic patients with documented CVD. What is unknown is if there were elevated levels of heavy metals in the TACT1 population in both diabetic and nondiabetic participants. Another unknown is if the presence of heavy metals alone singularly accelerated the cardiovascular damage in the diabetic subgroup of TACT1 with the chelating effect of disodium EDTA providing the benefit in cardiac outcomes. Also in question is whether TACT2 will be able to conclusively answer these questions. Unwinding the TACT1 results serves only to provide questions that TACT2 is not designed to answer. Specifically, are the infusion components additive or synergistic with disodium EDTA or independent? Is EDTA necessary in the infusion? What is the importance of pharmacologic ascorbate in diabetes, which is known to be deficient in diabetic populations[56]; low-circulating ascorbic acid concentrations are commonly associated with metabolic syndrome[57] and progression to type 2 diabetes.[58-63] That said, it is important that TACT2 proceed to determine if TACT1 findings can be replicated in diabetic patients as the reduction in cardiovascular events was profound.

What is urgently needed are preclinical models of diabetes with and without heavy metal burden investigating the individual components of the infusate alone and in combinations to try to tease out the importance of the solution called chelation. A phase I study in humans matching the TACT1 participants demographics and cardiovascular status using disodium EDTA alone in the infusion would be a necessary next step. This would be helpful in understanding if the heavy metal burden in the diabetic and nondiabetic populations are similar. It would also be important to design a randomized placebo-controlled blinded study using disodium EDTA alone and apart from the other components of the infusion in diabetic patients to determine if it is the actual practice of chelation that provides the cardiovascular effects.

For practitioners who care for patients with CVD, it is not important how future trials are developed especially since decades will elapse before conclusions are drawn. It is important that patients be rigorously evaluated for macro- and micronutrient status and corrections made accordingly with a healthful diet as the foundation. This must include an interprofessional team of integrative and functional practitioners including dieticians, advanced practice nurses, physicians, psychologists, coaches, and others as the clinic situation demands. No longer can single physicians in silos care for chronically ill patients.

Laboratory testing has evolved to include genetic testing along with micronutrient levels, conventional laboratory testing, endocrine evaluation, presence of environmental toxins, and heavy metal burden. This testing is imperative to give patients the opportunity to return to good health under care of the interprofessional team. When heavy metal testing is done appropriately with pre- and postchelation challenge specimen collection, decisions based on real-world evidence can be made about the use of chelators if heavy metal burden is present. Chelation has also evolved and is no longer limited to the use of EDTA,[4] although EDTA has its role. What the modern integrative and functional practitioner should seek out is appropriate training from organizations that provide broad detoxification techniques, not just heavy metal detoxification, as this expanded view leads to restoration of health (see appendix). When these tools are used and combined with the best of conventional medical interventions, patients are placed back at the center and true healing begins.

Additional Resources

1. American College for Advancement in Medicine www.acam.org Chelation education with certification and detoxification education
2. International College of Integrative Medicine https://icimed.com/ Chelation education with certification and detoxification education
3. American Academy of Environmental Medicine https://www.aaemonline.org/ detoxification education
4. Institute for Functional Medicine https://www.ifm.org/ detoxification education

References

1. Hodgson E. Chapter 1: Introduction to toxicology. In: Hodgson E, ed. *A Textbook of Modern Toxicology*. 3rd ed. Hoboken, NJ: John Wiley and Sons; 2004.
2. Rozema T. The protocol for the safe and effective administration of EDTA and other chelating agents for vascular disease, degenerative disease, and metal toxicity. *J Adv Med*. 1997;10(1):5-100.
3. Sears ME. Chelation: harnessing and enhancing heavy metal detoxification–a review. *Scientific World J*. 2013;2013:219840. doi:10.1155/2013/219840.
4. Aposhian HV. Mobilization of heavy metals by newer, therapeutically useful chelating agents. *Toxicology*. 1995;97(1-3):23-38.
5. Drisko JA. Chapter 107: chelation therapy. In: Rakel D, ed. *Textbook of Integrative Medicine*. 4th ed. Philadelphia, PA: Elsevier; 2018:1004-1015. doi:10.1016/B978-0-323-35868-2.00107-9.
6. Klaassen C. Heavy metals and heavy-metal antagonists. In: Brunton L, Lazo J, Parker K, Buxton I, Blumenthal DE, eds. *Goodmans and Gilman's the Pharmacological Basis of Therapeutics*. 11th ed. New York: McGraw Hill; 2006:1753-1775.
7. Flora SJS, Pachauri V. Chelation in metal intoxication. *Int J Environ Res Public Health*. 2010;7(7):2745-2788.
8. Flora SJS, Shrivastava R, Mittal M Chemistry and pharmacological properties of some natural and synthetic antioxidants for heavy metal toxicity. *Curr Med Chem*. 2013;20(36):4540-4574. doi:10.2174/09298673113209990146.
9. Andersen O. Principles and recent developments in chelation treatment of metal intoxication. *Chem Rev*. 1999;99(9):2683-2710. doi:10.1021/cr980453a.
10. Jones MM. *Chapter 35:* Design of new chelating agents for removal of intracellular toxic metals. In: Kauffman GB, ed. *Coordination Chemistry: A Century of Progress*. Washington, DC: American Chemical Society Publishing; 1994:427-438. doi:10.1021/bk-1994-0565.ch035.
11. Kosnett MJ. The Role of chelation in the treatment of arsenic and mercury poisoning. *J Med Toxicol*. 2013;9(4):347-354. doi:10.1007/s13181-013-0344-5.
12. McKay C. Public health department response to mercury poisoning: the importance of biomarkers and risks and benefits analysis for chelation therapy. *J Med Toxicol*. 2013;9(4):308-312. doi:10.1007/s13181-013-0340-9.
13. Crinnion WJ. The benefits of pre- and post-challenge urine heavy metal testing: Part 1. *Altern Med Rev*. 2009;14(1):3-8. PMID:19364190.
14. McKay C Jr. Introduction to special issue: use and misuse of metal chelation therapy. *J Med Toxicol*. 2013;9(4):298-300. doi:10.1007/s13181-013-0346-3.
15. Olmstead S. *A Critical Review of EDTA Chelation Therapy in the Treatment of Occlusive Vascular Disease*. Klamath Falls, Oregon: Merle West Medical Center Foundation; 1998.
16. Clarke CN, Clarke NE, Mosher RE. Treatment of angina pectoris with disodium ethylene diamine tetraacetic acid. *Am J Med Sci*. 1956;232(6):654-666. PMID:13372537.
17. Villarruz MV, Dans A, Tan F. Chelation therapy for atherosclerotic cardiovascular disease. *Cochrane Database Syst Rev*. 2002;(4):CD002785. doi:10.1002/14651858.CD002785/pdf/standard.
18. Seely DMR, Wu P, Mills EJ. EDTA chelation therapy for cardiovascular disease: a systematic review. *BMC Cardiovasc Disord*. 2005;5:32. doi:10.1186/1471-2261-5-32.
19. Kitchell JR, Meltzer LE, Seven MJ. Potential uses of chelation methods in the treatment of cardiovascular diseases. *Prog Cardiovasc Dis*. 1961;3:338-349. PMID:13756462.
20. Kitchell JR, Palmon F, Aytan N, Meltzer LE. The treatment of coronary artery disease with disodium EDTA. A reappraisal. *Am J Cardiol*. 1963;11:501-506. PMID:14033183.
21. Lewin MR. Chelation therapy for cardiovascular disease. Review and commentary. *Tex Heart Inst J*. 1997;24(2):81-89. PubMed:9205980.
22. Olszewer E, Sabbag FC, Carter JP. A pilot double-blind study of sodium-magnesium EDTA in peripheral vascular disease. *J Natl Med Assoc*. 1990;82(3):173-177. PubMed:2108254.
23. Chappell LT, Janson M. EDTA chelation therapy in the treatment of vascular disease. *J Cardiovasc Nurs*. 1996;10(3):78-86. PubMed:8820322.
24. Lamar CP. Chelation therapy of occlusive arteriosclerosis in diabetic patients. *Angiology*. 1964;15:379-395. PubMed:14210345.
25. American College for Advancement in Medicine. https://www.acam.org/.
26. International College of Integrative Medicine. https://icimed.com/.
27. http://www.fda.gov/Drugs/DrugSafety/PostmarketDrugSafetyInformationforPatientsandProviders/ucm113738.htm.

28. Meltzer LE, Kitchell JR, Palmon F. The long-term use, side effects, and toxicity of disodium ethylenediaminetetraacetic acid (EDTA). *Am J Med Sci.* 1961;242:11-17. doi:10.1097/00000441-196107000-00002.

29. Binns HJ, Campbell C, Brown MJ. Interpreting and managing blood lead levels of less than 10 microg/dL in children and reducing childhood exposure to lead: recommendations of the Centers for Disease Control and Prevention Advisory Committee on Childhood Lead Poisoning Prevention. *Pediatrics.* 2007;120(5):e1285-e1298. doi:10.1542/peds.2005-1770.

30. Schnur J, John RM. Childhood lead poisoning and the new Centers for Disease Control and Prevention guidelines for lead exposure. *J Am Assoc Nurse Pract.* 2014;26(5):238-247. doi:10.1002/2327-6924.12112.

31. Lin JL, Lin Tan DT, Hsu KH, Yu CC. Environmental lead exposure and progression of chronic renal diseases in patients without diabetes. *N Engl J Med.* 2003;348(4):277-286. doi:10.1056/NEJMoa021672.

32. Nash D, Magder L, Lustberg M, et al. Blood lead, blood pressure, and hypertension in perimenopausal and postmenopausal women. *JAMA.* 2003;289(12):1523-1532. doi:10.1001/jama.289.12.1523.

33. Knudtson ML, Wyse DG, Galbraith PD, et al. Chelation therapy for ischemic heart disease: a randomized controlled trial. *JAMA.* 2002;287(4):481-486. doi:joc11301 [pii].

34. Anderson TJ, Hubacek J, George Wyse D, Knudtson ML. Effect of chelation therapy on endothelial function in patients with coronary artery disease: PATCH substudy. *J Am Coll Cardiol.* 2003;41(3):420-425. doi:10.1016/S0735-1097(02)02770-5.

35. Lamas Ga, Goertz C, Boineau R, et al. Design of the trial to assess chelation therapy (TACT). *Am Heart J.* 2012;163(1):7-12. doi:10.1016/j.ahj.2011.10.002.

36. Lamas GA, Goertz C, Boineau R, et al. Effect of disodium EDTA chelation regimen on cardiovascular events in patients with previous myocardial infarction: the TACT randomized trial. *JAMA.* 2013;309(12):1241-1250. doi:10.1001/jama.2013.2107.

37. Lamas G, Boineau R, Goertz C, et al. EDTA chelation therapy alone and in combination with oral high-dose multivitamins and minerals for coronary disease: the factorial group results of the Trial to Assess Chelation Therapy. *Am Heart J.* 2014;168(1):37-44.e5. doi:10.1016/j.ahj.2014.02.012.

38. Escolar E, Lamas Ga, Mark DB, et al. The effect of an EDTA-based chelation regimen on patients with diabetes mellitus and prior myocardial infarction in the Trial to Assess Chelation Therapy (TACT). *Circ Cardiovasc Qual Outcomes.* 2014;7(1):15-24. doi:10.1161/CIRCOUTCOMES.113.000663.

39. Lamas GA, Ergui I. Chelation therapy to treat atherosclerosis, particularly in diabetes: is it time to reconsider? *Expert Rev Cardiovasc Ther.* 2016;14(8):927-938. doi:10.1080/14779072.2016.1180977.

40. Lamas GA, Navas-Acien A, Mark DB, Lee KL. Heavy metals, cardiovascular disease, and the unexpected benefits of chelation therapy. *J Am Coll Cardiol.* 2016;67(20):2411-2418. doi:10.1016/j.jacc.2016.02.066.

41. Alissa EM, Ferns GA. Heavy metal poisoning and cardiovascular disease. *J Toxicol.* 2011;2011:870125. doi:10.1155/2011/870125.

42. Chen YW, Yang CY, Huang CF, Hung DZ, Leung YM, Liu SH. Heavy metals, islet function and diabetes development. *Islets.* 2009;1(3):169-176. doi:10.4161/isl.1.3.9262.

43. Rani A, Kumar A, Lal A, Pant M. Cellular mechanisms of cadmium-induced toxicity: a review. *Int J Environ Health Res.* 2014;24(4):378-399. doi:10.1080/09603123.2013.835032.

44. Frizzell N, Baynes JW. Chelation therapy: overlooked in the treatment and prevention of diabetes complications? *Future Med Chem.* [Internet]. 2013;5(10):1075-1078. http://www.ncbi.nlm.nih.gov/pubmed/23795964.

45. Waters RS, Bryden NA, Patterson KY, Veillon C, Anderson RA. EDTA chelation effects on urinary losses of cadmium, calcium, chromium, cobalt, copper, lead, magnesium, and zinc. *Biol Trace Elem Res.* 2001;83(3):207-221. PMID:11794513.

46. Patrick L. Lead toxicity, a review of the literature. Part 1: exposure, evaluation, and treatment. *Altern Med Rev.* 2006;11(1):2-22. PMID:16597190.

47. Fiorim J, Ribeiro Júnior RF, Silveira EA, et al. Low-level lead exposure increases systolic arterial pressure and endothelium-derived vasodilator factors in rat aortas. *PLoS One.* 2011;6(2):e17117. PMID:21364020.

48. Stohs SJ, Bagchi D. Oxidative mechanisms in the toxicity of metal ions. *Free Radic Biol Med.* 1995;18(2):321-336. PMID:7744317.

49. Sanders T, Liu Y, Buchner V, Tchounwou PB. Neurotoxic effects and biomarkers of lead exposure: a review. *Rev Environ Health.* 2009;24(1):15-45.

50. Vaziri ND, Khan M. Interplay of reactive oxygen species and nitric oxide in the pathogenesis of experimental lead-induced hypertension. *Clin Exp Pharmacol Physiol.* 2007;34(9):920-925. PMID:17645641.

51. Hanna CW, Bloom MS, Robinson WP, et al. DNA methylation changes in whole blood is associated with exposure to the environmental contaminants, mercury, lead, cadmium and bisphenol A, in women undergoing ovarian stimulation for IVF. *Hum Reprod.* 2012;27(5):1401-1410. PMID:22381621.

52. Muntner P, Menke A, DeSalvo KB, Rabito FA, Batuman V. Continued decline in blood lead levels among adults in the United States: the National Health and Nutrition Examination Surveys. *Arch Intern Med.* 2005;165(18):2155-2161. PMID:16217007.

53. Navas-Acien A, Selvin E, Sharrett AR, Calderon-Aranda E, Silbergeld E, Guallar E. Lead, cadmium, smoking, and increased risk of peripheral arterial disease. *Circulation.* 2004;109(25):3196-3201.

54. Weisskopf MG, Jain N, Nie H, et al. A prospective study of bone lead concentration and death from all causes, cardiovascular diseases, and cancer in the Department of Veterans Affairs Normative Aging Study. *Circulation.* 2009;120(12):1056-1064. PMID:19738141.

55. Calderon Moreno R, Navas-Acien A, Escolar E, et al. Potential role of metal chelation to prevent the cardiovascular complications of diabetes. *J Clin Endocrinol Metab.* 2019;104(7):2931-2941. doi:10.1210/jc.2018-01484.

56. Schleicher RL, Carroll MD, Ford ES, Lacher DA, Serum vitamin C and the prevalence of vitamin C deficiency in the United States: 2003-2004 National Health and Nutrition Examination Survey (NHANES), *Am J Clin Nutr.* 2009;90:1252-1263. doi:10.3945/ajcn.2008.27016.

57. Wei J, Zeng C, Gong QY, Li XX, Lei GH, Yang TB. Associations between dietary antioxidant intake and metabolic syndrome. *PLoS One.* 2015;10:e0130876. doi:10.1371/journal.pone.0130876.

58. Donin AS, Dent JE, Nightingale CM, et al. Fruit, vegetable and vitamin C intakes and plasma vitamin C: cross-sectional associations with insulin resistance and glycaemia in 9-10 year-old children. *Diabet Med.* 2016;33:307-315. doi:10.1111/dme.13006.

59. Lamb MJ, Griffin SJ, Sharp SJ, Cooper AJ. Fruit and vegetable intake and cardiovascular risk factors in people with newly diagnosed type 2 diabetes, *Eur J Clin Nutr.* 2017;71:115-121. doi:10.1038/ejcn.2016.180.

60. Du H, Li L, Bennett D, et al. China Kadoorie Biobank Study. Fresh fruit consumption in relation to incident diabetes and diabetic vascular complications: a 7-y prospective study of 0.5 million Chinese adults. *Plos Med.* 2017;14:e1002279. doi:10.1371/journal.pmed.1002279.

61. Gudjinu HY, Sarfo B. Risk factors for type 2 diabetes mellitus among out-patients in Ho, the Volta regional capital of Ghana: a case-control study. *BMC Res Notes.* 2017;10: 324. doi:10.1186/s13104-017-2648-z.

62. Wilson R, Willis J, Gearry R, et al, Inadequate vitamin C status in prediabetes and type 2 diabetes mellitus: associations with glycaemic control, obesity, and smoking. *Nutrients.* 2017;9(9):pii:E997. doi:10.3390/nu9090997.

63. Harding AH, Wareham NJ, Bingham SA, et al, Plasma vitamin C level, fruit and vegetable consumption, and the risk of new-onset type 2 diabetes mellitus: the European prospective investigation of cancer–Norfolk prospective study. *Arch Intern Med.* 2008;168:1493-1499. doi:10.1001/archinte.168.14.1493.

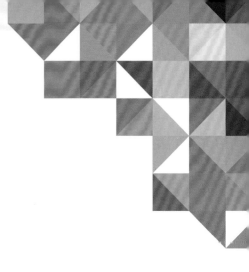

36

Heart Disease in Women

Stephen T. Sinatra, MD, FACC, FACN, CNS

2019 Considerations for a Gender Subspecialty

Gender-specific medicine may perhaps be the newest subspecialty in cardiology to emerge in the very near future. Almost 20 years ago in my book, *Heart Sense for Women*,[1] I discussed the differentiation of symptoms and presentation of heart disease for women, which we long thought to be the same as they were for men. The genders are definitely different not only in diagnosis and treatment, but prognosis as well.

Although women are generally better in touch with their physical and emotional pain than men are, they tend to experience more subtle or vague nondescript physical symptoms of heart disease compared to their male counterparts. As myocardial ischemia may be manifested as both typical and atypical symptoms in women, in my experience, making the diagnosis of angina—as well as myocardial infarction—is a more complex and a poorly understood process.

In general, most men may experience a dramatic crushing substernal pain in their chest—with or without radiation to the left shoulder and/or left elbow area—or extreme shortness of breath when having a myocardial infarction. But women's symptoms may be more vague including the following:

- Discomfort, pressure, or pain in the chest, arm, and/or back
- Tingling or pain in the jaw, elbow, or arm (both men and women collectively tend to feel pain in the left elbow or arm when having ischemia)
- Profound shortness of breath and/or dizziness with exertion
- Profound sudden fatigue
- Tightness or a strangling sensation in the throat
- Dizziness and/or vertigo
- Nausea and/or vomiting
- Indigestion (women often feel if they just "burp" they would feel better)

Although some men may have any of the above symptoms as well, they are more subtle in presentation for women. For example, I recently heard from a woman colleague in her 60s. She had called to share her experience of having a very recent and unexpected myocardial infarction in the middle of the night, she was awakened with profound nausea and vomiting. The unexplained symptoms dissipated. She realized that there was no apparent reason for the "attack": no real reason to suspect food poisoning or stomach flu. So, she went back to bed. A few days later she awoke again. The profuse sweating was then accompanied by some ill-defined chest discomfort. She experienced extreme dread, which can be another hallmark sign.

Dangerously, she drove herself to an urgent care center where both her electrocardiogram and blood tests confirmed the diagnosis of myocardial infarction. The damage was caused by a blockage in her circumflex coronary artery, a location much preferable to the left anterior descending, which would have resulted in more significant myocardial damage. She was successfully stented and fortunately had a "happy ending."

Although her prognosis remained good for the future, she was also placed on statin therapy, despite the fact that she had a cholesterol level within normal limits. Generally speaking, I am not a big fan of giving statin drugs to women because the risk/benefit ratio is just not in their favor. However, in situations of an acute coronary artery syndrome or preinfarction angina, continuation of statins in the coronary care unit (CCU) or intensive care unit (ICU) is strongly recommended as the pleotropic effects are especially noteworthy in overall survival. Although these blood thinning, antioxidant, and pleotropic properties of statins may be beneficial to some women, many more women compared to men develop intolerable side effects in the musculoskeletal system, developing weakness and myalgias.[2] In addition, calcification of the coronaries,[3] diabetes,[4] and even breast cancer[5] are all problematic for women on long-term statin therapy. In fact, a 2010 meta-analysis[6] found that statin therapy actually increased rather than decreased coronary artery disease (CAD) risk in women. Although it is well known that statins deplete precious nutrients like coenzyme Q10, vitamins D and E, zinc, and magnesium, to mention a few, the inhibition of vitamin K2, the cofactor for matrix and Gla-protein activation, and the decline in the biosynthesis of selenium-containing proteins (glutathione peroxidase) creates a possible ominous scenario.[7] Indeed this undesirable effect of artherosclerosis and heart failure by the pervasive use of statin drugs must be considered by the astute physician.[7] However, in men younger than 75 years with proven CAD, I do prefer a low-dose statin in combination with multivitamin/multimineral support and Coenzyme Q10 therapy. Like Coenzyme Q10, statins have favorable antioxidant, blood thinning, and anti-inflammatory properties which certainly appear promising for younger men. In my experience, the risk/benefit is worth the possible side effects, which is less intense than it is in women.[8] The use of statins warrants careful scrutiny as a gender-specific intervention. In the most recent study on statin therapy in the primary prevention of CAD, statin medications provided no clinical benefit when prior coronary artery calcium score was zero in a retrospective analysis of 13,644 patients.[9]

To further complicate the diagnosis and prognosis of heart disease in women, observational findings reported in a very recent medical communication how women physicians do a better job assessing other women presenting in urgent care centers who are experiencing chest pain than male physicians. Additionally, women patients are more likely to survive a myocardial infarction if their treatment is administered and overseen by female doctors.[10] This fact that women physicians have more success treating female patients is interesting. Perhaps women physicians are not only more intuitive, but more empathic as well than their male counterparts. Certainly, more research is needed in gender concordance situations.

Even though studies warrant that more consideration be given to females with heart disease symptoms, it still may take some time to help eradicate so many years of bias. For years, it has been generally thought that women are not serious candidates for CAD. For example, the difference in the use of percutaneous coronary artery (PTCA) intervention in acute MI in females demonstrated delay as the women in this study waited approximately 37 minutes longer before contacting emergency medical services.[11] In this study of 4360 patients (967 females) from 2006 to 2016, the 37-minute delay was costly in that the mortality rate in women was 5.9% versus that in men at 4.5%. Any invasive cardiologist knows that every minute counts when the blood supply in an area of the myocardium is obstructed. Since a woman's coronary anatomy is also somewhat smaller than a man's, PTCA and stenting may be more problematic with additional morbidity and mortality. In addition to realizing these gender-specific differences in myocardial ischemia between women and men, other major female cardiovascular concerns in this day and age include diastolic dysfunction (DD), hypertension, mitral valve prolapse (MVP), and peripheral artery disease (PAD).

Diastolic Dysfunction

In over 40 years of practicing cardiology, diastolic dysfunction (DD) is perhaps the most poorly understood pathological situation affecting both men and women. It is definitely the most impressive predisposing factor leading to systolic and eventually global left ventricular dysfunction. Most patients (females more so than males) with DD have normal or near-normal left ventricular ejection fractions.[12,13] Many of these patients experience the same signs and symptoms as patients with heart failure and reduced ejection fraction. Symptomatic suffering and unacceptable quality of life are reported in many of these patients.[14,15]

Diastolic heart failure results from compliance issues or a "stiffening of heart muscle." The left ventricle does not fill properly with blood and during diastole the filling cycle struggles and heart is somewhat energetically compromised. Patients may feel shortness of breath and fatigue and some even experience chest discomfort as well as peripheral edema. Their symptoms and physical findings are similar to patients with systolic heart failure caused by a weakened heart, and their prognosis remains guarded.[12,13] The mortality and morbidity caused by DD, which is also referred to as heart failure with well-preserved systolic function, is very similar to systolic heart failure. Approximately a decade ago, the estimated healthcare costs were $30 billion in the United States alone. Thus DD and systolic dysfunction place a great burden on our healthcare system.[16]

The identification of effective treatments for diastolic heart failure remains an important area of investigation and concern given the predominance of women with diastolic heart failure,[17] lack of specific therapies,[18,19] and high mortality and morbidity associated with this affliction.[12,13] A shocking projective occurrence statistic for this heart failure epidemic was estimated to be 20% in those older than 40 years.[14]

The treatment for DD continues to be disappointedly and severely limited as pharmaceutical drugs have been shown to be of little benefit in randomized clinical studies.[20] This Women's Health Coalition Report[20] also documented on the lack of effective treatments for DD and indicated that the prognosis has not changed for the last 15 years.

However, since the advent of the Treatment of Preserved Cardiac Function Heart Failure (TOPCAT) Trial (2014),[21] new pharmaceutical enthusiasm for spironolactone has emerged. Although treatment did not significantly reduce deaths for preserved ejection fraction,[21] in those patients at the lower end of the left ventricular ejection fraction (LVEF) spectrum (LVEF of 40%-50%), the effect of spironolactone was somewhat significant.[22]

Similar findings were seen in a *post hoc* subgroup in the PEACE Trial in which angiotensin-converting enzyme (ACE) inhibitors resulted in a benefit in patients with ischemic cardiomyopathy and midrange LVEF of 40% to 50%.[22,23] In another analysis of TOPCAT mineralocorticoid receptor antagonists can be considered to reduce risk of heart failure hospitalization in selected patients with preserved ejection fraction (HFpEF).[24] Although these recent trials suggest some benefit from pharmaceutical therapies on patient outcomes, clearly a more suitable alternative metabolic approach is needed to treat any patient with DD and/or systolic dysfunction.

An understanding of cardiac energetics and metabolic support with a focus on adenosine triphosphate (ATP) must be considered as a form of therapy for DD as well as global left ventricular failure.[25] Since muscle biopsies of cardiac tissues in heart failure patients reveal diminished quantities of ATP in their mitochondria, investigating therapies that promote cellular energetics and metabolism must be utilized. Myocytes contain the highest concentrations of mitochondria organelles necessary to generate the huge amounts of ATP required to fuel the high energy demand of cardiac energetics.[25,26]

The energetic imbalance of heart failure is characterized by an increase in energy demand and a decrease in energy production, transfer, and substrate utilization resulting in an ATP deficit. DD is the result of the heart muscle's inability to relax sufficiently after contraction because it cannot maintain the higher concentrations of ATP required to effectively activate the calcium pumps necessary to facilitate cardiac relaxation and diastolic filling.[25,27,28] All patients with heart failure have DD to some degree. Please see Figure 23.9 (Metabolic Cardiology Chapter).

Since the requirements of myocytes for ATP is absolute,[27] incorporating a metabolic approach with nutritional biochemical interventions that preserve and promote myocardial support and ATP production must be considered. In a randomized, controlled trial, 300 mg of Coenzyme Q10 reduced plasma pyruvate lactate ratios and improved endothelial function via reversal of mitochondrial dysfunction in patients with ischemic left ventricular systolic dysfunction.[29] Metabolic approaches do not create any adverse effects and are most supportive in patients with DD.

In my opinion, the most effective solution for failing ATP production involves nutraceutical support with Coenzyme Q10, L-carnitine, magnesium, and D-ribose. As discussed in the metabolic cardiology chapter, I prefer a high-quality ubiquinone over ubiquinol and would consider MITO-Q if the patient does not demonstrate clinical improvement despite an adequate blood level of Coenzyme Q10. In such a refractory patient, a trial of taurine 1 to 2 g two to three times a day is also recommended. When given on a daily basis, they provide essential raw materials that support cellular energy substrates needed by mitochondria to rebuild diminishing ATP levels. Treatment options that incorporate these metabolic interventions targeted to preserve ATP energy substrates (D-ribose) or accelerate ATP turnover (L-carnitine and Coenzyme Q10) are indicated for at-risk populations and patients undergoing cardiovascular surgery.[25,28] This metabolic approach does not create any adverse effects and may be also supportive in preventing atrial fibrillation occasionally seen in patients with DD after undergoing cardiac surgery[30] as well as in patients with hypertension where DD is also frequently seen.

Hypertension

In my early career as a heart specialist, I tended to treat men and women equally regarding blood pressure issues. Twenty years ago when I wrote *Heart Sense for Women*,[1] it became crystal clear to me that there are real gender-specific issues that exist, and blood pressure concern is one of them. More recently, a review article in the *Journal of Hypertension Research*[31] made some excellent points. Here are some of the conclusions from the article:

- After smoking cessation, hypertension control is the single most important intervention to reduce the risk of future cardiovascular events in women.
- Total life expectancy is almost 5 years less for women of age 50 years with high blood pressure compared to those without it.
- Early high blood pressure is considered if your level is over 130 (systolic) or 84 (diastolic). The most recent recommendations suggest optimal blood pressure readings of 120/80 and lower.
- In the elderly, high blood pressure affects more women than men and in general is underdiagnosed and undertreated.

The authors also indicated that the prevention of cardiovascular events by blood pressure control is "30% to 100% higher in women than in men" and that a mere 15-point rise in systolic blood pressure raises the risk of CVD by 56% in women compared with only 32% in men.[31] Women need to have knowledge of this especially if she is taking over-the-counter analgesics on a frequent basis.

A 2005 study[32] looked at nonnarcotic pain killers and the risk of incident hypertension in US women. The study found that women aged 51 to 77 years who took an average daily dose of 500 mg of acetaminophen or one Extra Strength Tylenol had about double the risk of developing high blood pressure in 3 years. Women in the same age range who took more than 400 mg of nonsteroidal anti-inflammatory drugs (NSAIDs), equal to about two ibuprofen, had a 78% risk of developing high blood pressure over those who did not take any nonsteroidal medications. Younger women, aged 34 to 53 years, who took an average of 500 mg of acetaminophen a day had a twofold higher risk of developing high blood pressure. Similar aged women who took 400 mg of NSAIDs had a 60% increased risk over those who did not take the meds. The study also demonstrated that aspirin did not increase these risks. The study involved 5123 women participating in the Nurse's Health Study at Harvard Medical School and Brigham and Women's Hospital in Boston.[32] Although none of the women had high blood pressure when the study began, higher doses of acetaminophen and NSAIDs independently increased the risk of hypertension in these women. Although NSAIDs increase renal sodium absorption, both acetaminophen and NSAIDs may impair endothelial function which may explain why blood pressure increases. Because the results of this study have confirmed previous investigations, it makes sense to educate women about the overzealous use of these analgesics.

Pregnancy may also create an undesirable situation for some women as hypertension can be observed in 6% to 8% of cases.[33] Eclampsia or high blood pressure during pregnancy can increase the risk of maternal as well as fetal mortality. Every pregnant woman needs to get her blood pressure evaluated as eclampsia can develop rapidly especially in the last trimester of pregnancy. Some women even need Rx following delivery.

Menopause is another phase of aging in which women need to have blood pressure evaluations especially if they are on pharmaceutical hormone replacement therapy (HRT).[34] I remember one striking case of a female in her late 50s who developed significant mitral regurgitation following a sudden increase in blood pressure. Although she had no prior history of high blood pressure, she became hypertensive following a treatment plan for menopausal symptoms with Premarin and medroxyprogesterone. After several months of treatment with HRT, her shortness of breath increased considerably and her quality of life was severely limited. After seeing several physicians and after taking multiple medications, she saw me in cardiovascular consultation as she was considering valvular replacement. Fortunately, the surgeon wanted her evaluated by a cardiologist prior to surgery. She indeed was hypertensive, and in my evaluation, I saw that she was taking medroxyprogesterone which is known to cause coronary artery constriction. After I suggested coming off HRT, I strongly advised that she delay surgery for the next few weeks. The blood pressure came down significantly, and the mitral regurgitation by echocardiographic analysis was significantly less. Several weeks after cessation of the hormonal therapy, she completely normalized with no quality of life issues. Her mitral regurgitation significantly decreased. She certainly did not need valvular surgery. It was a dramatic case to say the least. Hormonal therapy may be appropriate for many women; however, the side effects can overshadow situations in the myocardium that could result in limitation and quality of life issues. Diastolic dysfunction resulting from hypertension is something that we must consider in any woman who has shortness of breath or in women who have MVP where diastolic dysfunction is also frequently seen as well.

Mitral Valve Prolapse

MVP is a relatively benign condition of the mitral valve. Sometimes, the mitral valve leaflets become thickened, stretched, or even voluminous, which may cause a slight to even a profound leakage of the valve. Many times on physical evaluation, a mid- to late-systolic click may be heard followed by a late systolic murmur in most cases or a mid-systolic murmur in some. While most patients may not even know they have MVP, a few are particularly bothered by symptoms of atypical chest discomfort, shortness of breath, irregular heartbeats, or even fatigue. In rare cases, spontaneous rupture of the chordae tendineae may occur resulting in symptoms of severe shortness of breath, significant mitral regurgitation, and even left ventricular dysfunction or failure.

During my cardiovascular fellowship, the chief of cardiology at our institution authored the book on MVP.[35] As his senior cardiovascular fellow, I literally gathered enormous amounts of data on over 300 patients in our MVP clinic. MVP for many is not an affliction to worry about. Most people are asymptomatic, and they do not even know they have the problem. Although arrhythmias, atypical chest pain, clicks, and murmurs were present, several patients in our clinic had shortness of breath as their only symptom. This was both confusing and perplexing, so we proceeded to investigate and report our findings. After studying 20 patients with severe shortness of breath with MVP, pulmonary function studies were essentially normal. Although the clinical analysis was published in the pulmonary journal *Chest* in 1979,[36] we were unable to come up with a definitive reason why these patients with MVP had shortness of breath despite negative pulmonary function studies. It would take almost 20 years before sophisticated echocardiographic techniques were able to point out the phenomena of diastolic dysfunction (DD).[37] Looking back, I suspected that many of these patients had shortness of breath because of diastolic dysfunction. Although many patients with MVP symptoms were treated with β-blockers, my interest in metabolic cardiology was actually the most effective and therapeutic treatment in patients with MVP as many patients did not respond well on β-blocking meds. Interestingly, the conventional literature attests to the efficacy of magnesium.

Magnesium has shown efficacy in relieving symptoms of MVP. In a double-blind study of 181 participants, 80 serum magnesium levels were assessed in 141 patients with symptomatic MVP and compared to those of 40 healthy controls. While decreased magnesium levels were found in more than half (60% to be exact) of the patients with MVP, only 5% of the controlled subjects showed similar decreases.[38]

Participants with magnesium deficits were randomly assigned to receive magnesium supplement or placebo, and the results for the magnesium group were noteworthy. The mean (average) number of symptoms per patient was significantly reduced with magnesium supplementation. Weakness, chest pain, shortness of breath, palpitations, and even anxiety were assuaged. Laboratory analysis also demonstrated decreases in the amount of adrenalin-like substances in the urine. The researchers concluded that perhaps many patients with MVP have symptoms which may be related to low magnesium levels. In my experience, the most reliable and preferred magnesium test is the red blood cell analysis as it gives a more precise and truer picture of the body's magnesium levels. Additionally, with supplementation of the mineral, an improvement in symptoms and a decrease in adrenalin-like substances in the urine were realized.[38]

In my experience, treating the symptomatic patient with MVP with pharmaceutical drugs can be problematic. I especially saw this with β-blockers when many of my patients complained about side effects especially fatigue. When I started to utilize nutraceutical treatments including magnesium and Coenzyme Q10, many of my patients were able to experience an excellent quality of life despite echocardiographic correlations of moderate to severe MVP. On occasion, with some of my most refractory patients with MVP, the addition of 5 g of D-ribose and 1 to 2 g of L-carnitine was significant in the control of their symptoms. This metabolic approach also has been significant in the treatment of PAD—another significant clinical problem for women.

Peripheral Artery Disease

Peripheral artery disease (PAD) is the third leading cause of arteriosclerotic cardiovascular morbidity followed by CAD and stroke. In a broad-based review of the literature involving 34 studies worldwide,[39] PAD has become a global problem involving over 200 million people, with smoking, diabetes, and hypertension being the prevalent risk factors. In fact, when I was performing cardiac catheterization and saw plaque in the coronary arteries, I always knew it would show up elsewhere in the body. Frequently, it would show up in the arteries of the lower legs (PAD).

PAD has received very little public recognition, and it has always been considered a man's disease. In my practice, I saw many more men than women with PAD symptoms, most typically cramping and pain in the calves when walking (called intermittent claudication). Women do not seem to develop those symptoms as often unless they are smokers. They usually complain more of fatigue and functional decline in the legs. But the following revelations from a recent American Heart Association (AHA) "call to action" article published in the *Journal Circulation*[40] clearly illustrates how prevalent and serious a problem of PAD appears to be for women.

PAD increases with age for both men and women yet evidence suggests that over 40 years of age more women than men are affected. The summary statements by the authors indicate the following[40]:

- Most women with PAD, unlike men, do not have classic symptoms of intermittent claudication.
- Women with PAD have greater functional impairment and a more rapid functional decline than women without PAD.
- Women (and particularly African American females) are more likely than men to experience graft failure or limb loss.
- There is a need to identify women with or at risk for PAD, especially African American women, to lower cardiovascular ischemic event rates, loss of independent functional capacity, and ischemic amputation rates.

The evaluation of PAD is tedious and complex, involving a meticulous evaluation of peripheral pulses, targeted blood pressure measurements involving brachial and tibial arteries, duplex ultrasound, as well as advanced imaging studies in some patients. Although many successful treatments frequently involve pharmaceutical and surgical procedures including arterial stents, many patients without major obstructions to blood vessels continue to be symptomatic despite conventional methodologies. Frequently, small vessel disease is present and a metabolic approach can be very supportive in reducing pain and suffering in women.

My metabolic cardiology recommendations for women include the following targeted nutritional supplement program for PAD support:

- A high-quality multimineral/vitamin formula.
- A total of 100 to 300 mg of Coenzyme Q10 and 200 to 600 mg of magnesium, (what forms) both of which help to lower blood pressure and support endothelial function. I like Kreb Cycle magnesium components—citrate, glycinate, and taurinate to mention a few. I also prefer magnesium orotate as this varietal helps to drive ATP preferentially.
- A total of 1 to 2 g of L-carnitine or 2 g of glycine propionyl L-carnitine (GPLC), a proprietary form of L-carnitine. L-carnitine helps clear our metabolic wastes that aggravate vasoconstriction in small blood vessels generated by cellular energy production. Cellular efficiency and aerobic capacity are supported when toxic by-products or the β-oxidation of fats are shuttled out of the mitochondria. GPLC does the same and also helps to improve blood flow by boosting nitric oxide, a biochemical that keeps blood vessels relaxed.
- A total of 5 g D-ribose, three times daily and prior to exercise activities.
- A total of 1 to 2 g omega-3 fatty acid (fish or squid oil).
- Consider taurine 2 to 3 g, one to three times a day if above recommendations are not ideal.

Another simple and therapeutic intervention for diffuse distal vessel disease is earthing. Since it was introduced to me over 12 years ago, and after performing cardiovascular research, it became crystal clear that earthing will be a new therapeutic strategy for peripheral artery disease.[41] For a more detailed account of earthing and the cardiovascular system, see Chapter 33 of this book.

To summarize, the recognition and treatment of PAD is a widespread problem that is frequently undiagnosed and mismanaged. Remember that arteriosclerotic CVD is a diffuse process, and when lesions show up in one area of the body, it is most likely present in other areas as well. So, the diagnosis of PAD could literally tip off the physician that the carotid and coronary arteries are most likely involved. Although PAD was not considered to be a major pathology in women, it clearly has become a major problem afflicting women and especially African American women.

Summary and Conclusions

Women are vastly different than men. Their initial presenting symptoms may not be classic; their coronary circulation has arteries that are smaller and more difficult to navigate with stents and even bypass grafting, and this is probably why they have an increased mortality following acute MI, stent, and coronary artery bypass surgery interventions. They are also exposed to a number of life circumstances like pregnancy and menopause that influence classical cardiovascular risk factors. CAD goes up significantly when a women approaches perimenopausal and menopausal years.

Metabolic syndrome is another area where women need to be aggressively treated as women with type 2 diabetes or insulin resistance with higher triglyceride levels have more cardiac risk as opposed to men. DD, which is more prevalent in women with hypertension and occurring in MVP, frequently found in more women than men, is another area of marked concern given the fact that conventional medicine has very few options to offer.

Even painkillers in women can have a detrimental effect on their health. Acetaminophen and ibuprofen contribute to the high prevalence rate of hypertension in the United States which may be related to the overzealous use of these over-the-counter drugs.

CVD is the major leading cause of death in women today. Conducting appropriate gender-specific differences research and analysis of CVD trials has been difficult due to insufficient recruitment of women. Although this has contributed to a lack of understanding of gender differences in CVD, improved participation rates of women in new cardiovascular trials would yield more information concerning appropriate prevention, detection, accurate diagnosis, as well as proper treatment of all women with heart disease. In the near future, a new subspecialty of gender-specific medicine will probably be able to stand on its own and physicians will have a better understanding in the diagnosis and treatment of women with a wide range of cardiovascular concerns.

References

1. Sinatra ST. *Heart Sense for Women*. Washington, DC: Lifeline Press; 2000.
2. Golomb BA, Evans MA. Statin adverse effects: a review of the literature and evidence for a mitochondrial mechanism. *Am J Cardiovasc Drugs*. 2008;8:373-418.
3. Hecht HS, Harman SM. Relation of aggressiveness of lipid-lowering treatment to changes in calcified plaque burden by electron beam tomography. *J Am Coll Cardiol*. 2003;92(3):334-336.
4. Jones M, Tett S, Geeske M, et al. New-onset diabetes after statin exposure in elderly women: the Australian longitudinal study on women's health. *Drugs & Aging* 2017;34(3):203.
5. Goldstein MR, Mascitelli L, Pezzetta F. Do statins prevent or promote cancer? *Curr Oncol*. 2008;15(2):76-77.
6. Sattar N, Preiss D, Murray HM, et al. Statins and risk of incident diabetes: a collaborative meta-analysis of randomized statin trials. *Lancet*. 2010;375:735-742.
7. Okuyama H, Langsjoen PH, Hamazaki T, et al. Statins stimulate artherosclerosis and heart failure: pharmacological mechanisms. *Expert Rev Clin Pharmacol*. 2015;8(2):188-199.
8. Sinatra ST, Teter BB, Bowden J, et al. The saturated fat, cholesterol, and statin controversy a commentary. *J Am Coll Nutr*. 2014;33(1):79-88.
9. Mitchell JD, Fergestrom N, Gage BF, et al. Impact of statins on cardiovascular outcomes following coronary artery calcium scoring. *J Am Coll Cardiol*. 2018;72(25):3233-3242.
10. Greenwood BN, Carnahan S, Huang L. Patient-physician gender concordance and increased mortality among female heart attack patients. *PNAS*. 2018;115(34):8569-8574.
11. Meyer MR, Bernheim AM, Kurz DJ, et al. Gender differences in patient and system delay for primary percutaneous coronary intervention: current trends in a Swiss ST-segment elevation myocardial infarction population. *Eur Heart J Acute Cardiovasc Care*. 2019;8(3):283-290. doi:10.1177/2048872618810410.
12. Owan TE, Hodge DO, Herges RM, et al. Trends in prevalence and outcome of heart failure with preserved ejection fraction. *N Engl J Med*. 2006;355:251-259.
13. Bhatia RS, Tu JV, Lee DS, et al. Outcome of heart failure with preserved ejection fraction in a population-based study. *N Engl J Med*. 2006;355:260-269.
14. Redfield MM, Jacobsen SJ, Burnett JC, et al. Burden of systolic and diastolic ventricular dysfunction in the community: appreciating the scope of the heart failure epidemic. *JAMA*. 2003;289:194-202.
15. Hoekstra T, Lesman-Leegte I, van Veldhuisen DJ, et al. Quality of life is impaired similarly in heart failure patients with preserved and reduced ejection fraction. *Eur J Heart Fail*. 2011;13:1013-1018.
16. Roger VL, Go AS, Lloyd-Jones DM, et al. Heart disease and stroke statistics-2011 update: a report from the American Heart Association. *Circulation*. 2011;123(4):e18-e209.
17. Yancy CW, Lopatin M, Stevenson LW, et al. Clinical presentation, management, and in-hospital outcomes of patients admitted with acute decompensated heart failure with preserved systolic function: a report from the acute decompensated heart failure national registry (adhere) database. *J Am Coll Cardiol*. 2006;47:76-84.
18. Hunt SA, Abraham WT, Chin MH, et al. 2009 focused update incorporated into the ACC/AHA 2005 guidelines for the diagnosis and management of heart failure in adults a port of the American College of Cardiology Foundation/American Heart Association task force on practice guidelines developed in collaboration with the International Society for Heart and Lung Transplantation. *J Am Coll Cardiol*. 2009;53:e1-e90.
19. Paulus WJ, van Ballegoij JJ. Treatment of heart failure with normal ejection fraction: an inconvenient truth! *J Am Coll Cardiol*. 2010;55:526-537.
20. Wenger NK, Hayes SN, Pepine CJ, et al. Cardiovascular care for women: the 10-Q report and beyond. *Am J Cardiol*. 2013;112(4):S2.
21. Pitt B, Pfeffer MA, Assmann SF, et al. Spironolactone for heart failure with preserved ejection fraction. *N Engl J Med*. 2014;370:1383-1392.
22. Solomon SD, Claggett B, Lewis EF. Influence of ejection fraction on outcomes and efficacy of spironolactone in patients with heart failure with preserved ejection fraction. *Eur Heart J*. 2016;37(5):455-462.
23. Alzahrani T, Tiu J, Panjrath G, et al. The effect of angiotensin-converting enzyme inhibitors on clinical outcomes in patients with ischemic cardiomyopathy and midrange ejection fraction: a pot hoc subgroup analysis from the PEACE trial. *Ther Adv Cardiovasc Dis*. 2018;12(12):351-359.
24. Patel RB, Shah SJ, Fonarow GC, et al. Designing future clinical trials in heart failure with preserved ejection fraction: lessons from TOPCAT. *Curr Heart Fail Rep*. 2017;14(4):217-222.
25. Sinatra ST. Metabolic cardiology: an integrative strategy in the treatment of congestive heart failure. *Altern Ther Health Med*. 2009;15(3):44-52.
26. Bashore TM, Magorien DJ, Letterio J, et al. Histologic and biochemical correlates of left ventricular chamber dynamics in men. *J Am Coll Cardiol*. 1987;9(4):734-742.
27. Inwall JS, Weiss RG. Is the failing heart energy starve? On using chemical energy to support cardiac function. *Circ Res*. 2004;95(2):135-145.
28. Sinatra ST. Metabolic cardiology: the missing link in cardiovascular disease. *Altern Ther Health Med*. 2009;15(2):48-50.
29. Dai Y, Luk T, Yiu K, et al. Reversal of mitochondrial dysfunction by coenzyme Q10 supplement improves endothelial function in patients with ischemic left ventricular systolic dysfunction: a randomized controlled trial. *Atherosclerosis*. 2011;216:395-401.
30. Melduni RM, Suri RM, Seward JB, et al. Diastolic dysfunction in patients undergoing cardiac surgery: a pathological mechanism underlying the initiation of new-onset post-operative atrial fibrillation. *J Am Coll Cardiol*. 2011;58:953-961.

31. Engberding N, Wenger NK. Management of hypertension in women. *Hypertens Res.* 2012;35:251-260.

32. Forman JP, Stampfer MJ, Curhan GC. Non-narcotic analgesic dose and risk of incident hypertension in US women. *Hypertension.* 2005;46(3):500-507.

33. Medical researchers have found that birth control pills increase blood pressure in some women and According to the National Heart, Lung and Blood Institute (NHLBI), high blood pressure affects 6-8 percent of all pregnancies in the United States – The American Heart Association (AHA). High Blood Press Women. Heartorg. http://www.heart.org/HEARTORG/Conditions/HighBloodPressure/UnderstandYour RiskforHighBloodPressure/High-Blood-Pressure-and-Women_UCM_301867_Article.jspc. Accessed June 24, 2014.

34. Wassertheil-Smoller S, Anderson G, Psaty BM, et al. Hypertension and its treatment in postmeno-pausal women: baseline data from the Women's Health Initiative. *Hypertension.* 2000;36:780-789.

35. Jeresaty R. *Mitral Valve Prolapse.* New York, NY: Raven Press; 1979.

36. ZuWallack R, Sinatra S, Lahiri B, et al. Pulmonary function studies in patients with prolapse of the mitral valve. *Chest.* 1979;76(1):17-20.

37. Halley CM, Houghtaling PL, Khalil MK, et al. Mortality rate in patients with diastolic dysfunction and normal systolic function. *Arch Intern Med.* 2011;171(2):1082-1087.

38. Kitlinski M, Stepniewski M, Nessler J, et al. Is magnesium deficit in lymphocytes a part of the mitral valve prolapse syndrome? *Magnes Res.* 2004;17(1):39-45.

39. Fowkes FG, Rudan D, Rudan I, et al. Comparison of global estimates or prevalence and risk factors for peripheral artery disease in 2000 and 2010: a systematic review and analysis. *Lancet.* 2013;382(9901):1329-1340.

40. Hirsch AT, Allison MA, Gomes MS, et al. A call to action: women and peripheral artery disease: a scientific statement from the American Heart Association. *Circulation.* 2012;125(11):1449-1472.

41. Chevalier G, Sinatra ST, Oschman JL, et al. Earthing (grounding) the human body reduces blood viscosity: a major factor in cardiovascular disease. *J Altern Complement Med.* 2013;19(2):102-110.

37

Cross Talk Signaling and Networking—Improving Outcomes in the Cardiometabolic Patient

Andrew Heyman, MD, MHSA and James B. LaValle, RPh, DHM, MS, CCN, ND (trad)

Cardiovascular disease (CVD) is the leading cause of death in the United States and many parts of the world. A recent press release by the American Heart Association states that nearly 50% of all people have some form of CVD.[1] There are about 2200 deaths a day, averaging one death every 40 seconds, with almost one of every three deaths resulting from CVD.[2]

Considered a risk factor for CVD, the cardiometabolic syndrome is a metabolic disorder correlated in epidemiological studies with an increased risk of coronary heart disease, ischemic stroke, cardiovascular mortality, and total mortality. Cardiometabolic syndrome includes insulin resistance (prediabetes), impaired glucose tolerance, lipid imbalances, high blood pressure, and increased central adiposity. There is also evidence that the cardiometabolic syndrome is a risk factor for abnormalities in myocardial metabolism, cardiac dysfunction, and arrhythmias such as atrial fibrillation.[3]

Abdominal obesity is a key component of cardiometabolic (CM) risk, increasing the incidence of insulin resistance, vascular inflammation, dyslipidemia, and hypertension. Adipose tissue is recognized as an endocrine organ along with associated hormonal products. Adipose tissue appears to play a significant role in the regulation of fat and glucose metabolism throughout the body, and these mechanisms are clearly involved in the development of cardiovascular and CM disease.

The challenges of a strategy to treat the CM patient and to modify their risks are ever-evolving and should not be limited to drug therapy and surgery. On the surface, potentially modifiable risk factors include discontinuing tobacco use; improving physical inactivity; using drug therapy to control hypertension, blood glucose, and lipid imbalances; and changing some dietary habits. However, the CM patients generally have a cluster of symptoms that are also related to network biology problems that may not be so apparent initially, including involvement of insulin resistance and insulin signaling problems, hypothalamic-pituitary-adrenal (HPA) axis imbalances, and gut-heart axis (also encompasses the gut-immune-brain axis) involvement.

Understanding the effects and impact of systems biology networks, called TRIADs, on the cardiovascular system is essential in managing the CM patient. When these and other systems biology factors are taken into consideration, you can turn up the dial of response to treatments in these individuals, improving cardiovascular outcomes and improving the quality of life.

Background—What Are the TRIADs?

TRIADS are "categories" that group important organs/organ systems in your body together in "3s." The reason for the grouping is to show the interrelationship of various network biology systems that have a significant impact on your overall metabolic health. Understanding and acknowledging the interconnectivity of all the metabolic networks is essential in treating the cardiovascular and CM patient. Although any construct of relationships described is somewhat artificial because all organ systems and networks potentially can affect all others leading to metabolic disruption, the networks described are commonly published and described in the medical literature. There are five TRIADs in the Network Biology approach to medicine:

- TRIAD 1—consists of the adrenal, thyroid, and pancreas. TRIAD 1 encompasses HPA axis imbalances (stress and adrenals), sugar metabolism, and thyroid involvement in energy production and central network regulators of physiology. Imbalances manifest as fatigue, loss of vitality, and obesity.

- TRIAD 2—consists of the Gut-brain-immune network, their interrelationship and effects on metabolism. TRIAD 2 encompasses command and control, digestion and absorption of nutrients, defense and repair, memory and cognitive function, sleep regulation, mood, memory, and inflammatory responses. Imbalances include weight gain and overeating, digestive complaints, inflammatory bowel diseases, allergies/food intolerances, sinus/colds/flu, immune and autoimmune imbalances, chronic inflammatory responses, sleep disorders, and mood and memory problems.
- TRIAD 3—includes cardiovascular, pulmonary (cardiopulmonary), and neurovascular. TRIAD 3 includes the cardiopulmonary unit, autonomic and central nervous systems, and vascular tree. This triad reflects the relationship of cardiovascular health, cognition, mood, and stress. When TRIAD 3 organ systems are out of sync, the result is hypercholesterolemia, hypertension, increased resting heart rate, loss of vagal tone, increased fatigue, dyspnea or other pulmonary issues, and endothelial dysfunction. Of note, imbalances in TRIAD 1 and 2 in many cases will be the trigger to TRIAD 3 disturbances. In essence, chronic stress, elevated blood sugar, and low thyroid function lead to the eventual vasculopathy. The Network Biology approach helps map the complicated interconnected pathways of the brain-heart connection or in other words TRIAD 2 stacking with TRIAD 3. Again, looking at the metabolic network disturbances is essential.
- TRIAD 4 includes the organs of detoxification—the liver and gallbladder, lymphatic system, and kidneys. Imbalances will lead to fatigue, fluid retention, reduced detoxification capacity, sluggish metabolism, intolerance to fats, edema, body odor and halitosis, and profuse sweating even in cold temperatures. TRIAD 4 organs of detoxification imbalances such as nonalcoholic fatty liver disease (NAFLD) can lead to cardiovascular consequences.[4]
- TRIAD 5 is the metabolic network of the sex hormones—testosterone, estrogens, and progesterone. This TRIAD is potency and fertility. Imbalances can lead to impact on other networks, such as the cardiovascular and neurovascular. Weight gain, loss of muscle mass and strength, poor glucose regulation, inflammation, and disproportionate fat distribution are just a few of the issues when TRIAD 5 hormones are not in balance.

Cardiometabolic Disease—Underlying Factors

Obesity has been an epidemic for over a decade in both developed and developing nations and is the sixth most important risk factor contributing to the overall burden of disease worldwide.[5] The average American consumes over 135 lb of sugar per person per year, whereas the average German ingests 75 lb per person per year.[6] Central adiposity plays a critical role in the development of CM disease, and the extensive metabolic activity of visceral fat is increasingly recognized in the medical literature. Once thought of as merely a repository for excess calories, adipose tissue is now viewed as an endocrine gland capable of secreting numerous bioactive substances, including hormones, growth factors, and cytokines, that contribute directly to the development of heart disease and type 2 diabetes.[7,8] Additionally, research links these same biochemical factors, and in particular insulin resistance, with cancer.[9,10]

CM risk is an expansion of underlying risk factors linked to metabolic syndrome (MetS). Insulin resistance and visceral obesity are the hallmarks of MetS, with hypertension and hypertriglyceridemia (typically with abnormalities in high-density lipoprotein (HDL) cholesterol) also serving as important co-contributors. CM risk is also amplified by other known cardiovascular markers such as high-sensitivity C-reactive protein (hs-CRP), Lpa and Lp-PLA2, oxidized low-density lipoprotein (LDL) and LDL particle size, fibrinogen, myeloperoxidase and markers of oxidative stress, including 8-hydroxyguanosine (8-OHdG), ApoB, F2 isoprostanes, superoxide dismutase (SOD), and methyl malonic acid. Although a unified model of CM disease remains incomplete, it is now clear that inflammation, hormonal derangements, stress, central obesity, environmental burden, nutritional deficiencies, and high oxidative stress underlie the progression toward insulin resistance, diabetes, and heart disease.

Prevalence of Cardiometabolic Disease

The term CM disease is relatively new, and accurate estimates on prevalence are not well defined in the literature. In contrast, the statistics on MetS, diabetes, and heart disease provide insight into the problem because they act as proxies for the underlying features of CM risk. It is estimated that 20% of the US population has MetS and 50% of adults in the United States have prediabetes (insulin resistance) or type 2 diabetes. The Centers for Disease Control and Prevention report that diabetes is the sixth leading cause of death in the United States. Additionally, heart disease continues to be the primary cause of morbidity and mortality in the United States. The 2006 estimates show that 80 million people in the United States had one or more forms of CVD.[3]

Cardiometabolic Risk Key Considerations

- Visceral fat
- Insulin resistance
- Atherogenic dyslipidemia (triglycerides, ox-LDL, small dense LDL)
- Hypertension
- Glucose intolerance (IGT)
- Impaired fibrinolysis (plasminogen activator inhibitor-1 [PAI-1], fibrinogen)
- Inflammation (hs-CRP)
- Increased oxidative stress (8-OHdG, F2 isoprostanes, glutathione—total and reduced)

- Male—clinically or subclinically (trending) low free and total testosterone
- Female—polycystic ovary syndrome (PCOS) (sex hormone binding globulin [SHBG], free testosterone)
- NAFLD

Integrative Medicine

Nearly half of the US adult population utilizes integrative therapies to treat various medical conditions and modify disease risk, including risks for CM disease.[11] Patients demonstrate reliance on these modalities out of philosophical interest in "natural approaches" to augment conventional medical therapy and to improve their levels of well-being. Unfortunately, because of the negative stigma associated with "nontraditional" treatment approaches, 70% of patients do not tell their physician about use of integrative approaches.[9]

Integrative medicine is an evidence-based combination of conventional, alternative, and complementary therapies. Integrative medicine makes use of conventional medicine, surgery, and treatments in combination with herbs, supplements, manual therapies, mind-body techniques, and other modalities to allow patients to achieve optimal health and healing while being actively involved in their own care.[12]

Over 45 academic centers in the United States have established integrative medicine programs, and 75% of medical schools now teach these approaches to medical students. The annual budget of the National Center for Complementary and Alternative Medicine at the National Institutes of Health is now over $120 million.[13]

Pathophysiology of Cardiometabolic Disease

CM disease results from a complex combination of etiologies derived from hormonal derangements in principally insulin, cortisol, thyroid, and sex hormones. In addition, inflammatory mediators (eg, interleukin (IL)-6, tumor necrosis factor alpha (TNFα), leptin, resistin, transforming growth factor (TGF) beta-1, hs-CRP), nutritional deficiencies (magnesium, omega fatty acids, chromium, vitamin C and D, and coenzyme Q10), hypercoagulability (PAI-1,fibrinogen), oxidative stress, environmental toxins, genetic polymorphisms, poor lifestyle habits, disrupted sleep and apnea, and psychosocial stress also play an important role and many times are acting simultaneously on the individual. These pages will focus on the more influential hormonal derangements of insulin, cortisol, and testosterone amplifying the underlying CM risk and central obesity.

Visceral Obesity, Insulin Resistance, and Inflammation

Visceral adipocytes release inflammatory markers known as adipocytokines into the circulation. These adipocytokines include TNFα, IL-6, leptin, resistin, angiotensinogen, and nonesterified fatty acids (NEFAs), all of which contribute to insulin resistance and cardiovascular risk.[14] White adipose tissue is located around the viscera and has been shown to generate higher amounts of adipocytokines compared with subcutaneous fat, thereby highlighting its role in the development of central obesity and consequently type 2 diabetes and heart disease.[15]

Both hyperinsulinemia and insulin resistance have been implicated in CM disease. Elevated serum insulin is a well-recognized precursor to diabetes and heart disease, and it may be a stronger predictor of CVD and MetS than insulin resistance alone.[14] Perpetuation of receptor tissue resistance to insulin causes increased insulin production as a compensatory mechanism to sustain normoglycemia. Excess NEFAs are transported to the liver where they are converted into very-low-density lipoproteins and triglycerides, thereby inducing hyperlipidemia. Insulin elevation also stimulates the sympathetic nervous system thereby leading to sodium and water retention and vasoconstriction resulting in an increase in blood pressure.[9]

Insulin resistance in the myocardium can generate damage by at least three different mechanisms: (1) signal transduction alteration, (2) impaired regulation of substrate metabolism, and (3) altered delivery of substrates to the myocardium.[16]

Accumulation of adipose tissue in the abdominal area is associated with CVD as well.[3,17] Adipocytokines generated by these centralized adipocytes create a state of chronic systemic and local vascular inflammation, enhanced coagulation, and endothelial dysfunction.[3] Inflammatory markers contributing additional risk for atherogenesis include hs-CRP, PAI-1, ox-LDL, and fibrinogen. When combined with modifiable traditional risk factors such as hyperlipidemia, smoking, and hypertension, the potent mixture of visceral obesity, insulin abnormalities, and inflammation contribute directly to the development of CM disease.

Stress and Hypothalamic-Pituitary-Adrenal Axis Dysregulation

Stress is a critical mediator of increasing CM risk. Integrity of HPA axis function is essential for maintaining homeostasis.[18–20] Exposures to any stressors results in the stimulation of the "stress system" thereby inducing a myriad of adaptive hormonal responses designed to reestablish disrupted homeostasis and promote survival. These "fight or flight" responses are intended to ensure survival of the organism. Stress-induced HPA axis dysfunction has been reported to intensify insulin resistance, inflammation, endothelial dysfunction, neurological damage, and immunological damage.[21,22]

Under normal conditions, the HPA axis maintains a predictable pattern of diurnal variation under the influence of many factors. Cortisol is integral to normal HPA axis function and typically peaks before awakening and gradually decreases during the course of the day.[23] A growing body of research has positively correlated an association between alterations in rhythmicity of cortisol release and various comorbid conditions including posttraumatic stress disorder

(PTSD),[24] depression,[25] chronic fatigue syndrome/fibromyalgia,[26] metabolic syndrome,[27] CM disease (MetS),[28] cancer,[29] and memory impairment.[30]

It is not only the loss of the normal diurnal pattern of cortisol release but also flattening of the normal diurnal cortisol curve that negatively impacts multiple physiological systems, including the cardiovascular system, metabolic regulation of energy balance, and sites of fat deposition.[19,31–33]

Chronic stress has been linked to the development and/or exacerbation of diabetes and heart disease. Cortisol directly affects insulin release and glucose regulation.[19,33] Cortisol increases insulin levels, and the coelevation of these two hormones promotes visceral adipose deposition. Visceral fat has abundant glucocorticoid receptors and is very sensitive to the effects of cortisol and insulin.[34,35] This cycle of events inevitably plays a role in the development of insulin resistance, hyperlipidemia, hypertension, and ultimately CM disease.[3,36]

Although many of the deleterious effects of chronic stress have been attributed to elevated levels of cortisol, there is ample medical evidence also suggesting a link between chronic stress, hypocortisolism, and/or low cortisol releasing hormone (CRH) release.[3,37] Hypocortisolism is the paradoxical suppression of the HPA axis under conditions of chronic stress and is usually reported by patients as generalized fatigue. More commonly found in adults, hypocortisolism is thought to represent the cumulative effects of chronic stressors and mediates the progression of major chronic diseases such as CVD, cancer, cognitive and mood disorders, autoimmune diseases, as well as overall vitality and energy.[18]

Low cortisol production in response to chronic stress leads to loss of glucocorticoid receptor ligand activity[3] and an increase in proinflammatory cytokines, including IL-6.[38] The increase in inflammatory signaling due to loss of counterregulation by normal glucocorticoid activity is a crucial physiologic component of CM disease.

Although stress has long been associated with the development of diabetes and CVDs, the links between cortisol, insulin resistance, visceral adiposity, and increased inflammation have only recently been more fully appreciated. For the individual it does not matter whether they trigger high cortisol as a result of high insulin output due to excessive sugar and carbohydrate intake or trigger their metabolic dysfunction due to stress, the net result is the same as it relates to CM disruption. In the instance of systems biology network signaling, cortisol can lower the available free thyroid hormone, which in turns lowers signaling of insulin receptors as well as alterations in deposition of fat.

Testing for HPA Dysregulation

Although serum and urinary testing of cortisol and its metabolites has been traditionally utilized to diagnose the extremes of adrenal gland dysfunction, salivary cortisol testing has emerged as the preferred method of routine diagnostic testing.[39] Salivary cortisol levels have been reported to correlate predictably with serum levels and allow determination of free cortisol levels by

eliminating interference from serum cortisol binding globulin that precludes determination of the serum free cortisol fraction. Advantageous aspects to salivary testing include its noninvasive, convenient, and "stress-free" method of collection.[40] Typically, salivary testing includes four samples during the course of a single day to determine the slope of cortisol production. A 24-hour AM urine cortisol testing may also be used; however, this method does not allow for observation of the diurnal variation in cortisol. Of note is the issue of chronic elevation of cortisol and its impact on gonadotrophin releasing hormone, which in turn causes a downregulation of sex hormones. The downstream effect leads to hypertension, insulin dysregulation, bone and muscle loss, and hypogonadism.

Testosterone Dysregulation

Testosterone dysregulation in both men and women can lead to increased CM risk. For men, testosterone deficiency (free and total) is a significant contributing risk factor to CM disease.[41–43] It can result from any number of causes and affects men of all ages. The clinical signs and symptoms of this disorder depend on the age of the patient at onset and the degree of the deficiency. Testosterone deficiency in men typically manifests as symptoms of decreased erectile function and libido. Physiologically, testosterone plays a critical role in the regulation of normal growth, bone metabolism, and body composition.[44]

Testosterone in Men

Qualitative computed tomography (CT) imaging has confirmed that testosterone-deficient men have both a systemic increase in adipocyte deposits as well as alterations in adipocyte deposition. Studies have confirmed the significant relationship between serum free testosterone levels and the volume and distribution of body fat in both healthy and obese male subjects.[45] Free testosterone levels have been reported to be inversely correlated with obesity in a number of studies, and the link between low testosterone and central obesity has been particularly striking.[46,47]

The relationship between central obesity and total testosterone is even more pronounced when combined with the presence of low SHBG levels. Because SHBG binds free serum testosterone, an increase in serum SHBG leads to even lower free testosterone levels in obese men. In a subgroup of the men in the HERITAGE family study, low total testosterone and SHBG were predictors of greater obesity and visceral fat levels on CT scan.[48]

Hypogonadism in men plays an important adjunctive role with central adiposity in the development of glucose intolerance and cardiovascular risk.[49] Low serum testosterone levels are associated with both worsening insulin resistance as well as progression of atherosclerosis. Men with low testosterone levels have also been reported to be at higher risk for coronary artery disease, hypertension, and myocardial infarction.[50]

The use of total testosterone level as the initial assessment of hypogonadism in men has been advocated by the Institute of Medicine and in several recent guidelines.[51] No formal consensus exists on the presence of CM disease and how it is correlated with measurements of total testosterone, although low testosterone is present in 15% to 30% of men with obesity and diabetes. But free testosterone is the bioavailable testosterone.

The diagnostic threshold of hypogonadism in men remains a subject of debate. The American Association of Endocrinologists recommends 300 ng/dL (10.4 nmol/L) as the lower limit, and initiation of testosterone therapy is recommended when levels are 200 ng/dL (8 nmol/L) or less. Other guidelines recommend initiating testosterone replacement when serum testosterone levels are between 8 and 12 nmol/L and clinical signs and symptoms warrant therapy.[52] Serum testosterone levels, like the other sex hormones, have a circadian rhythm. Because testosterone levels tend to be the highest in the morning, it is recommended that testing be conducted at this time. However, several studies have shown that the circadian rhythm is often lost in elderly men.[53]

An assessment of serum SHBG levels is also important, particularly in elderly men, obese men, and men with underlying CM disease. The SHBG can then be used to calculate bioavailable testosterone levels when total testosterone levels are known. The bioavailable testosterone levels provide an assessment of both the free testosterone as well as the weakly bound to albumin portion that is readily available in tissue when needed.[53] Additional hormonal evaluations should include measurements of follicle stimulating hormone (FSH), luteinizing hormone (LH), and prolactin as indicated. If testosterone therapy is initiated, a baseline prostate specific antigen (PSA) and prostate examination should be performed. At the 3-month follow-up visit, repeat testing is recommended of total or bioavailable testosterone and SHBG, hematocrit, and PSA (free and total).[54]

Testosterone in Women

In women, testosterone also plays a key role in cardiovascular systems networking. A higher testosterone-to-estrogen ratio could be a strong risk factor for future CVD, coronary heart disease, and heart failure among postmenopausal women.[55] High free testosterone in women and low SHBG can lead to symptoms of polycystic ovary disease or PCOS.[56] PCOS increases CM risk, including hypertension, insulin resistance and insulin signaling problems, dyslipidemia, and obesity.[57,58]

A 2018 study in the *American Journal of Cardiology* reported these results from an average follow-up of 12.1 years in 2834 postmenopausal women participating in the MESA (Multi-Ethnic Study of Atherosclerosis) 2000 to 2002, using Cox hazard models to evaluate associations of sex hormones with CV outcomes[55]:

- Each standard deviation (SD) increase in total testosterone levels was associated with risk increases of 14% for CVD, 20% for coronary heart disease, and 9% for heart failure.

- Each SD increase in estradiol (an estrogen steroid hormone) was associated with risk reductions of 6% for CVD, 23% for coronary heart disease, and 22% for heart failure.

- Each SD increase in testosterone-estradiol ratio was linked to risk increases of 19% for CVD, 45% for coronary heart disease, and 31% for heart failure.

Another group used the MESA of 2000 to 2002 using 2759 postmenopausal women (ages 65 + 9 years) and reported that a more androgenic hormones profile in these women, higher free testosterone and lower SHBG, is associated with an increase in coronary artery calcification up to 10 years and a greater increase in left ventricular mass in men and women.[59] Women with higher free testosterone and SHBG also reported an increase in mass:volume ratio over the course of 9 years.[60]

Exogenous estrogen, particularly when administered orally, increases SHBG, which, in turn, reduces free T and estradiol (E2). Lower levels of testosterone in women can lead to clinical symptoms such as:

- Fatigue
- Decreased feeling of well-being
- Low motivation
- Muscle weakness
- Sleep problems
- Weight gain
- Decreased sexual libido

DIND/DIMD and Cardiometabolic Implications

One of the potential challenges facing heath care professionals today is the problem of drug-induced disease, including drug-induced nutrient depletion (DIND) and drug-induced microbiome disruption (DIMD).

DIND and DIMD in patients, including the cardiovascular patient, are important issues for the 21st century clinician to embrace and implement corrective measures into practice, which can be as simple as a multiple vitamin/mineral supplement. With over 48% of people in the United States taking prescription medications (up from 44% the previous decade), patients with CVD are placed a much higher risk for developing comorbid conditions and for increasing disease pathologies.[61] Polypharmacy prescribing is now occurring in younger and younger populations, so it is becoming increasingly important to assess nutrient depletion risks as they relate to increased drug side effects, future symptoms, comorbid health condition development, or progression of the underlying disease itself.

It is clear that a viable and thriving gut microbiome is essential for homeostasis. When this balance is disrupted, called dysbiosis, homeostasis is lost. One example of this is circulating endotoxin. As microflora is destroyed owing to reduced blood perfusion, high fat, low-fiber diets, or drug therapy, the cell wall fragments known as lipopolysaccharide (endotoxin) enter circulation potentially crossing the blood-brain barrier along with attaching to receptors of cells on other tissues. This triggers nuclear factor kappa-B and the full cascade of inflammatory cytokines. Elevated serum endotoxin has been associated with the progression of metabolic syndrome as well as an increased risk for cardiovascular events. An example of this could be elevated cortisol signaling from the brain, increased catecholamines, decreased blood perfusion to the gut leading to vascular inflammation, and reduced pliability. The network of brain-gut-heart becomes a driver for progression of CM disease.

The gut is now being called the "second brain." The gut-immune-brain axis helps control and is controlled by many body system networks, including the HPA axis, blood glucose and insulin regulation, sex hormone axes, detoxification systems, neurological disorders, and the cardiovascular system. Strong evidence exists supporting the fact that many chronic health conditions that are seen clinically are related to microbiome disruption—inflammatory bowel disease and other gastrointestinal (GI) conditions, liver cirrhosis, rheumatoid arthritis and autoimmune conditions (chronic inflammation), insulin resistance and type 2 diabetes, cognitive decline, depression, anxiety, schizophrenia and psychosis, cardiovascular conditions, and cancer.

There are many ways by which the gut microbiome network can become disrupted—poor food choices (high sugar/refined carb content, chemical food additives/preservatives/dyes, pesticide residues, acidic pH foods, and inflammatory foods like red meats), high levels of stress, infections, and many oral drugs that are taken can lead to dysbiosis.

In the medical management of individuals with CVD or comorbid conditions, several classes of prescription drugs may be employed with the potential for depletions of nutrients, which could induce metabolic changes and further the progression of any component of the underlying cardiovascular problems or comorbidities. Medications that are commonly used in the management of a patient with CVD include:

- Diuretics
- Angiotensin-converting enzyme inhibitors
- Angiotensin II receptor blockers
- Beta-blockers
- Calcium channel blockers
- Hypocholesterolemic agents
- Antidiabetic medications
- Anticoagulant/antiplatelet agents
- Nitrates
- Digitalis
- Pain medications, including opiates, acetaminophen, and nonsteroidal anti-inflammatory drugs
- Acid-reducing drugs, including H2 blockers or proton-pump inhibitors (PPIs)
- Antianxiety/sleep medications

Discussion of DIND is covered in another chapter, but an example of DIMD are PPIs. PPIs also are reported to significantly disrupt the human gut microbiome. PPIs lower gut acidity, which can lead to imbalances in the normal microflora—more species of nonhost microbes can thrive. Meta-analyses have reported that use of PPIs was associated with an increased incidence of *Clostridium difficile* infection if not treated aggressively.[62] Higher rates of *C difficile* recurrence in hospitalized patients and increased risk of other enteric infections and community-acquired *Streptococcus* pneumonia are also contributed to by the overuse of PPIs.[63,64] A recent study of 400 cirrhotic patients reported that PPI prescription was an independent predictor of infection.[64] Other studies suggest PPI microbiome disruption can lead to increases in esophageal and gastric cancers.[65]

Diagnosis and Evaluation of the CM Patient: A New Perspective

Evaluation of patients who may be at risk for CM disease includes not only identifying the presence of traditional cardiac risk factors but also delineation of underlying hormonal status. Identification of important hormonal abnormalities including insulin resistance and hyperinsulinemia, HPA axis dysregulation, and sex hormone (testosterone deficiency, estrogen imbalances) is essential. Furthermore, in patients who already have metabolic syndrome, evaluation of these hormones is particularly important in CM risk stratification. In essence it is important to get a thorough picture of what type of proinflammatory chemistry is present and more importantly what the systems biology factors driving the metabolic expression are.

Systems biology networking should be considered using laboratory analysis. These considerations are in addition to advanced markers directly related to CM risk such as Lpa, MPO, oxLDL, Kif 6, LpPLA2, LDL-p, and other markers mentioned throughout the text.

1. Stress levels (using five-point salivary cortisol OR in the least 8 AM serum cortisol) compared with DHEAs is important to determine HPA axis involvement.
2. Thyroid profile, including TSH, free and total T3 and T4, thyroid antibodies (ThyrAb), or thyroid peroxidase.
3. Fasting blood glucose, HbA1c and insulin, cystatin C. HDL, lactate dehydrogenase (LDH), vitamin D, red blood cell (RBC) chromium and magnesium, and serum potassium also impact blood glucose regulation.
4. Gut assessment—does the microbiome need support? Is the patient currently taking medications that can alter the microbiome? Are the patient's symptoms diarrhea/constipation, belching/burping, abdominal discomfort, feeling tired after eating large meals, weight gain, mental fogginess, immune dysregulation? Evaluating GI microflora and endotoxin may provide valuable insight into the inflammatory process.
5. Sex hormone analysis for men and women—serum free and total testosterone, estradiol, estrone, SHBG, DHT, and urinary metabolites of estrogen 4OH and 16-alpha derivatives.

Integrative Treatment Protocols

Once a patient with MetS has been identified by presenting with underlying hormonal derangements of insulin, cortisol, and/or testosterone, several integrative medicine treatment options can be considered. Conventional hormone replacement and medications may be considered as part of an overall treatment plan if necessary. However, bioavailable hormonal replacement therapies (HRTs) are preferred owing to side effects that can occur with the use of synthetics. Patients report greater satisfaction when using bioavailable HRT, especially with progesterone replacement, and not synthetic progestins.[66] Studies of both bioidentical estrogens and progesterone suggest a reduced risk of blood clots compared with nonbioidentical preparations.[67]

Dietary Supplements

Dietary supplementation that includes botanicals, nutrients, and nutraceuticals can help improve TRIAD balance and improve CM patient outcomes. Always use quality products from reputable manufacturers that follow strict good manufacturing practices.

TRIAD Network 1
Adrenal-Thyroid-Pancreas

Alpha-Lipoic Acid

α-Lipoic acid, also known as lipoic acid (ALA) or thioctic acid, and its reduced form, dihydrolipoic acid, are potent antioxidants and help improve glutathione levels. ALA is an essential cofactor for mitochondrial bioenergetic enzymes and functions as an antioxidant and anti-inflammatory agent.[68] ALA is reported in clinical studies to improve insulin sensitivity, improve glycemic control, and help improve symptoms and incidence of neuropathies.[69,70] ALA is reported to help activate AMP-K, which upregulates PGC-1 alpha, reducing insulin secretion, improving fatty acid and glucose utilization, and regulating cell growth.[71,72] ALA is also reported in laboratory animal studies to reduce the neurotoxic effects of heavy metal exposure, including lead, mercury, and cadmium.[73–75]

A general dose of ALA is 300 to 1200 mg daily.

Bitter Melon

Bitter melon (*Momordica charantia*) is a green, bitter vegetable from the gourd family, grown in tropical and subtropical regions throughout the Amazon, East Africa, Asia, the Caribbean, and South America and used as a food for diabetes and blood sugar control in these areas. Extracts are reported to contain poly-peptide P, similar in structure to bovine insulin. Laboratory studies have found that bitter melon may enhance insulin secretion by the islets of Langerhans, reduces glycogenesis in liver tissue, enhances peripheral glucose utilization, and increases serum protein levels.[76,77] Bitter melon activates PPAR gamma, an important metabolic pathway in glucose and weight control.[78] Clinical conditions for which bitter melon extracts are currently being used include diabetes, dyslipidemia, and microbial infections. It was found to decrease blood sugar levels when injected subcutaneously into type 1 diabetic patients.[79] Bitter melon supplements also help with obesity and symptoms of metabolic syndrome.

The dose is generally at 250 to 500 mg two times daily standardized to 10% charantins. Bitter melon is usually combined with other blood glucose supportive nutrients, including chromium, cinnamon, ALA, benfotiamine (a special form of thiamin B1), and pyrroloquinoline quinolone (PQQ, helps with mitochondrial energy production).

Chromium

Chromium supplementation has been reported in clinical trials for over 5 decades to improve insulin regulation and glucose tolerance in people with type 1 and 2 diabetes, gestational diabetes, and steroid-induced diabetes.[80,81] Chromium depletion can lead to hyperlipidemia, insulin resistance, fatigue, accelerated atherosclerosis, hypertension, anxiety, impaired wound healing, decreased glucose tolerance, and possibly infertility.[82] Some studies have reported negative clinical outcomes in patients supplementing chromium. However, low doses and poorly absorbable forms of chromium used in these studies may have negatively affected the therapeutic outcomes. Chromium is not found in sufficient amounts in food to replenish tissue stores or to affect clinically significant improvement in blood glucose control.[82]

Dose should be between 400 and 800 μg of folate daily; the form of 5-methylfolate is best, but one can also use folinic acid or a combination of 5-MTHF and folinic acid (400 μg each is optimal). Doses of up to 1200 μg daily can be used in severe blood glucose and insulin dysregulation.

Pyrroloquinoline-Quinone

PQQ is an antioxidant and redox cofactor for the membrane-bound dehydrogenases, leading to the growth and production of cells under stress.[83] PQQ helps support mitochondrial energy production and regulation. PQQ is reported in laboratory animal studies to be a protein tyrosine phosphatase 1B inhibitor, helping to activate insulin signaling and improve glucose tolerance and alter indicators of inflammation.[84,85]

Dose is 20 to 40 mg PQQ in the morning. Use a special microactive PQQ that is sustained release.

Benfotiamine (Lipid-Soluble Thiamin)

Thiamin (vitamin B1) is necessary for the metabolism of carbohydrates and amino acids to adenosine triphosphate (ATP), the primary source of energy in the human body. Thiamin is found in good amounts in milk, lean pork, legumes, rice bran, and the germ of cereal grains but is lost during food processing and cooking. Benfotiamine is a lipid-soluble form of thiamin (vitamin B1). Oral administration of benfotiamine raises thiamine levels in blood and tissues to a much higher degree than the water-soluble salts.[86] Several clinical studies support benfotiamine's use in diabetic patients. A 2006 clinical study reported that benfotiamine helped prevent macro- and microvascular endothelial dysfunction in patients with type 2 diabetes.[87] However, a 2013 clinical study reported that benfotiamine had no effect on postprandial vascular function in type 2 diabetic patients.[88] Other studies report that benfotiamine decreases advanced glycation end products (AGEs) and markers of endothelial dysfunction and inflammation.[89] Clinical studies also report that benfotiamine is beneficial in reducing symptoms associated with diabetic retinopathy.[90]

Dose is 50 to 100 mg daily. Regular thiamine HCl will work; benfotiamine is preferred but optional.

Botanical Adaptogens

A common category of adrenal and HPA axis supportive supplements includes plant *adaptogens,* which have long been touted to improve the ability of organisms to avoid systemic damage during periods of prolonged exposure to various stressors, including rhodiola (*Rhodiola rosea*) root, ashwagandha (*Withania somnifera*) root, and tongkat ali (*Eurycoma longifolia*) root.

Rhodiola Root

Rhodiola (*R rosea*) is used in traditional folk medicine in China, Serbia, and the Carpathian Mountains of the Ukraine as an herbal adaptogen. Rhodiola seems to enhance the body's physical and mental work capacity and productivity, working to strengthen the nervous system, fight depression, enhance immunity, elevate the capacity for exercise, enhance memorization, and improve energy levels. A clinical study reported that an extract of rhodiola significantly improved generalized anxiety disorder symptoms, with a reduction in HARS scores similar to that reported by pharmaceuticals in clinical trials.[91] Supplementation of rhodiola to physicians favorably influenced fatigue and mental performance during the first 2 weeks on night duty.[92] Students receiving a standardized extract of rhodiola demonstrated significant improvements in physical fitness, psychomotor function, mental performance, and general well-being. Subjects receiving rhodiola extract also reported statistically significant reductions in mental fatigue, improved sleep patterns, a reduced need for sleep, greater mood stability, and a greater motivation to study.[93]

A 2009 phase III clinical trial reported that a standardized rhodiola extract had antifatigue activity that increases mental performance, particularly the ability to concentrate, and decreases cortisol response to awakening stress in burnout patients with fatigue syndrome.[94] An extract of rhodiola in combination with vitamins/minerals was administered to 120 adults aged 50 to 89 years and reported to improve cognition in 81% of patients.[95] Rhodiola has also been reported to increase exercise endurance and performance in humans (n = 18 and n = 24).[96,97]

The adaptogenic properties, cardiopulmonary protective effects, and central nervous system activities of rhodiola have been attributed primarily to its ability to influence levels and activity of biogenic monoamines such as serotonin, dopamine, and norepinephrine in the cerebral cortex, brain stem, and hypothalamus. In addition to these central effects, rhodiola has been reported to prevent both catecholamine release and subsequent cyclic AMP elevation in the myocardium and the depletion of adrenal catecholamines induced by acute stress.[98]

Rhodiola's adaptogenic activity might also be secondary to induction of opioid peptide biosynthesis and through the activation of both central and peripheral opioid receptors.[99] Rhodiola may also help improve immune function through regulation of IL-2 in Th1 cells and IL-4, IL-6, IL-10 in Th2 cells.[100]

A review of the clinical studies supporting the effectiveness of rhodiola supplements was conducted in 2011.[101] Eleven randomized, placebo-controlled human studies were investigated. It was reported that rhodiola supplements may have beneficial effects on physical performance, mental performance, and mental health conditions like depression. The authors concluded that more research seems warranted.

Dose is 250 to 500 mg two times daily, standardized to 3% to 5% rosavins and 1% to 3% salidrosides.

Ashwagandha Root

Ashwagandha (*W somnifera*), also known as Indian ginseng and winter cherry, has been an important herb in Ayurvedic medicine for over 3000 years. Ashwagandha is used as an adaptogen, a plant that helps support the body during increased exposure to various stressors.[102–104] Ashwagandha contains alkaloids and steroidal lactones and is rich in iron. In human studies, ashwagandha is reported to have anti-inflammatory, anabolic, and analgesic activity that helps decrease fatigue and improve hemoglobin and RBC counts and physical performance.[105] Laboratory studies suggest that ashwagandha helps improve performance, decrease fatigue, and alter biochemical changes in the adrenal glands when under stress.[106]

A 2010 study in 75 infertile men reported that an extract of ashwagandha improved testosterone and LH, while decreasing oxidative stress, FSH, and prolactin.[107] A 2013 study (n = 100) reported that ashwagandha was effective in relieving fatigue and improving quality of life in patients with breast cancer.[108] A 2010 study (n = 40, mean age, 20.6 years) reported that an extract of ashwagandha improved physical performance and cardiorespiratory endurance, with the conclusion that ashwagandha may help improve generalized weakness and improve speed and lower limb muscular strength and neuromuscular coordination.[109]

Ashwagandha also has been reported in laboratory animal studies to help increase thyroid hormone production, particularly T4, which helps improve energy and metabolic performance.[110]

Use ashwagandha with caution if taking sedatives, as it has been reported to increase the effects of barbiturates. A case report exists of a patient developing thyrotoxicosis when using an extract of ashwagandha.[111]

Dose is 250 to 500 mg two times daily, standardized to 2.5% to 5% with anolides.

Eurycoma Root

Eurycoma (tongkat ali, *Eurycoma longifolia*), also known as Malaysian "ginseng" and long Jack, is an herb traditionally used in Southeast Asia for male reproductive health. Laboratory studies have supported these uses.[112] In clinical studies, Eurycoma is reported to increase male sexual vitality, along with increasing both total and free testosterone levels.[113–115] In a 2013 clinical study (n = 63, men and women), Eurycoma was reported to improve salivary cortisol levels and testosterone levels, along with improving symptoms of moderate stress, including tension, anger, and confusion.[116] Studies indicate that having healthy testosterone levels supports a healthy body composition in both men and women.[117,118]

Dose is 150 to 200 mg two times daily of a 100:1 or a 200:1 extract.

Thai Ginseng (*Kaempferia parviflora*) Root/Rhizome

Thai ginseng or black ginger is an herbaceous plant in the ginger family (*Zingiberaceae*) and is native to Thailand. Traditionally, Krachai-dum (*K parviflora*) is mainly used as an aphrodisiac and for male sexual function and is loosely referred to as "Thai Viagra." The 5,7-dimethoxyflavonoids in Thai ginseng have antioxidant, PDE5 inhibitory properties and SIRT-1 stimulating properties. Studied uses of *K parviflora* in humans include[119–122]:

- Weight loss supportive
- Improved thermogenesis
- Manages differentiation and adipogenesis of adipocytes
- Improves physical work capacity
- Antioxidant/anti-inflammatory
- Mitochondrial support—improves energy biogenesis
- Neuroprotection—flavonoids

Dose: Use 90 to 180 mg daily in divided doses of a 2% to 4% 5,7-dimethoxyflavone extract. Use with caution if taking PDE5 inhibitors concurrently.

TRIAD 2 Gut-Immune-Brain

Probiotics

As we have discussed, many factors can disrupt the gut microbiome, including diet, stress, and drugs. The word "probiotic" means "life" in Greek, and probiotics help directly decrease endotoxin release and effects. Recommending probiotic supplements to support microbiome health is one of the most important steps clinicians can take for their CM patient. Increased circulating endotoxin is commonly found in CM patients and leads to chronic inflammatory responses.

Bacteroidetes and **Firmicutes** are dominant (>90% of the total microbial population) in human intestine and play a significant role in nutrient absorption, mucosal barrier fortification, xenobiotic metabolism, angiogenesis, and postnatal intestinal maturation. Diet controls the composition of these bacteria, which are crucial in the development of metabolic disorders.[123]

Dose: 5 to 10 billion CFU two to three times daily (daily total of 15-20 billion CFU). Use heat- and acid-stable probiotic supplements, with a diverse microbial population containing several *Lactobacillus* and *Bifidobacterium* species. Probiotics should also contain prebiotics, or nondigestible food ingredients that benefit and increase the populations of friendly microbial in the gut. Examples of prebiotics include arabinogalactan and inulin. If diarrhea is present, *Saccharomyces* should be included.

Melatonin

Melatonin is a natural hormone produced by the pineal gland. Concentrations in serum, as well as urinary levels of its main metabolite, 6-sulphatoxymelatonin, decrease with age. The presence of vascular melatoninergic receptors/binding sites has been demonstrated; these receptors are functionally linked with vasoconstrictor or vasodilatory effects of melatonin.[124] The suprachiasmatic nucleus and, possibly, the melatoninergic system may also modulate cardiovascular rhythmicity. Also, people with hypertension have lower melatonin levels than those with normal blood pressure.[124] Melatonin may reduce blood pressure via the following mechanisms: (1) by a direct effect on the hypothalamus, (2) as an antioxidant that lowers blood pressure, (3) by decreasing the level of catecholamines, or (4) by relaxing the smooth muscle in the aorta wall.

Chronic depletion of melatonin can lead to systems biology network (TRIAD) imbalances. Chronic melatonin depletion directly influences daily rhythm of glucose, reduction in glucose transporter 4 (GLUT 4) levels, and suppression of insulin secretion.[125] The correlation may be that melatonin deficits lead to disrupted sleep and disrupted sleep can lead to increased insulin resistance. Melatonin may enhance insulin-receptor kinase and IRS-1 phosphorylation, which may improve insulin signaling and may actually counteract TNFα-induced insulin resistance in populations with type 2 diabetes and metabolic syndrome.[29] Melatonin also has significant antioxidant effects as it stimulates glutathione peroxidase, SOD, and catalase as well as NO synthase. Melatonin is reported to reduce oxidative stress in diabetic populations.

An evaluation of the National Health and Nutrition Examination Survey revealed that people who slept 5 hours a night had a 73% increased risk of becoming obese versus those who slept 7 to 9 hours per night.[126] Trials conducted at Stanford University found that people who slept an average of <5 hours per night had a 15.5% decrease in leptin, an increase of 14.9% of ghrelin, and higher body mass indexes (BMIs), regardless of the exercise and diet habits of the participants.[127] So with loss of sleep, the net effect was appetite centers were upregulated, BMI increased, and there was a shift in metabolic dysfunction toward metabolic syndrome. When melatonin levels are low, rapid eye movement (REM) sleep cycles are disturbed leading to increased wakefulness throughout the night, and studies have shown that administering melatonin in the late evening hours was significantly more effective than placebo at increasing REM sleep.[128,129]

Under conditions of high stress, cortisol levels increase, leading to a state of hyperarousal. Studies have shown that disturbed sleep as a result of hyperarousal can lead to its own effects on metabolic function (eg, ↑ TNFα,↑ IL-6,↑ visceral fat storage,↑ insulin resistance).[28] Other nutrient depletions such as reduced magnesium status and low folate status (↓ serotonin synthesis) can also simultaneously act on the sleep center and induce hyperarousal. All of this adds up to an increased risk for obesity, diabetes, and cardiovascular risk.

Lastly, melatonin seems to have a direct effect on inhibiting tumorigenesis. Melatonin helps to inhibit cellular proliferation and stimulated differentiation and apoptosis.[30] This is particularly interesting because people with insulin resistance and sleep disturbances are more prone to cancer owing to elevations of insulin-like growth factor 1 and increases in the immunologic shift toward chronic inflammatory chemistry leading to reduced activity of natural killer (NK) cells.

Melatonin is a potential drug nutrient depletion (DIND) of beta-blockers. Because of its potential to disrupt sleep and lead to further problems such as increased appetite, weight gain, insulin resistance, and increased inflammatory chemistry, it is an important nutrient to assess and administer if disrupted sleep is present. Cortisol levels should also be evaluated to determine if steps may be necessary to downregulate cortisol to further address hyperarousal as an underlying cause of insomnia.

Dose: 3 to 15 mg melatonin 1 hour before bedtime can help alleviate the symptoms of insomnia, with no worry of toxicity or dependence with chronic use.

TRIAD Network 3 Cardiovascular-Neurovascular-Pulmonary Supportive Supplements

Aged Garlic Extract

Aged garlic extract should be a hallmark of dietary supplementation for the CM patient. Aged garlic extract is a special fermentation of garlic that provides the health benefits of fresh garlic, without the pungent taste and halitosis or gastric distress. The fermentation of aged garlic generates high levels of *S*-allyl cysteine, the primary antioxidant compound. Aged garlic extract has been marketed for more than 50 years as an over-the-counter medicine in Japan and in more than 30 other countries for over 30 years. There are over 750 clinical studies directly using aged garlic extract for various uses, including hypertension, cardiovascular health, gut microbiome, and immune support.[130,131]

One of aged garlic's most promising uses is in the supportive treatment of hypertension. Aged garlic has reported in vitro antiglycation properties.[132] Aged garlic supports immune and inflammatory pathways and has been reported to decrease inflammatory mediators IL-6 and TNFα. Aged garlic is also reported to have microbiome enhancing properties, important in the CM patient.

Summary of aged garlic laboratory and clinical studies:

- Research reports aged garlic extract use is similar in effectiveness in reducing blood pressure in a large portion of hypertensive patients to first-line standard antihypertensive protocols using medication.[133]
- Hypertension has been linked to gut microbiome disruptions (dysbiosis), specifically an increase in the *Firmicutes* and *Bacteroidetes* sp.[134] Aged garlic is reported to improve the microbial richness and diversity with an increase in *Lactobacillus* and *Clostridia* species after 3 months of therapy.
- May protect against CVDs, reducing risk factors for atherosclerosis, myocardial infarctions, and stroke. Aged garlic extract may help lower LDL cholesterol and decrease LDL oxidation, glycation, reduce triglycerides, elevate HDL, reduce homocysteine and blood pressure, increase circulation in capillaries, provide antiplatelet activity, decrease vascular inflammation, and help prevent the formation of coronary atherogenic plaques.[135–138]
- A human study in 50 patients with uncontrolled hypertension reported aged garlic lowers systolic blood pressure as well as first-line conventional medical treatments.[130] A 2018 double-blind placebo-controlled study using 49 patients with uncontrolled hypertension taking 1.2 g daily aged garlic extract reported that mean BP reduced by 10 + 3.6 mm Hg systolic and 5.4 + 2.3 mm Hg diastolic. Aged garlic reduced central BP, pulse pressure, and arterial stiffness and improved gut microbiome diversity.
- Reported in human and laboratory studies to reduce homocysteine-induced endothelial dysfunction by inhibiting homocysteine-induced scavenger receptor CD36 expression and oxidized LDL cholesterol uptake in macrophages.[139]
- May decrease risks associated with certain cancers, including gastric and colon cancer. Antioxidant activity protects the body against free-radical- and carcinogen-induced DNA damage.[140]
- Provides antioxidant protection; may increase nitric oxide levels, improving vascular health.[141]
- Antioxidant activity helps protect against toxic effects of pollution, ultraviolet light, and drug toxicity by increasing hepatic glutathione levels.[142]
- May decrease protein glycation, decreasing complications associated with diabetes.[143]
- Helps improve immune activation; may help prevent viral, bacterial, and yeast infections and allergies.
- Reported to decrease the decline of NK cells in patients with advanced cancer.[144]
- Participants in a 2016 clinical study (n = 120, ages 21-50 years) took aged garlic for 90 days during cold/flu season.[145] At 45 days, NK and T cells were better proliferated and more activated than cells in the placebo group. At 90 days, patients who took aged garlic

reported less lost school and workdays and less severe symptoms of colds or flu than placebo.

- May enhance vigor, reduce fatigue and stress.[146]
- May inhibit the growth of *Helicobacter pylori* in the gastrointestinal tract.[147]
- Aged garlic's antioxidant activity may provide anti-aging and neuroprotective effects; prevent neuron death; enhance memory, learning, and cognition; and stimulate growth and branching of neurons of the hippocampus.[132,148]

Dose: The general dose for adults is 1 to 2 capsules, two times daily (600-1200 mg BID). Certainly, someone above 220 pounds or so would need the higher dosage. Aged garlic is reported NOT to interact with anticoagulants such as coumadin; regular garlic preparations have been reported to increase bleeding times.

Coenzyme Q10

One of the most frequently discussed depletions in drug-induced nutrient depletion is the area of coenzyme Q10 (CoQ10) depletion and the use of statin (3-hydroxyl 3-methylglutaryl coenzyme A reductase inhibitors or HMG CoA reductase inhibitors) medications. This depletion can also occur in the use of HMG CoA reductase inhibitors, centrally acting anti-hypertensive agents, fibrates, diuretics, beta-blockers, and second-generation sulfonylureas and biguanide drug therapies. It has been demonstrated that CoQ10 concentrations can fall as much as 54% in patients who are on HMG CoA reductase inhibitor therapy, with a dose-dependent drop in some patient populations.[149] Note that excessive and/or chronic alcohol consumption may also lead to CoQ10 depletion.[150]

CoQ10 is a cofactor in the electron transport chain, which is involved in cellular respiration and the generation of ATP. CoQ10 also plays an important role as an antioxidant and is a principle gene regulator in muscle tissue and plays a significant role in tissue metabolism. Clinical manifestations of CoQ10 depletion can include myalgias, rhabdomyolysis, cardiomyopathy, hypertension, angina, stroke, cardiac dysrhythmias, fatigue, leg weakness, decline in immune function, increase in neurodegenerative diseases, and loss of cognitive function.[151]

In one study, muscle fibers were examined in an elderly population preparing for hip surgery.[152] The findings, CoQ10-treated individuals had a lower proportion of type 1 (slow twitch) fibers and a higher concentration of type IIb (fast twitch) fibers compared with age-matched placebo-treated patients. This shift is consistent with fiber composition found in younger populations. In this study, significant change in gene expression of proteins was noted. The protective and regenerative effect of CoQ10 on skeletal muscle is promising, and it may be theorized that low CoQ10 status could accelerate aging and genetic changes in muscle tissue.

Another area of clinical concern in the patient with metabolic syndrome is the increased risk for Alzheimer disease. Disruption in mitochondrial ATP and an increase in hydrogen peroxide is one mechanism by which amyloid beta-peptide toxicity can take place. Disruptions in glucose metabolism and increased free radical damage have been implicated in the development of Alzheimer disease. In a promising study, isolated brain mitochondria from diabetic rats were treated with CoQ10. Treatment with CoQ10 attenuated the decreased oxidative phosphorylation efficiency and halted the hydrogen peroxide production induced by neurotoxic peptides. This indicates that CoQ10 treatment changed the mitochondrial alterations in Abeta 1-40, suggesting it could play a role in altering the cellular energy deficits correlated to diabetes and the progression of Alzheimer disease.[153] These findings suggest that it does not make sense to administer drugs that deplete CoQ10 without repletion when clearly mitochondrial energy deficits are involved in progression to Alzheimer disease.

The value of CoQ10 in hypertension was reported in one clinical trial where supplementing CoQ10 decreased systolic and diastolic blood pressure, decreased total cholesterol, and increased HDL cholesterol.[154] In another trial, supplementation of CoQ10 enabled hypertensive patients to reduce their medications. A mean dose of 225 mg in 109 patients led to discontinuation of 1 to 3 medications in 51% of patients within 6 months (average time 4.4 months), 80% of the individuals had been diagnosed for 9.2 years. Only 3% required addition of one more drug.[155] In another study, it was reported that drug-related myopathy, which is a complaint of CoQ10 therapy, was shown to be associated with a mild decrease in CoQ10 without presenting a histochemical or mitochondrial myopathy or even morphologic evidence of apoptosis in most patients examined. The net meaning of this is that significant cellular pathology may not exist and yet symptom expression could be likely.[156] Even though there may be no evidence of changes via creatine kinase concentrations, metabolic disruption of ATP production and cellular energetics is probable.

With several of the most common drugs used in metabolic syndrome depleting CoQ10 clinicians should consider the implications of chronic mild decreases of CoQ10 and its impact on the progression of the metabolic pathology as it relates to the cardiovascular component.

The CoQ10 serum reference range is 0.37 to 2.20 µg/mL. The recommended clinical dosage range for repletion of CoQ10 ranges from 30 to 300 mg/d of a solubilized form of coenzyme Q10. It should be noted that concomitant administration of CoQ10 supplements with anticoagulants such as warfarin is reported in several case studies to lead to decreased levels of the anticoagulant.[157,158] CoQ10 is chemically similar to the K vitamins, which may explain the interaction with warfarin.

The dosage of CoQ10 (ubiquinone) should be 50 to 100 mg daily, at night preferably.

CONDITIONS AND SYMPTOMS ASSOCIATED WITH COQ10 DEPLETION

- Myalgia
- Arthralgia
- Rhabdomyolysis
- Hypertension

- Angina
- Mitral valve prolapse
- Stroke
- Arrhythmias
- Cardiomyopathy
- Poor insulin production
- Low energy
- Gingivitis
- Weakened immunity

Magnesium

Magnesium is involved in over 300 enzymatic reactions in the body. It is needed for proper nerve transmission, production of energy, muscular activity, regulation of temperature, detoxification of cells, blood pressure regulation, and regulation of blood sugar and regulates vasospasm and helps with the building of healthy bones and teeth. Appropriate magnesium levels are especially important for the cardiovascular patient, and low levels of magnesium are associated with an increased risk of heart disease.[159,160]

It is reported that approximately 75% of Americans' intake of magnesium is below the recommended dietary allowance, and many may be clinically or subclinically deficient.[161] Because serum magnesium does not reflect intracellular magnesium, and the latter makes up more than 99% of total body magnesium, most cases of magnesium deficiency are undiagnosed. Many lifestyle factors such as stress and drinking alcohol can deplete magnesium, so it is easy to understand how with the addition of drug therapy a clinically significant low magnesium level can occur.

Hypomagnesemia and low dietary intake of magnesium are strongly related to cardiovascular risk factors among known subjects with coronary artery disease, including increasing the proinflammatory/pro-oxidant status and an increased risk of ischemic heart disease.[162–165] Also, one of the most significant and least discussed nutrients depleted from first-line drug therapy in hypertension is magnesium. A Japanese study of over 58,615 healthy men ages 40 to 79 years that lasted 14.7 years reported that increasing magnesium in the diet reduced CVD mortality risk by approximately 50%.[166]

In clinical practice, when patients are prescribed thiazide diuretics for hypertension, typically only potassium depletion is addressed, with patients advised to drink orange juice or eat a banana, which are rich sources of potassium. Often, no education in medical schools or allied health curriculums is given regarding the potential for magnesium depletion, although many of listed side effects of thiazide diuretics are also signs and symptoms of magnesium depletion. Although this topic may be controversial in the literature,[167] enough studies have reported a magnesium-depleting effect from thiazides (one report in 2000 suggested 20% of patients taking thiazide have hypomagnesaemia[168]) to at least justify a screening for magnesium depletion symptoms among thiazide users.[169,170] This is especially true when it is considered that the clinical manifestations of hypomagnesemia can be so severe.

Deficiency of magnesium is associated with increased incidence of atherosclerosis, hypertension, stroke, and myocardial infarction. Magnesium plays a role in inhibiting platelet aggregation, blood thinning, blocking of calcium and reuptake and relaxes blood vessels and increases oxygenation of the heart by improving contractility. Oral magnesium therapy is reported beneficial in patients with heart failure and those undergoing cardiovascular surgeries, improving blood pressure regulation via improved endothelial function and improving exercise heart rate, exercise tolerance, and myocardial function in general.[171–174]

It should be mentioned that serum magnesium is a poor measure of magnesium status because homeostatic mechanisms keep blood levels fairly constant by pulling magnesium from bone and other body tissues. It is often suggested that RBC levels are a more reliable indicator of magnesium status.[175] However, some researchers state that mid-normal magnesium levels could be indicative of an intracellular depletion. RBC levels of magnesium should be 4.2 to 6.8 mg/dL for most individuals. Likewise, levels do not always correspond with utilization in the body. Serum magnesium levels of 1.7 to 2.2 mg/dL are appropriate for most individuals.

POTENTIAL SYMPTOMS OF MAGNESIUM DEFICIENCY

- Muscle cramps and spasms, vasomotor spasms
- Anxiousness, nervousness, insomnia
- Hypertension, prehypertension
- Blood glucose imbalances/insulin resistance
- Depression/mood swings
- Fatigue
- Arrhythmias, dysrhythmias
- Migraines
- Constipation
- Osteoporosis/decreased bone density
- Kidney stones

MANIFESTATIONS OF MAGNESIUM DEFICIENCY

Even marginal magnesium deficiency can decrease myocardial magnesium, which can directly affect the contractility and excitability of the heart. The mechanism of action of this result is primarily by the reduced regulation of calcium ion channel. Even perfusion of the heart can be easily compromised. Studies have reported that low magnesium can lead to coronary vasospasm, reduced energy metabolism, changes in potassium homeostasis, and excessive induction of free radical generation.[176] In an animal study demonstrating this principle, a diet low in magnesium and high in sucrose progressively induced elevations in triglycerides and a reduction of insulin binding to erythrocyte insulin receptors (↑insulin resistance) over a 3-month period.[177]

Many of the symptoms and conditions that develop, progress, and are prescribed for in metabolic syndrome mimic the symptoms of magnesium depletion, primarily blood pressure regulation and blood sugar regulation. It should be noted that several of the listed side effects of thiazide diuretics are magnesium depletion symptoms, including arrhythmia, lower back pain, mood changes, muscle pain/weakness/cramps, constipation, headache, and fatigue.

An established potential consequence of long-term use of thiazide diuretics is development of type 2 diabetes, and because of this their use is controversial in those predisposed to blood glucose dysregulation.[178] The medical literature is clearly establishing the role of magnesium not only in insulin regulation but also in helping control inflammatory chemistry.[179] Drug-induced intracellular depletion of magnesium could be playing a significant role in the rapid induction into the complications of metabolic syndrome.

Dose: Clinical repletion dosage of magnesium as magnesium aspartate, citrate, or amino acid chelate is 300 to 800 mg/d. This dosage may induce loose stool, so titrate to larger doses if needed.

Dietary Factors

Several dietary interventions have been reported to decrease the risk of CHD. This review examines the role of dietary factors, including Mediterranean diet; fish and n-3 fatty acids; flavonoids and polyphenols (resveratrol, proanthocyanidins); fiber and whole grain; vitamins; and garlic (especially aged garlic) in the prevention of CHD.

The Mediterranean-style diet is a collection of traditional dietary habits in countries adjacent to the Mediterranean Sea—Greece, Spain, France, Monaco, Italy, Lebanon, Egypt, and others. These people eat higher amounts of fruit and vegetables (high antioxidants), legumes, and complex carbohydrates (high fiber) and low to moderate amounts of fish and poultry; they use a high amount of garlic; they use olive oil (omega-3 and omega-9) as the main source of dietary fats; and they consume a relatively low amount of red meat and low to moderate amount of red wine during meals. This "low inflammatory" diet is reported to reduce the risk of chronic health conditions including Alzheimer disease, cognitive impairment, stroke, and coronary heart disease.[180]

There are also studies supporting a plant-based diet for cardiovascular health.[181] This evidence includes several population-based cohort studies that have reported an inverse relationship between increased consumption of plant-based foods and incidence of heart failure.[182,183] Also, plant-based diets have been reported to improve blood pressure, glycemic control, and obesity, additional risk factors for heart failure.[184,185] Plant-based diets may slow the progression of atherosclerosis and may even reverse atherosclerosis.[186] Of interest is a 2015 case report that demonstrated a whole-food plant-based diet's ability to reverse angina without medical or invasive therapy.[187]

Plant-based diets are reported to decrease the formation of oxidized LDL-C. OxLDL is cytotoxic to endothelial cells and promotes chemotaxis of monocytes and T cells, which leads to endovascular inflammation and atherogenesis, and oxidized LDL-C attenuates the response of endothelial cells to nitric oxide.[188] Reactive oxygen species (ROS) induce myocyte hypertrophy, aortic stiffness, apoptosis, and interstitial fibrosis, potentially contributing to the progression of heart failure.[189] Furthermore, ROS may reduce myocardial contractility, and an inverse relationship between antioxidant uptake and heart failure has been described.[190] Plant-based diets are rich in antioxidants and in part by reducing ROS may improve myocardial contractility, whereas animal-based foods, with lower amounts of antioxidants, may lead to greater levels of ROS and may have the opposite effect. In addition, AGEs, which are less prevalent in plant-based foods than in high-fat, animal-rich foods, lead to the formation of ROS and may further contribute to systolic, diastolic, and vascular dysfunction.[191]

ROS may also deleteriously impact HDL-C, in part by decreasing HDL-C efflux capacity.[192] Improved HDL-C efflux capacity has been independently associated with improved cardiovascular outcomes. Although plant-based diets may lead to a minor lowering of HDL-C levels, they are associated with increased HDL-C efflux capacity.[193]

Plant-based diets are also reported to reduce inflammatory processes, which is associated with an increased incident of heart failure.[194] Plant-based diets are reported to decrease serum levels of inflammatory biomarkers, including CRP, soluble intercellular adhesion molecule-1, and IL-6.[195]

People eating a plant-based diet generally have lower levels of trimethylamine N-oxide (TMAO), which is formed via the interaction of the nutrients choline and L-carnitine with the gut microbiome and subsequent hepatic metabolism.[196,197] The microflora of vegans and vegetarians is such that they produce less trimethylamine, a precursor for TMAO when compared with omnivores. TMAO decreases reverse cholesterol transport and may promote platelet reactivity and vascular inflammation. Higher TMAO levels are associated with worse cardiovascular outcomes, including myocardial infarction, heart failure, and death.[198,199] This difference may account, in part, for their association with fewer cardiovascular events.

Conclusion

In conclusion, modern drug therapy and the emerging science of natural therapeutics together provide an integrative approach to management of chronic diseases as well as the best approach for prevention and wellness. After reading this chapter, it should be evident that managed care of the CM patient should include evaluation and treatment of dysregulated metabolic systems networks, the TRIADs. This knowledge and understanding enables clinicians to recommend optimal treatment protocols to prevent cardiovascular and metabolic morbidities. Is the patient overly stressed? Could their gut microbiome be dysbiotic? Is sleep a problem? Investigating these and other issues associated with TRIAD imbalances will help you create an integrative approach to your CM patient's care.

Current treatment protocols using drug therapy or surgery alone can offer only a fragmented approach to care. As CM risk factors tend to cluster, patients often have additional subclinical conditions that would be discovered through comprehensive evaluation for the entire constellation of risk factors. The end result should be improved patient care and improved quality of life.

References

1. American Heart Association. Available at: www.heart.org. Accessed January 2019.
2. CDC Centers for Disease Control. Available at: www.cdc.gov. Accessed January 2019.
3. Ash-Bernal R, Peterson LR. The cardiometabolic syndrome and cardiovascular disease. *J Cardiometab Syndr.* 2006;1(1):25-28.
4. Patil R, Sood GK. Non-alcoholic fatty liver disease and cardiovascular risk. *World J Gastrointest Pathophysiol.* 2017;8(2):51-58.
5. American Heart Association. Heart disease and stroke statistics-2009 update. A report from the American Heart Association Statistics Committee and Stroke Statistics Subcommittee. *Circulation.* 2008;119(3):e21-e181.
6. Masur K. *Janus face of glucose and glucos-regulating hormones.* In: *Diabetes and Cancer: Epidemiologic Evidence and Molecular Links. Frontiers in Diabetes.* Vol. 19. Karger; 2008:45.
7. Pi-Sunyer FX. The relation of adipose tissue to cardiometabolic risk. *Clin Cornerstone.* 2006;8(suppl 4):S14-S23.
8. McGown C, Birerdinc A, Younossi ZM. Adipose tissue as an endocrine organ. *Clin Liver Dis.* 2014;18(1):41-58.
9. Zanker KS. *The epidemiologic relationship between diabetes and cancer.* In: *Diabetes and Cancer: Epidemiologic Evidence and Molecular Links. Frontiers in Diabetes.* Vol. 19. Karger; 2008:85.
10. Ando S, Gelsomino L, Panza S, et al. Obesity, leptin and breast cancer: epidemiological evidence and proposed mechanisms. *Cancers (Basel).* 2019;11(1):pii:E62.
11. National Center for Complementary and Alternative Medicine, National Institutes of Health, U.S., Department of Health and Human Services. *The Use of Complementary and Alternative Medicine in the United States.* National Health Institute Survey; 2002.
12. Developed and Adopted by the Consortium of Academic Health Centers for Integrative Medicine (CAHCIM), May 2004 Edited May 2009. http://nccam.nih.gov/.
13. Deleted in review.
14. Thevenod F. *Pathophysiology of diabetes mellitus type 2: role of obesity, insulin resistance and β-cell dysfunction.* In: *Diabetes and Cancer: Epidemiologic Evidence and Molecular Links. Frontiers in Diabetes.* Vol. 19. Karger;2008:2-3.
15. Pouliot MC, Despres JR, Nadeau A, et al. Visceral obesity in men. Associations with glucose tolerance, plasma insulin, and lipoprotein levels. *Diabetes.* 1992;41:826-834.
16. Ormazabal V, Nair S, Elfeky O, Aguayo C, Salomon C, Zuñiga FA. Association between insulin resistance and the development of cardiovascular disease. *Cardio Diabetol.* 2018;17:122.
17. Gruzdeva O, Borodkina D, Uchasova E, Dyleva Y, Barbarash O. Localization of fat depots and cardiovascular risk. *Lipids Health Dis.* 2018;17(1):218.
18. Epel ES. Psychological and metabolic stress: a recipe for accelerated cellular aging? *Hormones.* 2009;8(1):7-22.
19. Parsons PA. The ecological stress theory of aging and hormesis: an energetic evolutionary model. *Biogerontology.* 2007;8:233-242.
20. Chrousos G, Gold P. The concepts of stress and stress system disorders. *JAMA.* 1992;267:1244-1252.
21. Stephens MAC. Stress and the HPA Axis. *Alcohol Res.* 2012;34(4):468-483.
22. Kassi E. HPA axis abnormalities and metabolic syndrome. *Endocr Abstr.* 2016;41(S4).
23. Posener JA, Schildkraut JJ, Samson JA, Schatzberg AF. Diurnal variation of plasma cortisol and homovanillic acid in healthy subjects. *Psychoneuroendocrinology.* 1996;21(1):33-38.
24. Yehuda R, Teicher MH, Trestman RL, Leven good RA, Siever LJ. Cortisol regulation in posttraumatic stress disorder and major depression: a chronobiological analysis. *Biol Psychiatry.* 1996;40:79-88.
25. Deuschle M, Schweiger U, Weber B, et al. Diurnal activity and pulsatility of the hypothalamus–pituitary– adrenal system in male depressed patients and healthy controls. *J Clin Endocrinol Metab.* 1997;82:234-238.
26. Nicolson NA, van Diest R. Salivary cortisol patterns in vital exhaustion. *J Psychosom Res.* 2000;49:335-342.
27. Bjorntorp P. "Portal" adipose tissue as a generator of risk factors for cardiovascular disease and diabetes. *Atherosclerosis.* 1990;10:493-496.
28. Brindley DN, Rolland Y. Possible connections between stress, diabetes, obesity, hypertension and altered lipoprotein metabolism that may result in atherosclerosis. *Clin Sci.* 1989;77:453-461.
29. Sephton S, Sapolsky R, Kraemer H, Spiegel D. Diurnal cortisol rhythm as a predictor of breast cancer survival. *J Natl Cancer Inst.* 2000;92:994-1000.
30. Abercrombie HC, Thurow ME, Rosenkranz MA, Kalin NH, Davidson RJ. Cortisol variation in humans affects memory for emotionally-laden and neutral information. *Behav Neurosci.* 2003;117:505-516.
31. Gunnar MR, Vazquez DM. Low cortisol and flattening of expected daytime rhythm: potential indices of risk in human development. *Dev Psychopathol.* 2001;13(3):515-538.
32. Maggio M, Lauretani F, Ceda GP, et al. Relationship between low levels of anabolic hormones and 6-year mortality in older men: the aging in the Chianti Area (InCHIANTI) study. *Arch Intern Med.* 2007;167:2249-2254.
33. Toussaint O, Michiels C, Raes M, Remacle J. Cellular aging and the importance of energetic factors. *Exp Gerontol.* 1995;30:1-22.
34. Dallman M, Pecoraro N, Akana S, et al. Chronic stress and obesity: a new view of comfort food. *PNAS.* 2003;100:11696-11701.
35. Rebuffe-Scrive M, Walsh U, McEwen B, Rodin J. Effect of chronic stress and exogenous glucocorticoids on regional fat distribution and metabolism. *Physiol Behav.* 1992;52:583-590.
36. Pou KM, Massaro JM, Hoffman U, et al. Visceral and subcutaneous adipose tissue volumes are cross-sectionally related to markers of inflammation and oxidative stress: the Framingham Heart Study. *Circulation.* 2007;116(11):1234-1241.
37. Fries E, Hesse J, Hellhammer J, Hellhammer DH. A new view on hypocortisolism. *Psychoneuroendocrinology.* 2005;30(10):1010-1016.
38. Bower JE, Ganz PA, Aziz N, Olmstead R, Irwin MR, Cole SW. Inflammatory responses to psychological stress in fatigued breast cancer survivors: relationship to glucocorticoids. *Brain Behav Immun.* 2007;21:251-258.
39. Papanicolaou DA, Mullen N, Kyrou I, Nieman LK. Nighttime salivary cortisol: a useful test for the diagnosis of Cushing's syndrome. *J Clin Endocrinol Metab.* 2005;90(10):5730-5736.
40. Arafah BM, Nishiyama FJ, Tlaygeh H, Hejal R. Measurement of salivary cortisol concentration in the assessment of adrenal function in critically ill subjects: a surrogate marker of the circulating free cortisol. *J Clin Endocrinol Metab.* 2007;92(8):2965-2971.
41. Morgentaler A. Testosterone deficiency and cardiovascular mortality. *Asian J Androl.* 2015;17(1):26-13.
42. Laughlin GA, Barrett-Connor E, Bergstrom J. Low serum testosterone and mortality in older men. *J Clin Endocrinol Metab.* 2008;93:68-75.
43. Malkin CJ, Pugh PJ, Morris PD, Asif S, Jones TH, et al. Low serum testosterone and increased mortality in men with coronary heart disease. *Heart.* 2010;96:1821-1825.
44. Maggi M, Schulman C, Quinton R, Langham S, Uhl-Hochgraeber K. The burden of testosterone deficiency syndrome in adult men: economic and quality of life impact. *J Sex Med.* 2007;4(pt 1):1056-1069.
45. Seidell JC, Bjorntorp P, Sjöström L, Kvist H, Sannerstedt R. Visceral fat accumulation in men is positively associated with insulin, glucose and C-peptide levels, but negatively with testosterone levels. *Metabolism.* 1990;39:897-901.
46. Fui MN, Dupuis P, Grossmann M. Lowered testosterone in male obesity: mechanisms, morbidity and management. *Asian J Androl.* 2014;16(2):223-231.

47. Tchernof A, Brochu D, Maltais-Payette I, et al. Androgens and the regulation of adiposity and body fat distributions in humans. *Compr Physiol*. 2018;8(4):1253-1290.

48. Couillard C, Gagnon J, Bergeron J, et al. Contribution of body fatness and adipose tissue distribution to the age variation in plasma steroid hormone concentrations in men: the HERITAGE Family Study. *J Clin Endocrinol Metab*. 2000;85:1026-1031.

49. Snyder PJ, Peachey H, Hannoush P, et al. Effect of testosterone treatment on body composition and muscle strength in men over 65 years of age. *J Clin Endocrinol Metab*. 1999;84:2647-2653.

50. Oskui PM, French WJ, Herring MJ, Mayeda GS, Burstein S, Kloner RA. Testosterone and the cardiovascular system: a comprehensive review of the clinical literature. *J Am Heart Assoc*. 2013;2(6):e000272.

51. Tostain JL, Blnac F. Testosterone deficiency: a common, unrecognized syndrome. *Nat Clin Pract*. 2008;5(7):388-396.

52. Kelleher S, Conway AJ, Handelsman DJ. Blood testosterone threshold for androgen deficiency symptoms. *J Clin Endorinol Metab*. 2004;89:3813-3817.

53. Crawford ED, et al. Diurnal serum testosterone variation in aging men: cross sectional analysis from a large national screening program reveals only a modest decline beginning in the mid-afternoon. *J Urol*. 2006;175:426.

54. The Endocrine Society. Testosterone therapy in adult men with androgen deficiency syndrome. *J Clin Endocr Metab*. 2006;91(6):1995-2010.

55. Zhao D, Guallar E, Ouyang P, et al. Endogenous sex hormones and incident of cardiovascular disease in post-menopausal women. *J Am Coll Cardiol*. 2018;71(22):2555-2556.

56. Torchen LC. Cardiometabolic risk in PCOS: more than a reproductive disorder. *Curr Diab Rep*. 2017;17(12):137.

57. Kakloy NS, Moran LJ, Teede HJ, Joham AE. Cardiometabolic risk in PCOS: a review of the current state of knowledge. *Expert Rev Endocrinol Metab*. 2019;14(1):23-33.

58. Studem LB, Pfeifer M. Cardiometabolic risk in polycystic ovary syndrome. *Endocr Connect*. 2018;7(7):R238-R251.

59. Subramanya V, Zhao D, Ouyang P, et al. Association of endogenous sex hormone levels with coronary artery calcium progression among post-menopausal women in the Multi-Ethnic Study of Atherosclerosis (MESA). *J Cardiovasc Comput Tomog*. 2018;13(1):41-47. [Epub ahead of print].

60. Subramanya V, Zhao D, Ouyang P, et al. Sex hormone levels and change in left ventricular structure among men and post-menopausal women: the multi-ethnic study of atherosclerosis (MESA). *Maturitas*. 2018;108:37-44.

61. Centers for Disease Control (CDC). Available at: www.cdc.gov. Accessed March 2019.

62. McDonald EG, Milligan J, Frenette C, Lee TC. Continuous proton pump inhibitor therapy and the associated risk of recurrent *Clostridium difficile* infection. *JAMA Intern Med*. 2015;175:784-791.

63. de Jager CPC, Wever PC, Gemen EFA, et al. Proton pump inhibitor therapy predisposes to community-acquired *Streptococcus pneumoniae* pneumonia. *Aliment Pharmacol Ther*. 2012;36:941-949.

64. Merli M, Lucidi C, Di Gregorio V, et al. The chronic use of beta-blockers and proton pump inhibitors may affect the rate of bacterial infections in cirrhosis. *Liver Int*. 2015;35:362-369.

65. Amir I, Konikoff FM, Oppenheim M, Gophna U, Half EE. Gastric microbiota is altered in esophagitis and Barrett's esophagitis and further modified by proton pump inhibitors. *Environ Microbiol*. 2014;16(9):2905-2914.

66. Holtorf K. The bioidentical hormone debate: are bioidentical hormones (estradiol, estriol, and progesterone) safer or more efficacious than commonly used synthetic versions in hormone replacement therapy? *Postgrad Med*. 2009;121(7):73-85.

67. Moskowitz D. A comprehensive review of the safety and efficacy of bioidentical hormones for the management of menopause and related health risks. *Altern Med Rev*. 2008;11(3):208-223.

68. Zhang Y, Han P, Wu N, et al. Amelioration of lipid abnormalities by α-lipoic acid through antioxidative and anti-inflammatory effects. *Obesity (Silver Spring)*. 2011;19(8):1647-1653.

69. Padmalayam I, Hasham S, Saxena U, Pillarisetti S. Lipoic acid synthase (LASY): a novel role in inflammation, mitochondrial function, and insulin resistance. *Diabetes*. 2009;58(3):600-608.

70. McIlduff CE, Rutkove SB. Critical appraisal of the use of alpha lipoic acid (thioctic acid) in the treatment of symptomatic diabetic polyneuropathy. *Ther Clin Risk Manag*. 2011;7:377-385.

71. Smith AR, Shenvi SV, Widlansky M, Suh JH, Hagen TM. Lipoic acid as a potential therapy for chronic diseases associated with oxidative stress. *Curr Med Chem*. 2004;11(9):1135-1146.

72. Henriksen EJ. Exercise training and the antioxidant alpha-lipoic acid in the treatment of insulin resistance and type 2 diabetes. *Free Radic Biol Med*. 2006;40(1):3-12.

73. Müller L. Protective effects of DL-alpha-lipoic acid on cadmium-induced deterioration of rat hepatocytes. *Toxicology*. 1989;58(2):175-185.

74. Anuradha B, Varalakshmi P. Protective role of DL-alpha-lipoic acid against mercury-induced neural lipid peroxidation. *Pharmacol Res*. 1999;39(1):67-80.

75. Gurer H, Ozgunes H, Oztezcan S, Ercal N. Antioxidant role of alpha-lipoic acid in lead toxicity. *Free Radic Biol Med*. 1999;27(1-2):75-81.

76. Fernandes NO, Laghisbetty CV, Panda VS, Naik SR. An experimental evaluation of the antidiabetic and antilipidemic properties of a standardized *Momordica charantia* fruit extract. *BMC Complement Altern Med*. 2007:7-29.

77. Day C, Cartwright T. Hypoglycemic effect of *Momordica charantia* extracts. *Planta Med*. 1990;56:426-429.

78. Alam MA, Uddin R, Subhan N, Rahman MM, Jain P, Reza HM. Beneficial role of bitter melon supplementation in obesity and related complications in metabolic syndrome. *J Lipids*. 2015;2015:496169.

79. Baldwa VS, Bhandari CM, Pangaria A, Goyal RK. Clinical trial in patients with diabetes mellitus of an insulin-like compound obtained from plant sources. *Upsala Med Sci*. 1977;82:39-41.

80. Kleefstra N, Houweling ST, Bakker SJ, et al. Effect of chromium supplementation on glucose metabolism and lipids: a systematic review of randomized controlled trials. *Diabetes Care*. 2007;30:2154-2163.

81. Lau F, Bagchi M, Sen C, Bagchi D. Nutrigenomic basis of beneficial effects of chromium (III) on obesity and diabetes. *Mol Cell Biochem*. 2008;317:1-10.

82. Langsjoen PH, Langsjoen AM. Supplemental ubiquinol in patients with advanced congestive heart failure. *Biofactors*. 2008;32(1-4):119-128.

83. Misra HS, Raipurohit YS, Khairnar NP. Pyrroloquinoline-quinone and its versatile roles in biological processes. *J Biosci*. 2012;37(2):313-325.

84. Harris CB, Chowanadisai W, Mishchuk DO, Satre MA, Slupsky CM, Rucker RB. Dietary pyrroloquinoline quinone (PQQ) alters indicators of inflammation and mitochondrial-related metabolism in human subjects. *J Nutr Biochem*. 2013;24(12):2076-2084.

85. Takada M, Sumi M, Maeda A, et al. Pyrroloquinoline quinone, a novel protein tyrosine phosphatase 1B inhibitor, activates insulin signaling in C2C12 myotubes and improves impaired glucose tolerance in diabetic KK-A(y) mice. *Biochem Biophys Res Commun*. 2012;428(2):315-320.

86. Bitsch R, Wolf M, Moller J, et al. Bioavailability assessment of the lipophilic benfotiamine as compared to a water-soluble thiamin derivative. *Ann Nutr Metab*. 1991;35:292-296.

87. Stirban A, Negrean M, Stratmann B, et al. Benfotiamine prevents macro- and microvascular endothelial dysfunction and oxidative stress following a meal rich in advanced glycation end products in individuals with type 2 diabetes. *Diabetes Care*. 2006;29(9):2064-2071.

88. Stirban A, Pop A, Tscheope D. A randomized, double-blind, cross-over, placebo-controlled trial of 6 weeks benfotiamine treatment on postprandial vascular function and variables of autonomic nerve function in Type 2 diabetes. *Diabet Med*. 2013;30(10):1204-1208.

89. Alkhalaf A, Kleefstra N, Groenier KH, et al. Effect of benfotiamine on advanced glycation end products and markers of endothelial dysfunction and inflammation in diabetic nephropathy. *PLoS One*. 2012;7(7):e40427.

90. Hammes HP, Du X, Edelstein D, et al. Benfotiamine blocks three major pathways of hyperglycemic damage and prevents experimental diabetic retinopathy. *Nat Med*. 2003;9:294-299.

91. Bystritsky A, Kerwin L, Feusner JD. A pilot study of *Rhodiola rosea* (Rhodax) for generalized anxiety disorder (GAD). *J Altern Complement Med.* 2008;14(2):175-180.

92. Darbinyan V, Kteyan A, Panossian A, Gabrielian E, Wikman G, Wagner H. Rhodiola rosea in stress induced fatigue–a double blind cross-over study of a standardized extract SHR-5 with a repeated low-dose regimen on the mental performance of healthy physicians during night duty. *Phytomedicine.* 2000;7(5):365-371.

93. Spasov AA, Wikman GK, Mandrikov VB, Mironova IA, Neumoin VV. A double-blind, placebo-controlled pilot study of the stimulating and adaptogenic effect of *Rhodiola rosea* SHR-5 extract on the fatigue of students caused by stress during an examination period with a repeated low-dose regimen. *Phytomedicine.* 2000;7(2):85-89.

94. Olsson EM, von Schéele B, Panossian AG. A randomised, double-blind, placebo-controlled, parallel-group study of the standardised extract shr-5 of the roots of *Rhodiola rosea* in the treatment of subjects with stress-related fatigue. *Planta Med.* February 2009;75(2):105-112. [Epub 2008 November 18.]

95. Fintelmann V, Gruenwald J. Efficacy and tolerability of a *Rhodiola rosea* extract in adults with physical and cognitive deficiencies. *Adv Ther.* 2007;24(4):929-939.

96. Noreen EE, Buckley JG, Lewis SL, et al. The effects of an acute dose of *Rhodiola rosea* on endurance exercise performance. *J Strength Cond Res.* 2013;27(3):839-847.

97. De Bock K, Eijnde BO, Ramaekers M, Hespel P. Acute *Rhodiola rosea* intake can improve endurance exercise performance. *Int J Sport Nutr Exerc Metab.* 2004;14(3):298-307.

98. Maslova LV, Kondrat'ev BI, Maslov LN, Lishmanov IB. The cardio-protective and antiadrenergic activity of an extract of *Rhodiola rosea* in stress. *Eksp Klin Farmakol.* 1994;57:61-63.

99. Lishmanov IB, Naumova AV, Afanas'ev SA, Maslov LN. Contribution of the opioid system to realization of inotropic effects of *Rhodiola rosea* extracts in ischemic and reperfusion heart damage in vitro. *Eksp Klin Farmakol.* 1997;60:34-36.

100. Li HX, Sze SC, Tong Y, Ng TB. Production of Th1- and Th2-dependent cytokines induced by the Chinese medicine herb, *Rhodiola algida*, on human peripheral blood monocytes. *J Ethnopharmacol.* 2009;123(2):257-266.

101. Hung SK, Perry R, Ernst E. The effectiveness and efficacy of Rhodiola rosea L.: a systematic review of randomized clinical trials. *Phytomedicine.* 2011;18(4):235-244.

102. Bhattacharya SK, Muruganandam AV. Adaptogenic activity of Withania somnifera: an experimental study using a rat model of chronic stress. *Pharmacol Biochem Behav.* 2003;75(3):547-555.

103. Singh N, Bhalla M, de Jager P, et al. An overview on ashwagandha: a Rasayana (rejuvenator) of Ayurveda. *Afr J Tradit Complement Altern Med.* 2011;8(5 suppl):208-213.

104. Chandrasekhar K, Kapoor J, Anishetty S. A prospective, randomized double-blind, placebo-controlled study of safety and efficacy of a high-concentration full-spectrum extract of ashwagandha root in reducing stress and anxiety in adults. *Indian J Psychol Med.* 2012;34(3):255-262.

105. Mishra LC, Singh BB, Dagenais S. Scientific basis for the therapeutic use of Withania somnifera (ashwagandha): a review. *Altern Med Rev.* 2000;5:334-346.

106. Singh B, Saxena AK, Chandan BK, et al. Adaptogenic activity of a novel, withanolide-free aqueous fraction from the roots of *Withania somnifera* Dun. *Phytother Res.* 2001;15(4):311-318.

107. Ahmad MK, Mahdi AA, Shukla KK, et al. *Withania somnifera* improves semen quality by regulating reproductive hormone levels and oxidative stress in seminal plasma of infertile males. *Fertil Steril.* 2010;94(3):989-996.

108. Biswal BM, Sulaiman SA, Ismail HC, et al. Effect of *Withania somnifera* (Ashwagandha) on the development of chemotherapy-induced fatigue and quality of life in breast cancer patients. *Integr Cancer Ther.* 2013;12(4):312-322.

109. Sandhu JS, Shah B, Shenoy S, et al. Effects of *Withania somnifera* (Ashwagandha) and *Terminalia arjuna* (Arjuna) on physical performance and cardiorespiratory endurance in healthy young adults. *Int J Ayurveda Res.* 2010;1(3):144-149.

110. Panda S, Kar A. Changes in thyroid hormone concentrations after administration of ashwagandha root extract to adult male mice. *J Pharm Pharmacol.* 1998;50(9):1065-1068.

111. Van der Hooft CS, Hoekstra A, Winter A, et al. *Ned Tijdschr Geneeskd.* 2005;149(47):2637-2638.

112. Bhat R, Karim AA. Tongkat Ali (Eurycoma longifolia Jack): a review on its ethnobotany and pharmacological importance. *Fitoterapia.* 2010;81(7):669-679.

113. Ismail SB, Wan Mohammad WM, George A, et al. Randomized clinical trial on the use of physta freeze-dried water extract of *Eurycoma longifolia* for the improvement of quality of life and sexual well-being in men. *Evid Based Complement Alternat Med.* 2012;2012:429268.

114. Henkel RR, Wang R, Bassett SH, et al. Tongkat Ali as a potential herbal supplement for physically active male and female seniors - a pilot study. *Phytother Res.* 2013;28(4):544-550. [Epub ahead of print].

115. Tambi MI, Imran ML, Henkel RR. Standardised water-soluble extract of *Eurycoma longifolia*, Tongkat ali, as testosterone booster for managing men with late-onset hypogonadism? *Andrologia.* 2012;44(suppl 1):226-230.

116. Talbott SM, Talbott JA, George A, et al. Effect of Tongkat Ali on stress hormones and psychological mood state in moderately stressed subjects. *J Int Soc Sports Nutr.* 2013;10(1):28.

117. Carcalliun L, Bianco C, Alonso-Bouzon C, et al. Sex differences in the association between serum levels of testosterone and frailty in an elderly population: the Toledo Study for Healthy Aging. *PLoS One.* 2012;7(3):e32401.

118. Morley JE. Andropause, testosterone therapy and quality of life in aging men. *Cleve Clin J Med.* 2000;67(12):880-882.

119. Temkithawon P, Hinds TR, Beavo JA, et al. Kaempferia parviflora, a plant used in traditional medicine to enhance sexual performance contains large amounts of low affinity PDE5 inhibitors. *J Ethnopharmacol.* 2011;137(3):1437-1441.

120. Nakata A, Koike Y, Matsui H, et al. Potent SIRT1 enzyme-stimulating and anti-glycation activities of polumethoxyflavonoids from *Kaemperfia parviflora.* Nat Prod Kcommun. 2014;9(9):1291-1294.

121. Promthep K, Eungpinichpong W, Sripanidkulchai B, et al. Effect of Kaempferia parviflora extract on physical fitness of soccer players: a randomized double-blind placebo-controlled trial. *Med Sci Monit Basic Res.* 2015;21:100-108.

122. Matsushita M, Yoneshiro T, Aita S, et al. Kaempferia parviflora extract increases whole-body energy expenditure in humans: roles of brown adipose tissue. *J Nutr Sci Vitaminol (Tokyo).* 2015;61(1):79-83.

123. Yoo JY, Kim SS. Probiotics and prebiotics: present status and future perspectives on metabolic disorders. *Nutrients.* 2018;8(3):173.

124. Sewerynek E. Melatonin and the cardiovascular system. *Neuro Endocrinol Lett.* 2002;23(suppl 1):79-83.

125. Picinato MC, Haber EP, Carpinelli AR, et al. Daily rhythm of glucose-induced secretion by isolated islets from the intact and pinealectomized rat. *J Pineal Res.* 2002;33(3):172-177.

126. NHANES I Data (Findings Reported at the Annual Scientific Meeting of North American Society for the Study of Obesity November 2004.).

127. Spiegel K, Tasali E, Penev P, Van Cauter E. Brief communication: sleep curtailment in healthy young men is associated with decreased leptin levels, elevated ghrelin levels, and increased hunger and appetite. *Ann Intern Med.* 2004;141(11):846-850.

128. Kunz D, Mahlberg R, Müller C, Tilmann A, Bes F. Melatonin in patients with reduced REM sleep duration: two randomized controlled trials. *J Clin Endocrinol Metab.* 2004;89(1):128-134.

129. Rajaratnam SM, Middleton B, Stone BM, Arendt J, Dijk D-J. Melatonin advances the circadian timing of EEG sleep and directly facilitates sleep without altering its duration in extended sleep opportunities in humans. *J Physiol.* 2004;561(pt 1):339-351.

130. Reid K, Frank OR, Stocks NP. Aged garlic extract lowers blood pressure in patients with treated but uncontrolled hypertension: a randomised controlled trial. *Maturitas.* 2010;67(2):144-150.

131. Elosta A, Slevin M, Rahman K, Ahmed N. Aged garlic has more potent antiglycation and antioxidant properties compared to fresh garlic extract in vitro. *Sci Rep.* 2017;7:39613.

132. Ried K, Travica N, Sali A. The effect of kyolic aged garlic on gut microbiota, inflammation and cardiovascular markers in hypertensives: the GarGIC Trial. *Front Nutr.* 2018;5:122.

133. Holick MF. Vitamin D deficiency. *N Engl J Med.* 2007;357:266-281.

134. Yang T, Santisteban MM, Rodriguez V, et al. GUT dysbiosis is linked to hypertension. *Hypertension.* 2015;65(6):1331-1340.

135. Steiner M, Li W. Aged garlic extract, a modulator of cardiovascular risk factors: a dose finding study on the effects of AGE on platelet functions. *J Nutr.* 2001;131:980S-4S.

136. Allison GL, Lowe GM, Rahman K. Aged garlic extract may inhibit aggregation in human platelets by suppressing calcium mobilization. *J Nutr.* 2006;136(3 suppl):789S-792S.

137. Budoff M. Aged garlic extract retards progression of coronary artery calcification. *J Nutr.* 2006;136(3 suppl):741S-744S.

138. Xu C, Mathews AE, Rodrigues C, et al. Aged garlic extract supplementation modifies inflammation and immunity of adults with obesity: a randomized double blind placebo controlled clinical trial. *Clin Nutr.* 2018;24:148-155.

139. Weiss N, Ide N, Abahji T, et al. Aged garlic extract improves homocysteine-induced endothelial dysfunction in macro and micro-circulation. *J Nutr.* 2006;136(3 suppl):750S-754S.

140. Milner JA. Preclinical perspectives on garlic and cancer. *J Nutr.* 2006;136(3 suppl):827S-831S.

141. Lau BH. Suppression of LDL oxidation by garlic. *J Nutr.* 2001;131:985S-8S.

142. Morihara N, Hayama M, Full H. Aged garlic extract scavenges super-oxide radicals. *Plant Foods Hum Nutr.* 2011;66(1):17-21.

143. Ahmad MS, Ahmed N. Antiglycation properties of aged garlic extract: possible role in prevention of diabetic complications. *J Nutr.* 2006;136(3 suppl):796S-799S.

144. Ishikawa H, Saeki T, Otani T, et al. Aged garlic extract prevents a decline of NK cell number and activity in patients with advanced cancer. *J Nutr.* 2006;138(3 suppl):816S-820S.

145. Percival SS. Aged garlic extract modifies human immunity. *J Nutr.* 2016;146(2):4335-4365.

146. Morihara N, Ushijima M, Kashimoto N. Aged garlic extract ameliorates physical fatigue. *Biol Pharm Bull.* 2006;29(5):962-966.

147. Zhang L, Gail MH, Wang YQ, et al. A randomized factorial study of the effects of long-term garlic and micronutrient supplementation and of 2 wk antibiotic treatment for *Helicobacter pylori* infection on serum cholesterol and lipoproteins. *Am J Clin Nutr.* 2006;84(4):912-919.

148. Mathew B, Biju R. Neuroprotective effects of garlic a review. *Libyan J Med.* 2008;3(1):23-33.

149. Kamikawa T, Kobayashi A, Yamashita T, Hayashi H, Yamazaki N. Effects of coenzyme Q10 on exercise tolerance in chronic stable angina pectoris. *Am J Cardiol.* 1985;56:247-251.

150. Vidyashankar S, Nandakumar KS, Patki PS. Alcohol depletes coenzyme-Q10 associated with increased TNF-alpha secretion to induce cytotoxicity in HepG2 cells. *Toxicology.* 2012;302(1):34-39.

151. Zozina VI, Covantev S, Goroshko OA, Krasnykh LM, Kukes VG. Coenzyme Q10 in cardiovascular and metabolic disease current state of the problem. *Curr Cardiol Rev.* 2018;14(3):164-174.

152. Linnane AW, Kopsidas G, Zhang C, et al. Cellular redox activity of coenzyme Q10 effect of CoQ10 supplementation on human skeletal muscle. *Free Radic Res.* 2002;36(4):445-453.

153. Moreira PL, Santos MS, Sena C, Nunes E, Seiça R, Oliveira CR. CoQ10 therapy attenuates amyloid beta-peptide toxicity in brain mitochondria isolated from aged diabetic rats. *Exp Neurol.* 2005;196(1):112-119.

154. Digiesi V, Cantini F, Oradei A, et al. Coenzyme Q10 in essential hypertension. *Mol Aspects Med.* 1994;15 suppl:s257-63.

155. Langsjoen P, Langsjoen P, Willis R, Folkers K. Treatment of essential hypertension with CoQ10. *Mol Aspects Med.* 1994;15 suppl:265-272.

156. Lamperti C, Nani AB, Lucchini V, et al. Muscle coenzyme Q10 level in statin related myopathy. *Arch Neurol.* 2005;62(11):1709-1712.

157. Spigset O. Reduced effect of warfarin caused by ubidecarenone. *Lancet.* 1994;344(8933):1372-1373.

158. Landbo C, Almdal TP. Interaction between warfarin and coenzyme Q10. *Ugeskr Laeger.* 1998;160(22):3226-3227.

159. Alon I, Gorelik O, Berman S, et al. Intracellular magnesium in elderly patients with heart failure: effects of diabetes and renal dysfunction. *J Trace Elem Med Biol.* 2006;20(4):221-226.

160. Gao XR, Wang MD, He XY, et al. Decreased intralympho-cytic magnesium content is associated with diastolic heart dysfunction in patients with essential hypertension. *Int J Cardiol.* 2011;147(2):331-334.

161. Alaimo K, McDowell MA, Briefel RR, et al. Dietary intake of vitamins, minerals and fiber of persons age 2 months and over in the United States: Third National Health and Nutrition Examination Survey, phase 1, 1988-91. *Adv Data Vital Health Stat.* 1994;258:1-26.

162. Chakraborti S, Chakraborti T, Mandal M, et al. Protective role of magnesium in cardiovascular disease: a review. *Mol Cell Biochem.* 2002;238(1-2):163-179.

163. Tejero-Taldo MI, Kramer JH, Mak Iu T, et al. The nerve-heart connection in the pro-oxidant response to Mg-deficiency. *Heart Fail Rev.* 2006;11(1):35-44.

164. Joosten MM, Gansevoort RT, Mukamai KJ, et al. Urinary and plasma magnesium and risk of ischemic heart disease. *Am J Clin Nutr.* 2013;97(6):1299-1306. [Epub ahead of print].

165. Del Gobbo LC, Song Y, Poirier P, et al. Low serum magnesium concentrations are associated with a high prevalence of premature ventricular complexes in obese adults with type 2 diabetes. *Cardiovasc Diabetol.* 2012;11:23.

166. Zhang W, Iso H, Ohira T, et al. Associations of dietary magnesium intake with mortality from cardiovascular disease: the JACC study. *Atherosclerosis.* 2012;221(2):587-595.

167. Atsmon J, Dolev E. Drug-induced hypomagnesaemia. *Drug Saf.* 2005;28(9):763-788.

168. Pak CY. Correction of thiazide-induced hypomagnesemia by potassium-magnesium citrate from review of prior trials. *Clin Nephrol* 2000;54:271-275.

169. Odvina CV, Mason RP, Pak CY. Prevention of thiazide-induced hypokalemia without magnesium depletion by potassium-magnesium-citrate. *Am J Ther.* 2006;13(2):101-108.

170. Palmer BF, Naderi AS. Metabolic consequences associated with thiazide diuretics. *J Am Soc Hypertens.* 2007;1(6):381-392.

171. Kass L, Weekes J, Carpenter L. Effect of magnesium supplementation on blood pressure: a meta-analysis. *Eur J Clin Nutr.* 2012;66(4):411-418.

172. Dorman BH, Sade RM, Burnette JS, et al. Magnesium supplementation in the prevention of arrhythmias in pediatric patients undergoing surgery for congenital heart defects. *Am Heart J.* 2000;139(3):522-528.

173. Shechter M, Sharir M, Labrador MJ, et al. Oral magnesium therapy improves endothelial function in patients with coronary artery disease. *Circulation.* 2000;102(7):2353-2358.

174. Pokan R, Hofmann P, von Duvillard SP, et al. Oral magnesium therapy, exercise heart rate, exercise tolerance and myocardial function in coronary artery disease patients. *Br J Sports Med.* 2006;40(9):773-778.

175. Bralley JA, Lord RS. *Laboratory Evaluations in Molecular Medicine.* Norcross, GA: The Institute for Advances in Molecular Medicine; 2001.

176. Nair RR, Nair P. Alteration of myocardial mechanics in marginal magnesium deficiency. *Magnes Res.* 2002;15(3-4):287-306 (ISSN:0953-1424). King DE, Mainous AG III, Geesey ME, Woolson RF. Dietary magnesium and C-reactive protein levels. *J Am Coll Nutr.* 2005;24:166-171.

177. Chaudhar DP, Boparai RK, Sharma R, et al. Studies on the development of an insulin resistant rat model by chronic feeding of low magnesium high sucrose diet. *Magnes Res.* 2004;17(4):293-300.

178. Shafi T, Appel LJ, Miller ER III, et al. Changes in serum potassium mediate thiazide-induced diabetes. *Hypertension.* 2008;52(6):1022-1029.

179. Nadler JL, Buchanan T, Natarajan R, Antonipillai I, Bergman R, Rude R. Magnesium deficiency produces insulin resistance and increased thromboxane synthesis. *Hypertension.* 1993;21:1024-1029.

180. Kochar J, Michael Gaziano J, Djoussé L. Dietary factors and the risk of coronary heart disease. *Aging Dis.* 2011;2(2):149-157.

181. Choi EY, Allen K, McDonnough M, et al. A plant-based diet and heart failure: case report and literature review. *J Geriatr Cardiol.* 2017;14(5):375-378.

182. Rautiainen S, Levitan EB, Mittleman MA, et al. Fruit and vegetable intake and rate of heart failure: a population-based prospective cohort of women. *Eur J Heart Fail.* 2015;17:20-26.

183. Djoussé L, Driver JA, Gaziano JM. Relation between modifiable lifestyle factors and lifetime risk of heart failure. *JAMA.* 2009;302:394-400.

184. Yokoyama Y, Nishimura K, Barnard ND, et al. Vegetarian diets and blood pressure: a meta-analysis. *JAMA Intern Med.* 2014;174:577-587.

185. Ingelsson E, Arnlöv J, Sundström J, et al. Novel metabolic risk factors for heart failure. *J Am Coll Cardiol.* 2005;46:2054-2060.

186. Esselstyn CB, Ellis SG, Medendorp SV, et al. A strategy to arrest and reverse coronary artery disease: a 5-year longitudinal study of a single physician's practice. *J Fam Pract.* 1995;41:560-568.

187. Massera D, Zaman T, Farren GE, et al. A whole-food plant-based diet reversed angina without medications or procedures. *Case Rep Cardiol.* 2015;2015:978906.

188. Witztum JL. The oxidation hypothesis of atherosclerosis. *Lancet.* 1994;344:793-795.

189. Münzel T, Gori T, Keaney JF, et al. Pathophysiological role of oxidative stress in systolic and diastolic heart failure and its therapeutic implications. *Eur Heart J.* 2015;36:2555-2564.

190. Holt EM, Steffen LM, Moran A, et al. Fruit and vegetable consumption and its relation to markers of inflammation and oxidative stress in adolescents. *J Am Diet Assoc.* 2009;109:414-421.

191. Uribarri J, Woodruff S, Goodman S, et al. Advanced glycation end products in foods and a practical guide to their reduction in the diet. *J Am Diet Assoc* 2010;110:911-916.e12.

192. de Souza Pinto R, Castilho G, Paim BA, et al. Inhibition of macrophage oxidative stress prevents the reduction of ABCA-1 transporter induced by advanced glycated albumin. *Lipids.* 2012;47:443-450.

193. Rohatgi A, Khera A, Berry JD, et al. HDL cholesterol efflux capacity and incident cardiovascular events. *N Engl J Med.* 2014;371:2383-2393.

194. Watzl B. Anti-inflammatory effects of plant-based foods and of their constituents. *Int J Vitam Nutr Res.* 2008;78:293-298.

195. Kardys I, Knetsch AM, Bleumink GS, et al. C-reactive protein and risk of heart failure. The Rotterdam Study. *Am Heart J.* 2006;152:514-520.

196. Koeth RA, Wang Z, Levison BS, et al. Intestinal microbiota metabolism of L-carnitine, a nutrient in red meat, promotes atherosclerosis. *Nat Med.* 2013;19:576-585.

197. Li XS, Obeid S, Klingenberg R, et al. Gut microbiota-dependent trimethylamine N-oxide in acute coronary syndromes: a prognostic marker for incident cardiovascular events beyond traditional risk factors. *Eur Heart J.* 2017;38:814-824.

198. Tang WHW, Wang Z, Fan Y, et al. Prognostic value of elevated levels of intestinal microbe-generated metabolite trimethylamine-N-oxide in patients with heart failure: refining the gut hypothesis. *J Am Coll Cardiol.* 2014;64:1908-1914.

199. Wang WHW, Hazen SL. The contributory role of gut microbiota in cardiovascular disease. *J Clin Invest.* 2014;124:4204-4211.

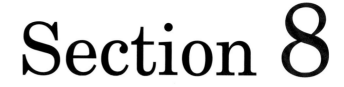

Section 8

Additional Topics

38

Consequences of Cardiovascular Drug-Induced Nutrient Depletion

James B. LaValle, RPh, DHM, MS, CCN, ND (trad)

Introduction

A challenge facing health care professionals today is the problem of drug-induced diseases, including drug-induced nutrient depletion (DIND) and drug-induced microbiome disruption (DIMD).

DIND and DIMD in patients, including the cardiovascular patient, are very important issues for the 21st-century clinician to embrace and implement corrective measures into practice—which can be as simple as a multiple vitamin/mineral supplement. This chapter will focus on DIND.

Background

With over 48% of people in the United States taking prescription medications (up from 44% the previous decade), patients with cardiovascular disease are placed a much higher risk for developing comorbid conditions and for increasing disease pathologies.[1] Polypharmacy prescribing is now occurring in younger and younger populations, so it is becoming increasingly important to assess nutrient depletion risks as they relate to increased drug side effects, future symptoms, comorbid health condition development, or progression of the underlying disease itself.

In the medical management of individuals with cardiovascular disease or comorbid conditions, several classes of prescription drugs may be employed with the potential for depletions of nutrients could induce metabolic changes and further the progression of any component of the underlying cardiovascular problems or comorbidities. Commonly used medications utilized in management of a patient with cardiovascular disease include:

- Diuretics
- ACE inhibitors (angiotensin-converting enzyme inhibitors)
- ARBs (angiotensin II receptor blockers)
- Beta-blockers
- Calcium channel blockers
- Hypocholesterolemic agents
- Antidiabetic medications
- Anticoagulant/antiplatelet agents
- Nitrates
- Digitalis
- Pain medications, including opiates, acetaminophen and nonsteroidal anti-inflammatory drugs (NSAIDs)
- Acid-reducing drugs including H2 blockers and proton-pump inhibitors (PPIs)
- Anti-anxiety/sleep medications

It is of scientific interest and clinical concern that the reported side effects of some of these commonly used medications in patients are actually manifestations of drug-nutrient depletion of these same medications. Drugs can inhibit nutrient absorption, synthesis, transport, storage, metabolism, or excretion of essential nutrients.

Table 38.1 lists some of the most commonly used medications in the cardiovascular patient, their potential short- and long-term side effects, potential nutrient depletions associated with these drugs, and some of the clinical effects often reported with the loss of one of these essential nutrients.

As an example, according to statistics, over 22 million patients in the United States take beta-blockers.[1] Beta-blockers have been reported to reduce the production of melatonin via specific inhibition of beta-1 adrenergic receptors.[2,3] Clinically, low levels of melatonin can lead to sleep disturbances, insulin resistance/impaired glucose tolerance, cardiovascular problems, increased cardiovascular events, immune imbalances, and increased oxidative stress and inflammation on various body systems.[4–6]

Several placebo-controlled studies have investigated the relationship between beta-blocker–induced central nervous system (CNS) side effects and the nightly urinary excretion of melatonin via the inhibition of the release of the enzyme

Table 38.1

DRUGS COMMONLY USED IN THE CARDIOVASCULAR PATIENTS THAT HAVE REPORTED NUTRIENT DEPLETIONS

Drug	Reported Potential Drug Side Effects (Short and Long Term)	Reported Potential Nutrient Depletion	Reported Potential Health Consequence(s) of Nutrient Depletion
Cardiac glycosides[96,97] Digoxin (Lanoxin, Lanoxicap)	*Potential Drug Side Effects (General)* *Short term* Nausea/vomiting Diarrhea Fatigue Dry mouth Dizziness Visual disturbances Headache Low pulse rate *Long term* Rash Depression Irregular heartbeat (arrhythmia) Cardiovascular problems Gynecomastia (enlarging of breast in males) Increased bone fractures Increased risk for osteoporosis	Calcium Magnesium Phosphorus Vitamin B$_1$ (thiamine)	Osteoporosis, heart and blood pressure problems, back or leg pain, nervousness, tooth decay Muscle cramps, weakness, fatigue, insomnia, restless leg syndrome, irritability, anxiety, insulin resistance, depression, high blood pressure, cardiovascular problems, Headaches Decreases calcium absorption, osteoporosis, brittle bones Depression, irritability, memory loss/confusion, indigestion, weight loss/anorexia, swelling, muscle weakness, irregular heartbeat, fatigue, numbness and tingling
Beta-blockers[97] Propranolol (Inderal), Inderal LA Metoprolol (Lopressor, Toprol, Toprol XL) Atenolol (Tenormin) Pindolol (Viskin) Bisoprolol (Monocor, Visken—w/HCTZ) Carvedilol (Coreg) Esmolol (Brevibloc) Labetalol (Normodyne) Nadolol (Corgard) Sotalol (Betapace) Timolol (Blocadren) Nebivolol (Bystolic)	*Short term* Nausea/vomiting Diarrhea Fatigue Dry mouth Dizziness Visual disturbances Headache Sexual side effects Dyspnea Insomnia Nightmares Arrhythmia *Long term* Depression Sexual side effects Decreased HDL Fatigue Blood glucose imbalances Increased risk of type 2 diabetes Increased risk of myocardial infarction/stroke	Coenzyme Q10 (CoQ10) Melatonin Testosterone	Hypertension Congestive heart failure Muscular fatigue, weakness Joint and muscle aches Rhabdomyolysis Decreased cognitive function/memory loss Gingivitis Arrhythmia Imbalanced immunity Insulin resistance/impaired glucose tolerance Sleep disturbances; insulin resistance/impaired glucose tolerance, cardiovascular problems imbalanced immune system; increased cancer risk, increased oxidative stress in the brain, decreased seizure threshold Loss of Libido, insulin signaling problems, type 2 diabetes, sleep disturbances, thyroid imbalances, loss of muscle mass, joint/muscle aches, increased cardiovascular problems, mood imbalances, memory and cognitive decline, weight gain, increased incidence of osteoporosis

Drug	Potential Drug Side Effects (Diuretics in General)	Nutrient	Symptoms
Thiazide diuretics[97] Hydrochlorothiazide (HCTZ, HydroDiuril) Methyclothiazide (Enduron) Indapamide (Lozol) Metolazone (Zaroxolyn)	*Short term* Nervousness/anxiousness Fatigue Increased urinary voiding Diarrhea Dizziness Loss of appetite Nausea/vomiting Headache Dry mouth and mucous membranes Constipation	Coenzyme Q10 (CoQ10)	High blood pressure Congestive heart failure Muscular/Joint fatigue/weakness Rhabdomyolysis Memory loss Gingivitis Irregular heartbeat Decreased immunity Insulin resistance
		Magnesium	Muscle cramps Weakness Fatigue Insomnia Restless leg syndrome Irritability Anxiety Insulin resistance depression High blood pressure Cardiovascular problems Headaches
	Long term Arrhythmia Breathing difficulty Numbness/tingling in extremities Confusion Nervousness Fatigue Muscle cramps Mood changes Blurred vision Poor wound healing Lowered immunity Increased risk of osteoporosis Cardiovascular problems Increased risk of birth defects	Phosphorus	Decreases calcium absorption, osteoporosis, brittle bones
		Potassium	Arrhythmia, poor reflexes, muscle weakness, fatigue, thirst, confusion, constipation, dizziness, nervousness
		Sodium	Muscle weakness, poor concentration, memory loss, dehydration, loss of appetite
		Zinc	Decreased immunity, decreased wound healing, smell and taste disturbances, anorexia, depression, night blindness, hair, skin and nail problems, menstrual irregularities, joint pain, nystagmus (involuntary eye movements), insulin resistance
Loop diuretics[97] Bumetanide (Bumex) Ethacrynic acid (Edecrin) Furosemide (Lasix)		Calcium	Osteoporosis, heart and blood pressure problems, back or leg pain, nervousness, tooth decay
		Magnesium	Muscle cramps, weakness, fatigue, insomnia, restless leg syndrome, irritability, anxiety, insulin resistance, depression, high blood pressure, cardiovascular problems, headaches
		Potassium	Irregular heartbeat, poor reflexes, muscle weakness, fatigue, thirst, confusion, constipation, dizziness, nervousness
		Sodium	Muscle weakness, poor concentration, memory loss, dehydration, loss of appetite

(Continued)

Table 38.1

DRUGS COMMONLY USED IN THE CARDIOVASCULAR PATIENTS THAT HAVE REPORTED NUTRIENT DEPLETIONS—CONT'D

Drug	Reported Potential Drug Side Effects (Short and Long Term)	Reported Potential Nutrient Depletion	Reported Potential Health Consequence(s) of Nutrient Depletion
		Vitamin B1 (thiamine)	Depression, irritability, memory loss/confusion, indigestion, weight loss/anorexia, swelling, muscle weakness, irregular heartbeat, fatigue, numbness and tingling
		Vitamin B6 (pyridoxine)	Depression, sleep disturbances, nerve inflammation, PMS, lethargy, decreased alertness, anemia, altered mobility, elevated homocysteine, nausea, vomiting, and seborrheic dermatitis
		Vitamin C	Loss of antioxidant potential, increased capillary fragility, muscle weakness, poor wound healing, bleeding gums, anemia, poor appetite, tender and swollen joints
		Zinc	Decreased immunity, decreased wound healing, smell and taste disturbances, anorexia, depression, night blindness, hair, skin and nail problems, menstrual irregularities, joint pain, nystagmus (involuntary eye movements), insulin resistance
Potassium-sparing diuretics[97] Triamterene (Dyrenium) Triamterene and HCTZ (Dyazide, Maxzide) Spironolactone (Aldactone)	*Potential Drug Side Effects (Diuretics in General)* *Short term* Nervousness/anxiousness Fatigue Increased urinary voiding Diarrhea Dizziness Loss of appetite Nausea/vomiting Headache Dry mouth and mucous membranes Constipation *Long term* Arrhythmia Breathing difficulty Numbness/tingling in extremities Confusion Nervousness Fatigue Muscle cramps Mood changes Blurred vision Poor wound healing Lowered immunity Increased risk of osteoporosis Cardiovascular problems Increased risk of birth defects	Calcium	Osteoporosis, heart and blood pressure problems, back or leg pain, nervousness, tooth decay
		Folic acid	Birth defects, cervical dysplasia, anemia, heart disease, elevated homocysteine, headaches, fatigue, insomnia, diarrhea, nausea, increased cancer risk, decreased methylation
		Zinc	Decreased immunity, decreased wound healing, smell and taste disturbances, anorexia, depression, night blindness, hair, skin and nail problems, menstrual irregularities, joint pain, nystagmus (involuntary eye movements), insulin resistance

Drug	Potential Drug Side Effects	Nutrient Depleted	Consequences of Depletion
Miscellaneous diuretics[97] Chlorthalidone (Hygroton, Thalitone)	*Short term* Nervousness/anxiousness Fatigue Increased urinary voiding Diarrhea Dizziness Loss of appetite Nausea/vomiting Headache Dry mouth and mucous membranes Constipation *Long term* Arrhythmia Breathing difficulty Numbness/tingling in extremities Confusion Nervousness Fatigue Muscle cramps Mood changes Blurred vision Poor wound healing Lowered immunity Increased risk of osteoporosis Cardiovascular problems Increased risk of birth defects	Magnesium Phosphorus Potassium Sodium Zinc	Muscle cramps, weakness, fatigue, insomnia, restless leg syndrome, irritability, anxiety, insulin resistance, depression, high blood pressure, cardiovascular problems, headaches Decreases calcium absorption, osteoporosis, brittle bones Arrhythmia, poor reflexes, muscle weakness, fatigue, thirst, confusion, constipation, dizziness, nervousness Muscle weakness, poor concentration, memory loss, dehydration, loss of appetite Decreased immunity, decreased wound healing, smell and taste disturbances, anorexia, depression, night blindness, hair, skin and nail problems, menstrual irregularities, joint pain, nystagmus, insulin resistance
ACE inhibitors (angiotensin-converting enzyme inhibitors)[97] Captopril (Capoten) Enalapril (Vasotec) Lisinopril (Zestril, Prinivil) Ramipril (Altace)	*Short term* Facial flushing Nausea/vomiting Headache Cough Insomnia Nasal congestion Sexual dysfunction *Long term* Edema Hypotension Kidney problems Increased potassium levels, which can lead to arrhythmias Immune imbalances	Zinc Sodium	Decreased immunity, decreased wound healing, smell and taste disturbances, anorexia, depression, night blindness, hair, skin and nail problems, menstrual irregularities, joint pain, nystagmus (involuntary eye movements), insulin resistance Muscle weakness, poor concentration, memory loss, dehydration, loss of appetite

(Continued)

Table 38.1

DRUGS COMMONLY USED IN THE CARDIOVASCULAR PATIENTS THAT HAVE REPORTED NUTRIENT DEPLETIONS—CONT'D

Drug	Reported Potential Drug Side Effects (Short and Long Term)	Reported Potential Nutrient Depletion	Reported Potential Health Consequence(s) of Nutrient Depletion
ARBs (angiotensin II receptor antagonists)[97] Losartan (Cozaar) Valsartan (Diovan) Telmisartan (Micardis) Irbesartan (Avapro) Azilsartan (Edarbi) Olmesartan (Benicar)	*Potential Drug Side Effects (in General)* *Short term* Facial flushing Nausea/vomiting Headache Cough Insomnia Nasal congestion Sexual dysfunction *Long term* Swelling (edema) Low blood pressure (hypotension) Kidney problems Increased potassium levels, which can lead to irregular heartbeat (arrhythmias) Immune imbalances	Zinc	Decreased immunity, decreased wound healing, small and taste disturbances, anorexia, depression, night blindness, hair, skin and nail problems, menstrual irregularities, joint pain, nystagmus (involuntary eye movements), insulin resistance
Centrally acting antihypertensive drugs[97] Clonidine (Catapres) Methyldopa (Aldomet)	*Potential Drug Side Effects (General)* *Short term* Nausea/vomiting Drowsiness Sedation Fatigue Dry mouth Sexual side effects Nasal congestion *Long term* Fever Blood sugar regulation problems Cardiovascular problems Psychotic reactions Depression Liver damage Anemia	Coenzyme Q10 (CoQ10)	Hypertension, congestive heart failure, muscular fatigue, joint and muscle aches, rhabdomyolysis, memory loss, gingivitis, muscle weakness, arrhythmia, imbalanced immunity, insulin resistance

HMG-CoA reductase inhibitors[97]	Potential Drug Side Effects (General)		
Atorvastatin (Lipitor) Lovastatin (Mevacor, Altocor) Fluvastatin (Lescol) Pravastatin (Pravachol) Simvastatin (Zocor)	*Short term* Nausea/vomiting Diarrhea Gas/bloating Blurred vision Constipation Heartburn Headache Dizziness *Long term* Elevated liver enzymes Muscle pain/weakness Memory loss Kidney failure	Coenzyme Q10 (CoQ10)	High blood pressure, congestive heart failure, fatigue, gingivitis, muscle weakness, irregular heartbeat, decreased immunity
		Vitamin E	Dry skin, dry hair, anemia, easy bruising, PMS, eczema, dermatitis, psoriasis, muscle weakness, decreased antioxidant capacity, poor wound healing/impaired immunity
		Vitamin D	Osteoporosis, increased risk of skeletal fractures, hearing difficulties, depression, hormonal imbalances, muscular weakness, hypertension, autoimmune diseases, multiple sclerosis, diabetes, schizophrenia and decrease immunity
		Carnitine	Elevated blood lipids, abnormal liver function, muscle weakness, fatigue, blood sugar imbalances, increased risk of cardiovascular disease
		Omega-3 fatty acids	Neurochemical imbalances, skin disorders, chronic inflammation, heart and blood vessel disorders, immune imbalances, autoimmune conditions, memory and cognitive impairment, joint and muscle pain, insulin resistance and increased risk of type 2 diabetes, increased risk of cancer
		Zinc	Decreased immunity, decreased wound healing, smell and taste disturbances, anorexia, depression, night blindness, hair, skin and nail problems, menstrual irregularities, joint pain, nystagmus (involuntary eye movements), insulin resistance
		Selenium	Decreased antioxidant protection, muscle aches, decreased immunity, red blood cell fragility, fatigue, anemia, and decreased conversion of T4 to T3
		Copper	Hair color loss, anemia, fatigue, low body temperature, cardiovascular problems, nervous system disorders, decreased immunity
		Testosterone	Increased mortality in men with CHD Insomnia Insulin resistance/Impaired glucose tolerance Obesity Type 2 diabetes Thyroid hormone imbalances Alzheimer disease Osteoporosis/decreased bone mineral density Immune imbalances

(Continued)

Table 38.1

DRUGS COMMONLY USED IN THE CARDIOVASCULAR PATIENTS THAT HAVE REPORTED NUTRIENT DEPLETIONS—CONT'D

Drug	Reported Potential Drug Side Effects (Short and Long Term)	Reported Potential Nutrient Depletion	Reported Potential Health Consequence(s) of Nutrient Depletion
Bile acid sequestrants[97] Cholestyramine (Questran)	***Potential Drug Side Effects (General)*** *Short term* Nausea/vomiting Diarrhea Gas/bloating Blurred vision Constipation Heartburn Headache Dizziness Loss of appetite Anxiety/nervousness *Long term* Elevated liver enzymes Muscle pain/weakness Memory loss Kidney failure Increased risk of osteoporosis Increased risk of bleeding Increased risk of night blindness Increased tooth decay	Beta-carotene (vitamin A)	Decreased immunity, night blindness, dry skin, brittle nails
		Calcium	Osteoporosis, heart and blood pressure problems, back or leg pain, nervousness, tooth decay
		Folic acid	Birth defects, cervical dysplasia, anemia, heart disease, elevated homocysteine, headaches, fatigue, insomnia, diarrhea, nausea, increased cancer risk, decreased methylation
		Iron	Anemia, fatigue, hair loss, brittle nails, decreased thyroid hormone production
		Magnesium	Muscle cramps, weakness, fatigue, insomnia, restless leg syndrome, irritability, anxiety, insulin resistance, depression, high blood pressure, cardiovascular problems, headaches
		Phosphorus	Decreases calcium absorption, osteoporosis, brittle bones
		Vitamin B_{12}	Fatigue, peripheral neuropathy, macrocytic anemia, depression, memory loss/confusion, easy bruising, loss of appetite, nausea, vomiting, increased cardiovascular disease risk, increased homocysteine levels, decreased methylation
		Vitamin D	Osteoporosis, increased risk of skeletal fractures, hearing difficulties, depression, hormonal imbalances, muscular weakness, hypertension, autoimmune diseases, multiple sclerosis, diabetes, schizophrenia and decrease immunity
		Vitamin E	Dry skin, dry hair, anemia, easy bruising, PMS, eczema, dermatitis, psoriasis, muscle weakness, decreased antioxidant capacity, poor wound healing/impaired immunity
		Vitamin K	Easy bleeding, osteoporosis and brittle bones
		Zinc	Decreased immunity, decreased wound healing, smell and taste disturbances, anorexia, depression, night blindness, hair, skin and nail problems, menstrual irregularities, joint pain, nystagmus (involuntary eye movements), insulin resistance

Drug	Potential Drug Side Effects	Nutrient	Consequences
Colestipol (Colestid, Welchol)[97]	*Short term* Nausea/vomiting Diarrhea Gas/bloating Blurred vision Constipation Heartburn Headache Dizziness Fatigue Loss of appetite Anxiety/nervousness *Long term* Anemia Cardiovascular problems Irregular heartbeat (arrhythmia) Musculoskeletal pain	Beta-carotene (vitamin A)	Decreased immunity, night blindness, dry skin, brittle nails
		Folic acid	Birth defects, cervical dysplasia, anemia, heart disease, elevated homocysteine, headaches, fatigue, insomnia, diarrhea, nausea, increased cancer risk
		Iron	Anemia, fatigue, hair loss, brittle nails
		Vitamin B_{12}	Fatigue, peripheral neuropathy, macrocytic anemia, depression, memory loss/confusion, easy bruising, loss of appetite, nausea, vomiting, increased cardiovascular disease risk, increased homocysteine levels, decreased methylation
		Vitamin E	Dry skin, dry hair, anemia, easy bruising, PMS, eczema, dermatitis, psoriasis, muscle weakness, decreased antioxidant capacity, poor wound healing/impaired immunity
		Coenzyme Q10 (CoQ10)	High blood pressure, congestive heart failure, muscular fatigue, joint and muscle aches, rhabdomyolysis, memory loss, gingivitis, muscle weakness, irregular heartbeat, decreased immunity, insulin resistance
Fibrates[97] Fenofibrate (Tricor) Gemfibrozil (Lopid)	*Short term* Headache Abdominal pain Nausea/vomiting Muscle aches Flu-like symptoms Asthenia Diarrhea Constipation Abnormal liver function tests *Long term* Respiratory problems Albuminuria Pancreatitis Retinopathy Pulmonary embolism Anemia	Vitamin E	Dry skin, dry hair, anemia, easy bruising, PMS, eczema, dermatitis, psoriasis, muscle weakness, decreased antioxidant capacity, poor wound healing/impaired immunity
		Coenzyme Q10 (CoQ10)	High blood pressure, congestive heart failure, muscular fatigue, joint and muscle aches, rhabdomyolysis, memory loss, gingivitis, muscle weakness, irregular heartbeat, decreased immunity, insulin resistance
		Vitamin D	Osteoporosis, increased risk of skeletal fractures, hearing difficulties, depression, hormonal imbalances, muscular weakness, hypertension, autoimmune diseases, multiple sclerosis, schizophrenia and decrease immunity
		DHEA	Increased risk of developing type 2 diabetes, heart disease, cancer, osteoporosis, depression, obesity, decreased immune function, loss of strength and muscle mass, and memory problems like Alzheimer disease, high blood pressure, elevated cholesterol levels, and increased platelet aggregation, increased risk of thrombosis

(Continued)

Table 38.1

DRUGS COMMONLY USED IN THE CARDIOVASCULAR PATIENTS THAT HAVE REPORTED NUTRIENT DEPLETIONS—CONT'D

Drug	Reported Potential Drug Side Effects (Short and Long Term)	Reported Potential Nutrient Depletion	Reported Potential Health Consequence(s) of Nutrient Depletion
Miscellaneous cholesterol-lowering drugs Ezetimibe (Zetia)	*Short term* Diarrhea Fatigue Joint pain Upper respiratory tract infections Sinus infection *Long term* Gallstones Muscle weakness Muscle breakdown/myopathy Liver problems	Vitamin D	Osteoporosis, increased risk of skeletal fractures, hearing difficulties, depression, hormonal imbalances, muscular weakness, hypertension, autoimmune diseases, multiple sclerosis, schizophrenia and decrease immunity
Salicylates Aspirin Choline and magnesium salicylates (Tricosal, Trilisate)	***Potential Drug Side Effects*** *Short term* GI ulcers Abdominal burning/pain/cramping Nausea Vomiting Ringing in the ears (tinnitus) Dizziness Rash *Long term* Fatigue Liver and kidney damage Black tarry stools Gastrointestinal bleeding Intestinal damage Increased risk of birth defects	Folic acid	Birth defects, cervical dysplasia, anemia, heart disease, elevated homocysteine, headaches, fatigue, insomnia, diarrhea, nausea, increased cancer risk, decreased methylation
		Iron	Anemia, fatigue, hair loss, brittle nails, decreased thyroid hormone production
		Potassium	Irregular heartbeat, poor reflexes, muscle weakness, fatigue, thirst, confusion, constipation, dizziness, nervousness
		Sodium	Muscle weakness, poor concentration, memory loss dehydration, loss of appetite

Drug	Potential Drug Side Effects	Nutrient	Consequences
Nonsteroidal anti-inflammatory drugs (NSAIDs) COX-1 inhibitors[97] including: Diclofenac (Cataflam, Voltaren) Diflunisal (Dolobid) Etodolac (Lodine, Lodine XL) Fenoprofen calcium (Nalfon) Flurbiprofen (Ansaid) Ibuprofen (Advil, Motrin) Ketoprofen (Actron, Orudis, Orudis KT, Oruvail) Meclofenamate sodium (Meclomen) Mefenamic acid (Ponstel) Meloxicam (Mobic) Nabumetone (Relafen) Naproxen (Aleve, Naprosyn) Oxaprozin (Daypro) Piroxicam (Feldene) Sulindac (Clinoril) Tolmetin sodium (Tolectin)	*Short term* GI ulcers Abdominal burning/pain/cramping Nausea/vomiting Diarrhea Constipation Edema Dizziness Sleep disturbances Rash Apnea (especially asthmatics) *Long term* Fatigue Liver and kidney damage Gastrointestinal bleeding Intestinal damage/dysbiosis Increased risk of birth defects	Folic acid Melatonin Sodium Zinc DHEA	Birth defects, cervical dysplasia, anemia, heart disease, elevated homocysteine, headaches, fatigue, insomnia, diarrhea, nausea, increased cancer risk, decreased methylation Sleep disturbances that may lead to insulin resistance and cardiovascular problems and a weakened immune system; increased cancer risk, increased oxidative stress in the brain, decreased seizure threshold Muscle weakness, poor concentration, memory loss, dehydration, loss of appetite Decreased immunity, decreased wound healing, smell and taste disturbances, anorexia, depression, night blindness, hair, skin and nail problems, menstrual irregularities, joint pain, nystagmus (involuntary eye movements), insulin resistance Fatigue, weight gain, depression, bone loss, musculoskeletal pain, immune imbalances, sleep disturbances
Opiate pain medications Morphine Hydrocodone (Lortab, Vicodin) Oxycodone (Percocet, Percodan, Oxycontin) Meperidine (Demerol) Codeine	*Potential Drug Side Effects (General)* *Short term* Euphoria Fatigue Somnolence *Long term* Liver and kidney damage Sleep disturbances Musculoskeletal pain Immune imbalances Fatigue Bone loss	DHEA	Fatigue, weight gain, depression, bone loss, musculoskeletal pain, immune imbalances, sleep disturbances

(Continued)

Table 38.1

DRUGS COMMONLY USED IN THE CARDIOVASCULAR PATIENTS THAT HAVE REPORTED NUTRIENT DEPLETIONS—CONT'D

Drug	Reported Potential Drug Side Effects (Short and Long Term)	Reported Potential Nutrient Depletion	Reported Potential Health Consequence(s) of Nutrient Depletion
Acetaminophen (Tylenol)[97]	*Potential Drug Side Effects (General)* *Short term* Liver toxicity Increased oxidative stress Increased sweating Nausea/vomiting Abdominal pain Gas/bloating *Long term* Liver damage Death from liver damage Anemia Fatigue Kidney damage Cardiovascular problems Itching, dry skin Increased sweating Irritability/mood swings Confusion	Glutathione	Decreased antioxidant capacity, liver damage, sweating, fatigue, decreased immunity, hair loss, dry skin, itching
Biguanides[97] Metformin (Glucophage)	*Potential Drug Side Effects* *Short term* Diarrhea Dizziness Drowsiness Fatigue Anxiety Headache Nausea Weight gain/hunger increase Fullness Heartburn Gas/bloating Hypoglycemia Edema (swelling) *Long term* Hypoglycemia Muscle weakness Tremor	Coenzyme Q10 (CoQ10) Folic acid Vitamin B$_{12}$	High blood pressure, congestive heart failure, muscle fatigue, joint and muscle aches, rhabdomyolysis, memory loss, gingivitis, muscle weakness, irregular heartbeat, decreased immunity, insulin resistance Birth defects, cervical dysplasia, anemia, heart disease, elevated homocysteine, headaches, fatigue, insomnia, diarrhea, nausea, increased cancer risk, decreased methylation Fatigue, peripheral neuropathy, macrocytic anemia, depression, memory loss/confusion, easy bruising, loss of appetite, nausea, vomiting, increased cardiovascular disease risk, decreased methylation

	Potential Drug Side Effects		
Sulfonylureas Glimepiride (Amaryl) Glipizide (Glucotrol) Glyburide (Diabeta, Glynase, Micronase) Tolbutamide (Orinase) Tolazamide (Tolinase)	*Short term* Dizziness Drowsiness Fatigue Anxiety Headache Nausea Weight gain/hunger increase Fullness Heartburn Gas/bloating Hypoglycemia Edema (swelling) *Long term* Hypoglycemia Muscle weakness Tremor Sleep disturbances Depression Arrhythmias Cardiovascular problems	Coenzyme Q10 (CoQ10)	Hypertension Congestive heart failure muscular and joint aches/fatigue Rhabdomyolysis Memory loss Gingivitis Imbalanced immunity Insulin resistance/impaired glucose tolerance
Potassium, timed release Micro K, Klor-Con, Kaon CL, others	**Potential Drug Side Effects (General)** *Short term* Nausea/vomiting Gas/bloating Abdominal pain Diarrhea *Long term* Muscle cramps Weakness Cardiovascular problems Swelling (edema) Dizziness Confusion	Vitamin B$_{12}$	Fatigue, peripheral neuropathy, macrocytic anemia, depression, memory loss/confusion, easy bruising, loss of appetite, nausea, vomiting, increased cardiovascular disease risk, elevated homocysteine levels, decreased methylation

(Continued)

Table 38.1

DRUGS COMMONLY USED IN THE CARDIOVASCULAR PATIENTS THAT HAVE REPORTED NUTRIENT DEPLETIONS—CONT'D

Drug	Reported Potential Drug Side Effects (Short and Long Term)	Reported Potential Nutrient Depletion	Reported Potential Health Consequence(s) of Nutrient Depletion
Magnesium and aluminum antacids[97]	*Potential Drug Side Effects (General)*		
	Short term		
	Loss of appetite	Calcium	Osteoporosis, heart and blood pressure problems, back or leg pain, nervousness, tooth decay
	Diarrhea	Folic acid	Birth defects, cervical dysplasia, anemia, heart disease, elevated homocysteine, headaches, fatigue, insomnia, diarrhea, nausea, increased cancer risk, decreased methylation
	Constipation		
	Nausea, vomiting	Phosphorus	Skeletal problems and anxiety or nervousness
	Long term		
	Mental confusion		
	Osteoporosis, bone loss		
	Weakness		
	Irregular heartbeat		
	Sleep disturbances		
	Increased risk of birth defects		
H2 blockers[97] Cimetidine (Tagamet) Ranitidine (Zantac) Famotidine (Pepcid) Nizatidine (Axid)	*Potential Drug Side Effects (General)*		
	Short term		
	Diarrhea	Calcium	Osteoporosis, heart and blood pressure problems, back or leg pain, nervousness, tooth decay
	Constipation	Folic acid	Birth defects, cervical dysplasia, anemia, heart disease, elevated homocysteine, headaches, fatigue, insomnia, diarrhea, nausea, increased cancer risk, decreased methylation
	Dizziness		
	Headaches	Iron	Anemia, fatigue, hair loss, brittle nails, decreased thyroid hormone
	Runny nose		
	Weakness		
	Long term		
	Irregular heartbeat (arrhythmia)		
	Depression		
	Liver damage		
	Swelling (edema)		
	Sexual dysfunction		
	Confusion		

Drug	Nutrient depleted	Symptoms	Potential Drug Side Effects (General)
	Vitamin B$_{12}$	Fatigue, peripheral neuropathy, macrocytic anemia, depression, memory loss/confusion, easy bruising, loss of appetite, nausea, vomiting, increased cardiovascular disease risk, decreased methylation	
	Vitamin D	Osteoporosis, increased risk of skeletal fractures, hearing difficulties, depression, hormonal imbalances, muscular weakness, hypertension, autoimmune diseases, multiple sclerosis, type 1 diabetes, schizophrenia and decrease immunity	
	Zinc	Decreased immunity, decreased wound healing, smell and taste disturbances, anorexia, depression, night blindness, hair, skin and nail problems, menstrual irregularities, joint pain, nystagmus (involuntary eye movements), insulin resistance	
Proton-pump inhibitors[97] Lansoprazole (Prevacid) Omeprazole (Prilosec) Pantoprazole (Protonix) Rabeprazole (Aciphex) Esomeprazole (Nexium)	Calcium	Osteoporosis, heart and blood pressure problems, back or leg pain, nervousness, tooth decay	*Short term* Diarrhea Constipation Dizziness Headaches Abdominal pain Nausea
	Folic acid	Birth defects, cervical dysplasia, anemia, heart disease, elevated homocysteine, headaches, fatigue, insomnia, diarrhea, nausea, increased cancer risk, decreased methylation	*Long term* Increased risk of osteoporosis and bone fractures Depression Weakness
	Iron	Anemia, fatigue, hair loss, brittle nails, decreased thyroid hormone	Numbness/tingling of hands/feet Increased risk of cardiovascular disease
	Sodium	Muscle weakness, poor concentration, memory loss, dehydration, loss of appetite	Irregular heartbeat (arrhythmia) Immune imbalances
	Vitamin C	Loss of antioxidant potential, increased capillary fragility, muscle weakness, poor wound healing, bleeding gums, anemia, poor appetite, tender and swollen joints	Increased risk of insulin resistance/type 2 diabetes Increased risk of cancer
	Vitamin D	Osteoporosis, increased risk of skeletal fractures, hearing difficulties, depression, hormonal imbalances, muscular weakness, hypertension, autoimmune diseases, multiple sclerosis, diabetes, schizophrenia and decrease immunity	
	Vitamin B$_{12}$	Fatigue, peripheral neuropathy, macrocytic anemia, depression, memory loss/confusion, easy bruising, loss of appetite, nausea, vomiting, increased cardiovascular disease risk, increased homocysteine levels, decreased methylation	
	Magnesium	Muscle cramps, weakness, fatigue, insomnia, restless leg syndrome, irritability, anxiety, insulin resistance, depression, high blood pressure, cardiovascular problems, headaches	

(Continued)

Table 38.1

DRUGS COMMONLY USED IN THE CARDIOVASCULAR PATIENTS THAT HAVE REPORTED NUTRIENT DEPLETIONS—CONT'D

Drug	Reported Potential Drug Side Effects (Short and Long Term)	Reported Potential Nutrient Depletion	Reported Potential Health Consequence(s) of Nutrient Depletion
Benzodiazepines including: Alprazolam (Xanax) Diazepam (Valium) Lorazepam (Ativan) Oxazepam (Serax)	***Potential Drug Side Effects*** *Short term* Loss of muscle coordination Dizziness Fatigue Drowsiness Blurred vision Upset stomach Mental fogginess Hangover effect Sleep disturbances *Long term* Tolerance and physical dependence Sleep disturbances Amnesia Vision changes Chest pain	Melatonin	Sleep disturbances that may lead to insulin resistance and cardiovascular problems and a weakened immune system; increased cancer risk, increased oxidative stress in the brain, decreased seizure threshold

Data from *Drug Induced Nutrient Depletion Handbook.* Lexi-Comp; 2001 and Pelton, LaValle et al. *Nutritional Cost of Drugs.* Morton Publishing; 2004.

serotonin-N-acetyltransferase.[7,8] Results report that the CNS side effects (including sleep disorders, nightmares) during beta-blocker therapy are related to a reduction of melatonin levels. Nighttime exogenous administration of melatonin as a dietary supplement is reported to reduce the incidence of beta-blocker–induced sleep disturbances.[8,9]

Of note, melatonin is also reduced by the administration of NSAIDs, commonly used in the cardiovascular patient with comorbid symptoms of joint/muscle pain. A recent cross-sectional, multicenter observational study of osteoarthritis patients reported that of the over 17,000 patients evaluated, over 90% were at an increased risk of GI and/or CV risk and that a large percentage of these patients (51%) were treated with an NSAID + PPI.[10]

Of interest is that PPI use, which are one of the most frequently prescribed drugs in the United States, also is reported to increase the risk of hospitalization for a CV event by 51%, and that individual PPIs each significantly raise that risk as well, ranging from 39% to 61%.[11] Other studies report similar results.[12,13] A 2018 systematic review of 37 clinical studies compared the effect of PPI use on mortality and/or cardiovascular morbidity. The study included 22,427 patients in mortality dataset and 354,446 patients in the morbidity datasets. The authors concluded that in patients using PPIs, there is a significant increase in morbidity because of CV disease.[14]

Also reported to be depleted by beta-blocker therapy is coenzyme Q10 (ubiquinol). Beta-blocker use is reported to deplete CoQ10 by interfering with the production of this essential enzyme for energy production.[15] CoQ10 is important in cardiovascular function, including production of cellular energy (ATP) via the electron transport chain. Depletion is CoQ10 from the body is clinically associated with myopathy (including cardiomyopathy), rhabdomyolysis, hypertension, angina, stroke, cardiac dysrhythmias, fatigue, leg weakness, immune imbalances, neurodegenerative disease, and cognitive decline.[16] Of interest is that the use of beta-blockers is reported to increase the risk of hospitalization in the elderly (45% in those using propranolol) because of myopathy.[17]

It is also widely reported that CoQ10 levels are decreased in congestive heart failure (CHF) patients.[18,19] The use of beta-blockers, although reported to deplete coenzyme Q10, is considered a standard of care in those with CHF. Using concomitant CoQ10 is reported to improve functional capacity, endothelial function, and LV contractility in CHF without side effects.[20] A 2013 meta-analysis reported that CoQ10 supplementation improved ejection fraction (EF) in those with CHF.[21] With the readmission rate of CHF patients within 6 months at approximately 30% to 40%, supplementation with CoQ10 may be an appropriate choice for the clinician and their patients.[22,23]

Also, genetic polymorphisms of substrates that metabolize cardiovascular medications may lead to specific nutrient depletions.[24] Only variations in VKORC1 (vitamin K epoxide reductase complex subunit 1) and CYP2C9 have consistently been associated with drug response (coumarins) that has clinical implications.

These polymorphisms include:
- Cyclooxygenase-1
- Vitamin D reductase complex subunit 1
- CYP2C9
- Alpha adducing
- 3-Hydroxy-3-methylglutaryl-CoA reductase

There are several factors that should be noted before discussing the relative impact of drug-induced depletions. Whether a nutrient depletion will occur is a complex and multifactorial issue. Variations in diet, genetic differences, individual stress, and activity levels all contribute to the nutritional status of the individual before drug therapy is administered. Therefore responses to drug therapy are highly individualized.

Potential Nutrient Depletions: A Review of Significant Findings

Rather than discuss the individual drugs used in the cardiovascular patient that may lead to nutrient depletion, a review of the principle nutrients depleted, their relationship to cardiovascular disease and comorbid conditions, and the associated risks of nutrient depletion will be covered. Because these are chronic conditions, the drugs are used long term and patients are on several of these drug therapies for many years. It is important to remember that metabolic disturbances build over time with subtle disturbances in enzyme function, leading to a cascade of metabolic disruption. Very often patients are displaying symptoms of a nutrient depletion. Rather than recommending the nutrient(s) that may be depleted, polypharmacy-prescribing habits are often used, which can mask metabolic problems that have been brought about by drug therapy.

Part of patient management should be assessing the overall nutritional status of the individual. In assessing individuals for possible drug-induced nutrient depletions, the prescribed medications may have no known nutrient depletions, but signs and symptoms of nutrient deficiencies should always be assessed, regardless, because many lifestyle factors such as smoking and drinking can also influence nutrient depletions. Addressing nutritional deficiencies is a foundation to good health care and in a health care environment where prevention is increasingly being mandated because of out-of-control health care costs, a very cost efficient way to improve the overall health and well-being of the patient and to prevent further comorbidities.

Magnesium

Magnesium is involved in over 300 enzymatic reactions in the body. It is needed for proper nerve transmission, production of energy, muscular activity, regulation of temperature, detoxification of cells, blood pressure regulation, regulation of blood sugar, and it regulates vasospasm and helps with the building of healthy bones and teeth. Appropriate magnesium levels are especially important for the cardiovascular patient, and low levels of magnesium are associated with an increased risk of heart disease.[25,26]

It is reported that approximately 75% of Americans' intake of magnesium is below the RDA.[27] In addition, many lifestyle factors such as stress and drinking alcohol can deplete magnesium, so it is easy to understand how with the addition of drug therapy a clinically significant low magnesium level can occur.

Hypomagnesemia and low dietary intake of magnesium are strongly related to cardiovascular risk factors among known subjects with coronary artery disease, including increasing the proinflammatory/pro-oxidant status and an increased risk of ischemic heart disease.[28–31] Also, one of the most significant and least discussed nutrients depleted from first-line drug therapy in hypertension is magnesium. A Japanese study of over 58,615 healthy men aged 40 to 79 years that lasted 14.7 years reported that increasing magnesium in the diet reduced CVD mortality risk by approximately 50%.[32]

In clinical practice, when patients are prescribed thiazide diuretics for hypertension, typically only potassium depletion is addressed, with patients advised to drink orange juice or eat a banana, which are rich sources of potassium. Often, no education in medical schools or allied health curriculums is given regarding the potential for magnesium depletion, despite the fact that many of listed side effects of thiazide diuretics are also signs and symptoms of magnesium depletion (see Table 38.1). Although this topic may be controversial in the literature,[33] enough studies have reported a magnesium-depleting effect from thiazides (one report in 2000 suggested 20% of thiazide patients have hypomagnesemia[34]) to at least justify a screening for magnesium depletion symptoms among thiazide users.[35,36] This is especially true when it is considered that the clinical manifestations of hypomagnesemia can be so severe.

Deficiency of magnesium is associated with increased incidence of atherosclerosis, hypertension, stroke, and myocardial infarction. Magnesium plays a role in inhibiting platelet aggregation, blood thinning, and blocking of calcium reuptake; relaxes blood vessels; and increases oxygenation of the heart by improving contractility. Oral magnesium therapy is reported beneficial in patients with heart failure and those undergoing cardiovascular surgeries, improving blood pressure regulation via improved endothelial function, and improving exercise heart rate, exercise tolerance, and myocardial function in general.[37–40]

It should be mentioned that serum magnesium is a poor measure of magnesium status because homeostatic mechanisms keep blood levels fairly constant by pulling magnesium from bone and other body tissues. It is often suggested that red blood cell levels are a more reliable indicator of magnesium status.[41] However, some researchers state that mid-normal magnesium levels could be indicative of an intracellular depletion. RBC levels of magnesium should be 4.2 to 6.8 mg/dL for most individuals. Likewise, levels do not always correspond with utilization in the body. Serum magnesium levels of 1.7 to 2.2 mg/dL are appropriate for most individuals.

Potential Symptoms of Magnesium Deficiency

- Muscle cramps and spasms, vasomotor spasms
- Anxiousness, nervousness, insomnia
- Hypertension, prehypertension
- Blood glucose imbalances/insulin resistance
- Depression/mood swings
- Fatigue
- Arrhythmias, dysrhythmias
- Migraines
- Constipation
- Osteoporosis/decreased bone density
- Kidney stones

Manifestations of Deficiency

Even marginal magnesium deficiency can decrease myocardial magnesium, which can directly affect contractility and excitability of the heart. The mechanism of action of this result is primarily by the reduced regulation of calcium ion channel. Even perfusion of the heart can be easily compromised. Studies have reported that low magnesium can lead to coronary vasospasm, reduced energy metabolism, changes in potassium homeostasis, and excessive induction of free radical generation.[42] In an animal study demonstrating this principle, a diet low in magnesium and high in sucrose progressively induced elevations in triglycerides, and a reduction of insulin binding to erythrocyte insulin receptors ($\uparrow$ insulin resistance) over a 3-month period.[43]

Many of the symptoms and conditions that develop, progress, and are prescribed for in metabolic syndrome mimic the symptoms of magnesium depletion, primarily blood pressure regulation and blood glucose regulation. It should be noted that several of the listed side effects of thiazide diuretics are magnesium depletion symptoms, including arrhythmia, lower back pain, mood changes, muscle pain/weakness/cramps, constipation, headache, and fatigue (see Table 38.1).

An established potential consequence of long-term use of thiazide diuretics is development of type II diabetes and because of this their use is controversial in those predisposed to blood glucose dysregulation.[44] Medical literature is clearly establishing the role of magnesium not only in insulin regulation, but in helping control inflammatory chemistry as well.[45] Drug-induced intracellular depletion of magnesium could be playing a significant role in the rapid induction into the complications of metabolic syndrome. Clinical repletion dosage of magnesium as magnesium aspartate, citrate, or amino acid chelate is 300 to 800 mg/d. This dosage may induce loose stool, so titrate to larger doses if needed.

Coenzyme Q10

One of the most frequently discussed depletions in drug-induced nutrient depletion is the area of CoQ10 depletion and the use of statin (3-hydroxy-3-methylglutaryl-coenzyme A reductase inhibitors or HMG-CoA reductase inhibitors) medications. This depletion can also occur in the use of

HMG-CoA reductase inhibitors, centrally acting antihypertensive agents, fibrates, diuretics, beta-blockers, and second-generation sulfonylureas and biguanide drug therapies. It has been demonstrated that CoQ10 concentrations can fall as much as 54% in patients who are on HMG-CoA reductase inhibitor therapy, with a dose-dependent drop in some patient populations.[46] Note that excessive and/or chronic alcohol consumption may also lead to CoQ10 depletion.[47]

CoQ10 is a cofactor in the electron transport chain, which is involved in cellular respiration and the generation of ATP. CoQ10 also plays an important role as an antioxidant and is a principle gene regulator in muscle tissue and plays a significant role in tissue metabolism. Clinical manifestations of CoQ10 depletion can include myalgias, rhabdomyolysis, cardiomyopathy, hypertension, angina, stroke, cardiac dysrhythmias, fatigue, leg weakness, decline in immune function, increase in neurodegenerative diseases, and loss of cognitive function.

In one study, muscle fibers were examined in an elderly population preparing for hip surgery.[48] The findings are that CoQ10-treated individuals had a lower proportion of type 1(slow twitch) fibers and a higher concentration of type IIb (fast twitch) fibers compared with age-matched placebo-treated patients. This shift is consistent with fiber composition found in younger populations. In this study, significant change in gene expression of proteins was noted. The protective and regenerative effect of CoQ10 on skeletal muscle is promising, and it may be theorized that low CoQ10 status could accelerate aging and genetic changes in muscle tissue.

Another area of clinical concern in the metabolic syndrome patient is the increased risk for Alzheimer disease. Disruption in mitochondrial ATP and an increase in hydrogen peroxide is one mechanism by with amyloid beta-peptide toxicity can take place. Disruptions in both glucose metabolism and increased free radical damage have been implicated in the development of Alzheimer disease. In a promising study, isolated brain mitochondria from diabetic rats were treated with CoQ10. Treatment with CoQ10 attenuated the decreased oxidative phosphorylation efficiency and halted the hydrogen peroxide production induced by neurotoxic peptides. This indicates that CoQ10 treatment changed the mitochondrial alterations in the Abeta 1 to 40, suggesting it could play a role in altering the cellular energy deficits correlated to diabetes and the progression of Alzheimer disease.[49] These findings suggest that it does not make sense to administer drugs that deplete CoQ10 without repletion when clearly mitochondrial energy deficits are involved in progression to Alzheimer disease.

The value of CoQ10 in hypertension was reported in one clinical trial where supplementing CoQ10 decreased systolic and diastolic blood pressure, decreased total cholesterol, and increased HDL cholesterol.[50] In another trial, supplementation of CoQ10 enabled hypertensive patients to reduce their medications. A mean dose of 225 mg in 109 patients led to discontinuation of one to three medications in 51% of patients within 6 months (average time 4.4 months); 80% of the individuals had been diagnosed for 9.2 years. Only

3% required addition of one more drug.[51] In another study it was reported that drug-related myopathy, which is a complaint of CoQ10 therapy, was shown to be associated with a mild decrease in CoQ10 without presenting a histochemical or mitochondrial myopathy or even morphologic evidence of apoptosis in most patients examined. The net meaning of this is that significant cellular pathology may not exist and yet symptom expression could be likely.[52] Even though there may be no evidence of changes via creatine kinase concentrations, metabolic disruption of ATP production and cellular energetics is probable.

With several of the most common drugs used in metabolic syndrome depleting CoQ10, clinicians should consider the implications of chronic mild decreases of CoQ10 and its impact on the progression of the metabolic pathology as it relates to the cardiovascular component.

CoQ10 serum reference range is 0.37 to 2.20 µg/mL. Recommended clinical dosage range for repletion of CoQ10 range from 30 to 300 mg/d of a solubilized form of coenzyme Q10. It should be noted that concomitant administration of CoQ10 supplements with anticoagulants such as warfarin is reported in several case studies to lead to decreased levels of the anticoagulant.[53,54] CoQ10 is chemically similar to the K-vitamins, which may explain the interaction with warfarin.

Conditions and Symptoms Associated With CoQ10 Depletion

- Myalgia
- Arthralgia
- Rhabdomyolysis
- Hypertension
- Angina
- Mitral valve prolapse
- Stroke
- Arrhythmias
- Cardiomyopathy
- Poor insulin production
- Low energy
- Gingivitis
- Weakened immunity

Zinc

Marginal zinc deficiencies are thought to be common in the United States. Because of zinc involvement in over 300 enzymatic reactions, the symptoms of deficiency can present itself in a wide array of physiologic dysfunction.

Conditions and diseases associated with of zinc deficiency can include:

- Loss of taste and smell
- Poor wound healing
- Anorexia
- Alterations in immunity including cytokine and T killer cell function
- Depression

- Photophobia
- Night blindness
- Frequent infections
- Disorders of skin, hair and nails
- Arthralgia
- Alteration in hormones including leptin, thyroid and insulin
- Kidney disease
- Celiac sprue and inflammatory bowel disorders
- Malignant melanoma
- Alcoholism
- Macular degeneration
- Prostate disorders

Zinc is depleted by several of the drugs listed in **Table 38.1**. One of the more significant findings related to zinc deficiency is the influence on mRNA and levels of cytokines on cell lines. Zinc deficiency decreased expression of IL-2 and IFN-gamma in the Th1 cell gene expression, and TNF-alpha, IL-1 beta, and IL-8 gene expression were upregulated.[55] This study clearly demonstrated the effects of zinc on genetic expression of cytokines and that the expression was specific to immune cells. Extrapolated to humans this would mean that zinc deficiency could increase the production of TNF-alpha, IL1-beta, and IL-8, which is associated with the development of chronic conditions such as cardiovascular disease, metabolic syndrome, cancer, and Alzheimer disease.[56]

In addition it has been shown that increased TNF-alpha induces insulin resistance and increased oxidative stress. Alterations in TNF-alpha have been associated with decreased HDL, increased LDL and triglycerides, and increases in C-reactive protein. As insulin resistance is increased by diet, mineral deficiencies (including magnesium, chromium, vitamin D), stress, lack of exercise, or other factors, the increase in adipocyte-driven TNF-alpha expression could be exacerbated by zinc-deficient chemistry.[57] Dosage for repletion of zinc is 10 to 50 mg/d.

B$_{12}$/Folic Acid

Vitamin B$_{12}$ (cyanocobalamin) and folate (folic acid) are often discussed together. Although the value of B$_{12}$ for reduction of anemia and regulation of DNA and neurologic changes is well understood, there are specific issues that relate to the depletion of B$_{12}$ and the progression of metabolic syndrome.

Depletion of folate and B$_{12}$ can elevate homocysteine levels. In a trial published in the *European Journal of Endocrinology*, folate and B$_{12}$ therapy was reported to reduce homocysteine levels, ameliorate insulin resistance, and help to resolve endothelial dysfunction in patients with metabolic syndrome.[58] In the treatment group, folate 5 mg and B$_{12}$ 500 µg/d for 1 month can lead to striking results with a decrease in homocysteine in homocysteine of 27.8%, significant decrease in insulin levels along with an improvement in endothelial dysfunction as evidenced by hyperemic vasodilatation of 29.8% and dimethylarginine levels decreased by

21.7%. Plasma homocysteine is clearly elevated and is used as a biomarker in metabolic syndrome. It is also an independent marker for the development of atherosclerotic disease. It is thought that folic acid facilitates and restores endothelial nitric oxide by acting as hydrogen and electron donor to tetrahydrobiopterin and through the lowering of total homocysteine along with B$_{12}$ by the enhancement of remethylation.[59]

Ironically, metformin, commonly used in metabolic syndrome to prevent progression to type II diabetes mellitus and hypertension, is reported to deplete vitamin B$_{12}$ and folate.[60,61] A study of 122 patients (59 taking metformin and 63 not taking the drug) reported that metformin administration was associated with B$_{12}$ depletion and an increase in homocysteine and an increase in peripheral neuropathy symptoms.[62] Metformin-treated patients had depressed Cbl levels and elevated fasting MMA and Hcy levels. Clinical and electrophysiological measures identified more severe peripheral neuropathy in these patients with the cumulative metformin dose correlated strongly with these clinical and paraclinical group differences.

Homocysteine, interleukin 6, and C-reactive protein can express more dramatically in a 677T mutation (MTHFR or methylene tetrahydrofolate reductase) and shows that innate immunity is involved when this cascade of atherosclerosis in patients with diabetes mellitus who are genetically predisposed.[63] Depletion of folic acid from drug therapy in an individual with the 677t mutation could accelerate the cascade of elevated homocysteine, increased IL-6 and increased C peptide that is associated with metabolic syndrome, cardiovascular disease, and type 2 diabetes. In these individuals who are homozygous for the TT genotype of 677T (MTHFR), supplementation with 5-methyltetrahydrofolate (5-MTHF, 1-5 mg daily) may be necessary to overcome genotypic barrier for absorption of folic acid.

Depression is a common comorbidity in cardiovascular disease and in metabolic syndrome.[64] Studies are reporting low folate levels, low B$_{12}$, and elevated homocysteine levels are correlated with depression.[65,66]

Folate and B$_{12}$ status should evaluated in cardiovascular patients. Dosage to replenish folate is 400 to 800 µg/d. Dosage to replenish B12 is 100 to 2000 µg/d (methylcobalamin is more readily absorbed and bioavailable with oral administration).

Conditions Associated With Folic Acid Depletion

- Elevated homocysteine
- Depression
- Cervical dysplasia
- Breast and colon cancer
- Anemia
- Fatigue
- Cardiovascular disease
- Birth defects

Vitamin D

Vitamin D is a fat-soluble vitamin also called the "sunshine vitamin." It is estimated that 1 billion people worldwide have vitamin D deficiency or insufficiency.[67]

Vitamin D is best known for its regulation, along with parathyroid hormone, of calcium and phosphorus metabolism. Vitamin D is primarily produced in the skin from 7-dehydrocholesterol through solar ultraviolet radiation.[68] Additional sources include the diet and oral supplementation. Independent of source, all vitamin D is converted in the liver to 25-hydroxyvitamin D, which is the major circulating form in the blood. The kidneys produce the final step to the active form 1,25-dihydroxyvitamin D. Most vitamin D is stored in the body as the 25-hydroxyvitamin D (25-OH-D).[68] Vitamin D receptors have been identified in virtually every tissue, including bone/teeth, kidney, skeletal, heart, adrenal, stomach, liver, skin, breast, pancreatic, immune, brain, prostate, ovaries, and testes.[69] Appropriate levels of vitamin D are necessary for the health of bones/teeth, cardiovascular system, including blood pressure and vascular health, insulin production, inflammatory balance, immune balance, and mood/cognitive function.[70-75]

A large study that looked at school children and adolescents in the United States found that approximately 50.8 million had low levels of vitamin D.[76] Age, season, northern latitudes, liver and kidney function, obesity, poor dietary intake, dark skin tone, and certain medications (corticosteroids, phenytoin) all contribute to low vitamin D levels.[77]

Vitamin D is deposited into fat stores, where it becomes less available for use in the body. This is a suggested mechanism leading to insulin resistance.[78] Vitamin D also helps improve immunity and has anti-inflammatory effects that may indirectly help improve insulin sensitivity.[71] Blood glucose control in people with type 2 diabetes has a seasonal variation, being worse in the winter, in part explained by variation in exposure to sunlight and vitamin D levels.[79] Research suggests that low levels of vitamin D may contribute to or be a cause of metabolic syndrome with associated hypertension, obesity, diabetes, and cardiovascular disease.[80]

In humans, low vitamin D has been strongly linked to heart and vascular problems including high blood pressure,[81] blood vessel problems,[82] atherosclerosis, myocardial infarction, and stroke.[83-86] In addition, low Vitamin D is linked to death associated with heart problems.[87] In a prospective observational study of adults older than 65 years participating in NHANES III, the risk of death was 45% lower in those with 25(OH)-D values greater than 40 ng/mL compared with those with values less than 10 ng/mL (hazard ratio [HR], 0.55; 95% CI, 0.34-0.88).[64]

Vitamin D deficiency is also linked to poor bone mineral density.[88] Vitamin D deficiency is prevalent in the United States, 60% of nursing home residents and 57% of hospitalized patients being vitamin D deficient.[89,90] Vitamin D supplementation has been reported to reduce bone fractures by at least 20% in individuals aged 65 and older.[91] 1000 to 5000 IU orally of vitamin D3 (25-hydroxyvitamin D) daily may help improve vitamin D levels, and some may require higher doses. Normal laboratory levels of 25-hydroxyvitamin D are 10 to 55 ng/mL.

There is some controversy whether oral vitamin K needs to be administered concurrently with oral vitamin D. Very high levels of vitamin D can lead to vascular calcification.[92] A 6-year clinical study of 25,567 patients reported that hypercalcemia due to vitamin D represented <4% of the total hypervitaminosis D detected in <0.1% of the tests performed. Although taking vitamin K (in the form of K2—menaquinone 180 μg/d) as a dietary supplement is generally a good idea, especially in the aging population to support cardiovascular health, it is not necessary, including if your patient is using vitamin D3 supplementation. Patients can eat more leafy greens like kale, broccoli, and cabbage to supply vitamin K1 (phylloquinone). Vitamin K2 is found in a few foods such as organ meats, egg yolks, cheeses (in particular Swiss Emmental and Norwegian Jarlsberg), and the Japanese condiment natto, but absorption is limited.

Melatonin

Chronic depletion of melatonin could directly influence daily rhythm of glucose, reduction in glucose transporter 4 aka GLUT 4 (the insulin-sensitive glucose transporter) levels, and suppression of insulin secretion.[93] The correlation may be that melatonin deficits lead to disrupted sleep, and disrupted sleep can lead to increased insulin resistance. Melatonin also has significant antioxidant effects as it stimulates glutathione peroxidase, SOD, and catalase as well as NO synthase. Melatonin is reported to reduce oxidative stress in diabetic populations.

An evaluation of the NHANES Survey revealed that people who slept 5 hours a night had a 73% increased risk of becoming obese versus those who slept 7 to 9 hours per night.[94] Trials conducted at Stanford University found that people who slept an average of <5 hours per night had a 15.5% decrease in leptin, an increase of 14.9% of ghrelin, and higher BMIs, regardless of the exercise and diet habits of the participants.[95] So with loss of sleep, the net effects were that appetite centers were up-regulated, BMI increased, and there was a shift in metabolic dysfunction toward metabolic syndrome. When melatonin levels are low, REM sleep cycles are disturbed leading to increased wakefulness throughout the night, and studies have shown that administering melatonin in the late evening hours was significantly more effective than placebo at increasing REM sleep.[96,97]

Under conditions of high stress, cortisol levels increase leading to a state of hyperarousal. Studies are showing that disturbed sleep as a result of hyperarousal can lead to its own effects on metabolic function (↑ TNF-alpha, ↑ IL-6, ↑ visceral fat storage, ↑ insulin resistance, etc).[32] Other nutrient depletions such as reduced magnesium status and low folate status (↓ serotonin synthesis) can also be simultaneously acting on the sleep center and inducing hyperarousal. All of this adds up to increased risk for obesity, diabetes, and cardiovascular risk. Melatonin may enhance insulin-receptor kinase and IRS-1 phosphorylation, which may improve insulin signaling and may actually counteract TNF-alpha–induced insulin resistance in type 2 and metabolic syndrome populations.[33] Lastly melatonin seems to have a direct effect on inhibiting tumorigenesis. Melatonin helps to inhibit cellular proliferation and stimulated differentiation and apoptosis.[34] This is particularly interesting because people with insulin resistance and sleep disturbances are more prone to cancer because of elevations of IGF-1 and increases in the immunologic shift toward chronic inflammatory chemistry leading to reduced activity of NK cells.

Melatonin is a potential drug-nutrient depletion of beta-blockers. Because of its potential to disrupt sleep and lead to further problems such as increased appetite, weight gain, insulin resistance, and increased inflammatory chemistry, it is an important nutrient to assess and administer if disrupted sleep is present. Cortisol levels should also be evaluated to determine if steps may be necessary to downregulate cortisol to further address hyperarousal as an underlying cause of insomnia. 3 to 15 mg melatonin 1 hour before bedtime can help alleviate the symptoms of insomnia.

Conclusion

After reading this chapter, it should be evident that nutrient depletions from many drug therapies used in the cardiovascular patient can have a profound effect on the progression of the diseases and the development of new comorbidities. Dysregulation of metabolic pathways should be evaluated to determine if nutrient depletions could be an underlying cause. This may help resolve common comorbidities in the cardiovascular patients, including restless leg syndrome, insomnia, low energy or depression, sexual dysfunction, and weight gain OR to determine if medication side effects could be linked to a nutrient depletion. Because many of the marginal nutrient deficiencies do not show up on traditional lab tests, the patient is left with another prescription to fill and/or decreased quality of life. Testing for nutrient deficiencies and then providing for these deficiencies in the form of vitamins, minerals, and other dietary supplements are relatively inexpensive and can provide significant margins of safety. They offer not only a solution to many of the comorbidities but they can reduce further progression of illness and improve patient quality of life.

As taught in medical school didactic training, vitamins, minerals, amino acids, and essential fatty acids are needed by every cell of the body to function. With depletion or genetic variation, metabolic consequences could lead to the initiation of chronic illness. Modern drug therapy and the emerging science of natural therapeutics together provide an integrative approach to management of chronic diseases as well as the best approach for prevention and wellness.

References

1. Centers for Disease Control (CDC). Available at: www.cdc.gov. Accessed March 2019.
2. Munoz-Hoyos A, Hubber E, Escames G, et al. Effect of propranolol plus exercise on melatonin and growth hormone levels in children with growth delay. *J Pineal Res*. 2001;30(2):75-81.
3. Stoschizky K, Sakotnik A, Lercher P, et al. Influence of beta-blockers on melatonin release. *Eur J Clin Pharmacol*. 1999;55(2):111-115.
4. Nishida S. Metabolic effects of melatonin on oxidative stress and diabetes. *Endocrine*. 2005;27(2):131-136.
5. Dominguez-Rodriguez A. Melatonin in cardiovascular disease. *Expert Opin Investig Drugs*. 2012;21(11):1593-1596.
6. Dominguez-Rodriguez A, Abreu-Gonzalez IP, Sanchez-Sanchez JJ, et al. Melatonin and circadian biology in human cardiovascular disease. *J Pineal Res*. 2010;49(1):14-22.
7. Brismar K, Mogensen L, Wetterberg L. Depressed melatonin secretion in patients with nightmares due to beta-adrenoceptor blocking drugs. *Acta Med Scand*. 1987;221:155-158.
8. Scheer FA, Morris CJ, Garcia JL, et al. Repeated melatonin supplementation improves sleep in hypertensive patients treat with beta-blockers: a randomized controlled trial. *Sleep*. 2012;35(10):1395-1402.
9. Fares A. Night-time exogenous melatonin administration may be a beneficial treatment for sleeping disorders in beta blocker patients. *J Cardiovasc Dis Res*. 2011;2(3):153-155.
10. Lanas A, Garcia-Tell G, Armada B, et al. Prescription patterns and appropriateness of NSAID therapy according to gastrointestinal risk and cardiovascular history in patients with diagnosis of osteoarthritis. *BMC Med*. 2011;9:38.
11. Mahabaleshwarkar RK, Yang Y, Datar MV, et al. Risk of adverse cardiovascular outcomes and all-cause mortality associated with concomitant use of clopidogrel and proton pump inhibitors in elderly patients. *Curr Med Res Opin*. 2013;29(4):315-323. [Epub ahead of print].
12. Lazaro AMP, Cristóbal C, Franco-Peláez JA, et al. Use of proton pump inhibitors predicts heart failure and death in patients with coronary artery disease. *PLoS One*. 2017;12(1):e0169826.
13. Bundhun PK, Teeluck AR, Bhurtu A, Huang WQ. Is the concomitant use of clopidogrel and Proton Pump Inhibitors still associated with increased adverse cardiovascular outcomes following coronary angioplasty?: A systematic review and meta-analysis of recently published studies (2012-2016). *BMC Cardiovasc Disord*. 2017;17:3.
14. Shiraev TP, Bullen A. Proton pump inhibitors and cardiovascular events: a systematic review. *Heart Lung Circ*. 2018;27(4):443-450.
15. Kishi T, Watanabe T, Folkers K. Bioenergetics in clinical medicine XV: inhibition of coenzyme Q10-enzymes by clinically used adrenergic blockers of beta-receptors. *Res Commun Chem Pathol Pharmacol*. 1977;17:157-164.
16. Potgieter M, Pretorius E, Pepper MS. Primary and secondary coenzyme Q10 deficiency: the role of therapeutic supplementation. *Nutr Rev*. 2013;71(3):180-188.
17. Setoguchi S, Higgins JM, Mogun H, et al. Propranolol and the risk of hospitalized myopathy: translating chemical genomics findings into population-level hypotheses. *Am Heart J*. 2010;159(3):428-433.
18. Fumagalli S, Fattirolli F, Guarducci L, et al. Coenzyme Q10 terclatrate and creatinine in chronic heart failure: a randomized, placebo-controlled, double blind study. *Clin Cardiol*. 2011;34(4):211-217.

19. Langsjoen PH, Langsjoen AM. Supplemental ubiquinol in patients with advanced congestive heart failure. *Biofactors.* 2008;32(1–4):119-128.

20. Belardinelli R, Mucai A, Lacalaprice F, et al. Coenzyme Q10 and exercise training in chronic heart failure. *Eur Heart J.* 2006;27(22):2675-2681.

21. Fotino AD, Thompson-Paul AM, Bazzano LA. Effect of coenzyme Q10 supplementation on heart failure: a meta-analysis. *Am J Clin Nutr.* 2013;97(2):268-275.

22. Hoyt R, Bowling LS. Reducing readmissions for congestive heart failure. *Am Fam Physician.* 2001;63(8):1593-1599.

23. Molyneux SL, Florkowski CM, Richards AM, et al. Coenzyme Q10; an adjunctive therapy for congestive heart failure?. *N Z Med J.* 2009;122(1305):74-79.

24. Johnson JA, Humma LM. Pharmacogenetics of cardiovascular drugs. *Brief Funct Genomic Proteomic.* 2002;1(1):66-79.

25. Alon I, Gorelik O, Berman S, et al. Intracellular magnesium in elderly patients with heart failure: effects of diabetes and renal dysfunction. *J Trace Elem Med Biol.* 2006;20(4):221-226.

26. Gao XR, Wang MD, He XY, et al. Decreased intralymphocytic magnesium content is associated with diastolic heart dysfunction in patients with essential hypertension. *Int J Cardiol.* 2011;147(2):331-334.

27. Alaimo K, McDowell MA, Briefel RR, et al. Dietary intake of vitamins, minerals and fiber of persons age 2 months and over in the United States: Third National Health and Nutrition Examination Survey, phase 1, 1988-91. *Adv Data Vital Health Stat.* 1994;258:1-26.

28. Chakraborti S, Chakraborti T, Mandal M, et al. Protective role of magnesium in cardiovascular disease: a review. *Mol Cell Biochem.* 2002;238(1-2):163-179.

29. Tejero-Taldo MI, Kramer JH, Mak Iu T, et al. The nerve-heart connection in the pro-oxidant response to Mg-deficiency. *Heart Fail Rev.* 2006;11(1):35-44.

30. Joosten MM, Gansevoort RT, Mukamai KJ, et al. Urinary and plasma magnesium and risk of ischemic heart disease. *Am J Clin Nutr.* 2013;97(6):1299-1306.[Epub ahead of print].

31. Del Gobbo LC, Song Y, Poirier P, et al. Low serum magnesium concentrations are associated with a high prevalence of premature ventricular complexes in obese adults with type 2 diabetes. *Cardiovasc Diabetol.* 2012;11:23.

32. Zhang W, Iso H, Ohira T, Date C, Tamakoshi A; JACC Study Group. Associations of dietary magnesium intake with mortality from cardiovascular disease: the JACC study. *Atherosclerosis.* 2012;221(2):587-595.

33. Atsmon J, Dolev E. Drug – induced hypomagnesaemia. *Drug Saf.* 2005;28(9):763-788.

34. Pak CY. Correction of thiazide-induced hypomagnesemia by potassium-magnesium citrate from review of prior trials. *Clin Nephrol.* 2000;54:271-275.

35. Odvina CV, Mason RP, Pak CY. Prevention of thiazide-induced hypokalemia without magnesium depletion by potassium-magnesium-citrate. *Am J Ther.* 2006;13(2):101-108.

36. Palmer BF, Naderi AS. Metabolic consequences associated with thiazide diuretics. *J Am Soc Hypertens.* 2007;1(6):381-392.

37. Kass L, Weekes J, Carpenter L. Effect of magnesium supplementation on blood pressure: a meta analysis. *Eur J Clin Nutr.* 2012;66(4):411-418.

38. Dorman BH, Sade RM, Burnette JS, et al. Magnesium supplementation in the prevention of arrhythmias in pediatric patients undergoing surgery for congenital heart defects. *Am Heart J.* 2000;139(3):522-528.

39. Shechter M, Sharir M, Labrador MJ, et al. Oral magnesium therapy improves endothelial function in patients with coronary artery disease. *Circulation.* 2000;102(7):2353-2358.

40. Pokan R, Hofmann P, von Duvillard SP, et al. Oral magnesium therapy, exercise heart rate, exercise tolerance and myocardial function in coronary artery disease patients. *Br J Sports Med.* 2006;40(9):773-778.

41. Bralley JA, Lord RS. *Laboratory Evaluations in Molecular Medicine.* Norcross, GA: The Institute for Advances in Molecular Medicine; 2001.

42. Nair RR, Nair P. Alteration of myocardial mechanics in marginal magnesium deficiency. *Magnes Res.* 2002;15(3-4):287-306 (ISSN:0953-1424). King DE, Mainous AG III, Geesey ME, Woolson RF. Dietary magnesium and C-reactive protein levels. *J Am Coll Nutr.* 2005;24:166-171.

43. Chaudhar DP, Boparai RK, Sharma R, et al. Studies on the development of an insulin resistant rat model by chronic feeding of low magnesium high sucrose diet. *Magnes Res.* 2004;17(4):293-300.

44. Shafi T, Appel LJ, Miller ER III, et al. Changes in serum potassium mediate thiazide-induced diabetes. *Hypertension.* 2008;52(6):1022-1029.

45. Nadler JL, Buchanan T, Natarajan R, Antonipillai I, Bergman R, Rude R. Magnesium deficiency produces insulin resistance and increased thromboxane synthesis. *Hypertension.* 1993;21:1024-1029.

46. Kamikawa T, Kobayashi A, Yamashita T, Hayashi H, Yamazaki N. Effects of coenzyme Q10 on exercise tolerance in chronic stable angina pectoris. *Am J Cardiol.* 1985;56:247-251.

47. Vidyashankar S, Nandakumar KS, Patki PS. Alcohol depletes coenzyme-Q10 associated with increased TNF-alpha secretion to induce cytotoxicity in HepG2 cells. *Toxicology.* 2012;302(1):34-39.

48. Linnane AW, Kopsidas G, Zhang C, et al. Cellular redox activity of coenzyme Q10 effect of CoQ10 supplementation on human skeletal muscle. *Free Radic Res.* 2002;36(4):445-453.

49. Moreira PL, Santos MS, Sena C, Nunes E, Seiça R, Oliveira CR. CoQ10 therapy attenuates amyloid beta-peptide toxicity in brain mitochondria isolated from aged diabetic rats. *Exp Neurol.* 2005;196(1):112-119.

50. Digiesi V, Cantini F, Oradei A, et al. Coenzyme Q10 in essential hypertension. *Mol Aspects Med.* 1994;15 suppl:s257-63.

51. Langsjoen P, Langsjoen P, Willis R, Folkers K. Treatment of essential hypertension with CoQ10. *Mol Aspects Med.* 1994;15 suppl:265-272.

52. Lamperti C, Nani AB, Lucchini V, et al. Muscle coenzyme Q10 level in statin related myopathy. *Arch Neurol.* 2005;62(11):1709-1712.

53. Spigset O. Reduced effect of warfarin caused by ubidecarenone. *Lancet.* 1994;344(8933):1372-1373.

54. Landbo C, Almdal TP. Interaction between warfarin and coenzyme Q10. *Ugeskr Laeger.* 1998;160(22):3226-3227.

55. Bao B, Prasad AS, Beck FW, Godmere M. Zinc modulates mRNA levels of cytokines. *Am J Physiol Endocrinol Metab.* 2003;285(5):E10 95-E1102.

56. Foster M, Samman S. Zinc regulation of inflammatory cytokines: implications for cardiometabolic disease. *Nutrients.* 2012;4(7):676-694.

57. Beletate V, El Dib RP, Atallah AN. Zinc supplementation for the prevention of type 2 diabetes mellitus. *Cochrane Database Syst Rev.* 2007;(1):CD005525.

58. Setola E, Monti LD, Galluccio E, et al. Insulin resistance and endothelial function are improved after folate and vitamin B12 therapy in patients with metabolic syndrome: relationship between homocysteine levels and hyperinsulinemia.. *Eur J Endocrinol.* 2004;151(4):483-489.

59. Hayden MR, Tyagi SC. Homocysteine and reactive oxygen species in metabolic syndrome, type 2 diabetes mellitus, and atherosderopathy: the pleiotropic effects of folate supplementation. *Nutr J.* 2004;3:4.

60. Derosa G, Cicero AF, Gaddi AV, et al. Long-term effects of glimepiride or rosiglitazone in combination with metformin on blood pressure control in type 2 diabetic patients affected by the metabolic syndrome: a 12-month, double-blind, randomized clinical trial. *Clin Ther.* 2005;27(9):1383-1391.

61. Peterson JL, McGuire DK. Impaired glucose tolerance and impaired fasting glucose – a review of diagnosis, clinical implications and management. *Diab Vasc Dis Res.* 2005;2(1):9-15.

62. Wile DJ, Toth C. Association of metformin, elevated homocysteine, and methylmalonic acid levels and clinically worsened diabetic peripheral neuropathy. *Diabetes Care.* 2010;33(1):156-161.

63. Akai A, Hosoi T, Ito H. Association of plasma homocysteine with serum interleukin 6 and C-peptide levels in patients with type 2 diabetes. *Metabolism.* 2005;54(6):809-810.

64. Bonnet F, Irving K, Terra JL, Nony P, Berthezène F, Moulin P. Depressive symptoms are associated with unhealthy lifestyle in hypertensive patients with the metabolic syndrome. *J Hypertens.* 2005;23(3):611-617.

65. Sachdev PS, Parslow RA, Lux O, et al. Relationship of homocysteine, folic acid and vitamin B12 with depression in a middle-aged community sample. *Psychol Med.* 2005;35(4):529-538.

66. Tiemeier H, van Tuijl HR, Hofman A, Meijer J, Kiliaan AJ, Breteler MM. Vitamin B-12, folate, and homocysteine in depression: the Rotterdam Study. *Am J Psychiatry.* 2002; 159(12):2099-2101.

67. Holick MF. Vitamin D deficiency. *N Engl J Med*. 2007;357:266-281.

68. Vieth R. Vitamin D supplementation, 25-hydroxyvitamin D concentrations, and safety. *Am J Clin Nutr*. 1999;69(5):825-826.

69. Nagpal S, Na S, Rathnachalam R. Noncalcemic actions of vitamin D receptor ligands. *Endocr Rev*. 2005;26:662-687.

70. Shoji T, Shinohara K, Kimoto E, et al. Lower risk for cardiovascular mortality in oral 1alpha-hydroxy vitamin D3 users in a haemodialysis population. *Nephrol Dial Transpl*. 2004;19:179-184.

71. Palomer X, Gonzalez-Clemente JM, Blanco-Vaca F, Mauricio D. Role of vitamin D in the pathogenesis of type 2 diabetes mellitus. *Diabetes Obes Metab*. 2008;10(3):185-197.

72. Mezawa H, Sugiura T, Watanabe M, et al. Serum vitamin D levels and survival of patients with colorectal cancer: post-hoc analysis of a prospective cohort study. *BMC Cancer*. 2010;10(1):347. [Epub ahead of print].

73. Holmøy T, Moen SM. Assessing vitamin D in the central nervous system. *Acta Neurol Scand Suppl*. 2010;(190):88-92.

74. Murphy PK, Wagner CL. Vitamin D and mood disorders among women: an integrative review. *J Midwifery Womens Health*. 2008;53(5):440-446.

75. Prince RL, Austin N, Devine A, et al. Effects of ergocalciferol added to calcium on the risk of falls in elderly high-risk women. *Arch Intern Med*. 2008;168(1):103-108.

76. Kumar J, Muntner P, Kaskel FJ, Hailpern SM, Melamed ML. Prevalence and associations of 25-hydroxyvitamin D deficiency in US children: NHANES 2001-2004. *Pediatrics*. 2009;124(3):e362-e370.

77. Webb AR, Kline L, Holick MF. Influence of season and latitude on the cutaneous synthesis of vitamin D3: exposure to winter sunlight in Boston and Edmonton will not promote vitamin D3 synthesis in human skin. *J Clin Endocrinol Metab*. 1988;67:373-378.

78. Liel Y, Ulmer E, Shary J, et al. Low circulating vitamin D in obesity. *Calcif Tissue Int*. 1998;43(4):199-201.

79. Dasgupta K, Chan C, Da Costa D, et al. Walking behaviour and glycemic control in type 2 diabetes: seasonal and gender differences–study design and methods. *Cardiovasc Diabetol*. 2007;6:1.

80. Beydoun MA, Boueiz A, Shroff MR, et al. Associations among 25-hydroxyvitamin D, diet quality, and metabolic disturbance differ by adiposity in United States adults. *J Clin Endocrinol Metab*. 2010;95(8):3814-3827.

81. Scragg R, Sowers MF, Bell C. Serum 25-hydroxyvitamin D, ethnicity, and blood pressure in the third national health and nutrition examination survey. *Am J Hypertens*. 2007;20:713-719.

82. Sugden JA, Davies JI, Witham MD, Morris AD, Struthers AD. Vitamin D improves endothelial function in patients with type 2 diabetes mellitus and low vitamin D levels. *Diabet Med*. 2008;25:320-325.

83. Melamed ML, Muntner P, Michos ED, et al. Serum 25-hydroxyvitamin D levels and the prevalence of peripheral arterial disease: results from NHANES 2001 to 2004. *Arterioscler Thromb Vasc Biol*. 2008;28:1179-1185.

84. Targher G, Bertolini L, Padovani R, et al. Serum 25 -hydroxyvitamin D3 concentrations and carotid artery intima-media thickness in type 2 diabetic patients. *Clin Endocrinol*. 2006;65:593-597.

85. Lindén V. Vitamin D and myocardial infarction. *Br Med J*. 1974;3:647-650.

86. Pilz S, Marz W, Wellnitz B, et al. Association of vitamin D deficiency with heart failure and sudden cardiac death in a large cross-sectional study referred for coronary angiography. *J Clin Endocrinol Metab*. 2008;93:3927-3935.

87. Dobnig H, Pilz S, Scharnagl H, et al. Independent association of low serum 25-hydroxyvitamin D and 1,25-dihydroxyvitamin D levels with all-cause and cardiovascular mortality. *Arch Intern Med*. 2008;168:1340-1349.

88. Harwood RH, Sahota O, Gaynor K, et al. A randomised, controlled comparison of different calcium and vitamin D supplementation regimens in elderly women after hip fracture: the Nottingham Neck of Femur (NONOF) Study. *Age Ageing*. 2004;33(1):45-51.

89. Hoeck HC, Li B, Qvist P. Changes in 25-Hydroxyvitamin D3 to oral treatment with vitamin D3 in postmenopausal females with osteoporosis. *Osteoporos Int*. 2009;20(8):1329-1335.

90. Elliott ME, Binkley NC, Carnes M, et al. Fracture risks for women in long-term care: high prevalence of calcaneal osteoporosis and hypovitaminosis D. *Pharmacotherapy*. 2003;23(6):702-710.

91. Bischoff-Ferrari HA, Willett WC, Wong JB, et al. Prevention of nonvertebral fractures with oral vitamin D and dose dependency: a meta-analysis of randomized controlled trials. *Arch Intern Med*. 2009;169(6):551-561.

92. Perez-Barrios C, Hernández-Álvarez E, Blanco-Navarro I, Pérez-Sacristán B, Granado-Lorencio F. Prevalence of hypercalcemia related to hypervitaminosis D in clinical practice. *Clin Nutr*. 2016;35(6):1354-1358.

93. Picinato MC, Haber EP, Carpinelli AR, et al. Daily rhythm of glucose-induced secretion by isolated islets from the intact and pinealectomized rat. *J Pineal Res*. 2002;33(3):172-177.

94. NHANES I Data (Findings Reported at the Annual Scientific Meeting of North American Society for the Study of Obesity November, 2004.).

95. Spiegel K, Tasali E, Penev P, Van Cauter E. Brief communication: sleep curtailment in healthy young men is associated with decreased leptin levels, elevated ghrelin levels, and increased hunger and appetite. *Ann Intern Med*. 2004;141(11):846-850.

96. Kunz D, Mahlberg R, Müller C, Tilmann A, Bes F. Melatonin in patients with reduced REM sleep duration: two randomized controlled trials. *J Clin Endocrinol Metab*. 2004;89(1):128-134.

97. Rajaratnam SM, Middleton B, Stone BM, Arendt J, Dijk DJ. Melatonin advances the circadian timing of EEG sleep and directly facilitates sleep without altering its duration in extended sleep opportunities in humans. *J Physiol*. 2004;561(pt 1):339-351.

39

The Role of Botanicals in Hypertension and Cardiovascular Disease

Tieraona Low Dog, MD

The role of botanicals, or herbal medicines, in the management of cardiovascular disease has been a long and distinguished one. Numerous plants with cardioactive glycosides were used to treat "dropsy," a folk term for congestive heart failure. One of the more famous was foxglove (*Digitalis purpurea*), written about as early as 1250 AD, which would eventually serve as the source for standardized digitalis, a drug still in use today.[1] The first truly effective antihypertensive drug, reserpine, was extracted from *Rauwolfia serpentina*, a plant with a long history of use in Ayurveda, the traditional medicine of India.

Botanical products are popular in the United States with sales topping $8 billion in 2017, growing at a rate of 8.5% since the previous year.[2] People use natural remedies for a variety of reasons including access, cost, and a perception that they are "safer" than pharmaceuticals.

Although many clinicians express interest in dietary supplements, including botanicals, they also voice legitimate concerns regarding efficacy, quality, safety, and potential drug interactions. Although it is beyond the scope of this chapter to discuss quality, clinicians should be cognizant of the tremendous variability that exists for botanical products in the US marketplace. Products that have been studied in controlled clinical trials are generally of higher quality and should be recommended when possible. Using clinically tested products also allows clinicians recommend an effective dose based on study results.

Clinicians concerns about the concomitant use of botanicals with prescription or over-the-counter medications, particularly in children, elders, and those with diminished renal or hepatic function, is justified. It is difficult to predict pharmacokinetic interactions. There are numerous herb-drug interaction checkers online: one that this author uses is Natural Medicines Comprehensive Database (www.naturalmedicines.therapeuticresearch.com). Clinicians input medications, vitamins, botanicals, and other supplements, and potential interactions will be displayed, the strength of the risk rated, and links to the primary research provided. Potential risks should be explained to patients and documented in the chart. If monitoring drug levels or serum tests (eg, liver function tests) would help mitigate risk, this should also be offered to the patient.

Although most plants have multimodal effects within the body, this chapter will solely focus on the role of specific botanicals in the management of hypertension.

Beet Root (*Beta vulgaris* L.)

Lifestyle modifications, particularly dietary, are the primary recommendation for those with prehypertension or stage 1 hypertension. These modifications include a reduction in salt and increase in fruit and vegetable intake. It is the latter, increasing vegetable consumption, that has grabbed the attention of researchers as they try to ascertain which constituents may be responsible for their hypotensive effects. One highly promising constituent is inorganic nitrate, which is found in leafy greens, spinach, beetroot, celery, and others.[3] For plasma nitrate to be successfully converted to nitric oxide (NO), the "enterosalivary circuit" plays a crucial role. Approximately 25% of the nitrate that enters the circulation from the gut becomes concentrated in the salivary glands through active uptake by the sialin transporter.[58] On interaction with oral bacteria, nitrate is reduced to nitrite, swallowed, and then absorbed, increasing plasma nitrite levels. Endogenous nitrite reductases in the circulation reduce plasma nitrite further to bioactive NO, which can then act as a vasodilator.[4] Of interest, daily use of an antiseptic mouthwash caused a decrease in salivary and plasma nitrite levels of healthy volunteers by 90% and 25%, respectively, an effect associated with an average increase in blood pressure of 3.5 mm Hg.[5] Alteration of the oral microflora may have broader significance to cardiovascular health than originally thought.

Gastric acid may also be an important part of the equation when it comes to dietary nitrates and blood pressure (BP). Proton pump inhibitors (PPIs), by suppressing gastric acidity, may prevent the formation of nitrous acid from inorganic nitrite after conversion by oral bacteria, blunting the release of NO.[6] PPIs also elevate levels of the NO synthase inhibitor asymmetric dimethylarginine (ADMA) via inhibition of dimethylarginine dimethylaminohydrolase, the enzyme responsible for the degradation of ADMA.[7] Elevation of ADMA is often seen in patients with cardiovascular disease. A randomized, double-blind, placebo-controlled crossover study of 15 healthy nonsmoking, normotensive subjects (19-39 years) who were pretreated with placebo or esomeprazole (3 × 40 mg) before ingesting sodium nitrite (0.3 mg/kg) found that systolic blood pressure (SBP) was reduced by a maximum of 6 ± 1.3 mm Hg when taken after placebo, whereas pretreatment with esomeprazole blunted this effect.[8] These effects could partially account for the growing body of evidence suggesting a link between these drugs and cardiovascular disease.[9]

Beetroot is naturally rich in inorganic nitrates and is gaining popularity for its purported benefits for the cardiovascular system and on athletic performance. Studies confirm that beetroot has a beneficial effect on endothelial function. A review of nine crossover trials and three parallel trails found that both inorganic nitrate and beetroot consumption were associated with an improvement in vascular function.[10] A meta-analysis found that inorganic nitrate and beetroot juice supplementation were associated with a significant reduction of blood pressure in adults.[11]

Additional studies have been published since these reviews, included two contradictory results in elder patients. A placebo-controlled, crossover trial in 12 healthy elders (mean age 64 years) randomized participants to receive 140 mL of nitrate-rich beetroot juice (12.9 mmol nitrate) or nitrate-depleted beetroot juice (≤0.04 mmol nitrate) after obtaining baseline data. Systolic, diastolic, and mean arterial blood pressure (MAP) decreased 3 hours relative to baseline only after ingestion of the high-nitrate beetroot juice ($P < .05$), with plasma nitrate and nitrite levels being elevated 3 and 6 hours post intake ($P < .05$). The number of blood monocyte-platelet aggregates decreased 3 hours after ingestion of only the high-nitrate beetroot juice ($P < .05$), indicating a reduction in platelet activation.[12] These results suggest that, in addition to a beneficial effect on blood pressure, beetroot may also exert antithrombotic activity in the aging population.

However, another randomized, double-blind, crossover, placebo-controlled study of 20 nonsmoking healthy participants aged 60 to 75 years (10 male and 10 female) with a body mass index (BMI) 20.0 to 29.9 kg/m^2 failed to note any beneficial effects on resting systolic or diastolic blood pressure after 7 days of nitrate-rich beetroot juice.[13] The study also failed to note any improvement in indexes of central and peripheral cardiac function during cardiopulmonary exercise training compared with nitrate-depleted beetroot as placebo.

Does beetroot supplementation have an "additive effect" in individuals already treated for hypertension? Researchers conducted a randomized, placebo-controlled, double-blind crossover study in 27 treated hypertensive men and women. Like other trials, this study assessed the effect of 1-week intake of nitrate-rich beetroot juice compared with 1-week intake of nitrate-depleted beetroot juice (placebo). Relative to placebo, 1-week intake of nitrate-rich beetroot juice resulted in a threefold increase in plasma nitrite and nitrate, a sevenfold increase in salivary nitrite, an eightfold higher salivary nitrate, and a fourfold increase in both urinary nitrite and nitrate ($P < .001$). However, no differences in home blood pressure and 24-hour ambulatory blood pressure were observed with 1-week intake of nitrate-rich beetroot juice in comparison with the placebo.[14] In those adequately treated for hypertension, the addition of beetroot did not impact blood pressure in this study.

Although there is well-documented biological rationale for the potential of beetroot to have a hypotensive effect, clinical trials have yielded varying results. This variance may be due to a variety of factors: dose of dietary nitrate and duration of supplementation, study design, measurement protocols of blood pressure, populations with low baseline blood pressures at start of trial, or its use in an aging population in which there is a decline in the reducing capacity to convert nitrates to nitrites.[13]

Dose: Most research trials used beetroot juice providing ~6.5 to 7.0 mmol NO$_3$ per 70 mL serving, with 2 to 3 servings taken per day. Studies included products from James White Drinks Ltd.: Beet It Sport (6.5-7.0 mmol NO$_3$ per 70 mL serving); Beet It Stamina Shot (6.0 mmol NO$_3$ per 70 mL serving), and Beet It (3.1 g nitrate/L and 0.1 g nitrite/L or 8.0-10.0 mmol NO$_3$ per 140 mL). Other juices studied include Love Beets Beetroot Juice (Gs Fresh Ltd) containing 210 mg nitrate per 250 mL and a standardized juice (Biotta AG) containing 350 mg nitrate per 80 mL.[15] A lozenge supplement Neo 40 (Neogenis Labs, Austin, TX, USA) containing beet root extract, hawthorn berry, vitamin C, L-citrulline, and sodium nitrite was also shown to lower SBP by an average of 6 mm Hg and diastolic blood pressure (DBP) by 6 mm Hg at 20 and 60 minutes post ingestion.[16]

Safety: There are no known safety issues with consumption of powdered beets or beet juice. Beeturia, a reddish hue in the urine, occurs in roughly 10% to 14% of the population and is harmless.[17]

Summary: The hypotensive effects of beetroot are modest but including beets in the diet, as nitrate-rich juice or standardized beet powder, can be healthy lifestyle recommendations. Patients wising to use beets for hypertension should be instructed to avoid the use of antibacterial mouthwash.

Dandelion Leaf (*Taraxacum officinale* G.H. Weber ex Wiggers)

Dandelion flower, leaf, and root have been consumed as food, beverage, and medicine since ancient times. Dandelion has been widely recognized as a diuretic for centuries. In fact, the French name *pissenlit*, from the verb *pisser* and the noun *lit*, translates to *piss in bed*, a nod to its diuretic activity, particularly when consumed later in the day. The German Commission E recognizes both the root and leaf of dandelion for the stimulation of diuresis,[18] although studies suggest the leaf is superior.[59] The European Medicines Agency recognizes dandelion as a "traditional herbal medicinal product to increase the amount of urine to achieve flushing of the urinary tract as an adjuvant in minor urinary complaints."[19]

In addition to preclinical animal data, a small pilot study examined the effects of fresh dandelion leaf hydroethanolic extract (1 g/mL, 43.5% EtOH final extract) in 28 healthy women aged 18 to 65 years. Subjects self-administered an 8-mL dose of dandelion leaf extract at 8:00 AM, 1:00 PM, and 6:00 PM on the study day. They were asked to measure fluid intake the day before and both fluid intake and urine output for 3 days starting on the study day. There was a significant ($P < .05$) increase in the frequency of urination for the study group on the day of the trial but not on the total daily urination volume.[20] Limitations of the study include significant drop-out (11 participants were unable to complete the study, citing difficulty collecting and measuring of fluid output and/or input) and lack of blinding and placebo group.

Clinicians should note that numerous botanicals have diuretic activity, such as parsley (*Petroselinum crispum*) and celery seed (*Apium graveolens*), and may be found in a variety of products designed for managing blood pressure and possibly for mild cases of congestive heart failure. Celery seed was shown in a rat model to reduce BP, likely through inhibition of intracellular calcium influx.[21]

Dose: 3 to 4 g/d of leaf three times daily.[18]

Safety: Dandelion has an excellent safety profile. Studies on rabbits, mice, and rats, with rabbits treated orally with dried dandelion plant (3-6 g/kg body) and mice treated with dandelion ethanolic extracts, showed no significant or visible signs of toxicity.[22] Contact dermatitis can occur in sensitive individuals when handling fresh dandelion.[23] When using large doses of dandelion leaf as a diuretic for a prolonged period, it would seem reasonable to periodically monitor potassium, sodium, magnesium levels.

Summary: Dandelion leaf has a long history of use as a diuretic with some data confirming its traditional use. There are no human clinical trials for dandelion in the management of hypertension.

Garlic (*Allium sativum* L.)

Garlic is widely consumed in many ethnic cuisines and has a long history as an herbal medicine. A member of the *Allium* family, which includes onions and leeks, garlic is popular as a dietary supplement. It is promoted for both immune and cardiovascular health, particularly for managing lipids and blood pressure. The mechanism by which it lowers blood pressure is biologically plausible owing to its interaction with hydrogen sulfide- and nitric oxide-signaling pathways.[24]

Garlic in various forms (eg, aged garlic, garlic powder) has been studied for its impact on blood pressure. A meta-analysis including 17 trials showed that garlic intake resulted in a 3.75-mm Hg reduction ($P < .001$) in SBP and a 3.39-mm Hg reduction ($P < .001$) in DBP compared with controls. When subgroups were examined, a significant reduction in SBP was seen in hypertensive (-4.4 mm Hg; $P = .004$) patients but not in normotensive participants. The authors concluded that "garlic supplements are superior to controls (placebo in most trials) in reducing BP, especially in hypertensive patients."[25]

An updated meta-analysis that included 20 trials reported a significant effect of garlic on blood pressure, with an average decrease in SBP of 8.6 mm Hg and in DBP of 6.1 mm Hg in participants with hypertension ($n = 14$ trial arms, $n = 468$ participants).[26]

Arterial stiffness is one of many other risk factors contributing to hypertension and is an important predictor of cardiovascular risk. To test whether garlic has an impact on arterial stiffness, as well as peripheral and central blood pressure, a 12-week randomized, double-blind, placebo-controlled trial of 88 participants with uncontrolled hypertension were given aged garlic extract (AGE; 1.2 g containing 1.2 mg *S*-allyl cysteine) or placebo. The mean BP was significantly reduced by 5.0 ± 2.1 mm Hg ($P = .016$) systolic, and in responders by 11.5 ± 1.9 mm Hg systolic and 6.3 ± 1.1 mm Hg diastolic compared with placebo ($P < .001$). Central hemodynamic measures tended to improve in the AGE group more than in the placebo group, including central blood pressure, central pulse pressure, mean arterial pressure, augmentation pressure, pulse-wave velocity, and arterial stiffness. Trends in beneficial effects of garlic on the inflammatory markers tumor necrosis factor -α, total cholesterol, low-density lipid cholesterol, and apolipoproteins were observed. The treatment was well tolerated, and there was no increase in bleeding risk in those taking blood-thinning medications.[27]

In 2018, a 12-week double-blind randomized placebo-controlled trial of 49 participants with uncontrolled hypertension found that AGE (1.2 g/d containing 1.2 mg *S*-allyl cysteine) significantly reduced SBP by 10 ± 3.6 mm Hg and DBP by 5.4 ± 2.3 mm Hg, compared with placebo. Garlic also significantly lowered central blood pressure, pulse pressure, and arterial stiffness ($P < .05$) Interestingly, this study also noted that the garlic extract increased microbial diversity in the gut, with a marked increase in *Lactobacillus* and *Clostridia* species.[28]

Dose: 600 mg AGE standardized to 0.6 mg of *S*-allyl cysteine 1 to 2 times daily (Kyolic; Wakunga/Wagner).

Standardized (1.3% allicin) garlic powder (Kwai; Lichtwer Pharma), 600 to 900 mg/d.

Dried garlic powder, 1000 to 1200 mg.

Safety: Mild gastrointestinal upset is reported in clinical trials. Animal studies show that garlic can impact platelet function, and case reports of postoperative bleeding in patients taking garlic before surgery have been reported.[25] A small, controlled study found no significant change in international normalized ratio (INR) values among patients stabilized on warfarin therapy (INR target, 2-3) given 1200 mg of AGE for 2 months compared with placebo.[29]

Another 12-week study of patients stabilized on warfarin given 1.525 g twice daily of AGE (Kyolic, Wakunaga Pharmaceutical Co.) failed to find any significant change in INR or increased risk of bleeding events.[60] In 2017, a systematic review failed to note any change in warfarin pharmacokinetic or pharmacodynamics with garlic.[30] Most studies were conducted in AGEs, and these results may not apply to other forms of garlic supplements. Clinicians should use common sense. Patients should discontinue most botanical supplements 7 to 10 days before an elective surgery, and patients taking warfarin should be monitored if a new supplement is added to their regimen.

Research found that oral aqueous extracts of garlic can significantly reduce isoniazid levels in rabbits. Oral administration of garlic extract decreased the bioavailability of isoniazid significantly with no change in the rate of elimination.[31] Clinicians should be aware of this interaction.

Summary: Garlic supplements, particularly those used in clinical trials, can be considered by clinicians for the management of prehypertension or stage 1 hypertension.

Grape Seed Extract (*Vitis vinifera* L.)

Grapes contain a variety of polyphenol compounds, including flavonoids, phenolic acids, and resveratrol. Grape seeds are a particularly rich source of these polyphenols, which have been found to exert a beneficial effect on blood pressure. Studies show that grape seed extracts (GSEs) increase prostacyclin (PGI2) and endothelium-derived nitric oxide,[32] which leads to vasodilation and inhibition of platelets, leukocyte adhesion to the endothelial surface, and proliferation of vascular smooth muscle cells.[33]

A meta-analysis of 16 clinical trials and 810 study subjects was published. The overall analyses found that GSE supplementation led to significant reductions in SBP (weighted mean difference [WMD] = −6.077; $P = .011$) and DBP (WMD = −2.803; $P = .001$). In subgroup analyses, there were significant reductions in three groups: younger subjects (mean age < 50 years) for SBP (WMD = −6.049; $P = .005$) and DBP (WMD = −3.116; $P < .001$), in obese participants (mean BMI≥ 25 kg/m) for SBP (WMD = −4.469; $P < .001$), and in patients with metabolic syndrome for SBP (WMD = −8.487; $P < .001$). The authors reported no indication of publication bias.[34]

An additional 12-week single-center, two-arm, double-blinded, placebo-controlled, parallel study randomized 36 middle-aged adults with prehypertension to 300 mg/d GSE or placebo. Twenty-nine participants completed the study (placebo = 17; GSE = 12). Subjects consumed a juice with no GSE (placebo) or juice containing 150 mg GSE twice daily for 6 weeks preceded by a 2-week placebo run-in and followed by 4-week follow-up. GSE significantly reduced SBP by 5.6% ($P = .012$) and DBP by 4.7% ($P = .049$) after 6 weeks of intervention period, which was significantly different (SBP; $P = .03$) or tended to be different (DBP; $P = .08$) from placebo. BP returned to baseline after the 4-week discontinuation period. Subjects with higher initial BP experienced

greater BP reduction, nearly double the effect size. No significant changes were observed with fasting plasma lipids, glucose, oxidized LDL, flow-mediated dilation, or vascular adhesion molecules. Total plasma phenolic acid concentrations were 1.6 times higher after 6 weeks of GSE versus placebo. GSE was found to be safe and to improve BP in people with prehypertension, supporting the use of GSE as a functional ingredient in a low-calorie beverage for blood pressure control.[35]

Dose: 150 to 300 mg/d (standardized to 90%-95% procyanidins).

Safety: GSEs appear to be well tolerated. There is a theoretical risk of bleeding if taken with anticoagulant or antiplatelet medications. A study of nine commercial GSE products found that there is little to no interaction with CYP3A4 and adverse effects are not likely to occur if GSE is taken concomitantly with drugs metabolized by this enzyme system.[61]

Summary: GSE can be considered for those with prehypertension or stage 1 hypertension.

Hibiscus Calyces (*Hibiscus sabdariffa* L.)

Hibiscus is a member of the Malvaceae family. Its calyces (outer parts of the flower) are deeply red in color and sour in taste, hence its other name, sour tea.[36] Hibiscus tea is consumed in the Middle East, Central and South America, India, and other areas, as both a flavorful beverage and as medicine. The calyces are a rich source of polyphenols, anthocyanins, and flavonoids, compounds that offer beneficial effects for the cardiovascular system.[37]

Data confirm that hibiscus inhibits calcium influx and angiotensin-converting enzyme, as well as exerts anti-inflammatory activity.[62] A review of 10 clinical trials found a significant decrease in SBP in participants taking hibiscus. The decrease in SBP ranged from 6.3 to 31.9 mm Hg in individual trials, whereas the decrease in DBP was significant in 9 of the 10 trials and ranged from 1.1 to 19.7 mm Hg. In comparative trials, a standardized extract of hibiscus (9.62 mg of total anthocyanins/dose/d) appeared to be as effective as captopril and hydrochlorothiazide (HCTZ) but not as effective as lisinopril.[38] Heterogeneity in trial design precluded combination of the results.

Given that hibiscus is widely consumed as a beverage, researchers have examined the antihypertensive activity when taken as a tisane (herbal tea). Tuft's researchers examined the antihypertensive effects of hibiscus tisane consumption in humans. A randomized, double-blind, placebo-controlled clinical trial was conducted in 65 pre- and mildly hypertensive adults (30-70 years), not taking blood pressure lowering medications, administered three 240-mL servings/d of brewed hibiscus tea (1.25 g hibiscus per 240 mL) or placebo beverage for 6 weeks. At 6 weeks, hibiscus tea lowered SBP compared with placebo (−7.2 ± 11.4 versus −1.3 ± 10.0 mm Hg; $P = .030$). DBP was also lower, although this change did not differ from placebo (−3.1 ± 7.0 versus −0.5 ± 7.5 mm Hg; $P = .160$). The change in MAP was of borderline significance compared with placebo (-4.5 ± 7.7 versus -0.8 ± 7.4 mm Hg; $P = .054$). Participants with higher SBP at baseline showed a greater response to hibiscus treatment (r = -0.421 for SBP change; $P = .010$). This study found that hibiscus tea, in an amount readily incorporated into the diet, lowers BP in pre- and mildly hypertensive adults.[39]

The use of hibiscus tea for hypertension has been studied in Nigeria, where it is commonly consumed as a refreshing beverage. Eighty newly diagnosed, untreated mild to moderate hypertensive subjects attending Medical Out-Patients clinic of Enugu State University Teaching Hospital, Enugu, were recruited for the study. They were randomized to receive 25 mg/d HCTZ, 150 mg/kg/d as hibiscus tisane, or 150 mg/kg/d of placebo (black currant tisane) for 4 weeks. Blood pressure, serum, and urine electrolytes were measured at baseline, weekly during treatment, and 1 week after treatment cessation. Both HCTZ and hibiscus significantly ($P < .001$) reduced SBP, DBP, MAP, and serum Na$^+$ compared with placebo. When compared with each other, HCTZ significantly ($P < .001$) reduced serum Na$^+$ and Cl$^-$ compared with *Hibiscus sabdariffa* and significantly ($P < .001$) increased K$^+$ and Cl$^-$ output in urine. No side effects were noted. This was an important study in that hibiscus was equivalent to HCTZ as an antihypertensive agent but did not cause electrolyte imbalance.[40]

This same research team in Nigeria conducted another study involving 78 patients (35-68 years) with newly diagnosed and untreated hypertension. Participants were randomized to receive 10 mg/d lisinopril, 150 mg/kg/d as hibiscus tisane, or 150 mg/kg/d of placebo (black currant tisane) each day before breakfast. At the end of the 4-week study, those in the hibiscus group had the greatest decrease in SBP (-17.08 ± 2.01 mm Hg), DBP ($-12.12 \pm$ mm Hg), and MAP (-13.68 ± 1.82 mm Hg), followed by reductions in SBP (-12.60 ± 1.15 mm Hg), DBP (-9.20 ± 1.10 mm Hg), and MAP (-10.31 ± 1.14 mm Hg) in the lisinopril group. Both hibiscus and lisinopril significantly increased ($P < .001$) urine volume compared with placebo, and hibiscus significantly ($P < .001$) increased urine volume more than lisinopril. Hibiscus significantly increased ($P < .001$) creatinine clearance compared with placebo, whereas lisinopril did not.[41] Two patients in the lisinopril group failed to complete the study owing to the development of cough, and one participant in the hibiscus group failed to complete the study owing to nonmedical reasons.

Another herb commonly used for hypertension in Africa is kinkeliba leaf (*Combretum micranthum*). Researchers in Senegal randomized 125 adult patients with untreated hypertension (140-175/90-110 mm Hg) to receive 190 mg twice daily of kinkeliba leaf capsules, 320 mg twice daily of hibiscus calyx capsules, or 5 mg/d of ramipril for four consecutive weeks. SBP and DBP decreased in all treatment groups ($P < .001$). For SBP, the mean decrease was higher with ramipril (-16.7 ± 8.4 mm Hg) than kinkeliba (-12.2 ± 6.6 mm Hg, $P = .016$) and hibiscus (-11.2 ± 3.3 mm Hg, $P = .001$). For DBP, the mean decrease with ramipril (-6.7 ± 3.6 mm Hg) was not statistically different from that with hibiscus (-6.0 ± 4.7 mm Hg, $P = .271$)

and was superior to kinkeliba. A significant natriuretic effect was observed in the kinkeliba and hibiscus groups but not in patients taking ramipril. At the end of the 4 weeks, 39% of patients in the ramipril group, 37% of patients in the kinkeliba group, and 21% of those taking hibiscus had normalized their blood pressure.[42]

Poorer countries shoulder a disproportionate part of the burden of morbidity and mortality associated with hypertension (and many other diseases), and researching plants that are part of the local pharmacopeia, such as hypertension and kinkeliba, that can be integrated into the system makes good economical and practical sense.[43]

Dose: Hibiscus tisane 1.25 to 10 g or 150 mg/kg, brewed in 150 to 500 mL of water and taken one to three times daily for 2 to 6 weeks, has been studied. Hibiscus extracts used in clinical research have been standardized to 3.6 mg anthocyanins/g, taken 2 to 3 times per day.

Safety: *H sabdariffa* preparations, predominantly the infusion and aqueous extracts, have a long-standing traditional use both in food and in medicine and are considered safe. A review of the toxicology studies suggest that doses of 200 mg/kg should be safe, and data from preclinical and clinical studies failed to provide substantiated evidence of any therapeutically relevant drug-interaction potential of commonplace teas or beverages containing hibiscus and its preparations.[44]

Summary: Hibiscus is widely used as a beverage in many areas of the world. It has an excellent safety profile and can be considered by clinicians for those with stage 1 to 2 hypertension. Hibiscus might be particularly beneficial in areas with limited health care dollars and access to medical care because of its wide acceptance as a beverage and minimal impact on electrolytes.

Motherwort Herb (*Leonurus cardiaca* L.)

Motherwort, a member of the mint family, has a long history of use in women's health as a relaxant for tension and anxiety and was highly valued for its beneficial effects on the heart, thus the species name "*cardiaca*." Today, it can be found in herbal formulae designed for those with nervous palpitations or elevated blood pressure accompanied by a nervous/anxious/stress component. Alkaloids in motherwort, stachydrine, and leonurine have been shown to be mildly sedating and hypotensive. Research suggests that leonurine is an inhibitor of vascular smooth muscle tone, probably acting by inhibiting Ca^{2+} influx and the release of intracellular Ca^{2+}.[45] Lavandulifolioside, another constituent, has also been shown to exert negative chronotropic and hypotensive effects.[46] Those with a "nervous heart" often find relief from palpitations and anxiety-provoked simple tachycardia.

An open prospective study enrolled 50 patients (ages 18-75 years) with stage 1 hypertension (140-159/90-99 mm Hg) or stage 2 hypertension (160-179/100-109 mm Hg) accompanied by anxiety and insomnia. The researchers examined the effects of motherwort administered in 300-mg soft gel capsules (1:10 soybean oil extract; 0.15 mg iridoids), two capsules taken twice daily. A statistically significant decrease and normalization in SBP and DBP were noted at 21 days of treatment. Anxiety was reduced in 61%, emotional liability in 53%, headache in 41%, and sleep disorders in 47% of participants. A tendency to a decrease in heart rate (from 81.7 to 75.4) was observed but was not statistically significant.[47] Although the study suffers from lack of blinding and placebo arm, it is consistent with the historical use of motherwort. More research is needed.

Clinicians should be aware that numerous botanicals have calmative and relaxant properties and may be included in formulations for managing hypertension. Some of the more commonly used relaxant botanicals include linden flowers (*Tilia europa*), saffron (*Crocus sativus*), valerian (*Valeriana officinalis*), cramp bark (*Viburnum opulus*), and kava (*Piper methysticum*). Of these, 400 mg of saffron resulted in a significant reduction in SBP and mean arterial pressure by 11 and 5 mm Hg, respectively, in a very small clinical trial.[48] The antihypertensive effect of saffron may be mediated through blockade of Ca^{2+} channels, opening of potassium channels, and antagonism of the β-adrenoceptors.[49]

Dose: The German Commission E lists the dose as 4.5 g/d of the cut herb.[18] Most products contain far less.

Safety: No documented side effects are known; however, it should not be used during pregnancy because of the potential for uterine stimulation.[50]

Summary: Motherwort has a long and distinguished history for nervous palpitations and is widely used by many herbalists in formulations for hypertension with an anxious component. Research should be considered preliminary.

Olive Leaf (*Olea europaea* L.)

Although most people are familiar with the fruits of the olive tree, far fewer realize that olive leaf has been used medicinally for millennia. Olive leaf extracts remain a popular remedy for hypertension in southern Europe. Preclinical studies demonstrate that olive leaf exerts antihypertensive activity, suppressing the L-type calcium channel directly and reversibly.[51]

A randomized, parallel, and active-controlled study in 162 patients with stage 1 hypertension was conducted to study the antihypertensive effect of olive leaf extract in comparison with captopril. After a 4-week run in (diet only), participants were randomized to receive 500 mg olive leaf extract (EFLA943; ethanolic extract of dried olive leaf standardized to 19.9% oleuropein) twice daily or 12.5 mg twice daily of captopril for 2 weeks. (Nonresponders were given a higher dose of 25 mg twice daily of captopril for study duration). The primary efficacy endpoint was reduction in SBP from baseline to week 8 of treatment. After 8 weeks of treatment, both groups experienced a significant reduction of SBP as well as DBP from baseline; the reductions were not significantly different between groups. Means of SBP reduction from baseline to the end of study were -11.5 ± 8.5 and -13.7 ± 7.6 mm Hg in olive leaf and captopril groups, respectively, and DBP reductions were

-4.8 ± 5.5 and -6.4 ± 5.2 mm Hg, respectively. Tolerability was similar between the two groups, with vertigo, muscle discomfort, and headache judged to be possibly related to both olive leaf extract and captopril, whereas cough was related primarily to captopril. In this study, olive leaf extract was found to be equivalent to captopril for lowering BP in patients with stage 1 hypertension, although it should be noted that the trial suffered from significant dropouts of 36.2%.[52]

Dose: 400 to 500 mg twice daily of olive leaf extract (EFLA 943, 20% oleuropein) was used in the clinical study. This extract is available in numerous products sold in the United States.

Safety: There are no significant safety issues reported for olive leaf extract.

Summary: There are limited data supporting the use of olive leaf for the management of hypertension.

Rauwolfia Root (*Rauwolfia serpentina* (L.) Benth. x Kurz.)

The roots from Rauwolfia, an evergreen shrub, have been used for millennia in Ayurvedic medicine to treat anxiety, insomnia, epilepsy, schizophrenia, and other ailments, with written records dating back 3000 years ago.[53] Reserpine, one of more than 50 alkaloids present in the root, was isolated in 1952. Reserpine is a selective inhibitor of the monoamine vesicular monoamine uptake transmitter that transports norepinephrine and epinephrine into presynaptic vesicles in sympathetic nerve terminals (as well as dopamine and serotonin into storage vesicles in the central nervous system).

This depletion of adrenergic neurons of norepinephrine explains its use in the management of certain psychiatric illnesses, as well as hypertension, and some of its adverse effects.

Reserpine revolutionized the management of hypertension in the 1950s. Even though it is seldom used anymore, a Cochrane review found that reserpine is effective in reducing SBP roughly to the same degree as other first-line antihypertensive drugs.[54] The primary drawbacks for reserpine were adverse effects (eg, sedation, depression), with one study noting adverse effects in 17.2% in the reserpine/diuretic group and 14.3% in the enalapril group.[55] Rauwolfia is still used by some naturopathic practitioners in the United States and abroad, who report less adverse effects with whole root than the isolated alkaloid.

Dose: 0.25 to 0.5 mg/d reserpine was typically used. In one review of Rauwolfia for the management of hypertension, the total daily dose should not exceed 500 mg of root and, in most cases, can be less than 250 mg/d.[56] Rauwolfia is currently available for sale online to the public in the United States in recommended daily intakes of 180 to 2500 mg of the root. Only a few products are standardized to alkaloid content.

Safety: Adverse side effects of reserpine include lethargy, sedation, psychiatric depression, hypotension, nausea, vomiting, abdominal cramping, gastric ulceration, bradycardia, bronchospasm, skin rash, itching, sexual dysfunction, and withdrawal psychosis in one case.[56] Possible interactions with other drugs include cardiac glycosides, alcohol, antipsychotic drugs, barbiturates, digoxin, diuretics, ephedrine, levodopa, monoamine oxidase inhibitors, propranolol, stimulant drugs, and tricyclic antidepressants.[56]

Summary: Rauwolfia and reserpine are highly effective for the reduction of BP as seen in clinical trials and decades of use. The eighth Joint National Committee (JNC8) recognized reserpine as an alternative drug for treating hypertension, although it was not recommended for initial treatment.[57] Drawbacks for its use have been due primarily to adverse effects and a possible link to cancer. It is concerning that Rauwolfia is readily available online without any clinical oversight at daily dosing recommendations of up to 2500 mg/d.

Summary

The first line of treatment of prehypertension and stage 1 hypertension is lifestyle modification. As part of that lifestyle modification, based on the current state of the science, clinicians may consider the use of hibiscus, GSE, and garlic extracts in patients who are amenable and interested in using natural products. There are no safety concerns with the use of beetroot or olive leaf extracts if patients choose to use them. If products contain botanicals with diuretic properties, clinicians should consider occasionally monitoring serum electrolytes. Clinicians should always guide patients toward high-quality products, monitor the effectiveness of the therapy, and be observant for potential adverse effects.

References

1. Norn S, Kruse PR. Cardiac glycosides: from ancient history through Withering's foxglove to endogenous cardiac glycosides. *Dan Medicinhist Arbog*. 2004;119-132. (Article in Danish).
2. Smith T, Kawa K, Eckl V, Morton C, Stredney R. Herbal supplement sales in US increased 8.5% in 2017, topping $8 billion. *HerbalGram*. 2018;119:62-71.
3. Gee LC, Ahluwalia A. Dietary nitrate lowers blood pressure: epidemiological, pre-clinical experimental and clinical trial evidence. *Curr Hypertens Rep*. 2016;18:17.
4. Lundberg JO, Weitzberg E, Gladwin MT. The nitrate-nitrite-nitric oxide pathway in physiology and therapeutics. *Nat Rev Drug Discov*. 2008;7:156-167.
5. Kapil V, Haydar SMA, Pearl V, Lundberg JO, Weitzberg E, Ahluwalia A. Physiological role for nitrate-reducing oral bacteria in blood pressure control. *Free Radic Biol Med*. 2013;55:93-100.
6. Pinheiro LC, Montenegro MF, Amaral JH, Ferreira GC, Oliveira AM, Tanus-Santos JE. Increase in gastric pH reduces hypotensive effect of oral sodium nitrite in rats. *Free Radic Biol Med*. 2012;53(4):701-709.
7. Ghebremariam YT, LePendu P, Lee JC, et al. Unexpected effect of proton pump inhibitors: elevation of the cardiovascular risk factor asymmetric dimethylarginine. *Circulation*. 2013;128(8):845-853.
8. Montenegro MF, Sundqvist ML, Larsen FJ, et al. Blood pressure-lowering effect of orally ingested nitrite is abolished by a proton pump inhibitor. *Hypertension*. 2017;69(1):23-31.
9. Sukhovershin RA, Cooke JP. How may proton pump inhibitors impair cardiovascular health? *Am J Cardiovasc Drugs*. 2016;16(3):153-161.
10. Lara J, Ashor AW, Oggioni C, et al. Effects of inorganic nitrate and beetroot supplementation on endothelial function: a systematic review and meta-analysis. *Eur J Nutr*. 2016;55(2):451-459.
11. Siervo M, Lara J, Ogbonmwan I, Mathers JC. Inorganic nitrate and beetroot juice supplementation reduces blood pressure in adults: a systematic review and meta-analysis. *J Nutr*. 2013;143:818-826. doi: 10.3945/jn.112.170233.
12. Raubenheimer K, Hickey D, Leveritt M, et al. Acute effects of nitrate-rich beetroot juice on blood pressure, hemostasis and vascular inflammation markers in healthy older adults: a randomized, placebo-controlled cross-over study. *Nutrients*. 2017;9(11). pii:E1270. doi:10.3390/nu9111270.
13. Oggioni C, Jakovljevic DG, Klonizakis M, et al. Dietary nitrate does not modify blood pressure and cardiac output at rest and during exercise in older adults: a randomised cross-over study. *Int J Food Sci Nutr*. 2018;69(1):74-83.
14. Bondonno CP, Liu AH, Croft KD, et al. Absence of an effect of high nitrate intake from beetroot juice on blood pressure in treated hypertensive individuals: a randomized controlled trial. *Am J Clin Nutr*. 2015;102(2):368-375.
15. Natural Medicines Database. Beets. https://naturalmedicines-therapeuticresearch-com.ezproxy4.library.arizona.edu/databases/food,-herbs-supplements/professional.aspx?productid=306. Accessed January 12, 2019.
16. Houston M, Hays L. Acute effects of an oral nitric oxide supplement on blood pressure, endothelial function, and vascular compliance in hypertensive patients. *J Clin Hypertens*. 2014;16(7):524-529.
17. Watts AR, Lennard MS, Mason SL, Tucker GT, Woods HF. Beeturia and the biological fate of beetroot pigments. *Pharmacogenetics*. 1993;3(6):302-311.
18. Blumenthal M, Busse WR, Goldberg A, Gruenwald J, Hall T, Riggins CW, eds. *The Complete German Commission E Monographs: Therapeutic Guide to Herbal Medicines*. Austin, TX: American Botanical Council; 1998.
19. EMA. European Medicines Agency Community herbal monograph on Taraxacum officinale Weber ex Wigg., radix cum herba EMA/HMPC/212895/2009 November 12, 2009. https://www.ema.europa.eu/documents/herbal-monograph/final-community-herbal monograph-taraxacum-officinale-weber-ex-wigg-radix-cum-herba_en.pdf. Accessed January 18, 2019.
20. Clare BA, Conroy RS, Spelman K. The diuretic effect in human subjects of an extract of *Taraxacum officinale* folium over a single day. *J Altern Complement Med*. 2009;15(8):929-934.
21. Moghadam MH, Imenshahidi M, Mohajeri SA. Antihypertensive effect of celery seed on rat blood pressure in chronic administration. *J Med Food*. 2013;16:558-563.
22. Wimgo FE, Lambert MN, Jeppesen PB. The physiological effects of dandelion (*Taraxacum officinale*) in type 2 diabetes. *Rev Diabet Stud*. 2016;13(2-3):113-131.
23. Paulsen E, Otkjaer A, Andersen KE. Sesquiterpene lactone dermatitis in the young: is atopy a risk factor? *Contact Dermatitis*. 2008;59(1):1-6.
24. Ried K, Fakler P. Potential of garlic (Allium sativum) in lowering high blood pressure: mechanisms of action and clinical relevance. *Integr Blood Press Control*. 2014;7:71-82.
25. Wang HP, Yang J, Qin LQ, Yang XJ. Effect of garlic on blood pressure: a meta-analysis. *J Clin Hypertens (Greenwich)*. 2015;17(3):223-231.
26. Ried K. Garlic lowers blood pressure in hypertensive individuals, regulates serum cholesterol, and stimulates immunity: an updated meta-analysis and review. *J Nutr*. 2016;146(2):389S-396S.
27. Ried K, Travica N, Sali A. The effect of aged garlic extract on blood pressure and other cardiovascular risk factors in uncontrolled hypertensives: the AGE at Heart trial. *Integr Blood Press Control*. 2016;9:9-21.
28. Ried K, Travica N, Sali A. The effect of kyolic aged garlic extract on gut microbiota, inflammation, and cardiovascular markers in hypertensives: the GarGIC trial. *Front Nutr*. 2018;5:122.

29. Rozenfeld V, Sisca TS, Callahan A, Crain J. *Double-blind, randomized, placebo-controlled trial of aged garlic extract in patients stabilized on warfarin therapy [abstract]. Presented at: American Society of Health-System Pharmacists (ASHP) Midyear Clinical Meeting*; December 3, 2000; Las Vegas, Nevada.

30. Choi S, Oh DS, Jerng UM. A systematic review of the pharmacokinetic and pharmacodynamic interactions of herbal medicine with warfarin. *PLoS One.* 2017;12(8):e0182794.

31. Dhamija P, Malhotra S, Pandhi P. Effect of oral administration of crude aqueous extract of garlic on pharmacokinetic parameters of isoniazid and rifampicin in rabbits. *Pharmacology.* 2006;77(2):100-104.

32. Pons Z, Margalef M, Bravo FI, Arola-Arnal A, Muguerza B. Acute administration of single oral dose of grape seed polyphenols restores blood pressure in a rat model of metabolic syndrome: role of nitric oxide and prostacyclin. *Eur J Clin Nutr.* 2016;55(2):749-758. doi:10.1007/s00394-015-0895-0.

33. Dohadwala MM, Vita JA. Grapes and cardiovascular disease. *J Nutr.* 2009;139(9):1788S-1793S.

34. Zhang H, Liu S, Li L, et al. The impact of grape seed extract treatment on blood pressure changes: a meta-analysis of 16 randomized controlled trials. *Medicine (Baltimore).* 2016;95(33): e4247. doi:10.1097/MD.0000000000004247.

35. Park E, Edirisinghe I, Choy YY, Waterhouse A, Burton-Freeman B. Effects of grape seed extract beverage on blood pressure and metabolic indices in individuals with pre-hypertension: a randomised, double-blinded, two-arm, parallel, placebo-controlled trial. *Br J Nutr.* 2016;115(2):226-238. doi:10.1017/S0007114515004328.

36. Asgary S, Soltani R, Zolghadr M, Keshvari M, Sarrafzadegan N. Evaluation of the effects of roselle (Hibiscus sabdariffa L.) on oxidative stress and serum levels of lipids, insulin and hs-CRP in adult patients with metabolic syndrome: a double-blind placebo-controlled clinical trial. *J Complement Integr Med.* 2016;13(2):175-180.

37. Aziz Z, Wong SY, Chong NJ. Effects of Hibiscus sabdariffa L. on serum lipids: a systematic review and meta-analysis. *J Ethnopharmacol.* 2013;150(2):442-450.

38. Walton R, Whitten DL, Hawrelak JA. The efficacy of Hibiscus sabdariffa (rosella) in essential hypertension: a systematic review of clinical trials. *Aust J Herbal Med.* 2016;28(2):48-51.

39. McKay DL, Chen CY, Saltzman E, Blumberg JB. *Hibiscus sabdariffa* L. tea (tisane) lowers blood pressure in prehypertensive and mildly hypertensive adults. *J Nutr.* 2010;140(2):298-303.

40. Nwachukwu DC, Aneke E, Nwachukwu NZ, Obika LF, Nwagha UI, Eze AA. Effect of Hibiscus sabdariffa on blood pressure and electrolyte profile of mild to moderate hypertensive Nigerians: a comparative study with hydrochlorothiazide. *Niger J Clin Pract.* 2015;18(6):762-770.

41. Nwachukwu DC, Aneke EI, Nwachukwu NZ, Azubike N, Obika LF. Does consumption of an aqueous extract of *Hibiscus sabdariffa* affect renal function in subjects with mild to moderate hypertension? *J Physiol Sci.* 2017;67(1):227-234.

42. Seck SM, Doupa D, Dia DG, et al. Clinical efficacy of African traditional medicines in hypertension: a randomized controlled trial with Combretum micranthum and Hibiscus sabdariffa. *J Hum Hypertens.* 2017;32(1):75-81.

43. World Health Organization. *WHO Traditional Medicine Strategy: 2014-2023.* Geneva: World Health Organization; 2013. http://apps.who.int/iris/bitstream/10665/92455/1/9789241506090_eng.pdf. Accessed December 2018.

44. Da-Costa-Rocha I, Bonnlaender B, Sievers H, Pischel I, Heinrich M. *Hibiscus sabdariffa* L. - a phytochemical and pharmacological review. *Food Chem.* 2014;165:424-443.

45. Chen CX, Kwan CY. Endothelium-independent vasorelaxation by leonurine, a plant alkaloid purified from Chinese motherwort. *Life Sci.* 2001;68(8):953-960.

46. Miłkowska-Leyck K, Filipek B, Strzelecka H. Pharmacological effects of lavandulifolioside from *Leonurus cardiaca. J Ethnopharmacol.* 2002;80(1):85-90.

47. Shikov AN, Pozharitskaya ON, Makarov VG, Demchenko DV, Shikh EV. Effect of *Leonurus cardiaca* oil extract in patients with arterial hypertension accompanied by anxiety and sleep disorders. *Phytother Res.* 2011;25(4):540-543.

48. Modaghegh MH, Shahabian M, Esmaeili HA, Rajbai O, Hosseinzadeh H. Safety evaluation of saffron (*Crocus sativus*) tablets in healthy volunteers. *Phytomedicine.* 2008;15:1032-1037.

49. Chrysant SG, Chrysant GS. Herbs used for the treatment of hypertension and their mechanism of action. *Curr Hypertens Rep.* 2017;19:77.

50. Bradley PR. *British Herbal Compendium: A Handbook of Scientific Information on Widely Used Plant Drugs.* Bournemouth, Dorset: British Herbal Medicine Association; 1992.

51. Scheffler A, Rauwald HW, Kampa B, Mann U, Mohr FW, Dhein S. *Olea europaea* leaf extract exerts L-type Ca(2+) channel antagonistic effects. *J Ethnopharmacol.* 2008;120(2):233-240.

52. Susalit E, Agus N, Effendi I, et al. Olive (Olea europaea) leaf extract effective in patients with stage-1 hypertension: comparison with Captopril. *Phytomedicine.* 2011;18(4):251-258.

53. Yarnell E, Abascal K. Treating hypertension botanically. *Altern Complement Ther.* 2001;7(5):284-290.

54. Shamon SD, Perez MI. Blood pressure-lowering efficacy of reserpine for primary hypertension. *Cochrane Database Syst Rev.* 2016;12:CD007655.

55. Griebenow R, Pittrow DB, Weidinger G, Mueller E, Mutschler E, Welzel D. Low-dose reserpine/thiazide combination in first-line treatment of hypertension: efficacy and safety compared to an ACE inhibitor. *Blood Press.* 1997;6(5):299-306.

56. Lobay D. Rauwolfia in the treatment of hypertension. *Integr Med.* 2015;14(3):40-46.

57. James PA, Oparil S, Carter BL, et al. Evidence-based guideline for the management of high blood pressure in adults report from the panel members appointed to the Eighth Joint National Committee (JNC 8). *JAMA.* 2014;311(5):507-520.

58. Gee LC, Ahluwalia A. Dietary nitrate lowers blood pressure: epidemiological, pre-clinical experimental and clinical trial evidence. *Curr Hypertens Rep.* 2016;18:17. doi:10.1007/s11906-015-0623-4.

59. Rácz-Kotilla E, Rácz G, Solomon A. Action of Taraxacum Officinale extracts on body-weight and diuresis of laboratory-animals. *Planta Med.* 1974;26:262–217.

60. Macan H, Uykimpang R, Alconcel M, et al. Aged garlic extract may be safe for patients on warfarin therapy. *J Nutr.* 2006;136 (3 Suppl):793S-795S.

61. Wanwimolruk S, Phopin K, Prachayasittikul V. Cytochrome P450 enzyme mediated herbal drug interactions (Part 2). *EXCLI J.* 2014;13:869–896.

62. Beltrán-Debón R, Rodríguez-Gallego E, Fernández-Arroyo S, et al. The acute impact of polyphenols from Hibiscus sabdariffa in metabolic homeostasis: an approach combining metabolomics and gene-expression analyses. *Food Funct.* 2015;6(9):2957–2966. doi:10.1039/c5fo00696a.

Index

Note: Page numbers followed by "f" indicate figures, "t" indicates tables.